Practical Anatomic Pathology

Series Editors

Fan Lin
Geisinger Health System
Danville, PA, USA

Ximing J. Yang
Feinberg School of Medicine
Northwestern University
Chicago, IL, USA

This Book Series is designed to provide a comprehensive, practical and state-of-the-art review and update of the major issues and challenges specific to each subspecialty field of surgical pathology in a question and answer (Q&A) format. Making an accurate diagnosis especially from a limited sample can be quite challenging, yet crucial to patient care. This Book Series, using the most current and evidence-based resources 1) focuses on frequently asked questions in surgical pathology in day-to-day practice; 2) provides quick, accurate, terse, and useful answers to many practical questions encountered in daily practice; 3) emphasizes the importance of a triple test (clinical, radiologic, and histologic correlation); 4) delineates how to appropriately utilize immunohistochemistry, in situ hybridization and molecular tests; and 5) minimizes any potential diagnostic pitfalls in surgical pathology. These books also include highly practical presentations of typical case scenarios seen in an anatomic pathology laboratory. These are in the form of case presentations with step-by-step expert analysis. Sample cases include common but challenging situations, such as evaluation of well-differentiated malignant tumors vs. benign/reactive lesions; distinction of two benign entities; sub-classification of a malignant tumor; identification of newly described tumor and non-tumor entities; workup of a tumor of unknown origin; and implementation of best practice in immunohistochemistry and molecular testing in a difficult case. The Q&A format is well accepted, especially by junior pathologists, for several reasons: 1) this is the most practical and effective way to deliver information to a new generation of pathologists accustomed to using the Internet as a resource and, therefore, comfortable and familiar with a Q&A learning environment; 2) it's impossible to memorialize and digest massive amounts of new information about new entities, new and revised classifications, molecular pathology, diagnostic IHC, and the therapeutic implications of each entity by reading large textbooks; 3) sub-specialization is a very popular practice model highly demanded by many clinicians; and 4) time is very precious for a practicing pathologist because of increasing workloads in recent years following U.S. health care reforms. This Book Series meets all of the above expectations. These books are written by established and recognized experts in their specialty fields and provide a unique and valuable resource in the field of surgical pathology, both for those currently in training and for those already in clinical practice at various skill levels. It does not seek to duplicate or completely replace other large standard textbooks; rather, it is a new, comprehensive yet concise and practical resource on these timely and critical topics.

More information about this series at http://www.springer.com/series/13808

Yi Ding • Linsheng Zhang
Editors

Practical Oncologic Molecular Pathology

Frequently Asked Questions

Springer

Editors
Yi Ding
Department of Laboratory Medicine
Geisinger Health
Danville, PA
USA

Linsheng Zhang
Department of Pathology and Laboratory Medicine
Emory University School of Medicine
Atlanta, GA
USA

Practical Anatomic Pathology
ISBN 978-3-030-73226-4   ISBN 978-3-030-73227-1 (eBook)
https://doi.org/10.1007/978-3-030-73227-1

This Springer imprint is published by the registered company Springer Nature Switzerland AG
The registered company address is: Gewerbestrasse 11, 6330 Cham, Switzerland

To Bing, Alivia, and Irene (Yi Ding).

Dedicated with love to my wife, Tianzhen, and with respect to my teachers and friends, Drs. Sumiko Watanabe, Rui Liu, and Rong Zeng, who opened the door for me to enter the field of molecular biology (Linsheng Zhang).

Preface

This book is a review and high-yield reference on the clinical molecular diagnostics of malignant neoplasms. We aim to address the practical questions frequently encountered in molecular oncology practice, as well as key points and pitfalls in the clinical interpretation of molecular tests in guiding precision cancer management. It uses the Q&A format and case presentations, with emphasis on understanding the molecular test methods, diagnosis, classification, risk assessment, and clinical correlation. Starting with an update on the molecular biology of cancer, the book focuses on topics related to molecular diagnostics and genetics-based precision oncology. The molecular methods used in clinical laboratories, from traditional single-gene, single-analyte methods to multiplex, cutting-edge, and high-throughput technologies, are reviewed. Separate chapters are dedicated to the discussion of bioinformatics for the analysis of genetic/genomic data generated from molecular assays and quality control (QC)/quality assurance (QA) programs in the clinical laboratories; both are critical in producing high-quality results for clinical care of cancer patients. These are followed by organ system–based reviews and discussions on molecular genetic abnormalities and related tests covering diverse types of common to rare malignant neoplasms.

In recent years, several professional societies have worked together to establish clinical practice guidelines for utilizing molecular genetic tests in clinical oncology practice, including molecular testing guidelines to select lung cancer patients for targeting therapy with tyrosine kinase inhibitors, molecular biomarker tests for evaluation of colorectal cancer, and guidelines for the initial workup of chronic myeloid neoplasms and acute leukemias. At the same time, there is also widely accepted consensus on how to utilize molecular tests in the diagnosis, classification, and staging of many other cancer types listed by the National Comprehensive Cancer Network (NCCN) , which is updated frequently. These are covered in detail in the chapters on specific types of cancer. Advances in biomedical research are continuously updating our understanding of the genetic and genomic landscape of malignancies and changing the diagnostic approaches and treatment options available for tumors which were previously considered terminal and untreatable. Newly identified genetic abnormalities could assist the establishment of specific criteria for new entities and newly discovered effective targeting therapies. The book provides up-to-date knowledge related to malignant neoplasms and discusses the established as well as evolving requirements for pathologic diagnosis of these malignancies. At the same time, as a practical manual, this book also discusses the cost-effective utilization of molecular tests in clinical oncology.

Although molecular test results are generally considered objective, correlation between histology and molecular results and utilization of these results in clinical management guidance are areas that still need much attention and consideration. This book emphasizes the interpretation of molecular results in the context of clinical management as well as the integration of molecular findings in the complete pathology evaluation. Special attention is also given to the selection of the "right" molecular test at the "right" clinical presentation. Due to the numerous newly discovered genetic and genomic abnormalities of clinical significance, the test menu in clinical molecular diagnostic laboratories is rapidly evolving. Although we cannot be sure where future biomedical and clinical studies will lead us, the best way to predict the future is to plan and create it. Pathologists and clinical oncologists are required to keep up with the most recent advances in the field in order to provide the best cancer care. To meet such needs, this book also covers those questions related to the most recent molecular findings and future directions.

There are many books published on molecular pathology. We hope the concise, clear descriptions and illustrations compiled by experts actively practicing molecular pathology will make it a valuable handbook and reference for you.

Danville, PA, USA Yi Ding
Atlanta, GA, USA Linsheng Zhang

Contents

Part III Molecular Hematopathology

Contributors

Khaleel I. Al-Obaidy, MD Department of Pathology and Laboratory Medicine, Indiana University School of Medicine, Indianapolis, IN, USA

Leomar Y. Ballester, MD, PhD Department of Pathology and Laboratory Medicine, McGovern Medical School, Houston, TX, USA

Cynthia Reyes Barron, MD Department of Pathology and Laboratory Medicine, University of Rochester Medical Center, Rochester, NY, USA

Andrew Campbell, PhD Department of Laboratory Medicine, Geisinger Health, Danville, PA, USA

Guoli Chen, MD, PhD Department of Pathology and Laboratory Medicine, Geisinger Medical Center, Danville, PA, USA

Liang Cheng, MD Department of Pathology and Laboratory Medicine, Indiana University School of Medicine, Indianapolis, IN, USA

Kristin K. Deeb, PhD Department of Pathology and Laboratory Medicine, Emory University School of Medicine, Atlanta, GA, USA

Yi Ding, MD, PhD Department of Laboratory Medicine, Geisinger Health, Danville, PA, USA

Deanna C. Fang, MD Department of Pathology, UC San Diego School of Medicine, San Diego, CA, USA

Juehua Gao, MD, PhD Department of Pathology, Northwestern University Feinberg School of Medicine, Chicago, IL, USA

Vikas A. Gupta, MD, PhD Department of Hematology and Medical Oncology, Emory University School of Medicine, Atlanta, GA, USA

David G. Hicks, MD Department of Pathology and Laboratory Medicine, University of Rochester Medical Center, Rochester, NY, USA

David L. Jaye, MD Department of Pathology and Laboratory Medicine, Emory University School of Medicine, Atlanta, GA, USA

Lawrence J. Jennings, MD, PhD Department of Pathology, Northwestern University Feinberg School of Medicine, Chicago, IL, USA

Nisha S. Joseph, MD Department of Hematology and Medical Oncology, Emory University School of Medicine, Atlanta, GA, USA

Mariana Kekis, PhD Laboratory Medicine and Genetics, Trillium Health Partners, Mississauga, ON, Canada

Julie Li, MD, PhD Pathology and Laboratory Medicine Department, Boston University/Boston Medical Center, Boston, MA, USA

Terrance J. Lynn, MD Department of Laboratory Medicine, Geisinger Health, Danville, PA, USA

Anthony P. Martinez, MD Department of Pathology and Laboratory Medicine, Department of Dermatology, Emory University School of Medicine, Atlanta, GA, USA

Mohammad K. Mohammad, MD Department of Pathology and Laboratory Medicine, Geisinger Medical Center, Geisinger Commonwealth School of Medicine, Danville, PA, USA

Zenggang Pan, MD, PhD Department of Pathology, Yale University School of Medicine, New Haven, CT, USA

Nathan Paulson, MD Department of Pathology and Laboratory Medicine, Yale University School of Medicine, New Haven, CT, USA

Matthew J. Schniederjan, MD Department of Pathology and Laboratory Medicine, Children's Healthcare of Atlanta – Scottish Rite and Egleston Hospitals, Emory University School of Medicine, Atlanta, GA, USA

Geoffrey H. Smith, MD Department of Pathology and Laboratory Medicine, Emory University School of Medicine, Atlanta, GA, USA

Bruce R. Smoller, MD Department of Pathology and Laboratory Medicine, University of Rochester Medical Center, Rochester, NY, USA

Harold C. Sullivan, MD, D(ABHI) Department of Pathology and Laboratory Medicine, Emory University School of Medicine, Atlanta, GA, USA

Patricia C. Tsang, MD Department of Pathology and Laboratory Medicine, Geisinger Commonwealth School of Medicine, Danville, PA, USA

Tatiana Tvrdik, PhD Department of Pathology and Laboratory Medicine, Emory University School of Medicine, Atlanta, GA, USA

José E. Velázquez Vega, MD Department of Pathology and Laboratory Medicine, Children's Healthcare of Atlanta – Scottish Rite and Egleston Hospitals, Emory University School of Medicine, Atlanta, GA, USA

Xi Wang, MD, PhD Department of Pathology and Laboratory Medicine, Yale University School of Medicine, New Haven, CT, USA

Guang Yang, MD, PhD Department of Pathology and Laboratory Medicine, University of Pennsylvania, Philadelphia, PA, USA

Huina Zhang, MD, PhD Department of Pathology and Laboratory Medicine, University of Rochester Medical Center, Rochester, NY, USA

Jennifer Q. Zhang, PhD, D(ABHI) UCLA Immunogenetics Center, Department of Pathology and Laboratory Medicine, David Geffen School of Medicine at UCLA, Los Angeles, CA, USA

Linsheng Zhang, MD, PhD Department of Pathology and Laboratory Medicine, Emory University School of Medicine, Atlanta, GA, USA

Xiaohui Zhang, MD, PhD Department of Pathology, H. Lee Moffitt Cancer Center and Research Institute, Tampa, FL, USA

Gang Zheng, MD, PhD Department of Laboratory Medicine and Pathology, Mayo Clinic, Rochester, MN, USA

Ruifang Zheng, MD, PhD Department of Pathology and Laboratory Medicine, Emory University School of Medicine, Atlanta, GA, USA

Part I

Molecular Methods and Data Analysis in Clinical Molecular Diagnostic Laboratories

The Molecular Pathobiology of Malignant Process and Molecular Diagnostic Testing for Cancer

1

Yi Ding and Linsheng Zhang

List of Frequently Asked Questions

1. What are the major cellular activities frequently involved in cancer development?
2. How are genes organized in the human cells?
3. What are oncogenes?
4. What are tumor suppressor genes?
5. How do epigenetic changes affect gene expression and cellular activity that may result in malignant transformation?
6. What are noncoding RNAs and microRNAs, and how are they involved in cancer development?
7. What is clonal diversity and how is this related to cancer development and progression?
8. What are the basic principles of tumorigenesis?
9. What are the frequent types of genetic abnormalities related to cancer development?
10. How are the types of mutations and combination of different genetic abnormalities associated with the targeted therapy strategy?
11. What are the purposes of molecular tests for cancers?
12. How to choose a molecular method for the detection of genetic abnormalities associated with cancer?
13. How to properly name different kinds of mutations or genetic abnormalities in a molecular pathology report?

Y. Ding
Department of Laboratory Medicine,
Geisinger Health, Danville, PA, USA
e-mail: yding1@geisinger.edu

L. Zhang (✉)
Department of Pathology and Laboratory Medicine,
Emory University School of Medicine, Atlanta, GA, USA
e-mail: linsheng.zhang@emory.edu

Frequently Asked Questions

1. **What are the major cellular activities frequently involved in cancer development?**
   - Cancer is now widely accepted as a genetic disease characterized by alterations of genes that regulate normal biologic process of the cells. Although current classification of cancer in clinical practice is still largely based on the phenotype and clinical presentation of malignant processes, cancer genomics are playing more and more important roles in the diagnosis, classification and guiding clinical management of cancer. With the progress of our understanding of the biologic basis of cancer, more genomic factors are integrated into the classification of malignancies, as we have already seen in the recently updated World Health Organization (WHO) classifications of hematopoietic and lymphoid, and central nervous system tumors.
   - The major characteristics of cancer include (1) unchecked proliferation irrespective of normal regulatory processes and unrestricted growth potential independent of growth factors (immortality); (2) arrested maturation/differentiation, failing to produce mature functional cells; (3) loss of the ability to remove dysfunctional and dysregulated cells through programed cell death (defective apoptosis); (3) a predominance when interacting with the environment, represented by invasive ectopic growth (metastasis) and enhanced angiogenesis for malignant growth. Therefore the cellular activities most relevant to cancer development are cell proliferation, differentiation, and apoptosis. Furthermore, the normal cells have molecular mechanisms to maintain the stability of the genome and repair the damages whenever possible; disruptions in the activities related to these mechanisms are often associated with increased cancer susceptibility.
   - Cell growth is a tightly controlled process, which is regulated when a cell enters and how fast it goes through

Y. Ding, L. Zhang (eds.), *Practical Oncologic Molecular Pathology*, Practical Anatomic Pathology,
https://doi.org/10.1007/978-3-030-73227-1_1

the proliferative cycle (cell cycle). A cell cycle progresses through four stages: G1 (growth), S (DNA synthesis), G2 (the second growth), and M (mitosis). Some cells (such as liver cells) can stay in a non-proliferative stage called G0 for a long time. The progression of each stage are regulated by activators, such as cyclin-dependent kinases (CDKs), and inhibitory factors, such as cyclin-dependent kinase inhibitors (CKIs). These regulators of cell cycles are themselves regulated by their production (transcription), activation (frequently phosphorylation-dephosphorylation), and controlled degradation through ubiquitins and proteasomes. The key obstacle of cell cycling is the G1 to S transition. Numerous factors involved in the diligently controlled switches of cell cycling, starting from growth factor receptors located on the cell surface, followed by signal transduction molecules in the growth factor pathway, to transcription factors, as well as CDKs/CDIs and ubiquitin and proteasome-related factors, are involved in the development of cancer, when they are mutated or somehow altered. The cell cycle checkpoints are also monitored and regulated by key tumor suppressor genes like *RB* and *TP53* (see discussion in question 4).

- Cells growing as a component of the tissue must mature to be functional through a differentiation process, which is mostly regulated by various transcription factors. The transcription factors turn on some protein production and shut off other proteins, shaping the phenotype and function of a cell. A cell that has lost the normal differentiation potential stays at the primitive stage. Cancer cells can retain some maturation mechanisms, even though not fully functional (well differentiated) or completely lose the differentiation potential (poorly differentiated).
- Programed cell death (apoptosis) is a physiologic process to remove the damaged, aged, or no-longer required cells, so as to keep the homeostasis of multicellular organisms, without triggering inflammatory reactions. There are two pathways, intrinsic and extrinsic, involving distinct factors associated with apoptosis. The intrinsic pathway is initiated by leaking of cytochrome c from mitochondria to cytoplasm; the extrinsic pathway is activated by death receptors such as FAS. Loss of elements promoting apoptosis, such as BAX, or accumulation of antiapoptotic proteins and inhibitors of apoptosis, such as BCL2, will render the cells survival advantage, resulting in immortality [1]. Another important cellular activity associated with apoptosis is cell senescence, regulated by the normal maintenance of telomere.
- Damages to the chromosome structure and mistakes in DNA replication occur due to extrinsic factors, such as ionizing radiation, or intrinsic errors of DNA polymerase activity. Normal cells carry robust mechanisms to correct DNA replication errors and remove cells damaged too much to resuscitate. The genes involved in DNA repair, such as *BRCA1/2*, *ATM*, and various mismatch repair (MMR) genes are "caretaker genes," maintaining the integrity of DNA. If these mechanisms are disrupted or lost, the cells will accumulate errors and chromosome abnormalities, referred to as genetic instability.
- In the multicellular organisms, all cells are part of a bigger machinery. Interactions with the microenvironment is a critical part of cellular activity and tissue development process. An abnormal interaction, if not inducing the cancerous process, can at least promote the development of malignancy. Alteration in the metabolism, cytoskeleton, and cellular adhesion as well as abnormal angiogenesis have all been confirmed to play a part in the tumor progression and metastasis. A classic example of an abnormal microenvironment promoting malignant cell growth is found in multiple myeloma. Cytokines, growth factors, and interleukins produced and secreted by cells in the bone marrow microenvironment create autocrine and paracrine loops to stimulate the growth of malignant myeloma cells. Therapeutic agents blocking the supportive effects of the microenvironment, such as thalidomide, lenalidomide, and bortezomib, have substantially changed the treatment regimens of multiple myeloma [2].

2. **How are genes organized in the human cells?**
    - The genetic blueprint of all living cells composes double-stranded DNA made from sequences of nucleotides with only four different nucleobases: adenine (A), guanine (G), cytosine (C), and thymine (T). As displayed in Fig. 1.1, the ribose and phosphate groups form the backbone of the DNA strand, and the nucleobases determine the complementary sequences of the double strand, with A paired to T, and C paired to G. In contrast, RNA is single stranded with an additional hydroxyl group at the 2′-position of the ribose. The chemical structure of DNA or RNA strands are directional, running from the 5′-phospate to 3′-hydroxyl group, which means in the process of DNA or RNA synthesis, adding a nucleotide only occurs at the 3′-end. The synthetic reaction of adding nucleotides to a DNA or RNA stand would not happen if the 3′-hydroxyl group is missing (di-deoxy nucleotide); this is the chemical basis of Sanger sequencing and some genotyping tests (chain-terminating method).
    - In a human cell, the genomic DNA molecules are packed in a highly organized and condensed architecture and enclosed in the nucleus. Each human cell contains 46 chromosomes, including 22 pairs of autosomes and 1 pair of sex chromosomes (XX, or XY). Each chromosome is a very long single linear DNA molecule that is packed with nuclear proteins and some RNAs. The tightly packed DNA together with the protein and RNA is referred to as chromatin.

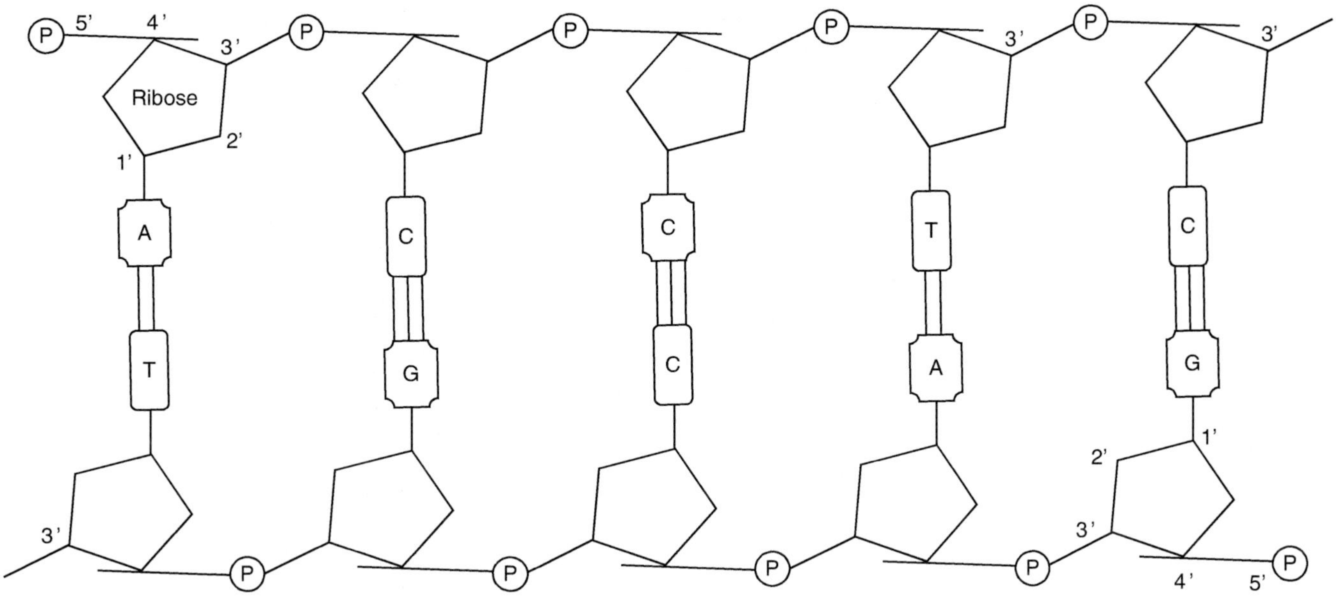

Fig. 1.1 **The chemical structure of double-stranded DNA.** See text for details

- Chromatins may change conformation in the different stages of cell cycle. The chromosomes are best organized and visible at the M stage (metaphase), at which the clinical karyotyping is obtained. Based on the morphology of the chromosomes, each chromosome contains a short (p) arm, a centromere, and a long (q) arm. The autosomes are numbered based on their sizes (chromosome 1 being the longest and chromosome 22 shortest).
- At each end of the chromosomes, there is a specialized chromatin called telomere that functions to protect the integrity of the chromosome ends, preventing them from loss or fusing with other DNA molecules.
- Many different types of chromosomal abnormalities have been identified in malignant cells, from a simple copy number change to complex abnormalities resulting from chromothripsis. The commonly seen abnormalities are:
  - Polyploidy: extra complete set(s) of chromosomes. The normal 23 pairs of chromosomes are 2N; addition of one complete set, therefore, creates 3N (triploidy), and addition of two sets is 4N (tetraploidy).
  - Aneuploidy: abnormal loss or gain of a single or multiple whole chromosome(s). For example, monosomy 5 and 7 are frequently seen in myelodysplastic syndrome (MDS): 44,XY,−5,−7.
  - Translocation: abnormal break and rearrangement in a chromosome, e.g., inv(16);*CBFB-MYH11*, or between chromosomes, e.g., t(11;22)(q24;q12) *EWSR1-FLI1*.
  - Insertions or deletions: loss or gain of part of the chromosome regions (e.g., −5q in MDS; dup(21q) amplifies *RUNX1* in B-lymphoblastic leukemia). The detection sensitivity (size of insertion or deletion) is determined by the method used for karyotyping.
  - Complex abnormalities with multiple different changes occur in one set of chromosomes. In tumor cells with complex abnormalities, it is not rare to see diversified changes with a stemline (abnormalities in all cells) and subclones (different additional abnormalities present in separate subpopulations of tumor cells).
- A human genome comprises 6.4 billion (3.2 X 2) nucleotides in the 23 pairs of chromosomes. However, only approximately 30,000 genes are recognized in the genome. Like all the eukaryotic cells, within the human DNA sequences that we call "genes," the coding regions (exons) containing messages to transcribe into functional RNA are interrupted by noncoding sequences (introns), which could be much longer than the coding exons. After transcribing double-stranded DNA to single-stranded RNA (transcription), the early RNA is modified by splicing out the exon regions and other posttranscriptional modifications (such as adding poly-adenine tail to the 3′ end for the messenger RNA). For any given cell, the size of total RNA (whole transcriptome) is less than 6% of the total human genome [3].
- Each and every different cell in the living body contains the same genomic DNA sequence (genotype). However, they are vastly different in their appearances and function (phenotype). The phenotype is determined by the on and off regulation of different genes, which is usually controlled via the noncoding, regulatory DNA sequences (regulatory elements). Because the default state of eukaryotic genes within the packed chromatin is in the "off" state, the most important reg-

ulatory elements are activator sequences including promoters and enhancers.

- Promoters are DNA sequences recognized and bound by universal transcription factors and RNA polymerases, to turn on the transcription process. They are usually located near and upstream (to the 5′-end) of the coding sequences. A negative regulatory element similar and related to a promoter is a repressor. On the other hand, enhancers are usually located relatively distant from the coding sequences. They bind to more tissue-specific transcription factors responsible to turn on specific genes. The regulatory elements that are similar but functioning opposite to enhancers are called silencers. The positive and negative regulatory elements can be brought together by the proteins binding to the corresponding sequences.
- The regulatory DNA sequences are on the same DNA strand, near or far, with the regulated genes. Therefore, they are called *cis*-regulatory elements. On the other hand, the regulatory proteins (e.g., transcription factors) binding to the regulatory elements can be encoded anywhere in the genome. The gene sequences for these protein factors are collectively referred to as "*trans*-regulatory elements."
- Many other noncoding sequences function as regulatory elements. To prevent regulatory elements from activating nearby unrelated genes, there are DNA sequences that compartmentalize the genome into discrete domains. On a large scale, the barrier sequences mark the border of chromatin accessible to regulatory proteins; on a smaller scale, the insulator limits the *cis*-regulatory elements functioning within the related genes. However, depending on the proteins binding to the insulators, the regulated genes limited by insulators can be different in variable cell or tissue types, increasing the versatility of the regulatory elements.

Alterations/mutations occur in the regulatory sequences may result in aberrant expression of genes and changes of the phenotype. This is one of the important molecular mechanisms of tumorigenesis. See more discussions under questions 5 and 6.

3. **What are oncogenes?**
   - Oncogenes are cellular genes that cause cancer development when they are abnormally hyperactive. The hyperactive state can be a result of mutation of the gene or overexpression of a normal gene.
   - Although classified as oncogenes due to their obnoxious effect in driving transformation to malignancy, oncogenes are usually critical for normal cellular activity. To distinguish the normal activity from malignant activity of these genes, the normal version of these genes are sometimes referred to as "proto-oncogenes." When a virus picks up cellular oncogene and integrates it in the viral genome, that version becomes the viral oncogene. For example, the *SRC* gene (named after "sarcoma in chicken") carried by the Rous sarcoma virus is v-*SRC* and the cellular version is c-*SRC*.
   - In a normal cell, the proto-oncogenes are essential directors or regulators of basic cellular activities including cell proliferation, survival, and blocking of terminal differentiation and adhesion/motility. When abnormally activated, the affected cells are transformed, gaining features of malignancy, including unregulated growth, immortal survival potential, arrested differentiation, and unlimited motility.
   - The well-known oncogenes include those involved in growth factor receptor signal transduction pathways (e.g., *EGFR*, *RAS*, *RAF*, *MYC*), blocking apoptotic process (e.g., *BCL2*), and driving or promoting cell cycle progression (e.g., *CCND1*) and transcription factors (e.g., *JUN*, *FOS*, *STAT3*, and *STAT5*).
   - Oncogenes usually collaborate with each other and with defective tumor suppressor genes in driving cancer development. Inhibiting the hyperactivity of the proteins encoded by the aberrant oncogenes, with either antibodies or small molecule inhibitors, is the most frequent targeted therapy strategy in precision cancer treatment.
   - Depending on the activity level and the background cellular activity, some oncoproteins may become tumor suppressors when the expression level is overly high or the mutations create an excessively active protein.
4. **What are tumor suppressor genes?**
   - Tumor suppressor genes are gene-encoding products that, when functioning normally, prevent the malignant transformation of cells.
   - As each human cell has two alleles of each gene/locus, and expression of one normal copy of a gene is usually sufficient for the normal function, it usually takes aberrations in more than one locus to disrupt the tumor suppressor activity. These can happen when there are biallelic mutations, deletions, or downregulations. However, sometimes aberrancy in only one copy of a tumor suppressor gene can result in cancer development due to haploinsufficiency (one copy is not enough for the full function) or dominant effect (the mutant protein blocks the function of its normal counterpart). For example, deletion or mutation of one copy of *GATA2* is sufficient to drive a *GATA2* deficiency syndrome; a mutant p53, when forming dimers/tetramers with normal p53 proteins, may create an inactive protein complex due to its dominant effect. In these situations, a homozygous mutation or compound heterozygous abnormality is not required for cancer development.

- Tumor suppressor genes encode products (protein or noncoding RNA) blocking the progression of cell cycle when the cell contains damaged DNA, promoting cell apoptosis or senescence; they may also be components of the DNA-repairing complex. The most important tumor suppressor genes are *RB*, *TP53*, and those encoding proteins for DNA repairing machineries.
- The *RB* gene, which was discovered and is frequently mutated in retinoblastoma, encodes the RB protein that binds to transcription factors, most importantly E2Fs, to regulate cell cycle progression. Only in a phosphorylation state, RB releases transcription factors that promote the initiation of DNA synthesis. The normal RB protein functions as a brake to the cell cycle, sequestering transcription factors and preventing the start of DNA replication. Mutant RB gene loses the brake function, so it is related to the development of a variety of cancer types, not limited to retinoblastoma. Disrupting the RB function in cell cycle regulation is also one of the important molecular mechanisms that human papilloma virus (HPV) drives malignant transformation. The E7 protein encoded by high-risk HPVs binds to and impairs the normal function of RB protein, mimicking the binding of cyclin D family proteins [4]. HPV E6 and E7 proteins also have other activities in promoting cell cycle progression.
- The p53 protein encoded by *TP53* is activated by many different mechanisms related to malignant transformation, e.g., DNA damage induced by irradiation. When activated, p53 blocks the cell cycle progression and induces apoptosis through transcription control of multiple genes.
- The genes involved in the regulation of either *RB* or *TP53* expression, or encoding factors in the RB/p53 activity complex, are also associated with cancer development and, therefore, can be either oncogenes or tumor suppressor genes.
- In recent years, many genes involved in the DNA mismatch repair or other DNA-repairing mechanisms have been identified. Inability to repair damaged DNA resulting in accumulation of mutations, thus, significantly decreases the stability of the genome and increases the chance of malignant transformation. The well-known examples include *BRCA1/2* genes, and mismatch repair genes *MLH1*, *MSH2*, *MSH6*, and *PMS2*, of which the loss of function can be detected by the consequent microsatellite instability (more discussions in Chap. 8).

5. **How do epigenetic changes affect gene expression and cellular activity that may result in malignant transformation?**

- The term "epigenetic regulation" refers to the control of gene expression without changing the genomic DNA sequence. Epigenetic regulation as we understand now includes changes at three different levels: dynamic transformation of the patterns of chromatin structure, modification of the proteins (e.g., histones) involved in the nucleosome architecture, and methylation of DNA that usually happens in the regulatory sequences.
- Based on the pattern and the density seen under the electron microscope, chromatins are recognized as euchromatin and heterochromatin. The euchromatin is loosely packed and available for active transcription; the heterochromatin, in contrast, is more tightly packed and not transcribed. Chromatins are not static; they transform dynamically according to the cell activity status through epigenetic regulation.
- In chromatin, the genomic DNA forms nucleosome complexes with histones, in which approximately 150 bp length of DNA is wrapped around histone scaffolds. Due to this structural pattern, when genomic DNA is released into the blood circulation from apoptotic or necrotic cells, the nucleosomes are relatively protected from enzymatic digestion. Therefore, circulation cell-free DNA (cfDNA) usually has a size range between 130 to 210 bp (peak at 167 bp [5]). Modification of histone proteins may change the availability of DNA sequences for transcription; therefore, it is an important mechanism of epigenetic regulation.
- DNA methylation is covalent addition of a methyl group to the 5-position of the cytosine base, which usually occurs in the context of the cytidine-guanosine dinucleotide (CpG), and is frequently seen in small stretches of DNA called CpG islands associated with promoter regions of genes. After methylation, the CpG is modified to mCpG; and presence of multiple mCpGs in a CpG island is referred to as hypermethylation. Hypermethylation occurring in the promoter region, together with some modification of the histones, shuts off the promoter.
- Methylation of DNA is induced by the "writer" enzymes, DNA methyltransferases (DNMTs), and the methyl group can be removed by the "eraser" enzymes, the ten-eleven translocation proteins (TETs). Mutations in these enzymes are frequently found in myeloid neoplasms, and hypomethylation therapy has been established as an effective treatment for myelodysplastic syndrome. Silencing of DNA mismatch repair gene *MLH1* by promoter region hypermethylation is well recognized in sporadic colorectal cancer, with a similar phenotype to Lynch syndrome (see Chap. 8).
- Some cancers are found to have CpG island methylator phenotype (CIMP), exhibiting hypermethylation

of usually unmethylated regions in up to half of all human gene promoters, resulting in aberrant silencing of hundreds of genes [6–8].

- The modifications of histone proteins include acetylation and methylation. They are also mediated by "writer" enzymes and "eraser" enzymes, of which mutations are frequently associated with malignancies. Effective treatment of malignancies targeting these proteins have also started to gain attention in clinical trials.
  - Currently found histone acetylation "writers" (lysine acetyltransferases, KATs) include GNAT, p300/CBP, MYST, SRC, etc.; three classes of "erasers" (histone deacetylases, HDACs) have been identified. HDAC inhibitors have been approved for the treatment of some lymphoid malignancies [9, 10].
  - Methylation of histone proteins are mediated by "writer" enzymes lysine methyltransferases (KMTs) and protein arginine methyltransferases (PRMTs). Multiple "eraser" enzymes (lysine demethylase, KDMs) have also been identified [11].
  - Modification of non-histone proteins also occurs as epigenetic regulations. However, these are less well studied [12].
- Regulator proteins (sometimes called "readers") recognizing DNA methylation, lysine acetylation, and methylation most likely integrate all the epigenetic signals together to effectively control gene expression. In recent years, mutations of several proteins/enzymes active in the metabolic pathways have been recognized as driver mutations of certain malignancies through modification of the epigenetic signals. For example, mutant isocitrate dehydrogenase (IDH1/2) converts alpha-ketoglutarate (α-KG), a normal metabolite of citric acid cycle, to 2-hydroxyglutarate (2-HG), an antagonist of α-KG and inhibitor of histone and DNA demethylases, disrupting the normal epigenetic control of gene expression and cell differentiation [13]. Targeting *IDH* mutations is effective in treating *IDH1/2* mutated acute myeloid leukemia.
- Epigenetic modifications are not maintained in germ cells; therefore, they are not inheritable to the second generation. However, these modifications can be passed on to the progeny of somatic cells; a silenced gene will remain silent in the whole clonal population of tumor cells.
- Noncoding areas in the genome previously alleged to be "junk" may transcribe to regulatory RNA, playing important roles in gene regulation (see question 6 below). In addition, posttranscriptional modification of mRNA, posttranslational modification of proteins, and degradation of proteins are also highly regulated, and any abnormalities in these processes may be associated with cancer development.

6. **What are noncoding RNA and microRNA, and how are they involved in cancer development?**
   - RNA molecules have been found to function much beyond being the intermediate coding template between DNA and protein. Although only approximately 1% of the genome is coding sequences, studies have found that >90% of the genome is transcribed [14]. In addition to the well-studied tRNA, rRNA, and small nucleolar RNA (snoRNA), the cells also have abundant other noncoding RNA molecules (ncRNA), including long ncRNA (lncRNA, >200 up to thousands of nucleotides (nt)), small ncRNA (up to 200 nt), and circular RNA (circRNA).
   - MicroRNAs (miRNAs) are defined as endogenously expressed single-stranded ncRNAs of approximately 20 nt. MiRNA can be transcribed from the introns, sequences spanning intron-exons, within the regulatory elements (promoter, enhancer), antisense sequence, or intergenic regions (with independent promoters). The transcribed precursor RNA goes through a maturing process and eventually becomes the single-stranded mature functional miRNA [15].
   - MiRNAs bind to the sequence-complementary mRNA, most frequently in the 3′-untranslated region (UTR), to affect the stability by accelerating the deadenylation and degradation of targeted mRNAs [16, 17]. The sequence specificity and the secondary architecture of the RNA interactions both affect the functional consequence of the interaction, which is facilitated by miRNA-induced silencing complex (miRISC). MiRNAs are actively involved in regulating gene expression on the posttranscriptional level, functioning as oncogenes or tumor suppressor genes. For example, *miR-21* and *miR-31* suppress RAS–MEK–ERK signaling via multiple targets and can be considered a tumor suppressor gene; on the other hand, *miR-155* and *miR-221* targeting SHIP1 and PTEN can be considered as oncogenes. The sequence complementary specificity of miRNA is usually not very restrictive; therefore, miRNAs simultaneously target many mRNAs, likely yielding suppression on multiple targets.
   - The diverse and complex biologic functions of lncRNA have not been well characterized yet. However, studies have found lncRNAs to be involved in maintaining genome architecture, genomic imprinting or regulating epigenetic mechanisms in a large scale, and affecting posttranscriptional RNA modification. The structure rather than the primary sequence determines the function of many lncRNA. Interestingly, some

lncRNA can serve both as a coding template and ncRNA functions [18].

- The miRNA molecules are released to and relatively stable in blood circulation with the protection of protein carriers. The circulating miRNAs may serve as biomarkers when a unique signature can be associated with a specific disease condition, including cancer. Detection of ncRNA is now performed by NGS-based RNA sequencing, and the findings are usually verified by quantitative (real-time) reverse transcription polymerase chain reaction (RT-qPCR) [19].

7. **What is clonal diversity and how is this related to cancer development and progression?**
   - Following Darwinian evolution, cell competition or cellular fitness plays an essential role in not only normal but also cancer cell biology. By creating a high degree of genetic and phenotypic diversity through somatic evolution, cancer cells compete among themselves and with their surrounding microenvironment to gain maximum proliferation and growth advantage. This process, which is also called clonal evolution, promotes survival and spread of oncogenic cells as well as eliminates the intratumoral cells and surrounding nontumor cells with suboptimal fitness traits [20].
   - Different models of cancer evolutional biology exist, primarily including the branching model (multiple phenotypically distinct cancer clones evolves in parallel) and the linear progression model (the cancer cells pass through multiple rounds of genetic changes sequentially). The accumulated mutations during clonal evolution result in spatial intratumoral heterogeneity (ITH) and provide the sources of genetic diversity in cancers. For example, as one of the most common and aggressive primary brain tumors in adults, glioblastoma (GBM), has shown remarkable ITH and intertumoral heterogeneity between patients. It is not only because of the diverse origin of tumor cells such as astrocytes, oligodendrocytes, and ependymal cells, GBM also demonstrates heterogeneous molecular profile through *IDH1/IDH2*, *ATRX*, *EGFR*, *H3K27M*, *PDGFRA*, *TP53*, and chromosomal aberration such as 1p/19q deletion, chromosomal 7 insertion, and chromosomal 10 deletion [21].
   - Because the fitness of clonal cancer cells can affect tumor growth and metastasis, tumorigenesis is a highly dynamic process affected by many factors, such as inherent genomic instability, clonal diversity or tumor heterogeneity, tumor microenvironment, treatment pressure, host metabolic status, etc. [22]. The complex interaction/competition determines the fate of tumor progression over the realms of space and time, which suggests the importance of monitoring tumor mutational profile [23, 24].
   - Advances in the understanding of the molecular mechanisms of tumorigenesis is reshaping the tumor subclassification and helping us to treat cancer more efficiently. Cancer mutation profiling, including mutation testing of different "space" (sampling of one tumor mass at multiple locations) and time (serial sampling of a malignancy in the disease process) for some tumors with high clonal diversities, can provide critical information in guiding personalized cancer treatment.
8. **What are the basic principles of tumorigenesis?**
   - Cancer formation is a process of somatic evolution that resulted from the accumulation of genomic alterations conferring a selective advantage [25, 26]. Driver mutations are those major recurrent somatic alterations that not only induce the proliferation and differentiation of malignancy but also play a "fate-determination" role. For example, mutations in *KRAS*, *EGFR*, *ALK*, *BRAF*, *MET*, and *PI3KCA* are well-accepted drivers in non-small cell lung carcinoma whereas *FGFR1*, *PIK3CA*, *PTEN*, *PDGFRA*, *MET*, and *DDR2* mutations are known drivers in squamous cell lung cancer [27].
   - Compared to driver mutations, passenger mutations are less critical, usually having no effect on the clonal fitness but playing a role in cancer growth and expansion. They are also known as a hitchhikers in evolutionary biology. Although passenger mutations are larger by number, their pathological and clinical significances largely remain unknown.
   - It is important to understand the difference between a driver gene and a driver mutation. A driver gene is the gene that can generate driver mutations, but it can also produce passenger mutations.
   - Besides the classic driver mutation model in which the clonal and subclonal mutations arise early and the tumor grows as an intermixed population depending on the growth advantage of tumor cells, the "two-hit model" or "multi-hit model" for tumorigenesis is also commonly known. Different from the clonal evolutional model, the first hit (mutation) does not confer cell survival fitness. There will be no cumulative effect until the combination of two or multiple hits (mutations) occur [28, 29].
   - Clinically, somatic mutations are classified into four different tiers using an evidence-based categorization system [30, 31]. Based on the therapeutic, prognostic, and diagnostic impacts, the four tiers are:
   - **Tier I: Variants of strong clinical significance**
     - Level A evidence: FDA-approved therapy or included in professional guidelines
     - Level B evidence: Well-powered studies with consensus from experts in the field

- **Tier II: Variants of potential clinical significance**
  - Level C evidence: FDA-approved therapies for different tumor types or investigational therapies or multiple small published studies with some consensus
  - Level D evidence: Preclinical trials or a few case reports without consensus
- **Tier III: Variants of unknown clinical significance** include variants which are not observed at a significant allele frequency in the general or specific subpopulation databases, or pan-cancer or tumor-specific variant databases. There is no convincing published evidence of cancer association.
- **Tier IV: Benign or likely benign variants** include variants that are observed at a significant allele frequency in the general or specific subpopulation databases. There is no existing published evidence of cancer association. Tier IV variants are usually not included in the clinical molecular test reports.

9. **What are the frequent types of genetic abnormalities related to cancer development?**
   - Many different kinds of genetic alterations are found in cancer cells. Mutations in the coding DNA segments can affect the structure, function, and amount of the corresponding proteins and change a cell's behavior from normal to cancerous. Based on their effect upon the transcript, it can be categorized as missense, nonsense, silent, frameshift mutations, and chromosome rearrangements. Their definition and consequences are summarized in Table 1.1 with representative examples listed.
   - Noncoding DNA (ncDNA) segments that do not directly code for proteins consist of introns, repetitive DNA, and regulatory DNA and account for more than 98% of the human genome. A large portion of ncDNA is transcribed to ncRNA. Mutations in the ncDNA and alterations in ncRNA have also been found to play a significant role in cancer pathogenesis (see question 6). For example, emerging evidence has shown that lncRNAs can function through modulating liver microenvironment, and dysregulation of lncRNA plays a critical role in chronic hepatitis and development of hepatocellular carcinoma [32, 33].
   - Cancer epigenetics is a rapidly expanding field (see question 5). Combined with genetic mutations, alterations in epigenetic regulations play a critical role in

Table 1.1 Major genetic abnormalities in cancer

Mutation		Definition	Consequence	Example
Missense		A substitution of a nucleotide that changes a codon and results in a different amino acid.	Depending on the amino acid changed; sometimes can greatly alter the protein's function.	A single point mutation in *KRAS* with nucleotide substitution of G to T at position 34 (c. 34G > T) which results glycine-to-cysteine substitution at codon 12 (p.G12C). This is the most frequent *KRAS* mutation in non-small-cell lung cancer.
Nonsense		A change that could be nucleotide substitution, deletion, or insertion that creates a pre-mature stop codon, which terminates translation.	A shortened protein that may not function or that may have an abnormal or even dominant function.	A single nucleotide from CAG to TAG in DNA which results in a stop codon UAG and causes premature termination of translation. A truncated p53 protein may have a dominant negative effect.
Silent		A nucleotide substitution that results in codon alteration without changing its encoded amino acid.	Usually none.	If the codon AAA is changed to AAG, there is no change of its encoded amino acid, lysine (Lys).
Frameshift		The insertion or deletion of nucleotides that shifts both the codon and the corresponding amino acid sequence.	Alteration of sequence, structure and function of the protein.	DNA amino acid Normal CAG CCC ACT Gln-Pro-Thr Frameshift CAG TCC CAC T Gln-Ser-His (Frameshift mutation caused by a single nucleotide insertion of T)
Chromosome rearrangement	Deletion	A fragment of or the entire chromosome breaks and is lost.	Can change several critical genes' functions at the same time.	Chromosome 3p deletion in clear cell RCC
	Translocation	A fragment of a chromosome breaks and moves to a different chromosomal location.		t(21;22)(q22.3;q12.2) in Ewing's sarcoma
	Inversion	A fragment of a chromosome breaks and flips directions.		inv(16)(p13.1;q22) in AML
	Duplication	A fragment of or the entire chromosome is repeated.		7q34 duplication in pilocytic astrocytoma

RCC renal cell carcinoma, *AML* acute myeloid leukemia

tumorigenesis. For example, there are usually 3–6 key driver mutations (e.g., *APC*, *KRAS*, *BRAF*, *PIK3CA*, *SMAD4*, *TP53*) and 30–70 passenger mutations in a typical colorectal carcinoma ("driver and passenger mutations" are discussed more detailed in question 8); however, there are about 600–800 hypermethylated CpG islands in promoter regions of genes that could be epigenetically regulated [34]. Of note, epigenetic modification and genetic alterations function in an interactive networking manner and should not be considered as isolated events and processes.

10. **How are the types of mutations and combinations of different genetic abnormalities associated with the targeted therapy strategy?**
    - Different types of mutations can create the same or similar pathologic activity in a malignant process. For example, constitutive EGFR tyrosine kinase activity is a result of gain of function mutations in the tyrosine kinase domain; on the other hand, enhanced EGFR activity can be achieved through increased expression level resulting from amplification or copy gains of *EGFR* [35].
    - Although there are usually multiple mutations orchestrating a tumorigenic process, the majority of malignancies start from a single driver mutation event. Generally, the driver mutations, especially those occurring in genes involved in the same functional pathway, are mutually exclusive because one mutation in that pathway is sufficient to disrupt the biologic process. For example, *JAK2*, *CALR*, and *MPL* mutations rarely occur together in one patient; similarly, *ALK1* translocation very rarely happens in *EGFR*-mutated lung cancer.
    - The type of genetic alterations and at which point a mutant protein functions in the signal transduction pathway are critical in determining the strategy of targeted therapy. For example, when EGFR function is enhanced by overexpression of the protein, antibodies blocking the EGFR ligand binding can be effective in sabotaging the tumorigenic activity [36]. However, the antibodies would not affect the constitutive activity of a mutant EGFR; in this situation, small molecule inhibitors suppressing the mutated and hyperactive kinase have been confirmed to be very effective in targeted therapy for lung adenocarcinoma [37]. Another example from lung-cancer-related genetic alterations is the mutations of *KRAS*, the second most commonly mutated genes in lung cancer (see Chap. 7). RAS is located downstream of the EGFR signal pathway to promote cell growth and survival [38]. Therefore, if the *RAS* gene or any other genes located at the downstream of the EGFR signal transduction pathway (see Fig. 8.1 in Chap. 8) are mutated, targeting EGFR either by antibodies or kinase inhibitors will not break the active mutagenic process.
    - Given the complexity of the cell signal transduction and interconnection of different pathways, secondary mutations compensating the pathway blocked by the inhibitors, developed under the selection pressure of targeted therapies, frequently result in secondary resistance to targeted therapy. This is one of the common mechanisms of drug resistance [35, 39].

11. **What are the purposes of molecular tests for cancers?**
    Identification of certain genes or gene mutations can be helpful in diagnosing cancer, learning about prognosis, triaging treatment, and monitoring the effects of treatment.
    - Diagnosis and classification
      Although cancer diagnosis is a multilayer process usually including routine laboratory tests, imaging studies, and biopsy, some gene mutations are now known to be strongly associated with certain neoplasms and being integrated in the disease diagnosis or subclassification.
      For example, 90–95% of chronic myeloid leukemia (CML) cases have t(9;22)(q34.1;q11.2) translocation (also called Philadelphia chromosome) that forms a *BCR-ABL1* fusion gene at diagnosis. It not only becomes the major diagnostic criteria for CML, a negative result is also required to diagnose other non-CML myeloproliferative neoplasms, such as primary myelofibrosis (PMF), essential thrombocythemia (ET), etc. The genetic alterations now are used to define several subtypes of acute myeloid leukemia and central nervous system tumors.
    - Prognosis and treatment decisions
      Once a cancer is diagnosed, understanding the cancer prognosis is likely the next important question. Besides classic factors that affect cancer prognosis such as the tumor type, anatomic site, pathology grade, and the clinical stage, the molecular profile of the cancer is gaining lots of attention in association with prognosis and treatment decisions.
      For example, in acute myeloid leukemia (AML), *FLT3* internal tandem duplication (ITD) and nucleophosmin 1(*NPM1*) mutations provide prognostic information with clinical relevance through the choice of treatment.
    - Targeted therapy selection and drug resistance monitoring
      Targeted therapy is a type of chemotherapy that uses drugs designed to "target" only cancer cells without affecting other normal cells.
      For example, approximately 50% of malignant melanomas carry the *BRAF* mutation in codon V600. On July 30, 2020, the US Food and Drug

Administration (FDA) approved the combo use of atezolizumab, cobimetinib, and vemurafenib for the treatment of patients with *BRAF* V600-mutation-positive unresectable or metastatic melanoma.

In cases where patients received target treatments, molecular tests can also be used in mutation detection associated with drug resistance. See more discussion in Chap. 7 for the lung-cancer-targeted therapy and detection of secondary resistant mutations.

- Disease monitoring
  For diseases with known detectable biomarkers, molecular tests can be used to monitor the treatment response and residual disease. It is important to understand the lower limit of detection (LLOD) of the assay for these purposes.

  The t(9;22)(q34.1;q11.2) translocation or the *BCR-ABL1* fusion gene is a great example for CML monitoring during tyrosine kinase inhibitor (TKI) treatment and is now part of standard practice. However, the LLODs of different test methods are different; the disease response levels determined by different tests are summarized in Table 1.2.

12. **How to choose a molecular method for the detection of genetic abnormalities associated with cancer?**
    - For a molecular diagnostic laboratory to build a test menu, a comprehensive mechanism to assess cost versus impact for each potential new test or technology is required. The cost includes instrument, reagent, storage, quality controls (QC), proficiency tests (PT), facility, labor, and maintenance. The impact of the test includes patient/member experience, financial health, markets, and workforce impact.
    - Like all other laboratory tests, the selection of different methods should be based on the clinical indications, the analytic and diagnostic sensitivities, and specificities of the methods. The method of choice for initial diagnosis and classification may not be appropriate for posttreatment follow-up and disease monitoring. The performances and clinical utilities of various methods used in clinical laboratories for molecular diagnosis are discussed in Chap. 2 of this book.
    - In general, molecular methods can be divided into different categories depending on the targets of interests (Table 1.3).

– Mutations such as single-nucleotide variants (SNVs), small insertions/deletions (indels)

– Large chromosomal or structural abnormalities such as translocations/fusions, large insertions/deletions and copy number variants (CNVs)

– Epigenetic changes such as methylation, etc.

- It is critical to understand the differences between clinical diagnostic sensitivity and analytic sensitivity. For example, a FISH method is sufficient and has higher diagnostic sensitivity than a PCR-based method for a sample of chronic myeloid leukemia or follicular lymphoma at initial diagnosis. However, RT-qPCR is required for the follow-up of chronic myeloid leukemia, and the PCR-based method has higher analytic sensitivity for follicular lymphoma when a bone marrow sample with low-level involvement is being tested. The selection of test methods for different clinical situations is discussed in the chapters of specific tumor types.
- For the mutation tests of solid tumor and sarcoma, the tumor biopsy or resection specimen with sufficient tumor content is the sample of choice. However, testing blood samples (liquid biopsy) has become a feasible approach with expanding indications. Currently tumor mutation tests using blood samples (excluding hematolymphoid neoplasms for which blood is frequently the major tumor site) can be considered in the following situations:

– Unable to get tumor tissue due to the anatomic location of the tumor or the patient's clinical condition.

– In some tumor types, there are significant intratumoral clonal diversity and clonal evolution. Testing blood samples might provide a better overall mutation profile.

– Liquid biopsy provides a convenient noninvasive sampling method for clinical follow-up to assess the treatment response and residual disease.

– Deep sequencing with high analytic sensitivity and specificity is now being studied to detect very low level mutations at early stages of malignancies or posttreatment minimal residual disease. However, the clinical sensitivity of these tests is not yet optimal for routine clinical practice.

Table 1.2 Treatment response criteria in CML

Level of response		Definition
Complete hematologic response		Normal CBC and differential counts
Cytogenetic response	Minor	35–90% Ph chromosome identified in metaphases
	Major	1–34% Ph chromosome identified in metaphases
	Complete	0% Ph chromosome identified in metaphases
Molecular response	Major	≥ 3-log IS reduction of *BCR-ABL1* mRNA
	Complete	≥ 4.5-log IS reduction of *BCR-ABL1* mRNA

CBC: complete blood count, Ph: Philadelphia chromosome, IS: International Scale

For a cytogenetic response, fluorescence in situ hybridization (FISH) is used, and at least 20 metaphases must be analyzed

For a molecular response, quantitative real-time PCR (RT-qPCR) is used

Table 1.3 Molecular methods for the detection of genetic abnormalities in cancer

	SNVs	Small indels	Translocation	Large indels	CNVs	DNA methylation	Gene expression profiling
Karyotyping	**No**	**No**	**Yes**	**Yes**	**Yes**	**No**	**No**
FISH	**No**	**No**	**Yes**	**Yes**	**Yes**	**No**	**No**
aCGH	**No**	**No**	**No**	**Yes**	**Yes**	**No**	**No**
RT-qPCR	**Yes**	**Yes/no**	**Yes**	**No**	**No**	**No**	**Yes (confirmatory)**
Fragment analysis	**Yes**	**Yes**	**No**	**Yes**	**No**	**Yes**	**No**
Allele-specific PCR	**Yes**	**Yes**	**Yes/No**	**No**	**No**	**Yes (modification required)**	**No**
Sanger sequencing	**Yes**	**Yes**	**Yes**	**Yes/No**	**No**	**Yes (modification required)**	**No**
NGS	**Yes**	**Yes**	**Yes**	**Yes**	**Yes**	**Yes**	**Yes**

- Despite quick development of molecular methods and several significant drawbacks related to conventional karyotyping, chromosome analysis of cultured cells is still the best method to directly display complex structural abnormalities that are difficult to map onto the chromosomes from sequencing and other molecular test results. In this regard, there is still no optimal method to replace chromosome analysis.

13. **How to properly name different kinds of mutations or genetic abnormalities in a molecular pathology report?**
    - Our understanding of the human genome and their regulations is ever evolving, posting substantial challenges to reporting variants in a uniform way. However, it is important for the clinical diagnostic laboratories to use standardized nomenclature so that the report can be communicated consistently between healthcare providers and interpreted correctly.
    - Nomenclature of sequence variants are generally based on the guidelines published by Genome Variation Society (HGVS: http://varnomen.hgvs.org/) [40]. The Association for Molecular Pathology has also published a special article to standardize the mutation nomenclature [41]. See more discussion in Chap. 3, Q&A 13, Fig. 3.13, and case 1. Many well-defined mutations are known for their published names given at the time when they were first discovered. Including these generally accepted labels (e.g., *BRAF* V600E, *EGFR* exon 19 deletion, *FLT3*-ITD), in addition to the standardized nomenclature, in the report will help the oncologists to cognize the significant mutations.
    - It is common for a gene to have several different transcripts after RNA processing. For example, in the Ensembl genome browser, five protein coding transcripts are listed for the *BRAF* gene (ENSG00000157764). Whenever possible, it is advised to use the most Locus Reference Genomic (LRG) transcript number [42] with a RefSeq ID to report the variants (see more discussion in Chap. 3, Q&A 14 and Fig. 3.14). As an example, unless a detected sequence variant is out of range, the BRAF variants should be reported based on the LRG transcript NM_004333.4 (in Ensembl transcript table, BRAF-220, CCDS5863). It is also recommended to include the transcript or RefSeq ID (with version number, see Chap. 3, Q&A 15) when reporting the variants [31]; this is especially critical when a variant is detected at a nucleotide position not in the LRG transcript or reported based on a transcript other than LRG.
    - It is not uncommon to see substitutions involving two or more consecutive nucleotides located on the same strand of DNA, which is referred to as a multinucleotide variant (MNV). One good example is *BRAF* V600K. The coding sequence for valine (V) at codon 600, GTG, is mutated to AAG to encode a lysine (K). Based on the HGVS guidelines, two adjacent substitutions should be described as a single deletion-insertion variant instead of two SNVs (http://varnomen.hgvs.org/recommendations/DNA/variant/substitution/). Therefore, instead of writing as separate *BRAF* (NM_004333.4) c.1798G > A, and *BRAF* c.1799T > A, the correct nomenclature should be *BRAF* (NM_004333.4) c.1798_1799delGTinsAA).
    - A study based on the whole-exon and whole-genome sequencing data identified numerous MNVs in the human genome and more than 18,000 of them have a novel combined effect on the protein sequence [43]. MNV represents a challenge to the bioinformatics pipelines for the variant calling and annotation. Incorrect nomenclature may lead to misinterpretation of the variant and the pathologic effect [44]. When the sequencing panel is relatively small, manual assessment of the sequencing alignment can be routinely performed to avoid potential misinterpretation (see case 5). However, in clinical laboratories performing cancer mutation profiling with large panel NGS tests, the base calling is completely relied on the automated tools. Special attention to the base calling and annotation of MNVs is required when validating the bioinformatics pipelines [44].

Case Presentations

The clinical histories of these cases are slightly modified to simplify the presentation and avoid the potential association of any protected patient information.

Case 1

Learning Objectives

- Understand the sequential acquisition mechanism of genetic alteration in colorectal cancer (CRC)
- Familiarize the molecular biomarker testing guideline recommendations for the evaluation of CRC

Case History

A 59-year-old male presented to the emergency room for periumbilical pain for the past 6 months and acute blood loss per rectum. Patient's past medical history includes gastroesophageal reflux disease and no history of nonsteroidal antiinflammatory drug (NSAIDs) use. His last colonoscopy was 7 years ago and had two colonic polyps removed that were diagnosed as tubular adenoma by pathology.

Initial Work-up

An abdomen/pelvis CT revealed a 6 cm mass at the cecum involving the ileocecal valve, with upstream small bowel obstruction which was highly concerning for colon cancer. Right hemicolectomy was performed.

Histologic Findings

The surgical specimen showed well-differentiated invasive adenocarcinoma of the cecum, measuring 8.5 cm in the greatest dimension and invading into the pericolonic fat (Fig. 1.2a–b). Metastatic adenocarcinoma was identified in 5 of 36 lymph nodes. Immunohistochemical stains show normal (intact) expression of mismatch repair proteins MLH1, MSH2, MSH6, and PMS2 in both adenocarcinoma cells and normal tissue. Patient is being considered for anti-EGFR therapy.

Molecular Genetic Study

NGS-based colorectal tumor assay was performed on the tumor tissue, and multiple variants, including *APC* Q1429*, *APC* S644fs*6, *KRAS* G13D, *SMAD4* S411*5, and *TP53* R273C, were detected.

Final Diagnosis

Invasive adenocarcinoma of the cecum (pT3N2a) and microsatellite stable

Discussion

For patients with CRC being considered for anti-EGFR treatment, it is recommended to test for extended *RAS* genes, including at least *KRAS* and *NRAS* codons 12 and 13 of exon 2, 59 and 61 of exon 3, and 117 and 146 of exon 4 [45]. These tests, at least for *KRAS* codons 12 and 13 exon 2, used to be most often done by a single-gene mutation assay such as real-time PCR or Sanger sequencing. With the expanded gene and exon coverage recommendation for prognosis and treatment purpose, multigene NGS panel testing has gained its popularity in clinical molecular oncology practice. In this case, a hotspot missense mutation *KRAS* G13D was identified in the tumor. KRAS normally functions as a GTPase involved in signal transduction, but as a result of the somatic p.G13D mutation, the protein constitutively signals downstream effectors leading to unregulated tumor cell proliferation [46, 47]. Panitumumab and cetuximab are antibodies binding to the extracellular domain of EGFR and are effective therapies for metastatic colorectal cancer with improved progression-free survival (PFS) and overall survival (OS) in patients with advanced staged CRC and wild-type *KRAS* [48–51].

Besides *KRAS* G13D mutation, we also observed other mutations in *APC*, *SMAD4*, and *TP53* genes, which suggested that the CRC could result from the progressive accumulation of multiple mutations within cells. We next reviewed and sequenced the patient's previous colonic biopsy sample from 7 years ago. The H&E section shows a tubular adenoma in which low-grade dysplasia is seen in the surface glands, while the deeper glands are uninvolved. NGS-based colorectal tumor assay on the tubular adenoma tissue revealed the same variants in *APC* Q1429* and *KRAS* G13D as detected in this patient's CRC sample; however, *APC* S644fs*6, *SMAD4* S411*5 and *TP53* R273C were not detected in the tubular adenoma.

CRC is a group of heterogeneous diseases, and growing research evidences suggest that the progression from benign colonic adenoma to carcinoma is mainly caused by three genetic pathways, including chromosomal instability (CIN), microsatellite instability (MSI), and CpG island methylator phenotype (CIMP) [52–55]. This process may take years to decades to escape the normal cell regulatory mechanisms and develop into malignancy. CIN, as the most common type of genetic instability in CRC, was proposed by Fearon and Vogelstein and is observed in approximately 85% of adenoma-to-carcinoma transformation [56]. It is characterized by an increased rate of chromosomal gain or loss or the accumulation of oncogenic mutations. The CIN model of colorectal carcinogenesis consists of multiple steps, which start with the inactivation of tumor suppressor gene *APC*,

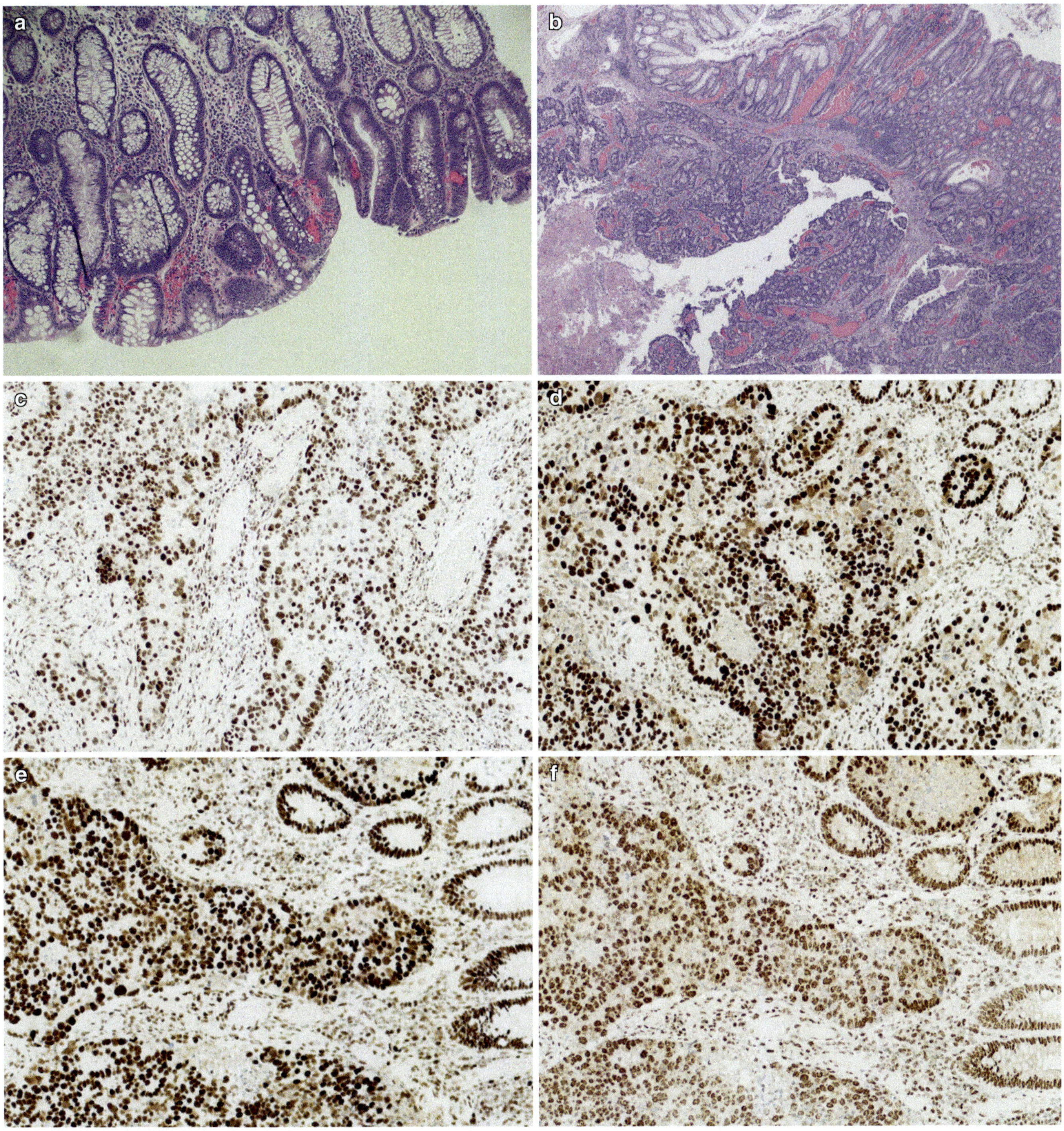

Fig. 1.2 **Histomorphologic findings.** (**a**) A tubular adenoma was diagnosed in the patient's colonic biopsy seven years ago. The section shows an early tubular adenoma in which low-grade dysplasia is seen in the surface glands, while the deeper glands are uninvolved (H&E stain, 40×). (**b**) Invasive adenocarcinoma. Poorly formed glands and single cells infiltrate through a desmoplastic stroma (H&E stain, 20×). (**c**) Immunohistochemistry stain for MLH1 (100×), (**d**) MSH2 (100×), (**e**) MSH6 (100×), and (**f**) PMS2 (100×)

followed by oncogenic *KRAS* mutations in the adenomatous stage, deletion of chromosome 18q, and inactivation of the tumor suppressor gene *TP53* in the malignant transformation stage.

Case 2

Learning Objectives

- Clonal evolution resulting in clonal diversity in a cancer lesion.
- *TP53* mutation is associated with poor clinical outcome in lung cancer.

Case History

A 73-year-old male with a past medical history of chronic obstructive pulmonary disease is found to have a right lower lobe lung mass. A wedge resection is performed. Representative histomorphologic images are displayed in Fig. 1.3a, b. Immunohistochemical stains show the neoplastic cells are positive for TTF1. The lesion is diagnosed as lung adenocarcinoma.

Molecular Genetic Studies

Fluorescence in situ hybridization reveals no rearrangement involving *ALK1*, *ROS1*, *RET*, and no *MET* amplification. A targeted panel next-generation sequencing mutation profiling detected two mutations:

KRAS (NM_004985.3) c.531_533del (p. Lys178del) in 32% of alleles

TP53 (NM_000546.5) c.1024C > T (p.Arg342Ter) in 6% of alleles

Final Diagnosis

Lung adenocarcinoma, acinar/cribriform with micropapillary and solid areas

Clinical Follow-Up

The patient received chemotherapy, radiation therapy, and nivolumab. One year later, CT reveals no new lung lesions; however, multiple bone lesions are identified at L1 vertebrae and ribs, considered to be metastasis. Given the patient's overall performance, no further treatment is considered.

Discussion

The diagnosis of lung adenocarcinoma is straightforward based on the morphologic and immunophenotypic features. Although the *KRAS* mutation detected in this case is not a hotspot mutation (not documented in the somatic mutation database), it is somatic and clonal based on the variant allele frequency. There are two common molecular features seen in this case: (1) Lung cancers harboring *KRAS* mutations generally lack other drive mutations (*EGFR, ALK1*), indicating that the *KRAS* mutation itself is sufficient as a driver for malignancy. (2) The *TP53* truncation mutation is detected at a significantly lower percentage, suggesting that this is only present in a subpopulation of malignant cells, representing clonal evolution of this tumor. Most clinical studies suggest that non-small-cell lung carcinoma (NSCLC) with *TP53* alteration carries a worse prognosis and may be relatively more resistant to chemotherapy and radiation. The presence of clonal evaluation with a subpopulation harboring *TP53* mutation is likely associated with the patient's poor clinical outcome.

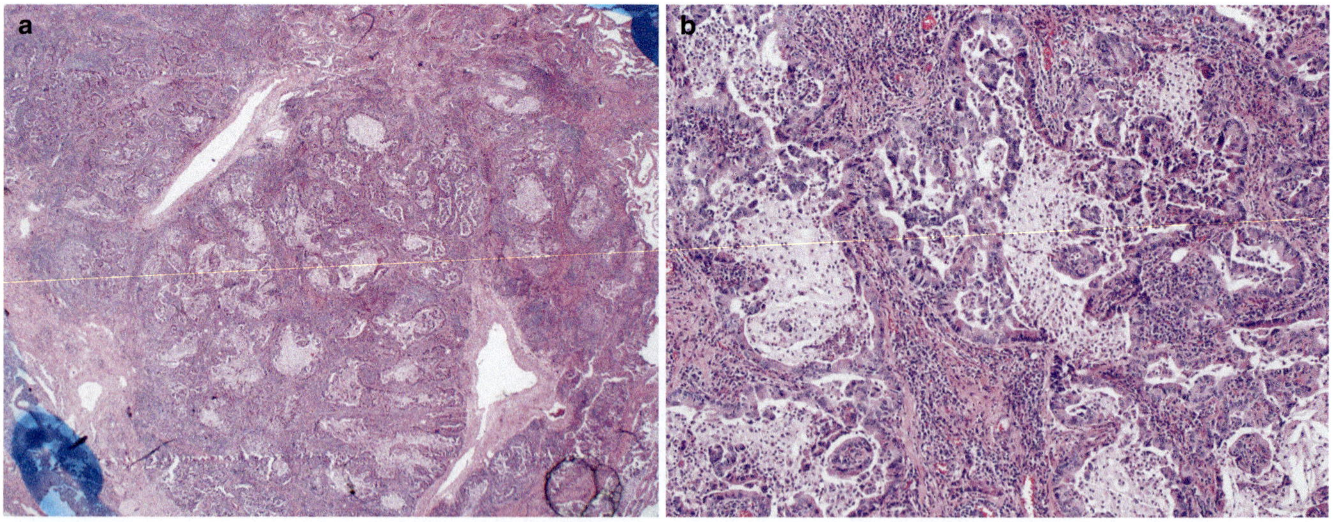

Fig. 1.3 Histomorphologic features of the lung adenocarcinoma. The glandular structure is disorganized, with cribriform and micropapillary components. There is also a lymphoid rich infiltrate. H&E stain. (**a**). 20×; (**b**). 100×

Case 3

Learning Objectives

- A therapy-related myeloid neoplasm frequently harbors *TP53* mutation.
- A hemizygous *TP53* mutation can be detected at an unusually high allele frequency.

Case History

A 70-year-old male was diagnosed with multiple myeloma, IgA kappa type 7 years ago. At that time, fluorescence in situ hybridization reported three copies of 1q21 and three copies of *TP53* in 10–15% of cells (no *TP53* deletion). After systemic therapy with bortezomib/dexamethasone ×10 cycles, he was considered for hematopoietic stem cell transplantation. However, flow cytometric analysis of the collected stem cell collection detected approximately 25% monotypic plasma cell population. He developed persistent cytopenia that progressed to pancytopenia 3 years after completing multiple cycles of combined chemotherapy and lenalidomide.

Laboratory Findings

White blood cell count: 1.5 × 10^3/μL (Ref: 4.2 – 9.1) with myelocyte 4%, metamyelocyte 4%, neutrophil/band 17%, lymphocyte 48%, monocyte 27%; red blood cell count: 2.62 × 10^6/μL (Ref: 4.63 – 6.08), hemoglobin: 9.4 g/dL (Ref: 12.9 – 16.1), hematocrit: 29.5% (Ref: 37.7 – 46.5), MCV: 112.6 fL (Ref: 79.0 – 92.2); and platelet count: 9 × 10^3/μL (Ref: 150.0 – 400.0).

Serum protein electrophoresis and immunofixation reveal no abnormal paraprotein.

A bone marrow sampling (aspirate and biopsy) is performed. There are no significant morphologic abnormalities in trilineage hematopoietic components although the bone marrow is mildly hypocellular. Blasts are not increased by morphologic evaluation and flow cytometric analysis. Plasma cells are polytypic.

Molecular Genetic Studies

Chromosome analysis reveals complex abnormal karyotype (see Fig. 1.4a, b):

42~45,XY,−4,−7,add(7)(q22),−13,+16,−17,add(17)(p13),- 21,add(21)(q21),add(22)q11.2),+1~2mar[cp20]

A 75-gene targeted next-generation sequencing for myeloid -neoplasm-associated mutations identified *TP53* (NM_000546.5) c.659A > G (p.Y220C) in 74.7% alleles.

Final Diagnosis

Therapy-related myeloid neoplasm (myelodysplastic syndrome)

Clinical follow-up

Treated with decitabine and supportive care, clinically stable

Discussion

Although morphologically inconspicuous, the complex karyotypic abnormalities, especially presence of monosomy 7, add(7)(q22), together with high frequency *TP53* mutation, indicate therapy-related myelodysplastic syndrome. In MDS patients, *TP53* mutations strongly correlate with complex karyotype and poor overall survival. *TP53* mutations are considered as early initiating drivers in myeloid neoplasms; they can be detected in the "pre-leukemic" clones, and studies have found that *TP53* mutations are not acquired during cytotoxic therapy in therapy-related myeloid neoplasms but preexisted in hematopoietic cells; the mutant clone(s) expand preferentially after treatment [57].

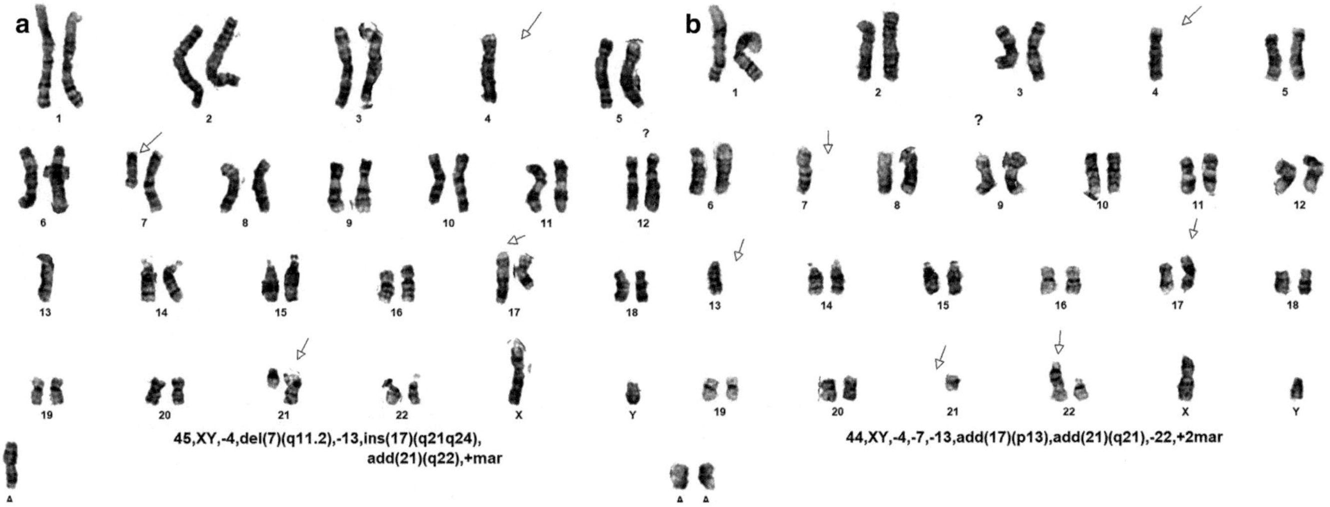

Fig. 1.4 The complex karyotypic abnormalities detected in bone marrow cells. Two representative G-band karyotyping images are displayed. The abnormal findings are denoted in the image

It is not unusual to detect *TP53* mutations at high allele frequency in cancer cells. In this case, a *TP53* deletion resulting in a hemizygous state as seen in the abnormal karyotype add(17)(p13) explains the allele frequency over 50%. A skewed allele frequency, significantly higher than the tumor cell percentage in the sample, may also be detected in cancer with abnormal duplication/amplification of the *TP53* allele.

Case 4

Learning Objective

- A specific molecular abnormality is very helpful to establish a definitive diagnosis even when the sample is limited.

Case History

A 53-year-old female has a right fifth metacarpal mass. X-ray reveals a bone cyst lesion. A biopsy of the lesion is received. The histomorphologic features are displayed in Fig. 1.5. Given the limited sample size and non-specific morphology, a next-generation-sequencing-based fusion gene test (Archer™ FusionPlex™ Sarcoma Panel) is performed.

Molecular Genetic Studies

An inframe fusion transcript of *THRAP3* (exon 2) to *USP6* (exon 1) is detected.

Final Diagnosis

Aneurysmal bone cysts

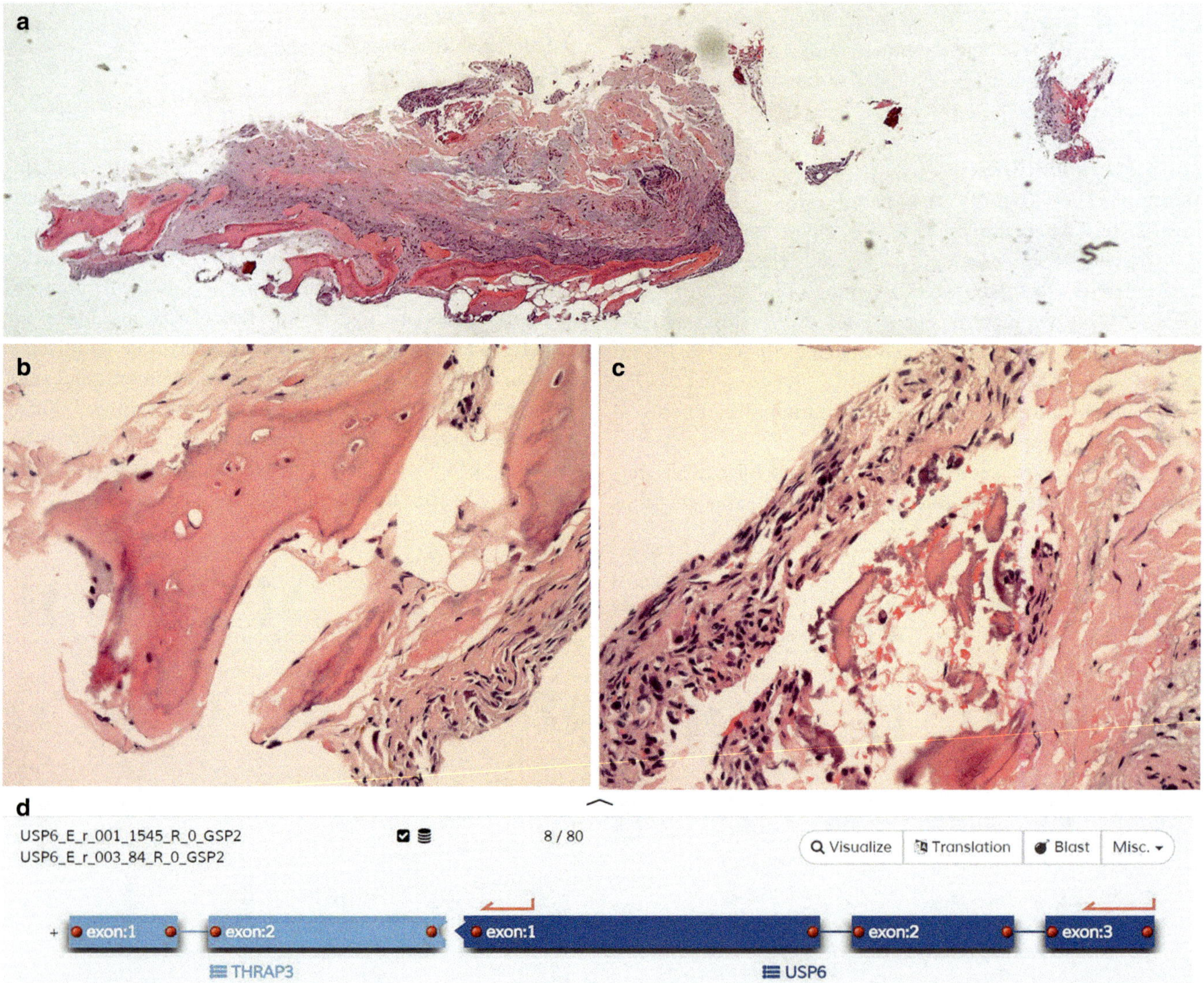

Fig. 1.5 Histomorphologic and molecular findings. (**a–c**) A very limited biopsy of the bone lesion with bone and fibrotic tissue; clusters of slightly atypical spindle cells are present, raising the concerns of a malignant process (H&E stain a, 40×; b and c, 200×). Next-generation sequencing (NGS)-based RNA sequencing (26 gene FusionPlex Sarcoma panel, ArcherDx, Boulder, CO) reveals *THRAP3-USP6* fusion (**d**, screenshot from Archer informatics pipeline). The red arrow bar denotes where specific primers (GSP) used to amplify the targeted sequences in this amplicon-based NGS library. In the 80 sequencing unique reads containing the *USP6* gene-specific sequences, 8 reads represent the fusion transcript

Discussion

The diagnosis of this case is challenging due to limited sample size and atypical spindle cell proliferation. The malignant potential would not be confidently addressed based on the morphologic evaluation. *THRAP3-USP6* fusion has been documented specifically associated with aneurysmal bone cysts. Detection of the *THRAP3-USP6* fusion is critical for the final diagnosis and to rule out the possibility of malignancy in this case. The fusion is believed to upregulate *USP6* transcription by promoter swapping [58, 59].

Case 5

Learning Objectives

- Interpretation of multinucleotide variants (MNVs) can be a challenge to the bioinformatics pipeline.
- Examining the alignment to confirm whether the MNVs are in the same sequencing read is critical to reach a correct nomenclature.

Case History

A 37 –year-old male is diagnosed with acute myeloid leukemia by smear review and flow cytometric analysis of a blood sample (blasts comprise 56% of leukocytes). The blood cells are submitted for next-generation sequencing of a 75-gene panel for myeloid-neoplasm-associated mutations (Archer® VariantPlex® Myeloid panel).

Molecular Genetic Studies

A *PFH6* mutation is detected at codon 20 (cysteine), displayed in Fig. 1.6. The bioinformatics pipeline named three different mutations:

- *PHF6* c.58_59insAG;p.C20*
- *PHF6* c.59delGinsAGT;p.C20*
- *PHF6* c.59G > T;p.C20F

The image shows in the integrative genomics viewer (IGV) in 93% of the reads.

Final Diagnosis

Acute myeloid leukemia

Discussion

Nomenclature of multinucleotide variants in NGS results can be challenging in the bioinformatics analysis, as illustrated in this case, because the computer program may not be able to combine all the *cis* variants together into one variant call. The MNV of three nucleotides are next to each other in the same DNA reads (*cis* variants); they should be combined in interpretation. The correct nomenclature of this MNV should

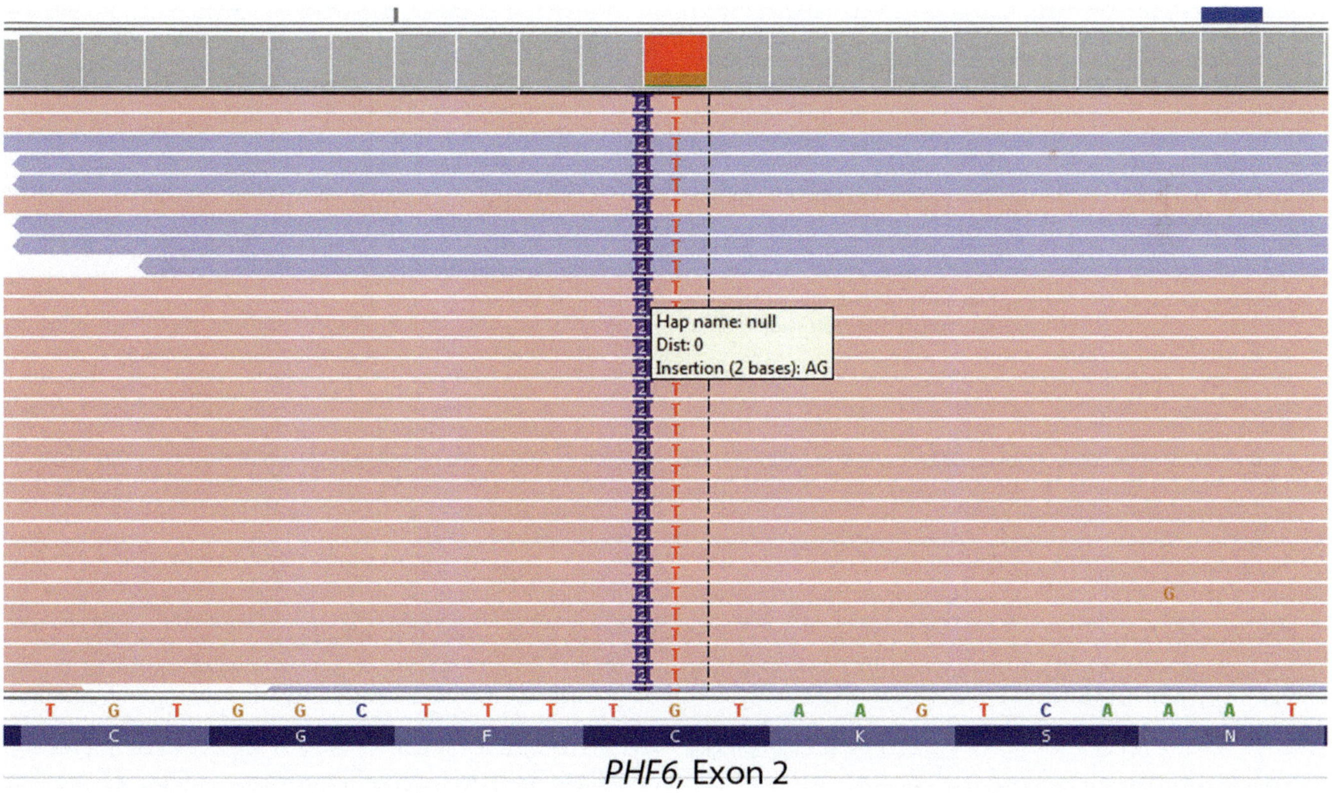

Fig. 1.6 The alignment of a portion of the *PHF6* exon 2 sequencing reads as displayed in the integrative genomics viewer (IGV, Broad Institute). The pink and blue colors show different read directions. Insertion of the two nucleotides (AG) is displayed as numbers but is revealed in the small yellow box. The nucleotide variants are next to each other and present in the same reads, indicating *cis*-variants

be *PHF6* c.59delGinsAGT;p.C20*. Separating the MNV to two different calls with a p.C20F is misleading in this case. If the interpretation completely relies on the automatic annotation from the informatics pipeline, there is a risk of misinterpretation.

References

1. Cavalcante GC, et al. A cell's fate: an overview of the molecular biology and genetics of apoptosis. Int J Mol Sci. 2019;20(17):4133.
2. Raab MS, et al. Multiple myeloma. Lancet. 2009;374(9686):324–39.
3. Pertea M. The human transcriptome: an unfinished story. Genes (Basel). 2012;3(3):344–60.
4. Ghittoni R, et al. The biological properties of E6 and E7 oncoproteins from human papillomaviruses. Virus Genes. 2010;40(1):1–13.
5. Snyder MW, et al. Cell-free DNA comprises an in vivo nucleosome footprint that informs its tissues-of-origin. Cell. 2016;164(1–2):57–68.
6. Issa JP. CpG island methylator phenotype in cancer. Nat Rev Cancer. 2004;4(12):988–93.
7. Kang GH. Four molecular subtypes of colorectal cancer and their precursor lesions. Arch Pathol Lab Med. 2011;135(6):698–703.
8. Malta TM, et al. Glioma CpG island methylator phenotype (G-CIMP): biological and clinical implications. Neuro-Oncology. 2018;20(5):608–20.
9. Audia JE, Campbell RM. Histone modifications and cancer. Cold Spring Harb Perspect Biol. 2016;8(4):a019521.
10. West AC, Johnstone RW. New and emerging HDAC inhibitors for cancer treatment. J Clin Invest. 2014;124(1):30–9.
11. McCabe MT, et al. Targeting histone methylation in cancer. Cancer J. 2017;23(5):292–301.
12. Narita T, Weinert BT, Choudhary C. Functions and mechanisms of non-histone protein acetylation. Nat Rev Mol Cell Biol. 2019;20(3):156–74.
13. Ye D, Xiong Y, Guan KL. The mechanisms of IDH mutations in tumorigenesis. Cell Res. 2012;22(7):1102–4.
14. Birney E, et al. Identification and analysis of functional elements in 1% of the human genome by the ENCODE pilot project. Nature. 2007;447(7146):799–816.
15. Lee Y, et al. The nuclear RNase III Drosha initiates microRNA processing. Nature. 2003;425(6956):415–9.
16. Bartel DP. MicroRNAs: target recognition and regulatory functions. Cell. 2009;136(2):215–33.
17. Eichhorn SW, et al. mRNA destabilization is the dominant effect of mammalian microRNAs by the time substantial repression ensues. Mol Cell. 2014;56(1):104–15.
18. Beermann J, et al. Non-coding RNAs in development and disease: background, mechanisms, and therapeutic approaches. Physiol Rev. 2016;96(4):1297–325.
19. Drula R, et al. MicroRNAs from liquid biopsy derived extracellular vesicles: recent advances in detection and characterization methods. Cancers (Basel). 2020;12(8):2009.
20. Zhou H, Neelakantan D, Ford HL. Clonal cooperativity in heterogenous cancers. Semin Cell Dev Biol. 2017;64:79–89.
21. DeCordova S, et al. Molecular heterogeneity and immunosuppressive microenvironment in glioblastoma. Front Immunol. 2020;11:1402.
22. Stanta G, Bonin S. A practical approach to tumor heterogeneity in clinical research and diagnostics. Pathobiology. 2018;85(1–2):7–17.
23. Ellsworth RE, et al. Molecular heterogeneity in breast cancer: state of the science and implications for patient care. Semin Cell Dev Biol. 2017;64:65–72.
24. Uhlen M, et al. A pathology atlas of the human cancer transcriptome. Science. 2017;357(6352):eaan2507.
25. Bozic I, et al. Accumulation of driver and passenger mutations during tumor progression. Proc Natl Acad Sci U S A. 2010;107(43):18545–50.
26. Vogelstein B, et al. Cancer genome landscapes. Science. 2013;339(6127):1546–58.
27. Tessema M, et al. Common cancer-driver mutations and their association with abnormally methylated genes in lung adenocarcinoma from never-smokers. Lung Cancer. 2018;123:99–106.
28. Nowell PC. The clonal evolution of tumor cell populations. Science. 1976;194(4260):23–8.
29. Spencer SL, et al. Modeling somatic evolution in tumorigenesis. PLoS Comput Biol. 2006;2(8):e108.
30. Amaral PP, et al. The eukaryotic genome as an RNA machine. Science. 2008;319(5871):1787–9.
31. Li MM, et al. Standards and guidelines for the interpretation and reporting of sequence variants in cancer: a joint consensus recommendation of the Association for Molecular Pathology, American Society of Clinical Oncology, and College of American Pathologists. J Mol Diagn. 2017;19(1):4–23.
32. Nishida N, et al. Aberrant methylation of multiple tumor suppressor genes in aging liver, chronic hepatitis, and hepatocellular carcinoma. Hepatology. 2008;47(3):908–18.
33. Yang Y, et al. Recurrently deregulated lncRNAs in hepatocellular carcinoma. Nat Commun. 2017;8:14421.
34. Jung G, et al. Epigenetics of colorectal cancer: biomarker and therapeutic potential. Nat Rev Gastroenterol Hepatol. 2020;17(2):111–30.
35. Ono M, Kuwano M. Molecular mechanisms of epidermal growth factor receptor (EGFR) activation and response to Gefitinib and other EGFR-targeting drugs. Clin Cancer Res. 2006;12(24):7242–51.
36. Martinelli E, et al. Implementing anti-epidermal growth factor receptor (EGFR) therapy in metastatic colorectal cancer: challenges and future perspectives. Ann Oncol. 2020;31(1):30–40.
37. Reckamp KL. Targeted therapy for patients with metastatic non-small cell lung Cancer. J Natl Compr Cancer Netw. 2018;16(5s):601–4.
38. Sigismund S, Avanzato D, Lanzetti L. Emerging functions of the EGFR in cancer. Mol Oncol. 2018;12(1):3–20.
39. Dulgar O, Kutuk T, Eroglu Z. Mechanisms of resistance to BRAF-targeted melanoma therapies. Am J Clin Dermatol. 2020;22:1.
40. den Dunnen JT, et al. HGVS recommendations for the description of sequence variants: 2016 update. Hum Mutat. 2016;37(6):564–9.
41. Ogino S, et al. Standard mutation nomenclature in molecular diagnostics: practical and educational challenges. J Mol Diagn. 2007;9(1):1–6.
42. MacArthur JAL, et al. Locus reference genomic: reference sequences for the reporting of clinically relevant sequence variants. Nucleic Acids Res. 2014;42(Database issue):D873–8.
43. Wakeling MN, et al. Misannotation of multiple-nucleotide variants risks misdiagnosis. Wellcome Open Res. 2019;4:145.
44. Wang Q, et al. Landscape of multi-nucleotide variants in 125,748 human exomes and 15,708 genomes. Nat Commun. 2020;11(1):2539.
45. Sepulveda AR, et al. Molecular biomarkers for the evaluation of colorectal cancer: guideline from the American Society for Clinical Pathology, College of American Pathologists, Association for Molecular Pathology, and American Society of Clinical Oncology. J Mol Diagn. 2017;19(2):187–225.
46. Stolze B, et al. Comparative analysis of KRAS codon 12, 13, 18, 61, and 117 mutations using human MCF10A isogenic cell lines. Sci Rep. 2015;5:8535.
47. Jancik S, et al. Clinical relevance of KRAS in human cancers. J Biomed Biotechnol. 2010;2010:150960.

48. Grothey A. EGFR antibodies in colorectal cancer: where do they belong? J Clin Oncol. 2010;28(31):4668–70.
49. Hecht JR, et al. Extended RAS analysis for anti-epidermal growth factor therapy in patients with metastatic colorectal cancer. Cancer Treat Rev. 2015;41(8):653–9.
50. De Roock W, et al. Effects of KRAS, BRAF, NRAS, and PIK3CA mutations on the efficacy of cetuximab plus chemotherapy in chemotherapy-refractory metastatic colorectal cancer: a retrospective consortium analysis. Lancet Oncol. 2010;11(8):753–62.
51. Karapetis CS, et al. K-ras mutations and benefit from cetuximab in advanced colorectal cancer. N Engl J Med. 2008;359(17):1757–65.
52. Lengauer C, Kinzler KW, Vogelstein B. Genetic instabilities in human cancers. Nature. 1998;396(6712):643–9.
53. Markowitz SD, Bertagnolli MM. Molecular origins of cancer: molecular basis of colorectal cancer. N Engl J Med. 2009;361(25):2449–60.
54. Tsang AH, et al. Current and future molecular diagnostics in colorectal cancer and colorectal adenoma. World J Gastroenterol. 2014;20(14):3847–57.
55. Tejpar S, Van Cutsem E. Molecular and genetic defects in colorectal tumorigenesis. Best Pract Res Clin Gastroenterol. 2002;16(2):171–85.
56. Fearon ER, Vogelstein B. A genetic model for colorectal tumorigenesis. Cell. 1990;61(5):759–67.
57. Wong TN, et al. Role of TP53 mutations in the origin and evolution of therapy-related acute myeloid leukaemia. Nature. 2015;518(7540):552–5.
58. Oliveira AM, et al. Aneurysmal bone cyst: a neoplasm driven by upregulation of the USP6 oncogene. J Clin Oncol. 2006;24(1):e1; author reply e2.
59. Oliveira AM, et al. Aneurysmal bone cyst variant translocations upregulate USP6 transcription by promoter swapping with the ZNF9, COL1A1, TRAP150, and OMD genes. Oncogene. 2005;24(21):3419–26.

Molecular Diagnostic Methods

2

Terrance J. Lynn and Andrew Campbell

List of Frequently Asked Questions

I. **Pre-analytical Variables, Sample Integrity, and Nucleic Acid Extraction**
   1. What types of tissue or samples can be tested using molecular techniques?
   2. What are the specimen requirements for molecular testing?
   3. What factors will affect the yield and quality of nucleic acids extracted from samples?
   4. What methods are commonly used for nucleic acid extraction?
   5. Can cells be selectively sampled to increase molecular diagnostic sensitivity?
   6. How are DNA and RNA qualities assessed after extraction?

II. **Single-Gene Molecular Profiling**
   1. What are the benefits of single-gene molecular profiling?
   2. What components and conditions are standard for conventional polymerase chain reaction (PCR)?
   3. What are nucleic acid analogs, and how are they used in PCR reactions?
   4. What methods are used to resolve and detect nucleic acids after PCR/qPCR reactions?
   5. What components and conditions are typical for a quantitative polymerase chain reaction (qPCR)?
   6. What detection methods are commonly used in qPCR?
   7. What does the delta C_t value in qPCR mean?
   8. How does droplet digital PCR (ddPCR) contrast with qPCR? How does ddPCR provide absolute quantification in the absence of standard curves or sample calibrations?
   9. Sanger sequencing is considered the "gold standard" sequencing method. What are the advantages and limitations?
   10. What methods can resolve suspected cross-contamination or sample identification issues?
   11. What is allele dropout?
   12. How do you detect DNA methylation?
   13. What common molecular applications require RNA analysis and reverse transcription?
   14. How are RNA-based analyses used to detect translocations?
   15. How are translocations involving proto-oncogenes and cis-regulatory elements detected using DNA-based analysis?
   16. What molecular techniques do not require DNA or RNA target amplification? What are the advantages of these techniques?

III. **Multiplex and High-Throughput Molecular Testing**
   1. What is multiplex PCR?
   2. How is microsatellite instability measured by PCR? If immunohistochemistry is available for mismatch repair proteins, is microsatellite instability testing still useful?
   3. What is next-generation sequencing (NGS) and why has it been adopted in molecular diagnostics?
   4. What is the workflow for NGS and how long does testing take? Can urgent results be expediated?
   5. What are the benefits and limitations of hybrid-capture-based and multiplex-PCR-amplicon-based NGS target enrichment strategies?
   6. What sequencing chemistries are used for the most common NGS platforms, and how do they work?

T. J. Lynn · A. Campbell (✉)
Department of Laboratory Medicine, Geisinger Health, Danville, PA, USA
e-mail: tjlynn2@geisinger.edu; acampbell4@geisinger.edu

Y. Ding, L. Zhang (eds.), *Practical Oncologic Molecular Pathology*, Practical Anatomic Pathology,
https://doi.org/10.1007/978-3-030-73227-1_2

7. What wet bench processes cause NGS errors and sequencing artifacts?
8. What is the relationship between sequencing depth and confident mutation identification at varying allele frequencies?
9. What is a liquid biopsy for cancer?

Frequently Asked Questions

I. **Pre-analytical Variables, Sample Integrity, and Nucleic Acid Extraction**

1. **What types of tissue or samples can be tested using molecular techniques?**
- Molecular diagnostics is a collection of techniques used in the detection and analysis of DNA and RNA. In oncology, molecular techniques can be used for the detection of pathogens linked to cancer (HPV, EBV, HBV, HCV, HIV, HHV-8, HTLV-1, MCV, *Helicobacter pylori, Schistosoma haematobium, Opithorchis viverrini, Clonorchis sinensis*) [1] and genetic analysis of human cells to provide information for diagnosis, treatment, and prognosis.
- Nucleic acids can be isolated from a variety of sources including blood, bone marrow, buccal swabs, cultured cells, solid tissue (fresh, frozen, fixed), body fluids (nasal mucus, pleural, saliva, urine, cerebrospinal, peritoneal), and feces. Because isolation of DNA and RNA is nearly ubiquitous, the appropriate sample types and extraction methods for each molecular assay need to be selected and validated prior to clinical testing.

2. **What are the specimen requirements for molecular testing?**
- The application of molecular techniques depends on the quantity and quality of nucleic acid that can be isolated from a sample, which are highly dependent on the source and quality of the starting material. Due to the heterogeneity of samples, the quantity of nucleic acids isolated from samples is influenced by several factors including size/volume, cellularity, and necrosis.
- Inhibitory substances and nucleic acid degradation are significant factors for molecular testing. Hemoglobin, heparin, triglycerides, and endogenous proteins are some of the factors that may impair molecular analysis or cause false-negative results (see Table 2.1). Nucleic acid extraction procedures are optimized to remove or limit inhibitory substances. In some cases, this can be corrected by diluting the sample after nucleic acid extraction. Carryover of extraction reagents might also inhibit molecular analysis. The best way to detect inhibition from extraction carryover would be to use internal positive controls for extraction and analysis.

Table 2.1 Inhibitory substances in PCR and their mechanism of inhibition

Substance	Mechanism of inhibition
Calcium	Inhibits polymerase activity Competitively binds to DNA polymerase and prevents binding of magnesium
Complex polysaccharides	Reduce ability to resuspend precipitated DNA/RNA Disturb enzymatic process through mimicking nucleic acidstructure
Detergents	Directly denature DNA polymerase
Hemoglobin	Reduces activity of DNA polymerase Quenches fluorescence
Heparin	Binds to DNA and DNA polymerase, and DNA polymerase cofactors Suppresses DNA amplification in a dose-dependent manner
Humic acids	Interact with template DNA and DNA polymerase Prevents enzymatic reaction
Melanin	Forms complex with DNA polymerase
Metal ions	Reduction in specificity of primers
Phenols	Denature DNA polymerases
Tannic acid	Depletes magnesium needed as cofactor for polymerase
Triglycerides	Reduce ability to resuspend precipitated DNA/RNA
Urea	Denature DNA polymerases

3. **What factors will affect the yield and quality of nucleic acids extracted from samples?**
- In addition to sample specific factors, the procedures used for sample collection, processing, storage, and DNA/RNA extraction will affect the yield and quality of nucleic acids extracted from each sample type differently.
- Nucleic acid degradation decreases the quality of the DNA and RNA polymers through many processes including enzymatic hydrolysis (nucleases), damaged bases, cross-linkage, and phosphodiester backbone strand breaks. Several factors including nuclease activity, pH, ionic concentration, temperature, and exogenous chemical compounds will affect the degradation rate of nucleic acids (Table 2.2). Optimal conditions maximize sample quality during collection and limit sample degradation before extraction.
  - For nucleated cells in suspension (e.g., blood and bone marrow aspirates, cytology) samples are stored at 4–8 °C to reduce extracellular nuclease activity. Over time, however, cells become unstable and cell lysis allows nucleases access to DNA and RNA. Cells in suspension should not be stored at 4–8 °C for longer than 7 days before DNA extraction. RNA should be extracted from cell suspensions within 2–3 days when stored at 4–8 °C immediately after collection. Alternatively, blood RNA collection tubes containing proprietary additives that stabilize intracellular RNA

Table 2.2 **Factors affecting nucleic acid stability**

Factor	Mechanism
Ionic concentration	High concentrations disrupt DNA helix causing denaturation
Nuclease activity	Cleaves phosphodiester bonds between nucleotides
pH	Low pH decreases solubility and causes depurination and strand breakage High pH causes denaturation
Temperature	Cold temperatures can cause physical shear through formation of ice crystals and cutting through nucleic acid strands RNA spontaneously degrades at high temperatures

for up to 3 days at room temperature or 5 days at 4–8 °C.

- Snap freezing may be used to preserve tissue samples prior to DNA and RNA extractions. For optimal preservation of nucleic acids, particularly RNA, specimens should be frozen within 30 min of surgical resection and stored at −80 °C or below [2]. Embedding samples in optimal cutting temperature compound provides both a convenient matrix for sectioning and preserves DNA, RNA, and protein quality [3].
- Formalin-fixed, paraffin-embedded tissue is the standard method of tissue preservation in pathology. Many factors including postmortem interval, specimen size, decalcification method, and time post fixation alter the DNA/RNA integrity and subsequent molecular testing. Ideal specimens for FFPE fixation and subsequent DNA analysis are 3–10 mm^3 in size and fixed in neutral buffered formalin within 24 h of collection. Samples should be fixed for less than 72 h at 4–23 °C and embedded in beeswax-free paraffin [4]. Formalin fixation will decrease the length of amplifiable DNA fragments over time, making maximum storage length assay dependent. This occurs through the generation of apurinic/apyrimidinic sites through hydrolysis which leaves free pyrimidine and purine residues. There is also slow hydrolysis of phosphodiester bonds that leads to short chains of polydeoxyriboses. For RNA analysis, samples should be fixed within 12 h of collection. Fixation duration should be limited to 8–48 h in neutral buffered formalin at 4–23 °C [4]. Any specimen requiring decalcification should be processed using EDTA, as other methods result in highly fragmented nucleic acids and low yields [5, 6].
- Zinc or mercury fixatives (e.g., B5), highly acidic, or prolonged decalcification processes in acidic conditions do not consistently yield sufficient quantities of high-quality nucleic acid for molecular diagnostic testing.
- Accurate identification of circulating tumor DNA requires a minimum release of genomic DNA from leukocytes during collection, transport, and processing. Cell rupture is minimized when using smaller (20–21) gauge needles and avoiding extra tubing (e.g., butterfly needles). Preservatives in cell-free DNA collection tubes stabilize circulating DNA and blood cells, preventing the release of genomic DNA for up to 14 days at room temperature.

• When extracting nucleic acids from samples, pretreatment is often necessary. For blood and bone marrow specimens, red blood cells are removed by differential lysis or centrifugation. Tissue samples must be dissociated before extraction and deparaffinized for FFPE sections. Omitting these steps my lead to inhibitor carryover or significantly decreased nucleic acid quality and yield.

4. **What methods are commonly used for nucleic acid extraction?**

• The process of extraction releases DNA and RNA from cells and purifies nucleic acids from contaminating cell debris, proteins, lipids, and carbohydrates. Nucleic acid extraction can be divided into three steps: cell lysis, purification, and resuspension/stabilization in solution. The methods used for these steps include organic, inorganic, or solid-phase isolation.

- Organic isolation – For DNA, cells are lysed using sodium dodecylsulfate (SDS) and proteinase K. A mixture of phenol:chloroform:isoamyl alcohol is used to separate the hydrophobic components (lipids and cellular debris) from the hydrophilic DNA in the aqueous phase. DNA is then precipitated using alcohol precipitation. Organic RNA extraction commonly uses single-step acid-guanidinium thiocyanate-phenol-chloroform extraction. A solution of phenol and guanidine isothiocyanate (e.g., TRIzol) is used to lyse the sample. Addition of chloroform and centrifugation separate the solution, retaining RNA in the aqueous phase. The RNA is then precipitated using isopropanol and resuspended in nuclease-free water.
- Inorganic isolation – Cells are first lysed and mixed with low pH, high salt concentration solution (Salting-out method). The saturated salt solution precipitates the proteins out of solution, and nucleic acid is then precipitated from the supernatant using alcohol. DNase or RNase can be used to remove either nucleic acid from the sample. An advantage of this method is the use of non-toxic chemicals. Nucleic acid extracts, however, may not be as pure as organic isolation.
- Solid-phase isolation – Nucleic acids are bound to solid matrices based on optimized absorption conditions. This method is used in most commercial extraction kits and is often based on silica, glass, or carboxyl-coated particles in columns or paramagnetic beads. Common methods use high concentrations of chaotropic salts or crowding agents such as a polyethylene glycol/salt mix to drive nucleic acid binding to the matrix. Nucleic acids are then eluted from the solid matrix in low salt buffers such as TE or water.

Chaotropic salts inhibit DNA polymerase; so rigorous wash steps are required to purify nucleic acids.

5. **Can cells be selectively sampled to increase molecular diagnostic sensitivity?**

- The minimum percentage of tumor cells in a sample required to avoid a false-negative result will depend on the sensitivity of the downstream molecular assay. In order to detect 5% mutant alleles, a sample must contain at least 10% viable tumor cells. For samples with limited viable tumor percentage, macrodissection is often used to extract nucleic acids for molecular studies.
- Using an H&E slide as a guide, the pathologist should estimate the percentage of tumor cells present in slide-mounted tissue sections. The areas containing non-necrotic neoplastic cells can be marked on multiple unstained slides. Areas of tissue containing the tumor cells are then dissected in the molecular laboratory using sterile techniques.

6. **How are DNA and RNA qualities assessed after extraction?**

- The four main techniques for nucleic acid quantification are UV spectrophotometry, fluorometry, electrophoresis, and quantitative PCR (Table 2.3).
- UV spectrophotometry (Fig. 2.1) – Nucleic acids absorption peaks at 260 nm due to the nitrogenous bases in their structure. The concentration of nucleic acid in solution can be estimated based on the absorbance at 260 nm (A_{260}). An A_{260} of 1.0 in a 1 cm path length = 50 ng/μL pure dsDNA, 33 ng/μL pure ssDNA, and 40 ng/μL pure RNA. The A_{260}/A_{280} ratio can be used to estimate nucleic acid purity. Contaminating proteins have an absorption maximum of 280 nm due to tryptophan residues. The A_{260}/A_{280} ratio should be 1.6-2 for high-purity nucleic acid samples. Other contaminants such as carbohydrates, EDTA, guanidine HCl used in DNA extractions, and TRIzol used in RNA extractions have absorbances near 230 nm. The A_{260}/A_{230} ratio should be 2-2.2 for high purity nucleic acid samples. If present in the eluted sample, guanidine isothiocyanate (A_{260} absorption) and phenol (A_{230} and A_{270} absorption) will also cause erroneously high nucleic acid measurements. Advantages of UV spectrophotometry include rapid measurement of concentration and purity, low sample volume input, no additional reagents or accessories, and a wide detection range (2-15000 ng/μL) depending on the

Table 2.3 **How are DNA and RNA qualities assessed after extraction?**

Method	Sensitivity	Specificity	Advantages	Disadvantages	How it works
Automated electrophoresis	High sensitivity (<5 pg/μL)	High specificity	Low sample input Fast analysis (1–2 min/sample)	Does not provide information of sample purity	Nucleic acids are separated in a porous matrix and subjected to electric current Visualized with binding dyes or fluorophores Concentration and yield of DNA determined by comparing to reference standard
Fluorometry	High sensitivity (0.1 ng/μL to 1 μg/μL)	High target specificity	More accurate determination of nucleic acid concentration (compared to UV spectrophotometric)	Does not distinguish between fragmented and unfragmented nucleic acids Provides no information on purity	Fluorophores or dye molecules designed to bind different species of nucleic acid (dsDNA, ssDNA, RNA) are combined with extracted specimens. Fluorescence emitted when excited by light source
qPCR	Most sensitive	Most specific	Can be used to quantitate very low picogram quantities of nucleic acids	Degraded samples will not be measured Time consuming, heavily affected by sample purity and PCR inhibitors	Thermal cycling *n* times yields 2^n PCR products Uses real-time fluorescence reporters to determine quantity of amplifiable DNA
UV spectrophotometry	Dependent on concentration	Accuracy concern due to contaminants and close absorbance at similar wavelengths	Rapid measurement of concentration and purity Low sample volume input No need for additional reagents or accessories needed, wide detection range	Decreased accuracy at low concentrations Cannot distinguish between fragmented and unfragmented nucleic acids or nucleotides from each other in a sample	Uses Beer-Lambert law, $A = \varepsilon cl$, and extinction coefficients. Nucleic acid absorption peaks at 260 nm

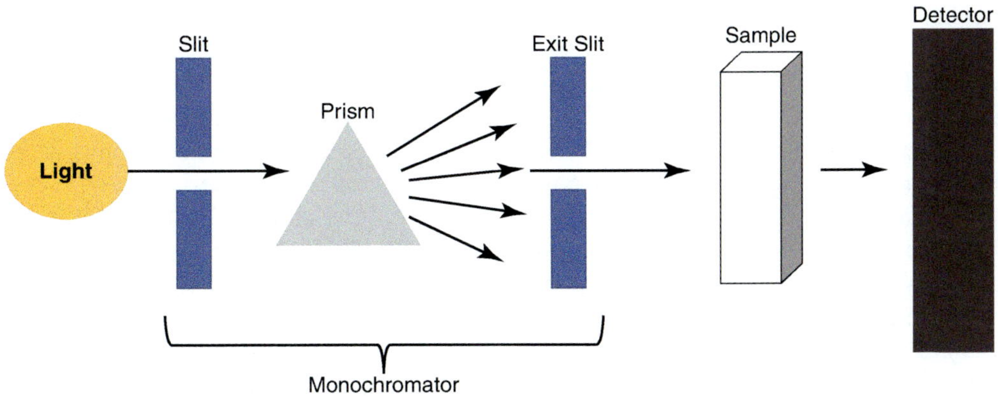

Fig. 2.1 Diagram of UV spectrophotometry instrument: The UV spectrophotometry instrument is composed of a light source, a monochromator, and a detector. The monochromator is composed of an entrance slit, a prism, and an exit slit. As light enters, the monochromator is manipulated to allow light of a specific wavelength to exit. This light then passes through the sample and then hits the detector that generates a spectrum

instrument. Disadvantages include decreased accuracy at low concentrations (i.e., 2 ng/μL) and an inability to distinguish between fragmented and unfragmented nucleic acids.

- Fluorometry – Fluorophores or dye molecules designed to bind different species of nucleic acid (dsDNA, ssDNA, RNA) are combined with extracted specimens. Unbound dye molecules have extremely low background fluorescence while nucleic acid binding results in conformation shifts in the fluorophore, producing fluorescence when excited by a light source (see Fig. 2.2). The amount of fluorescent signal is directly proportional to the amount of nucleic acid in the sample. For quantification, the fluorescent signal must be compared to a set of standards. Advantages of fluorometry include a broad range, high sensitivity (0.1 ng/μL to 1 μg/μL) and target specificity. Fluorometry does not provide information on sample purity and does not distinguish between fragmented and unfragmented nucleic acid.
- Electrophoresis – Nucleic acids are separated in a porous matrix subjected to electric current and visualized with binding dyes or fluorophores. The concentration and yield of the sample can be determined by comparing the sample to a reference standard. Commercial systems offer the benefits of low sample input (1–2 μL), fast analysis (1–2 min per sample), high sensitivity (<5 pg/μL), nucleic acid specificity, and measurement of nucleic acid integrity. Electrophoretic based quantification does not provide information on sample purity.
- Real-time PCR – qPCR uses real-time fluorescent measurements to determine the quantity of amplifiable DNA present in a sample. An unknown sample concentration can be determined by comparison to a standard curve. This method can be used to quantitate low picogram quantities of nucleic acid. The PCR primers can be designed for sequence-specific targets, allowing measurements of nucleic acids of interest. qPCR only measures amplifiable nucleic acid, so degraded samples will not be measured. The accuracy of the measurement depends on amplification efficiency and can also be affected by low sample purity or PCR inhibitors. This method is significantly more time consuming and labor intensive than other quantification methods.

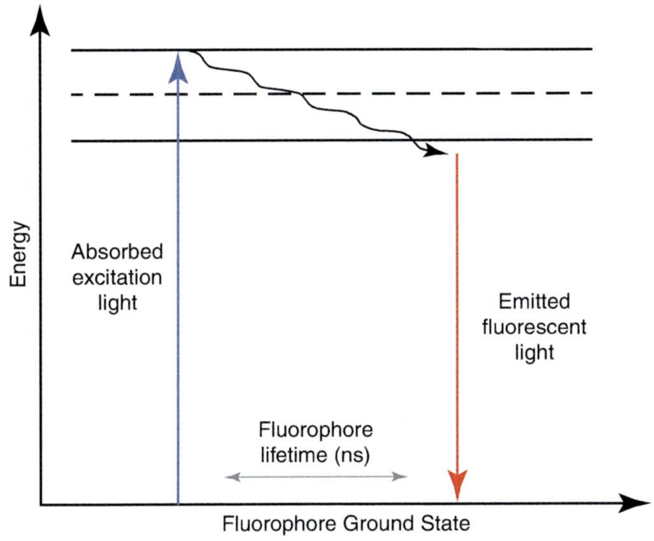

Fig. 2.2 Principle of utilizing fluorometry in nucleic acid quantitation: When nucleic acids and fluorophores bind, there is a conformational shift in the fluorophore. The fluorophore has minimal background fluorescence and is at its ground state until acted upon. A light source is used, and the fluorophore absorbs the light and eventually emits fluorescent light. The emitted fluorescence is then detected by the analyzer and the fluorophore returns to its ground state

II. **Single-Gene Molecular Profiling**

1. **What are the benefits of single-gene molecular profiling?**

- Testing in molecular diagnostics should be guided by clinical utility. Laboratories should screen for all mutations with evidence of clinical efficacy, including diagnostic, prognostic, and therapeutic decisions. In some cancers, clinically actionable mutations are in a limited number of hotspots and rarely found elsewhere in the gene. Single-gene testing may be more cost-effective by minimizing the analysis of genes or regions that are not of clinical interest.
- Although NGS-based testing allows the simultaneous analysis of large gene panels, it is a costly and complex methodology with significantly higher turnaround times than standard single-gene testing (12.5 versus 5.6 days, respectively) [7]. Analysis and interpretation of NGS data are also a challenge as curated databases with comprehensive clinical information remain limited.

2. **What components and conditions are standard for conventional polymerase chain reaction (PCR)?**

- PCR assays require a template, oligonucleotide primers, DNA polymerase, dNTPs, and magnesium.
- Standard PCR reactions generally contain 1 ng to 1 μg of genomic DNA or 1 pg −1 ng of plasmid or viral DNA per 20–100 μL reaction. cDNA input can vary due to variability in reverse transcription efficiency, but typically a corresponding RNA amount of 10–100 ng and 0.2–5 ng is used for PCR and qPCR, respectively.
- Oligonucleotide primers are short, single-stranded DNA sequences that hybridize to the desired DNA region and allow DNA synthesis. Primer pairs are typically 15–40 nucleotides in length with a GC content of 40–60% and complimentary to the DNA on opposing strands. When designing primers, avoiding runs of ≥ 4 nucleotides helps prevent formation of secondary structures such as G quadruplexes. The T_m of the primers should be +/− 2 °C. A formula to estimate short oligonucleotide melting temperature: $T_m = 4(G + C) + 2(A + T)$.
- BLAST potential primer sequences to avoid repeated sequences and limit non-specific amplification. Primer concentrations may range from 50–1000 nM, but a final concentration of 100–500 nM for each primer is optimal for most reactions.
- DNA polymerase is required for PCR reactions due to its ability to synthesize new DNA strands. There is a large variety of DNA polymerase enzymes, and the correct polymerase is dictated by the assay design. Factors to consider when selecting a polymerase include specificity, thermostability, fidelity, and processivity.
  - Polymerases with low specificity will amplify primer-dimers and mis-primed targets at higher rates. One solution is using hot-start DNA polymerase to prevent synthesis of targets before the PCR reaction initiates.
  - Although DNA polymerases are relatively stable at high temperatures, they can become depleted after extended incubation periods. DNA polymerases with higher thermostability might be considered when using prolonged high heat temperatures to denature GC-rich sequences or secondary structures.
  - Fidelity refers to the proofreading capability of DNA polymerases. High-fidelity enzymes more accurately replicate the template DNA sequence, leading to low-error sequences. Fidelity = 1/error rate, with error rate referring to the number of mis-incorporated nucleotides relative to the total number of nucleotides polymerized.
  - DNA polymerases with high processivity add more nucleotides before dissociating from the DNA. High-fidelity enzymes generally have low processivity, taking more time to amplify DNA targets.
- dNTPs (deoxynucleotide triphosphates) are the nucleotides that are incorporated into the newly synthesized DNA strand by DNA polymerase. The concentrations of dNTP (dATP, dCTP, dGTP, dTTP) are provided in excess in the reaction, and the concentration of each is usually 200 μM. Alternatively, dUTP may be used as a substitute for dTTP. Single- and double-stranded DNA containing dUTP will be sensitive to uracil-N-glycosylase (UNG) digestion. Treating PCR reactions with UNG prior to amplification will eliminate carry-over contamination.
- Free magnesium ions (Mg^{2++}) are required as a co-factor by forming complexes with the dNTP to form the substrate for DNA polymerase. Excess Mg^{2++} can increase the T_m of double-stranded DNA and decrease the specificity of the reaction. Optimal magnesium concentrations are generally 1–5 mM.
- Amplification of difficult targets such as those with high GC content may be improved with additives seen in Table 2.4
- A standard PCR reaction (Fig. 2.3) consists of the following parameters:
  - Initial denaturation: 94–98 °C for 30 s-10 min
  - Denaturation: 94–98 °C for 15–30 s
  - Annealing: 45–60 °C for 15–60 s
  - Extension: 68–72 °C, 1 min per kb of amplicon
  - Repeat denaturation, annealing, extension 25–40 cycles
  - Final extension: 68–72 °C for 5–15 min
  - Hold: 4–10 °C

- Initial denaturation ensures separation of double-stranded DNA from amplification and activation of DNA polymerase if using hot-start enzymes.

Table 2.4 Additives that improve amplification of targets with high GC content

Substance	Mechanism
DMSO (2–8%)	Binds the major and minor grooves of DNA Destabilizes the double helix and intermolecular secondary structures 10% DMSO can reduce Taq polymerase activity by up to 50%
Glycerol (5–10%)	Increases thermostability of polymerase Reduces secondary structure
0.1–3.5 M Betaine monohydrate	Reduces the T_m and secondary structure formation
7-deaza-2′deoxyguanosine	dGTP analog used at 3:1 ratio Prevents DNA secondary structure in GC-rich regions
15–100 mM Tetramethyl ammonium chloride (TMAC)	Increases hybridization specificity and T_m Reduces non-specific priming
0.01–0.1 μg/μl BSA	Negates effects of PCR inhibitors in DNA samples Enhances amplification of GC-rich regions when combined with DMSO or formamide

- Annealing allows binding of the primers to template DNA. Annealing temperature typically 3–5 °C below calculated T_m. Additives and modified nucleotides may alter the T_m (e.g., 10% DMSO decreasing T_m 5.5–6 °C) [8].
- Extension temperature is based on optimal DNA polymerase activity. The extension time depends on the synthesis rate of the target and the length of the target DNA.
- If the primer annealing temperature is within 3 °C of the extension temperature, the annealing and extension steps may be combined (two-step PCR).
- The number of PCR cycles depends on the amount of input DNA and desired yield of PCR product. More than 45 cycles will lead to increased accumulation of non-specific byproducts and depletion of PCR components. Lower cycle numbers are preferred for unbiased amplification (NGS) and accurate DNA replication (cloning).
- Final extension allows DNA polymerase to complete partial amplicons, clear DNA polymerase from the amplicons, and allow re-annealing of the PCR product into double-stranded DNA.

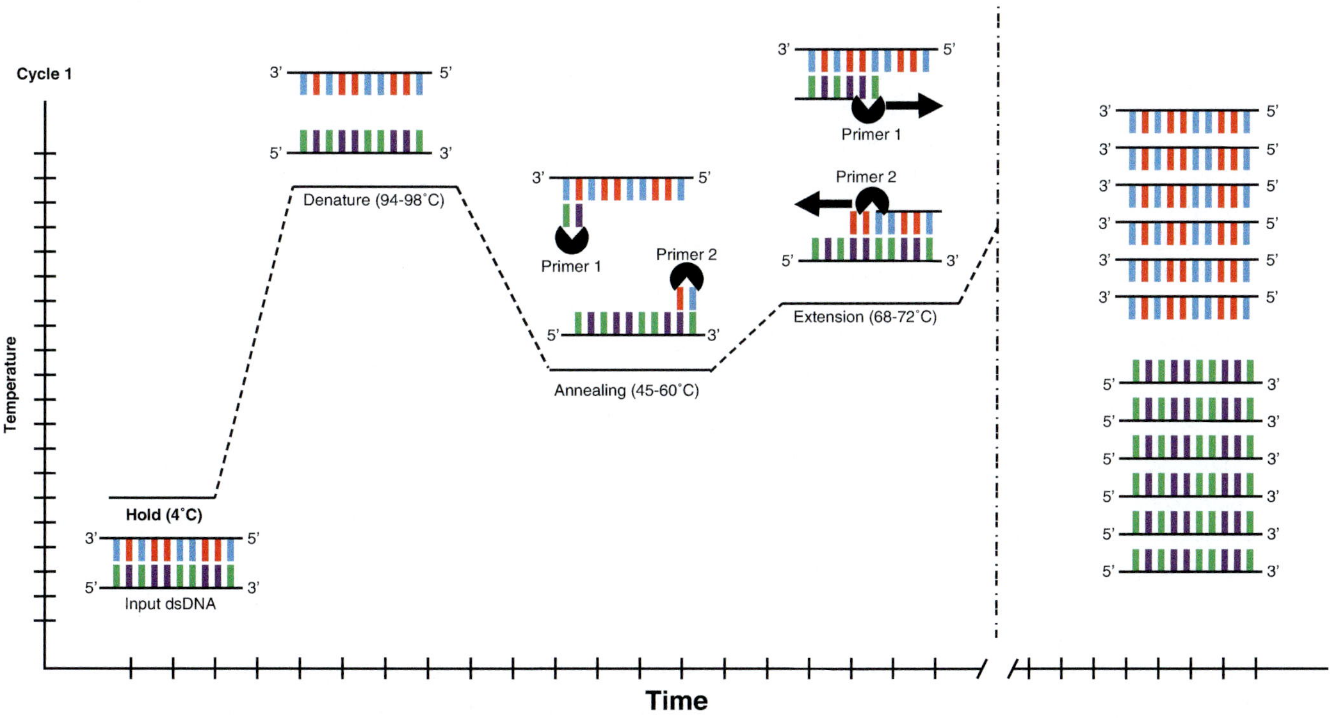

Fig. 2.3 Illustration of a standard PCR reaction: Input dsDNA sample is heated up to a denaturation temperature of 94–98 °C and then is cooled to 45–60 °C for annealing. During annealing, the primers bind to each strand and then the reaction is heated to 68–72 °C for the extension phase where the complementary strand is synthesized. The process repeats for an additional 25–40 cycles in which additional amplicons are synthesized

3. **What are nucleic acid analogs and how are they used in PCR reactions?**

   - Nucleic acid analogs mimic the native nucleotides adenine, thymine, guanine, cytosine, and uracil but have chemical modifications in their nucleobase, pentose sugar, or phosphate backbone. These modifications can be used in PCR applications where Watson-Crick base pairing is necessary, but they can modulate the oligonucleotide hybridization properties such as T_m and target specificity. Examples include peptide nucleic acid (PNA), locked nucleic acid (LNA), and 8-aza-7-deazaguanosine. Other nucleic acid analogs such as dideoxynucleotides are used in chain-terminating reactions.
   - PNA – The phosphate backbone in PNA nucleotides is replaced by a neutral charge peptide backbone while incorporating the nucleobases A/G/C/T. These oligonucleotides maintain correct intra-molecular spacing to allow for Watson-Crick base pairing. Due to the uncharged backbone, no electrostatic repulsion exists with the complementary DNA, resulting in a higher binding affinity with DNA and RNA. The T_m is around 1 °C higher per base pair compared to native nucleotide complexes. The higher affinity allows the use of shorter oligomers, which are more sensitive to base mismatches such as mutations and SNPs.
   - LNA – RNA analogs contain a methylene bridge connecting the 2′ oxygen and 4′ carbon of the ribose ring, locking the ribose in the ideal conformation for Watson-Crick binding with DNA or RNA. LNA oligonucleotides consist of mixtures of LNA monomers and DNA and RNA, and each LNA base can increase the T_m of the oligonucleotide duplex by 2–8 °C. This is useful in mismatch discrimination incorporation into AT-rich nucleotides with low melting temperatures.
   - 8-aza-7-deazaguanosine – This lacks the N-7 nitrogen atom, preventing the formation of non-canonical base pairs. This eliminates secondary structure formation that impairs the synthesis of oligonucleotides containing poly G tracts. Super G bases also do not quench fluorophore dyes as occurs with guanosine.
   - Dideoxynucleotides – Nucleotides without the 3′-OH group necessary for nucleic acid elongation, i.e., chain terminating. In Sanger sequencing, fluorescently labeled dideoxynucleotides are randomly incorporated by DNA polymerase according to Watson-Crick base pairing during DNA replication, producing a mixture of extension products of different lengths. Electrophoresis and fluorescent detection are then used to reconstruct the sequence.

4. **What methods are used to resolve and detect nucleic acids after PCR/qPCR reactions?**
   - For traditional PCR, nucleic acids are commonly analyzed through gel or capillary electrophoresis after completion of the PCR reaction (endpoint detection). In the case of quantitative or real-time PCR, nucleic acid amplification and detection are combined in one application.
   - Agarose gel electrophoresis is the most widely used technique for separating nucleic acid fragments due to its low cost, ease of use, and large separation range. By varying the agarose concentration, gel pore size can be controlled to separate nucleic acids based on their size and charge. Nucleic acid stains are necessary for agarose gel electrophoresis, allowing visualization of the product using UV transilluminators, LED light, black light, or white light systems. Stains may be added to loading dyes before electrophoresis, pre-cast in the separation medium, or used in a post-staining process. dsDNA stains are highly sensitive, allowing detection of low picogram quantities of DNA. Depending on nucleic acid polymer size and electrophoresis conditions, agarose gel electrophoresis can resolve differences of ~5 bp. Alternatively, polyacrylamide gel electrophoresis can resolve single base pair DNA differences under the right conditions. Sample loading and cleanup of standard gel electrophoresis instruments pose a high risk for laboratory and sample cross-contamination. Good laboratory practice recommendations for reducing contamination include restricting electrophoresis apparatus to defined post-PCR work areas.
   - Capillary gel electrophoresis (CGE) is another common analytical method that separates nucleic acid polymers according to their size in submillimeter diameter capillaries. In contrast to gel electrophoresis, capillary systems are run with high electrical fields to produce high separation efficiency and resolution (<1 bp) in shorter analysis times. Other advantages of CGE include minimal sample volume requirements (1–10 μL), on-capillary detection, automation, and high-throughput sample analysis. Multiplex PCR with dye-labeled primers is widely used to measure fragment length in CGE. Similarly, dye-labeled chain-terminating dideoxynucleotides are used to label and analyze DNA fragments from Sanger sequencing reactions.
   - Real-time PCR (qPCR) detection systems consist of a reaction module, where thermocycling occurs, and an optical system to excite and measure the fluorescent intensity of DNA-binding dyes or fluorescent probes in each reaction. The amount of DNA is measured after each amplification cycle, with the fluores-

cent signal increasing in direct proportion to the number of amplicons generated. When using compatible primer/dye sets, qPCR assays are often multiplexed to simultaneously detect multiple targets. Although qPCR does not necessarily offer increased analytical sensitivity, it does provide advantages in speed, reproducibility, and a lower contamination risk over conventional PCR.

- Summarized in Table 2.5.

5. **What components and conditions are typical for a quantitative polymerase chain reaction (qPCR)?**
   - Like conventional PCR, qPCR reactions require template, oligonucleotide primers, DNA polymerase, dNTPs, and magnesium. Unlike conventional PCR where DNA is measured after the final amplification, qPCR measures the amount of DNA present after each cycle using fluorescent dyes. These fluorescent reporters include double-stranded DNA binding dyes, labeled primers, or probes that hybridize with PCR product during amplification. Some qPCR thermal detection systems also require a loading dye such as ROX or fluorescein in each reaction to control for variability in the optical detection system differences in signal intensity, compensate for volume variations, and optimize detection precision.
   - In general, the considerations for primer design in PCR reactions apply to qPCR with the following caveats:
     - qPCR master mixes containing buffer, dNTPs, polymerase and dyes (when necessary) are frequently used for qPCR. Different PCR assays will perform differently with different master mixes and each must be optimized and validated.
     - Most probe-based qPCR assays are designed to run under two-step cycling conditions (95 °C denature, 60 °C anneal/elongation). The optimal primer annealing temperature (T_a) is typically 63 ± 2 °C. Primer concentrations vary between assays and primer pairs. SYBR I Green assays tend to be 100–400 nM while probe-based assays are 300–900 nM.
     - In most applications, probe T_a should be 4–10 °C higher than the primers to allow for annealing to the template as amplification begins. Probe concentrations may range from 50–500 nM, with 250 nM sufficient for most assays.
     - Probe lengths are generally less than 30 bases when using dual-labeled probes, unless they contain an internal quencher.
     - Target amplicons of 80–150 bp and 60–90 bp are optimal for SYBR Green and probe-based assays, respectively, as shorter amplicons amplify with higher efficiency.
   - Optimal qPCR conditions should be sensitive and specific. The optimal annealing temperature and efficiency of the reaction should be determined for each assay and reagent mix. The reaction amplification

Table 2.5 Methods to detect amplification products

Method	Sensitivity	Resolution	Advantages	Disadvantages	How it works
Agarose gel electrophoresis	Highly sensitive, low picogram quantities	Can resolve differences of approximately 5 bp	Low cost Ease of use Large separation range dsDNA stains are highly sensitive which allow for low picogram quantity detection	Cannot resolve differences smaller than 5 bp Sample loading and cleanup are high risk for lab contamination	Gel pore size is controlled to separate nucleic acids based on size and charge
Capillary electrophoresis	Variable	Less than 1 bp	Minimal sample volume needed (1–10 μL) On-capillary detection Automated High throughput	Small diameter of capillary causes heat dissipation, thus increasing diffusion and can cause resolution issues	Uses high electrical fields to produce high separation efficiency and resolution Separates nucleic acid polymers according to their size in submillimeter diameter capillaries
Fluorescent real-time detection	High technical sensitivity (<5 copies)	Detection is capable down to two-fold change	Speed Reproducibility Lower contamination risk than traditional PCR Wide dynamic range of quantification High precision No post-PCR processing Increase in reporter fluorescent signal directly proportional to number of amplicons generated	At very high and low levels of DNA, precision can suffer Requires high technical skill and support High equipment cost Not ideal for multiplexing	Thermocycling occurs and optical system excites and measure the fluorescent intensity of DNA-binding dyes or fluorescent probes in reaction DNA is measured after each amplification cycle

efficiency, E, should be 90–105% and is calculated from the slope of the standard curve.

$E = 10^{-1/\text{slope}}$ % Efficiency = (E – 1) x 100%

6. **What detection methods are commonly used in qPCR?**
   - The two main methods to perform qPCR are dye-based (non-specific) and probe-based (specific) detections. The chemistry used for detection depends largely on the use of single or multiplex experiments and the assay specificity.
   - DNA dyes used in qPCR adhere nonspecifically to double-stranded DNA by intercalation, minor and major groove binding, and external binding. SYBR Green I is commonly used for qPCR and exhibits 1000-fold more fluorescence when bound to dsDNA than when in solution. When using dsDNA-binding dyes, fluorescent signal proportional to the amount of dsDNA present is measured after each extension step.
   - Assays requiring dsDNA-binding dyes require only two primers (simple assay design), and the specificity of the reaction can be checked using melt-curve analysis. DNA-binding dyes, however, lack specificity so non-specific target amplification and primer dimers may contribute to fluorescent signal. DNA-binding dyes also cannot be used in multiplex reactions.
   - Probe-based detection methods use sequence-specific DNA-based fluorescent reporter probes in combination with target specific primers. This allows for quantification of only the sequence of interest. Probe chemistry is based on either the combination of a fluorescent fluorophore and a quencher, or a donor and acceptor fluorophore. In both cases, the increase in fluorescent signal is directly correlated to the amplification of the target sequence.
   - The common qPCR probe designs are based on two general methods: linear probes (hydrolysis and hybridization) and structured probes (e.g., Molecular beacons and scorpions)
   - Hydrolysis probes – Dual-labeled fluorescent probes or TaqMan. Probes contain a 5′ fluorophore and 3′ quencher. The fluorophore is released from the quencher when polymerase displaces and degrades the probe following probe binding and DNA replication.
   - Hybridization probes – Two probes designed to anneal in a head-to-tail arrangement on the target. A donor probe carries a donor dye on its 3′ end and the acceptor probes carry an acceptor dye on its 5′ end. Annealing of the probe to the target results in fluorescence energy transfer and detection of fluorescent signal. Hybridization probes are not hydrolyzed and are commonly used in melt curve SNP detection where one of the probes is positioned over the polymorphic site and will dissociate at a different temperature than the fully complimentary amplicon. These probes generally avoid placing the fluorophore adjacent to G bases, as it can have a quenching effect.
   - Molecular beacon probes – Designed with target specific binding sequence flanked by short inverted repeat sequences that will form a hairpin loop structure. The hairpin-loop brings a 5′ fluorophore in proximity to a 3′ quencher, limiting fluorescence. When bound to target DNA, the hairpin loop is opened and the 5′ fluorophore is separated from the 3′ quencher. Molecular beacon probes are not hydrolyzed and are released from the target before the primer annealing step.
   - Scorpion probes – Variation of molecular beacons probes. Incorporate a target-specific primer that results in probe incorporation into the amplicon. The primer is extended and synthesizes the complementary strand of the target sequence. During the next cycle the hairpin-loop unfolds and hybridizes to a new complementary strand, separating the reporter dye from the quencher.
7. **What does the delta C_t value in qPCR mean?**
   - C_t, or threshold cycle, is the cycle number at which the fluorescent signal from the amplification reaction reaches a significant level above the background fluorescence. Assuming that the qPCR reaction is performing at 100% efficiency, the amount of product doubles during each reaction cycle, and there is a corresponding increase in fluorescent signal. Initially the increases in fluorescence is not detectable, although the product is accumulating exponentially.
   - The C_t is inversely related to the amount of target amplicon present at the start of the reaction. Reactions with more target will have a lower C_t value, and reactions with less starting target will have higher C_t values.
   - Absolute quantification of a target is determined using a standard curve. The log of each known concentration (x-axis) in a dilution series is plotted against the C_t value (y axis) for that concentration. The equation for the linear regression line of the standard curve
- (y = mx + b) can be used to determine the quantity of an unknown sample:
- Quantity = 10 x ([C_t – b]/m)
   - In relative quantification the result is calculated as a ratio, or the relative amount/fold change of a target in different samples. This method is used to compare gene expression analysis. For relative quantification, a normalizer must be used to control for experimental or sample variability. One form of normalization is unit mass (cell number or input nucleic acid). This method requires accurate quantification of the starting material. The ratio of the experimental and control sample is:

- $Ratio_{(test: control)} = 2^{(Ct\ control\ -\ Ct\ test)}$. Alternatively, relative quantification is often normalized to a reference target ($2^{\Delta\Delta Ct}$ Method). First, the C_t of the control and experimental sample are normalized to the reference target: $\Delta C_t = C_t$ (target) – C_t (reference). The ΔC_t of the experimental sample is then normalized to the ΔC_t of the control sample:
- $\Delta\Delta C_t = \Delta C_t$ (experimental) – ΔC_t (control). The expression ratio is then calculated as: normalized expression ratio = $2^{-\Delta\Delta Ct}$

8. **How does droplet digital PCR (ddPCR) contrast with qPCR? How does ddPCR provide absolute quantification in the absence of standard curves or sample calibrations?**
   - In qPCR, fluorescence is measured with each cycle to determine quantification. This methodology is subject to poor assay optimization and differences in the reaction efficiencies of both the primer pairs and samples. Like qPCR, ddPCR uses fluorescent detection of primer/probe assays but relies on end-point measurements to determine target concentration independent of reaction efficiency [9].
   - Compared to qPCR, ddPCR can be much more sensitive and precise. Unlike qPCR where precision decreases with copy number due to variability in sampling, the ddPCR method works by distributing the target molecules into many reactions. This mitigates the presence of sample contaminants and is also necessary for target quantification.
   - Accurate quantification by ddPCR depends on the random distribution of the target molecules so that each reaction gets any number of targets (0, 1, 2, etc.) according to a Poisson distribution. Following PCR amplification, end-point detection results in positive reactions (1+ target) or negative reactions (no target) [10]. Using Poisson statistics, the fraction of positive reactions is then used to determine the average number of molecules per reaction and converted to absolute quantification.
   - Precision in ddPCR is dependent on input sample concentration and the total number of reactions. For rare targets, samples can be divided into multiple replicate samples to increase the number of reactions used in the Poisson analysis. Unlike qPCR where detection of rare events might be impeded by amplification of other targets, each target in ddPCR is clonally amplified within its own reaction. Absolute quantification is then dependent on the distribution of positive and negative reactions.
9. **Sanger sequencing is considered the "gold standard" sequencing method. What are the advantages and limitations?**
   - Sanger sequencing requires short targets (<1000 bp) and samples to be analyzed in separate reactions using unique primer sets. Compared to NGS approaches where samples and primers are combined into single sequencing reactions, Sanger sequencing has a much higher cost per-base read. When it is necessary to look only at a small number of target areas or limited number of samples, then the low cost per sample of Sanger sequencing is beneficial.
   - In addition to the high cost per-base cost, the individual target approach of Sanger sequencing is limited by low sensitivity (limit of detection ~15–20%), low scalability due to sample input requirements (10 ng DNA produce ~1 kb with Sanger or ~300 kb with targeted NGS sequencing), and is time consuming.
   - For testing and validation, Sanger is easily adapted to new targets. Once the procedure is validated for a few targets of interest, new regions of can be interrogated simply by designing new primer sets. The capital costs of capillary sequencer instruments and reagents are also much cheaper than NGS equipment, and the analysis of Sanger sequencing data is much less complicated.
10. **What methods can resolve suspected cross-contamination or sample identification issues?**
    - Due to the high number of sample and nucleic acid processing steps required for molecular testing, there is a risk for sample cross-contamination. Likewise, analysis of hematopoietic chimerism after allogenic stem cell transplantation is important for monitoring the health of the graft and predicting disease relapse. Both require sensitive and specific molecular techniques to detect and quantify mixed specimens.
    - Traditional methods of sample cross-contamination and chimerism utilized genomic regions known as short tandem repeats (STR). These genetic loci consist of 3–5 nucleotide repeating units of DNA sequence and are highly polymorphic. As the ability to detect mixed samples depends on the variability of the STR markers, using several highly polymorphic regions increases the chances of identification. Samples containing only one genetic contributor should exhibit one or two STR repeat lengths for each tested locus, while mixed samples are identified by the presence of three or more peaks at any of the tested loci. Standard methods for STR analysis include conventional multiplex PCR followed by fragment analysis using capillary electrophoresis. This technique can detect low level mixtures or chimerism in samples greater than 1% minor allele fraction [11].
    - Recent applications for sample identification include quantitative PCR and digital PCR. In contrast to STR detection and fragment analysis, most methods of qPCR and ddPCR detect single-nucleotide polymor-

phisms or short deletions/insertions. Detection is based on primer and probe hybridization, which allows 0.1% sensitivity in qPCR and as low as 0.008% sensitivity in ddPCR. Sample discrimination, however, is restricted by the reduced number of polymorphisms per loci compared to STR analysis and, therefore, require much larger target sets for confident sample identification (up to 52 versus 12-16 for STR) [11].

- Next-generation sequencing is routinely used for genetic analysis and produces millions of reads covering thousands of polymorphic loci. This makes NGS ideal for simultaneous detection of both minimal residual disease and sample cross-contamination. The sensitivity of detection depends on the read depth achieved during sequencing but variant allele frequencies ranging from 0.001–0.1% can be detected [12]. In contrast to conventional PCR, qPCR, and ddPCR that can analyze samples in hours to days, NGS testing typically takes several days to weeks for results.

11. **What is allele dropout?**
    - Allele dropout refers to the loss or greatly diminished amplification/detection of one allele when using PCR-based applications. Allele dropout can result from either sequence-independent factors or allele-specific sequence variations. Sequence-independent factors include variations in the nucleic acid extraction quantity or quality, presence of PCR inhibitors, variations in pipetting volumes of reagents or templates, and variations in thermocycler temperatures. These factors occur independently of the patient's genotype and are expected to affect either of the two alleles of a genome with equal probability. In contrast, nonrandom amplification failures will predominantly affect a single allele and are generally caused by poor primer or probe design that does not account for sequence polymorphisms, secondary structures, GC content, or other sequence variants occurring with the target amplicon [13].
    - Due to the nature of genotyping tests being conducted once in an individual's lifetime, it is unlikely that erroneous results will be detected or corrected. Although the process of validating and implementing molecular assays includes rigorous testing of specimens containing a variety of target genotypes, it is not possible to account for all sources of sequence-dependent allele dropout. When designing assays, it is therefore critical to allow for the ability to detect both unpredictable and sequence-specific allele dropout [13].
    - Allele dropout due to sequence-independent factors can be addressed by running test and control samples in duplicates. Variations in allele detection will be inconsistent between replicate samples. For sequence-dependent allele dropout, assays may be designed using multiple neighboring sets of independent primers/probes for each target or confirming the results with additional testing such as DNA sequencing [13].
12. **How do you detect DNA methylation?**
    - DNA methylation of cytosine and adenine is an epigenetic form of regulation that is heritable, sample specific, and correlated with regulating gene expression. Global or gene-specific analysis of DNA methylation has applications in facilitating the detection/diagnosis of disease, treatment selection, and prediction of prognosis. Although DNA methylation is a reversible process, methylation profiles of human samples are only negligibly affected by variations in ex vivo sample processing and storage conditions [14–16].
    - There are three primary methods to identify and quantify DNA methylation: differential enzymatic cleavage of methylated DNA, sodium bisulfite conversion, and affinity capture of methylated DNA. Selection of the optimal method will depend on the purpose of the test, amount, and quality of DNA sample, sensitivity and specificity requirements, robustness and simplicity of the method, equipment availability, bioinformatics expertise, and cost [17].
    - Differential enzymatic methylation assays rely on the application of methylation-sensitive restriction enzymes, where cleavage may be blocked or impaired at methylated DNA restriction sites. This method is useful when target genes or loci are known and can be combined with other molecular techniques such as PCR, microarrays, or sequencing to assess the methylation status of specific sites or the whole genome.
    - Treatment of DNA with bisulfite mediates the deamination of cytosine to uracil, which will be converted to thymine-adenine base pairs during PCR amplification. Selective amplification of converted sites or sequencing can be used to determine the proportion of methylated DNA in the sample.
    - Enrichment of methylated DNA regions can also be performed using pull down of methylated DNA using anti-methyl-binding proteins (MBD) or anti-methyl antibodies (MAb). In contrast to the restriction-based methods, immunoprecipitation does not require high-quality DNA and is not limited to enzymes' restriction sites [17]. Alternatively, target-specific oligonucleotide probes may be used to capture and enrich the targets of interest, reducing the complexity of the DNA that is analyzed in downstream applications.

13. **What common molecular applications require RNA analysis and reverse transcription?**
    - In molecular diagnostics, RNA analysis is a common technique for the detection and quantification of infectious agents including viruses, bacteria, fungi, and parasites. In order to analyze RNA by PCR-based methods, the nucleic acid must first be converted to DNA in the process of reverse transcription. Often this step is combined in a single reaction containing both the reverse transcriptase and DNA polymerase (reverse-transcriptase PCR, RT-PCR). The RNA template undergoes reverse transcription at an appropriate temperature (25–58 °C) [18] depending on the reverse transcriptase and oligonucleotide primers (amplicon-specific, oligodT, random hexamers). Following the 10–30 min reverse transcription incubation, a denaturation step (94–98 °C) destroys the enzyme activity and activates the DNA polymerase. Next, multi-cycle PCR is used for exponential amplification and detection.
    - Traditionally, RNA must first be isolated from the sample in order to remove PCR inhibitors from the reaction. The combination of inhibitor-tolerant polymerases, PCR enhancers, and optimized direct RT-PCR conditions allows the application of direct RT-PCR. These procedures remove the time- and labor-intensive sample pretreatment process of nucleic acid extraction.
    - Chromosomal rearrangements that lead to the generation of fusion transcripts are frequently found and used for targeted therapy various cancer types. Fluorescent in situ hybridization (FISH) and RT-PCR are both used to detect common cancer fusion translocations and rearrangements. FISH can detect cytogenetic abnormalities in the histopathological context while RT-PCR-based methods offer high sensitivity. Both methods are tailored to the detection of specific abnormalities and rely on other diagnostic indications for testing. NGS-based fusion detection overcomes these limitations by allowing the simultaneous detection of large sets of targets and the identification of unknown fusion combinations.
14. **How are RNA-based analyses used to detect translocations?**
    - Chromosomal translocations can function as both drivers of tumorigenesis and therapeutic targets. Oncogenic translocations function by generating productive fusion transcripts or bringing proto-oncogenes in proximity with the regulatory elements of actively transcribed genes. Many of these fusion-generating translocations involve one or two intergenic breakpoints, making them more difficult to detect by DNA-based molecular analysis due to both the variability in breakpoint locations and large intronic regions included in the target [19]. RNA-based analysis can also provide information on non-genomic factors such as alternative splicing, trans-splicing, and read through events [20].
    - Translocations with limited and well-known breakpoints generating productive RNA fusion transcripts such as *BCR-ABL* are amendable to rapid and sensitive detection by quantitative reverse transcriptase PCR (qRT-PCR). Nearly all *BCR-ABL* RNA transcripts contain *BCR* exon1 (e1), exon 13 (e13 or b2), exon 14 (e14 or b3), or exon 19 (e19 or c3) and *ABL* exon 2 (a2) junctions (m-BCR p190 e1a2, M-BCR p210 e13a2/b2a2 or e14/b3a2, μ-BCR p230 e19a2/c3a2) [21–23]. Therefore, primer/probe sets containing exonic primers at either end of the fusion breakpoint (e.g., *BCR* e1, e13, e14, e19 and *ABL* a2) can be used for rapid and sensitive detection of most *BCR-ABL* translocations [24]. Since qRT-PCR primers and probes are designed to detect the most common breakpoints and require knowledge of the fusion partners, false-negative results may occur in samples with atypical transcripts or non-productive rearrangements.
    - For fusion translocations with unknown partners or challenging rearrangements such as the highly variable 5′ fusion partners of *NTRK1/2/3*, multiplex NGS assays are better suited to detect rearrangements [25]. In addition to interrogating multiple targets simultaneously, NGS-based analysis can detect both established and novel fusions, leading to the identification of more than 90% of the known fusions [26–27]. Unlike qRT-PCR-based fusion detection where defined target sets require prior diagnostic indications to select the appropriate test, fusion detection by NGS provides an unbiased approach for identifying mutations. This is beneficial in heterogenous diseases that are challenging to diagnose such as sarcoma where about one-third of cases express fusion transcripts [28].
    - RNA-based analysis techniques are preferable for identifying fusion translocation events because they have a higher likelihood of being functionally relevant in oncology. Challenges of using RNA-based techniques for translocation detection include higher likelihood of false-negative results due to poor RNA quality, susceptibility to low expression and transcriptional silencing, and the inability to detect translocations without fusion transcripts such as those involving proto-oncogenes and *cis*-regulatory elements.

15. **How are translocations involving proto-oncogenes and *cis*-regulatory elements detected using DNA-based analysis?**
    - Translocations involving proto-oncogenes and *cis*-regulatory elements do not produce fusion transcripts and can only be detected by directly analyzing DNA or inferred through mRNA expression level analysis. These types of rearrangements are common in lymphoproliferative disorders as recombination of the antigen receptor loci may increase the risk of translocations with proto-oncogenes [29]. Examples include *IGH* with *c-MYC*, *BCL-2*, *CCND1*, and *BCL-6*, and the TCR locus with *TLX1*, *TLX3*, *LMO2*, *c-MYC*, and *LYL1*.
    - Several PCR-based methods have been used to detect these translocated sequences, but the sensitivity of the assay will be limited by the complexity of the breakpoints and the genetic coverage of the assay. For example, *IGH-BCL2* PCR assays typically focus on the common *IgH* JH translocations involving the *BCL2* major breakpoint region (MBR), 3′MBR, and minor cluster region (mcr). This approach leaves some breakpoint regions uncovered, such as those involving *IgK* or *IgL*, leading to false-negative PCR results [30, 31]. Although traditional FISH techniques might be more sensitive at detecting breakpoints outside regions covered by PCR, it can be negatively affected by probe coverage, tissue handling, specimen age, and fixative [31, 32]. A combination of complementary techniques such as FISH and PCR might be necessary to comprehensively detect these translocations [32].
    - Like RNA-based fusion analysis, DNA-based multiplex NGS assays are better suited to overcome the coverage limitations of PCR-based translocation analysis. Using DNA-based targeting techniques, it is possible to detect both known and unknown rearrangements using the target genes such as *BCL2* to capture the translocation fragments. Rare breakpoints, uncommon translocation partners, and low-complexity sequence regions, however, could still lead to false-negative results by NGS [31].
16. **What molecular techniques do not require DNA or RNA target amplification? What are the advantages of these techniques?**
    - Hybridization technologies include various methodologies used to detect nucleic acids without target amplification. Northern and Southern blot analyses use RNA or fragmented DNA (respectively) that is separated by electrophoresis and transferred to a solid support such as nitrocellulose. The fragments are then incubated with a labeled probe, specific to the target region. The first methods used radiolabeled probes to detect the nucleic acid targets, but several non-radioactive methods including biotin and digoxigenin combined with colorimetric or luminescent detection provide sensitive alternatives. Although PCR, microarrays, and NGS have largely replaced the need for blotting techniques, they can be useful for detecting chromosomal rearrangements and determining the copy number of genes.
    - Microarray technology is another type of hybridization analysis that can detect DNA and RNA targets in the background of other nucleic acids. Microarrays consist of thousands of defined target probes attached to a solid substrate at defined locations. Nucleic acids are labeled with fluorescent dyes and hybridized to their complementary probes on the microarray. Microarrays are used for mRNA expression analysis, mutation analysis, and comparative genomic hybridization. As with blotting analysis, array technology utilization has declined due to RNA and DNA next-generation sequencing.
    - Another alternative to the target-based amplification method is signal amplification. These methods amplify the signal bound to the target sequence. Commonly used signal amplification technologies include branched DNA amplification and hybrid capture assays. Branched DNA amplification is based on a series of hybridizations involving capture probes, extender probes, and amplifier probes. The signal enhancement is achieved by the branched DNA molecules that contain many reporter molecules for colorimetric or luminescent detection.
    - Hybrid capture assays use target-specific DNA or RNA signal probes that are mixed with the sample. The DNA/RNA complexes that form are recognized by hybrid-specific antibodies labeled with molecules such as alkaline phosphatase to mediate signal detection. An alternative to enzymatic-based detection methods is hybridization to target and signal probes to electrodes for electrochemical detection.
    - Methods using signal amplification can be highly specific for the target sequence and can be used for RNA species without first performing reverse transcription. Since the target is not amplified, these techniques are also less prone to inhibitory substances in the sample and PCR product cross-contamination.

III. Multiplex and High-Throughput Molecular Testing

1. **What is multiplex PCR?**
    - Multiplex PCR is the simultaneous amplification of targets in a single reaction, using different primer pairs for each target. In order to distinguish the amplicons, the method requires two or more probes or fluorophore-conjugated primers.

Alternatively, amplicons with adequate size separation may also be analyzed using non-fluorescent methods such as gel electrophoresis. In the case of NGS, nucleic acid fragments are individually sequenced.

- When performing multiplex PCR, it is important to ensure that all primer pairs, probes, and fluorophores are compatible. Ideally all primer pairs will have similar melting temperatures and optimized individually before multiplexing. This includes determining the efficiency and limit of detection for each assay individually. If one target is amplified more in a multiplex reaction, primer concentration may be adjusted to balance target amplification. Adjusting the magnesium concentration may be necessary in the multiplex reaction to limit mis-priming events and primer-primer interactions.
- Multiplex reactions can also be limited by the spectral overlap of the dyes and detection capability of the instrument. Fluorophores with narrow excitation/emission are preferred to limit signal crosstalk between targets.

2. **How is microsatellite instability measured by PCR? If immunohistochemistry is available for mismatch repair proteins, is microsatellite instability testing still useful?**
   - Microsatellites are 10–60 bp regions containing 1–5 bp repetitive DNA sequences. Mutations in or loss of mismatch repair protein expression can lead to expansion or contraction of these repeat sequences and is correlated with overall tumor mutation burden and PD-L1 expression in cancer cells [33].
   - Traditional methods of MSI analysis rely on IHC detection of MMR proteins MLH1, MSH2, MSH6, and PMS2. Alternatively, PCR-based assays targeting least five microsatellites of mononucleotide and dinucleotide repeats are also used in MSI analysis. For PCR analysis, DNA from a tumor sample is usually paired with a non-malignant specimen from the patient. Following PCR amplification of the MSI markers, the fragments are resolved by capillary electrophoresis. Tumor samples with alterations in 40% or more of the markers are defined as MSI-high, no alterations are MSI-stable, and the remaining as MSI-low.
   - Either IHC or MSI may be used as a screening method for MMR status, but there are limitations for each. Not all pathogenic mutations in MMR proteins will result in changes to IHC staining. Although IHC for MLH1, MSH2, MSH6, and PMS2 will detect most germline MMR mutations, MSI causing mutations can also occur in other genes. These mutations would not be detected by standard IHC testing. Conversely, PCR-based MSI screening takes longer to perform and does not identify the responsible underlying gene.
3. **What is next-generation sequencing and why has it been adopted in molecular diagnostics?**
   - Next-generation sequencing refers to several sequencing technologies that use high-throughput testing to generate large amounts of sequencing data by simultaneously profiling large sample or target sets. In NGS the individual sequence of millions of molecules is captured simultaneously, in contrast to standard sequencing technology where the signal is the sum of a pool of molecules.
   - Profiling comprehensive sets of target genes provides clinical utility in many cancers. For example, mutations in *KRAS, EGFR, BRAF, ALK/ROS*, and *NTRK*1-3 occur at different frequencies in non-small-cell lung cancer. Conducting parallel or sequential single-gene tests for each gene would be time consuming and cost ineffective. Less nucleic acid or tissue is also needed to analyze a sample using a multi-gene panel compared to multiple single-gene tests. This conserves valuable sample, especially in disease types where the tissue is limited.
   - NGS panels also provide increased information, flexibility, and clinical options. Unlike many standard single-gene molecular tests, NGS panels provide information regarding variant allele frequency and in some cases if mutations are in cis or in trans. This can be helpful for identification of tumor heterogeneity and tracking responses to treatment. Multi-gene panels are also increasingly used to guide patient participation in clinical trials, providing more treatment options beyond genes with established clinical utility. As new treatments are developed, NGS panels also allow laboratories to integrate new genes/targets into their panels relatively quickly.
4. **What is the workflow for NGS and how long does testing take? Can urgent results be expediated?**
   - The NGS workflow contains four basic steps: sample preparation, library preparation, sequencing, and data analysis. NGS is a high-complexity workflow that requires skilled personnel to perform testing, an IT support system to enable the analysis and interpretation of massive amounts of data, and the expertise of laboratory directors for variant interpretation. The turnaround time for

NGS testing will vary widely for each test and depends on several factors including sample batching, library preparation methodology, gene content, sequencing equipment, staffing, bioinformatics support, and the complexity of variant interpretation. The testing algorithms and clinical needs of the system are carefully considered prior to assay selection and implementation to ensure the optimal balance of resource allocation and shortest feasible turnaround times.

- Sample preparation is a critical step for NGS as samples are finite resources and accurate; reproducible data depends on the quality of the input material. The sample preparation must take into account the type of nucleic acid needed and the material from which it will be extracted. This will affect the sample collection, handling, and nucleic acid extraction techniques. Similarly, nucleic acid quantification can have a significant impact on NGS assay performance. An optimized workflow for the qualifications of DNA preparations should be part of every NGS workflow, including the suitability of the method for the specific downstream application.
- Numerous kits and workflows are available for NGS library preparation. This generally entails the addition of adapters and barcodes to the input nucleic acid. Adapters are the platform-specific nucleic acid sequences that are required for fragment identification and sequencing on the NGS instrument. Sample barcoding, or indexing, facilitates the multiplexing of different samples for sequencing and analysis. Molecular barcoding involves the labeling of each nucleic acid fragment with a distinct sequence. This allows sequencing reads and errors to be de-duplicated to form a consensus read for each input fragment. Most NGS library preparation methods also utilize target capture or PCR amplification prior to sequencing in order to enrich for specific regions of interest. NGS library cleanup is used to remove adapters, PCR primers, dNTPs, enzymes, unwanted buffers, or library molecules that are above or below the optimal size range for the sequencing platform. Accurate quantification and quality check are also necessary for successful sequencing runs.
- Sequencing requires any number of specialized instruments that are heterogeneous regarding technology, throughput (sample number and speed), read length, accuracy, cost per base, size, and capital costs. The clinical application and throughput requirements determine the instrument that is best suited.
- NGS data analysis is complex and divided into multiple analysis steps: quality assessment of the raw data, read alignment to a reference genome, variant identification, annotation of the variants, and data review/interpretation. Many commercial and custom bioinformatics platforms have been developed to complete each of these analysis steps. In order to produce accurate and meaningful results, the analysis workflow must be carefully considered and optimized at each step.
- Summarized in Fig. 2.4.

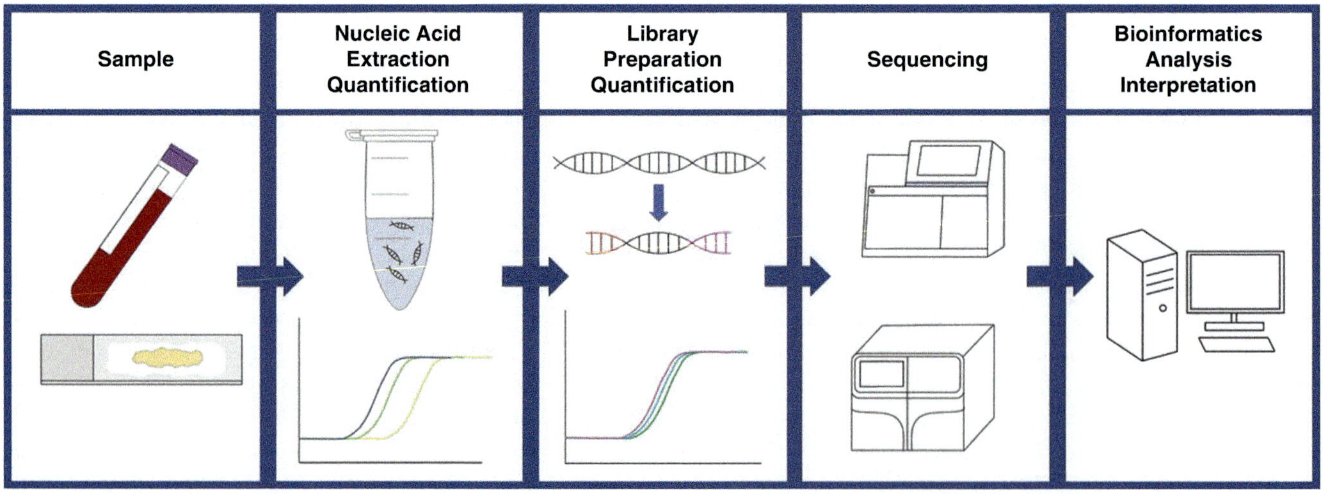

Fig. 2.4 Next-generation sequencing workflow: The NGS workflow contains four basic steps: sample preparation (including collection, processing, and nucleic acid extraction), library preparation, sequencing, and data analysis (bioinformatics analysis, variant review, and interpretation)

5. **What are the benefits and limitations of hybrid-capture-based and multiplex-PCR-amplicon-based NGS target enrichment strategies?**
   - In order to decrease the time and costs associated with sequencing, targeted NGS is employed for an in-depth analysis of regions of clinical diagnostic interest. Targeted NGS also generally requires less sample input and produces more manageable data sets. Hybrid capture and multiplex PCR amplicon are the standard methods for NGS library preparation. The basic principles of these methods are summarized in Fig. 2.5.
   - In general, hybrid-capture-based enrichment strategies are advantageous for their ability to provide more uniform coverage. This increases the accuracy and sensitivity of the assay, especially in difficult regions containing high GC content or repetitive sequences. Hybrid-capture-based assay probes are also easier to design, accommodate larger target regions, and are less sensitive to sample contaminants. These assays require higher input DNA (>10 ng, typically 50–500 ng) and are more time consuming than amplicon-based approaches. Hybrid capture is more expensive because of the higher number of probes used for enrichment.
   - PCR-based enrichment strategies generally provide less uniform coverage as a result of primer competition and non-uniform amplification of target regions due to variations in GC content or amplicon length. PCR-based enrichments require lower DNA input (1–10 ng), making them more amendable to cases where clinical sample availability is limited. These assays also have shorter and/or less complex workflows and generally a lower cost per sample.
6. **What sequencing chemistries are used for the most common NGS platforms, and how do they work?**
   - The most common NGS platforms are based on the detection of clonally amplified DNA through sequencing by synthesis (SBS). Sequencing base calls are determined through optical detection following reversible termination (Illumina) or detection of hydrogen ions during the polymerization reaction (Thermo Fisher Scientific Ion Torrent).
   - In the Illumina sequencing platforms, single-stranded fragments from DNA libraries are hybridized to a solid-surface flow cell at low molar quantities to ensure physical separation between strands. The fragments then undergo bridge amplification to generate millions of anchored clonal clusters. Sequencing is then performed using reversible terminator (RT) nucleotides that contain a blocker at the 3′-OH groups and a unique fluorescent label. In each sequencing cycle the four RT nucleotides are added, and a single base is incorporated using the anchored DNA clones as the template. The identity of the fluorescently labeled nucleotide incorporated into each cluster is then detected optically. The terminator and fluorescent dyes are then cleaved from the 3′-OH group, allowing the sequencing cycle to repeat. Illumina platforms support paired-end sequencing, where each DNA molecule (cluster) is sequenced from both ends, improving alignments [34]. These instruments are less prone to errors resulting from homopolymer tracts and have low overall error rates (0.1–2.6%) [35]. Optical imaging is relatively time consuming however, leading to longer run times compared to other platforms.
   - For sequencing on the traditional Ion Torrent systems, DNA library is amplified using emulsion PCR. In this process a single-stranded DNA fragment is captured by an ion sphere particle and undergoes amplification on the surface of the bead. After amplification, the ion spheres are separated from the emulsion oil and the clonally enriched beads are loaded on an ion semiconductor chip. A single nucleotide is added to the chip during each cycle and results in the release of a hydrogen ion when incorporated into the growing strand. The change in pH is converted to a digital signal which is used to determine the DNA sequence. Ion torrent systems have been associated with higher error rates than Illumina sequencers (0.46–2.4%) [36]. They also suffer from sequencing errors in homopolymer regions and lower coverage in AT-rich or GC-rich regions [37]. Ion torrent systems provide automated workflow solutions for emulsion PCR and fast sequencing times.
7. **What wet bench processes cause NGS errors and sequencing artifacts?**
   - NGS artifacts and errors can be introduced during any step of the process including nucleic acid damage introduced during sample preservation or preparation, adapter ligation and cleanup, and PCR errors during library preparation, templating, and sequencing [38].
   - FFPE specimens are a major source of both testing material and artifactual variation in NGS. FFPE-induced fragmentation in DNA reduces the number of targets for analysis and can introduce sequence variants not seen in the

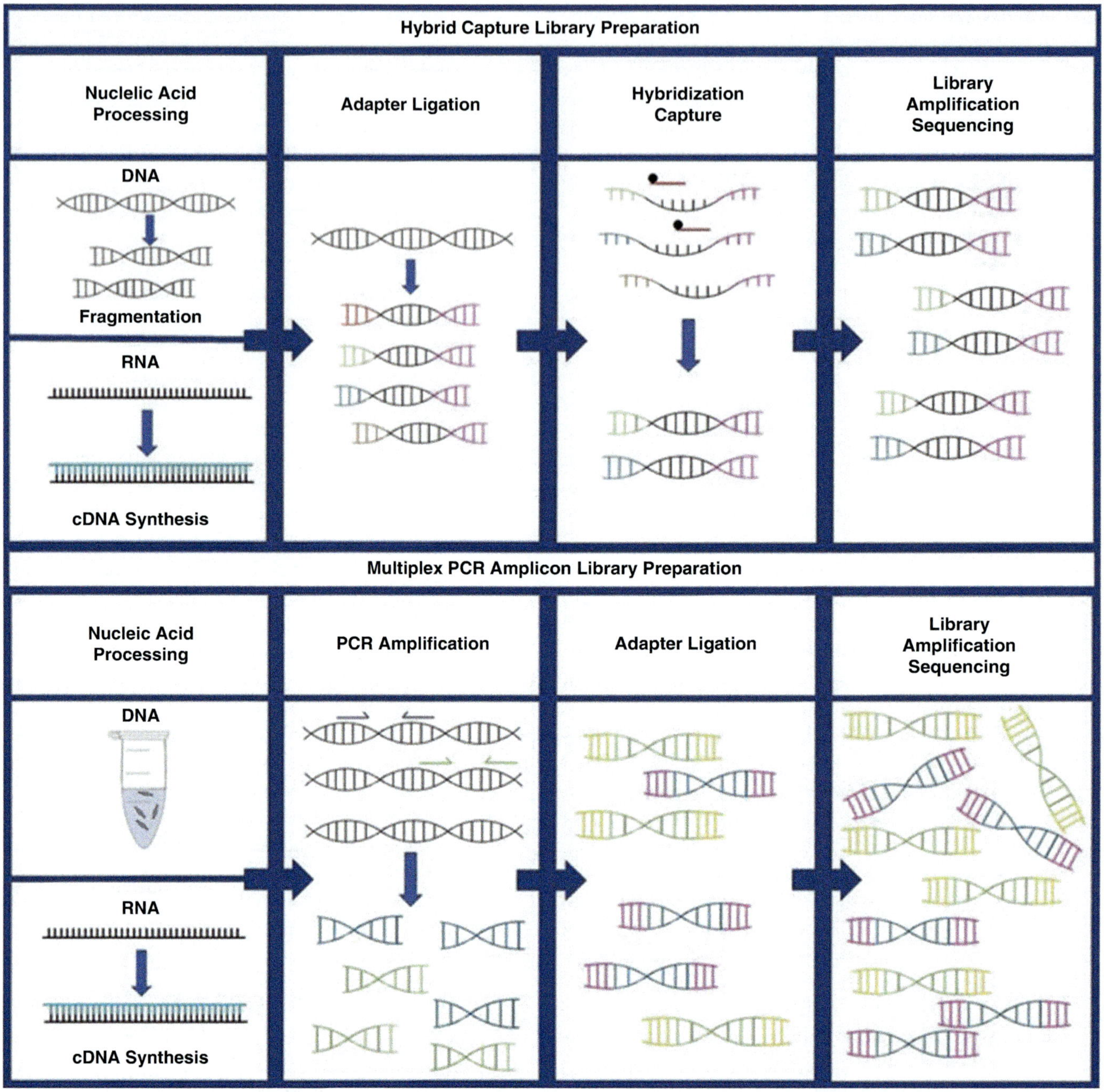

Fig. 2.5 Hybrid capture and multiplex PCR amplicon library preparation: In hybrid capture library preparations, randomly sheared DNA or intact cDNA fragments are denatured and subjected to hybridization with overlapping DNA or RNA oligonucleotides (probes or baits) specific to the regions of interest. Unbound molecules are washed away, and the enriched pools containing ligated adapters undergo limited library amplification before sequencing. In multiplex PCR amplicon library preparations, target specific primers are used to amplify the region of interest in DNA or cDNA. The adapter-ligated pools undergo limited library amplification before sequencing

original sample such as Strand-split artifact reads [39]. FFPE can also cause formation of abasic sites, leading to guanine substitutions or 1–3 bp deletions. Uracil lesions are a major source of sequence artifacts in DNA, causing high levels of C: G>T: A SNV artifacts in FFPE samples [38]. Stochastic bias, capture bias, primer bias, and allele dropout are also potential sources of error.

- Adapters are required for library capture and template amplification in the Illumina and Ion Torrent platforms but adding these sequences to the ends of DNA molecules through ligation or PCR during library preparation is a common source of sequence artifact. Self-ligation or self-priming of adapter oligonucleotides will generate dimers without any library sequence. These fragments hybridize efficiently to the templating matrices and will generate sequencing data. Using insufficient starting material, poor quality nucleic acid, and inefficient clean-up methods can all increase adapter dimers in the library pool. Improperly trimmed adapter sequence at the ends of sequence reads can also interfere with mapping. If the adapter sequence is included in the data, it must be identified and trimmed appropriately [40].

- NGS errors are frequently attributed to PCR errors during sample preparation, templating, or sequencing, but the effect during sample preparation is negligible if the target itself is not problematic for PCR (such as AT-rich or repetitive sequences) [35]. Although it is shown that PCR may increase substitution errors by as much as sixfold, computational analysis can reduce the error rate to 10^{-5}–10^{-4}, which is enough to detect more than 70% of hotspot variants at 0.1–0.01% allele frequency [41].
- The DNA polymerases commonly used in sequencing by synthesis platforms have also been identified as a significant source of error. Modification of the polymerase to increase efficiency of ddNTP incorporation leads to preferential ddGTP addition and bias toward motifs ending in "GG" [42]. Fluorometric detection methods can also introduce error. Spectral overlap between fluorophores used in the Illumina four-channel sequencing by synthesis platforms has been shown to lead to miscalling of A/C and G/T nucleotides [35]. Overlap of clusters on the flow cell surface, dimming, and phasing can cause intrinsic errors. Pre-phasing occurs when two or more nucleotides are incorporated in one cycle due to the presence of residual non-incorporated nucleotides. Post-phasing is caused by incomplete removal of the terminator [35]. Accumulation of phasing problems compounds sequencing errors, particularly at the end of reads [42]. In addition to the homopolymer associated errors in the Ion Torrent platform, there are also context-dependent indel errors and an overall higher error rate and poorer coverage in GC-poor sequences [43].

8. **What is the relationship between sequencing depth and confident mutation identification at varying allele frequencies?**
   - Sequencing depth refers to the number of aligned reads that contain a given nucleotide position. Factors that influence sequencing depth include the sample quantity/quality, library preparation, sequence complexity of the target region, sequencing platform (including total reads generated and pooled samples per run), and read processing/mapping by the bioinformatics pipeline.
   - A greater number of high-quality sequence reads increase the confidence of a base called at a position. The probability of detecting true positives and false positives at a given allele burden can be calculated using binomial calculations [44]. For example, as shown in Fig. 2.6 at a mutant allele frequency of 5%, the probability of detecting the mutant allele at greater than 4% allele frequency (10+ mutant reads) when achieving 250 read sequencing depth is 80.5%. The probability

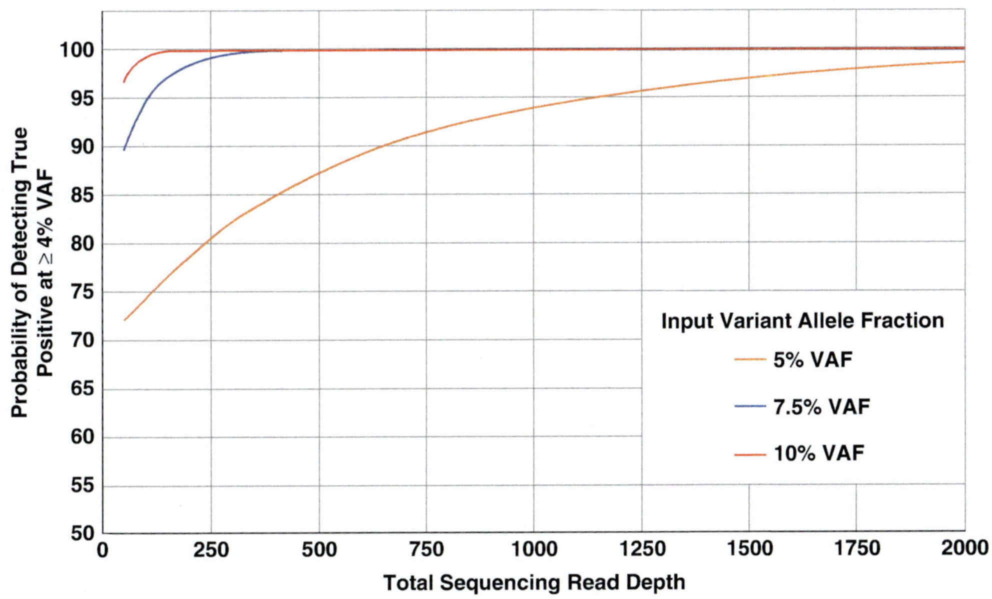

Fig. 2.6 Probability of detecting true-positive events using binomial calculations: Using binomial calculations, the probability of detecting true-positive events at different variant allele frequencies and sequencing depths can be calculated. In this example, the probability that the total sequencing reads contain at least 4% variant allele fraction is calculated using 5, 7.5, and 10% input variant allele fraction. Lower input variant allele fraction (e.g., 5%) requires significantly higher sequencing depth to achieve the same probability of detection

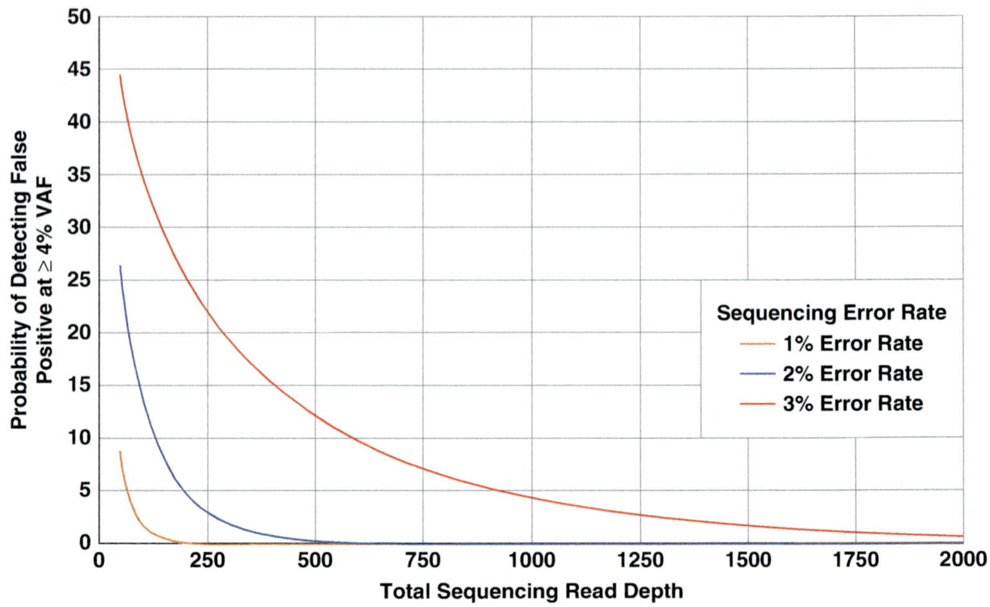

Fig. 2.7 Probability of detecting false-positive events using binomial calculations: Using binomial calculations, the probability of observing false-positive events at different sequencing error rates and sequencing depths can be calculated. In this example, the probability that the total sequencing reads contain at least 4% false-positive variant allele fraction is calculated using 1, 2, and 3% sequencing error rates. Higher sequencing error rates significantly increase the probability of false-positive events but to a limited degree can be mitigated by higher sequencing depth

increases to 87.3% and 98.5% when the read depth is 500 and 2000, respectively.

- Likewise, as shown in Fig. 2.7 the probability of false positives at specific sequence error rates can also be calculated. Using a sequence error rate of 1% and sequence depth of 250, the probability of detecting ≥ 4% false positives at a given position is 0.025%. Increasing the sequence error rate to 3% results in a 22.1% probability of detecting ≥ 4% false-positive events. At read depths of 500 and 2000, the probability of detecting ≥ 4% false-positive events with a sequence error rate of 3% are 12.1% and 0.7%, respectively.
- As discussed above, sequence errors are not random. Sample, library, target, and platform-specific sequence errors occur. A determination of the false-positive and false-negative rates for a given depth and allele threshold should be validated for each methodology and sequencing platform [44].

9. **What is a liquid biopsy for cancer?**
   - Human body fluids including blood, urine, saliva, sputum, pleural, and cerebrospinal contain cell-free tumor DNA (ctDNA) [45]. These small DNA fragments are released from apoptotic and necrotic tumor cells and carry the tumor specific alterations such as point mutations, DNA methylation, and copy number variations that can be identified by molecular testing [46].
   - Liquid biopsies offer an alternative tool for invasive biopsies, especially those with limited access. Liquid biopsy also circumvents the need for multi-sampling to adequately characterize the heterogenous tumor [45]. This technique also has the potential to be used for early diagnostic results and therapeutic targets, monitoring therapy in real time, and monitoring metastatic relapse and progression.
   - Current applications of liquid biopsy include both monitoring total cfDNA and quantification of tumor-specific mutations. The levels of cfDNA have been shown to distinguish lung cancer patients from controls, and the level of cfDNA concentration is associated with both tumor volume and overall survival [47].
   - A technical challenge of using liquid biopsy for detection of tumor specific mutations is the high variability in concordance between the tumor sample and the measurement of cfDNA. The tumor fraction of cfDNA can vary widely by tumor type, location, size, and vascularity and impacts the detectability of somatic alterations in the sample. The tumor fraction can also be affected by the techniques and time delay before extracting the cfDNA. Overall, the concordance between liquid biopsy and solid tumor samples has been 10–100% depending on the cancer type, mutation panel, and method of detection [47].

Case Examples

Case #1

Learning Objectives

1.) Recognize PCR fragment length analysis and assess for *FLT3* D835/I836 and ITD mutations in AML.

Case History

The patient is a 75-year-old female who presented to the clinic with shortness of breath. Routine lab work demonstrated a leukocytosis of 300 K/μL and 90% blasts on peripheral smear review. Flow cytometry confirmed AML. The provider requested rapid *FLT3* testing.

Final Diagnosis

A *FLT3* ITD mutation is present. There is no evidence of a mutation at *FLT3* codons 835 and 836 in this specimen within the sensitivity limit of 3%.

Discussion

FLT3 encodes a cell surface tyrosine kinase that functions as a growth factor receptor for myeloid and lymphoid hematopoietic progenitors [48–50]. *FLT3* internal tandem duplications (ITD) of 3–400+ base pairs result in constitutively active kinase activity and occur in 5–35% of AML cases [51–62]. *FLT3* ITD mutations are associated with significantly increased relapse risk and decreased overall survival [51, 52]. Mutations at codons D835 and I836 occur in 7–14% of AML cases and produce constitutively active tyrosine kinase activity [51, 53, 57, 63, 64]. Integration of *FLT3* inhibitors in induction and consolidation therapy significantly improves outcomes in *FLT3* mutated AML, making early identification of these mutations essential. Unlike next-generation sequencing which can take weeks to report results, assessment of *FLT3* D835/I836 and ITD mutations can be performed within days.

This case illustrates the finding of *FLT3* ITD in a patient with AML using PCR fragment length analysis. The isolated DNA sample is PCR amplified using two fluorescently labeled primer pairs targeting the D835/I836 and ITD regions. The wild-type D835/I836 codon contains an EcoRV restriction site and is detected by digestion with EcoRV enzyme. To monitor restriction digestion, a novel EcoRV site is incorporated into the D835/I836 primer pair. For the *FLT3* ITD amplicon, the PCR product will be larger than the wild-type fragment. The products are separated by capillary electrophoresis and compared to the expected values for known wild-type and mutant sequences (Fig. 2.8).

Case #2

Learning Objectives

1.) Understand the use of NGS for myeloid neoplasms to facilitate the disease subclassification 2.) Communicate NGS results in a clear and concise report to clinicians

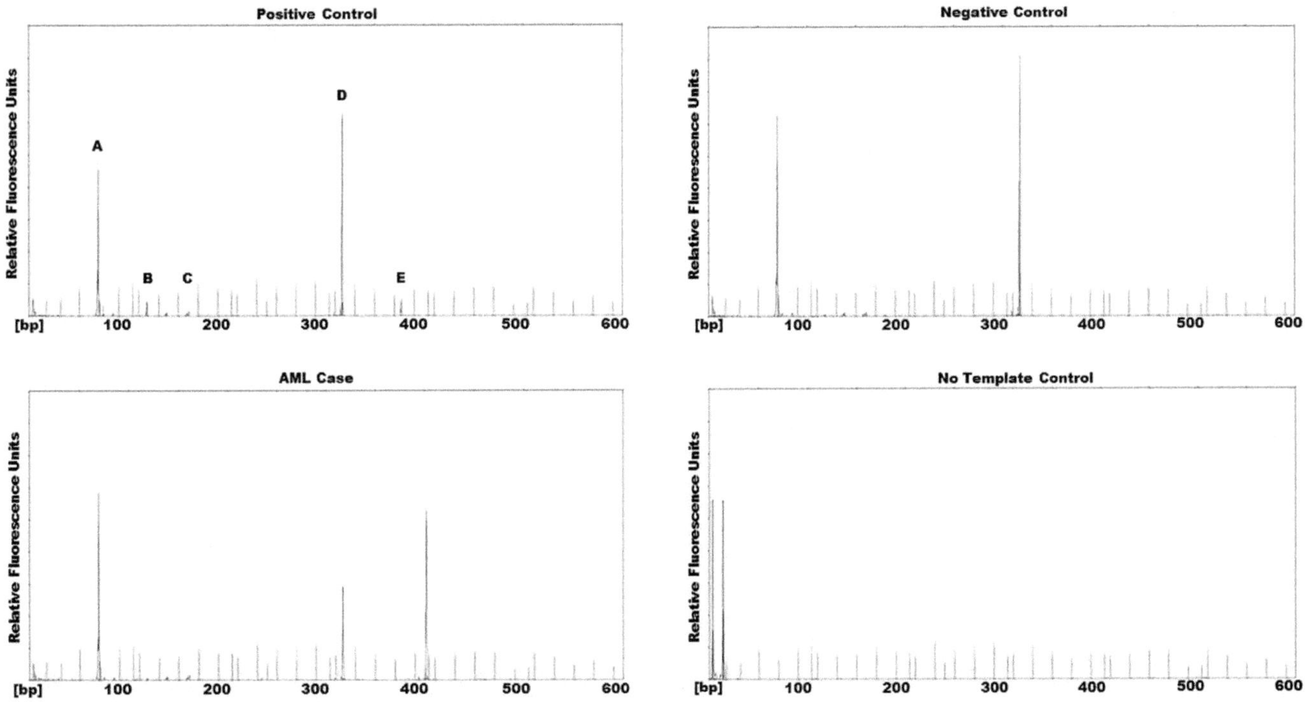

Fig. 2.8 ***FLT3*** **D835/I836 and ITD fragment analysis:** In each assay run, a positive control (D835/I836 and *FLT3* ITD mutations), negative control, and no template control are required. Amplicons are combined with a size marker (orange peaks) for the calibration of the fragment sizes. In the positive control, the wild-type amplicon digested with EcoRV is represented by peak (**A**) at 79 bp. Peak (**C**) at 148 bp represents incomplete digestion of the PCR amplicon, and peak (**B**) at 128 bp represents a D835/I836 mutation. Peak (**D**) at 327 bp illustrates the wild-type amplicon for the *FLT3* ITD primer pair, and peak (**E**) at 387 bp represents a *FLT3* ITD. The AML case contains no detectable D835/I836 mutation and an 84 bp *FLT3* ITD

Case History

The patient is a 60-year-old female who has a history of multiple myeloma that was previously treated with stem cell transplant. The patient presented with generalized weakness and worsening low back pain.

Laboratory Work-up

Her laboratory studies are seen in Table 2.6 that showed leukocytosis. The patient also underwent a bone marrow aspiration and biopsy.

Question 1: After reviewing this preliminary information, which hematologic diseases are in the differential diagnosis?

Patient's CBC data between January 2020 and October 2020 demonstrates progressive leukocytosis with neutrophilia and some circulating neutrophil precursors. There is no increase of blasts in the peripheral blood. Based on the described findings, there are two primary considerations: reactive leukocytosis and a primary bone marrow disorder. A clearly defined secondary cause of leukocytosis, such as infections, inflammation, and autoimmune reactions, is not identified. Thus, a bone marrow biopsy is performed to rule out a primary myeloid disorder, such as myeloproliferative neoplasm (MPN).

Histologic Findings

There is marked increase in the number of granulocytes with left-shifted maturation, including myelocytes and metamyelocytes in the peripheral blood smear (Fig. 2.9). Bone marrow aspirates are hypercellular for age with hyperplastic granulopoiesis and maturation (Fig. 2.10a). There is no increase in myeloblasts (1%). Marrow biopsy sections are hypercellular with >90% cellularity. Myeloid elements are increased. Erythroid elements and megakaryocytes are present with orderly maturation (Fig. 2.10b). Molecular genetic studies, including karyotype, FISH panel for MPN and NGS hematology panel, are ordered to aid diagnosis.

Molecular Genetic Studies

Cytogenetics study showed 46,XX [20] and normal female karyotype. FISH analysis for MPN was negative for t(9;22), and chromosomal rearrangement of *PDGFRA*, *PDGFRB*, and *FGFR1*. NGS-based hematology panel identified multiple mutations including *CSF3R*, *ASXL1*, *SETBP1*, and *SRSF2* (Table 2.7).

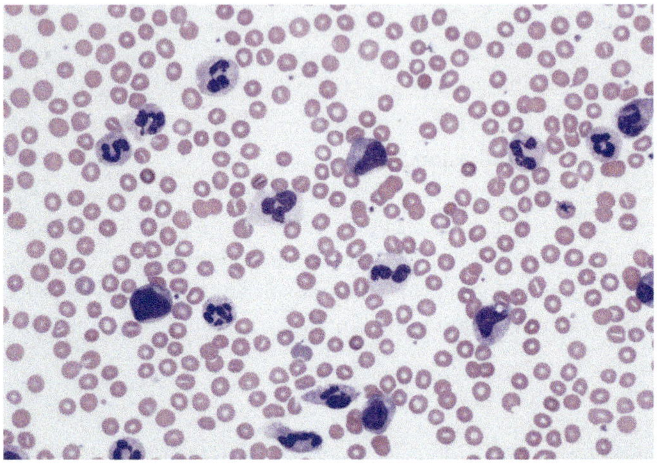

Fig. 2.9 Peripheral blood smear shows characteristic neutrophilia. There are segmented neutrophils mixed with some neutrophil precursors (myelocytes and metamyelocytes). Wright-Giemsa stain, 400×

Table 2.6 Complete blood count with differential demonstrating persistent leukocytosis

	January 2020	February 2020	September 2020	October 2020	October 2020 (2 weeks later)
WBC (K/uL)	15.2	19.2	63.5	96.2	179.7
Hgb (g/dL)	11.1	8.9	11	9.5	10.5
HCT (%)	36.7	31.3	36	31.2	31.5
MCV (fL)	93.6	92	94	94.3	91.3
MCH (pg)	28.3	29.2	29	28.7	30.4
RDW (%)	15.4	15	16	16.3	16.1
Platelet (K/uL)	382	346	326	223	275
MPV (fL)	12.5	12.7	11.8	11.2	11.5
Differential (absolute)					
Neutrophils (K/uL)	11.4	15.5	50.76	73.12	155.66
Lymphocytes (K/uL)	1.5	2.5	3.63	3.85	0
Monocytes (K/uL)	0.5	0.37	0.6	5.77	2.58
Eosinophils (K/uL)	0.7	0.37	4.23	0.96	0
Basophils (K/uL)	0.2	0.24	0	1.92	0
Metamyelocytes (K/uL)	0	0.24	4.23	3.85	12.88
Promyelocyte (K/uL)	0	0	1.21	0	0
Myelocytes (K/uL)	0	0	0	6.73	8.59
Blasts (K/uL)	0	0	0	0	0

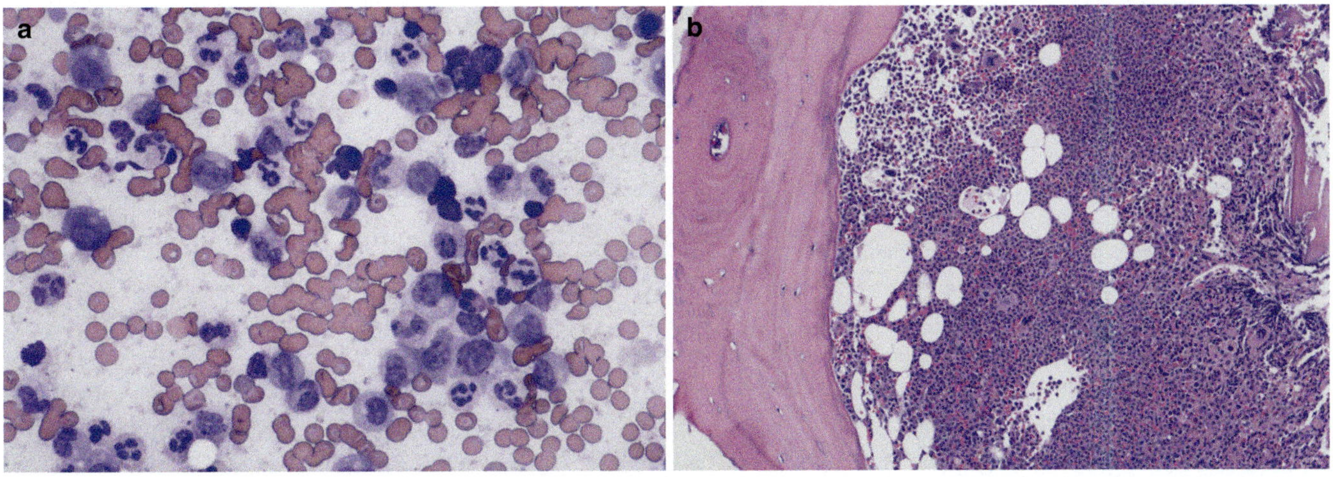

Fig. 2.10 (**a**) Bone marrow aspirate smear demonstrates neutrophil proliferation of different maturation stages with no increase in myeloblasts. Wright-Giemsa staining, 400×. (**b**) The bone marrow biopsy specimen is hypercellular, showing a significantly increased number of neutrophils and myeloid-to-erythroid ratio. Hematoxylin and eosin staining, 100×

Table 2.7 Patient results from next-generation sequencing

Gene	Variant	Amino Acid change	Nucleotide change	Consequence	Variant allele frequency (%)	Read Depth
CSF3R	T618I	p.Thr618Ile	NM_000760.3: c.1853C>T	Missense	39.2	1815
ASXL1	C730*	p.Cys730Ter	NM_015338.5: c.2190C>A	Nonsense	53.1	1924
SETBP1	I871T	p.Ile871Thr	NM_015559.2: c.2612T>C	Missense	47.3	4650
SRSF2	P95L	p.Pro95Leu	NM_003016.4: c.284C>T	Missense	48.9	932

Final Diagnosis

Chronic neutrophilic leukemia (CNL) with *CSF3R* T618I mutation

Discussion

Chronic neutrophilic leukemia usually occurs in the sixth decade and has a strong male predominance (70%) and may present as neutrophilia, hepatosplenomegaly, and fatigue. However, majority of patients are asymptomatic. Important laboratory testing includes a CBC, peripheral blood and bone marrow examination, molecular analysis, and cytogenetics. Majority (>90%) of these patients are cytogenetically normal. On sequencing, the *CSF3R* mutation is present in almost all cases. The most critical region to examine is in the membrane proximal region which is coded by exon 14. The missense mutation T618I in *CSF3R* is the most commonly seen variant in CNL [65]. Other myeloid associated mutations such as *SRSF2*, *TET2*, *U2AF1*, and *NRAS* may be identified [65]. In rare cases, *SETBP1* mutations may be seen. A mutation in ASXL1 is associated with a poor prognosis.

To detect the *CSF3R* mutation, methodologies such as Sanger sequencing, pyrosequencing, high-resolution melting curve analysis, and next-generation sequencing can be performed. NGS is useful because the individual sequence of millions of molecules is captured simultaneously. Therefore, the number of genes sequenced in the NGS panel are dependent on the library. In contrast to the single-gene assay, NGS offers additional information such as VAF and if the mutation is in *cis-* or in *trans* or the presence of multiple gene mutations. In this case, the analysis was based on the detection of clonally amplified DNA through SBS. The sequencing of base calls was then determined by optical detection after reversible chain termination.

NGS Sequencing Results

Mutations in *CSF3R, ASXL1, SRSF2,* and *SETBP1* were identified. *CSF3R*, a granulocyte colony-stimulating factor is located on Chromosome 1, p34.3 and is composed of 17 exons and codes for an 813-amino-acid protein [66]. It encodes a transmembrane receptor that is responsible for proliferation, differentiation, survival, and function of granulocytes [65]. Activating missense mutations that effect the extracellular domain are responsible for CNL. The signature mutation in CNL is the *CSF3R T618I* [65]. This mutation leads to a sustained mature neutrophil proliferation, hepatosplenomegaly, and bone marrow granulocytic hyperplasia.

To obtain the mutational data, a major bioinformatics analysis is required. This process begins with the raw data after sequencing completion. The raw short reads are resulted in a plain text format called a FASTQ file. A FASTQ file is a text-based format that contains the nucleotide sequence and the quality score. The FASTQ file is then uploaded to a bioinformatics platform in which automated sequence analysis and mutation detection are performed. The reads and alignment are performed and mapped to a known reference sequence (as seen in Fig. 2.11). Next, variant identification and annotation of the variants occurs, and then final step of data review/interpretation can occur.

After review of this data and review of the literature to examine for new updates to the clinical implications of the mutation, the final report can be created. The report is clear, concise, and follows the joint consensus recommendations from the Association of Molecular Pathology, American College of Medical Genetics and Genomics, American Society of Clinical Oncology, and College of American Pathologists. The gene name should be reported as defined by HUGO gene nomenclature committee. If there are SNVs or indels, they should be reported using the p. and c. notation (as seen in Table 2.7). CNVs should be reported with clear communication of "loss" or "gain." Other important report elements are the transcript reference sequences (e.g., NM_000760.3). Finally, it is recommended to use the tier system to define genomic findings since there is clinical management decisions that can be made. Tier 1 and 2 should always be communicated, while tier 3 may be communicated but could detract from the clarity of the report. The most important caveat is that the amount of information should not affect the clear and concise communication of results.

Case #3

Learning Objectives

1.) Understand the use of qPCR and its components such as the calibration curve, amplification curve, and multicomponent plot.

Case History

The patient is a 63-year-old female who presented with fever and weakness for the past few days. The CBC demonstrated a white count of 75 K/μL and a differential that was predominantly blasts. Flow cytometry demonstrated a B-lymphoblastic leukemia. A bone marrow biopsy demonstrated sheets of lymphoblasts. The bone marrow specimen was submitted for further workup including *BCR-ABL1* by quantitative reverse transcriptase PCR (qRT-PCR).

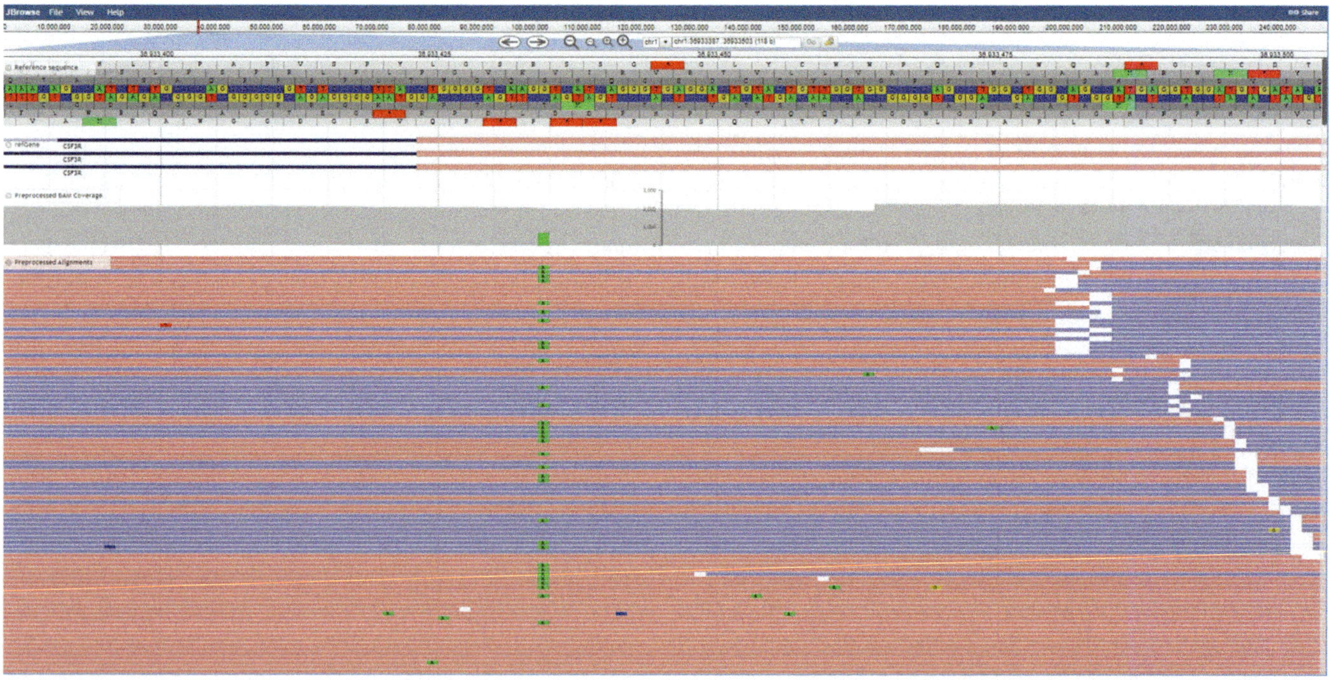

Fig. 2.11 NGS data alignment and visualization: Genome visualization and analysis are used to view mutations and assess variant calling by the bioinformatics pipeline. In this case, the sequence data is loaded into JBrowse [67] and aligned to the reference genome. Variants are highlighted in the preprocessed BAM coverage as a colored bar in the grey coverage plot, with the height representing the fraction of reads with alternate alleles at that genomic position (711 variant reads/1815 total reads, 39.2%). The preprocessed alignment tracks show the NM_000760.3:c.1853C>T single-nucleotide variant as a green "A" in both DNA strands (red and blue tracks). The reference sequence illustrates that the potential causes of PCR and sequencing error such as homopolymers and nucleotide repeats are not present in this genomic region. The surrounding sequence shows negligible variants, supporting the identification of the CSF3R c.1853C>T p.T618I mutation

Final Diagnosis

B-Lymphoblastic leukemia with *BCR-ABL1* (p190) fusion

Discussion

The *BCR-ABL1* fusion occurs in approximately 60–70% of adult B-ALL cases. This minor (m) breakpoint results in the generation of the transcript e1-a2, which corresponds to a fusion protein size of 190 kDa. To detect this m breakpoint, qPCR is utilized. An important component of qPCR is the standard calibration curve that contains the information about the calibrators and the controls. This curve is needed to quantify the product of interest in the patient sample. The calibration curve for this case is seen in Fig. 2.12. The amplification plot (Fig. 2.13) shows the relation of the normalized reporter value in relation to cycle. The normalized reporter value is the difference between the fluorescence of the reporter dye signal (FAM *BCR-ABL1,* CY5 *ABL1*) to the fluorescence signal of the passive reference dye. The multicomponent plot (Fig. 2.14) demonstrates the amount of fluorescence per PCR cycle. Each of these components are required for the quantification of the product of interest. In cases where the value is higher than the controls, the quantification cannot be performed. The *BCR-ABL1* fusion can be followed over the course of treatment to determine the level of response. The International Scale (IS) and the log reduction are used to quantify the response to therapy. The %IS the ratio of the *BCR-ABL1* to *ABL1*. To calculate this, the standard curve must be used. The standard curve is a linear regression curve that plots known concentrations of a template at various dilutions (*x*-axis) and their corresponding C_t (*y*-axis) generated during qPCR. The unknown concentration of the amplicon of interest will generate a C_t. Using this C_t, a horizontal line can be drawn and at the point it intersects the standard curve, a vertical line drawn to the *x*-axis will reveal the number of copies of the amplicon. If the C_t of the unknown sample does not fall on the linear regression curve between the high and low standards, this will result in a copy number that is above or below the limit of quantification, respectively.

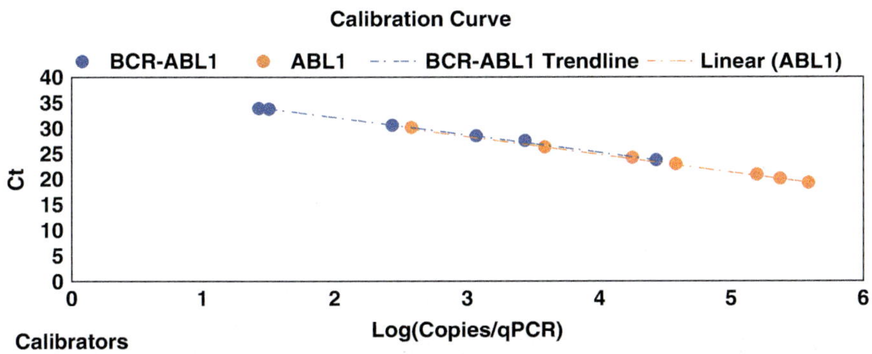

ABL 1	BCR-ABL 1
y = mx + b	y = mx + b
m = −3.55	m = −3.317
b = 39.25	b = 38.70
R^2 = 0.999	R^2 = 0.999

Calibrators

Well	Calibrator	ABL1 Ct mean	BCR-ABL1 minor Ct mean	ABL1 Copies/qPCR	BCR-ABL1 minor Copies/qPCR
B2,B3	CAL1	19.3	23.9	380,000	27,000
C2,C3	CAL2	23.1	27.5	38,000	2,700
D2,D3	CAL3	26.3	30.7	3,800	270
E2,E3	CAL4	30.1	33.9	380	27

Controls

Well	Control	ABL1 Ct	BCR-ABL1 minor Ct	ABL1 Copies/qPCR	BCR-ABL1 minor Copies/qPCR	%ratio
F2	CONH	24.1	28.5	17,962	1,157	6.4387
G2	CONL	20.2	33.7	230,331	32	0.0137
F3	CONN	20.8	N/D	155,842	N/D	N/A

Well	Specimen Name	ABL1 Ct	BCR-ABL1 minor Ct	ABL1 Copies/qPCR	BCR-ABL1 minor Copies/qPCR	%ratio	Comments
B4	Patient 1	16.1	18.1	2,280,869	1,645,739	72.154	Positive (above LOQ)

Fig. 2.12 ***BCR-ABL1* and *ABL1* calibration curve and control analysis:** This calibration curve utilizes a series of *ABL1* and *BCR-ABL1* calibrators that are in a series of tenfold dilutions. The controls in this analysis are a negative control (no *BCR-ABL1* copies), a low positive control, and a high positive control. The patient's result demonstrates a *BCR-ABL1* minor product with a C_t of 18.1 and a %IS ratio of 72.154. While the result is positive, it is above the limit of quantification as it is off the curve

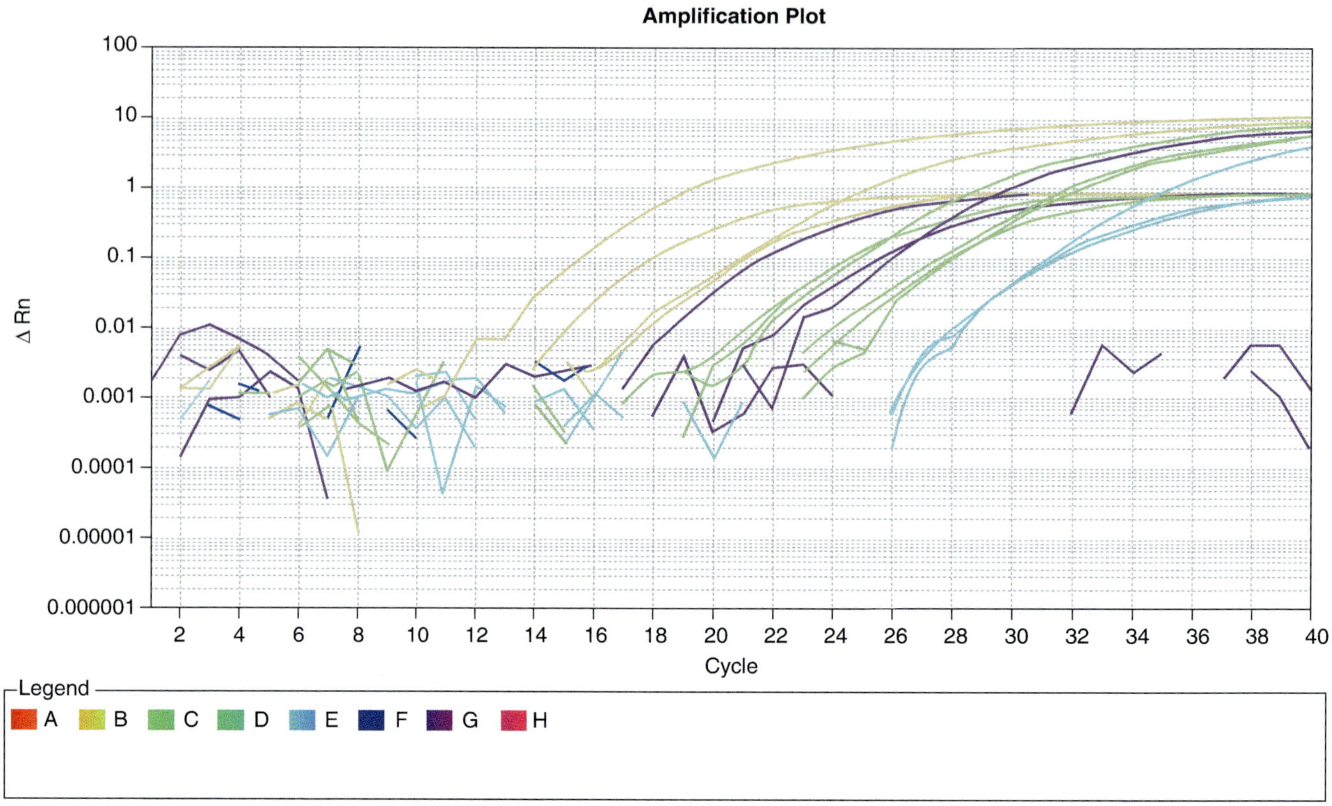

Fig. 2.13 ***BCR-ABL1*** **and** ***ABL1*** **qPCR amplification plot:** The amplification plot of a series of eight dilutions is shown. The curve is a log view (*y*-axis is a log scale) with a normalized reporter value on the *y*-axis. The *x*-axis is the cycle number of the PCR. The initial PCR cycles produce a low background level of fluorescent signals that cannot be detected. Eventually, the reaction progresses into the exponential phase in which the level of fluorescence is linear and can be detected above the background fluorescence, and thus the PCR products have doubled. The amount of product doubles each cycle. The flat portion of the curve demonstrates minimal fluorescent signal increase. This signifies the depletion of primers and dNTPs

Case #4

Learning Objectives

1.) Understand the use of endpoint PCR and recognize an electropherogram.

Case History

The patient is a 60-year-old female who underwent an inguinal excisional lymph node biopsy after non-response to antibiotic therapy. Microscopic examination of the lymph node revealed effacement of the architecture and a proliferation of densely packed uniform neoplastic follicles and was characteristic of follicular lymphoma. However, the BCL2 immunohistochemical assay was negative in the follicles. The specimen was sent for endpoint PCR for assessment of a *BCL2-IGH* translocation.

Final Diagnosis

Follicular lymphoma with *BCL2-IGH* translocation

Discussion

Identification of a *BCL2-IGH* translocation through endpoint PCR is complicated for many reasons. First, the translocation must be detected at the DNA level due to lack of a fusion transcript, which makes this analysis complicated. Also, the variable regions of the *IGH* gene undergo extensive mutations and, thus, require multiple primers sets. Without multiple primer sets, the result could be falsely negative due to the gene rearrangements in *IGH*. Additionally, *BCL2* has multiple breakpoints and thus they each must be individually assessed. Approximately 50–60% of follicular lymphomas with t(14;18) will have the major breakpoint cluster region (MBR). The intermediate cluster

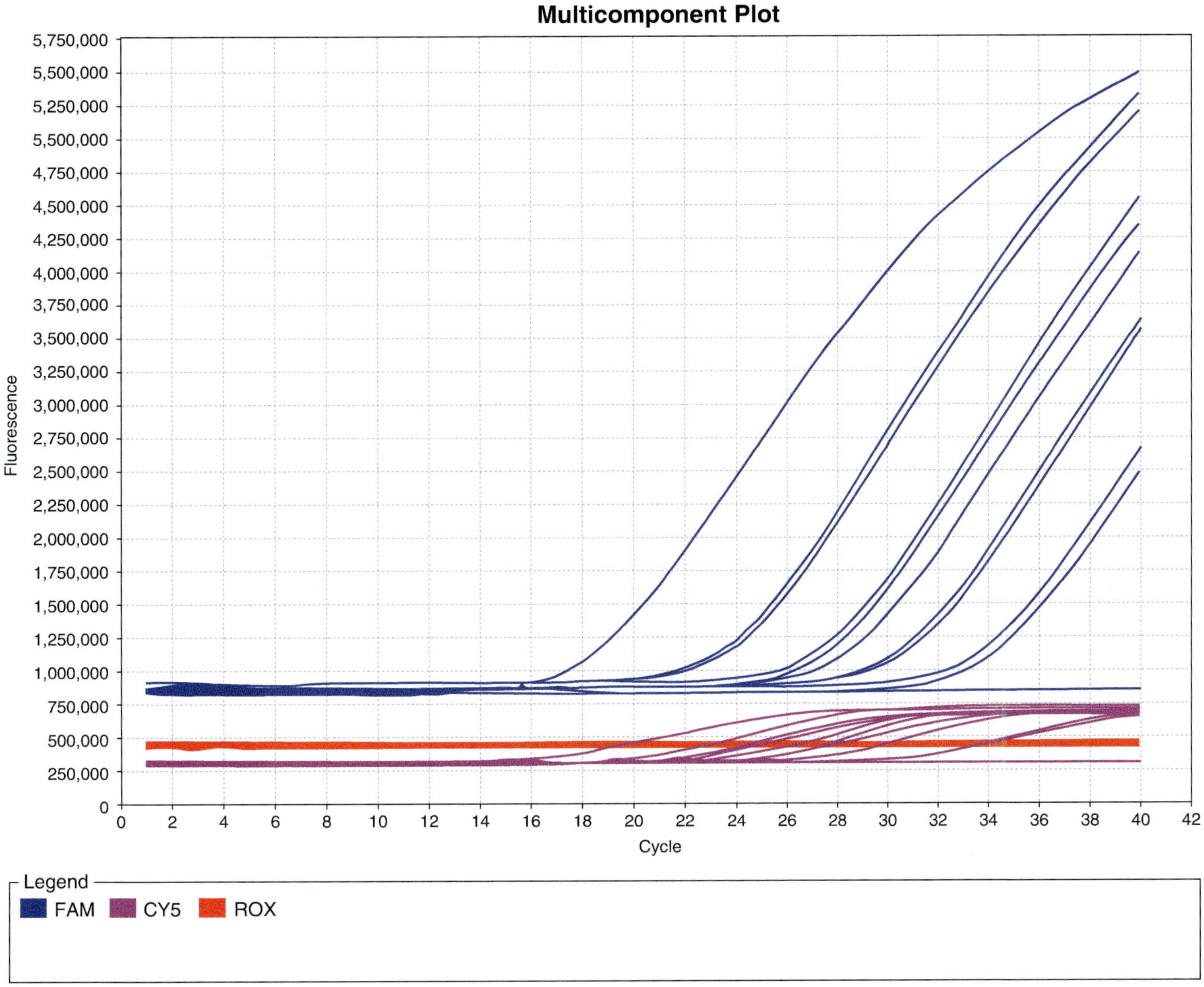

Fig. 2.14 ***BCR-ABL1* and *ABL1* qPCR multicomponent plot:** The multicomponent plot is a raw amplification plot that shows the spectral contribution of each dye per well during each PCR cycle. The fluorescence values are on the *y*-axis and the cycle number is on the *x*-axis

region (ICR) is seen in approximately 10–15% of follicular lymphomas. Less commonly, a minor breakpoint cluster region (mcr) is seen in only 5–10% of follicular lymphomas. In rare cases, approximately 5% of follicular lymphomas will possess the 5′ breakpoint region. In B-lymphocytes, the *IGH* gene is actively transcribed. Thus, when *BCL2* is translocated adjacent to the *IGH* locus enhancer, *BCL2* is expressed at the same level. In contrast to qPCR in which quantification occurs during the exponential phase, end-point PCR utilizes the plateau phase after the PCR is completed.

In this case, to detect the *BCL2-IGH* rearrangement, four master mixes were utilized. Of these master mixes, three targeted distinct regions of *BCL2* and the joining region of the *IGH* gene. These master mixes are able to detect the MBR, 3′MBR, and mcr of the t(14;18) *BCL2-IGH* translocations. The fourth master mix contains a control size ladder. This master mix utilizes a multiplex reaction and generates amplicons of varying sizes of multiple genes, which range in size from 100 to 600 base pairs. The PCR products were then subjected to capillary electrophoresis. The results are seen in Figs. 2.15, 2.16, and 2.17 and confirm the diagnosis of follicular lymphoma.

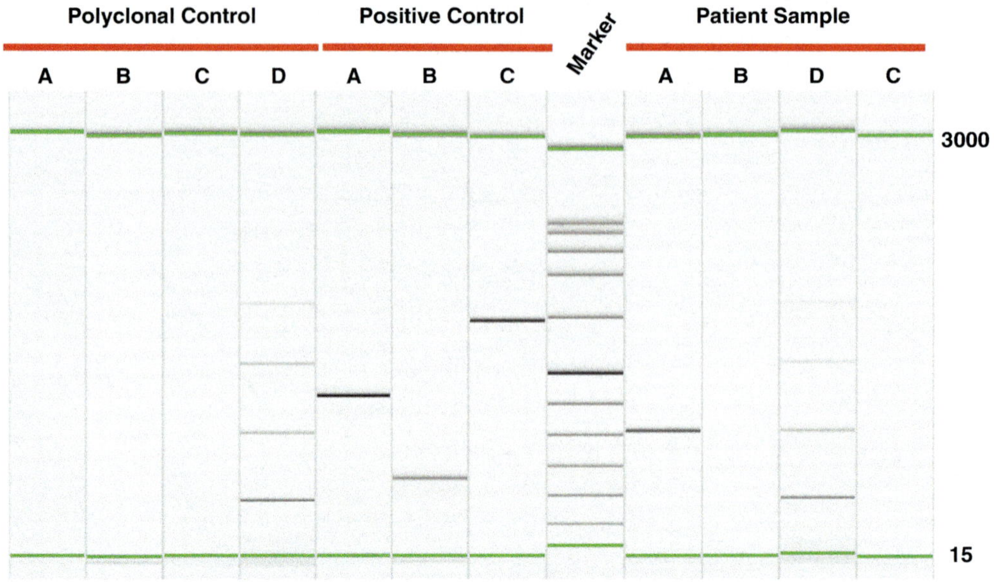

Fig. 2.15 **Simulated *BCL2-IGH* gel image**: The first three lanes, A, B, C, are the three master mixes for the MBR, 3′MBR, and mcr (respectively). The fourth lane, D, is the control size ladder. A fragment size marker is utilized for calibration of the amplicon lengths. In each run, no amplicons (polyclonal controls) and amplicons at different sizes (positive controls) are required. The band present in lane A of the patient sample indicates a positive t(14;18); *BCL2-IGH* fusion in the major breakpoint cluster region (MBR). Figure provided by Dr. Linsheng Zhang

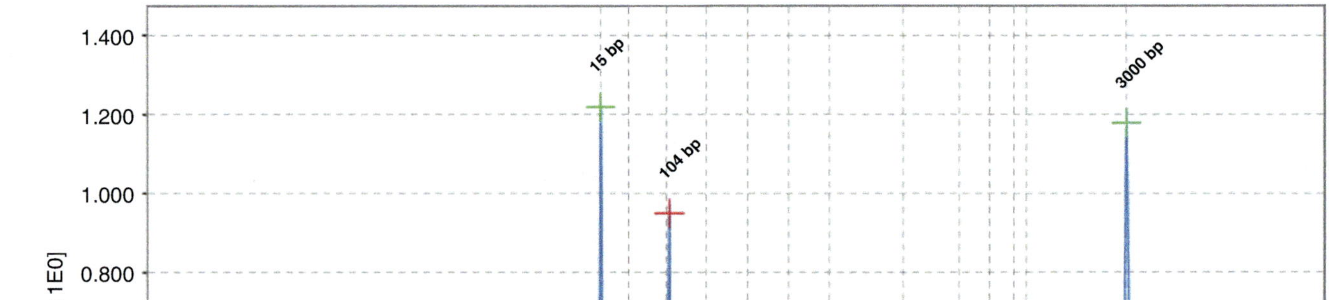

Fig. 2.16 **Control size ladder electropherogram:** The largest amplifiable fragment from the sample is greater than 400 base pairs. Alignment markers are also present for the lower and upper ranges of the electrophoresis (15 bp and 3000 bp). In this case, the DNA in the FFPE nodal tissue is preserved. However, if the DNA were to have been heavily fragmented in this sample, the amplification process would have failed. Figure provided by Dr. Linsheng Zhang

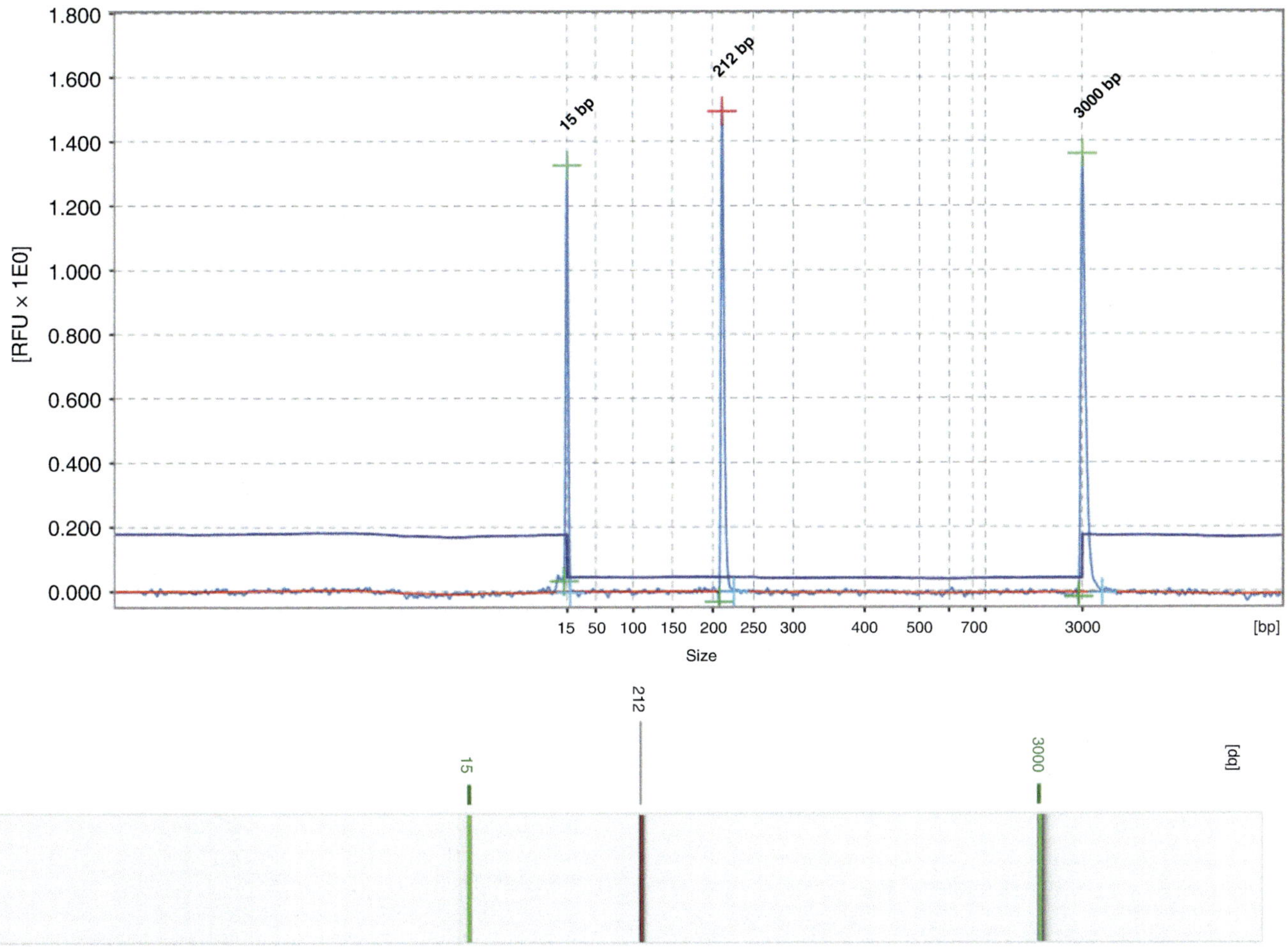

Fig. 2.17 ***BCL2-IGH* electropherogram:** The electropherogram of the patient sample demonstrates a peak of 212 bp, which indicates the presence of the fusion. Figure provided by Dr. Linsheng Zhang

References

1. Vandeven N, Nghiem P. Pathogen-driven cancers and emerging immune therapeutic strategies. Cancer Immunol Res. 2014;2(1):9–14. Available from: https://cancerimmunolres.aacrjournals.org/content/2/1/9.full. https://doi.org/10.1158/2326-6066.CIR-13-0179.
2. Medeiros F, Rigl T, Anderson G, Becker S, Halling K. Tissue handling for genome-wide expression analysis: a review of the issues, evidence, and opportunities. Arch Pathol Lab Med. 2007;131(12):1805–16. Available from https://meridian.allenpress.com/aplm/article/131/12/1805/63021. https://doi.org/10.1043/1543-2165(2007)131[1805:THFGEA]2.0.CO;2.
3. Wang Y, Zheng H, Chen J, Zhong X, Wang Y, Wang Z, et al. The impact of different preservation conditions and freezing-thawing cycles on quality of RNA, DNA, and proteins in cancer tissue. Biopreserv Biobank. 2015;13(5):335–47. Available from https://www.liebertpub.com/doi/10.1089/bio.2015.0029. https://doi.org/10.1089/bio.2015.0029.
4. Bass BP, Engel KB, Greytak SR, Moore HM. A review of pre-analytical factors affecting molecular, protein, and morphological analysis of formalin-fixed, paraffin-embedded (FFPE) tissue: how well Do you know your FFPE specimen. Arch Pathol Lab Med. 2014;138(11):1520–30. Available from: https://meridian.allenpress.com/aplm/article/138/11/1520/128727. https://doi.org/10.5858/arpa.2013-0691-RA.
5. Wickham CL, Boyce M, Joyner MV, Sarsfield P, Wilkins BS, Jones DB, Ellard S. Amplification of PCR products in excess of 600 base pairs using DNA extracted from decalcified, paraffin wax embedded bone marrow trephine biopsies. Mol Pathol. 2000;53(1):19–23. Available from: https://www.ncbi.nlm.nih.gov/pmc/articles/PMC1186897. https://doi.org/10.1136/mp.53.1.19.
6. Sarsfield P, Wickham CL, Joyner MV, Ellard S, Jones DB, Wilkins BS. Formic acid decalcification of bone marrow trephines degrades DNA: alternative use of ETA allows the amplification and sequencing of relatively long PCR products. Mol Pathol. 2000;53(6):336. Available from: https://www.ncbi.nlm.nih.gov/pmc/articles/PMC1186990. https://doi.org/10.1136/mp.53.6.336.
7. Tsongalis G, Al-Turkmani MR, Suriawinata M, Babcock MJ, Mitchell K, Ding Y, et al. Comparison of tissue molecular biomarker testing turnaround times and concordance between standard of care and the biocartis idylla platform in patients with colorectal cancer. Am J Clin Pathol. 2020;154(2):266–76. Available from: https://academic.oup.com/ajcp/article/154/2/266/5856048. https://doi.org/10.1093/ajcp/aqaa044.
8. Chester N, Marshak DR. Dimethyl sulfoxide-mediated primer tm reduction: a method for analyzing the role of renaturation temperature in the polymerase chain reaction. Anal Biochem. 1993;209(2):284–90. Available from: https://www.sciencedirect.com/science/article/abs/pii/S0003269783711218?via%3Dihub. https://doi.org/10.1006/abio.1993.1121.
9. Taylor SC, Laperriere G, Germain H. Droplet digital PCR versus qPCR for expression analysis with low abundant targets: from variable nonsense to publication quality data. Sci Rep. 2017;7:2409. Available from: https://www.nature.com/articles/s41598-017-02217 x. https://doi.org/10.1038/s41598-017-02217-x.

10. Majumdar N, Banerjee S, Pallas M, Wessel T, Hegerich P. Poisson plus quantification for digital PCR systems. Sci Rep. 2017:9617. Available from: https://www.nature.com/articles/s41598-017-09183-4. https://doi.org/10.1038/s41598-017-09183-4.
11. Andrikovics H, Orfi Z, Meggyesi N, Bors A, Varg L, Kovy P, et al. Current trends in applications of circulatory microchimerism detection in transplantation. Int J Mol Sci. 2019;20(18):4450. Available from: https://www.mdpi.com/1422-0067/20/18/4450/htm. https://doi.org/10.3390/ijms20184450.
12. Sanchez R, Ayala R, Martinez-Lopez J. Minimal residual disease monitoring with next-generation sequencing methodologies in hematological malignancies. Int J Mol Sci. 2019;20(11):2832. Available from: https://www.mdpi.com/1422-0067/20/11/2832. https://doi.org/10.3390/ijms20112832.
13. Blais J, Lavoie SB, Giroux S, Bussieres J, Lindsay C, Dionne J, et al. Risk of misdiagnosis due to allele dropout and false-positive PCR artifacts in molecular diagnostics: analysis of 30769 genotypes. J Mol Diagn. 2015;17(5):505–14. Available from: https://www.sciencedirect.com/science/article/abs/pii/S1525157815001208?showall%3Dtrue%26via%3Dihub. https://doi.org/10.1016/j.jmoldx.2015.04.004.
14. Sasaki A, Kim B, Murphy KE, Matthews SG. Impact of ex vivo sample handling on DNA methylation profiles in human cord blood and neonatal dried blood spots. Front Genet. 2020;11:224. Available from: https://www.ncbi.nlm.nih.gov/pmc/articles/PMC7106936/. https://doi.org/10.3389/fgene.2020.00224.
15. Groen K, Lea RA, Maltby VE, Scott RJ, Lechner-Scott J. Letter to the editor: blood processing and sample storage have negligible effects on methylation. Clin Epigenetics. 2018;10:22. Available from: https://clinicalepigeneticsjournal.biomedcentral.com/articles/10.1186/s13148-018-0455-6. https://doi.org/10.1186/s13148-018-0455-6.
16. Moran B, Das S, Smeets D, Peutman G, Klinger R, Fender B, et al. Assessment of concordance between fresh-frozen and formalin-fixed paraffin embedded tumor DNA methylation using a targeted sequencing approach. Oncotarget. 2017;8(29):48126–37. Available from: https://www.oncotarget.com/article/18296/text. https://doi.org/10.18632/oncotarget.18296.
17. Kurdyukov S, Bullock M. DNA methylation analysis: choosing the right method. Biology. 5(1):3. Available from: https://www.mdpi.com/2079-7737/5/1/3/htm. https://doi.org/10.3390/biology5010003.
18. Gerard GF, Potter RJ, Smith MD, Rosenthal K, Dhariwal G, Lee J, et al. The role of template-primer in protection of reverse transcriptase from thermal inactivation. Nucleic Acids Res. 2002;30(14):3118–29. Available from: https://academic.oup.com/nar/article/30/14/3118/2904298. https://doi.org/10.1093/nar/gkf417.
19. Yun JW, Yang L, Park HY, Lee CW, Cha H, Shin HT, et al. Dysregulation of cancer genes by recurrent intergenic fusions. Genome Biol. 2020;21(1):166. Available from: https://genomebiology.biomedcentral.com/articles/10.1186/s13059-020-02076-2. https://doi.org/10.1186/s13059-020-02076-2.
20. Ozsolak F, Milos PM. RNA sequencing: advances, challenges, and opportunities. Nat Rev Genet. 2011;12(2):87–98. Available from: https://www.nature.com/articles/nrg2934. https://doi.org/10.1038/nrg2934.
21. Chasseriau J, Rivet J, Bilan F, Chomel JC, Guilhot F, Bourmeyster N, Kitzis A. Characterization of the different BCR-ABL transcripts with a single multiplex RT-PCR. J Mol Diagn. 2004;6(4):343–7. Available from: https://www.sciencedirect.com/science/article/pii/S1525157810605302?via%3Dihub. https://doi.org/10.1016/S1525-1578(10)60530-2.
22. Torres F, Ivanova-Dragoeva A, Pereira M, Veiga J, Rodrigues AS, Sousa AB, et al. An e6a2 BCR-ABL fusion transcript in a CML patient having an iliac chloroma at initial presentation. Leuk Lymphoma. 2007;48(5):1034–7. Available from: https://www.tandfonline.com/doi/abs/10.1080/10428190701216402. https://doi.org/10.1080/10428190701216402.
23. Piedimonte M, Ottone T, Alfonso V, Ferrari A, Conte E, Divona M, et al. A rare BCR-ABL1 transcript in Philadelphia-positive acute myeloid leukemia: case report and literature review. BMC Cancer. 2019;19(1):50. Available from: https://bmccancer.biomedcentral.com/articles/10.1186/s12885-019-5265-5. https://doi.org/10.1186/s12885-019-5265-5.
24. Gabert J, Beillard E, van der Velden V, Grimwade D, Pallisgaard N, Barbany G, et al. Standardization and quality control studies of 'real-time' quantitative reverse transcriptase polymerase chain reaction of fusion gene transcripts for residual disease detection in leukemia – a Europe against cancer program. Leukemia. 2003;17:2318–57. Available from: https://www.nature.com/articles/2403135. https://doi.org/10.1038/sj.leu.2403135.
25. Marchiò C, Scaltriti M, Ladanyi M, Iafrate AJ, Bibeau F, Dietel M, et al. ESMO recommendations on the standard methods to detect NTRK fusions in daily practice and clinical research. Ann Oncol. 2019;30(9):1417–27. Available from: https://www.sciencedirect.com/science/article/pii/S0923753419459929?via%3Dihub. https://doi.org/10.1093/annonc/mdz204.
26. Teixidó C, Giménez-Capitán A, Molina-Vila MA, Peg V, Karachaliou N, Rodríguez-Capote A, et al. RNA analysis as a tool to determine clinically relevant gene fusions and splice variants. Arch Pathol Lab Med. 2018;142(4):474–9. Available from: https://meridian.allenpress.com/aplm/article/142/4/474/194239/RNA-Analysis-as-a-Tool-to-Determine-Clinically. https://doi.org/10.5858/arpa.2017-0134-RA.
27. Bruno R, Fontanini G. Next generation sequencing for gene fusion analysis in lung cancer: a literature review. Diagnostics (Basel). 2020;10(8):521. Available from: https://www.mdpi.com/2075-4418/10/8/521. https://doi.org/10.3390/diagnostics10080521.
28. Racanelli D, Brenca M, Baldazzi D, Goeman F, Casini B, De Angelis B, et al. Next-generation sequencing approaches for the identification of pathognomonic fusion transcripts in sarcomas: the experience of the Italian ACC sarcoma working group. Front Oncol. 2020;10:944. Available from: https://www.frontiersin.org/articles/10.3389/fonc.2020.00489/full. https://doi.org/10.3389/fonc.2020.00489.
29. Zheng J. Oncogenic chromosomal translocations and human cancer. Oncol Rep. 2013;30(5):2011–9. Available from: https://www.spandidos-publications.com/10.3892/or.2013.2677. https://doi.org/10.3892/or.2013.2677.
30. Espinet B, Bellosillo B, Melero C, Vela MC, Pedro C, Salido M, et al. FISH is better than BIOMED-2 PCR to detect IgH / BCL 2 translocation in follicular lymphoma at diagnosis using paraffin-embedded tissue sections. Leuk Res. 2008;32(5):737–42. Available from: https://www.clinicalkey.com/#!/content/journal/1-s2.0-S0145212607003517. https://doi.org/10.1016/j.leukres.2007.09.010.
31. Szankasi P, Bolia A, Liew M, Schumacher JA, Gee EPS, Matynia AP, et al. Comprehensive detection of chromosomal translocations in lymphoproliferative disorders by massively parallel sequencing. J Hematop. 2019;12:121–33. Available from: https://link.springer.com/article/10.1007/s12308-019-00360-0#citeas. https://doi.org/10.1007/s12308-019-00360-0.
32. Selvi N, Kosova B, Hekimgil M, Gunduz C, Kaymaz BT, Karaca E, et al. Molecular evaluation of t(14;18)(bcl-2/IgH) translocation in follicular lymphoma at diagnosis using paraffin-embedded tissue sections. Turk J Haematol. 2012;29(2):126–34. Available from: https://www.ncbi.nlm.nih.gov/pmc/articles/PMC3986950/. https://doi.org/10.5505/tjh.2012.93898.
33. Bonneville R, Krook MA, Chen H, Smith A, Samorodnitsky E, Wing MR, et al. Detection of microsatellite instability biomarkers via next-generation sequencing. Methods Mol Biol.

2020;2055:119–32. Available from: https://link.springer.com/protocol/10.1007%2F978-1-4939-9773-2_5. https://doi.org/10.1007/978-1-4939-9773-2_5.
34. Levy SE, Myers RM. Advancements in next generation sequencing. Annu Rev Genom Hum G. 2016;17:95–115. Available from: https://www.annualreviews.org/doi/full/10.1146/annurev-genom-083115-022413. https://doi.org/10.1146/annurev-genom-083115-022413.
35. Pfeiffer F, Grober C, Blank M, Handler K, Beyer M, Schultze JL, Mayer G. Systematic evaluation of error rates and causes in short samples in next-generation sequencing. Sci Rep. 2018;8:10950. Available from: https://www.nature.com/articles/s41598-018-29325-6. https://doi.org/10.1038/s41598-018-29325-6.
36. Song L, Huang W, Kang J, Huang Y, Ren H, Ding K. Comparison of error correction algorithms for ion torrent PGM data: application to hepatitis B virus. Sci Rep. 2017;7:8106. Available from: https://www.nature.com/articles/s41598-017-08139-y. https://doi.org/10.1038/s41598-017-08139-y.
37. Kwong JC, McCallum N, Sintchenko V, Howden BP. Whole genome sequencing in clinical and public health microbiology. Pathology. 2015;47(3):199–210. Available from: https://www.clinicalkey.com/#!/content/journal/1-s2.0-S003130251630126X. https://doi.org/10.1097/PAT.0000000000000235.
38. Do H, Dobrovic A. Sequence artifacts in DNA from formalin-fixed tissues: causes and strategies for minimization. Clin Chem. 2015;61(1):64–71. Available from: https://academic.oup.com/clinchem/article/61/1/64/5611545. https://doi.org/10.1373/clinchem.2014.223040.
39. Haile S, Corbett RD, Bilobram S, Bye MH, Kirk H, Pandoh P, et al. Sources of erroneous sequences and artifact chimeric reads in next-generation sequencing of genomic DNA from formalin-fixed paraffin-embedded samples. Nucleic Acids Res. 2018;47(2):e12. Available from: https://academic.oup.com/nar/article/47/2/e12/5173669. https://doi.org/10.1093/nar/gky1142.
40. Kircher M, Heyn P, Kelso J. Addressing challenges in the production and analysis of illumina sequencing data. BMC Genomics. 2011;12:382. Available from: https://bmcgenomics.biomedcentral.com/articles/10.1186/1471-2164-12-382. https://doi.org/10.1186/1471-2164-12-382.
41. Ma X, Shao Y, Tian L, Flasch DA, Mulder HL, Edmonson MN, et al. Analysis of error profiles in deep next-generation sequencing data. Genome Biol. 2019;20:50. Available from: https://genomebiology.biomedcentral.com/articles/10.1186/s13059-019-1659-6. https://doi.org/10.1186/s13059-019-1659-6.
42. Schirmer M, D'Amore R, Ijaz UZ, Quince C. Illumina error profiles: resolving fine-scale variation in metagenomic sequencing data. BMC Bioinf. 2016;17:125. Available from: https://bmcbioinformatics.biomedcentral.com/articles/10.1186/s12859-016-0976-y. https://doi.org/10.1186/s12859-016-0976-y.
43. Abnizova I, Boekhorst R, Orlov YL. Computational errors and biases in short read next generation sequencing. J Proteomics Bioinform. 2017;10(1):1–17. Available from: https://www.longdom.org/open-access/computational-errors-and-biases-in-short-read-next-generationsequencing-jpb-1000420.pdf. https://doi.org/10.4172/jpb.1000420.
44. Jennings LJ, Arcila ME, Corless C, Kamel-Reid S, Lubin IM, Pfeifer J, et al. Guidelines for validation of next-generation sequencing-based oncology panels: a joint consensus recommendation of the Association for Molecular Pathology and College of American Pathologists. J Mol Diag. 2017;19(3):341–65. Available from: https://www.jmdjournal.org/article/S1525-1578(17)30025-9/fulltext. https://doi.org/10.1016/j.jmoldx.2017.01.011.
45. Peng M, Chen C, Hulbert A, Brock MV, Yu F. Non-blood circulating tumor DNA detection in cancer. Oncotarget. 2017;8(40):69162–73. Available from: https://www.oncotarget.com/article/19942/text/. https://doi.org/10.18632/oncotarget.19942.
46. Di Meo A, Bartlett J, Cheng Y, Pasic MD, Yousef GM. Liquid biopsy: a step towards precision medicine in urologic malignancies. Mol Cancer. 2017;16:80. Available from: https://molecular-cancer.biomedcentral.com/articles/10.1186/s12943-017-0644-5. https://doi.org/10.1186/s12943-017-0644-5.
47. Jahangiri L, Hurst T. Assessing the concordance of genomic alterations between circulating-free DNA and tumour tissue in cancer patients. Cancers. 2019;11(12):1938. Available from: https://www.mdpi.com/2072-6694/11/12/1938. https://doi.org/10.3390/cancers11121938.
48. Lyman SD, Jacobsen SEW. C-kit ligand and Flt3 ligand: stem/progenitor cell factors with overlapping yet distinct activities. Blood. 1998;91(4):1101–34. Available from: https://ashpublications.org/blood/article/91/4/1101/139529/c-kit-Ligand-and-Flt3-Ligand-Stem-Progenitor-Cell. https://doi.org/10.1182/blood.V91.4.1101.
49. Small D, Levenstein M, Kim E, Carow C, Amin S, Rockwell P, et al. STK-1, the human homolog of Flk-2/Flt-3, is selectively expressed in CD34+ human bone marrow cells and is involved in the proliferation of early progenitor/stem cells. Proc Natl Acad Sci U S A. 1994;91(2):459–63. Available from: https://www.pnas.org/content/91/2/459. https://doi.org/10.1073/pnas.91.2.459.
50. Mackarehtschian K, Hardin JD, Moore KA, Boast S, Goff SP, Lemischka IR. Targeted disruption of the Flk2/Flt3 gene leads to deficiencies in primitive hematopoietic progenitors. Immunity. 1995;3(1):147–61. Available from: https://www.cell.com/immunity/pdf/1074-7613(95)90167-1.pdf. https://doi.org/10.1016/1074-7613(95)90167-1.
51. Patnaik MM. The importance of FLT3 mutational analysis in acute myeloid leukemia. Leuk Lymphoma. 2018;59(10):2273–86. Available from: https://www.tandfonline.com/doi/full/10.1080/10428194.2017.1399312. https://doi.org/10.1080/10428194.2017.1399312.
52. Schranz K, Hubmann M, Harin E, Vosberg S, Herold T, Metzeler KH, et al. Clonal heterogeneity of FLT3-ITD detected by high-throughput amplicon sequencing correlates with adverse prognosis in acute myeloid leukemia. Oncotarget. 2018;9(53):30128–45. Available from: https://www.oncotarget.com/article/25729/text/. https://doi.org/10.18632/oncotarget.25729.
53. Annesly CE, Brown P. The biology and targeting of FLT3 in pediatric leukemia. Front Oncol. 2014;4:263. Available from: https://www.frontiersin.org/articles/10.3389/fonc.2014.00263/full. https://doi.org/10.3389/fonc.2014.00263.
54. Horiike S, Yokota S, Nakao M, Iwai T, Sasai Y, Kaneko H, et al. Tandem duplications of the FLT3 receptor gene are associated with leukemic transformation of myelodysplasia. Leukemia. 1997;11:1442–6. Available from: https://www.nature.com/articles/2400770. https://doi.org/10.1038/sj.leu.2400770.
55. Yokota S, Kiyoi H, Nakao M, Iwai T, Misawa S, Okuda T, et al. Internal tandem duplication of the FLT3 gene is preferentially seen in acute myeloid leukemia and myelodysplastic syndrome among various hematological malignancies. A study on a large series of patients and cell lines. Leukemia. 1997;11(10):1605–9. Available from: https://www.nature.com/articles/2400812. https://doi.org/10.1038/sj.leu.2400812.
56. Xu F, Taki T, Yang HW, Hanada R, Hongo T, Ohnishi H, et al. Tandem duplication of the FLT3 gene is found in acute lymphoblastic leukaemia as well as acute myeloid Leukaemia but not in myelodysplastic syndrome or juvenile chronic myelogenous leukaemia in children. Br J Hematol. 1999;105(1):155–62. Available from: https://onlinelibrary.wiley.com/doi/full/10.1111/j.1365-2141.1999.01284.x. https://doi.org/10.1111/j.1365-2141.1999.01284.x.
57. Thiede C, Steudel C, Mohr B, Schaich M, Schäkel U, Platzbecker U, et al. Analysis of FLT3-activating mutations in 979 patients with acute myelogenous leukemia: association with FAB subtypes and identification of subgroups with poor prognosis. Blood. 2002;99(12):4326–35. Available from: https://ashpublications.org/

blood/article/99/12/4326/105972/Analysis-of-FLT3-activating-mutations-in-979. https://doi.org/10.1182/blood.V99.12.4326.
58. Nakao M, Yokota S, Iwai T, Kaneko H, Horiike S, Kashima K, et al. Internal tandem duplication of the Flt3 gene found in acute myeloid leukemia. Leukemia. 1996;10(12):1911–8. Available from: https://pubmed.ncbi.nlm.nih.gov/8946930/
59. Schnittger S, Schoch C, Dugas M, Kern W, Staib P, Wuchter C, et al. Analysis of FLT3 length mutations in 1003 patients with acute myeloid leukemia: correlation to Cytogenetics, FAB subtype, and prognosis in the AMLCG study and usefulness as a marker for the detection of minimal residual disease. Blood. 2002;100(1):59–66. Available from: https://ashpublications.org/blood/article/100/1/59/133972/Analysis-of-FLT3-length-mutations-in-1003-patients. https://doi.org/10.1182/blood.V100.1.59.
60. Hayakawa F, Towatari M, Kiyoi H, Tanimoto M, Kitamura T, Saito H, et al. Tandem-duplicated Flt3 constitutively activates STAT5 and MAP kinase and introduces autonomous cell growth in IL-3-dependent cell lines. Oncogene. 2000;19:624–31. Available from: https://www.nature.com/articles/1203354. https://doi.org/10.1038/sj.onc.1203354.
61. Kiyoi H, Towatari M, Yokota S, Hamaguchi M, Ohno R, Saito H, et al. Internal tandem duplication of the FLT3 gene is a novel modality of elongation mutation which causes constitutive activation of the product. Leukemia. 1998;12:1333–7. Available from: https://www.nature.com/articles/2401130. https://doi.org/10.1038/sj.leu.2401130.
62. Fenski R, Flesch K, Serve S, Mizuki M, Oelmann E, Kratz-Albers K, et al. Constitutive activation of FLT3 in acute myeloid leukaemia and its consequences for growth of 32D cells. Br. J. Hematol. 2000;108(2):322–30. Available from: https://onlinelibrary.wiley.com/doi/full/10.1046/j.1365-2141.2000.01831.x. https://doi.org/10.1046/j.1365-2141.2000.01831.x.
63. Abu-Duhier FM, Goodeve AC, Wilson GA, Care RS, Peake IR, Reilly JT. Identification of novel FLT-3 Asp835 mutations in adult acute myeloid Leukaemia. Br J Haematol. 2001;113(4):983–8. Available from: https://onlinelibrary.wiley.com/doi/full/10.1046/j.1365-2141.2001.02850.x. https://doi.org/10.1046/j.1365-2141.2001.02850.x.
64. Yamamoto Y, Kiyoi H, Nakano Y, Suzuki R, Kodera Y, Miyawaki S, et al. Activating mutation of D835 within the activation loop of FLT3 in human hematologic malignancies. Blood. 2001;97(8):2434–9. Available from: https://ashpublications.org/blood/article/97/8/2434/53253/Activating-mutation-of-D835-within-the-activation. https://doi.org/10.1182/blood.V97.8.2434.
65. Maxson JE, Tyner JW. Genomics of chronic neutrophilic leukemia. Blood. 2017;129(6):715–22. Available from: https://www.ncbi.nlm.nih.gov/pmc/articles/PMC5301820. https://doi.org/10.1182/blood-2016-10-695981.
66. Szuber N, Tefferi A. Chronic neutrophilic leukemia: new science and new diagnostic criteria. Blood Cancer J. 2018;8(2):19. Available from: https://www.nature.com/articles/s41408-018-0049-8. https://doi.org/10.1038/s41408-018-0049-8.
67. Buels R, Yao E, Diesh CM, Hayes RD, Munoz-Torres M, Helt G, et al. JBrowse: a dynamic web platform for genome visualization and analysis. Genome Biol. 2016;17:66. Available from: https://genomebiology.biomedcentral.com/articles/10.1186/s13059-016-0924-1. https://doi.org/10.1186/s13059-016-0924-1.

3 Bioinformatics Analysis in Molecular Pathology

Geoffrey H. Smith

List of Frequently Asked Questions

1. What is bioinformatics and how is it distinguished from similar terms like informatics, biomedical informatics, and clinical informatics?
2. I am a physician, not an information technology expert. Why is bioinformatics important for me?
3. What does a typical bioinformatics pipeline for processing DNA sequenced using an NGS method look like?
4. What does a base call look like?
5. What does a FASTQ file look like?
6. Why do the names of all of my FASTQ files end with ".gz?"
7. Why do I have so many FASTQ files for each specimen?
8. What does a BAM file look like?
9. You showed me what a BAM file looks like in IGV. But how do I view BAM files from the command line?
10. How are molecular bar codes represented in FASTQ and BAM files?
11. What does a VCF file look like?
12. Do the bioinformatics pipelines we use to process short reads generated from NGS cancer panels involve any other standard bioinformatics file formats I should know about?
13. How are small variants described by the annotator?
14. Which gene transcript should I clinically report for a gene?
15. Is the version number in a RefSeq accession number important?
16. What does the annotator do besides generate the HGVS nomenclature for small variants?
17. How should I report clinical significance for a variant?
18. What does a clinical report look like?
19. My clinical laboratory is inspected by the College of American Pathologists (CAP). What should I know?
20. You have not talked much about actually running a bioinformatics pipeline.

G. H. Smith (✉)
Department of Pathology and Laboratory Medicine, Emory University School of Medicine, Atlanta, GA, USA
e-mail: geoffrey.smith@emory.edu

Frequently Asked Questions

1. **What is bioinformatics and how is it distinguished from similar terms like informatics, biomedical informatics, and clinical informatics?**
   - *Informatics* is the art and science of turning data into useful information [1]. The term *information science* might also be reasonably used to refer to this discipline. The word is borrowed from the French term for computer science: *informatique*. There is a distinction between *informatics*, which is a discipline, and *information technology*, which is a tool.
   - *Biomedical informatics* is the basic science concerned with informatics in the biomedical domain, or "the interdisciplinary field that studies and pursues the effective uses of biomedical data, information, and knowledge for scientific inquiry, problem solving, and decision making, driven by efforts to improve human health [Fig. 3.1]" [2].
   - *Clinical informatics* (CI) is the subdomain of biomedical informatics concerned with transforming health care using information and communication systems like electronic health records [3]. This discipline is distinguished by the fact that it was recognized as a boarded medical discipline in 2014. Certification is available to physicians boarded in another discipline who have completed an ACGME-accredited CI fellowship and passed a written examination [4]. Physicians with CI certification are well positioned to assume the role of chief medical information officer (CMIO) in a health care organization. CI certification does not demonstrate bioinformatics competence, but there are certainly synergies between the disciplines.
   - *Bioinformatics* is the subdomain of biomedical informatics concerned with molecular and cellular processes. This chapter is concerned with the applications bioinformatics in the analysis of molecular data collected in the clinical laboratory. For all practical purposes, this chapter is about the tools we use to detect

Y. Ding, L. Zhang (eds.), *Practical Oncologic Molecular Pathology*, Practical Anatomic Pathology,
https://doi.org/10.1007/978-3-030-73227-1_3

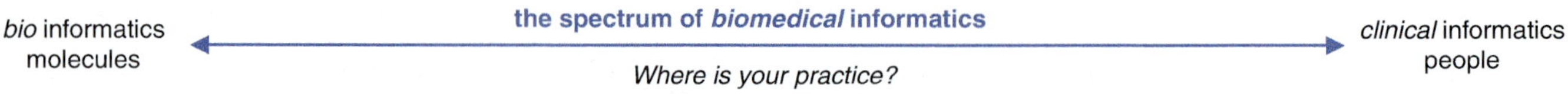

Fig. 3.1 Bioinformatics is a subdomain of biomedical informatics. Although this chapter is concerned with bioinformatics, as clinical laboratorians, we all practice somewhere on this continuum in the clinical molecular laboratory

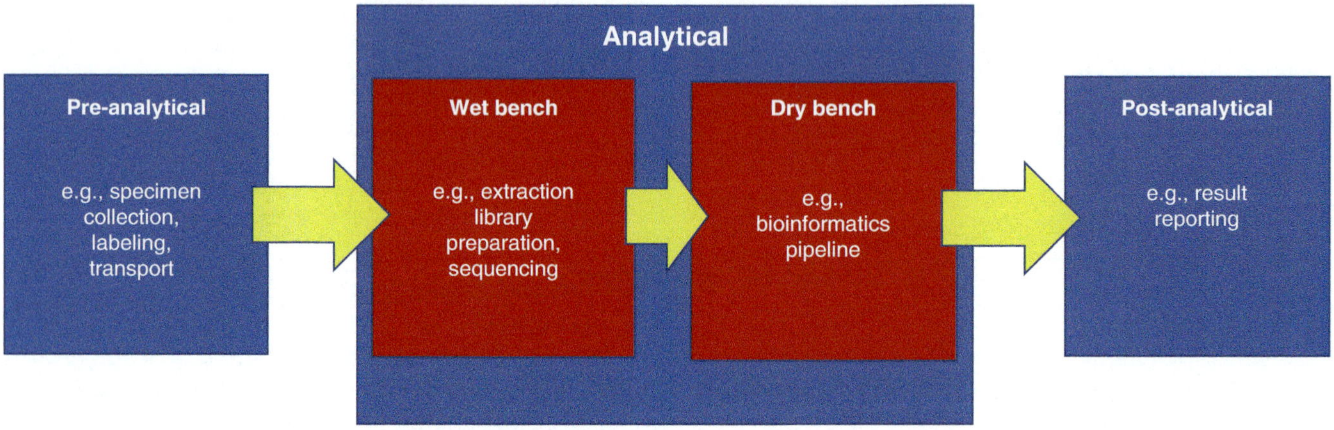

Fig. 3.2 The three phases of laboratory testing: pre-analytical, analytical, and post-analytical. The bioinformatics component of the analytical phase of laboratory testing is frequently called the "dry bench"

genetic variants associated with cancer (i.e., somatic variants) in molecular data generated by high-throughput massively parallel sequencing methods, or so-called next-generation sequencing (NGS).

2. **I am a physician, not an information technology expert. Why is bioinformatics important for me?**
   - Clinical laboratory workflow is traditionally divided into pre-analytic, analytic, and post-analytic phases [5]. In the clinical molecular laboratory, bioinformatics is a component of the analytical phase of laboratory testing [Fig. 3.2].
   - The discipline of bioinformatics is separate and distinct from the information technology tools we currently use to practice the discipline. We exist in the age of the digital electronic computer and bioinformatics analysis in the molecular laboratory depends on software programs that run on these devices. An information scientist of the early twentieth century working with paper records could not conceive of a digital electronic computer. Hopefully, an information scientist of the early twenty-second century will look back on our age and remark on the primitiveness of our tools.
   - The bioinformatics component of the analytical phase of laboratory testing is frequently referred to as the "dry bench" to distinguish it from the "wet" operations performed at a traditional laboratory bench [6].
   - As a clinical pathologist with bioinformatics domain expertise, your role is to medically direct your laboratory's dry bench operations. In this capacity, you are legally, ethically, and morally responsible for the integrity of the bioinformatics pipelines that your lab uses to process molecular data.

3. **What does a typical bioinformatics pipeline for processing DNA sequenced using an NGS method look like?**
   - A pipeline consists of a series of bioinformatics operations [Fig. 3.3].
   - **Step 1: nucleotide sequence generation.** Base calls from the sequencer are converted into nucleotide sequences and stored using the text-based FASTQ (fast-all with quality) file format. Most NGS methods interrogate a limited number of bases located at the ends of short DNA fragments (100-200 bp), so these nucleotide sequences are sometimes called "short reads."
   - **Step 2: alignment.** Short reads are mapped – or "aligned" – to a reference genome and stored using the binary BAM (binary sequence alignment/map) file format. My laboratory uses the Genome Reference Consortium Human Build 37 (hg19/GRCh37), which was released in 2009 and consists of approximately three billion bases agreed to by consensus. The alignment of a short read to the reference genome is frequently imperfect because of expected variation between the consensus-derived reference genome and the individual you sequenced [7].
   - **Step 3: variant calling.** Differences between aligned short reads and the reference genome are identified and stored using the text-based VCF (variant call format) file format. Each line in the VCF file represents an instance of nucleotide variation between the subject of your sequencing and the reference genome.
   - **Step 4: annotation.** Variants are functionally annotated to facilitate interpretation by a subject matter expert and stored using various spreadsheet file formats like CSV (comma separated values). With cancer pan-

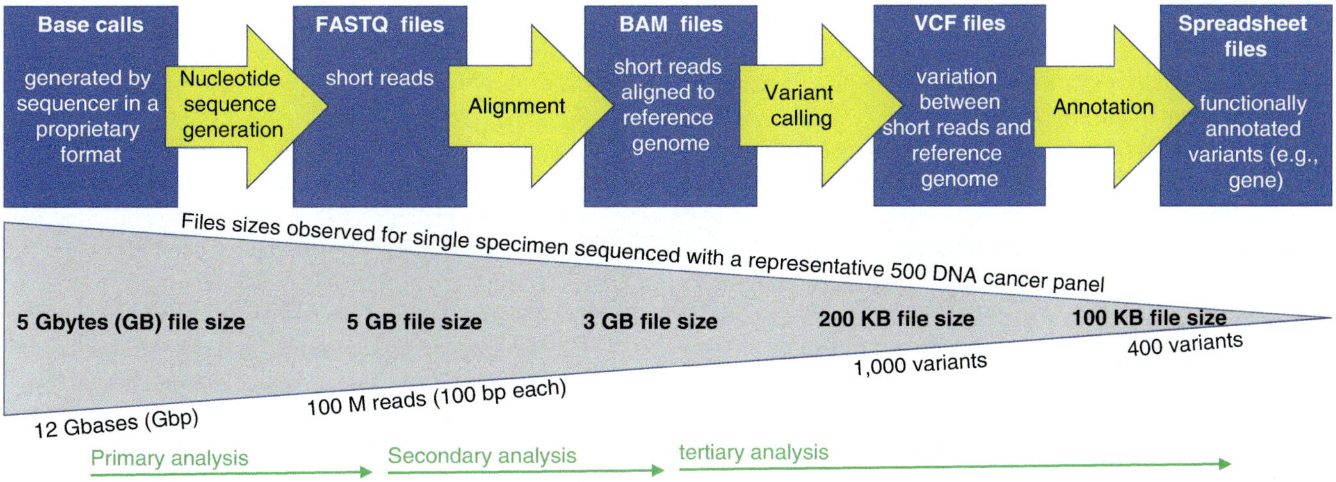

Fig. 3.3 A typical bioinformatics pipeline for processing DNA sequenced using an NGS method. The file sizes generally decrease as you advance through the pipeline. The file sizes shown here are for a specimen sequenced using a clinically validated 500 gene DNA cancer panel in my laboratory. The terms primary, secondary, and tertiary analysis are sometimes used to refer to pipeline operations [8]

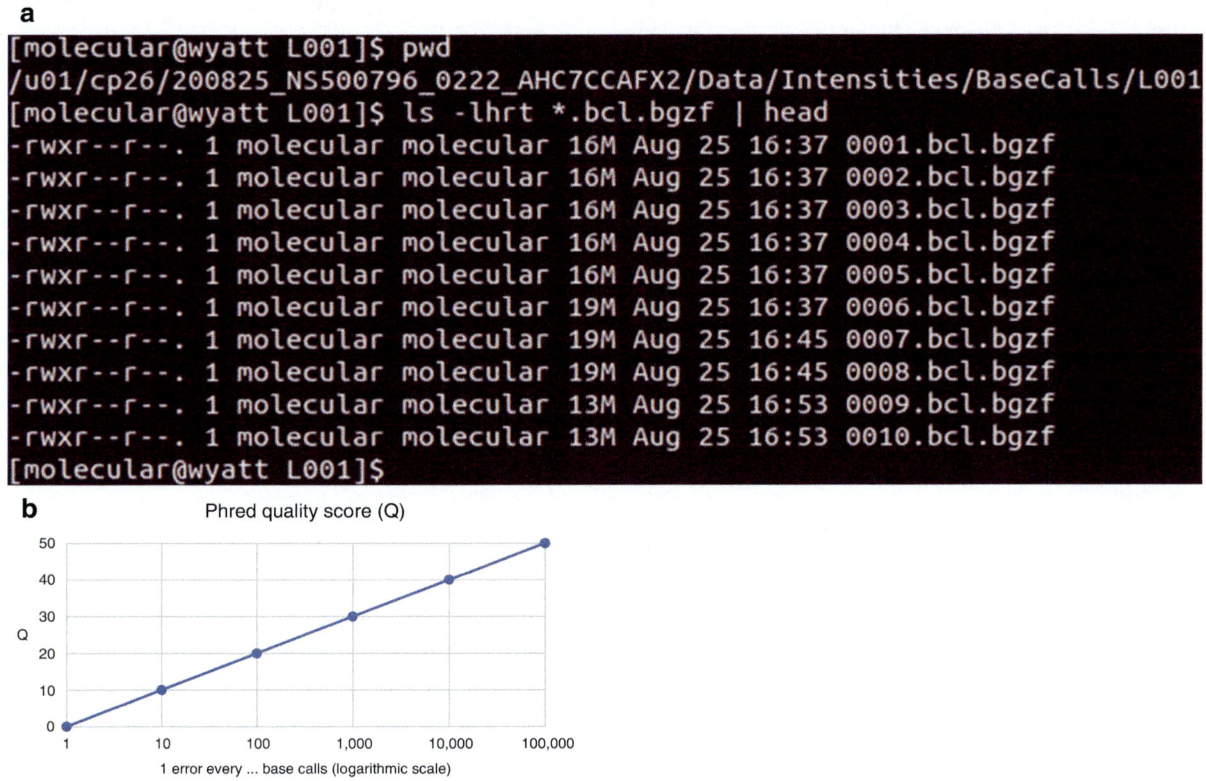

Fig. 3.4 (**a**) The files representing the base calls for the first 10 cycles of an NGS run on an Illumina NextSeq sequencer as they appear from the Linux command line. These files are generated in a proprietary format and processed to FASTQ files using software provided by the hardware vendor. You can infer cycle time from the file timestamps. (**b**) Each base call includes quality information that is used generate a Phred quality score. Q30 (1 error every 1000 base calls) is frequently used as a threshold for an acceptable base call in clinical cancer panels [10]

els, functional annotation of a variant usually consists of at least the identity of the gene, the coding position within the gene, the protein change, and a consequence (e.g., synonymous, missense). Robust annotation systems provide significantly more information than that.

4. **What does a base call look like?**
   - High-throughput massively parallel sequencing instruments infer bases from electronically measurable signals, such as light color, and store this information as base calls [9].
   - Base calls are stored in a proprietary format and are intended to be processed to FASTQ files using nucleotide sequence generation software provided by the hardware vendor (e.g., Illumina bcl2fastq, Illumina bcl-convert) [Fig. 3.4a].

- The sequencer encodes quality information with each base call. The quality information is used to generate a Phred quality score during FASTQ file generation according to the expression $Q = -10\log_{10}P$ where Q is the Phred quality score and P is the probability of an incorrect base call [Fig. 3.4b].

5. **What does a FASTQ file look like?**
   - FASTQ files store nucleotide sequences and their associated quality data. The FASTQ nomenclature derives from the terms FASTA and quality, where FASTA is the name of a sequence alignment software package that defined this now ubiquitous format for storing sequence data and metadata.
   - The FASTA format is the FASTQ format without quality data. Or, conversely, the FASTQ format is the FASTA format with quality data.
   - A FASTQ file is simply a text file that typically contains millions of four-line records [Fig. 3.5] [11].
   - **Line 1:** The read header. This starts with an at sign ("@") and uniquely identifies the physical location of the read on the flow cell, the read direction, etc. In paired-end sequencing, the read headers for read pairs differ only in the read direction (read 1/read 2 or R1/R2). The length of this line cannot exceed your sequencer's read length.
   - **Line 2:** The nucleotide sequence read 5' to 3'.
   - **Line 3:** A plus sign ("+"). This separates the nucleotide sequence in line 2 from the encoded Phred quality scores line 4.
   - **Line 4:** The encoded Phred quality scores. Each nucleotide in line 2 is associated with a quality score at the same position in line 4, so line 2 and line 4 are always the same length.
6. **Why do the names of all of my FASTQ files end with ".gz?"**
   - Since the FASTQ file format is a text-based file format, it tends to create bulky files.
   - Text files are generally highly compressible.
   - GNU Gzip is a popular lossless file compression program and a standard component of Linux distributions.

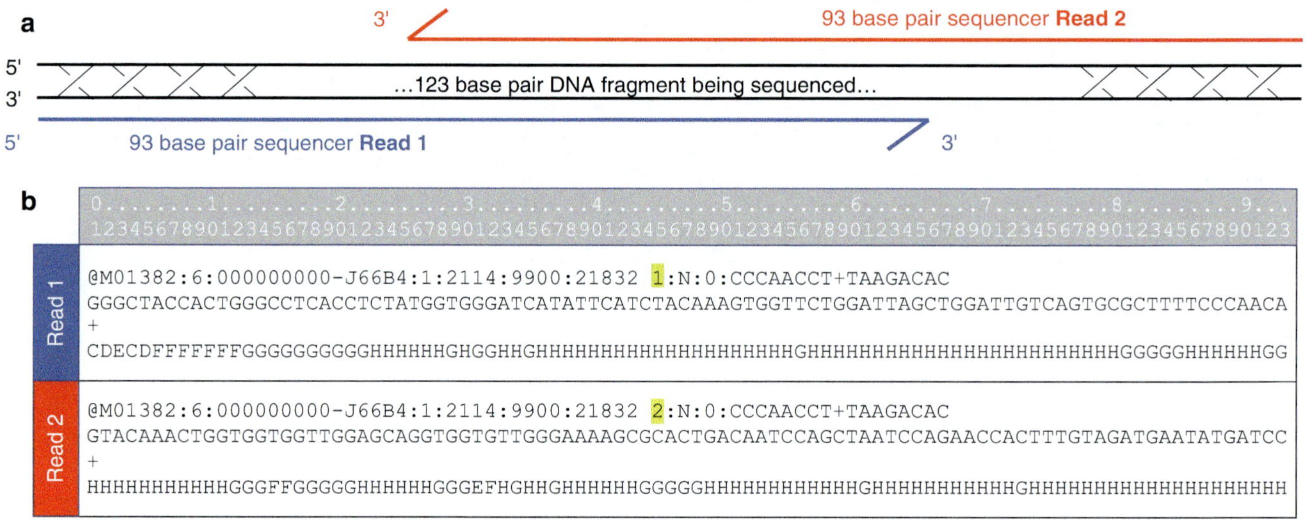

Fig. 3.5 (**a**) A schematic representation of a paired-end sequencing. In this example, a 123-base-pair DNA fragment is sequenced from both ends using a sequencer read length of 93 base pairs. The 30 bases at each end of the fragment are only present in one read (123 − 93 = 30). The 63 bases in the middle of the fragment are present in both reads (123 − 60 = 63). This figure shows just one of three possible read 1/read 2 relationships, where there is *partial* overlap of the mate pairs; the other two possibilities are *no* overlap, where there are un-sequenced bases between the reads, and *complete* overlap, where all bases are present in both reads. (**b**) A 93-nucleotide read pair in FASTQ format from an Illumina MiSeq run. A single FASTQ file might contain millions of records that look like this. The first line of every FASTQ record starts with an at sign (@) and is followed by a read identifier that typically includes things like the sequencer serial number and read direction (highlighted in yellow). The second line represents the nucleotide sequence. With NGS methods, the nucleotide sequence is usually short and each record in a FASTQ file might be called a "short read." The third line is always a plus sign (+) and represents a delimiter between the nucleotide sequence and the associated quality scores. The fourth line represents the encoded Phred quality scores for the corresponding nucleotide in the second line. The nucleotides are read 5' to 3'

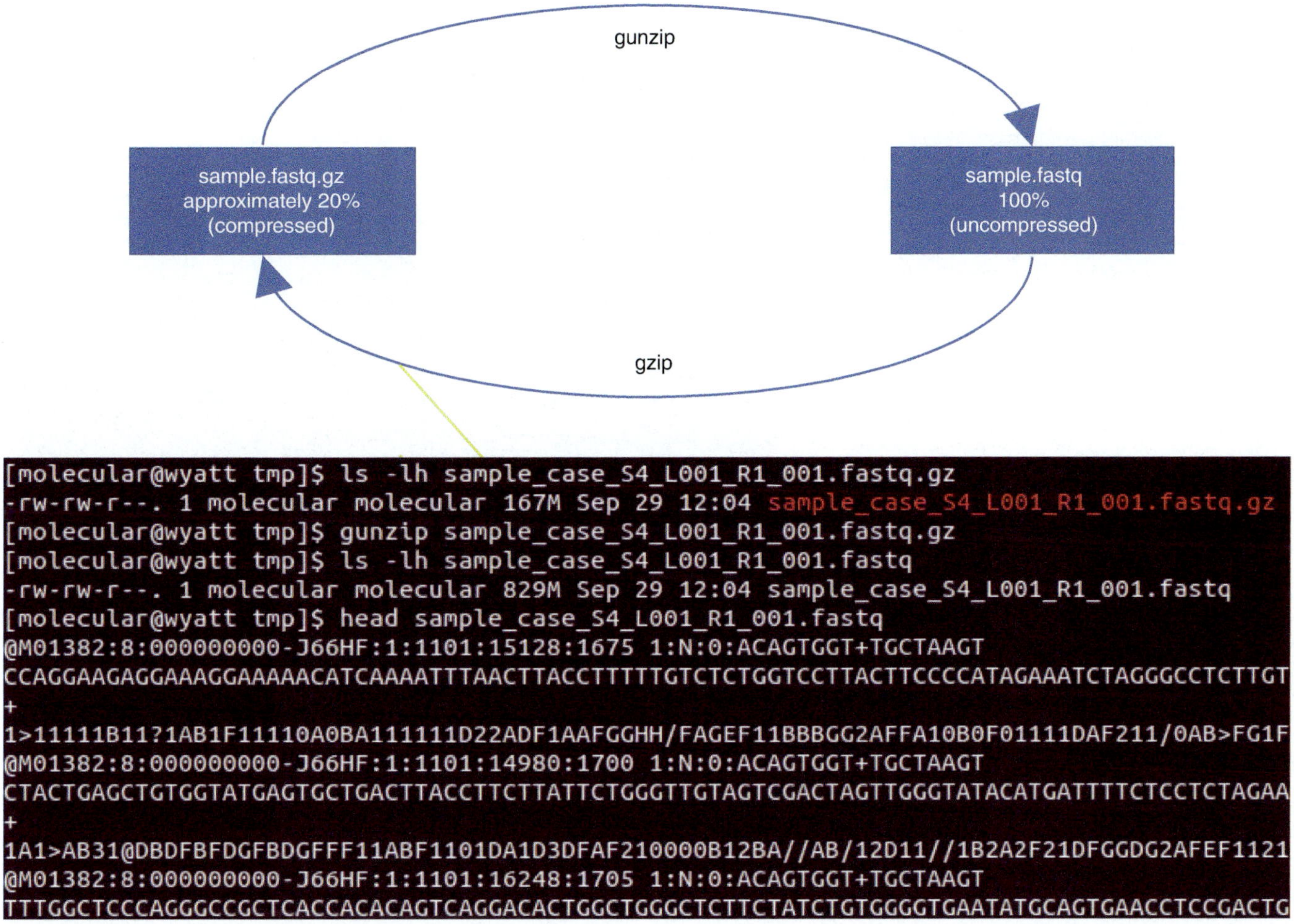
gunzip
sample.fastq.gz
approximately 20%
(compressed)
sample.fastq
100%
(uncompressed)
gzip
[molecular@wyatt tmp]$ ls -lh sample_case_S4_L001_R1_001.fastq.gz
-rw-rw-r--. 1 molecular molecular 167M Sep 29 12:04 sample_case_S4_L001_R1_001.fastq.gz
[molecular@wyatt tmp]$ gunzip sample_case_S4_L001_R1_001.fastq.gz
[molecular@wyatt tmp]$ ls -lh sample_case_S4_L001_R1_001.fastq
-rw-rw-r--. 1 molecular molecular 829M Sep 29 12:04 sample_case_S4_L001_R1_001.fastq
[molecular@wyatt tmp]$ head sample_case_S4_L001_R1_001.fastq
@M01382:8:000000000-J66HF:1:1101:15128:1675 1:N:0:ACAGTGGT+TGCTAAGT
CCAGGAAGAGGAAAGGAAAAACATCAAAATTTAACTTACCTTTTTGTCTCTGGTCCTTACTTCCCCATAGAAATCTAGGGCCTCTTGT
+
1>11111B11?1AB1F11110A0BA111111D22ADF1AAFGGHH/FAGEF11BBBGG2AFFA10B0F01111DAF211/0AB>FG1F
@M01382:8:000000000-J66HF:1:1101:14980:1700 1:N:0:ACAGTGGT+TGCTAAGT
CTACTGAGCTGTGGTATGAGTGCTGACTTACCTTCTTATTCTGGGTTGTAGTCGACTAGTTGGGTATACATGATTTTCTCCTCTAGAA
+
1A1>AB31@DBDFBFDGFBDGFFF11ABF1101DA1D3DFAF210000B12BA//AB/12D11//1B2A2F21DFGGDG2AFEF1121
@M01382:8:000000000-J66HF:1:1101:16248:1705 1:N:0:ACAGTGGT+TGCTAAGT
TTTGGCTCCCAGGGCCGCTCACCACACAGTCAGGACACTGGCTGGGCTCTTCTATCTGTGGGGTGAATATGCAGTGAACCTCCGACTG

Fig. 3.6 GNU Gzip decompression of a representative compressed FASTQ file (fastq.gz). The compressed file is 167 MB. The uncompressed file is 829 MB. The compression ratio is 5:1. Or, in other words, the compressed version of the file only uses 20% as much disk drive as the uncompressed version of the file. This compression ratio is typical for FASTQ files and significantly reduces the storage burden at the expense of increased bioinformatics pipeline run time

- Compression and decompression are computationally intensive operations and contribute to the execution time for bioinformatics pipelines, but this contribution is relatively small.
- Most bioinformatics pipelines automatically decompress and compress FASTQ files to minimize disk utilization, so if you want to inspect the contents of a FASTQ file from the command line you will probably have to manually decompress it using the GNU Gzip utility [Fig. 3.6].

7. **Why do I have so many FASTQ files for each specimen?**
   - The bioinformatics pipelines in my laboratory generally create eight FASTQ files per specimen [Fig. 3.7].
   - The number of FASTQ files you generate in your laboratory per specimen depends on which vendor and platform you are using and how you have configured the nucleotide sequence generation phase of your bioinformatics pipeline.
   - Rigorous FASTQ file naming conventions are critical in the clinical laboratory since they represent specimen identity and the name of the FASTQ file is usually used for downstream processes in the bioinformatics pipeline like naming a VCF created by a variant caller. In my laboratory, we use two patient identifiers in our specimen names.

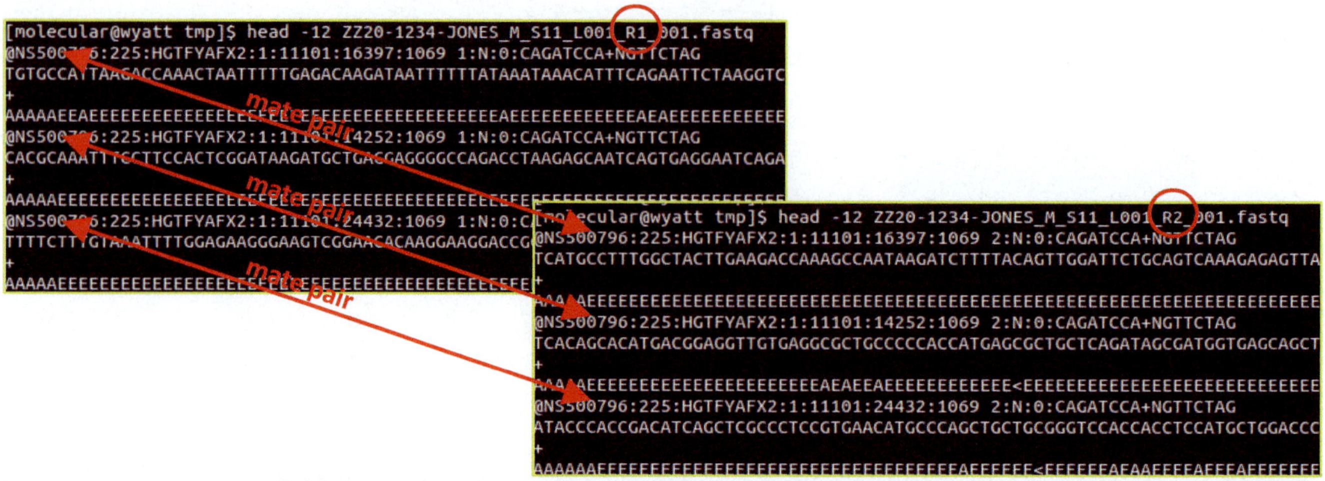

	Read 1	Read 2
Lane 1	ZZ20-1234-JONES_S11_L001_R1_001.fastq.gz	ZZ20-1234-JONES_S11_L001_R2_001.fastq.gz
Lane 2	ZZ20-1234-JONES_S11_L002_R1_001.fastq.gz	ZZ20-1234-JONES_S11_L002_R2_001.fastq.gz
Lane 3	ZZ20-1234-JONES_S11_L003_R1_001.fastq.gz	ZZ20-1234-JONES_S11_L003_R2_001.fastq.gz
Lane 4	ZZ20-1234-JONES_S11_L004_R1_001.fastq.gz	ZZ20-1234-JONES_S11_L004_R2_001.fastq.gz

Fig. 3.7 The FASTQ naming conventions used in my laboratory for a sample with laboratory accession number *ZZ20-1234* and patient last name "Jones" that was in the eleventh (S11) position in the sample sheet. We use instruments that have four lanes (L001–L004). Much of the naming convention for FASTQ files is imposed by your sequencer vendor, but you typically have flexibility with the sample name. In my laboratory, the mate pairs are in the same sequence in the read 1 (R1) and read 2 (R2) files, so the first read in the read 1 file is mated with the first read in the read 2 file, the second read in the read 1 file is mated with the second read in the read 2 file, and so on. It is also possible to determine the mate pairs using the read headers, but it might be more convenient to do it positionally

8. **What does a BAM file look like?**
   - The "B" in "BAM" stands for binary: binary sequence alignment/map (BAM). The corresponding text format is sequence alignment/map (SAM) [12].
   - The distinction between a BAM and a SAM file is similar to the distinction between a compressed and uncompressed FASTQ file. The BAM is smaller and you use a software utility to convert between the two formats. SAMtools is a popular conversion utility and a standard component of Linux distributions [13]. SAM:BAM file size ratios are similar to those observed with uncompressed:compressed FASTQ files, around 5:1 in my experience, but BAM files can be consumed by bioinformatics pipelines in their native form without any file conversion.
   - You cannot render a binary file from the command line without using special software. By analogy, consider the problem of trying to view a JPG image without an image viewer. The archetype for rendering BAM files is the excellent Integrative Genomics Viewer (IGV), a product of the Broad Institute [Fig. 3.8] [14, 15].

9. **You showed me what a BAM file looks like in IGV. But how do I view BAM files from the command line?**
   - You can use the SAMTools view function to see the SAM (text) records in a BAM (binary) file [Fig. 3.9a] [13].
   - The SAM record format is arcane, but you should generally be able to trace a short read from a FASTQ file to an alignment in a BAM file using the read header [12].
   - Unlike in the FASTQ file, where sequence is read 5′ to 3′, sequence in a SAM record is aligned to the positive DNA strand. This means that reads from the FASTQ file that align to the negative strand are represented by their reverse complement in the SAM record [Fig. 3.9b].

10. **How are molecular bar codes represented in FASTQ and BAM files?**
    - Template molecules can be uniquely identified prior to amplification using short oligonucleotide sequences [16]. These sequences have various names, such as molecular bar codes and unique molecular identifiers (UMI). All the cancer pipelines in my laboratory use some form of UMI.

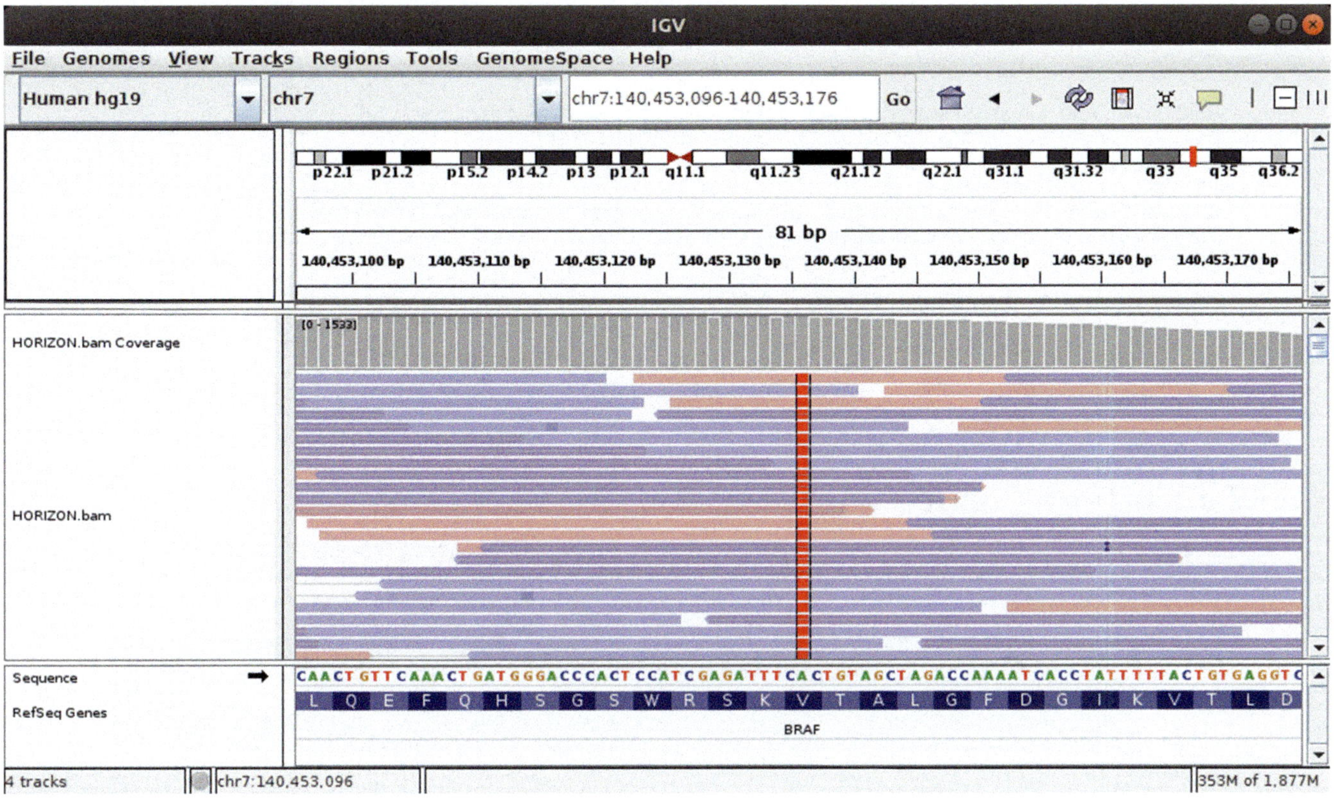

Fig. 3.8 Alignments in a BAM file rendered in the Broad Institute's IGV desktop application showing a *BRAF* V600E variant. There are many examples of bioinformatics track viewers. This is the track viewer we use in my laboratory. The hg19/GRCh37 reference sequence is shown at the bottom. The forward reads are light red and the reverse reads are light blue; purple corresponds to overlapping forward and reverse reads. The bright-red base in the middle represents an A (reference) to T (specimen) variant at nucleotide position chr7:140,453,136. Since *BRAF* has a negative orientation, this corresponds to a T to A variant in the mRNA. There is a read-depth histogram labeled "coverage" near the top that reflects how many reads include each nucleotide position

- The UMI sequences are used as the basis for error correction algorithms and to mitigate the impact of amplification bias in quantitative determinations like variant allele frequency (VAF).
- This effectively introduces an additional step to the bioinformatics pipeline, where multiple reads with the same UMI that align to the same locus are "collapsed" into a single consensus read.
- Pipelines that involve UMIs and read collapsing typically generate metrics to help you understand the how much read collapsing is occurring with a specimen (e.g., average uncollapsed:collapsed read ratio).
- The representation of UMI sequences and read collapsing in FASTSQ and BAM files depends on the platform you are using [Fig. 3.10].
- Read collapsing reduces the number of reads considered by downstream steps in the bioinformatics pipeline.

11. **What does a VCF file look like?**
    - The variant call file format (VCF) is a text-based format originally associated with the 1000 Genomes Project [17, 18].
    - The file consists of header information followed by variant data in a tab-separated-values (TSV) format. The file is self-documenting in the sense that the codes used in the variant section are described in the header section. The header lines all appear at the beginning of the VCF file and start with a pound sign ("#") [Fig. 3.11].
    - Unfortunately, if you have seen one VCF file then you have seen one VCF file, because there is considerable variability in how different variant callers use the QUAL, FILTER, INFO, and FORMAT columns.
12. **Do the bioinformatics pipelines we use to process short reads generated from NGS cancer panels involve any other standard bioinformatics file formats I should know about?**
    - The FASTQ-BAM-VCF bioinformatics file formats discussed so far are commonly encountered with NGS cancer panels that detect so-called "small variants": single-nucleotide variants (SNV) and short multi-nucleotide variants (MNV) from DNA. Your panel may be more complicated.

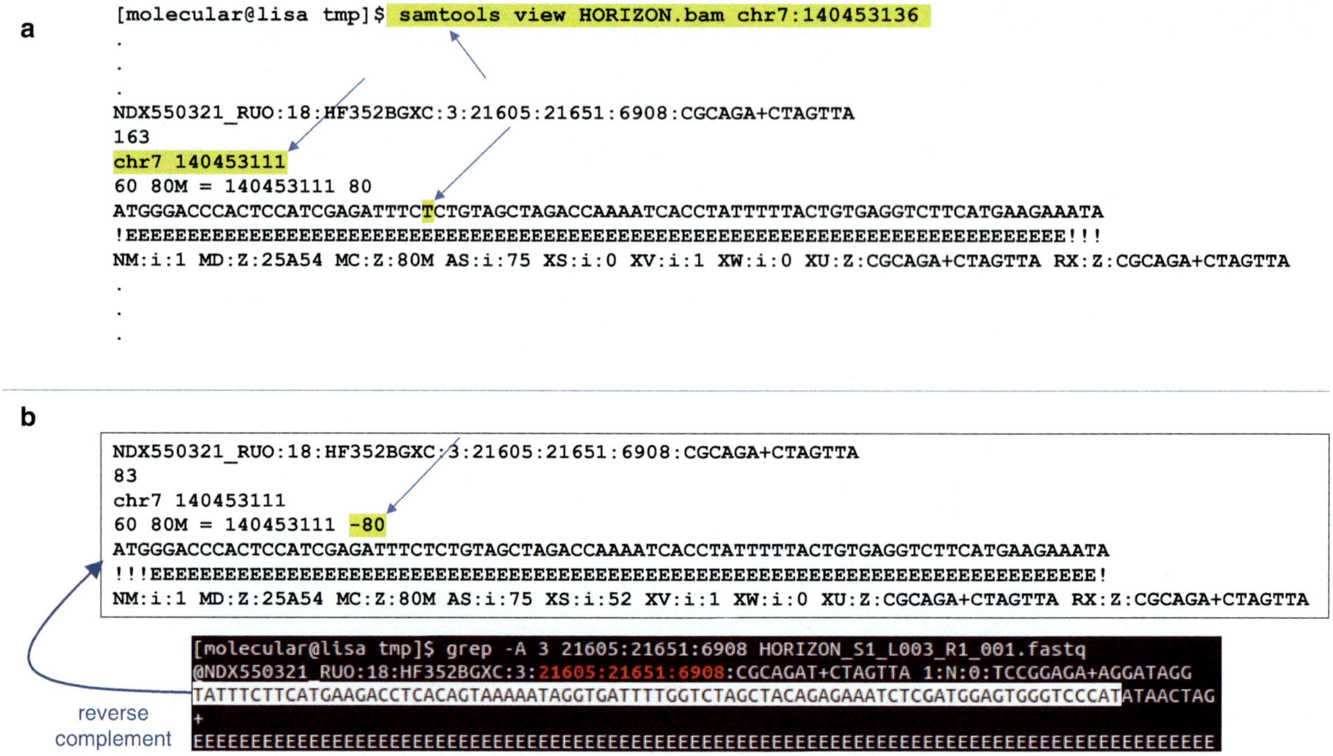

Fig. 3.9 (**a**) An example usage of the SAMTools view function to view all alignments in a BAM file that include chr7:140,453,136, which is the location of the *BRAF* V600E variant from the previous topic. For clarity, only a single alignment is shown, and it consists of an 80-base-pair short read that aligns to the reference sequence at chr7:140,453,111. The 26th nucleotide from the beginning of the short read represents chr7:140,453,136 (140,453,136–140,453,111 + 1 = 26) and is a T, which diverges from the reference sequence (although that divergence is not evident in this representation). (**b**) This figure demonstrates the relationship between a short read in a FASTQ file (*bottom*) and its corresponding SAM record (*top*) when the read is from the negative strand. The SAM record is oriented to the positive strand and is the reverse complement of the sequence in the FASTQ file. This happens to be the mate pair for the alignment shown in the prior figure. The negative TLEN attribute in the SAM record (−80) is the clue that this alignment corresponds to the read from the negative strand. Note that last 8 nucleotides from the short read in the FASTQ file (not highlighted: ATAACTAG) were "clipped" from the alignment by the aligner. Another interesting feature here is that the read from the negative strand was found in the read 1 (R1) FASTQ file, which nicely demonstrates that read 1 and read 2 are not synonyms for forward/positive and reverse/negative

- Modern NGS cancer panels use sophisticated bioinformatics approaches to detect classes of genetic variation in DNA and RNA well beyond SNVs and MNVs. The latest commercial NGS cancer panel we clinically validated in my laboratory detects SNV, MNV, tumor mutational burden (TMB) expressed in variants per megabase, microsatellite instability (MSI) expressed as a percentage of unstable sites, and copy number variation (CNV) expressed as a gene copy fold change from DNA. The same panel detects fusions and splice-site variants from RNA. To be clear, we did not clinically validate all of these classes of variation and do not clinically report them all, but there are bioinformatics outputs associated with all of them. Some are based on evolving existing standards (e.g., representing fusions in a VCF file) and some appear entirely novel (e.g., TMB metrics in a vendor-defined TSV file). Because of the heterogeneity in these file formats, we can't discuss them in any detail here.
- If there is another specific bioinformatics file format to know about, it is probably the ubiquitous browser extensible data (BED) file format. The BED format simply defines named intervals in a TSV format and is frequently encountered in NGS bioinformatics pipelines as either an input or an output [Fig. 3.12] [19].

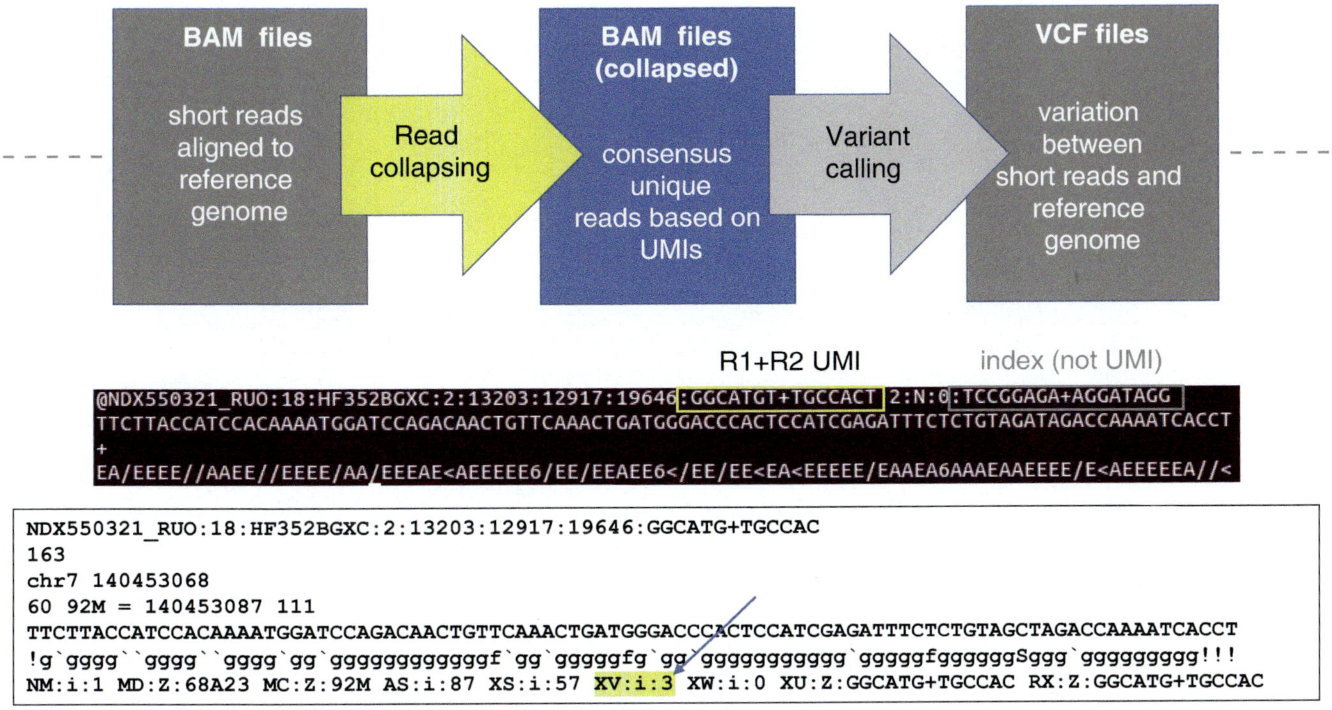

Fig. 3.10 The representation of UMIs and read collapsing in one of the pipelines run in my laboratory. A FASTQ record is shown at the top and a SAM record is shown at the bottom. Different pipelines do this in different ways, but read collapsing introduces an additional step to the pipeline. In this example, the seven-nucleotide UMI sequence from the read is inserted into the FASTQ read header during nucleotide sequence generation along with the seven-nucleotide UMI sequence from the read's mate pair (do not confuse the UMI with the index sequence further to the right; the index sequence identifies the specimen, and all reads in a FASTQ file generally have the same index sequence). During read collapsing, the number of reads used to generate the consensus read is inserted into the SAM record as the XV attribute. In this case, XV = 3, so three reads were collapsed to generate the consensus read. Most bioinformatics track viewers like IGV display read attributes like XV in a much more user-friendly fashion (e.g., double-click on a read)

13. **How are small variants described by the annotator?**
    - The annotator reports small variants using Human Genome Variation Society (HGVS) nomenclature [20].
    - There are different forms of HGVS nomenclature for describing genomic (nucleotide), transcript (mRNA), and protein (amino acid) variations with respect to a consensus normal reference sequence. With NGS cancer panels, variation is usually described as transcript variation with respect to a coding DNA reference sequence (HGVS C-dot nomenclature) or protein reference sequence (HGVS P-dot nomenclature) [Fig. 3.13].
    - HGVS syntax consists of an NCBI RefSeq accession number identifying the chromosome (NC_xxxx), the mRNA (NM_xxxx) or the protein (NP_xxxx), the coordinates of the variation, and the reference and alternate nucleotide or amino acid.

14. **Which gene transcript should I clinically report for a gene?**
    - The annotation systems in my laboratory generate HGVS C-dot and P-dot nomenclature using a single transcript for each gene. The transcript used for each gene is stipulated when an assay is clinically validated and then used for the life of the assay. The gene-transcript information is stored in a configuration file associated with the annotation system.
    - The best transcripts to clinically report for a gene are generally the transcripts that everybody else is reporting. In some cases this is the longest, or "canonical" transcript for a gene. In other cases this is the transcript that appears in the literature. Using the canonical transcript is appealing since it maximizes the number of coding bases considered, but the canonical transcript might omit clinically relevant exons.

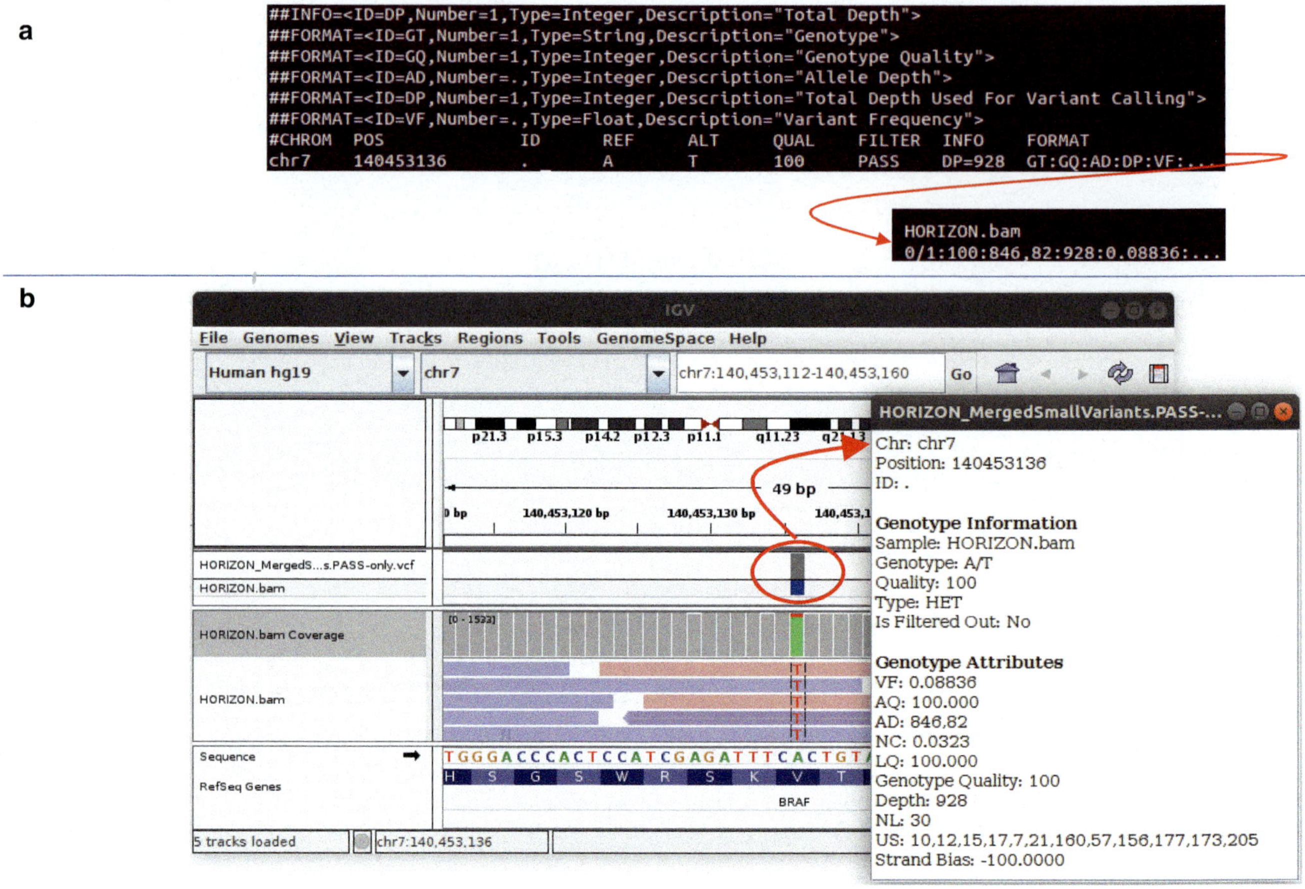

Fig. 3.11 (a) A BRAF V600E variant in a typical VCF file. VCF files usually contain more than a single variant, but only one is shown here. The file tells us that this call is supported by 928 reads, 846 reference reads, and 82 alternate reads for a variant allele frequency of 8.8%. The header and the FORMAT column have been truncated for clarity. (b) The VCF file from the previous figure rendered in IGV and showing the BRAF V600E variant details

- The Locus Reference Genomic (LRG) database (https://lrg-sequence.org) is an excellent source of stable and clinically relevant consensus transcripts for reporting variants [21, 22]. Most LRG records designate a single RefSeq transcript for each gene, although this is not always the case [Fig. 3.14].
- HGVS recommends using LRG sequences to report variants [23]. This is an excellent idea, although we still clinically report using RefSeq transcripts (NM_xxxx) in my laboratory. An example of HGVS nomenclature using an LRG reference is shown in the figure for the previous topic.
- Sophisticated annotation systems are capable of reporting multiple transcripts per gene.

15. **Is the version number in a RefSeq accession number important?**
    - RefSeq accession numbers in clinical reports should always include a version number. The version number is the integer that follows the decimal point. For example, in NC_000007.13, the version number is 13.
    - In some cases, the significance of the version number is obvious. For example, NC_000007.13 is chromosome seven in reference genome hg19/GRCh37, and NC_000007.14 is chromosome seven in reference genome hg38/GRCh38.
    - In some cases, the significance of the version number is more subtle. An excellent example of this is *BRAF*

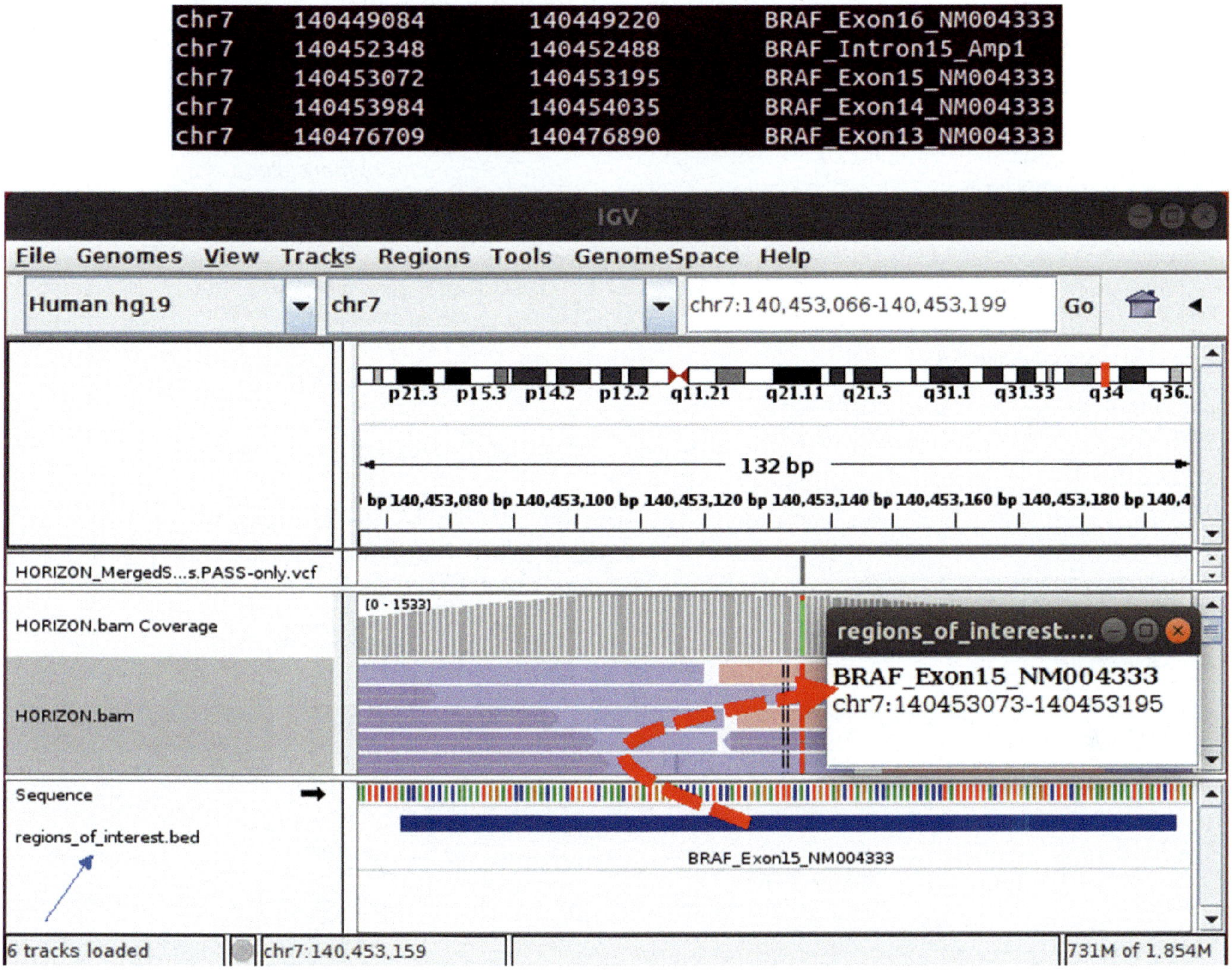

Fig. 3.12 (**a**) Some representative intervals from a BED file. Although this is a simple format, try to remember that the BED format uses a zero-based numbering scheme, where the first base in a chromosome is 0 – this is inconvenient for pathologists but convenient for software engineers! (**b**) The BED file above rendered as a track in IGV and displaying the *BRAF_Exon15_NM004333* interval as a thick blue line. Note that IGV converts the coordinates to a more user-friendly1-based numbering scheme (i.e., 140,453,072 in the BED is rendered as 140,453,073 in IGV)

V599E, which is illustrated in the figure accompanying this topic [Fig. 3.15].

- The fact that RefSeq accession numbers are versioned is another excellent reason to consider clinically reporting using Locus Reference Genomic (LRG) references instead of RefSeq accession numbers, but – as I said in the previous topic – we continue to clinically report using RefSeq accession numbers in my laboratory.

16. **What does the annotator do besides generate the HGVS nomenclature for small variants?**
    - At a minimum, most small variant annotations include the HGVS C-dot & P-dot nomenclatures, the variant allele frequency (VAF), the mutation type (e.g., synonymous, missense, frameshift), and a reference to the variant in one or more public variant databases (e.g., dbSNP, COSMIC).

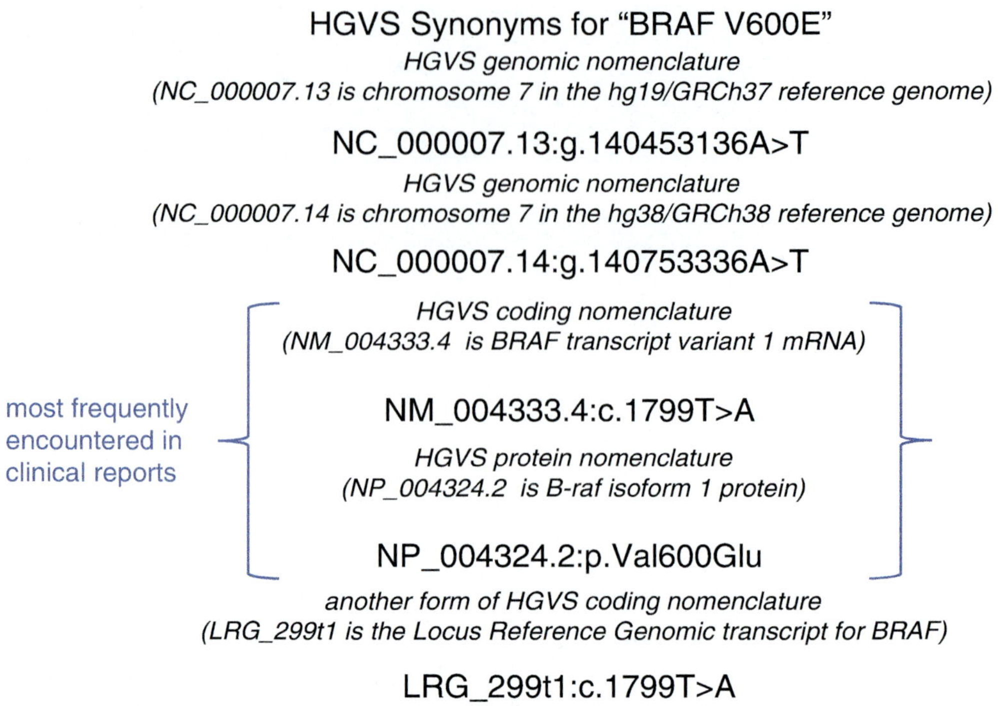

Fig. 3.13 These examples of HGVS nomenclature are all synonyms for the well-known *BRAF* V600E variant. The change from reference may be described in terms of the nucleotide on chromosome 7 (G-dot), the nucleotide in the coding sequence of the mRNA (C-dot), or the translated protein (P-dot). Since *BRAF* has a negative strand orientation, the G-dot and C-dot nomenclature are reverse complements (i.e., the positive strand nucleotide change is from reference A to variant T, but the negative strand change, which reflects the mRNA orientation, is from reference T to variant A). The Locus Reference Genomic nomenclature is discussed in the next topic

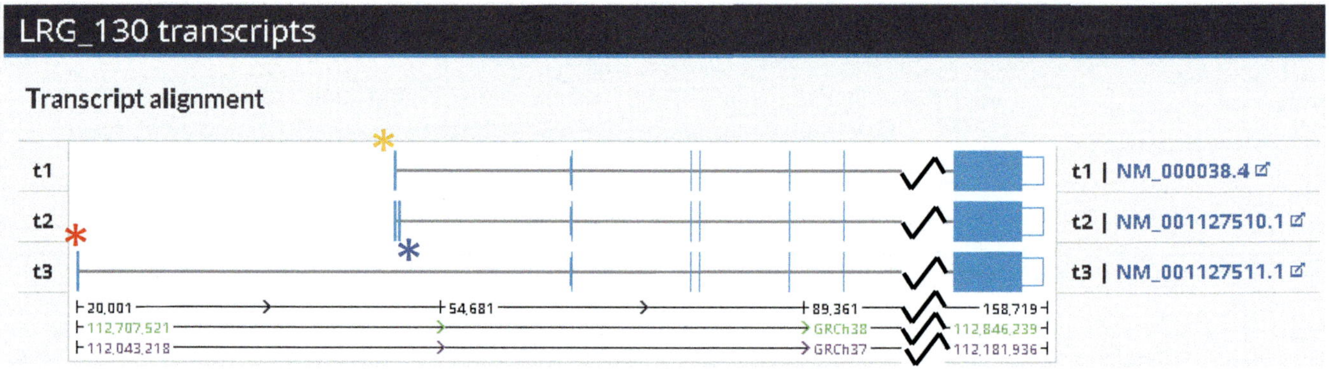

Fig. 3.14 Unfortunately, some genes have multiple transcripts, even in the LRG database. Reporting multiple transcripts might present challenges for your annotation system. This figure shows the three transcripts for LRG_130 (*APC*) in the elegant transcript alignment viewer on the LRG web site (https://lrg-sequence.org, accessed October 22, 2020). The vertical blue lines correspond to exons numbered from *left* (exon 1) to *right*. The first exon in *t3* (red star) does not correspond to any exon in *t1* or *t2*. The first exon in *t1* (yellow star) corresponds to the first exon in *t2* and no exon in *t3*. The second exon in *t2* (blue star) does not correspond to any exon in *t1* or *t3*

- Annotation systems used in clinical laboratories are generally sophisticated interactive software systems that go far beyond providing the minimal set of annotations described above. These systems are intended to make the clinical interpretation process both high quality and efficient.
- An example of an annotation for a small variant in one of the annotation systems used in my laboratory is illustrated in the figure accompanying this topic [Fig. 3.16].
- Our annotation system also maintains a database of narrative variant interpretations with references to the literature. The first time we encounter a variant we spend considerable time writing the interpretation for that variant, but when we encounter the same variant later the system automatically applies the interpretation we previously used. Portions of our interpretations may be organized by disease; so a different interpretation may be used for the same variant in different diseases.

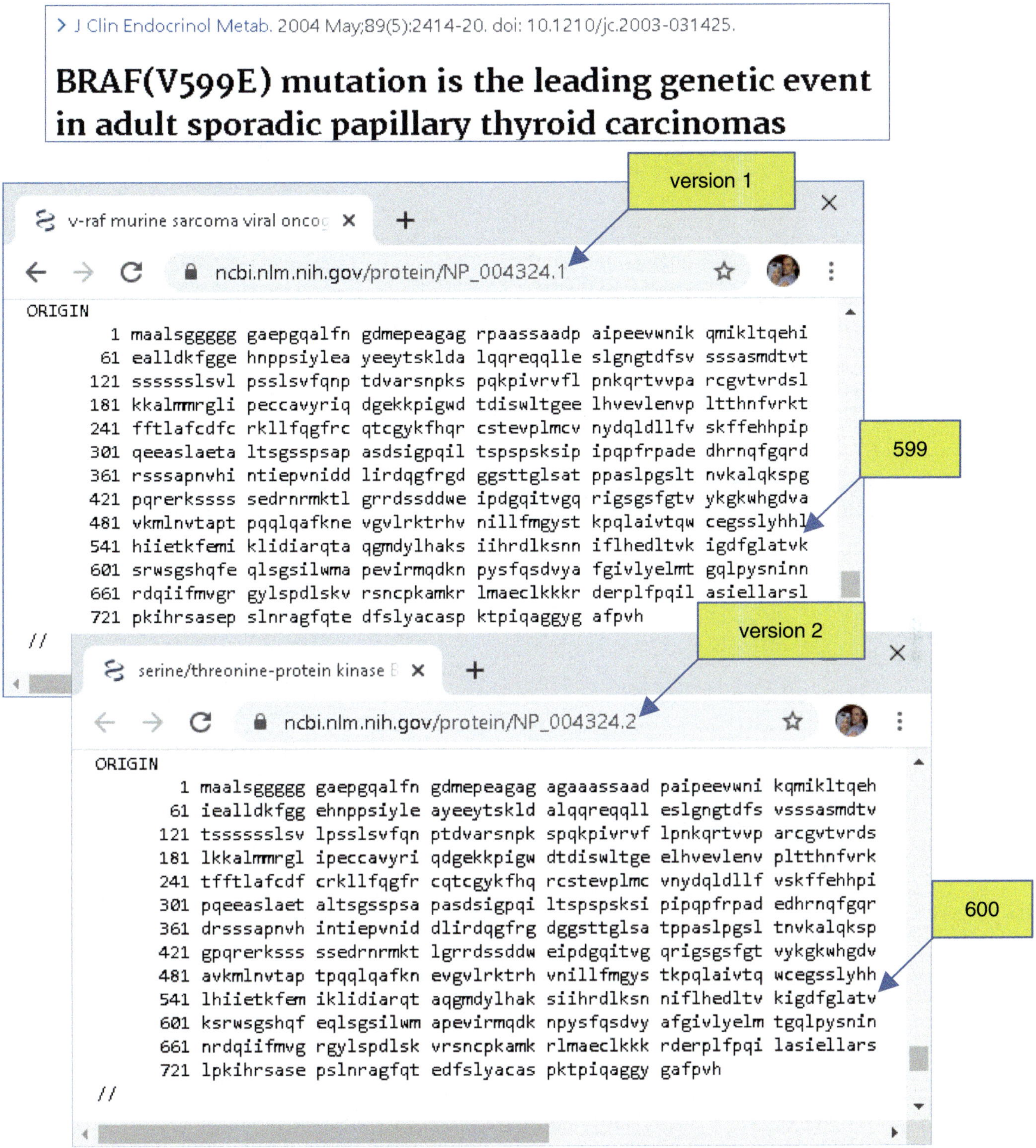

Fig. 3.15 Prior to July 24, 2003, BRAF V600E was BRAF V599E [24]. On that date, NP_004324.1 was replaced by NP_004324.2 in the NCBI protein database. It took a while for the literature to catch up. The version 2 protein included an additional amino acid that moved the valine involved in what we now know as the BRAF V600E mutation from position 599 to position 600. This illustrates the importance of using RefSeq version numbers in your clinical reporting to ensure that your clinical reports represent durable historical documents

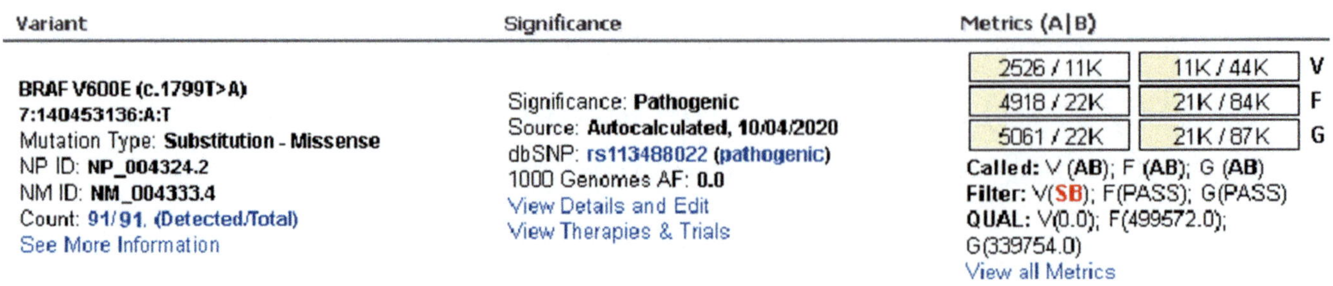

Fig. 3.16 A nicely annotated variant in one of the annotation systems used in my laboratory. The "Variant" section includes the HGVS nomenclatures, mutation type, and a count of how many times this variant has been clinically called (i.e., marked as detected by the pathologist) in prior cases where the same variant was reported by the variant caller. The "Significance" section includes the clinical significance of the variant, the source of the clinical significance, the identity of the variant in the dbSNP database, and the allele frequency (AF) of the variant in the 1000 Genomes database. The "Metrics" section graphically shows the number of alternate and reference reads reported by three different variant callers (i.e., VarScan, FreeBayes, and GATK) in two different DNA libraries A and B (i.e., samples for this assay are run in replicate) from which we can infer that the variant allele frequency (VAF) is around 25% and that all three variant callers and sample replicates are in agreement. This is an interactive annotation system; so hyperlinks can be clicked to expose many more annotations and deep-links to the variant's record in various databases

Laboratory significance	AMP/ASCO/CAP Tier	Clinically Reported?
Pathogenic	Tier I	Yes
Likely pathogenic		
Potential significance	Tier II	Yes
Uncertain significance	Tier III	Yes, but with minimal or no narrative interpretation
Likely benign	Tier IV	No
Benign		
Technical artifact	Not applicable	No

Fig. 3.17 The levels of clinical significance in the annotation system used in my laboratory and how those levels map to the four AMP/ASCO/CAP tiers. The "Likely Pathogenic" and "Likely Benign" classifications are used as markers for variants where there is uncertainty in the classification and that should be reviewed on a regular basis. The "Technical Artifact" classification is used for non-pathogenic variants that are repeatedly reported by the variant caller at a low allele frequency in genomic regions that are challenging to sequence (e.g., homopolymer regions, short repeat regions, regions near the ends of amplicons)

17. **How should I report clinical significance for a variant?**
    - The clinical significance of somatic variants should be reported using the joint Association for Molecular Pathology (AMP), American Society of Clinical Oncology (ASCO), and College of American Pathologists (CAP) standards [Fig. 3.17] [25]. These guidelines describe an evidence-based four-tiered system:
    - Tier I. Variants of Strong Clinical Significance
    - Tier II. Variants of Potential Clinical Significance
    - Tier III. Variants of Unknown Clinical Significance
    - Tier IV. Benign or Likely Benign Variants
    - Your annotation system may define more than four levels of significance for operational or technical reasons, but it should be possible to map from the levels of significance in your annotation system to the AMP/ASCO/CAP tiers described above. The figure accompanying this topic illustrates how we do this in my laboratory.
    - Good annotation systems will attempt to automatically attach significance to variants by looking them up in databases like ClinVar.

Interpretation

Tier 1. Variants of knowm clinical significance:
JAK2 c.1849G>T (p.V617F) detected in approximately 28% of alleles.

Tier 2. Variants of potential clinical significance:
None detected

Tier 3. Variants of uncertain clinical significance:
None detected

Copy Number Abnormalities
None detected

Comment

JAK2 c.1849G>T (p.V617F) [NM_004972.3]
About this gene: *JAK2* (Janus kinase 2) encodes a non-receptor protein tyrosine kinase that regulates STAT transcription factors in response to cytokine receptor signaling (PMID: 21442038).
Pathways: JAK-STAT signaling
Mutation location: Pseudokinase domain (exon 14); PMID: 15793561
Effect of mutation: The JAK2 V617F mutation results in an amino acid substitution at position 617 in exon 14, from a valine (V) to a phenylalanine (F). Crystallography studies hve shown that V617F is located within the JAK2 JH2 domain, which exerts an inhibitory effect on the JH1 kinase (PMID: 22820988). The JAK2 V617F mutation disables this inhibitory effect, leading to constitutive activation of JAK2 (PMID: 22820988, 24918545, 24013208. The mutant JAK2 acts on STAT5, a downstream transcription factor that targets multiple oncogenes leading to increased proliferation, cell cycling, and excessive myeloid diffeentiation (PMID: 18843287, 18216297). This particular JAK2 mutation (p.V617F) occurs in the pseudokinase (JH2) domain and leads to activation of the JAK-STAT pathway signaling. PMF patients with JAK2 mutation have a worse outcome compared to PMF patients with CALR mutations but a better outcome compared to the group of so-called 'triple negative' patients who lack JAK2, CALR and MPL mutations (PMID: 24986690).
Gene prevalence in disease: Somatic m utations of JAK2, almost always JAK2 p.V617F, are commonly found in patients with
Geme prevalence in disease: Somatic mutations of JAK2, almost always JAK2 p.V617F, are commonly found in patients with myeloproliferative neoplasms (MPN) including 95-99% of patients with polycythemia vera (PV), 50-70% of patients with essentail thrombocythemia (ET), and 40-50% of patients with primary myelogibrosis (PMF) (PMID: 15781101, 15739561, 15858187, 15837627, 17984312, 17267906).
About this mutation: Frequency of JAL2 p.V617F mutation in JAK2-mutated MPNs is 75% in JAK2-mutated PV (PMID: 15837627, 17597810, 24325359), ~100% in JAK2-mutated ET (PMID: 22160036)., and ~ 100% in JAK2-mutated PMF (PMID: 22160036).

The reference assembly is hg19, GRCh37.

Results

JAK2 c.1849G>T (p.V617F) [NM_004972.3]

Variant Frequency: 27.7%
Genomic Coordinates: chr9:5073770:G:T

Fig. 3.18 A representative clinical report from my laboratory. The "Interpretation" is an easy-to-read high-level summary, the "Comment" includes the lengthy narrative interpretation with extensive references, and the "Results" contains the required reporting elements for each variant. Not included in this report, but sometimes included in reports like this, are sections for drugs and clinical trials associated with the reported variants

18. **What does a clinical report look like?**
    - An example of a variant reported using one of the annotation and interpretation systems used in my laboratory is illustrated in the figure accompanying this topic [Fig. 3.18].
19. **My clinical laboratory is inspected by the College of American Pathologists (CAP) [Fig. 3.19]. What should I know?**

    - **MOL.35865 NGS Data Transfer Confidentiality:** *The laboratory ensures that internal and external storage and transfer of NGS data maintains patient confidentiality, security, and data integrity* [26].
    Most clinical laboratories take advantage of cloud services in their bioinformatics pipelines and access these services over public data networks, so this requirement is highly relevant. If your laboratory

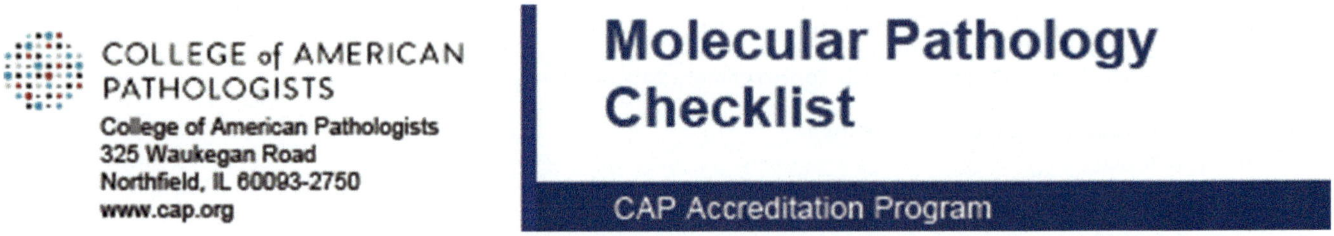

Fig. 3.19 If you are a CAP lab, become familiar with the bioinformatics content in the checklist

engaged your cloud service provider under the terms of HIPAA Business Associate Agreement (BAA), there is a pretty good chance that you are in compliance with this requirement since BAAs are typically vetted by your organization's legal and technical organizations.

- **MOL.35870 NGS Data Storage:** *There is a written policy for retention of NGS data necessary to support primary results generation and re-analysis* [26].
  In general, you must keep primary bioinformatics outputs like FASTQ files for 2 years. Remember that an old FASTQ file is only useful for if you also have the old bioinformatics pipeline that is needed to process it! So do not forget to keep track of your old bioinformatics pipelines, too.
- **MOL.36105 NGS Analytical Bioinformatics Procedure:** *There is a written procedure that describes the steps included in recording the bioinformatics process (also termed bioinformatics pipeline) used to analyze, interpret, and report NGS test results* [26].
  This requirement has an enormous note section that cannot be repeated here. The bioinformatics pipelines in my laboratory are largely composed of commercial software components that we integrate into our workflow. In general, the commercial vendors in the clinical NGS space are cognizant of these requirements and can help you demonstrate compliance.
- **MOL.36108 Analysis of Tumor Cell and Sequencing Lower Limit of Detection:** *For NGS assays involving analysis of tumor cells, the laboratory considers the tumor cell percentage in cells, tissues, or the area of the slide from which the DNA is extracted…* [26].
  When working from FFPE specimens, estimate the tumor percentage on the slide and maintain it as a structured data field somewhere in your laboratory information system.
- **MOL.36115 NGS Analytical Bioinformatics Process Validation:** *The laboratory validates the analytical bioinformatics process…* [26].
  The wide scope of this requirement will not surprise a clinical laboratorian. To date, all the NGS panels in my laboratory are research-use-only (RUO) commercial kits that we have validated as lab-developed tests (LDT). These validation exercises have become progressively more difficult as the size of the panels and the classes of variation they detect has expanded.
- **MOL.36125 NGS Bioinformatics Process/ Pipeline – Quality Management Program:** *The laboratory follows a written quality management (QM) program for the NGS bioinformatics process/ pipeline* [26].
  Beyond the obvious record keeping involved here, the commercial bioinformatics pipelines used in my laboratory generate quality outputs at the run and sample level. Our annotation system is aware of these quality outputs and will reject annotating a run and/or sample that does not meet quality criteria established during clinical validation. We also participate in a proficiency testing program.
- **MOL.36155 Sequence Variants – Interpretation and Reporting:** *Interpretation and reporting of sequence variants follow professional organization recommendations and guidelines* [26].
  As discussed in the previous two topics, make sure you are clinically reporting using AMP/ASCO/CAP guidelines and being fastidious with your HGVS nomenclatures [25].

20. **You have not talked much about actually running a bioinformatics pipeline.**
    - Unless your clinical laboratory has access to a large bioinformatics organization, you are probably going to run bioinformatics pipelines provided by the same commercial vendor that supplied your test kit. Your vendor might give you the option to install the software locally or use it in the cloud. If they give you software to install locally, it can come in many different forms, although these days vendors usually supply either a heavyweight virtual machine image (e.g., for deployment under a VMware hypervisor) or a lightweight container image (e.g., for deployment under Docker). I

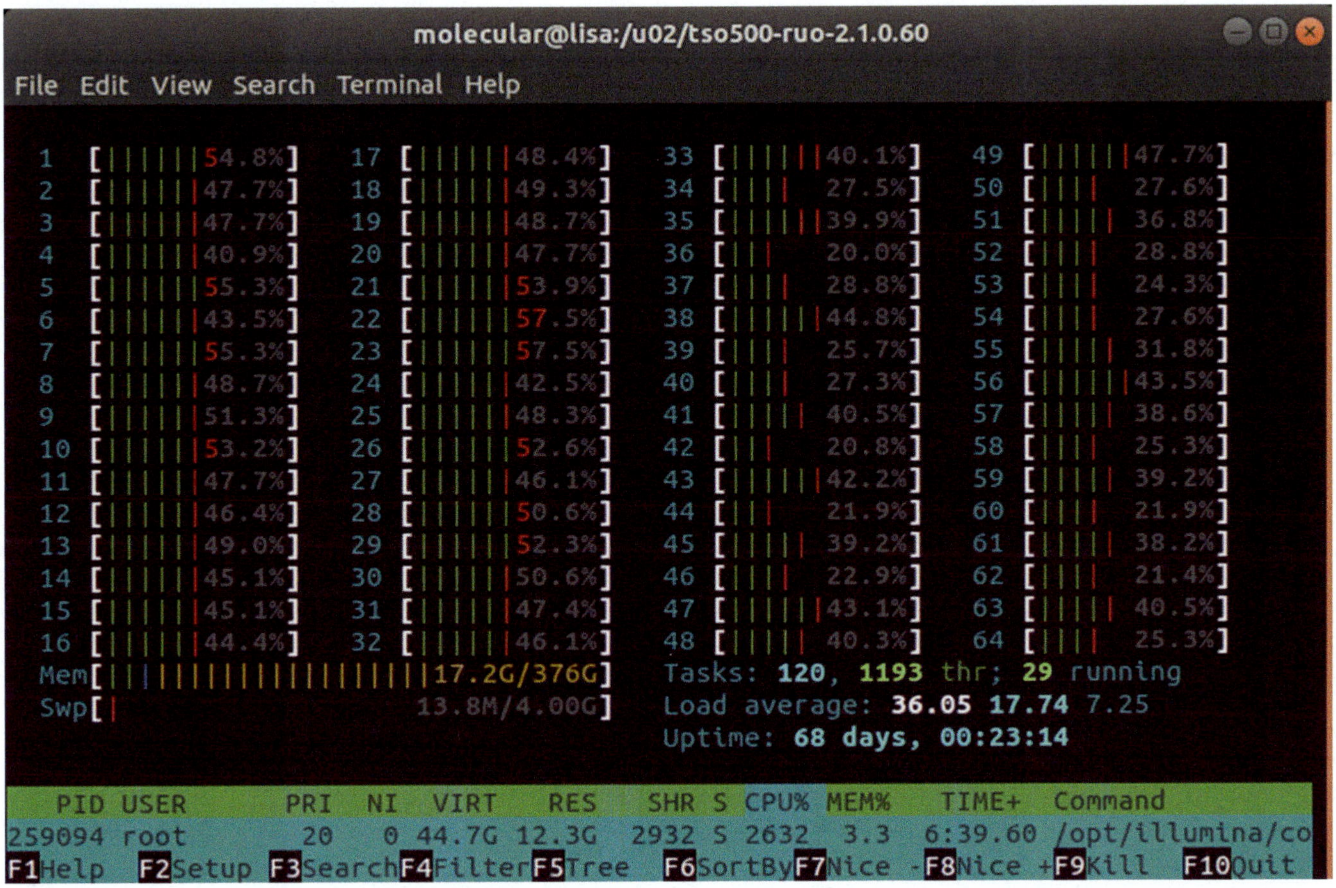
molecular@lisa:/u02/tso500-ruo-2.1.0.60
File Edit View Search Terminal Help
1 [||||||54.8%] 17 [||||||48.4%] 33 [||||||40.1%] 49 [||||||47.7%]
2 [||||||47.7%] 18 [||||||49.3%] 34 [|||| 27.5%] 50 [|||| 27.6%]
3 [||||||47.7%] 19 [||||||48.7%] 35 [||||||39.9%] 51 [||||| 36.8%]
4 [||||||40.9%] 20 [||||||47.7%] 36 [||| 20.0%] 52 [|||| 28.8%]
5 [||||||55.3%] 21 [||||||53.9%] 37 [|||| 28.8%] 53 [|||| 24.3%]
6 [||||||43.5%] 22 [||||||57.5%] 38 [||||||44.8%] 54 [|||| 27.6%]
7 [||||||55.3%] 23 [||||||57.5%] 39 [|||| 25.7%] 55 [||||| 31.8%]
8 [||||||48.7%] 24 [||||||42.5%] 40 [|||| 27.3%] 56 [||||||43.5%]
9 [||||||51.3%] 25 [||||||48.3%] 41 [||||| 40.5%] 57 [||||| 38.6%]
10 [||||||53.2%] 26 [||||||52.6%] 42 [||| 20.8%] 58 [|||| 25.3%]
11 [||||||47.7%] 27 [||||||46.1%] 43 [||||||42.2%] 59 [||||| 39.2%]
12 [||||||46.4%] 28 [||||||50.6%] 44 [||| 21.9%] 60 [|||| 21.9%]
13 [||||||49.0%] 29 [||||||52.3%] 45 [||||| 39.2%] 61 [||||| 38.2%]
14 [||||||45.1%] 30 [||||||50.6%] 46 [|||| 22.9%] 62 [|||| 21.4%]
15 [||||||45.1%] 31 [||||||47.4%] 47 [||||||43.1%] 63 [||||| 40.5%]
16 [||||||44.4%] 32 [||||||46.1%] 48 [||||| 40.3%] 64 [|||| 25.3%]
Mem[||||||||||||||||||||17.2G/376G] Tasks: 120, 1193 thr; 29 running
Swp[| 13.8M/4.00G] Load average: 36.05 17.74 7.25
Uptime: 68 days, 00:23:14
PID USER PRI NI VIRT RES SHR S CPU% MEM% TIME+ Command
259094 root 20 0 44.7G 12.3G 2932 S 2632 3.3 6:39.60 /opt/illumina/co
F1Help F2Setup F3SearchF4FilterF5Tree F6SortByF7Nice -F8Nice +F9Kill F10Quit

Fig. 3.20 Processor utilization during the nucleotide sequence generation phase of a well-engineered commercial bioinformatics pipeline running on a Linux machine with 64 processors. The software is using of all the machine's 64 processors in parallel, numbered 1–64 in the figure. This is a good example of symmetric multiprocessing (SMP)

favor cloud-based bioinformatics components in my laboratory, although the cloud-based components do involve additional compliance considerations, such as the negotiation of a HIPAA business associate agreement (BAA) with the vendor. In all these scenarios, you are going to function more as a systems integrator than a bioinformatician as you figure out how to run your vendor's bioinformatics pipeline in your clinical laboratory workflow. Although this might seem unsatisfying at first, I assure you that systems integration is extremely challenging and having a good working knowledge of NGS bioinformatics file formats – the standards that tie everything together – makes the systems integration process far easier.

- A final topic that deserves consideration is *time*. These bioinformatics pipelines can take a long time to run, even on powerful computers. In my laboratory, the bioinformatics run times vary from 6 h to 48 h depending on the NGS panel and, to some extent, how many different samples are in the run. Vendors use different strategies to reduce bioinformatics run time, but they almost always involved parallel processing, where a large task is divided into many smaller tasks that are run at the same time. In some cases, the smaller tasks run on different processor cores of a single computer (i.e., symmetric multiprocessing – SMP) [Fig. 3.20]. In other cases, the smaller tasks run on entirely different computers in a clustered computing environment (i.e., massively parallel processing – MMP). In either case, the technical infrastructure required to support the bioinformatics pipeline may be considerable and require a lot of technical care-and-feeding, which is one of many reasons that I favor cloud-based bioinformatics components in my laboratory. Finally, the throughput of a bioinformatics pipeline is as much or more dependent on the quality of the software engineering than the amount of hardware that you throw at it, so running a poorly engineered bioinformatics pipeline on more performant hardware may not be very helpful.

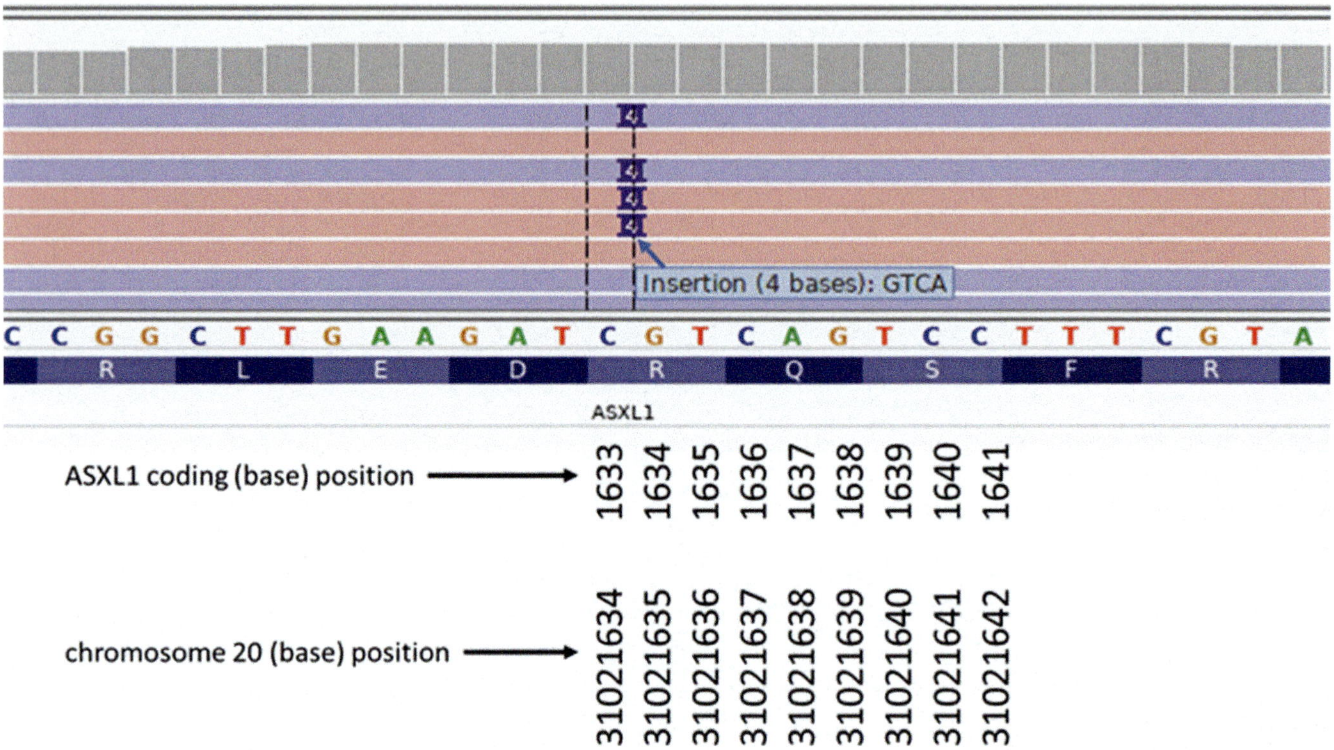

Fig. 3.21 A four nucleotide insertion in gene *ASXL1*

Cases

Case 1: HGVS Nomenclature and Rules

Your two molecular genetic pathology fellows, Fellow 1 & Fellow 2, interpret a case involving a four-base GTCA insertion in gene *ASXL1*. The insertion is in chromosome 20 at position 31,021,634 (hg19/GRCh37) and is shown in the figure below in the Broad Institute's Integrative Genomics Viewer (IGV) along with the reference sequence at that position [Fig. 3.21]. Each fellow reports a different HGVS C-dot nomenclature for the insertion. Which fellow is more correct?

Fellow 1 says the HGVS C-dot nomenclature for the insertion is: **ASXL1 NM_015338.5:c.1634_1637dupGTCA**.

Fellow 2 says the HGVS C-dot nomenclature for the insertion is: **ASXL1 NM_015338.5:c.1637_1640dupAGTC**.

Discussion for Case 1

Both HGVS C-dot nomenclatures describe the same four-base insertion, but Fellow 2's nomenclature is more correct because her nomenclature is compliant with the HGVS 3′ rule which states that *for all descriptions the most 3′ position possible of the reference sequence is arbitrarily assigned to have been changed* [27]. This case illustrates that HGVS nomenclature is not always canonical. There are subtle rules that must be followed if we want to make sure everyone uses the same HGVS nomenclature for the same variant. This is important to remember because using different forms of HGVS nomenclature for the same variant might confound your search of the literature or unnecessarily fragment a database you are building.

Case 2: Read Depth and Molecular Bar Coding

Your two molecular genetic pathology fellows, Fellow 1 & Fellow 2, interpret a case involving *PTCH1* NP_000255.2:T728M (NM_000264.3:c.2183C > T). The NGS panel uses molecular bar codes; so the bioinformatics pipeline produces two BAM files, which are shown below in the Broad Institute's Integrative Genomics Viewer (IGV) [Fig. 3.22]. The upper alignments represent the reads prior to read collapsing and the lower alignments represent the reads

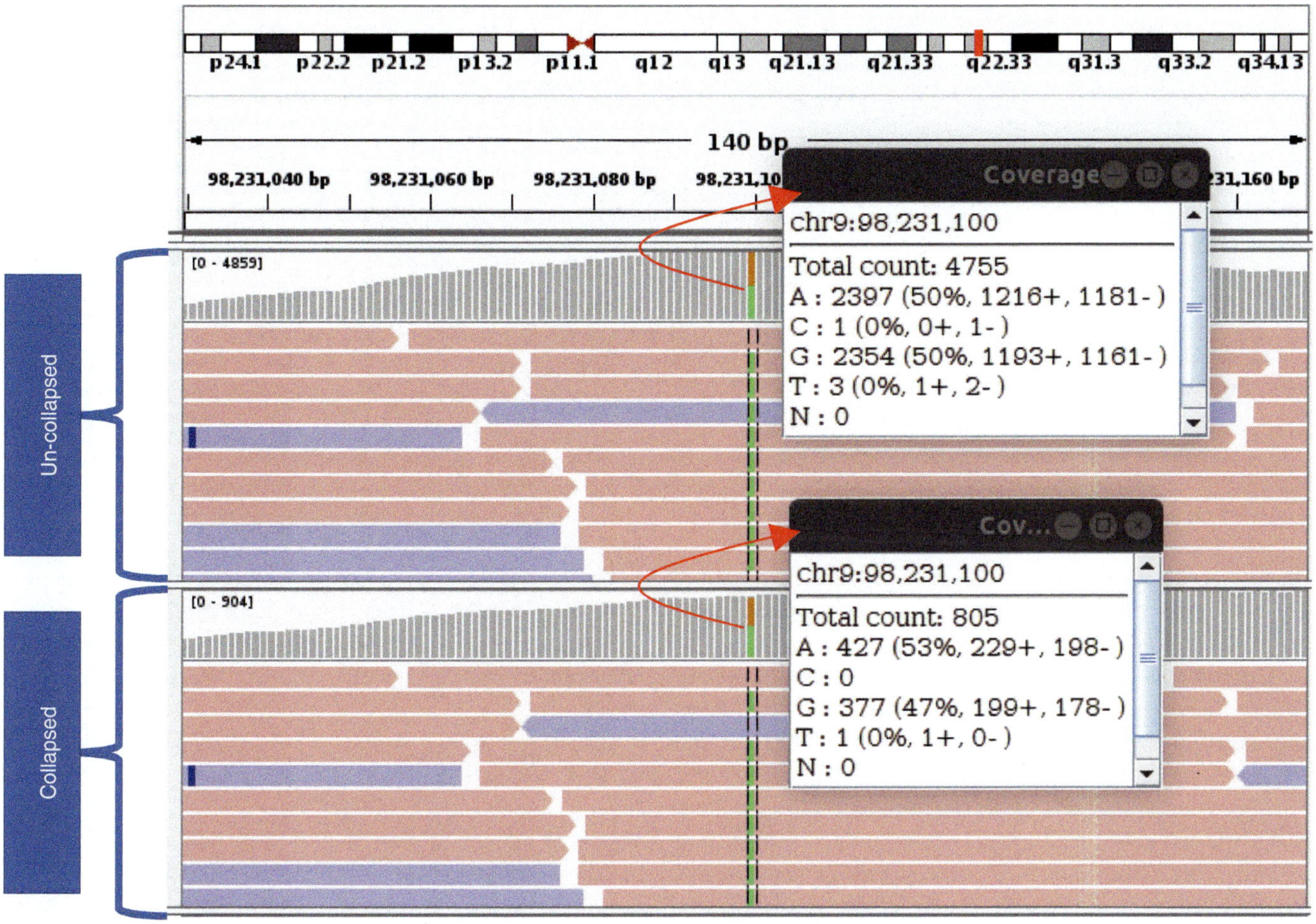

Fig. 3.22 Un-collapsed and collapsed short read alignments in IGV for an NGS panel that uses UMIs

after read collapsing. Each fellow reports a different read depth. Which fellow is more correct?

Fellow 1 says the read depth at the variant position is 4755 reads.

Fellow 2 says the read depth at the variant position is 805 reads.

Discussion for Case 2

As always, both of your fellows are correct, but I would go with the read depth reported by Fellow 2, 805, which represents the read depth after the unique molecular identifiers (UMI) are used to collapse and error correct reads at the locus that share the same UMI sequences. In general, the bioinformatics pipelines in my laboratory apply quality criteria (e.g., median coverage thresholds) to the collapsed reads. At the variant position there are 4755 un-collapsed reads and 805 collapsed reads, so, on average, each collapsed read represents a consensus of 4755/805 = 5.9 un-collapsed reads. This is actually a bit high for this panel which usually operates at uncollapsed:collapsed read ratios of around 3.

Case 3: FASTQ Format and Mate-Pairs

The following FASTQ records represent a mate-pair from a paired-end DNA NGS panel. The reads shown are highly representative of the reads in the FASTQ file in terms of their length and the underlying DNA fragment size.

What is the sequencer read length probably set to?

What is a good estimate for the average DNA fragment size for this library?

Read 1 (record from R1 FASTQ file):

```
@NDX550321_RUO:17:HN7NKBGXF:1:11101:18193:1456 1:N:0:ACTGCTTA+AGAGGCGC
CCTTCACAATTTATTTTCTCAAACAAAGGTGTGTTGTCATTCAAGTTATTGAGAGTAATTGTAGCAAGGACTTCGACTTCCCGGCGGTACGGC
+
EEEEEEEEEEEEEEEEAEEEEEEEEEEEEEEEAEE<EEEEEEEEEEEAEEEEEEEEEEEEEEAEEEEEEEEEAEEEEEEEAEEEEEAEEEEEEAEEEEEEA
```

Read 2 (record from R2 FASTQ file that is mate-pair of above):

```
@NDX550321_RUO:17:HN7NKBGXF:1:11101:18193:1456 2:N:0:ACTGCTTA+AGAGGCGC
CTGATGCCTCGGGTTTATACTCTGAGGATTCGTGCATCAGACTGGGGCTTGCCGTACCGCCGGGAAGTCGAAGTCCTTGCTACAATTACTCTC
+
EEEEEEEEEEAAEAEEEEEEEEE/EEEEEEEAAEEAEEEEEAE6EEEE<EEEEEEEEEAEEEEEEEEEEEEEEEAEEAA<EEEEE<EEEE/EEEEEEE
```

Discussion for Case 3
Every bioinformatician must know how to use a text editor and some basic web services.

The first question is easy to answer. Assuming these are representative reads, then the sequencer read length is approximately the length of either line 2 (nucleotide sequence) or line 4 (encoded Phred quality scores) in the FASTQ records. Those lines are 93 characters long, and that is also the sequencer read length, or something close to it.

The second question is a little harder to answer and requires us to assume that at least some of the DNA fragment is sequenced in both read 1 and read 2 (i.e., the reads overlap in the middle of the fragment). If there is overlap, then we should be able to reverse complement one of the reads using a web service (e.g., https://www.bioinformatics.org/sms/rev_comp.html) and find a contiguous stretch of identical sequence in both reads. In this case, the reverse complement of read 2 matches read 1 starting at position 51, as shown in the figure below (the reads have been split across two lines so they will fit on the page), resulting in a fragment length of 143 bases [Fig. 3.23].

Another consideration is whether read 1 represents the forward or reverse read. This is easy to determine using a web service like BLAST (https://blast.ncbi.nlm.nih.gov/Blast.cgi), where read 1 matches the plus strand in NC_000004.12.

Case 4: Variant Filtering

Your two molecular genetic pathology fellows, Fellow 1 & Fellow 2, come to your office complaining about their variant interpretation workload. Their daily work includes reviewing variants in your laboratory's clinical variant interpretation system and marking them as *detected* or *not detected* for clinical reporting purposes. Your fellows say that the signal-to-noise ratio of your laboratory's commercial NGS cancer panel is low and they have to review too many variants that are likely artifactual (e.g., sequencing artifacts near homopolymers) or not clinically reportable (e.g., silent) and represent noise. They want to implement more aggressive variant filtering so they do not have to review so many variants in the interpretation system. Your NGS panel uses

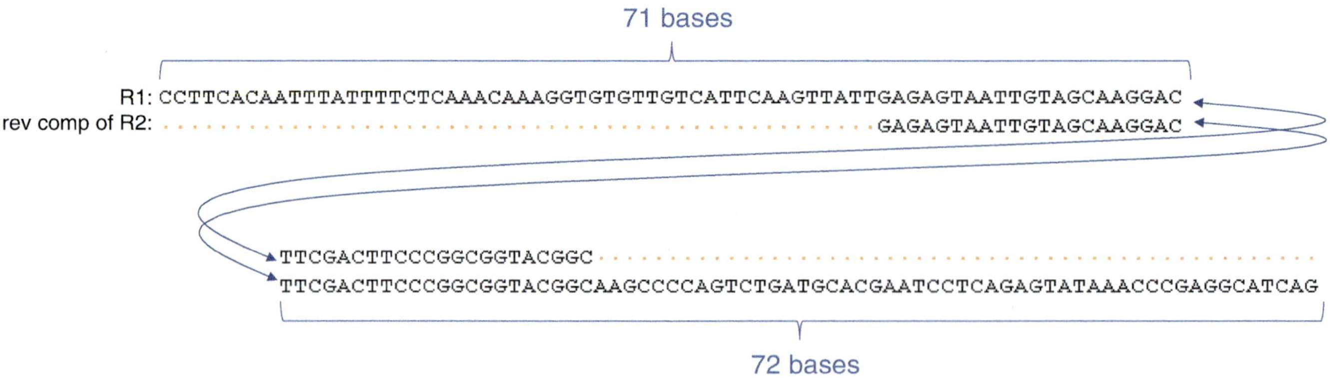

Fig. 3.23 The reads from case 3 with read 2 reverse complemented and aligned to read 1

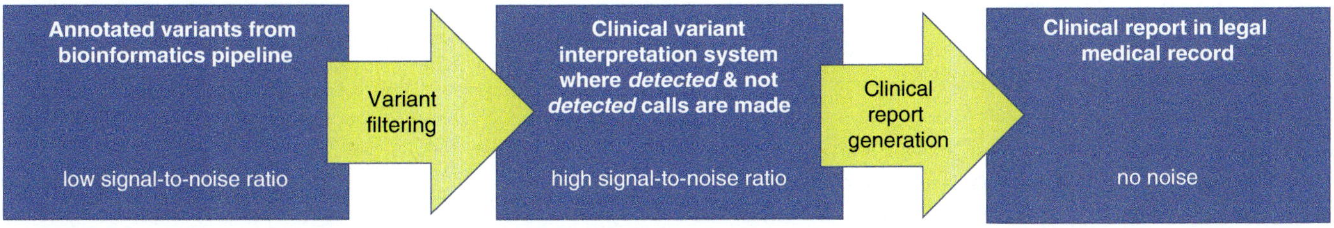

Fig. 3.24 Some bioinformatics pipeline have a low signal-to-noise ratio. Sophisticated variant filtering rules can make your clinical interpretation process more efficient

molecular bar codes and is clinically validated for reporting variants with variant allele frequencies (VAF) down to 3%. Both fellows have proposals for how to do more aggressive variant filtering.

Fellow 1 suggests filtering out all variants with VAFs below 5% since she has determined this would eliminate much of the noise.

Fellow 2 suggests reviewing all the variant annotations reported by the bioinformatics pipeline, beyond just the VAF, to determine if there are more sophisticated annotations that might be used to develop a nuanced filtering strategy.

Discussion for Case 4

Although Fellow 1's proposal is compelling in its directness and simplicity, it would reduce the sensitivity of your NGS cancer panel for detecting low-VAF variants. Fellow 2's proposal is better and illustrates how important it is for you to learn the outputs of your bioinformatics pipeline and the capabilities of your interpretation system. My laboratory uses a variety of filtering strategies beyond a simple VAF threshold to increase the signal-to-noise ratio in our interpretation system, including [Fig. 3.24]:

- Filtering out variants with high allele frequencies in population databases (e.g., ExAC, gnoMAD)
- Filtering out variants with *sequence direction bias* (disagreement between R1 and R2)
- Filtering out variants with *sample strand bias* (disagreement between fragment originating from the plus strand and fragment originating from the minus strand)
- Filtering out variants that are not statistical outliers ($p > 0.05$) with respect to a set of normal control cases,
- Filtering out low VAF variants that are not at known hotspots and that have been reported by the variant caller but not marked as *detected* in at least 100 prior cases
- Filtering out highly intronic variants while being careful to avoid splice sites
- Listing known pathogenic (AMP/ASCO/CAP Tier I) variants for a case first in the variant interpretation system so they are the first thing you see when opening a new case

This is a partial list and what you can do with filtering in your laboratory depends on your bioinformatics pipeline and the capabilities of your interpretation system.

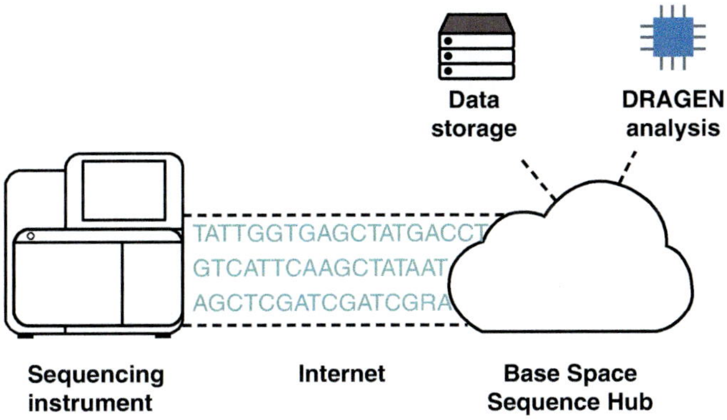

Fig. 3.25 An example of one major sequencer vendor's cloud architecture. The sequencer streams the base calls from the run to the vendor's cloud service in real time (while the run is in progress)

Case 5: Protected Health Information and Cloud Services

You are making plans to clinically validate a commercial 1000 gene NGS cancer panel in your clinical laboratory. The panel has enormous bioinformatics resource requirements. Your local information technology organization does not have the resources to support the project locally, so you plan to use the vendor's cloud services for both data storage and to run the bioinformatics pipeline. The vendor's cloud services are accessible over the public Internet on a subscription basis and the rates are reasonable. You are concerned about compliance with privacy rules, such as the Health Insurance Portability and Accountability Act (HIPAA) privacy rule, because your normal practice is to name NGS samples using two patient identifiers (e.g., accession number and last name – an excellent practice) and you know that these identifiers represent protected health information (PHI) that should not be transferred outside of your organization. You wonder if you can achieve compliance with privacy rules by changing your sample naming conventions to avoid using patient identifiers in the sample names. The figure below shows one major sequencer vendor's cloud service architecture [Fig. 3.25].

Discussion for Case 5

Genetic information is covered by the HIPAA privacy rule; so simply using sample names that do not include PHI is not adequate to allow genetic information to leave your HIPAA covered entity unless you have engaged your cloud service provider under the terms of a HIPAA business associated agreement (BAA) [28]. The BAA is negotiated along with the contract for the cloud services and basically requires the cloud service provider to treat your clinical data as if they were you. This usually requires additional subscription fees (e.g., some kind of upgraded subscription level) since the vendor becomes subject to onerous HIPAA auditing requirements and liability in the event of a data breach. Do not forget to consider the BAA in your plans because the associated legal review can considerably extend the time required to execute the contract.

References

1. Jones R, O'Connor J. Information management and informatics: need for a modern pathology service. Ann Clin Biochem. 2004;41(Pt 3):183–91.
2. Shortliffe EH. Biomedical informatics. London: Springer; 2014.
3. Gardner RM, Overhage JM, Steen EB, Munger BS, Holmes JH, Williamson JJ, et al. Core content for the subspecialty of clinical informatics. J Am Med Inform Assoc. 2009;16(2):153–7.
4. Lehmann CU, Gundlapalli AV, Williamson JJ, Fridsma DB, Hersh WR, Krousel-Wood M, et al. Five years of clinical informatics board certification for physicians in the United States of America. Yearb Med Inform. 2018;27(1):237–42.
5. The National Acadamies of Sciences EM. In: Balogh EP, Miller BT, Ball JR, editors. Improving diagnosis in health care. Washington, DC; 2015.
6. Aziz N, Zhao Q, Bry L, Driscoll DK, Funke B, Gibson JS, et al. College of American Pathologists' laboratory standards for next-generation sequencing clinical tests. Arch Pathol Lab Med. 2015;139(4):481–93.
7. Rodríguez-Ezpeleta N, Hackenberg M, Aransay AM. Bioinformatics for high throughput sequencing. New York: Springer; 2012. xii, 255 p
8. Di Resta C, Galbiati S, Carrera P, Ferrari M. Next-generation sequencing approach for the diagnosis of human diseases: open challenges and new opportunities. EJIFCC. 2018;29(1):4–14.
9. Ledergerber C, Dessimoz C. Base-calling for next-generation sequencing platforms. Brief Bioinform. 2011;12(5):489–97.
10. Fisher KE, Zhang L, Wang J, Smith GH, Newman S, Schneider TM, et al. Clinical validation and implementation of a targeted next-generation sequencing assay to detect somatic variants in non-small cell lung, melanoma, and gastrointestinal malignancies. J Mol Diagn. 2016;18(2):299–315.
11. File Format Guide: National Center for Biotechnology Information; 2020. Available from: https://www.ncbi.nlm.nih.gov/sra/docs/submitformats
12. Sequence Alignment/Map Format Specification: The SAM/BAM Format Specification Working Group; 2020. Available from: https://samtools.github.io/hts-specs/SAMv1.pdf
13. Li H, Handsaker B, Wysoker A, Fennell T, Ruan J, Homer N, et al. The Sequence Alignment/Map format and SAMtools. Bioinformatics. 2009;25(16):2078–9.
14. Robinson JT, Thorvaldsdottir H, Winckler W, Guttman M, Lander ES, Getz G, et al. Integrative genomics viewer. Nat Biotechnol. 2011;29(1):24–6.
15. Thorvaldsdottir H, Robinson JT, Mesirov JP. Integrative Genomics Viewer (IGV): high-performance genomics data visualization and exploration. Brief Bioinform. 2013;14(2):178–92.
16. Kou R, Lam H, Duan H, Ye L, Jongkam N, Chen W, et al. Benefits and challenges with applying unique molecular identifiers in next generation sequencing to detect low frequency mutations. PLoS One. 2016;11(1):e0146638.
17. The Variant Call Format (VCF) Version 4.2 Specification: The GitHub samtools Project Contributors; 2020. Available from: https://samtools.github.io/hts-specs/VCFv4.2.pdf
18. Danecek P, Auton A, Abecasis G, Albers CA, Banks E, DePristo MA, et al. The variant call format and VCFtools. Bioinformatics. 2011;27(15):2156–8.
19. Data File Formats: University of California Santa Cruz; 2020. Available from: http://genome.ucsc.edu/FAQ/FAQformat
20. den Dunnen JT, Dalgleish R, Maglott DR, Hart RK, Greenblatt MS, McGowan-Jordan J, et al. HGVS recommendations for the description of sequence variants: 2016 update. Hum Mutat. 2016;37(6):564–9.
21. Dalgleish R, Flicek P, Cunningham F, Astashyn A, Tully RE, Proctor G, et al. Locus Reference Genomic sequences: an improved basis for describing human DNA variants. Genome Med. 2010;2(4):24.
22. MacArthur JA, Morales J, Tully RE, Astashyn A, Gil L, Bruford EA, et al. Locus Reference Genomic: reference sequences for the reporting of clinically relevant sequence variants. Nucleic Acids Res. 2014;42(Database issue):D873–8.
23. A Reference Sequence – Discussions and FAQs: Human Genome Variation Society; 2020. Available from: https://www.hgvs.org/mutnomen/refseq.html#general
24. Puxeddu E, Moretti S, Elisei R, Romei C, Pascucci R, Martinelli M, et al. BRAF(V599E) mutation is the leading genetic event in adult sporadic papillary thyroid carcinomas. J Clin Endocrinol Metab. 2004;89(5):2414–20.
25. Li MM, Datto M, Duncavage EJ, Kulkarni S, Lindeman NI, Roy S, et al. Standards and guidelines for the interpretation and reporting of sequence variants in cancer: A Joint Consensus Recommendation of the Association for Molecular Pathology, American Society of Clinical Oncology, and College of American Pathologists. J Mol Diagn. 2017;19(1):4–23.
26. Molecular Pathology Checklist. College of American Pathologists; 2020.
27. Sequence Variant Nomenclature – DNA Recommendations – Duplication 2020. Available from: https://varnomen.hgvs.org/recommendations/DNA/variant/duplication/
28. Clayton EW, Evans BJ, Hazel JW, Rothstein MA. The law of genetic privacy: applications, implications, and limitations. J Law Biosci. 2019;6(1):1–36.

Quality Assurance and Quality Control in Molecular Diagnostic Laboratories

4

Juehua Gao and Lawrence J. Jennings

List of Frequently Asked Questions

J. Gao (✉) · L. J. Jennings
Department of Pathology, Northwestern University Feinberg School of Medicine, Chicago, IL, USA
e-mail: j-gao@northwestern.edu; l-jennings@northwestern.edu

Frequently Asked Questions

1. **What is the role of the US Food & Drug Administration in clinical laboratory testing?**
    - In 1976, federal regulation of clinical laboratory tests began with the Medical Device Amendments to the Food, Drug, and Cosmetic Act.
    - This amendment covered all reagents, tests, and equipment manufactured for the diagnosis or treatment of disease and was intended to provide reasonable assurance of safety and effectiveness. It created the three-class, risk-based classification (low-, moderate-, and high-risk), and established the regulatory pathway by which new tests would be evaluated before introducing them to the market (i.e., Premarket Approval (PMA) and premarket notification (510(k)) (https://www.fda.gov/media/102367/download).
    - The FDA maintains its regulatory oversight of all clinical laboratory tests although it has largely exercised a policy of enforcement discretion for laboratory-developed tests (LDTs), which they define as an in vitro diagnostic test that is designed, manufactured, and used within a single laboratory.
    - However, the FDA retains the right to enforce premarket review for any LDT and may exercise that right if it deems that test a significant risk to patients. For example, they may require review of an LDT that is widely marketed, marketed with deceptive promotion, not adequately validated, or has a reasonable probability of causing death or serious injury. For all LDTs, a disclaimer must be included on clinical reports to clearly state that the performance of the test had not been evaluated by the FDA [1, 2].
2. **What is an analyte-specific reagent (ASR)?**
    - In 1997, the FDA published three rules that were intended to reduce the risks associated with reagents used in LDTs.

Y. Ding, L. Zhang (eds.), *Practical Oncologic Molecular Pathology*, Practical Anatomic Pathology,
https://doi.org/10.1007/978-3-030-73227-1_4

- These rules defined and classified analyte-specific reagents (ASRs) such as antibodies, nucleic acid sequences, and similar reagents that were essential to ensure the accuracy of LDTs. Since LDTs were not subject to premarket review, ensuring good manufacturing production of ASRs was deemed necessary.
- The rules restricted the sale, distribution, and use of ASRs and established requirements for ASR labeling. These rules are collectively known as the "ASR Rule."

3. **Can research-use-only reagents, instruments, and systems be used in clinical laboratory testing?**
   - In 2011, the FDA provided a draft guidance entitled, "Commercially Distributed in Vitro Diagnostic Products Labeled for Research Use Only or Investigational Use Only: Frequently Asked Questions" (https://asm.org/ASM/media/Policy-and-Advocacy/LRN/FDA-IVGuidance6-2011.pdf). This draft document prohibited the sale of all RUO/IUO reagents, instruments or systems to clinical laboratories even when used as part of a laboratory test.
   - However, CAP presented a response stating, "use of RUO and IUO reagents, instruments, and systems, as components of LDTs, should be permissible in clinical diagnosis and patient management when reasonable substitutes are not available" (https://documents.cap.org/documents/2011-fda-research-use-only-draft-guidance-faqs.pdf).
   - CAP provided an argument for the need of these reagents and systems for patient access and quality of care. It also highlighted the current regulation of LDTs through CLIA and organizations with deemed status such as CAP.
   - The final FDA guidance document was issued in 2013 and cautioned manufacturers about inappropriate labeling or distribution of RUO/IUO products for clinical laboratory testing but did not prohibit the sale to clinical laboratories (https://www.fda.gov/media/87374/download).
4. **What is the role of CLIA in clinical laboratory testing?**
   - The need for laboratory regulation became apparent soon after Medicare and Medicaid went into effect to prevent fraud and abuse. Minimum quality requirements for clinical laboratories were first established for laboratories doing business across state lines that wished to collect Medicare dollars. These requirements were collectively known as the Clinical Laboratory Improvement Act of 1967 (CLIA '67).
   - However, most labs were not doing business across state lines and, therefore, not subject to the requirements. Many laboratories self-regulated through professional organizations such as the College of American Pathologists but this was completely voluntary.
   - Over the next two decades, additional requirements including those for professional qualifications were added but the most significant amendment occurred in 1988. In 1988, Congress passed the Clinical Laboratory Improvement Amendment (CLIA) to establish quality standards for all aspects of clinical laboratory testing and extend these standards to all clinical laboratories. The CLIA is overseen by the Centers for Medicare & Medicaid Services (CMS), which publishes regulations and assumes primary responsibility for financial management operations of the CLIA program. The FDA has primary responsibility for categorizing the complexity of laboratory tests into one of three CLIA regulatory categories: waived for simple tests, and moderate or high complexity for other tests based on their potential risk to public health. The Centers for Disease Control serves an advisory role and provides scientific support.
5. **What are the CLIA requirements?**
   - CLIA regulations require certification of all laboratories performing clinical testing of any kind and provide both general guidelines and subspecialty-specific standards. Although there is a cytogenetic subspecialty under CLIA, there is no molecular pathology subspecialty, but the general guidelines and requirements still apply and are considered sufficient.
   - CLIA requirements for test validation vary by test complexity and FDA premarket review. Waived tests require no analytical validation whereas FDA-approved (PMA) or FDA-cleared (510(k)) tests that are of moderate or high complexity require verification of performance specifications established by the manufacturer. The performance specifications that must be addressed include accuracy, precision, reference range and reportable range.
   - If an FDA-approved or cleared test is modified even slightly (e.g., different sample source) or is entirely laboratory-developed, performance specifications must be established by the laboratory. The performance specifications that must be addressed include accuracy, precision, reference range and reportable range as well as analytical sensitivity, analytical specificity and any other specification considered important for the performance of the test (e.g., cross-contamination).
   - How and to what extent performance specifications should be verified or established is ultimately under the purview of medical laboratory professionals and is overseen by the CLIA certification process most commonly through an organization with deemed status. Minimum requirements as defined by accrediting organization standards and published guidelines vary

and should be determined at the start of any validation to define required performance criteria.

6. **What is the difference between analytical validation and clinical validation?**
   - Analytical validation focuses on the analytes targeted by the assay and is intended to identify and quantify potential sources of technical variation in the analysis of patient samples. Clinical validation is intended to identify and quantify potential sources of biologic variation in the analysis of a given sample. Only by limiting and quantifying the technical variation can the biological variation be ascertained.
   - The performance specifications that should be addressed for analytical validation are listed in the CLIA requirements for validation (see Table 4.1). Note that not all performance specifications apply to each test and many molecular tests may have other unlisted parameters (e.g., in silico sensitivity and specificity, carryover, robustness, etc.)
   - The performance specifications for clinical validation most commonly include clinical (or diagnostic) sensitivity and specificity as well as positive and negative predictive values. However, many other performance specifications are also used including positive and negative likelihood ratios, relative risk, and probabilities. Even the establishment of the "normal range" or "reference range" is part of the clinical validation since it defines the range of "normal" biological variation for a population. The relationship of these to one another is shown in Table 4.2. Note that presence or absence of disease is not always obvious and defining that may require multiple sources of clinical information (e.g., other tests, radiography, clinical history and exam) to create a combined "gold standard" for comparison.

Table 4.1 CLIA requirements for analytical validation

	Definition	FDA approved/cleared	LDTs and modified FDA tests
Accuracy	Closeness of agreement between a single test result and the accepted reference value (modified from ISO 5725-1)	20–40 samples	At least 40 samples
Precision	Closeness of agreement between independent test results from the same sample obtained under prescribed (stipulated) conditions (modified from ISO 5725-1)	2–3 samples at clinical decision points run daily for 5 days	Replicates over at least 20 days
Analytic sensitivity	In genotyping or DNA sequencing, the limit of detection is the lowest concentration of the target nucleic acid that can be reproducibly measured which exceeds the blank sample with no analyte. It may be below the linear range of the assay	Verification; may use literature or manufacture documentation	Validation
Analytic specificity (interferences or cross reactivity)	Ability of a measurement procedure to determine solely the quantity it purports to measure (ISO 15193)	Verification; may use literature or manufacture documentation	Validation
Reportable range	The range of test result values over which the laboratory can establish or verify the accuracy of the instrument, kit, or test system measurement response	Three points near low end midpoint, and high end	Three points near low end, midpoint, and high end
Reference range	Interval between, and including, the lower reference limit to the upper reference limit of the reference population (e.g., 95% of persons presumed to be healthy [or normal])	20 samples	20–40 samples

Table 4.2 A 2×2 contingency table for clinical performance characteristics in diagnostic tests

		Disease			
Diagnostic results test		Present	Absent	Total	
	Positive	A True positive (TP)	B False positive (FP)	A+B	**Positive predictive value (PPV)**= TP/(TP+FP)=A/(A+B)
	Negative	C False negative (FN)	D True negative (TN)	C+D	**Negative predictive value (NPV)**= TN/(FN+TN)=D/(C+D)
	Total	A+C	B+D	A+B+C+D	
		Sensitivity=TP/(TP+FN) =A/(A+C)	**Specificity**=TN/(FP+TN) =D/(B+D)	**Prevalence**=(A+C)/(A+B+C+D) **Accuracy**= (A+D)/(A+B+C+D)	**Likelihood ratio positive** =sensitivity/(1-specficity)=A/(A+C)/B/(B+D) **Likelihood ratio negative** = (1-sensitivity)/specificity=C/(A+C)/D/(B+D)

7. **What is the role of the College of American Pathologists (CAP) and other professional organizations in clinical laboratory testing?**
   - Professional organizations or state agencies demonstrating that their accreditation requirements meet or exceed those specified by CLIA have "deemed status" from CMS to accredit laboratories. Some of the larger professional organizations with deemed status include The Joint Commission, American Osteopathic Association, American Association of Blood Banks, American Association of Laboratory Accreditation, College of American Pathologists (CAP), Commission of Laboratory Accreditation, or American Society for Histocompatibility and Immunogenetics [3].
   - CAP accredits most molecular pathology laboratories and other high-complexity laboratories. CAP requirements largely reflect the performance specifications outlined by CLIA, but in some circumstances CAP requirements exceed those of CLIA. The CAP standards for molecular pathology were created in 1991 and have been periodically updated to modernize the requirements for test validation in the face of changing technologies and applications (www.cap.org).
8. **What is the CAP Laboratory Accreditation program? What are the requirements of laboratory accreditation?**
   - The CAP Laboratory Accreditation program provides a reciprocal, peer-based inspection to assess the overall quality of the laboratory.
   - The requirements for laboratory accreditation comprise of documents known as checklists. The checklists are guidelines used by laboratories and inspectors to ensure quality and patient safety. The CAP checklists are updated annually to reflect the latest best practices.
   - An on-site laboratory inspection occurs every 2 years. Following the inspection, the inspection team provides a summary of findings. The laboratory has 30 days to address the deficiencies identified. In the years when an on-site inspection does not occur, the laboratory performs a self-inspection using materials provided by the CAP.
   - The checklists a molecular laboratory commonly uses include a molecular pathology checklist, cytogenetics checklist, microbiology checklist, all common checklist, and laboratory general checklist.
9. **What are the quality control challenges for next-generation sequencing (NGS) tests in the clinical laboratory?**
   - Many laboratories are moving away from single-gene assays toward panel testing, particularly next-generation sequencing that has the advantage of simultaneously testing a large number of genes of interest. The quality of data may be affected by many factors in the NGS process. All measurable parameters should remain within acceptable limits as defined in the validation report for the test.
   - The parameters may reflect quality control in each of the steps including DNA extraction (OD 260/280 ratio), library generation (fragment size), sequencing (cluster density, error rate, total reads, number of reads pass filter), and bioinformatics analysis (percentage of read on target, average coverage, minimal coverage/base, library complexity, strand bias, GC/AT bias).
   - Many laboratories may have single-gene assays for particular genes, and the results should be in concordance. Although technical difference should be taken into consideration. For example, next generation sequencing is sensitive to low-level genetic alteration, which may not be detectable by pyrosequencing or Sanger sequencing. The percentage of mutations for specific tumor types can vary depending on the patient population tested, but frequency significantly out of the reported range should raise question and be investigated. Formalin or extraction-induced artifacts in DNA may mimic mutations such as deamination (C>T, G>A) or guanine oxidation (G>T, C>A) and usually occur at a low allele frequency (e.g., <5% VAF).
   - Most of the bioinformatics pipelines provides tools for quality check and filtering of the sequencing output. Sequence artifacts, including read errors, poor quality reads, and primer/adaptor contamination, need to be filtered and removed by bioinformatic tools before downstream sequence analysis. It is important during the validation process to recognize the common artifacts in the specific NGS platform the assay runs [4].
10. **What are the quality control samples?**
    - To ensure the end-to-end performance of a test, quality control materials are used within each test run.
    - Quality control samples should be similar to the patient's samples to monitor the testing process. Both positive and negative control samples should be used along with the patient's samples. Some quality control samples may be commercially available. Laboratory can also use previously tested patients' samples. However, rare genetic variants are difficult to obtain.
    - The CDC Genetic Testing Reference Material Coordination Program (GeT-RM) distributes a wide range of reference materials to the genetics community for quality control, proficiency testing, test

development, and validation (https://www.cdc.gov/labquality/get-rm/).

11. **What is quality assurance? What are the main quality assurance areas in a clinical molecular laboratory?**
    - Quality assurance is a procedure involving the entire testing process in the clinical laboratory to ensure the lab produces test results without any error. Laboratory errors may occur and fall into several categories. Misidentification at any stage of the testing process could result in incorrect assignment of the test result to the wrong patient. Technical errors do occur, often as a failure in the test system or failure to follow the SOP. Interpretation errors are less common.
    - When laboratory errors occur, it is important to perform a root-cause analysis and to improve the process. Quality assurance covers the entire testing process including pre-analytical, analytical, and post-analytical stages. For example, in the pre-analytical stage, the patient information and proper test ordered are double checked to avoid misidentification. In the analytical stage, proper SOPs should be followed to produce correct results. And in the post-analytical stage, if samples are analyzed by instruments, instruments should have routine calibration and maintenance.
12. **What is a standard operation procedure (SOP) manual? What are the important components of a standard operation procedure (SOP) manual?**
    - A standard operation procedure (SOP) is a document that provides step-by-step instructions on a laboratory process that can be performed in a consistent manner by laboratory personnel. SOPs should be written with sufficient details that someone else with limited experience can reproduce the procedure.
    - An SOP manual may include scope of the assay, summary of the method, equipment and suppliers, computer hardware or software, procedure for sample preparation, data acquisition, interpretation, and trouble shooting. Specific criteria for quality control data and prompted actions should also be included.
    - For clinical testing, document control of SOPs is essential and an electronic database of SOPs and policies can be prove very useful for the storage of active SOPs and archiving of retired SOPs.
13. **What are quality management and improvement initiatives? What are the challenges of quality improvement measures?**
    - Quality management and improvement initiatives help to establish a culture of quality in the organization.
    - There are major steps of quality management and improvement initiatives.
    - First is to recognize and identify areas for improvement, for example, to identify work flow issues contributing to long turnaround time or barriers to timely communication of critical values.
    - Next is to collect and analyze data. The data help to identify critical areas for improvement and to establish measurable goals and quality metrics.
    - After data analysis, changes in the process could be evaluated. Final decisions could be made to implement changes and hold the gains. It is important to recognize that quality improvement is an ongoing effort, and this cycle is repeated continuously.
14. **What are proficiency tests? What are the recommendation and regulatory requirements for molecular proficiency tests?**
    - Proficiency testing (PT) determines the performance of individual laboratories for specific tests and offer some inter-laboratory comparison. PT is used to monitor laboratories' continuing performance as part of verification for tests and/or as part of process improvement. Under Clinical Laboratory Improvement Amendments (CLIA), all accredited laboratories that perform non-waived testing are required to enroll in and perform PT using one of the CMS-approved PT programs at least twice each year. For some common analytes, PT needs to be done at least three times each year. For tests that have no formal proficiency test program, laboratories are required to identify an alternative approach such as exchanging samples with other clinical laboratories or internal testing of known samples.
    - Per CLIA, PT specimens must be tested with the laboratory's regular patient workload, using routine methods and testing the PT specimens the same way the laboratory routinely tests patient specimens. The PT specimens cannot be sent to a reference lab with a different CLIA identification number. And repeated testing PT samples is also not appropriate unless that is the normal workflow for patient samples.
    - The rapidly developing technology and expanding test menu in the diagnostic molecular laboratory is challenging for both laboratories conducting PT testing and PT program providers. PT does not covers all the tests performed in the clinical laboratory, nor does it always correlate how the clinical specimens are handled. College of American Pathologists recently published a couple of studies comparing Proficiency Testing for clinically relevant somatic single-nucleotide variants for oncology specimens in laboratories using different test methods, kit manufacturers, and pre-analytic and post-analytic practices. These studies showed a high degree of accuracy and comparable performance across all laboratories,

regardless of methodology [5, 6]. Proficiency testing of standardized samples shows very high inter-laboratory agreement for clinical next-generation-sequencing-based oncology assays. These studies highlight the importance of establishing high inter-laboratory agreement, particularly for clinically relevant variants as these test results impact clinical decisions [7].

15. **What is an individualized quality control plan (IQCP)? How to develop an IQCP?**
    - An individualized quality control plan (IQCP) is a risk-based approach that allows each laboratory flexibility in achieving regulatory QC requirements. It is intended to be a laboratory-specific tailored plan instead of a standardized one-size-fits-all approach: http://www.cms.gov/Regulations-and-Guidance/Legislation/CLIA/Individualized_Quality_Control_Plan_IQCP.html
    - The use of IQCPs is under the CMS regulation 42 CFR 493.1256 Standard: Control Procedures and applies to most CMS-certified current and new non-waived tests. It does not apply to waived tests.
    - The IQCP consists of three parts: risk assessment (RA), quality control plan (QCP), and quality assessment (QA). Risk assessment identifies potential failures and sources of errors in the five components: specimen, test system, reagent, environment, and testing personnel. For example, an inadequate specimen volume than manufacturer's instruction may result in the test kit reagents performing improperly. Based on the identified risks, a quality control plan (QCP) could be developed to prevent and monitor errors. QCP includes all control procedures to reduce risk and to immediately detect errors. For example, to reduce the potential error associated with inadequate specimen volume, a QCP procedure requires verify each specimen for acceptability upon receipt in the laboratory, and follows the laboratory specimen rejection policy. Quality assessment (QA) provides constant monitoring and reviewing to determine if the quality activities work or not.

CDC and CMS have developed a step-by-step guide for developing an IQCP in clinical laboratories: https://www.cms.gov/Regulations-and-Guidance/Legislation/CLIA/Downloads/IQCP-Workbook.pdf

Case Presentations

Case 1

Learning Objective

Understand the potential sources of error that can lead to a false positive result

Case History

A 29-year-old man presented with fatigue and petechia. CBC reported anemia with hemoglobin of 9 g/dL, elevated white blood cell count (45.6 K/uL) and moderate thrombocytopenia (37 K/uL). A peripheral blood smear review showed many circulating blasts. Flow cytometric analysis demonstrated a large B lymphoblast population that was bright CD34+, CD19+, CD10+, and TdT+. The morphology (see Fig. 4.1a) and immunophenotype were consistent with B lymphoblastic leukemia. A sample was collected and sent to a molecular lab for *BCR-ABL1* fusion transcript. The qualitative RT-PCR for *BCR-ABL1* (see Fig. 4.1b) revealed a p190 fusion peak. These results would indicate a diagnosis of B lymphoblastic leukemia with t(9;22), *BCR-ABL1*. However, FISH analysis for *BCR-ABL1* using dual-fusion probes did not identify any fusion signal (see Fig. 4.1c). A quick analysis of five metaphase cells reported a normal male karyotype. Given to the discrepant molecular and cytogenetic/FISH results, a quantitative RT-PCR was performed from the specimen in the lab, which resulted positive results and a high *BCR-ABL1/ABL1* copy number of 56.2%. Positive control, negative control, and blank were appropriate. RT-PCR analysis was performed on another freshly collected sample and was negative for *BCR-ABL1*.

Diagnosis: B lymphoblastic leukemia, NOS

Discussion: This example of a false-positive result may render a wrong diagnosis and subject the patient to ineffective treatment. The reasons for discrepant molecular and cytogenetic/FISH results include the following possibilities: (1) Sample mix up at the time of collection or during transportation to the lab. (2) Sample mix up during extraction or at the time of setting up RT-PCR. (3) Cross-contamination with a positive sample or positive control. (4) Low-level positivity picked up by RT-PCR but not by FISH or cytogenetics. RT-PCR is far more sensitive than FISH although follow-up quantitative RT-PCR showed 56% fusion transcripts as compared to the *ABL1* housekeeping gene making this fourth possibility very unlikely.

Because a false-positive RT-PCR result can be caused by sample or reagent contamination, appropriate negative and blank controls should be set up in each run to identify possible contamination. When there is discrepant lab result, a different test methodology can be used to confirm the results as was done in this case with quantitative RT-PCR, which showed there was no sample mix-up or contamination after the time of extraction. Since sample mix up can occur during collection, transportation, and assay set up, it is important to use two sets of identifiers for each step. Use of automation or multi-channel pipettes during the assay set up may eliminate some error prone steps.

Follow-up: Additional STR identity testing was performed that confirmed the false-positive sample was from a different individual due to a sample mislabeling at the time of collection or during transportation to the lab.

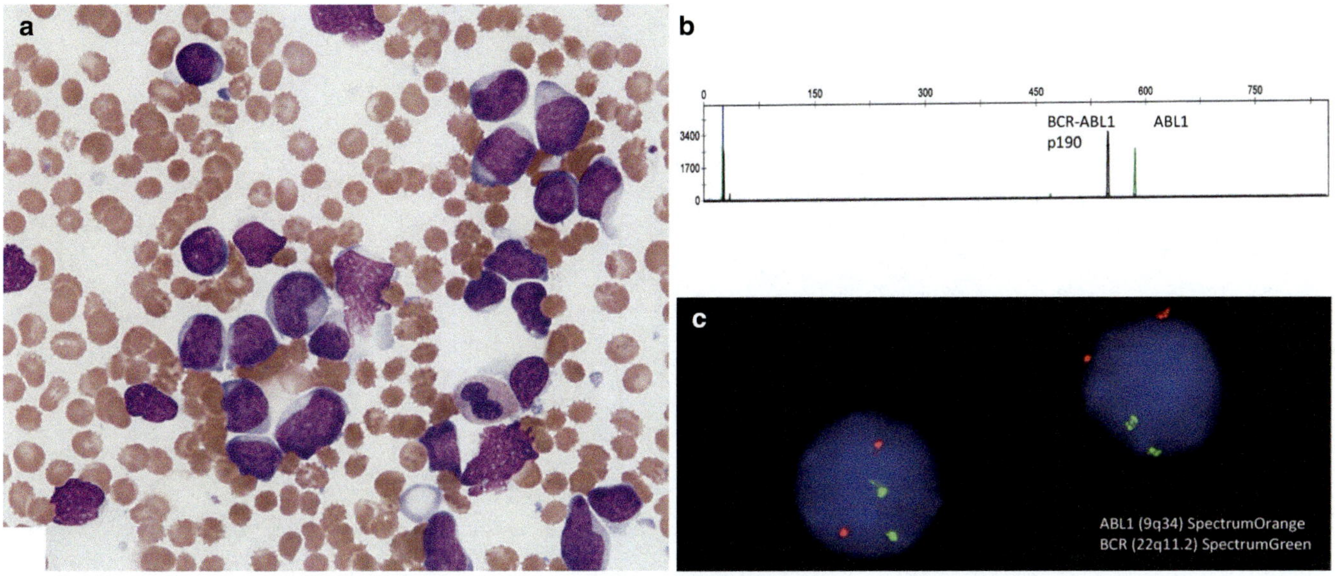

Fig. 4.1 **Case 1.** The bone marrow aspirate revealed frequent blasts (**a**. Wright-Giemsa, ×1000). Flow cytometric analysis confirmed the presence of a large B-lymphoblast population (data not shown). Qualitative RT-PCR showed a *BCR-ABL1 p190* fusion transcript together with the longer amplified transcript of the housekeeping gene, *ABL1* (**b**). FISH analysis was negative for *BCR-ABL1* fusion signal using a Vysis dual-fusion probe set (**c**). FISH picture courtesy of Madina Sukhanova, PhD

Case 2

Learning Objective

Understand the potential sources of error that can lead to a false-negative result

Case History

A 30-year-old female with a thyroid nodule presented for a fine needle aspiration (FNA). The FNA cytology revealed benign follicular cells, along with occasional cells with nuclear enlargement and irregular nuclear contours, with very rare intranuclear inclusions (Fig. 4.2a, b). The FNA was interpreted as atypia of undetermined significance (AUS). A Roche Cobas 4800 *BRAF* V600 mutation assay was performed on the FNA cell block and reported negative for *BRAF* V600 mutation. The patient had an additional FNA along with a core biopsy, which showed papillary thyroid carcinoma (Fig. 4.2c). The Roche Cobas 4800 *BRAF* V600 mutation assay was again performed on the core biopsy with over 50% of tumor cells and was positive for *BRAF* V600E mutation.

Final diagnosis: Papillary thyroid carcinoma with *BRAF* V600E mutation.

Discussion: This is an example of a false-negative molecular result probably due to inadequate sampling, which may delay the diagnosis or lead to a misdiagnosis. The activating mutation of the *BRAF* gene, T1799A, is the most common and specific genetic alteration in papillary thyroid carcinoma. The *BRAF* mutational status could be used as a "ruled-in" marker for malignancy. The risk factors for false-negative *BRAF* V600E mutation results include the presence of a PCR inhibitor or low tumor percentage. Studies also reported that false-negative results were observed more often in old age and certain subtypes of papillary thyroid carcinoma (conventional and tall-cell variant subtypes) [8]. In addition, rare variants that are not specifically targeted (e.g., V600R, V600K) may not be detected by a test specifically designed and validated for *BRAF* V600E.

Follow-up: The patient had a hemithyroidectomy with the final pathology diagnostic for papillary thyroid carcinoma. Next-generation sequencing confirmed the presence of *BRAF* V600E mutation (Fig. 4.2d).

Case 3

Learning Objective

Understand the potential sources of error that can lead to a QNS result

Case History

A 39-year-old male presented to his primary care physician with fatigue and frequent nose bleeds. His complete blood cell count showed white blood cell count 1.7 K/uL, hemoglobin 7.6 g/dL, and platelet of 42 K/uL. A peripheral blood smear review showed pancytopenias with rare circulating immature cells that were medium to large in size, with bilobed nuclei, cytoplasmic granules, and occasional Auer rods (Fig. 4.3a).

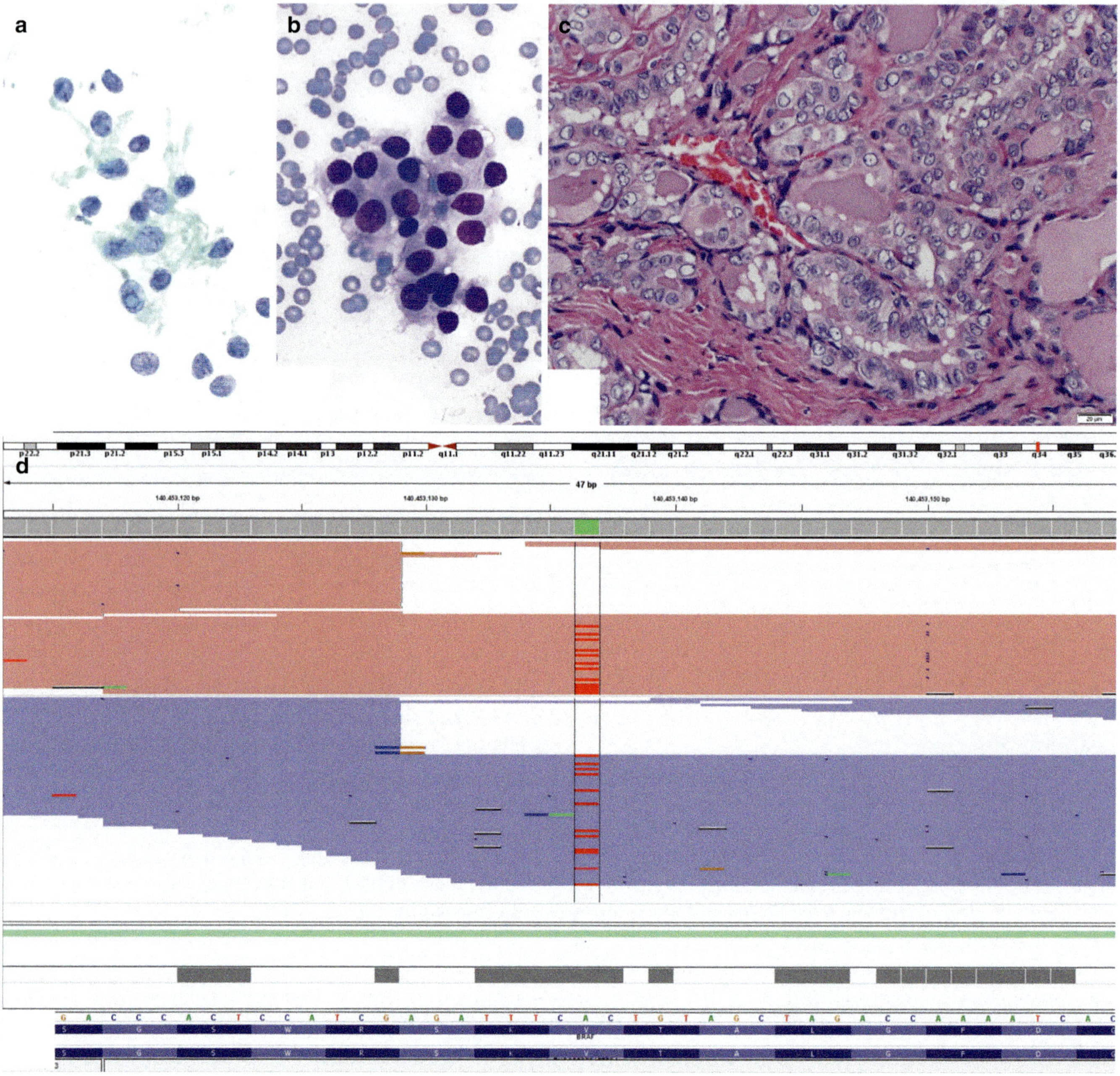

Fig. 4.2 **Case 2.** The FNA cytology revealed occasional cells with nuclear enlargement and irregular nuclear contours, with very rare intranuclear inclusions. (**a**. PAP ×600, **b**. DiffQuik ×600). A Roche Cobas 4800 BRAF V600 mutation assay reported negative for *BRAF* V600 mutation (data not shown). The patient's surgical resection showed papillary thyroid carcinoma (**c**. H&E, ×400). Next generation sequencing revealed *BRAF* V600E (**d**). (**a-c**. Pictures courtesy of Daniel Johnson, MD)

The morphologic findings are suspicious for acute promyelocytic leukemia. This critical finding was communicated to the patient's physician by the on-call pathology resident. The patient was asked to come to ER for further evaluation. In the meantime, the left over CBC sample was sent to the molecular lab for confirmatory testing. The on-call pathology resident reviewed the data for the *PML-RARα* RT-PCR assay and noted there was no amplification using all sets of primers (long, short, and variable, see Fig. 4.3b) and considered this was a negative result which could exclude a diagnosis of acute promyelocytic leukemia with t(15;17), *PML-RARα*. The senior technologist pointed out that there was no amplification for the *ABL1* gene as well, which indicated sample degradation. This was communicated to the ER physician who was evaluating the patient. A new sample was sent to the molecular lab. The repeated RT-PCR assay showed amplification of *PML-RARα* using the short-form primer sets and amplification of the *ABL1* gene (see Fig. 4.3c).

Final diagnosis: Acute promyelocytic leukemia with t(15;17), *PML-RARα*

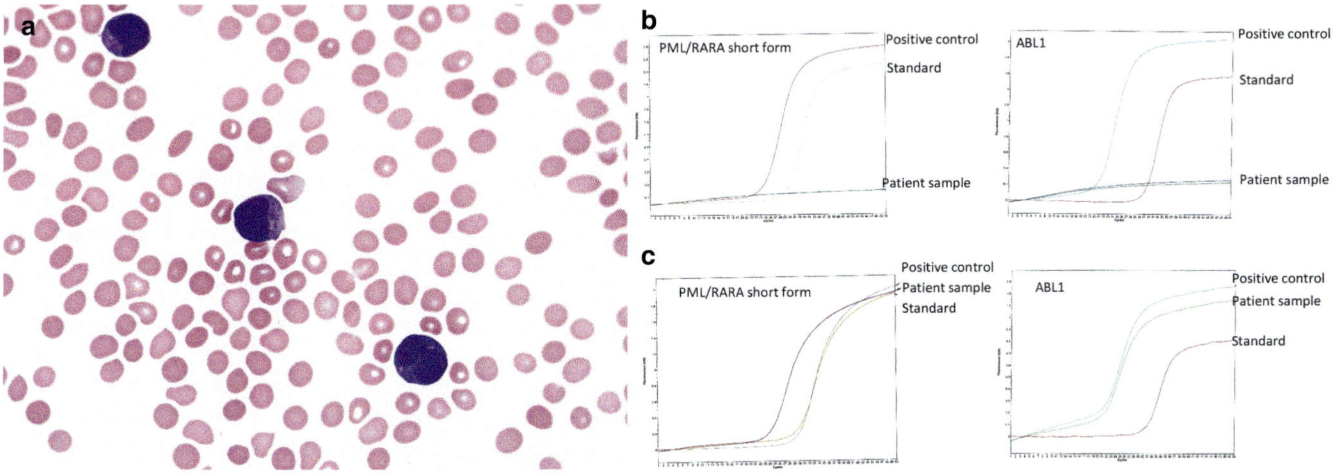

Fig. 4.3 **Case 3.** (**a**). The peripheral blood smear reveals scattered abnormal promyelocytes with bilobed nuclei, and cytoplasmic granules (Wright-Giemsa, ×1000). (**b**). RT-PCR analysis did not reveal amplification of *PML-RARα* and *ABL1* genes. (**c**). RT-PCR performed on a fresh sample revealed amplification for both *PML-RARα* and *ABL1* genes

Discussion: RT-PCR assay remains the most sensitive and rapid technique for the detection of *PML-RARα*. The quality of the template is arguably the most important determinant of the subsequent RT-PCR results. The RNA should have the highest quality, free of DNA, without inhibitor to interfere with the RT or PCR steps, and without nucleases to cause degradation during testing or RNA storage. The most common problem is degradation of the RNA. The use of housekeeping genes, such as *ABL1*, has been widely used as internal reference for RT-PCR assays to demonstrate amplifiable RNA. The housekeeping gene should be expressed and degraded at about the same rate as the target fusion transcript and the amplified product should be longer to demonstrate RNA integrity.

Follow-up: The patient started ATRA treatment. A bone marrow biopsy revealed typical morphologic findings of APL. Conventional karyotyping revealed t(15;17). *PML-RARα* was detected in the bone marrow aspirate by RT-PCR. The patient achieved a complete morphologic remission at the end of the induction phase, and molecular remission at 6 weeks of therapy with no detectable *PML-RARα* by RT-PCR.

References

1. Genzen JR. Regulation of laboratory-developed tests. Am J Clin Pathol. 2019;152:122–31.
2. Jennings L, Van Deerlin VM, Gulley ML, College of American Pathologists Molecular Pathology Resource C. Recommended principles and practices for validating clinical molecular pathology tests. Arch Pathol Lab Med. 2009;133:743–55.
3. Schreier J, Feeney R, Keeling P. Diagnostics reform and harmonization of clinical laboratory testing. J Mol Diagn. 2019;21:737–45.
4. Roy S, Coldren C, Karunamurthy A, Kip NS, Klee EW, Lincoln SE, Leon A, Pullambhatla M, Temple-Smolkin RL, Voelkerding KV, Wang C, Carter AB. Standards and guidelines for validating next-generation sequencing bioinformatics pipelines: a joint recommendation of the Association for Molecular Pathology and the College of American Pathologists. J Mol Diagn. 2018;20:4–27.
5. Moncur JT, Bartley AN, Bridge JA, Kamel-Reid S, Lazar AJ, Lindeman NI, Long TA, Merker JD, Rai AJ, Rimm DL, Rothberg PG, Vasalos P, Kim AS. Performance comparison of different analytic methods in proficiency testing for mutations in the BRAF, EGFR, and KRAS genes: a study of the College of American Pathologists Molecular Oncology Committee. Arch Pathol Lab Med. 2019;143:1203–11.
6. Surrey LF, Oakley FD, Merker JD, Long TA, Vasalos P, Moncur JT, Kim AS. Next-generation sequencing (NGS) methods show superior or equivalent performance to non-NGS methods on BRAF, EGFR, and KRAS proficiency testing samples. Arch Pathol Lab Med. 2019;143:980–4.
7. Zehnbauer B, Lofton-Day C, Pfeifer J, Shaughnessy E, Goh L. Diagnostic quality assurance pilot: a model to demonstrate comparative laboratory test performance with an oncology companion diagnostic assay. J Mol Diagn. 2017;19:1–3.
8. Paek SH, Kim BS, Kang KH, Kim HS. False-negative BRAF V600E mutation results on fine-needle aspiration cytology of papillary thyroid carcinoma. World J Surg Oncol. 2017;15:202.

Part II

Molecular Pathology of Solid and Soft Tissue Tumors

Breast and Gynecologic Tumors

5

Huina Zhang and David G. Hicks

List of Frequently Asked Questions

I **Breast tumor**

1. What are the roles of molecular testing in breast pathology?
2. What are the most common hereditary mutations associated with breast cancer?
3. What are the main pathologic features of breast cancer associated with hereditary disease?
4. When should we consider recommending breast cancer patients for genetic testing for hereditary breast cancer?
5. What is the significance of identifying breast cancer patients with hereditary mutations?
6. Which genes should be included in genetic testing for hereditary breast cancer?
7. What are the testing methods for *BRCA* mutations?
8. What are the limitations of the genetic testing for hereditary breast cancer?
9. What is the molecular subclassification of breast cancer? What are the clinicopathologic features of breast cancers by molecular subclassification?
10. What is the relationship between triple-negative and basal-like subtype breast cancers?
11. When should the biomarkers in breast cancers be assessed?
12. Why does the ASCO/CAP recommend testing PR status in breast cancers although there is no targeted therapy?
13. When should we consider repeating biomarker testing in breast cancers on the resection specimen?
14. Should the biomarker status be repeated in the breast specimen status/post neoadjuvant therapy?
15. What are the key points of ASCO/CAP recommendations for pre-analytic variables for biomarker assessment in breast cancers? What are the common pre-analytic, analytic, and post-analytic factors that could affect the biomarker testing in breast cancer?
16. How to handle a bone specimen if it is suspicious for metastatic breast cancer?
17. Do the ASCO/CAP guidelines for biomarker tests in breast cancer exclude testing of cytology specimens (fluids and aspirates) that have been fixed in 95% ethanol rather than formalin?
18. How should we interpret the ER/PR staining results in breast cancers?
19. What are the semiquantitative scoring methods for immunohistochemical assessment of ER and PR in breast cancers?
20. What is the significance of the ER low positivity in breast cancer?
21. Are other ER expression assays acceptable for identifying patients likely to benefit from endocrine therapy?
22. What are the possible causes for the discordant ER status by IHC and RT-PCR (Oncotype Dx result)?
23. Which method is better for HER2 testing in breast cancers, immunohistochemistry (IHC), or in situ hybridization (ISH)?
24. When should the breast cancer case be considered for HER2 ISH testing if using IHC as the primary test?
25. What are single-probe and dual-probe assays in HER2 in situ hybridization assays? Which assay is better?
26. What are the HER2 ISH groups in breast cancers on dual-probe assays? What are the unusual HER2 groups?
27. What are the possible causes for the discordant HER2 results between IHC and ISH analyses?
28. What are the common discordances of biomarker status with histology or other clinicopathologic findings?

H. Zhang (✉) · D. G. Hicks
Department of Pathology and Laboratory Medicine,
University of Rochester Medical Center, Rochester, NY, USA
e-mail: Huina_Zhang@urmc.rochester.edu;
David_Hicks@urmc.rochester.edu

Y. Ding, L. Zhang (eds.), *Practical Oncologic Molecular Pathology*, Practical Anatomic Pathology,
https://doi.org/10.1007/978-3-030-73227-1_5

What are the possible causes for these discordances? How to solve these discordances?

29. What are the possible causes of discordant biomarker status between primary and metastatic breast tumors?
30. What are gene signature and molecular profiling of cancers? What are the roles of molecular profiling tests in early stage ER+ breast cancers? What are the commercially available molecular profiling tests for prognostication in early stage ER+ breast cancers?
31. When should we raise the suspicion for a major discordance between pathologic findings and Oncotype recurrence risk result? What shall we do if there is major discordance between the pathology result and Oncotype DX recurrence score (RS) result?
32. What is the role of testing the *PIK3CA* mutation in breast cancer?
33. How can molecular testing help in the diagnosis of breast tumors?

II **Gynecologic tumors**

1. What are the roles of molecular testing in gynecologic pathology?
2. Why testing *BRCA1* and *BRCA2* genomic status is important in patients with ovarian carcinomas?
3. What is homologous recombination deficiency (HRD)?
4. How to diagnose HRD?
5. In which individual should risk evaluation, counseling, and genomic testing for germline and somatic tumor alterations in ovarian cancer be performed?
6. What is the best approach for testing *BRCA* mutations in patients with ovarian/tubal/primary peritoneal carcinomas?
7. What is the significance of detecting deficient mismatch repair (dMMR) in patients with ovarian carcinomas?
8. What are the pathologic features of Lynch syndrome-associated endometrial cancer?
9. Why testing for mismatch repair protein is important in patients diagnosed with endometrial carcinomas?
10. Who should be screened for Lynch syndrome on tissue when diagnosed with endometrial cancer?
11. What are the common testing methods for screening Lynch syndrome?
12. How to interpret the immunohistochemical stains for MMR proteins? What are the pitfalls in the interpretation of MMR on IHC? How to resolve these pitfalls?
13. Should the mismatch repair protein testing be repeated in cases of tumor recurrence?
14. What is microsatellite instability (MSI)? What are the MSI testing methods? What are MSI-high, MSI-low, and MSI stable?
15. What is *MLH1* promoter methylation? How to test *MLH1* promoter methylation?
16. What are the possible causes for normal tissue testing result in patients with known MMR gene mutations? What are the possible causes for abnormal MSI/IHC results with non-detectable MMR gene mutations?
17. What are the advantages and disadvantages of IHC method, PCR-based MSI testing, and NGS-based MSI testing for Lynch syndrome screening?
18. What is the TCGA molecular classification of endometrial carcinomas?
19. What are the roles of molecular testing in endometrial stromal tumors?
20. What are the biomarker tests in endometrial carcinoma? How should these biomarkers be reported?
21. What is the role of HER2 testing in uterine serous carcinoma?
22. What is molecular human papillomavirus (HPV) testing in the cervical cytology specimen?
23. When should p16 immunostaining be performed in the lower anogenital squamous lesions?
24. What are the roles of molecular testing in sex cord stromal tumors of the ovary?
25. What are the roles of molecular testing in the diagnosis of gestational trophoblast disease?

Frequently Asked Questions

I **Breast tumor**

1. **What are the roles of molecular testing in breast pathology?**
   - Molecular testing for genetic and genomic variations has become an integral part of breast cancer management. The applications of molecular testing in breast pathology include the following:
     - Testing for hereditary DNA mutation in patients with breast cancer to define hereditary cancer syndrome and identify patients for selected therapy
     - Subclassifying molecular tumor types
     - Identifying biomarkers that can predict the response to treatment
     - Testing for genomic signatures in early stage estrogen receptor (ER) positive breast cancers for prognostication of cancers and predicating benefit from adjuvant chemotherapy
     - Testing for tumor genomic mutations to identify mutations for targeted therapy in metastatic breast cancer or other experimental therapy for precision medicine purpose

– Testing for specific translocations/markers to facilitate the diagnosis of certain breast cancers

2. **What are the most common hereditary mutations associated with breast cancer?**
   - Approximately 5–10% of breast cancers are linked to a specific inherited high penetrance germline mutation in a breast cancer susceptibility gene [1].
   - The common hereditary mutations in breast cancers include *BRCA1/2, PALB2*, Li-Fraumeni syndrome (*TP53* pathologic variant), Cowden syndrome (*PTEN* pathologic variant), hereditary diffuse gastric cancer syndrome (*CDH1* pathologic variant), and Peutz-Jeghers syndrome (*STK11* pathologic variant). Among them, more than 50% of these pathologic germline variants are mutations of *BRCA1* and *BRCA2* genes, and women have a 57–60% and 49–55% lifetime risk of developing breast cancer if they carry a *BRCA1* or *BRCA2* mutation, respectively [2–5].

3. **What are the main pathologic features of breast cancer associated with hereditary disease?**
   - The majority (~75%) of *BRCA1/2* associated breast cancer is ductal carcinoma.
   - When compared to the sporadic breast cancer, a significant higher frequency of *BRCA1/2*-associated tumors are present in younger patients, having higher histologic grade with medullary pathologic features (circumscribed border, high histologic grade, brisk host immune cell response) and somatic *TP53* mutations. The tumor is usually ER negative/progesterone receptor (PR) negative/human epidermal growth factor receptor 2 (HER2) negative/epidermal growth factor receptor (EGFR) positive in *BRCA1*-associated cancers (see Fig. 5.1), while in the *BRCA2*-associated breast cancers, the biomarker expressions are similar to those in the sporadic breast cancers [5, 6].

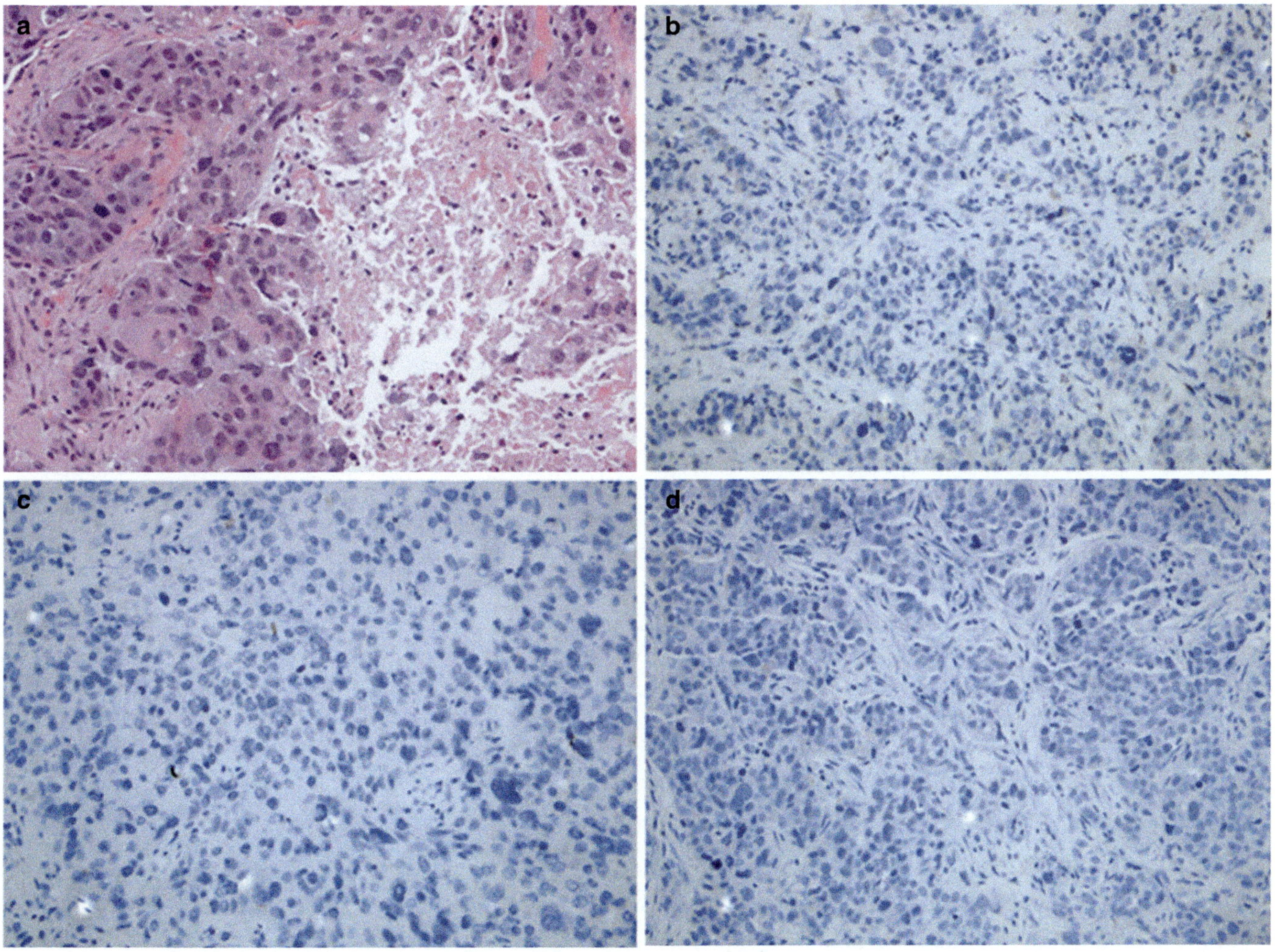

Fig. 5.1 Invasive ductal carcinoma in a 38-year-old woman with known *BRCA1* deleterious mutation. H&E section shows high-grade morphology with frequent mitotic figures and focal necrosis (**a**, ×200). The tumor cells are negative for ER (**b**, ×200), PR (**c**, ×200), and HER2 (**d**, ×200)

- The pathologic features of breast cancer associated with other pathologic germline mutations are less characterized.

4. **When should we consider recommending breast cancer patients for genetic testing for hereditary breast cancer?**
   - According to the National Comprehensive Cancer Network (NCCN) guidelines [7], clinicians should consider genetic testing for breast cancer patients in:
     - 50 years old or younger
     - Triple-negative breast cancer at an age younger than 60 years old
     - Male patients with breast cancer
     - Bilateral or a second primary breast cancer
     - Prior history of ovarian cancer
     - For individuals without the personal history and additional family history criteria must be met including:
   - At least one relative with breast cancer diagnosed at 50 years old or younger
   - One relative with ovarian cancer
   - More than two relatives with breast cancer, prostate cancer (Gleason score≥7 or metastatic disease), or pancreatic cancer.
   - The recent guidelines from the American Society of Breast Surgeons recommended that genetic testing should be offered to all breast cancer patients, both newly diagnosed and those with a previous personal history, or patients without breast cancer but who otherwise meet NCCN guidelines [8].
5. **What is the significance of identifying breast cancer patients with hereditary mutations?**
   - Identification of patients with pathologic variants of these hereditary mutations can impact patient management in terms of high-risk testing, surveillance, risk reduction, and therapeutic intervention related to surgery, radiation, and system therapy including the application of poly(ADP-ribose) polymerase (PAPR) inhibitors.
   - It also has potential impact on the patient's family member health and management.
6. **Which genes should be included in genetic testing for hereditary breast cancer?**
   - A wide variety of genetic testing panels are available with different genes on different panels.
   - There is lack of consensus among professional societies and experts regarding which genes should be tested in different clinical scenarios, but it is recommended that the panel should include at least *BRCA1/BRCA2* and *PALB2*, with other genes as appropriate for the clinical scenarios and family history.
   - A survey among clinicians and clinical scientists in UK recommended gene panel with majority agreement (>75%) for breast cancer should include *BRCA1*, *BRCA2*, *PALB2*, *PTEN*, *STK11*, *TP53*, *CHEK2* (truncating variants), and *ATM* (truncating variants plus ATM c.7271T>G, p.(Val2424Gly) [9].
7. **What are the testing methods for *BRCA* mutations?**
   - The predominant genetic test for *BRCA1* and *BRCA2* mutations was BRACA*nalysis* (Myriad Genetic Laboratories, Utah, USA):
     - The testing is performed via forward and reverse sequencing of amplified DNA aliquots obtained from patient's buccal mucosa or peripheral blood sample.
     - Variants of the BRACA*nalysis* test include (1) BRACA*nalysis* rearrangement test, which is indicated for patients who are suspected of having a *BRCA* mutation; (2) single-site BRACA*nalysis*, which is indicated for patients with a known familial mutation; and (3) multisite 3 BRACA*nalysis*, which is indicated for patients with Ashkenazi Jewish heritage.
   - Since 2013, genetic options to include gene mutation panels have been expanded by university-based and private laboratories.
   - The standard method for the laboratory assessment of BRCA genes includes comprehensive sequencing and testing of broad genomic rearrangements including next-generation multi-gene sequencing.
   - If the patient has a relative with a particular mutation, a single-site targeted mutation analysis can also be performed.
   - The results are broadly described in three ways: (1) positive for a deleterious mutation, (2) genetic variant, and (3) no deleterious mutations.
8. **What are the limitations of the genetic testing for hereditary breast cancer** [8, 9]**?**
   - It is only one of several tools for assessing breast cancer risk and the result is not always straightforward with clear guideline. The negative result does not necessarily mean that they are not at increased risk for developing breast cancer, and other contributing factors such as age, medical history, family history, life style, and exposure should also be considered.
   - Testing a larger number of genes will result in finding more variants of uncertain significance, which causes difficulty in interpreting and explaining the results, and can leave families with more questions than answers.
   - Finding a pathogenic variant in a moderate-risk gene in the context of a high-risk family history does not

always aid clinical management since the variant cannot be assumed to account for all of the genetic risks in the family.

9. **What is the molecular subclassification of breast cancer? What are the clinicopathologic features of breast cancers by molecular subclassification?**
   - Breast cancers have traditionally been classified based on clinicopathological features, mainly histologic type, histologic grade, and tumor stage. With the advancement in detecting biomarker expression profile, breast cancer can be classified into ER positive, ER negative, HER2 positive, HER2 negative, and triple-negative categories. This simplified molecular classification system remains the most important and informative molecular breast cancer taxonomy to date for clinical management in routine practice [10].
   - In 2000, Perou and colleagues [11] studied 8,102 human genes on 65 breast specimens by using complementary DNA (cDNA) microarray and unsupervised cluster analysis. Their results indicated each tumor was unique and had distinct gene expression signatures, which led to a selection of 496 "intrinsic gene subset" and subsequently revealed five distinct classes of breast carcinomas: luminal A, luminal B, ERBB2 (HER2)-enriched, basal-like, and normal breast-like in an extended analysis [12, 13].
     - The luminal tumors were named as such because of the high expression of genes normally expressed by luminal epithelium of the breast. These luminal tumors also express ER and ER-related genes.
     - The ERBB2 (HER2)-enriched tumors were characterized by high expression of several genes in the *ERBB2* amplicon at 17q22.24 including ERBB2, GRB7, and TRAP100.
     - The basal-like tumors were named due to the high expression of KRT5, KRT17, annexin 8, CX3CL1, and TRIM29 and were completely negative for the luminal/ER cluster of genes.
     - The normal breast-like group has been shown to have the highest expression of many genes known to be expressed by adipose tissue and other non-epithelial cell types, and it is unclear whether these tumors represent poorly sampled tumor tissue or a distinct, clinically important group [14].
   - In addition, other molecular subtypes including claudin-low and molecular apocrine types have later been identified, and both groups are considered defined molecular subgroups of triple negative breast cancer [15–17].
   - Each of these molecular subtypes is characterized by different clinical features such as significant difference in overall survival, relapse-free survival, and pattern of recurrence, independent of traditional pathologic features. Table 5.1 lists the clinicopathologic characteristics and key molecular features of most common molecular subtypes of breast cancer.
10. **What is the relationship between triple-negative and basal-like subtype breast cancers?**
    - The triple-negative breast cancers (TNBC) are characterized by the absence of ER and PR expression and lack of overexpression/amplification of HER2.
    - Basal-like subtype of breast cancer in the abovementioned molecular subclassification refers to a distinct gene expression signature characterized by high expression of basal epithelial markers such as cytokeratin 5, 6, and 17. Both TNBCs and triple-like breast cancers are associated with poor prognosis and show disproportionally higher prevalence in African women.
    - The majority (~70%) of TNBCs are found to be basal-like by gene expression, and recent studies using hierarchical clustering have identified four stable TNBC subtypes including two basal-like, mesenchymal, and luminal androgen receptor subtypes [23, 24].
    - Most basal-like cancers (50–77%) are triple negative in nature [25, 26].
11. **When should the biomarkers in breast cancers be assessed?**
    - According to the American Society of Clinical Oncology (ASCO)/College of American Pathologists (CAP) guidelines [27, 28]:
      - The evaluation of biomarkers including ER, PR, and HER2 should be performed in all patients with newly diagnosed invasive breast cancer and in recurrent and metastatic breast cancers when the tissue sample is available.
      - The evaluation of ER in cases of newly diagnosed ductal carcinoma in situ (DCIS, without association invasion) is recommended and PR testing is considered optional in DCIS.
12. **Why does the ASCO/CAP recommend testing PR status in breast cancers although there is no targeted therapy?**
    - Upon binding by progesterone, the progesterone receptors dimerize, bind progesterone responsive elements (PRE) in the promoters of a number of genes, and thus induce transcription of these genes including those regulating proliferation.
    - PR status serves as an indicator of intact ER function since PR expression can be regulated by ER. The possible mechanisms of PR loss in the ER positive breast cancers include the aberrant

Table 5.1 The clinicopathologic characteristics and key molecular features of most common molecular subtypes of breast cancer

Molecular subtypes	Luminal A	Luminal B	HER2 enriched	Basal-like
% of breast cancer	~30–40%	~20–30%	10–15%	15–20%
Age	Older age	Younger	Younger	Younger
Histologic grade	1–2	2–3	2–3	Typically 3
Common histologic types	IC-NST(well-differentiated), classic lobular, tubular, cribriform, mucinous, neuroendocrine	IC-NST, micropapillary	IC-NST, apocrine, pleomorphic lobular	IC-NST, medullary features, metaplastic, adenoid cystic, secretory
ER status by IHC	Positive (high)	Positive (maybe low)	Negative	Mostly negative
PR status by IHC	Usually positive	Negative or low positive	Negative	Mostly negative
HER2 by IHC or FISH	Negative	Positive in ~40% (luminal HER2)	Positive (Classic HER2)	Negative
Ki-67	Low (<10%)	Typically high (>14%)	Typically high (>20%)	Typically very high (>50%)
CK5/6 or EGFR	Negative	Negative	Occasionally positive	50–85% positive
Key molecular features [1, 18]	*PIK3CA* mutations, *MAP3K1* mutations, *ESR1* high expression, *XBP1* high expression, *GATA* mutations, *FOXA1* mutations; quiet genomes, gain of 1q, 8q, loss of 8p, 16q	*TP53* mutations, *PIK3CA* mutations, *Cyclin* D1 amplifications, *MDM2* amplifications, *ATM* loss, enhanced genomic instability, focal amplifications	*ERBB2* amplifications, *TP53* mutations, *PIK3CA* mutations, *FGFR4* high expression, *EGFR* high expression, *APOBEC* mutations, *Cyclin D1* amplifications, high genomic instability	*TP53* mutations, *RB1* loss, *BRCA1* loss, high expression of DNA repair proteins, *FOXM1* activation, high genomic instability, focal amplifications (e.g., 8q24)
Natural history	Indolent, possible late recurrence	More aggressive than luminal A	Worse natural history; sensitive to HER2-targeted therapy	Worse natural history except for some special types, early recurrence more likely
Local recurrence [19]	0.8–8%	1.5–8.7%	4–15% (without HER2 targeted therapy)	3–17%
Neoadjuvant response (pCR rate) [20, 21]	~2%	~6%	≥ 57%	~34%
Type of therapy [22]	Endocrine therapy alone	Endocrine ± systemic chemotherapy Luminal HER2: Add HER2-targeted therapy	Systemic chemotherapy+ targeted therapy	Systemic chemotherapy

EGFR epidermal growth factor receptor, *FISH* fluorescent in situ hybridization, *ER* estrogen receptor, *HER2* human epidermal growth factor receptor 2, *IC-NST* invasive carcinoma of no special type, *IHC* immunohistochemistry, *pCR* pathologic complete response, *PR* progesterone receptor

ER-alpha signaling pathway, loss of PR gene, or downregulation by HER2 [29, 30].

- PR status has predominant prognostic values in the ER-positive breast cancers. When ER-positive invasive breast carcinoma has low or negative PR expression, it is usually high-grade tumor with higher mitotic activity (luminal type B), and the prognosis is worse than the ER+/PR+ breast cancers and is less responsive to hormonal therapy.
- Therefore, although only ER should be used as a predictor of benefit from adjuvant endocrine therapy, the ASCO/CAP updated ER/PR testing guidelines continue to recommend routine PR testing in invasive breast cancers [27].

13. **When should we consider repeating biomarker testing in breast cancers on the resection specimen?**
    - Initial core biopsy shows borderline, insufficient, equivocal, unusual, or discordant with clinicopathologic findings.
    - The invasive tumor shows high grade morphology with negative HER2 result on the initial core.
    - Tumor shows morphologic heterogeneity or high grade on the resection specimen.
    - Limited tumor cells on core biopsy.
    - Any suspicions on the tissue handling or testing errors on core biopsy.

14. **Should the biomarker status be repeated in the breast specimen status/post neoadjuvant therapy?**
    - Neoadjuvant chemotherapy (NAC) has been increasingly used for breast cancer. Studies have reported that the discordance rates between pre- and post-neoadjuvant therapy were up to 46% for ER and up to 43% for HER2 [see Reviews 31, 32]. The possible explanations for these discrepancies include intra-tumoral heterogeneity, treatment effect of targeted therapy, different antibody clones or methods, specimen handling/processing, and result interpretation variability.
    - Currently there are no guidelines regarding whether the biomarker studies should be repeated in the residual tumor after NAC. Whether to retest the biomarkers after NAC is an institutional-dependent decision or on a case by case basis.
    - Retesting of these biomarkers must be performed if previously unknown or if required by clinical trial. One may consider retesting if the pre-therapy results were negative, the pre-therapy tumor sample was insufficient, residual tumor shows heterogenous morphology, there are multiple tumors with different morphologic appearance, or if requested by clinicians [33].
    - It needs to be noted that a few studies have suggested that fluorescence in situ hybridization (FISH) analysis is preferred to immunohistochemistry (IHC) when retesting for HER2 because FISH analysis is more stable than IHC [34, 35].
15. **What are the key points of ASCO/CAP recommendations for pre-analytic variables for biomarker assessment in breast cancers? What are the common pre-analytic, analytic, and post-analytic factors that could affect the biomarker testing in breast cancer?**
    - According to the most updated ASCO/CAP recommendations, the key points for pre-analytic variables for biomarker (ER, PR and HER2) assessment in breast cancers include [27, 28]:
      - Minimize cold ischemic time (time intervals between tissue removal from patient to exposure to formalin fixation) to 1 h or less.
      - Use 10% neutral buffered formalin as the standard fixative.
      - Tissue fixation time is at least 6 h, but no more than 72 h. This applies to both core biopsy and resection specimens. For specimens fixed longer than 72 h in which negative test results are obtained, the report should state that prolonged fixation could be a possible cause for the negative result, and alternative testing methods should be considered (e.g., FISH for HER2; gene expression assay for ER). For HER2 testing, labs should also consider confirming by FISH on any specimen fixed longer than 72 h, especially when it is not HER2 positive by IHC (score of 3+).
      - Unstained slides cut more than 6 weeks should not be used for analysis.
      - The common pre-analytic, analytic, and post-analytic factors that could affect the biomarker testing in breast cancer include prolonged cold ischemic times (>1 h), strong decalcification process or inadequate fixation, test methodology differences and standards or test interpretation criteria and methods, and under/over interpretation.
16. **How to handle a bone specimen if it is suspicious for metastatic breast cancer?**
    - Bone is the most common site of breast cancer involvement and the bone specimen always requires decalcification.
    - The current ASCO/CAP guidelines do not recommend a specific decalcification process for biomarker testing. The guidelines state that the sample with decalcification artifacts should be rejected, and the sample that was decalcified in a strong acid solution may be rejected [28].
    - It has been demonstrated that EDTA decalcification is the preferred method since it has been shown to be molecular friendly and that it minimally affects the biomarker expression results [36].
17. **Do the ASCO/CAP guidelines for biomarker tests in breast cancer exclude testing of cytology specimens (fluids and aspirates) that have been fixed in 95% ethanol rather than formalin?**
    - According to CAP [37], fixatives other than formalin are not precluded by the guidelines.
    - For tissue specimens, laboratories that choose to use a fixative other than neutral buffered formalin must validate that fixative's performance against the results of testing of the same samples fixed in neutral buffered formalin and tested with the identical assay.
    - Since cytology specimens are not ordinarily fixed in formalin such concordance studies are not practical, but labs performing testing on such specimens must document that they validated their methods and achieved acceptable concordance, perhaps by comparing staining of alcohol-fixed cytology specimens with subsequently excised routinely processed, formalin-fixed, surgical pathology specimens.

18. **How should we interpret the ER/PR staining results in breast cancers?**
    - According to the ASCO/CAP guidelines, ER/PR in breast invasive cancers and carcinoma in situ should be interpreted [27]:
      – ER- or PR-positive cancer is one in which ≥1% of invasive carcinoma/carcinoma in situ cell nuclei show immunoreactivity. If 1–10% of invasive tumor cell nuclei are immunoreactive for ER, the sample should be reported as ER low positive with a recommended comment (This does not apply to PR).
      – ER- or PR-negative cancer is one in which <1% or 0% of invasive carcinoma/carcinoma in situ cell nuclei show immunoreactivity, regardless of staining intensity.
      – ER and/or PR status is not interpretable if the sample is inadequate (insufficient cancer or severe artifacts present), if the external and internal controls do not show appropriate and acceptable staining, or if pre-analytic variables have interfered with the assay's accuracy.
      – Interpretation of any ER result should include evaluation of the concordance with the histologic findings of each case.
      – For cases without internal controls present and with positive external controls, an additional report comment is recommended.
19. **What are the semiquantitative scoring methods for immunohistochemical assessment of ER and PR in breast cancers?**
    - The H score is also called "histo" score and is a method of assessing the extent of nuclear immunoreactivity. The score is calculated by the formula: 3 × percentage of strongly staining nuclei +2 × percentage of moderately staining nuclei +1 × percentage of weakly staining nuclei +0 × percentage of no staining nuclei, giving a range of 0–300.
    - The Allred score is calculated by adding the proportion score (PS, score 0–5 depends on the proportion of tumor cells which are stained) and the intensity score (IS, score 0–3 depends on the intensity of staining), giving a final score of 0–8.
    - The Quickscore is similar to the Allred score system, but the final score is calculated by multiplying the percentage score (score 0–6 depends on the proportion of tumor cells which are stained) and intensity score (score 0–3 depends on the intensity of staining), together giving a final score of 0–18.
20. **What is the significance of the ER low positivity in breast cancer?**
    - The newly released ASCO/CAP updated ER/PR testing guidelines specifically addressed the low ER-expressing breast cancers.
    - Low ER positive breast cancer refers to the tumor cells showing 1–10% ER expression by immunohistochemistry, which accounts for ~2–3% of breast cancers [38].
    - Recent studies showed that the breast cancers with low ER positivity is a heterogenous group, more often to have basal-like intrinsic subtype than luminal subtype including high-grade morphology, sheet-like growth pattern, and the presence of tumor necrosis. These low-ER positivity breast cancers usually fail to show survival benefit from hormonal therapy although the overall prognosis is slightly better than the ER negative breast cancers [27, 39, 40].
    - When one encounters such a case, other clinicopathologic variables such as age, histologic grade, tumor size, PR status, and molecular assays such as PAM50 or BluePrint may be helpful in making clinical decisions.
21. **Are other ER expression assays acceptable for identifying patients likely to benefit from endocrine therapy?**
    - According to the ASCO/CAP updated ER/PR testing guidelines [27], validated IHC is the recommended gold standard test for predicting benefit from endocrine therapy in patients with breast cancer, and no other assay types are recommended as the primary screening test.
    - Data on the ability of new methods of ER testing such as mRNA testing in the panel-based gene expression assays to predict endocrine therapy benefit for breast cancer as an initial screening test are limited.
22. **What are the possible causes for the discordant ER status by IHC and RT-PCR (Oncotype Dx result)?**
    - Earlier studies have demonstrated good agreement (93–98.9%) for ER status between RT-PCR-based methods and IHC, with IHC being slightly more sensitive [41, 42]. However, the tumor rarely can be ER positive by IHC and negative by RT-PCR quantitative result on an Oncotype DX assay.
    - The possible causes for this discordance include low ER positive/borderline result, false positive IHC result due to mis-interpretation, or low cancer cellularity (such as what might be seen with invasive lobular carcinoma) that causes false negative RT-PCR results.
    - It is always important to correlate the ER-testing results with other histopathologic features.
23. **Which method is better for HER2 testing in breast cancers, immunohistochemistry (IHC), or in situ hybridization (ISH)?**
    - Currently, there are several FDA-approved methods to evaluate HER2 status in breast cancer including

IHC assessment of HER2 protein expression and in situ hybridization (ISH) for gene amplification, most commonly FISH.

- Both IHC and ISH are clinically validated to help predict the response of the tumor to the HER2-targeted therapy, and each method has its own advantages and disadvantages.
- The ASCO/CAP guidelines do not recommend one test over the other, and both assays could be used to assess the HER2 status of breast cancers if the test had been appropriately validated and the laboratory follows the recommendations of the guidelines.
- Worldwide, most laboratories use IHC as the primary test with reflex FISH analysis in the equivocal cases or discordant cases. It is also acceptable to do ISH testing as first-line testing method (with appropriate reflex IHC testing) or to do IHC and ISH co-testing in all cases.
- The main advantages of IHC are that it is easy to perform, is relatively inexpensive, and has permanent storage. The major disadvantages of IHC include considerable interobserver variability, less reliability since IHC can be significantly affected by specimen handling, antigen retrieval methods, and antibody specificity and sensitivity. These disadvantages have largely decreased since the introduction of the highly standardized Hercep test, the use of fully automated staining system, and the published ASCO/CAP testing guidelines [43].
- The main advantages of FISH include more objective and quantitative results, more accurate and less impacted by pre-analytical factors. The major disadvantages of FISH include being labor intensive and costly, more time-consuming, requirement of costly equipment, faded signals, and possible missed tumor heterogeneity [43].

24. **When should the breast cancer case be considered for HER2 ISH testing, if using IHC as the primary test?**
    - HER2 is scored 2+ by IHC.
    - HER2 IHC shows granular, cytoplasmic staining that is difficult to interpret the extent of membranous staining.
    - Cases with significant crush artifact that disrupts the membranous staining.
    - HER2 IHC shows moderate-strong but incomplete staining or basolateral pattern.
    - HER2 IHC shows heterogeneity.
25. **What are single-probe and dual-probe assays in HER2 in situ hybridization assay? Which assay is better?**
    - In breast cancer, the ISH assay is used to quantify the HER2 gene copy number within tumor cell nuclei. ISH can be performed either as a single-probe assay (HER2 probe only) or dual-probe assay (using differentially labeled HER2 and chromosome 17 centromere probes simultaneously).
    - Single-probe assays: If single-probe assays are used, only the average HER2 signals per cell are counted. If the average HER2 signals per cell$\geq$ 6, the tumor is considered as HER2 positive; if the average HER2 signals per cell<4, the tumor is considered as HER2 negative. For cases with $\geq$4 but <6 average HER2 signals per cell, the concurrent HER2 IHC on the same block need to be reviewed. If the concurrent IHC shows positive (3+), then it is considered as ISH positive; if the concurrent IHC shows negative (0 or 1+), it is ISH negative. If the concurrent IHC shows equivocal (2+), then a dual-probe ISH needs to be performed for a final result.
    - Dual-probe assays: When using the dual-probe assays, one probe for the HER2 gene and one probe for the control gene in chromosome 17 will be counted. The interpretations for dual-probe ISH are based on the HER2/CEP17 ratio and the average HER2 signals/cell, and the result will fall into one of five result groups (see detailed below in Question 26).
    - The current ASCO/CAP testing guidelines also recommend the use of dual-probe instead of single-probe methods, although it recognizes that several single-probe ISH assays have regulatory approval in many parts of the world.
26. **What are the HER2 ISH groups in breast cancers on dual-probe assays? What are the unusual HER2 groups?**
    - There are five HER2 ISH groups in breast cancers when using dual-probe assays:
      - Group 1 (positive): HER2/CEP17 ratio$\geq$2.0 and average HER2 signals per cell $\geq$4.0
      - Group 2: HER2/CEP17 ratio $\geq$ 2.0 and average HER2 copy number < 4.0 signals per cell
      - Group 3: HER2/CEP17 ratio <2.0 and average HER2 copy number $\geq$ 6.0 signals per cell
      - Group 4: HER2/CEP17 ratio < 2.0 and average HER2 copy number $\geq$ 4.0 and < 6.0 signals per cell
      - Group 5 (negative): HER2/CEP 17 ratio <2.0 and average HER2 signals per cell <4.0
    - The unusual HER2 ISH groups refer to groups 2, 3, and 4 on dual-probe assays (see Table 5.2).
    - ISH workup of an IHC HER2 equivocal (2+) breast carcinoma case using a dual-probe assay. Between 2013 and 2018, cases with equivocal HER2 ISH results were often sent for additional testing using alternative probes. However, this strategy was challenged based on the evidence that the indiscriminate use of alternative control probes to calculate

Table 5.2 HER2 ISH unusual group by dual-probe assay

HER2 ISH result	Group 2 (Monosomy)	Group 3 (Co-amplified/polysomy)	Group 4
Incidence (ISH testing)	0.4–3.7%	0.4–3.0%	1.9–14.2%
Reasons	Amplification of the *HER2* gene and an associated increased HER2 copy number, with a loss of chromosome 17 copy number	Either polysomy of chromosome 17 or more commonly co-amplification of both the *HER2* and *CEP17* genes	Mainly heterozygous deletions
Histologic features	Usually ER+ (~80%) Majority histologic grade 2 and 3	Typically ER+ (75%) Majority histologic grade 2 and 3	Usually ER+ (~82%) Majority histologic grade 2 and 3
HER2 IHC	Negative to equivocal:~88% IHC3+: ~12.4%	Negative to equivocal:~48% IHC3+:~31.7%	Negative to equivocal:~92.7% IHC3+:~7.3%

ER estrogen receptor, *IHC* immunohistochemistry, *ISH* in situ hybridization

HER2 ISH ratios in HER2-equivocal breast cancers may lead to false-positive interpretations of HER2 status, resulting from unrecognized heterozygous deletions of these alternative control genomic sites and incorrect HER2 ratio determinations [44, 45]. The 2018 ASCO/CAP guidelines discontinued the recommendation for using an alternative control probe to resolve ISH equivocal cases. Figure 5.2 illustrates the ISH workup of an IHC HER2 equivocal (2+) breast carcinoma case using a dual-probe assay, according to the most recent ASCO/CAP guidelines.

27. **What are the possible causes for the discordant HER2 results between IHC and ISH analyses?**
    - False-negative IHC results due to tissue handling.
    - False-positive IHC results due to analytic and post-analytic errors.
    - Unusual ISH positive group (such as HER2/CEP17 ratio>2 and the average HER2 copy number between 4–6, group 1b) or tumor heterogeneity.
    - It has been recommended to use HER2 IHC slides as the guide map for ISH analysis and to coordinate between IHC and ISH results for HER2 interpretation.
28. **What are the common discordances of biomarker status with histology or other clinicopathologic findings? What are the possible causes for these discordances? How to solve these discordances?**
    - ER negative or HER2 positive (score 3+, by IHC) results in a grade 1 invasive ductal or lobular cancers, pure tubular, cribriform, or mucinous cancers.
    - The possible causes include, but are not limited to, incorrect initial histologic classification, false negative/positive result, or specimen mix-up.
    - When this discordance occurs, reviewing the original H&E slide for confirmation of histologic discordance, repeating testing on the same or different blocks, sending the specimen for HER2 ISH analysis, or exploring the possible pre-analytic, analytic, and post-analytic causes can be helpful.
    - It needs to be noted that rare low-grade breast cancers can be HER2 positive, such as ~5–6% of classical or nonpleomorphic invasive lobular carcinomas are HER2 positive [46, 47]. Fig. 5.3 demonstrates a classical invasive lobular carcinoma with positive HER2 expression.
29. **What are the possible causes of discordant biomarker status between primary and metastatic breast tumors?**
    - It is widely accepted that receptor conversion occurs during metastatic progression of breast cancer and the reported incidence is variable. For example, Schrijver et al. reported in their meta-analysis that the pooled percentage of positive to negative conversion during metastasis in ER, PR, and HER2 was 22.5%, 49.4%, and 21.3%, respectively; conversely, the percentage of negative to positive conversion was 21.5%, 15.9%, and 9.5% [48]. In the study of Woo et al., positive to negative conversion was found in 5.3%, 24.3%, and 5.9% while negative to positive conversion was found in 0.7%, 2.0%, and 2.0% for ER, PR, and HER2, respectively [49].
    - The possible causes of discordance of biomarker status between primary and metastatic breast tumors include heterogeneity for the biomarker expression in tumor cells, loss of ER expression due to clonal selection and disease progression, treatment effect of targeted therapy, unusual or borderline/equivocal results for HER2, false-negative result for ER in the metastatic tumor due to tissue handling, false-negative initial HER2 result, or different testing methods for HER2.

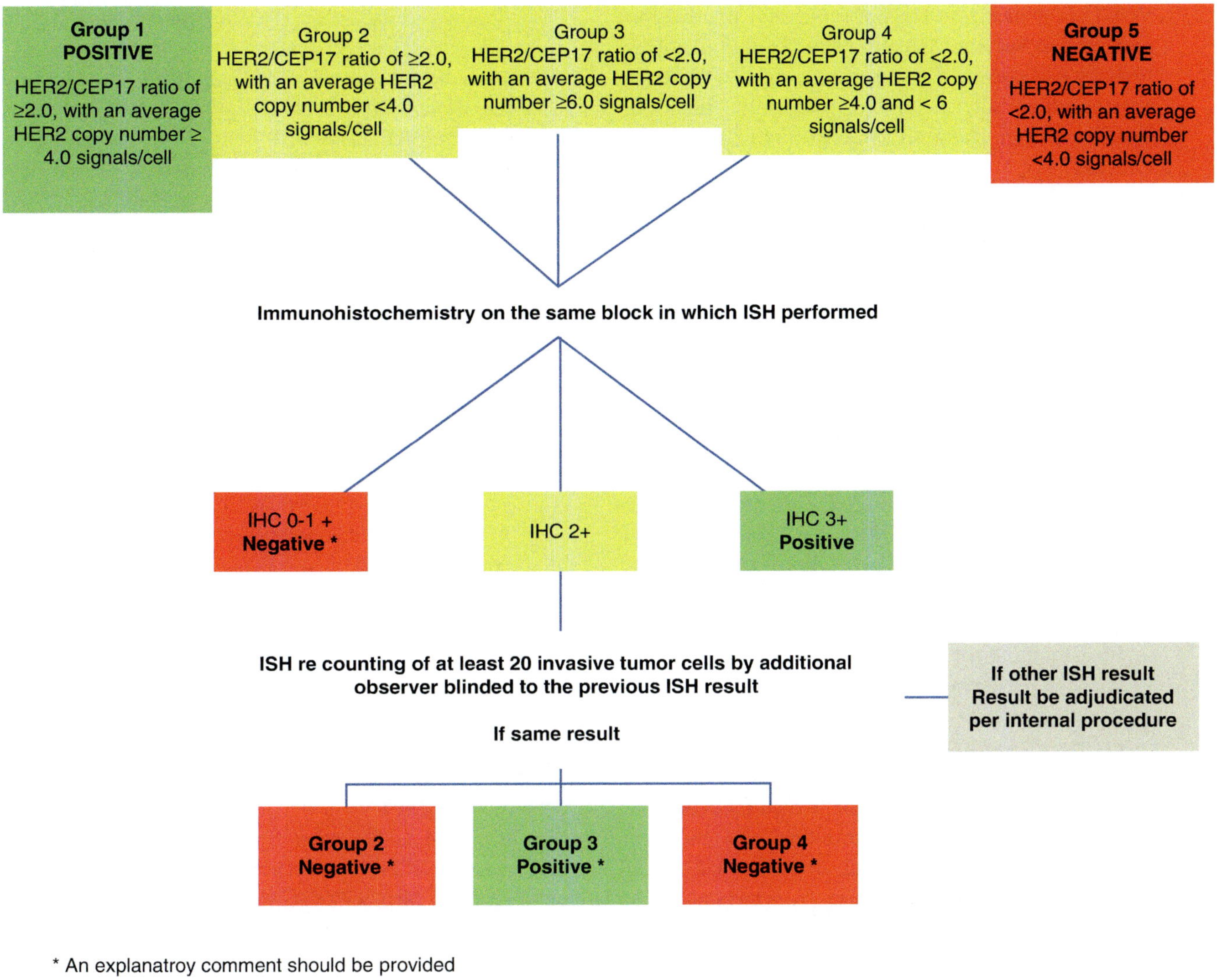

Fig. 5.2 The ISH workup of an IHC HER2 equivocal (2+) breast carcinoma case using a dual-probe assay. Used with permission: Zhang H, Moisini I, Ajabnoor RM, Turner BM, Hicks DG. Applying the New Guidelines of HER2 Testing in Breast Cancer. Curr Oncol Rep. 2020;22:51

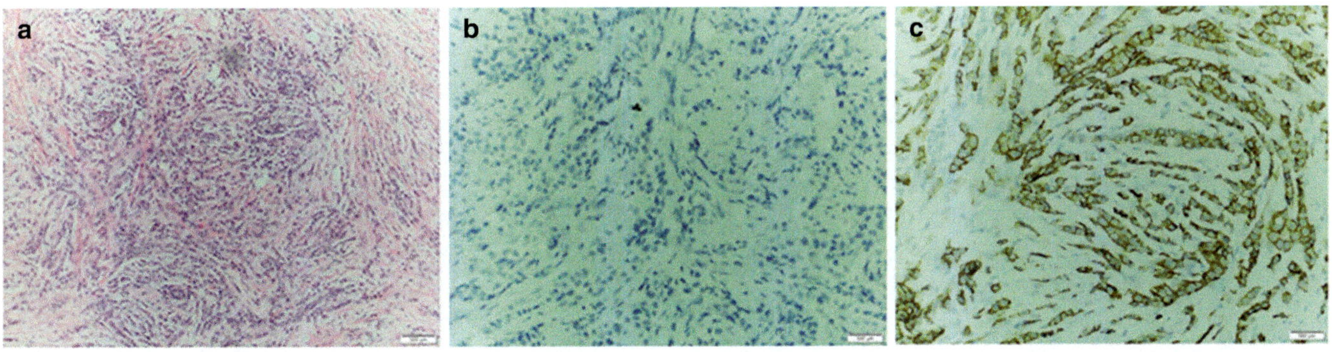

Fig. 5.3 Classical invasive lobular carcinoma with positive HER2 expression. (**a**) H&E: ×200; (**b**) Tumor cells are negative for E-cadherin (×200); (**c**) Tumor cells are positive for HER2 by immunohistochemistry (score 3+, ×200)

30. **What are gene signature and molecular profiling of cancers? What are the roles of molecular profiling tests in early-stage ER+ breast cancers? What are the commercially available molecular profiling tests for prognostication in early-stage ER+ breast cancers?**
    - A gene signature refers to a group of genes in a cell whose combined expression pattern is uniquely characteristic of a biological phenotype or medical condition. Molecular profiling refers to the assessment of DNA, RNA, and/or protein within an individual patient's tumor using cells obtained from a tumor biopsy or through the capture of tumor cells circulating in the bloodstream. The results of molecular profiling test can (1) reveal the genetic characteristics and any unique biomarkers; (2) give the risk score and the recurrence free survival rate for each patient; and (3) identify and create targeted therapies that are designed to work better for a specific cancer tumor profile.
    - In clinical practice, ER positive/HER2 negative breast cancer is the most commonly encountered but also the most challenging group for treatment due to significant clinical heterogeneity. It is crucial to identify those tumors with more aggressive biology that may benefit from additional chemotherapy from those tumors that can be treated by endocrine therapy alone. Molecular profiling tests can help determine the prognosis for an individual cancer patient with ER positive cancer, which is either node negative (largest group) or node positive, with the goal being to identify the low-risk group, in whom risks of adjuvant systemic chemotherapy outweigh the predicted benefit. Molecular profiling also identifies the patients with high risk, who are likely to respond to systemic chemotherapy. The result of molecular profiling tests plays an important role in clinical decision making in the era of precision medicine.
    - The commercially available molecular profiling tests for ER positive breast cancer include Oncotype Dx test, MammaPrint test, Prosigna test, EndoPredict test, Breast Cancer Index test, Mammostrate, and IHC4 (see Table 5.3).
    - When choosing the block for molecular profiling tests, the most ideal sample should have the largest area of invasive carcinoma available (usually resection specimen is preferred), avoiding the areas of biopsy site changes, inflammation, carcinoma in situ, or normal tissue as much as possible. Cases with only microinvasion or blocks from metastatic carcinoma in a lymph node are generally not appropriate for molecular profiling test due to the interference of non-cancer tissue and the potential to skew the assay results.
31. **When should we raise the suspicion for a major discordance between pathologic findings and Oncotype recurrence risk result? What shall we do if there is major discordance between the pathology result and Oncotype DX recurrence score (RS) result?**
    - The major discordance between pathologic findings and oncotype recurrence risk result should be concerned:
      - When the recurrence score of a tumor is higher than the expected such as a high RS score in a low-grade tumor with low proliferation index
      - When the quantitative ER result on Oncotype DX is negative or much lower compared to IHC result
    - If such major discordance is present, the pathologist can:
      - Review the original H&E section for the tested block to see whether there is large areas of biopsy site changes or inflammation
      - Retesting on additional material, either from different block without biopsy site changes or inflammation, or the biopsy material
32. **What is the role of testing *PIK3CA* mutation in breast cancer?**
    - *PIK3CA* is the most frequently mutated gene in ER+/HER2– breast cancer and up to 40% of these cancers carry a *PIK3CA* mutation [50].
    - In results from the phase III SOLAR-1 study, patients with *PIK3CA* mutations and prior endocrine therapy had significantly improved progression-free survival when treated with PI3K alpha-specific inhibitors alpelisib and fulvestrant compared to fulvestrant alone (11.0 vs. 5.7 months) [51].
    - *PIK3CA* mutation CDx testing is an FDA-approved qualitative companion diagnostic assay performed on DNA extracted from FFPE breast tissue to detect 11 mutations in exons 8, 10, and 21 of the *PIK3CA* gene (NM_006218.4; transcript ID: ENST00000263967.4), and this test is intended to identify *PIK3CA* mutations in patients with advanced HR+/HER2– breast cancer who may be candidates for therapy with alpelisib.
33. **How can molecular testing help in the diagnosis of breast tumors?**
    - In addition to providing prognostication and treatment response predication, molecular markers are also used to help the diagnosis of breast lesions.
      - Immunohistochemical stain for ER has been utilized frequently in differentiating between usual

Table 5.3 Comparison of selected commercially available molecular profiling tests for prognostication in ER-positive breast cancer

Test	Material	Method	Centralized	Component genes	Indication	Molecular subtyping	Result	AJCC staging	ASCO/NCCN recommendation	Involved in score assessment
Oncotype DX (Genomic Health, Redwood City, CA, USA)	FFPE	RT-PCR	Yes	21 genes	ER+, HER2- and 0-3 positive nodes	No	Low risk (RS < 18), intermediate risk (RS 18-31), high risk (RS > 31)	Yes	Yes (strong)	No
MammaPrint (Agendia, Amsterdam, The Netherlands)	Fresh or FFPE	Microarray	Yes	70 genes	ER+/−, HER2-, Stage 1-2, 0-3 positive nodes	Yes (BluePrint, 80 genes)	Low risk and high risk	Yes	Yes (strong)	Yes (Adjuvant! online)
Prosigna (NanoString Technologies Inc. Seattle, WA, USA)	FFPE	RT-PCR	No	50 genes	ER+, HER2-, Stage 1-2, 0-3 positive node	Yes	Node -: Low risk (0–40); intermediate risk (41–60); high risk (61–100) Node +: Low risk (0–40); High risk (41–100)	Yes	Yes (moderate)	Yes (Proliferation score, tumor size)
EndoPredict (Sividon Diagnostics GmbH, Koln, Germany)	FFPE	RT-PCR	No	12 genes	ER+, HER2-, 0-3 positive nodes	No	Low risk: EPclin Risk score <3.3287; High risk: EPclin Risk score >3.3287	Yes	Yes (moderate)	Yes (tumor size and nodal status EPclin Risk score)
Breast Cancer Index (Biotheranostic, San Diego, CA, USA)	FFPE	RT-PCR	Yes	Combine 2 independent biomarkers (HOXB13:IL17BR [H/I] and the 5 gene molecular grade index (MGI)	ER/PR+, HER2-, node 0-3 positive	No	BCI prognostic score: Low or high risk; BCI predictive score: High or low likelihood of benefit from extended endocrine therapy	Yes	Yes (moderate)	No

AJCC American Joint Committee on Cancer, *ASCO* American Society of Clinical Oncology, *ER* estrogen receptor, *FFPE* formalin fixed paraffin embedded, *HER2* human epidermal growth factor receptor 2, *NCCN* National Comprehensive Cancer Network, *RS* recurrence score, *RT-PCR* reverse transcription polymerase chain reaction ductal hyperplasia and neoplastic clonal epithelial proliferation (atypical ductal hyperplasia/low grade ductal carcinoma in situ), between microglandular adenosis and well-differentiated carcinoma and in determination of tumor origin.

- As the product of the *CDH1* gene, immunohistochemical stain for E-cadherin helps distinguish the ductal and lobular phenotype of breast lesions due to the *CDH1* gene aberrations in lobular lesions, as well as serves as a prognostic marker in breast cancers.
- Some uncommon, special type mammary carcinomas show specific translocations which characterize these tumors and can be used as diagnostic adjunct. Secretory carcinoma of the breast is characterized by a balanced translocation of genetic material between chromosomes 12 and 15 [t(12:15)] which produce *ETV6-NTRK3* fusion gene [52]. Adenoid cystic carcinomas show a specific translocation [t(6:9)(q22-23;p23-24)] and create *MYB-NFIB* transfusion gene [53].

II **Gynecologic tumors**

1. **What are the roles of molecular testing in gynecologic pathology?**
   - Same as in breast pathology, molecular testing has become increasingly important in the diagnosis and management of gynecologic tumors in the era of precision medicine. The applications of molecular testing in gynecologic pathology include:
     - Helping in the understanding of the tumor pathogenesis especially in ovarian, endometrial, and cervical carcinomas.
     - Testing for hereditary DNA mutation in patients with endometrial and ovarian/fallopian tube/peritoneal cancers to define hereditary cancer syndrome and identify patients for selected therapy.
     - Subclassifying molecular tumor types in endometrial cancers.
     - Identifying biomarkers that can predict or monitor the response to treatment.
     - Testing for specific markers and translocations to facilitate the diagnosis of certain gynecologic tumors.
2. **Why testing *BRCA1* and *BRCA2* genomic status is important in patients with ovarian carcinomas?**
   - *BRCA1* and *BRCA2* encode essential proteins for DNA homologous recombination repair (HRR) (see question 3 below).
   - Germline mutations in *BRCA1* and *BRCA2* have been identified in approximately 17% of high-grade ovarian serous carcinomas and somatic mutations in additional 3% [54].
   - Women with non-serous ovarian carcinomas including endometrioid, clear cell, low-grade serous, or carcinosarcoma subtypes also have appreciable rates of carrying *BRCA* mutations [55].
   - In additional to identifying patients with hereditary *BRCA* mutations for high-risk surveillance and management for patients and their affected family members, *BRCA*-mutated ovarian cancer displays enhanced sensitivity to DNA-damaging agents (platinum-based chemotherapy) or to novel agents that block parallel DNA repair pathways, including PARP inhibitors [55–58]. PARP inhibition blocks the repair of DNA single-strand breaks and results in stalling of replication fork progression by trapping PARP on the DNA break [59].
3. **What is homologous recombination deficiency (HRD)?**
   - DNA double-strand break (DSB) is one of the most cytotoxic DNA lesions and causes chromosomal aberration and ultimately cell death if not adequately repaired. The ability to restore DSBs depends on the activity of HRR apparatus, which copies the respective undamaged, homologous DNA of the sister chromatid to reconstruct the corrupted double strand during S and G2 phases. If HRR fails, the process is ended by the so-called non-homologous end joining, an error-prone process of random end-to-end fusion of damaged strands, and leads to accumulation of additional mutations and chromosomal stability, as well as increasing risk of malignant transformation.
   - The function of this HRR apparatus relies on the interaction of a complex set proteins such as the BRCA1, BRCA2, RAD51C, RAD51D, BRIP1, PALB2, and the MMR proteins.
   - Any dysfunctional protein involved may induce phenotypical homologous recombination deficiency (HRD).
   - The Cancer Genome Atlas (TCGA) data showed that approximately half of the high-grade ovarian serous cancers have aberrations in HRR and a majority of them harbor *BRCA1* or *BRCA2* germline or somatic mutations [54]. However, approximately 30% of high-grade serous carcinomas show *BRCA* wild-type status but are associated with alteration of HRR apparatus and cause the phenotypical-deficient cell behavior [54, 60, 61].

4. **How to diagnose HRD?**
   - Testing for HRD can define a subset of high-grade serous carcinoma patients who are most likely to benefit from PARP inhibitor therapy in the first-line and recurrent settings. Currently, there are several different strategies to test for HRD. Since all proposed methods lack broad prospective validation, currently no specific assay may be generally recommended.
     - Germline mutation testing of genes related to HRR.
     - Somatic mutation screening of genes related to HRR.
     - Genomic scarring assays: These assays aim to quantify large genomic aberrations, which represent the genomic instability secondary to HRD, by next-generation whole genome sequencing. The "CDx BRCA LOH" (Foundation Medicine, Cambridge, MA, USA) detects the percentage of loss of heterozygosity throughout the genome and mutations in *BRCA1* or *BRCA2*. The "myChoice" HR deficiency test (Myriad Genetics Inc., Salt Lake City, UT, USA) calculates a score based on the presence of heterozygosity, large scale transitions, and telomeric allelic imbalance. All the clinical trials relied on these genomic scarring assays.
     - HRDetect test: A whole-genome sequencing-based classifier designed to predict *BRCA1* and *BRCA2* deficiency based on six HRD-associated mutational signatures, this test identifies *BRCA1/BRCA2*-deficient tumors with 98.7% sensitivity [62]. Limitations include the need for whole-genome sequencing and, therefore, increased expense, possibly longer turn-around time, and the requirement of a tumor cell percentage greater than 50%.
     - RAD51 foci assays: A functional assay for detecting HRD in tumor samples by immunohistochemistry or immunofluorescence. *RAD51* encodes a recombinase with an essential role in HRR. RAD51 forms distinct subnuclear foci after DNA damage, and the inability to form RAD51 foci is a common feature of HRD. HRD scores based on RAD51 foci formation assays have been shown to correlate to chemosensitivity, PARP inhibitor sensitivity, and overall survival [63, 64].
5. **In which individual should risk evaluation, counseling, and genomic testing for germline and somatic tumor alterations in ovarian cancer be performed?**
   - According to the recent ASCO guidelines [65], the following patients are recommended to have genomic testing for germline and somatic alterations:
     - All women diagnosed with epithelial ovarian cancer should be offered germline genetic testing for *BRCA1*, *BRCA2*, and other ovarian cancer susceptibility genes, irrespective of their clinical features or family cancer history.
     - Somatic tumor testing for *BRCA1* and *BRCA2* pathogenic or likely pathogenic variants should be performed in women who do not carry a germline pathogenic or likely pathogenic *BRCA1/2* variant.
     - Women diagnosed with clear cell, endometrioid, or mucinous ovarian cancer should be offered somatic testing for mismatch repair deficiency (dMMR).
     - Testing for dMMR may be offered to women diagnosed with other histologic types of epithelial ovarian cancer.
     - First- or second-degree blood relatives of a patient with ovarian cancer with a known germline pathogenic cancer susceptibility gene mutation or variant should be offered individualized genetic risk evaluation, counseling, and genetic testing.
6. **What is the best approach for testing *BRCA* mutations in patients with ovarian/tubal/primary peritoneal carcinoma?**
   - Women with ovarian/fallopian tube/primary peritoneal carcinomas should be offered testing at the time of diagnosis. If the patients have not had testing at the time of diagnosis, they should be offered germline genetic testing if possible.
   - The most sensitive approach for *BRCA* mutation in patients with ovarian/tubal/primary peritoneal carcinoma is the sequencing of germline DNA.
   - If germline mutation DNA is negative for *BRCA* mutation, the DNA from tumor tissue should be sequenced since additional 5–6% of patients have somatic *BRCA* mutations [54, 65–67].
   - Due to the less sensitivity of somatic testing, the decision to sequence germline DNA should not depend on finding a mutation in tumor tissue. Up to 5% of germline mutations will be missed if using tumor somatic mutation results to determine whether to sequence germline DNA [65].
   - The expert panel from the ASCO guidelines recommends that germline sequencing of *BRCA1* and *BRCA2* can be performed in the context of a multigene panel that includes, at minimum, *BRCA1, BRCA2, RAD51C, RAD51D, BRIP1, MLH1, MSH2, MSH6, PMS2*, and *PALB2* [65].

7. **What is the significance of detecting deficient mismatch repair (dMMR) in patients with ovarian carcinomas?**
   - Overall dMMR has been identified in approximately 10–12% of unselected epithelial ovarian cancers. It is more common in endometrioid ovarian cancer (~13–20%) but can also be found in clear cell carcinomas (~2.4%) [68–70].
   - The identification of dMMR status can provide additional treatment options such as immunotherapy for patients with recurrent ovarian, fallopian tube, or primary peritoneal cancers [65].
8. **What are the pathologic features of Lynch syndrome-associated endometrial cancer?**
   - The experience with the pathologic features of Lynch syndrome-associated endometrial cancer is less compared to those of colorectal cancer. It has been found that endometrial cancer associated with Lynch syndrome tends to show the following pathologic features:
     - Histologically diverse and include a much greater proportion of mixed and nonendometrioid morphologies, and frequent dedifferentiated/biphasic morphology in Lynch syndrome-related endometrial cancer [71–73].
     - Present in a relatively young age with a mean age of 46.4 years at the diagnosis.
     - Cancer arising from the lower uterine segment (LUS). A large series of endometrial cancers demonstrated that the prevalence of Lynch syndrome in patients with LUS endometrial carcinoma (29%) is much greater than that of the general endometrial cancer patient population (1.8%) or in endometrial cancer patients younger than age 50 years (8–9%) [74].
     - Presence of prominent tumor-infiltrating lymphocytes and peritumoral lymphocytes.
9. **Why testing for mismatch repair protein is important in patients diagnosed with endometrial carcinomas?**
   - Appropriately 2–5% of endometrial cancers are due to Lynch syndrome, which results from germline mutation in one of mismatch repair protein genes: *MLH1*, *MSH2*, *MSH6*, *PMS2*, and *EPCAM*.
   - Patients with Lynch syndrome have 40–60% lifetime risk for endometrial and colon cancers and are at risk for other cancers in the ovary, stomach, small bowel, and liver.
   - Among women with Lynch syndrome who have both colon and endometrial cancers, about half present first with endometrial cancer, which makes endometrial cancer the most common sentinel cancer in Lynch syndrome [75, 76].
   - Identification of patients with Lynch syndrome may allow for screening and prevention strategies for patients themselves and their affected family members.
   - US FDA-approved PD-L1 inhibitor pembrolizumab for the treatment of unresectable or metastatic dMMR cancers including endometrial cancer.
10. **Who should be screened for Lynch syndrome on tissue when diagnosed with endometrial cancer?**
   - Currently, the practice of tissue testing for screening of Lynch syndrome in endometrial cancer is highly variable across institutions and countries. There are three approaches for assessing the possibility of Lynch syndrome in a woman with a diagnosis of endometrial cancer [77]:
     - Perform tissue testing on endometrial cancer from a woman identified to be at risk through a systemic screen that includes a focused personal and family history.
     - Perform tumor testing on all endometrial cancers irrespective of age of diagnosis.
     - Perform tumor testing on all endometrial cancers diagnosed before age 60 years.
     - A universal Lynch-syndrome-screening algorithm has been proposed by Mills and Longacre [78].
11. **What are the common testing methods for screening Lynch syndrome?**
   - Immunohistochemistry method to assess the expression status of key MMR proteins including MLH1, MSH2, MSH6, and PMS2. It is simple, cost-effective, and is the most-commonly used first-line method. The major disadvantage of the IHC method is to miss dMMR tumors due to mutations that lead to loss of MMR function but still maintain antigenicity [79].
   - Polymerase chain reaction (PCR)-based microsatellite instability testing. Microsatellite instability testing has been shown to be less sensitive than IHC, which is due to the failure to detect many *MSH6* germline mutation carriers and fails to identify the putative causative gene/protein deficiency.
   - Both IHC and MSI tests have high sensitivity. The false-negative rates in both tests are 5–10%.
   - *MLH1* promoter methylation analysis: *MLH1* promoter methylation accounts for up to 96.9% of endometrial cancer occurrences that have an absence of MLH1 and PMS2 on IHC [75]. If the tumor demonstrates an absent expression of MLH1 and PMS2 on IHC, an *MLH1* promoter methylation needs to be done before germline genetic testing.
   - Germline mutation testing is the most conclusive method. Next-generation sequencing has also been

used to predict microsatellite status by focusing on targeted sequencing of known microsatellite loci or analysis of microsatellite regions using novel informatics algorithms [80, 81].

12. **How to interpret the immunohistochemical stains for MMR proteins? What are the pitfalls in the interpretation of MMR on IHC? How to resolve these pitfalls?**
    - Immunohistochemical stains for MMR proteins are performed on a tumor sample.
    - The result should be reported as either positive or negative.
    - Unequivocal nuclear staining of MMR protein in viable tumor cells in the presence of appropriate internal positive controls is considered as intact protein expression. Strong nuclear staining in the surrounding endometrial stroma, myometrium, lymphocytes, or normal endometrium should serve as an internal positive control. The absence of nuclear staining of MMR protein in viable tumor cells in the presence of appropriate internal positive controls is considered as negative for the MMR protein.
    - The presence of dot-like nuclear, cytoplasmic, and other potentially "artifactual" staining patterns should be disregarded in the interpretation of status.
    - Figure 5.4 shows a representative case of MMR intact endometrial cancer by immunohistochemistry. Figure 5.5 shows heterogenous expression of MMR by immunohistochemistry on a dedifferentiated endometrial cancer with loss of nuclear expression of MLH1 and PMS2 in the undifferentiated carcinoma component, while intact expression of MLH1 and PMS2 in the well-differentiated endometrioid component.
    - When interpreting the MMR status using IHC method, there are some pitfalls:
    - False-negative nuclear staining in the tumor cells occurs in the setting of inadequate internal positive controls. This may be resolved by repeating the IHC with consideration of increasing antigen exposure time or using different tissue blocks from the same specimen.
    - Presence of endometrial stromal cells or lymphocytes on the IHC sections may cause difficulties in MMR interpretation. Correlation with the corresponding H&E sections should resolve this problem.
    - Heterogenous staining of MSH6 expression was reported in 0.17% cases of colorectal, endometrial, and sebaceous tumors [82]. This is not a typical feature of Lynch syndrome; however, a possibility of germline mutation in the other MMR genes cannot be excluded.
    - Subclonal loss of MMR protein: Predominantly MLH1 is identified by recognizing an area with retained expression of MMR in tumor cell nuclei

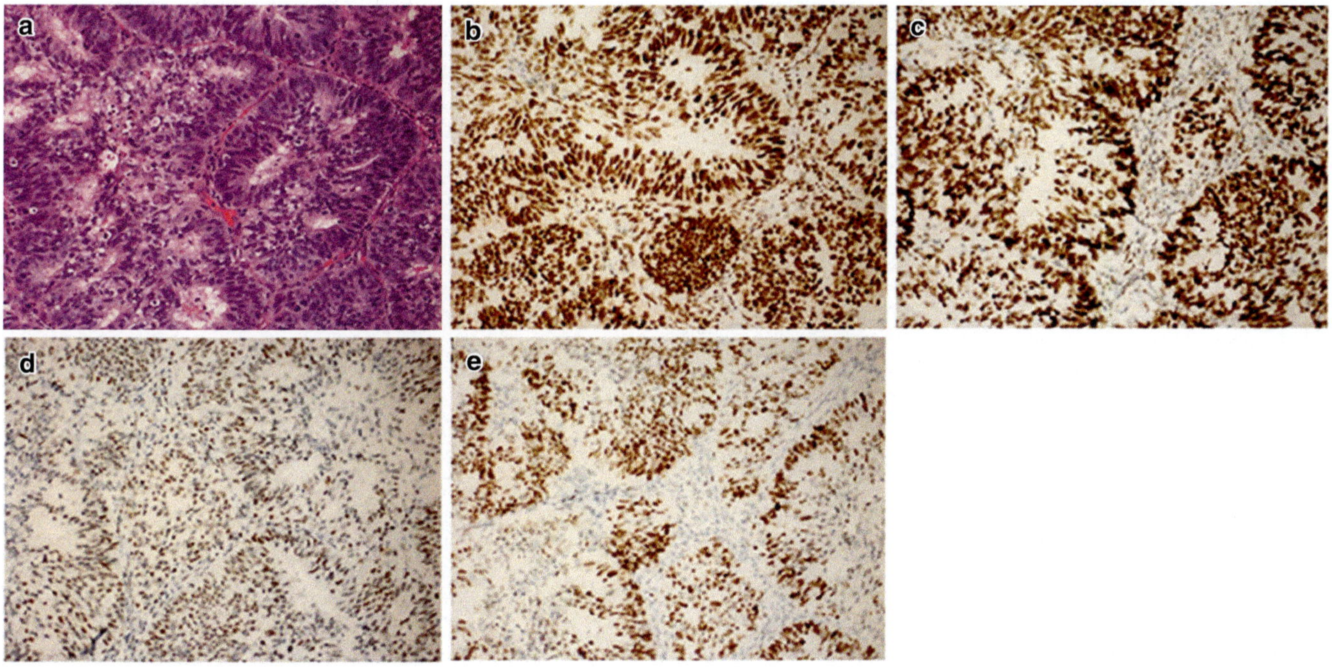

Fig. 5.4 A 68-year-old woman with endometrial adenocarcinoma. The tumor shows endometrioid histotype (**a**, H&E, ×100) and intact MLH1(**b**, ×100), MSH2 (**c**, ×100), PMS2 (**d**, ×100), and MSH6 (**e**, ×100)

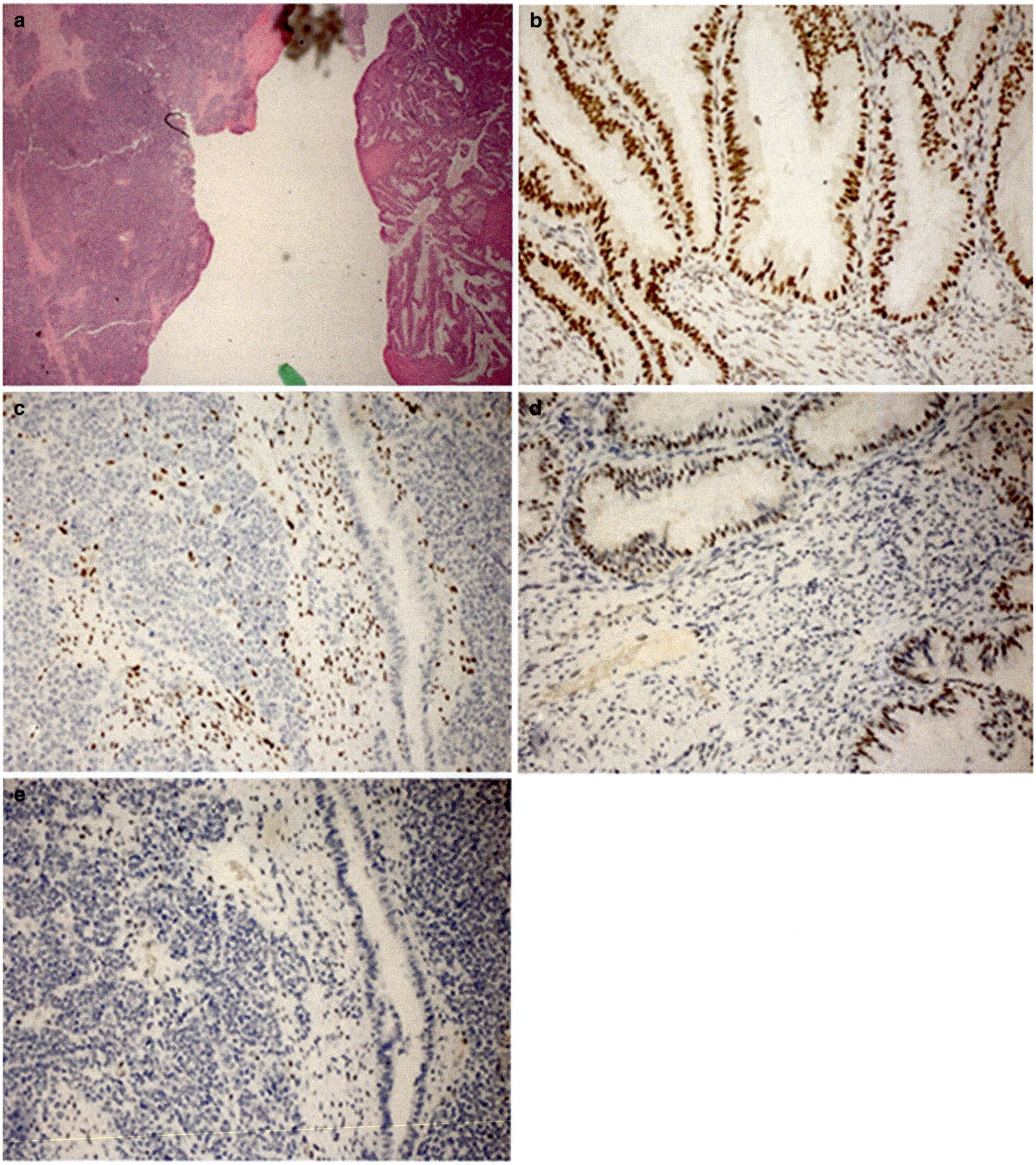

Fig. 5.5 A 56-year-old woman with endometrial adenocarcinoma. The tumor shows dedifferentiated histotype with well-differentiated endometrioid adenocarcinoma and abrupt transition into solid growth of medium-sized, discohesive tumor cell population (**a**, H&E, ×20). MMR immunohistochemistry shows heterogenous expression with loss of nuclear expression of MLH1 (**c**, ×200) and PMS2 (**e**, ×200) in the undifferentiated carcinoma component, while intact expression of MLH1 (**b**, ×200) and PMS2 (**d**, ×200) in the well-differentiated endometrioid component. *MLH1* promoter methylation by PCR shows positive *MLH1* promoter methylation, indicating sporadic endometrial cancer

and an abrupt transition to a clearly delineated regional area with complete loss of expression. The subclonal loss of MMR protein can be seen in appropriately 7% of endometrial carcinomas and it is associated with epigenetic silencing of the *MLH1* promoter by methylation rather than a germline *MLH1* mutation [83]. Subclonal loss can be distinguished from the inadequate fixation or an error in the staining process by identifying staining in positive internal control cells. In exceptional cases, heterogeneous MLH1 loss can be due to mutations in DNA polymerase epsilon (*POLE*) gene [84].

13. **Should the mismatch repair protein testing be repeated in cases of tumor recurrence?**
    - The role of MMR testing has evolved from identifying Lynch syndrome patients to predicting response to the immune checkpoint inhibitors. This may lead to request from clinical providers to retest recurrences of MMR-proficient primary tumors in the hope that the recurrence may show a different MMR status and may qualify the patient for additional treatment.
    - Aird et al. recently evaluated recurrent tumors from 137 patients with MMR-proficient primary tumors of the gynecological and gastrointestinal tracts, and they did not identify any cases with a genuine discordance between the primary and recurrent cases. Therefore, the authors do not advocate repeating MMR IHC on recurrences when the primary tumor shows intact MMR staining [85].
    - Ta et al. found that advanced endometrial cancer may rarely (~7%) exhibit discordant somatic MMR loss compared to primary tumor and the discordant metastatic endometrial carcinoma may be derived from an MMR-deficient subclone. Their results indicated MMR testing of recurrent tumor or metastasis should be considered for guiding immunotherapy if primary uterine tumor exhibits abnormal subclonal MMR loss [86].
14. **What is microsatellite instability (MSI)? What are the MSI testing methods? What are MSI-high, MSI-low, and MSI stable?**
    - Microsatellites are short-repeated sequences of DNA that are composed of repeating sequence of nucleotides of one to six base pairs in length (e.g., AAAAA or CGCGCGCG).
    - Microsatellite instability (MSI) is a form of genomic instability resulting in the accumulation of insertions or deletions (indels) in microsatellites during replication due to an impaired MMR protein function.
    - MSI can be tested by PCR-based technology and next-generation sequencing.
    - The PCR-based analysis is the commonly used method for screening MSI in patients with endometrial cancer. It compares the sizes of microsatellite marker sets in tumor DNA with corresponding DNA isolated from a normal tissue sample from the same patients via electrophoresis. A range of markers may be used but the core panel recommended five microsatellite markers consisting of three dinucleotide repeats (D2S123, D5S346, D17S250) and two mononucleotide repeats (BAT26, BAT25) [87].
    - Next-generation sequencing-based analyses have comprehensively characterized MSI-positive cancers, and different panels demonstrated the clinical validity of specific methodology and the NGS approach for detection of MSI for Lynch syndrome [88–91].
    - Definition of MSI-high varies by the panel used and the reference standard depends upon the purpose of the test. By using PCR-based MSI testing method, tumor with ≥2 of core panel, or >30% of markers for other panels showing instability is considered as MSI-high. Tumor with 1 of core markers, or <30% of markers for other panels showing instability is considered as MSI-low. MSI-stable refers to the tumor with 0 marker showing instability.
15. **What is *MLH1* promoter methylation? How to test *MLH1* promoter methylation?**
    - Gene inactivation through an epigenetic process marked by promoter region hypermethylation associated with transcriptional loss is an alternative mode for cancer development.
    - In endometrial cancers with loss of MLH1 protein expression, approximately 65–96.9% of these tumors are due to MLH1 promoter methylation [92–94].
    - MLH1 promoter methylation analysis is used to distinguish sporadic endometrial cancers from Lynch syndrome in tumors that are MLH1-deficient by IHC staining and/or high level of MSI-H.
    - MLH1 promotor methylation is detected by methylation specific real-time PCR. In this assay, extracted tumor tissue DNA (typically from the same block in the IHC/MSI assay) is exposed to a bisulfate compound, which converts unmethylated cytosines to uracil, whereas methylated cytosines are resistant to this conversion, allowing for creation of different PCR reaction primers that can differentiate these two types of sequences. The absence of *MLH1* promotor methylation in tumors demonstrating loss of MLH1 protein expression and/or MSI-H may suggest a *MLH1* mutation associated with Lynch syndrome and genetic testing for

germline *MLH1* mutation is recommended. The presence of *MLH1* promotor hypermethylation in tumor tissue is suggestive of sporadic MSI and not associated with Lynch syndrome.

- Rare cases of co-*MLH1* promotor methylation and *MLH1* germline mutations have been reported [95, 96]. Constitutional epimutations that result in heritable *MLH1* germline mutation has also been reported, which cause Lynch syndrome phenotype in the absence of primary sequence alterations in the *MLH1* gene [97]. If there is a clinical suspicion of germline *MLH1* promotor methylation, a germline *MLH1* promotor methylation testing on peripheral blood is recommended.

16. **What are the possible causes for normal tissue testing result in patients with known MMR gene mutations? What are the possible causes for abnormal MSI/IHC results with non-detectable MMR gene mutations?**
    - In some endometrial cancer patients with known MMR gene mutations, the MMR IHC or MSI testing shows normal results. The possible causes include:
      - Patients with full-length but non-functional MMR protein resulting from missense mutations in MMR genes [98].
      - In endometrial cancer, the proportion of unstable microsatellite marker is lower (0.27 for endometrium vs 0.45 for colon per average tumor), the allelic shifts in BAT loci is shorter, and a greater proportion of tumor shows MSS [98, 99].
      - Patients with *MSH6* germline mutation tend to have tumors that are disproportionally MSI-low or MSS [100–102].
    - In some patients with abnormal MSI/IHC results indicative of Lynch syndrome, while the genetic analysis fails to reveal a pathologic mutation in the MMR gene, the possible causes include the following:
      - The presence of MMR gene variants of undetermined significance
      - The presence of MSH2 inversion (exons 1–7) [103]
      - The presence of EPCAM germline mutation, resulting in hypermethylation of the MSH2 promoter and subsequent transcriptional silence of an otherwise normal MSH2 gene [104]
      - The presence of bi-allelic somatic DNA mutations in MMR genes [105, 106]

17. **What are the advantages and disadvantages of IHC method, PCR-based MSI testing, and NGS-based MSI testing for Lynch syndrome screening?**
    - The advantages of IHC method for Lynch syndrome screening include:
      - High sensitivity and nearly perfect specificity
      - Cheap and available in most laboratories
      - Only requires tumor sample (not matched tumor/normal samples as required by PCR for MSI)
      - Can identify the candidate protein/gene most likely to be affected

      The disadvantages of IHC method for Lynch syndrome screening include:
      - Presence of false-negative results where protein function is impaired but still present such as MLH1 promoter hypermethylation cases which may show loss of nuclear staining for MLH1 and PMS2
      - Variation in tissue fixation and other pre-analytic and analytic issues
      - Presence of tumor heterogeneity in endometrial cancer
      - Less reliable on small tissue
    - The advantages of PCR-based MSI testing for Lynch syndrome testing include:
      - Complementary with IHC
      - Identifies MSI status regardless of protein function
      - Can be performed on small samples
      - High reproducibility

      The disadvantages of PCR-based MSI testing for Lynch syndrome testing include:
      - Time consuming due to microdissection and subsequent molecular analysis
      - Require both tumor tissue and normal tissue
      - Additional testing needed to identify the candidate gene
      - dMMR tumor detection depends on the proposed cut-off and not all tumors with dMMR are necessarily MSI-H, especially in *MSH6* and *PMS2* mutated tumors
    - The advantages of NGS-based MSI testing for Lynch syndrome testing include the following:
      - Does not require tumor microdissection
      - Can be performed on small samples
      - Potentially faster result than PCR-based methods
      - Potentially more accurate result than MSI PCR-based method for detection of MSI-H status in some cancers

- Can perform large-scale testing, especially when looking for dMMR in the low-incidence cancers
- Can integrate results such as MSI status, tumor mutation burden within the same test

The disadvantages of NGS-based MSI testing for Lynch syndrome testing include:

- Clinical utility as a pan-tumor assay is not widely-established
- Currently, no evidence available directly in support of predicative purpose for immunotherapy

18. **What is the TCGA molecular classification of endometrial carcinomas?**
    - Endometrial carcinoma is a clinically heterogenous disease with diverse underlying molecular alterations.
    - The Cancer Genome Atlas (TCGA) Research Network performed an integrated genomic, transcriptomic, and proteomic characterization of endometrial carcinomas, using array- and sequencing-based assays. The study included 307 endometrioid, 53 serous, and 13 mixed histology cases and classified these endometrial carcinomas into four distinct molecular subtypes based on the somatic copy number alterations and tumor mutational burden: polymerase epslon (*POLE*) ultramutated, microsatellite instability hypermutated, copy-number low, and copy-number high [107].
    - This molecular classification provides clinically relevant and prognostic information, with the potential to influence the clinical management [107–109]. Table 5.4 shows the clinicopathological features, outcomes, and clinical management of high-risk endometrial cancers by the molecular subtypes.

Table 5.4 The clinicopathological features, outcomes, and clinical management of high-risk endometrial cancers by the molecular subtypes

Molecular subgroups	*POLE* ultramutated	Microsatellite instability hypermutated	Copy number low (NSMP)	Copy number high (p53 aberrant)
Incidence	12.4%	33.4%	31.5%	22.7%
Molecular alterations	*POLE , DMD, CSMD1, FAT4, PTEN*	*PTEN,PIK3CA,PIK3R1, RPL22,ARID1A*	*PTEN, PIK3CA,CTNNB1, ARID1A*	Frequently *TP53;* Focal amplifications of *MYC, ERBB2*,and *CCNE1*
Somatic copy number alterations	Very low	Low	Low	High
Mutation frequency	High	Moderate to High	Low	Low
Diagnostic test	NGS; Sanger sequencing	See question 11		P53 IHC; NGS
Histology	Typically, high grade endometrioid type or morphologically ambiguous, superficially broad front invasion, scattered tumor giant cells, prominent TILS	Mostly endometrioid type, abundant TILs, "MELF" pattern of invasion may present	Usually endometrioid type with squamous differentiation and ER/PR positivity	Most serous and mixed histology, a minority of endometrioid type
Surrogate IHC markers		MMR protein		P53
Prognosis	Excellent	Intermediate	Mixed	Poor
Potential utility in surgical planning	May skip the lymphadenectomy			More aggressive surgery with lymph node assessment and omentectomy
Adjuvant treatment	No benefit of CTRT over RT	No significant benefit of CTRT vs CT	No significant benefit of CTRT vs CT, although a trend toward benefit from CTRT	Significant benefit from CTRT
Suggested Treatment in recurrent/ metastatic disease	Checkpoint inhibitors	Checkpoint inhibitors	Hormonal therapy/mTOR inhibitors	HER2-targeted therapy in serous carcinoma

CTRT combined adjuvant chemotherapy and radiotherapy, *ER* estrogen receptor, *MELF* microcystic elongated and fragmented, *NGS* next-generation sequencing, *NSMP* non-specific molecular profile, *POLE* polymerase epslon; PR: progesterone receptor, *RT* radiotherapy, *TILs* tumor-infiltrating lymphocytes

19. **What are the roles of molecular testing in endometrial stromal tumors?**
    - The understanding of endometrial stromal sarcomas has evolved dramatically since the discovery of several recurrent cytogenetic aberrations occurring in low- and high-grade endometrial stromal sarcomas.
    - Low-grade endometrial stromal sarcomas bear close histopathological resemblance to proliferative-type endometrial stroma and approximately 50% of cases harbor gene rearrangement of t(7:17)(p15;q21), which causes *JAZF1-SUZ12* fusion [110, 111]. Less common rearrangements involving PHD finger protein-1 (PHF1) and multiple fusion partners, including JAZF1, EPC1, EPC2, MRAF6, and MBTD1, have also been reported [112].
    - The term "high-grade endometrial stromal sarcoma" was recently re-introduced in the classification of endometrial stromal tumors after the discovery of t(10;17)(q22;p13) resulting in *YWHAE-NUTM2A/B* fusion and is associated with distinct morphological characteristics [113–115].
20. **What are the biomarker tests for endometrial carcinoma? How should these biomarkers be reported?**
    - The biomarker tests for endometrial carcinomas includes ER, PR, HER2, MMR proteins/MSI, and p53.
    - CAP offers the templates for reporting results of biomarker testing in specimens from patients with endometrial carcinoma.
21. **What is the role of HER2 testing in uterine serous carcinoma?**
    - The HER2 overexpression in the uterine serous carcinoma is variable, between 14% and 80%, and HER2 overexpression/amplification has been linked to poor prognosis in endometrial cancer [116].
    - The gynecologic oncologists request HER2 testing in uterine serous carcinomas given the proven benefit of adding Trastuzumab to the traditional regimen of carboplatin-paclitaxel increased the progression-free survivals in patients with advanced or recurrent uterine serous carcinoma [117].
    - Currently, there are no HER2 testing guidelines for endometrial cancer, and CAP offers a template for prognosis marker reporting results for cases with uterine carcinomas, by using the breast guideline.
22. **What is molecular human papillomavirus (HPV) testing in the cervical cytology specimen?**
    - Approximately 95% cervical cancers are caused by 12–15 high-risk human papillomavirus (hr-HPV) infections.
    - Molecular HPV testing on liquid-based cervical cytology specimens has been approved by the US FDA since 2001 from initially being as a reflex testing, to a routine co-tests in women aged 30 years and above, and to a primary screening test.
    - The molecular HPV testing is performed using assays that detect viral DNA or RNA within the cells.
    - There are at least 254 distinct commercial HPV tests and at least 425 testing variants on the global market in 2020. These tests include hr-HPV DNA screening tests, hr-HPV DNA screening tests with concurrent partial genotyping tests (HPV16/18/45), HPV DNA full genotyping tests, HPV DNA type- or group-specific genotyping tests, hr-HPV E6/E7 mRNA tests, in situ hybridization DNA in mRNA-based HPV tests, and HPV DNA tests targeting miscellaneous HPV types [118].
    - The US FDA has approved five testing modalities for the detection of HPV in cervical cytology specimens [119]: Hybrid Capture 2 HPV DNA test by Qiagen (Hilden, Germany, 2001), Cervista HPV DNA test by Hologic (Marlborough, Massachusetts, 2009), Cobas 4800 HPV DNA test by Roche (Basel, Switzerland, 2011), Aptima HPV RNA assay by Gen Probe (San Diego, California, 2011, purchased by Hologic in 2012), and BD Onclarity HPV DNA assay by Becton Dickinson (Franklin Lakes, New Jersey, 2018). Table 5.5 lists the comparisons among FDA-approved hrHPV testing platforms.
23. **When should p16 immunostaining be performed in lower anogenital squamous lesions?**
    - The Lower Anogenital Squamous Terminology (LAST) Standardization Project only recommended immunostaining of p16, a biomarker that is recognized in the context of HPV biology to reflect the activation of E6/E7-driven cell proliferation can be used as an adjunctive diagnostic tool in the lower anogenital squamous lesions [120]:
      – When the H&E morphologic differential diagnosis is between precancer (high-grade squamous intraepithelial lesion, -IN2 or –IN3) and its mimics such as immature squamous metaplasia, atrophy, reparative epithelial changes, tangential cutting.
      – To clarify the situation if the pathologist is entertaining an H&E morphologic interpretation of -IN2, the equivocal lesions falling between low grade lesions and precancer lesions.
      – When there is a professional disagreement in histologic specimen interpretation, with the caveat that the differential diagnosis includes a precancerous lesion (-IN2 or-IN3).

Table 5.5 Comparisons among FDA-approved hrHPV testing platforms

HPV testing	HC2	Cervista	Cobas 4800	Aptima	Onclarity
Manufacturer	Qiagen	Hologic	Roche	Hologic	Becton Dickinson
Approval in ASC-US triage	2001	2009	2011 (TP) 2016 (SP)	2011	2018
Primary screening, co-testing	Yes	Yes	Yes	Yes	Yes
Primary screening, HPV alone	N/A	N/A	Yes	N/A	Yes
Preparation	TP	TP	TP and SP	TP	SP
Method	DNA (non-PCR based); signal amplification: full-genome probe	DNA (non-PCR based) signal amplification: L1, E6, and E7 gene targets	DNA (PCR based); target amplification: L1 gene target	mRNA (PCR based); target amplification: E6/E7 gene target	DNA (PCR based); target amplification: E6/E7 gene target
Genotype detected	13 genotypes (16, 18, 31, 33, 35, 39, 45, 51, 52, 56, 58, 59, 68)	14 genotypes (13 genotypes as HC2, adding 66)	14 genotypes (same as Cervista with genotyping of 16 and 18)	14 genotypes (same as Cervista; genotyping [16,18/45] as separate test	14 genotypes (same as Cervista; simultaneous identification of 16, 18, and 45)
Clinical validation	Extensive	Limited	Limited	Limited	Limited
Sensitivity for CIN2/3	63.6–100%	92.8–100%	71.1–99%	55.3–100%	85.7–100%
Specificity for CIN2/3	6.2–98.4%		24–86.2%	28.8–99.2%	17–98.8%
Built-in internal control	No	Yes (HIST2H2BE)	Yes (ß-globin)	Yes	Yes (ß-globin)
Main limitations	Cross-reactivity with low-risk HPV types and bacterial plasmid pBR322 False-negative due to low levels of HPV infection, insufficient cellular material, high concentrations of anti-fungal cream, contraceptive jelly, or douche	Cross-reactivity with HPV 67/70 False-negative due to presence of high levels of contraceptive jelly and/or anti-fungal creams False-positive due to high levels of human DNA	False negative due to high concentration of blood contamination False positive due to cross-contamination Non-epithelial cell-specific internal control	Interfered by the presence of lubricants containing polyquaternium 15 or anti-fungal medications containing tioconazole	False negative due to high concentration of mucin acyclovir cream, or clindamycin vaginal cream

CIN cervical intraepithelial neoplasia, *HC2* hybrid capture 2, *Hr-HPV* high-risk human papillomavirus, *N/A* not applicable, *PCR* polymerase chain reaction, *SP* SurePath (BD, Franklin Lakes, NJ, USA), *TP* ThinPrep (Hologic, Marlborough, MA, USA)

- When biopsy specimens interpreted as ≤-IN1 that are at high risk for missed high-grade disease, which is defined as a prior cytologic interpretation of HSIL, ASC-H, ASC-US/HPV16+ or AGC (NOS).
- In these scenarios, the strong and diffuse block-positive p16 results support a categorization of precancerous disease and negative or non-block-positive staining favors an interpretation as low-grade disease (low-grade squamous intraepithelial lesion, -IN1) or a non-HPV-associated pathology.
- Positive p16 IHC (strong and diffuse block) is defined as "continuous strong nuclear or nuclear plus cytoplasmic staining of the basal cell layer with extension upward involving at least one third of the epithelial thickness."
- Negative p16 IHC is defined as "focal or patchy nuclear staining, and all other staining patterns, including cytoplasmic only, wispy, blob-like, puddled, scattered, single cells."

24. **What are the roles of molecular testing in sex cord-stromal tumors of the ovary?**
    - Molecular testing has potential roles in the pathological diagnosis of some ovarian sex-cord stromal tumors and helps to recognize patients with inherited cancer susceptibility syndromes (see review article [121]).

- *FOXL2* mutation testing: *FOXL2* (chromosome 3q23) encodes a transcription factor that is a member of the forehead box (FOX) family of proteins. A somatic missense mutation (402 C→G) (C134W) of *FOXL2* was reported in the majority (61–97%) of adult granulosa cell tumors (AGCT), 5–10% of thecomas, and less than 10% of juvenile GCT cases, but not in other ovarian tumors. The methods used to test for the FOXL2 C134W missense mutation include Sanger sequencing, targeted next-generation sequencing, and allele-specific quantitative amplification assays such as Taqman.
- *DICER1* mutation testing: *DICER1* (chromosome 14q32.13) encodes an RNA endoribonuclease that cleaves (i.e., dices) microRNA precursors to create mature miRNAs, which subsequently regulate the translation of a broad array of endogenous and exogenous RNAs. Germline mutation of *DICER1* gene is associated with DICER1 syndrome. This condition causes benign and malignant tumors in the lungs, kidneys, ovaries, and thyroid. In the gynecologic tumors, somatic mutation of *DICER1* is commonly found in ovarian moderately or poorly differentiated Sertoli-Leydig cell tumors (SLCTs) and cervical embryonal rhabdomyosarcomas as well as in a minority of juvenile granulosa cell tumor (JGCTs), gynandroblastomas, and germ cell tumors. Determining *DICER1* mutation status in SLCT cases can assist with the diagnosis and risk assessment for DICER1 syndrome. Sanger sequencing or targeted NGS of the relevant exons is the mainstay of DICER1 mutation testing.
- *CTNNB1* mutation testing: *CTNNB1* (chromosome 3p22.1) encodes β-catenin, which is an adherens junction protein that is critical for the establishment and maintenance of epithelial layers. Mutations in *CTNNB1* are seen in a wide range of cancers, including hepatocellular carcinoma, colorectal carcinoma, breast cancer, and glioblastoma. In the gynecologic tumors, a somatic mutation of *CTNNB1* exon 3 has been reported in 73% of microcystic stromal tumors (MCSTs). Interestingly, immunohistochemical expression of β-catenin did not perfectly correlate with mutation status. The presence of nuclear staining in MCSTs is associated with *CTNNB1* mutation in approximately three-quarters of cases, and nearly all MCSTs with *CTNNB1* mutations show β-catenin nuclear staining. Sanger sequencing or targeted NGS of exon 3 is the mainstay of *CTNNB1* mutation testing.

25. **What are the roles of molecular testing in the diagnosis of gestational trophoblast disease?**
    - The diagnostic accuracy of various gestational trophoblast disease (GTDs) has been significantly improved by the application of molecular testing. An algorithmic approach combining histology and the ancillary tests has been proposed by Buza and Hui to provide the best practice in the diagnosis of hydatidiform moles [122].
    - Ploidy analysis: By determining the number of complete haploid sets of chromosomes, ploidy analysis can separate diploid gestations from triploid, tetraploid, or other aneuploid ones. It can be performed by conventional karyotyping, flow cytometry, or polymorphic deletion probe (PDP) fluorescent in situ hybridization. The results cannot separate triploid partial moles from non-molar digynic triploidy, and diploid complete moles from diploid non-molar hydropic abortions.
    - Short tandem repeat (STR) genotyping: By comparing the alleles of maternal and villous tissue at each STR locus, the presence and relative proportion (copy number) of maternal and paternal alleles in the villous tissue can be determined. The genotypic profile of a complete hydatidiform mole contains exclusively paternal alleles of either homozygous or heterozygous pattern in at least two informative STR loci. Monospermic (homozygous) partial moles show one maternal allele and a duplicate quantity of one paternal allele at every STR locus, while two unique paternal alleles in addition to one maternal allele in at least two loci is diagnostic of dispermic (heterozygous) partial hydatidiform mole. A balanced biallelic profile of both maternal and paternal genetic contributions is seen in non-molar hydropic abortions.
    - P57 immunohistochemistry: p57 is paternally imprinted and expressed from the maternal allele. In a complete hydatidiform mole, the cytotrophoblasts and villous trophoblasts lack p57 immunoreactivity while its expression is retained in intervillous intermediate trophoblasts, villous endothelial cells, and maternal decidua. P57 IHC can separate a complete hydatidiform mole from its mimics including partial moles, hydropic non-molar abortions, and trisomies.

Case Presentations

Case 1

Case History

A 70-year-old woman with vague hypoechoic mass on screening mammogram

Histologic Finding

H&E sections show small uniform, round glands haphazardly distributed in the fibrofatty stroma with luminal eosinophilic secretions. The glands are lined by a monolayer of flat to cuboidal epithelial cells that lack a myoepithelial layer (see Fig. 5.6a–b).

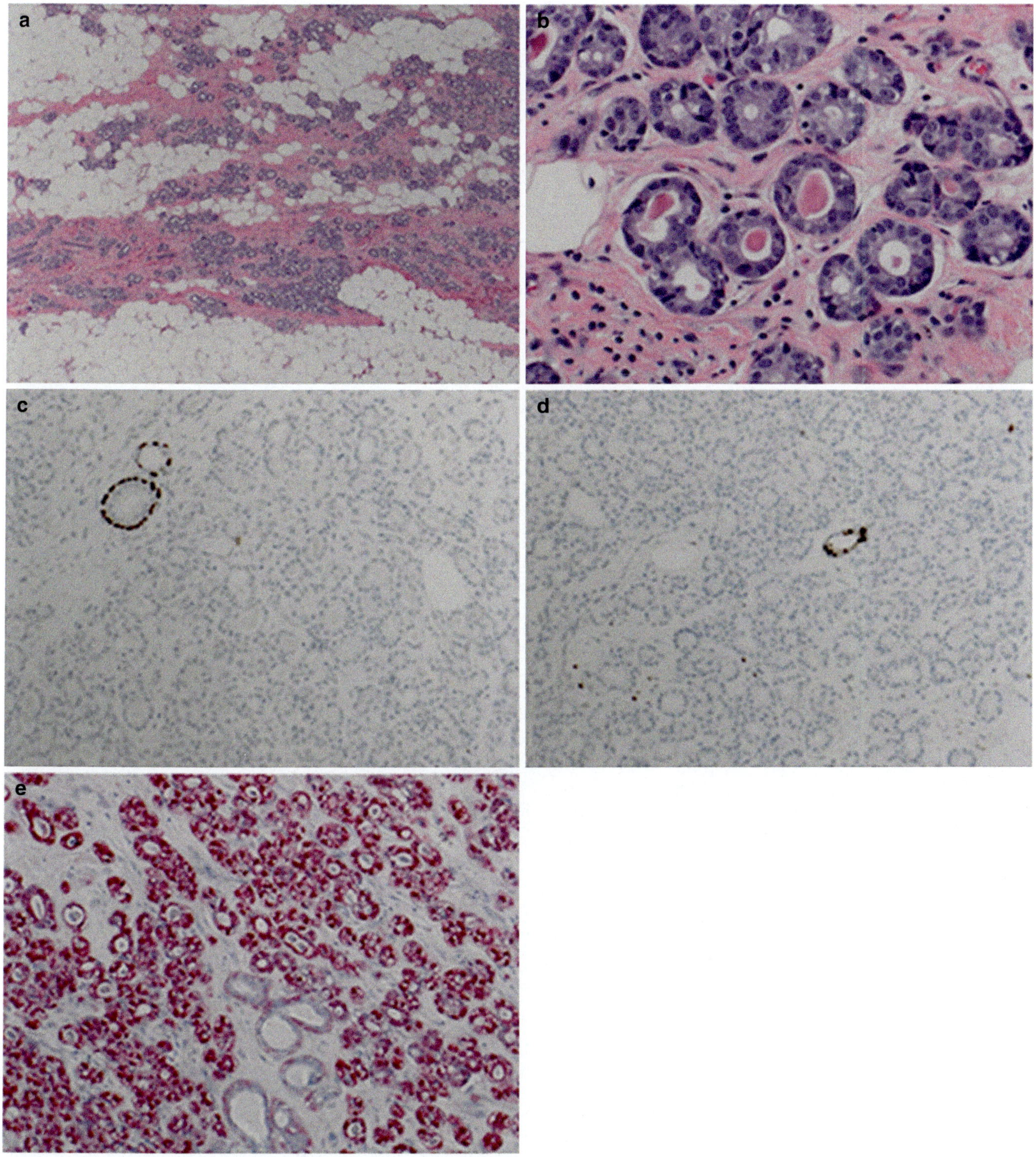

Fig. 5.6 A case of microglandular adenosis demonstrating the diagnostic value of ER/PR. A and B: Morphology of the lesion (**a** H&E, ×40 and **b**, H&E, ×400). The areas of interest are negative for p63 (**c**, ×200), ER (**d**, ×200), and PR and are positive for S100 (**e**, ×200)

Differential Diagnosis

Well-differentiated carcinoma (tubular carcinoma), microglandular adenosis

Ancillary Studies

The areas of interest are negative for p63, ER, and PR and positive for S100 (see Fig. 5.6c–e).

Final Diagnosis

Microglandular adenosis

Discussion

This case demonstrates that microglandular adenosis can closely mimic well-differentiated breast cancer both clinically and pathologically. Immunohistochemistry for ER/PR may be very helpful in this scenario since negative ER and PR expressions are very unusual in the well-differentiated breast carcinoma. Expression of S100 protein is additional information supporting a diagnosis of microglandular adenosis. An absence of the myoepithelial cell layer needs to be interpreted with caution since both well differentiated carcinomas and microglandular adenosis will show a lack of staining for myoepithelial cells.

Case 2

History

A 59-year-old woman was found to have a mass on a screening mammogram. The core biopsy shows invasive ductal carcinoma, histologic grade 3 (see Fig. 5.7a).

HER2 Testing

- **Immunohistochemistry:** Initial HER2 IHC shows ~40% of tumor cells with complete, strong intensity and ~40% with complete moderate to strong intensity (score 3+); however, there is weak to moderate staining in the benign breast glands. A repeated HER2 IHC shows absent staining in the benign breast glands and negative HER2 staining in the tumor cells (score 1+). A reflex HER2 FISH analysis was performed (see Fig. 5.7b–c).

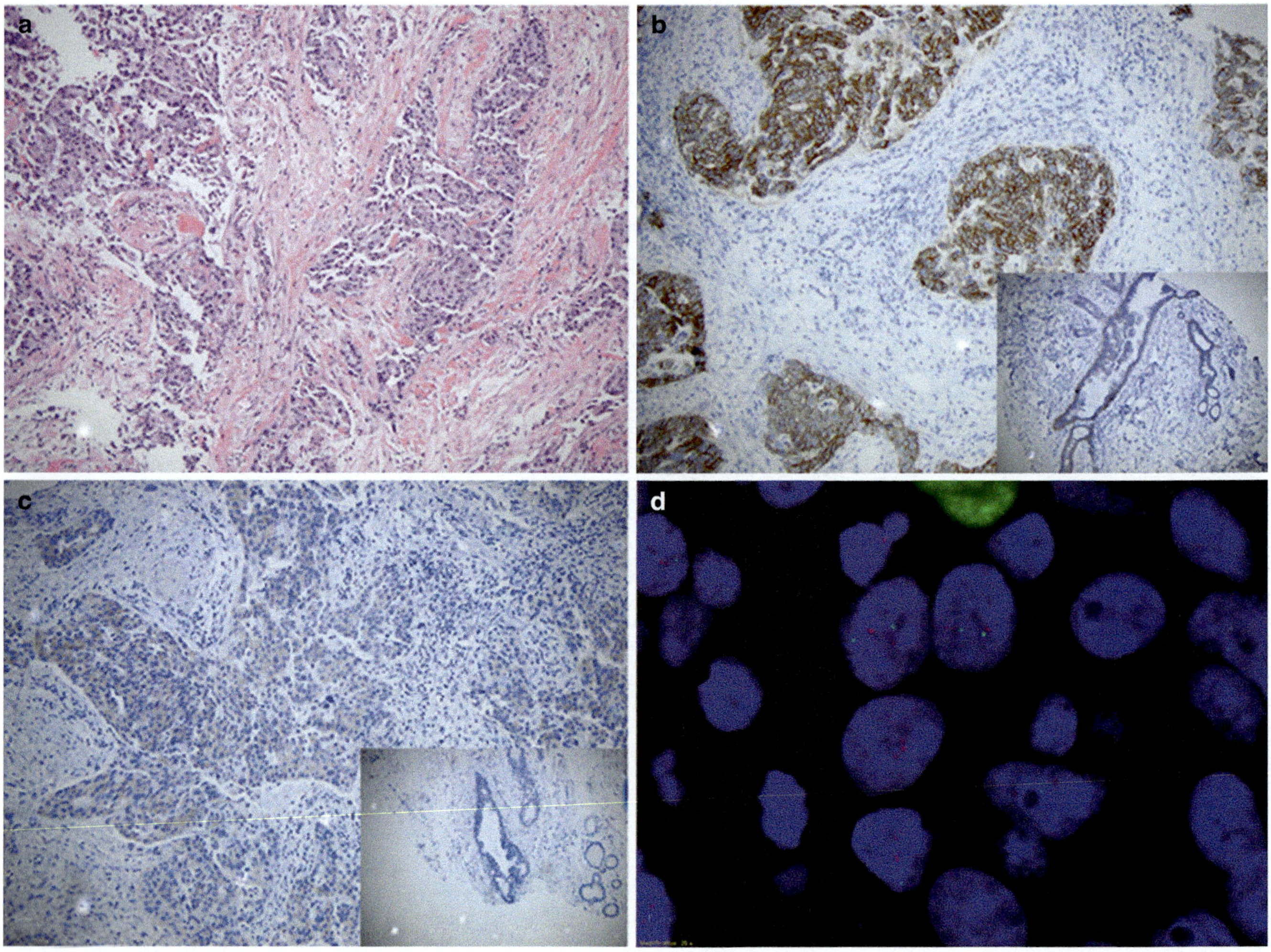

Fig. 5.7 Interpretation of HER2 immunohistochemistry. **a**: H&E (×100); **b**: Initial HER2 IHC (inlet: benign breast ducts) (×200); **c**: Repeated HER2 IHC (inlet: benign breast ducts) (×200), and D: FISH: non-amplified (**d**, ×1,000)

- **FISH:** Non-amplified (HER2 copy number: 3.7/cell and HER2/CEP17 ratio: 1.5) (see Fig. 5.7d).

Final HER2 Interpretation

Negative

Discussion

Accurate assessment of HER2 status in breast cancer is critically important and clinically relevant. This case demonstrates the importance of knowing IHC rejection criteria when interpreting HER2 IHC, which include (1) controls are not as expected, (2) artifact involves most of the sample, and (3) sample has strong membrane staining of normal breast ducts (internal controls). If the sample meets the IHC rejection criteria, repeating IHC or sending for FISH analysis can be performed to assure the accurate interpretation of HER2 status.

Case 3

History

A 55-year-old female presented with bloating and pelvic pressure. Pelvic ultrasound revealed a 3 cm cystic mass within the uterus that had been persistent over at least 4 months, suggestive of a possible hemangioma or arteriovenous malformation. A definitive surgical management with a hysterectomy and bilateral salpingo-oophorectomy was performed.

Gross Findings

There is a 4 × 4 cm purple-gray, irregularly shaped, ill-defined, cystic membranous lesion in both the anterior and posterior aspects of the uterus serosa and the left paraovarian tissue, extending 1.2 cm into the myometrium from the lateral aspect and comes within 0.1 cm from the endometrial lining. The endometrial cavity is not grossly involved.

Histologic Findings

H&E sections show small, monotonous ovoid cells inflitrate between bundles of myometrium, in the background of prominent arterioles (see Fig. 5.8a–b).

Differential Diagnosis

Vascular lesion, smooth muscle tumor (vascular leiomyoma), endometrial stromal tumor

Ancillary Studies

- Immunohistochemistry: The cells of interest are positive for CD10 and ER and are negative for CAM5.2, AE1/AE3, PAX8, CD31, CD34, desmin, h-caldesmon, SMA, and beta-catenin (see Fig. 5.8c–e).
- FISH analysis: The result indicates an unbalanced rearrangement involving the *PHF1* gene region with loss of the 5'PHF1 probe. Rearrangement of the *PHF1* gene at 6p21 has been observed in endometrial stromal sarcoma and ossifying fibromyxoid tumor. No rearrangement involving the *JAZF1* and *YWHAE* gene regions was identified.

Final Diagnosis

Low-grade endometrial stromal sarcoma

Discussion

Molecular testing can be very helpful in some challenging cases in gynecologic pathology. In this case, due to the unusual gross and morphologic findings, it would be difficult to render the diagnosis of endometrial stromal sarcoma without the FISH findings.

Case 4

History

A 54-year-old female with history of ductal carcinoma in situ of breast, s/p partial mastectomy, and hormonal therapy presented with postmenopausal bleeding. Pelvic ultrasound revealed a mildly thickened endometrium. Endometrial biopsy showed atypical hyperplasia. A hysterectomy and bilateral salpingo-oophorectomy was performed.

Histologic Findings

Endometrioid adenocarcinoma, FIGO grade 1 (see Fig. 5.9a)

MMR Studies

The tumor demonstrates loss of expression of PMS2. There is retained nuclear expression of MLH1, MSH2, and MSH6 (see Fig. 5.9b–e).

Genetic Testing

Sequence analysis identified one copy (heterozygous) of *PMS2* mutation S46I(137G > T) (genetic variant, suspected deleterious).

Follow-up

- Patient developed urothelial carcinoma 3 years later.
- Genetic follow-up detected a variant of unknown significance in the *ATM* gene, and negative *BRCA1/2*, *CDH1*, *CHECK2*, *PALB2*, *PTEN*, and *TP53*.

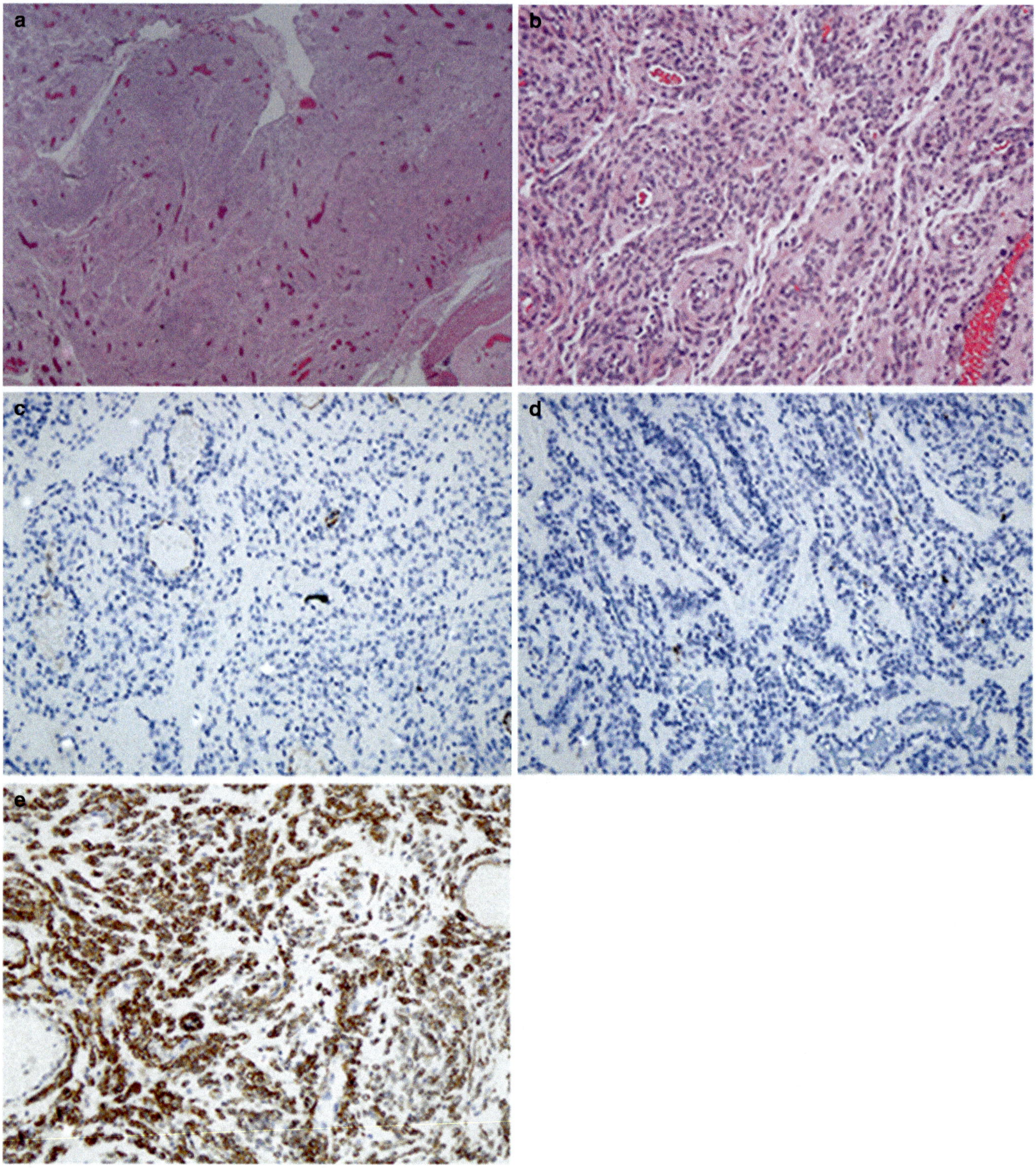

Fig. 5.8 A case of low-grade endometrial stromal sarcoma, demonstrating the diagnostic value of molecular testing. **a** and **b**: Morphology of the lesion (**a**, H&E, ×20; **b**, H&E, ×200). The cells of interest are positive for CD10 (**e**, ×200) and are negative for CD34 (**c**, ×200) and caldesmon (**d**, ×200)

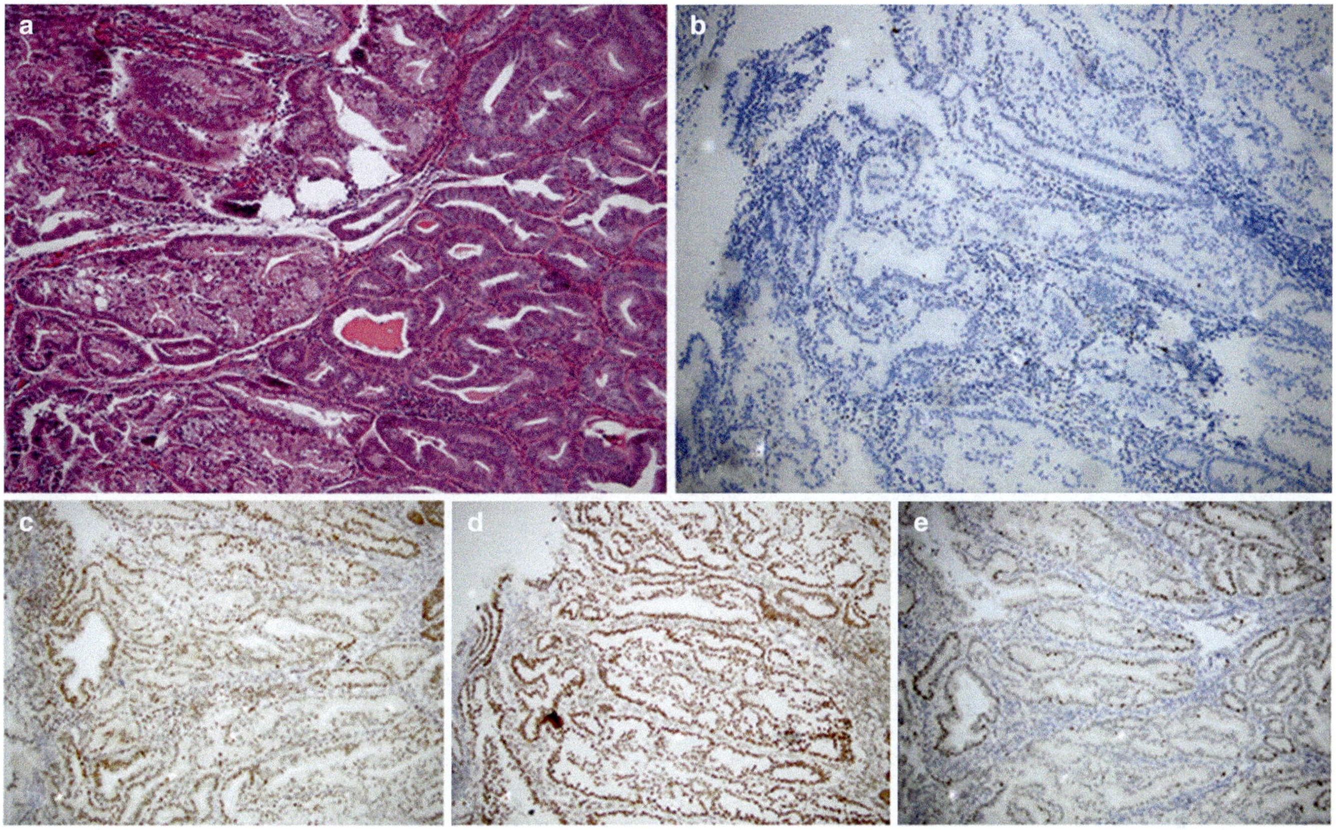

Fig. 5.9 A case of endometrioid adenocarcinoma, demonstrating the significance of routine MMR testing in women with endometrial cancer. **a**: Morphology of tumor (H&E, ×100); the tumor cells show loss of expression of PMS2 (**b**, ×200) and retained nuclear expression of MLH1 (**c**, ×200), MSH2 (**d**, × 200), and MSH6 (**e**, ×200)

- Normal surveillance colonoscopy, gastric and pancreatic cancer screenings.
- The patient's daughter also showed *PMS2* mutation S46I(137G > T) and undergoes surveillance.

Discussion

Identification of patients with Lynch syndrome may allow for screening and prevention strategies for patients themselves and their affected family members. This case illustrates the importance of routine MMR testing in women with endometrial cancer. As mentioned in Part 1, immunohistochemistry of MMR proteins is a simple and cost-effective method for Lynch syndrome screening.

References

1. The Cancer Genome Atlas Network. Comprehensive molecular portraits of human breast tumours. Nature. 2012;490:61–70.
2. Castera L, Krieger S, Rousselin A, et al. Next-generation sequencing for the diagnosis of hereditary breast and ovarian cancer using genomic capture targeting multiple candidate genes. Eur J Hum Genet. 2014;22:1305–13.
3. Walsh T, Lee MK, Casadei S, et al. Detection of inherited pathogenic variants for breast and ovarian cancer using genomic capture and massively parallel sequencing. Proc Natl Acad Sci U S A. 2010;107:12629–33.
4. Walsh T, King MC. Ten genes for inherited breast cancer. Cancer Cell. 2007;11:103–5.
5. van der Groep P, van der Wall E, van Diest PJ. Pathology of hereditary breast cancer. Cell Oncol (Dordr). 2011;34:71–88.
6. Honrado E, Benítez J, Palacios J. Histopathology of BRCA1- and BRCA2-associated breast cancer. Crit Rev Oncol Hematol. 2006;59:27–39.
7. NCCN Clinical Practice Guidelines in Oncology-Breast Cancer Version 2020. https://www.nccn.org/professionals/physician_gls/pdf/breast.pdf. Accessed 10 Dec 2020.
8. Manahan ER, Kuerer HM, Sebastian M, et al. Consensus guidelines on genetic testing for hereditary breast cancer from the American Society of Breast Surgeons. Ann Surg Oncol. 2019;26:3025–31.
9. Taylor A, Brady AF, Frayling IM, et al. Consensus for genes to be included on cancer panel tests offered by UK genetics services: guidelines of the UK Cancer genetics group. J Med Genet. 2018;55:372–7.
10. Harris LN, Ismaila N, McShane LM, et al. Use of biomarkers to guide decisions on adjuvant systemic therapy for women with early-stage invasive breast Cancer: American Society of

Clinical Oncology clinical practice guideline. J Clin Oncol. 2016;34:1134–50.
11. Perou CM, Sørlie T, Eisen MB, et al. Molecular portraits of human breast tumours. Nature. 2000;406:747–52.
12. Sørlie T, Perou CM, Tibshirani R, et al. Gene expression patterns of breast carcinomas distinguish tumor subclasses with clinical implications. Proc Natl Acad Sci U S A. 2001;98:10869–74.
13. Sorlie T, Tibshirani R, Parker J, et al. Repeated observation of breast tumor subtypes in independent gene expression data sets. Proc Natl Acad Sci U S A. 2003;100:8418–23.
14. Sørlie T. Molecular classification of breast tumors: toward improved diagnostics and treatments. Methods Mol Biol. 2007;360:91–114.
15. Hennessy BT, Gonzalez-Angulo AM, Stemke-Hale K, et al. Characterization of a naturally occurring breast cancer subset enriched in epithelial-to-mesenchymal transition and stem cell characteristics. Cancer Res. 2009;69:4116–24.
16. Prat A, Parker JS, Karginova O, et al. Phenotypic and molecular characterization of the claudin-low intrinsic subtype of breast cancer. Breast Cancer Res. 2010;12:R68.
17. Farmer P, Bonnefoi H, Becette V, et al. Identification of molecular apocrine breast tumours by microarray analysis. Oncogene. 2005;24:4660–71.
18. Vuong D, Simpson PT, Green B, Cummings MC, Lakhani SR. Molecular classification of breast cancer. Virchows Arch. 2014;465:1–14.
19. Fragomeni SM, Sciallis A, Jeruss JS. Molecular subtypes and local-regional control of breast cancer. Surg Oncol Clin N Am. 2018;27:95–120.
20. Groenendijk FH, Treece T, Yoder E, et al. Estrogen receptor variants in ER-positive basal-type breast cancers responding to therapy like ER-negative breast cancers. NPJ Breast Cancer. 2019;5:15.
21. Beitsch P, Whitworth P, Baron P, et al. Pertuzumab/Trastuzumab/CT versus Trastuzumab/CT therapy for HER2+ breast cancer: results from the prospective neoadjuvant breast registry symphony trial (NBRST). Ann Surg Oncol. 2017;24:2539–46.
22. Goldhirsch A, Wood WC, Coates AS, Gelber RD, Thürlimann B, Senn HJ, Panel members. Strategies for subtypes--dealing with the diversity of breast cancer: highlights of the St. Gallen international expert consensus on the primary therapy of early breast Cancer 2011. Ann Oncol. 2011;22:1736–47.
23. Lehmann BD, Bauer JA, Chen X, et al. Identification of human triple-negative breast cancer subtypes and preclinical models for selection of targeted therapies. J Clin Invest. 2011;121:2750–67.
24. Lehmann BD, Jovanović B, Chen X, et al. Refinement of triple-negative breast cancer molecular subtypes: implications for neoadjuvant chemotherapy selection. PLoS One. 2016;11:e0157368.
25. Bertucci F, Finetti P, Cervera N, et al. How basal are triple-negative breast cancers? Int J Cancer. 2008;123:236–40.
26. Alluri P, Newman LA. Basal-like and triple-negative breast cancers: searching for positives among many negatives. Surg Oncol Clin N Am. 2014;23:567–77.
27. Allison KH, Hammond MEH, Dowsett M, et al. Estrogen and progesterone receptor testing in breast cancer: ASCO/CAP guideline update. J Clin Oncol. 2020;38:1346–66.
28. Wolff AC, Hammond MEH, Allison KH, et al. Human epidermal growth factor receptor 2 testing in breast cancer: American Society of Clinical Oncology/College of American Pathologists clinical practice guideline focused update. J Clin Oncol. 2018;36:2105–22.
29. Cui X, Schiff R, Arpino G, Osborne CK, Lee AV. Biology of progesterone receptor loss in breast cancer and its implications for endocrine therapy. J Clin Oncol. 2005;23:7721–35.
30. Allison KH. Ancillary prognostic and predictive testing in breast cancer: focus on discordant, unusual, and borderline results. Surg Pathol Clin. 2018;11:147–76.
31. van de Ven S, Smit VT, Dekker TJ, Nortier JW, Kroep JR. Discordances in ER, PR and HER2 receptors after neoadjuvant chemotherapy in breast cancer. Cancer Treat Rev. 2011;37:422–30.
32. Zhang H, Moisini I, Ajabnoor RM, Turner BM, Hicks DG. Applying the new guidelines of HER2 testing in breast cancer. Curr Oncol Rep. 2020;22:51.
33. Sahoo S, Dabbs DJ, Bhargava R. Pathology of neoadjuvant therapeutic response of breast carcinoma. In: Dabbs, editor. Breast pathology. 2nd ed. Philadelphia: Elsevier Inc. 2016.
34. Kasami M, Uematsu T, Honda M, et al. Comparison of estrogen receptor, progesterone receptor and HER-2 status in breast cancer pre- and post-neoadjuvant chemotherapy. Breast. 2008;17:523–7.
35. Li P, Liu T, Wang Y, et al. Influence of neoadjuvant chemotherapy on HER2/neu status in invasive breast cancer. Clin Breast Cancer. 2013;13:53–60.
36. van Es SC, van der Vegt B, Bensch F, et al. Decalcification of breast cancer bone metastases with EDTA does not affect ER, PR, and HER2 results. Am J Surg Pathol. 2019;43:1355–60.
37. Frequently Asked Questions for Human Epidermal Growth Factor Receptor 2 (HER2) Testing in Breast Cancer: ASCO/CAP Clinical Practice Guideline Focused Update. https://www.cap.org/protocols-and-guidelines/cap-guidelines/current-cap-guidelines/recommendations-for-human-epidermal-growth-factor-2-testing-in-breast-cancer. Accessed 10 Dec 2020.
38. Zhang Z, Wang J, Skinner KA, et al. Pathological features and clinical outcomes of breast cancer according to levels of oestrogen receptor expression. Histopathology. 2014;65:508–16.
39. Raghav KP, Hernandez-Aya LF, Lei X, et al. Impact of low estrogen/progesterone receptor expression on survival outcomes in breast cancers previously classified as triple negative breast cancers. Cancer. 2012;118:1498–506.
40. Gloyeske NC, Dabbs DJ, Bhargava R. Low ER+ breast cancer: is this a distinct group? Am J Clin Pathol. 2014;141:697–701.
41. Kraus JA, Dabbs DJ, Beriwal S, Bhargava R. Semi-quantitative immunohistochemical assay versus oncotype DX(®) qRT-PCR assay for estrogen and progesterone receptors: an independent quality assurance study. Mod Pathol. 2012;25:869–76.
42. Badve SS, Baehner FL, Gray RP, et al. Estrogen- and progesterone-receptor status in ECOG 2197: comparison of immunohistochemistry by local and central laboratories and quantitative reverse transcription polymerase chain reaction by central laboratory. J Clin Oncol. 2008;26:2473–81.
43. Furrer D, Sanschagrin F, Jacob S, Diorio C. Advantages and disadvantages of technologies for HER2 testing in breast cancer specimens. Am J Clin Pathol. 2015;144:686–703.
44. Press MF, Seoane JA, Curtis C, et al. Assessment of ERBB2/HER2 status in HER2-equivocal breast cancers by FISH and 2013/2014 ASCO-CAP guidelines. JAMA Oncol. 2019;5:366–75.
45. Sneige N, Hess KR, Multani AS, Gong Y, Ibrahim NK. Prognostic significance of equivocal human epidermal growth factor receptor 2 results and clinical utility of alternative chromosome 17 genes in patients with invasive breast cancer: a cohort study. Cancer. 2017;123:1115–23.
46. Yu J, Dabbs DJ, Shuai Y, Niemeier LA, Bhargava R. Classical-type invasive lobular carcinoma with HER2 overexpression: clinical, histologic, and hormone receptor characteristics. Am J Clin Pathol. 2011;136:88–97.
47. Zhang H, Moisini I, Ajabnoor RM, et al. Frequency, clinicopathologic characteristics, and follow-up of HER2-positive nonpleomorphic invasive lobular carcinoma of the breast. Am J Clin Pathol. 2020;153:583–92.

48. Schrijver WA, Suijkerbuijk KP, van Gils CH, van der Wall E, Moelans CB, van Diest PJ. Receptor conversion in distant breast cancer metastases: a systematic review and meta-analysis. J Natl Cancer Inst. 2018;110:568–80.
49. Woo JW, Chung YR, Ahn S, et al. Changes in biomarker status in metastatic breast cancer and their prognostic value. J Breast Cancer. 2019;22:439–52.
50. Sabine V, Crozier C, Brookes C, et al. Mutational analysis of PI3K/AKT signaling pathway in tamoxifen exemestane adjuvant multinational pathology study. J Clin Oncol. 2014;32:2951–8.
51. Andre F, Ciruelos E, Rubovszky G, et al. Alpelisib for PIK3CA-mutated, hormone receptor-positive advanced breast cancer. N Engl J Med. 2019;380:1929–40.
52. Tognon C, Knezevich SR, Huntsman D, et al. Expression of the ETV6-NTRK3 gene fusion as a primary event in human secretory breast carcinoma. Cancer Cell. 2002;2:367–76.
53. Persson M, Andren Y, Mark J, et al. Recurrent fusion of MYB and NFIB transcription factor genes in carcinomas of the breast and head and neck. Proc Natl Acad Sci U S A. 2009;106:18740–4.
54. Cancer Genome Atlas Research Network. Integrated genomic analyses of ovarian carcinoma. Nature. 2011;474:609–15.
55. Pennington KP, Walsh T, Harrell MI, et al. Germline and somatic mutations in homologous recombination genes predict platinum response and survival in ovarian, fallopian tube, and peritoneal carcinomas. Clin Cancer Res. 2014;20:764–75.
56. Farmer H, McCabe N, Lord CJ, et al. Targeting the DNA repair defect in BRCA mutant cells as a therapeutic strategy. Nature. 2005;434:917–21.
57. Fong PC, Boss DS, Yap TA, et al. Inhibition of poly(ADP-ribose) polymerase in tumors from BRCA mutation carriers. N Engl J Med. 2009;361:123–34.
58. Veeck J, Ropero S, Setien F, et al. BRCA1 CpG island hypermethylation predicts sensitivity to poly(adenosine diphosphate)-ribose polymerase inhibitors. J Clin Oncol. 2010;28:e563–4.
59. O'Connor MJ. Targeting the DNA damage response in cancer. Mol Cell. 2015;60:547–60.
60. Pennington KP, Swisher EM. Hereditary ovarian cancer: beyond the usual suspects. Gynecol Oncol. 2012;124:347–53.
61. Norquist BM, Harrell MI, Brady MF, et al. Inherited mutations in women with ovarian carcinoma. JAMA Oncol. 2016;2:482–90.
62. Davies H, Glodzik D, Morganella S, et al. HRDetect is a predictor of BRCA1 and BRCA2 deficiency based on mutational signatures. Nat Med. 2017;23:517–25.
63. Cruz C, Castroviejo-Bermejo M, Gutiérrez-Enríquez S, et al. RAD51 foci as a functional biomarker of homologous recombination repair and PARP inhibitor resistance in germline BRCA-mutated breast cancer. Ann Oncol. 2018;29:1203–10.
64. Castroviejo-Bermejo M, Cruz C, Llop-Guevara A, et al. A RAD51 assay feasible in routine tumor samples calls PARP inhibitor response beyond BRCA mutation. EMBO Mol Med. 2018;10:e9172.
65. Konstantinopoulos PA, Norquist B, Lacchetti C, et al. Germline and somatic tumor testing in epithelial ovarian cancer: ASCO guideline. J Clin Oncol. 2020;38:1222–45.
66. Dougherty BA, Lai Z, Hodgson DR, et al. Biological and clinical evidence for somatic mutations in BRCA1 and BRCA2 as predictive markers for olaparib response in high-grade serous ovarian cancers in the maintenance setting. Oncotarget. 2017;8:43653–61.
67. Merajver SD, Pham TM, Caduff RF, et al. Somatic mutations in the BRCA1 gene in sporadic ovarian tumours. Nat Genet. 1995;9:439–43.
68. Fraune C, Rosebrock J, Simon R, et al. High homogeneity of MMR deficiency in ovarian cancer. Gynecol Oncol. 2020;156:669–75.
69. Rambau PF, Duggan MA, Ghatage P, et al. Significant frequency of MSH2/MSH6 abnormality in ovarian endometrioid carcinoma supports histotype-specific Lynch syndrome screening in ovarian carcinomas. Histopathology. 2016;69:288–97.
70. Leskela S, Romero I, Cristobal E, et al. Mismatch repair deficiency in ovarian carcinoma: frequency, causes, and consequences. Am J Surg Pathol. 2020;44:649–56.
71. Rabban JT, Calkins SM, Karnezis AN, et al. Association of tumor morphology with mismatch-repair protein status in older endometrial cancer patients: implications for universal versus selective screening strategies for Lynch syndrome. Am J Surg Pathol. 2014;38:793–800.
72. Garg K, Soslow RA. Lynch syndrome (hereditary non-polyposis colorectal cancer) and endometrial carcinoma. J Clin Pathol. 2009;62:679–84.
73. Broaddus RR, Lynch HT, Chen LM, et al. Pathologic features of endometrial carcinoma associated with HNPCC: a comparison with sporadic endometrial carcinoma. Cancer. 2006;106:87–94.
74. Westin SN, Lacour RA, Urbauer DL, et al. Carcinoma of the lower uterine segment: a newly described association with Lynch syndrome. J Clin Oncol. 2008;26:5965–71.
75. Hampel H, Frankel W, Panescu J, et al. Screening for Lynch syndrome (hereditary nonpolyposis colorectal cancer) among endometrial cancer patients. Cancer Res. 2006;66:7810–7.
76. Lu KH, Dinh M, Kohlmann W, et al. Gynecologic cancer as a "sentinel cancer" for women with hereditary nonpolyposis colorectal cancer syndrome. Obstet Gynecol. 2005;105:569–74.
77. Practice Bulletin No. 147. Lynch syndrome. Obstet Gynecol. 2014;124:1042–54.
78. Mills AM, Longacre TA. Lynch syndrome screening in the gynecologic tract: current state of the art. Am J Surg Pathol. 2016;40:e35–44.
79. McConechy MK, Talhouk A, Li-Chang HH, et al. Detection of DNA mismatch repair (MMR) deficiencies by immunohistochemistry can effectively diagnose the microsatellite instability (MSI) phenotype in endometrial carcinomas. Gynecol Oncol. 2015;137:306–10.
80. Gan C, Love C, Beshay V, et al. Applicability of next generation sequencing technology in microsatellite instability testing. Genes (Basel). 2015;6(1):46–59.
81. Salipante SJ, Scroggins SM, Hampel HL, Turner EH, Pritchard CC. Microsatellite instability detection by next generation sequencing. Clin Chem. 2014;60:1192–9.
82. Graham RP, Kerr SE, Butz ML, et al. Heterogenous MSH6 loss is a result of microsatellite instability within MSH6 and occurs in sporadic and hereditary colorectal and endometrial carcinomas. Am J Surg Pathol. 2015;39:1370–6.
83. Watkins JC, Nucci MR, Ritterhouse LL, Howitt BE, Sholl LM. Unusual mismatch repair immunohistochemical patterns in endometrial carcinoma. Am J Surg Pathol. 2016;40:909–16.
84. Stelloo E, Jansen AML, Osse EM, et al. Practical guidance for mismatch repair-deficiency testing in endometrial cancer. Ann Oncol. 2017;28:96–102.
85. Aird JJ, Steel MJ, Chow C, et al. Should you repeat mismatch repair testing in cases of tumour recurrence? An evaluation of repeat mismatch repair testing by the use of immunohistochemistry in recurrent tumours of the gastrointestinal and gynaecological tracts. Histopathology. 2020;76:521–30.
86. Ta RM, Hecht JL, Lin DI. Discordant loss of mismatch repair proteins in advanced endometrial endometrioid carcinoma compared to paired primary uterine tumors. Gynecol Oncol. 2018;151:401–6.
87. Boland CR, Thibodeau SN, Hamilton SR, et al. A National Cancer Institute workshop on microsatellite instability for cancer detection and familial predisposition: development of international criteria for the determination of microsatellite instability in colorectal cancer. Cancer Res. 1998;58:5248–57.

88. Salipante SJ, Scroggins SM, Hampel HL, Turner EH, Pritchard CC. Microsatellite instability detection by next generation sequencing. Clin Chem. 2014;60:1192–9.
89. Middha S, Zhang L, Nafa K, et al. Reliable pan-cancer microsatellite instability assessment by using targeted next-generation sequencing data. JCO Precis Oncol. 2017;2017:PO.17.00084.
90. Gan C, Love C, Beshay V, et al. Applicability of next generation sequencing technology in microsatellite instability testing. Genes (Basel). 2015;6:46–59.
91. Pang J, Gindin T, Mansukhani M, Fernandes H, Hsiao S. Microsatellite instability detection using a large next-generation sequencing cancer panel across diverse tumour types. J Clin Pathol. 2020;73:83–9.
92. Simpkins SB, Bocker T, Swisher EM, et al. MLH1 promoter methylation and gene silencing is the primary cause of microsatellite instability in sporadic endometrial cancers. Hum Mol Genet. 1999;8:661–6.
93. Bruegl AS, Djordjevic B, Urbauer DL, et al. Utility of MLH1 methylation analysis in the clinical evaluation of Lynch syndrome in women with endometrial cancer. Curr Pharm Des. 2014;20:1655–63.
94. Peterson LM, Kipp BR, Halling KC, et al. Molecular characterization of endometrial cancer: a correlative study assessing microsatellite instability, MLH1 hypermethylation, DNA mismatch repair protein expression, and PTEN, PIK3CA, KRAS, and BRAF mutation analysis. Int J Gynecol Pathol. 2012;31:195–205.
95. Yokoyama T, Takehara K, Sugimoto N, et al. Lynch syndrome-associated endometrial carcinoma with MLH1 germline mutation and MLH1 promoter hypermethylation: a case report and literature review. BMC Cancer. 2018;18:576.
96. Rahner N, Friedrichs N, Steinke V, et al. Coexisting somatic promoter hypermethylation and pathogenic MLH1 germline mutation in Lynch syndrome. J Pathol. 2008;214:10–6.
97. Crucianelli F, Tricarico R, Turchetti D, et al. MLH1 constitutional and somatic methylation in patients with MLH1 negative tumors fulfilling the revised Bethesda criteria. Epigenetics. 2014;9:1431–8.
98. Djordjevic B, Broaddus RR. Laboratory assays in evaluation of Lynch syndrome in patients with endometrial carcinoma. Surg Pathol Clin. 2016;9:289–99.
99. Kuismanen SA, Moisio AL, Schweizer P, et al. Endometrial and colorectal tumors from patients with hereditary nonpolyposis colon cancer display different patterns of microsatellite instability. Am J Pathol. 2002;160:1953–8.
100. Berends MJ, Wu Y, Sijmons RH, et al. Molecular and clinical characteristics of MSH6 variants: an analysis of 25 index carriers of a germline variant. Am J Hum Genet. 2002;70:26–37.
101. Wagner A, Hendriks Y, Meijers-Heijboer EJ, et al. Atypical HNPCC owing to MSH6 germline mutations: analysis of a large Dutch pedigree. J Med Genet. 2001;38:318–22.
102. Wu Y, Berends MJ, Mensink RG, et al. Association of hereditary nonpolyposis colorectal cancer-related tumors displaying low microsatellite instability with MSH6 germline mutations. Am J Hum Genet. 1999;65:1291–8.
103. Rhees J, Arnold M, Boland CR. Inversion of exons 1-7 of the MSH2 gene is a frequent cause of unexplained Lynch syndrome in one local population. Familial Cancer. 2014;13:219–25.
104. Rumilla K, Schowalter KV, Lindor NM, et al. Frequency of deletions of EPCAM (TACSTD1) in MSH2-associated Lynch syndrome cases. J Mol Diagn. 2011;13:93–9.
105. Geurts-Giele WR, Leenen CH, Dubbink HJ, et al. Somatic aberrations of mismatch repair genes as a cause of microsatellite-unstable cancers. J Pathol. 2014;234:548–59.
106. Haraldsdottir S, Hampel H, Tomsic J, et al. Colon and endometrial cancers with mismatch repair deficiency can arise from somatic, rather than germline, mutations. Gastroenterology. 2014;147:1308–1316.e1.
107. Cancer Genome Atlas Research Network, Kandoth C, Schultz N, et al. Integrated genomic characterization of endometrial carcinoma. Nature. 2013;497:67–73.
108. León-Castillo A, de Boer SM, Powell ME, et al. Molecular classification of the PORTEC-3 trial for high-risk endometrial Cancer: impact on prognosis and benefit from adjuvant therapy. J Clin Oncol. 2020;38:JCO2000549.
109. McAlpine J, Leon-Castillo A, Bosse T. The rise of a novel classification system for endometrial carcinoma; integration of molecular subclasses. J Pathol. 2018;244:538–49.
110. Koontz JI, Soreng AL, Nucci M, et al. Frequent fusion of the JAZF1 and JJAZ1 genes in endometrial stromal tumors. Proc Natl Acad Sci U S A. 2001;98:6348–53.
111. Nucci MR, Harburger D, Koontz J, Dal Cin P, Sklar J. Molecular analysis of the JAZF1-JJAZ1 gene fusion by RT-PCR and fluorescence in situ hybridization in endometrial stromal neoplasms. Am J Surg Pathol. 2007;31:65–70.
112. Hoang L, Chiang S, Lee CH. Endometrial stromal sarcomas and related neoplasms: new developments and diagnostic considerations. Pathology. 2018;50:162–77.
113. Lee CH, Ou WB, Mariño-Enriquez A, et al. 14-3-3 fusion oncogenes in high-grade endometrial stromal sarcoma. Proc Natl Acad Sci U S A. 2012;109:929–34.
114. Lee CH, Ali RH, Rouzbahman M, et al. The clinicopathologic features of YWHAE-FAM22 endometrial stromal sarcomas: a histologically high-grade and clinically aggressive tumor. Am J Surg Pathol. 2012;36:1562–70.
115. Conklin CM, Longacre TA. Endometrial stromal tumors: the new WHO classification. Adv Anat Pathol. 2014;21:383–93.
116. Buza N, Roque DM, Santin AD. HER2/neu in endometrial cancer: a promising therapeutic target with diagnostic challenges. Arch Pathol Lab Med. 2014;138:343–50.
117. Fader AN, Roque DM, Siegel E, et al. Randomized phase II trial of carboplatin-paclitaxel versus carboplatin-paclitaxel-Trastuzumab in uterine serous carcinomas that overexpress human epidermal growth factor receptor 2/neu. J Clin Oncol. 2018;36:2044–51.
118. Poljak M, Oštrbenk Valenčak A, Gimpelj Domjanič G, Xu L, Arbyn M. Commercially available molecular tests for human papillomaviruses: a global overview. Clin Microbiol Infect. 2020;26:1144. S1198-743X(20)30179-8
119. Salazar KL, Duhon DJ, Olsen R, Thrall M. A review of the FDA-approved molecular testing platforms for human papillomavirus. J Am Soc Cytopathol. 2019;8:284–92.
120. Darragh TM, Colgan TJ, Cox JT, et al. The lower Anogenital squamous terminology standardization project for HPV-associated lesions: background and consensus recommendations from the College of American Pathologists and the American Society for Colposcopy and Cervical Pathology. Arch Pathol Lab Med. 2012;136:1266–97.
121. Rabban JT, Karnezis AN, Devine WP. Practical roles for molecular diagnostic testing in ovarian adult granulosa cell tumour, Sertoli-Leydig cell tumour, microcystic stromal tumour and their mimics. Histopathology. 2020;76:11–24.
122. Buza N, Hui P. Immunohistochemistry and other ancillary techniques in the diagnosis of gestational trophoblastic diseases. Semin Diagn Pathol. 2014;31:223–32.

Tumors of the Central Nervous System

6

José E. Velázquez Vega, Leomar Y. Ballester, and Matthew J. Schniederjan

List of Frequently Asked Questions

1. How has an accelerated understanding of molecular genetics impacted the diagnosis of central nervous system (CNS) tumors?
2. What are some of the most common molecular methods utilized in brain tumor diagnostics?
3. What is the significance of identifying an *IDH1* or *IDH2* mutation by immunohistochemistry or sequencing analysis in a glial proliferation?
4. Is *IDH1* and *IDH2* gene sequencing necessary in GBMs arising in patients aged 55 years and older that are negative for the IDH1 R132H immunostain?
5. What is the utility of *ATRX* and *TP53* mutations in the classification of an IDH-mutant infiltrating glioma?
6. What is the current consensus on grading of IDH-mutant astrocytomas and what is the clinical significance of incorporation of molecular genetic parameters into grading algorithms?
7. What is the molecular signature of oligodendrogliomas?
8. What is a disadvantage of FISH test for 1p/19q codeletion in infiltrating gliomas?
9. What is the significance of identifying a concurrent gain of chromosome 7 and loss of chromosome 10, an *EGFR* amplification, and/or *TERT* promoter mutation in a diffuse astrocytic glioma without microvascular proliferation and necrosis?
10. What is the significance of finding an H3 K27M mutation in a diffuse midline glioma?
11. What is the significance of finding an H3.3 G34 mutation in a hemispheric diffuse glioma and what are some of the clinicopathologic features of this tumor?
12. What is the clinical utility of *MGMT* methylation analysis and what are the recommended methods to assess it?
13. What is the frequency and distribution of the *KIAA1549-BRAF* fusion and other MAPK pathway alterations in pilocytic astrocytomas?
14. What are some of the most common genetic alterations in pediatric low-grade neuroepithelial tumors?
15. What is the best diagnosis for an infiltrative appearing glioma with perivascular affinity and a *MYB-QKI* fusion?
16. What is the frequency of *BRAF* mutation and *CDKN2A/B* homozygous deletion in PXA and what is the significance of these findings in the differential diagnosis?
17. What are some of the most common genetic alterations in pediatric high-grade gliomas?
18. What are recent advances in the molecular classification of ependymal tumors?
19. What is the clinical significance of detecting a *C11orf95-RELA* fusion in a pediatric supratentorial ependymoma?
20. What CNAs differentially characterize posterior fossa ependymomas groups A and B and how can they be diagnosed in daily practice?
21. What are some of the hallmark genomic alterations most commonly utilized in medulloblastoma diagnostics?
22. The finding of loss of nuclear expression of INI1 (SMARCB1) immunostain in an embryonal appearing neoplasm arising in a young child is diagnostic of what entity?
23. What emerging CNS tumor entities are characterized by *BCOR*, *MN1*, *FOXR2*, and *CIC* gene alterations?
24. The finding of a focal amplification or fusion at chromosome 19q13.42 is characteristic of which family of CNS tumors?

J. E. Velázquez Vega (✉) · M. J. Schniederjan
Department of Pathology and Laboratory Medicine, Children's Healthcare of Atlanta – Scottish Rite and Egleston Hospitals, Emory University School of Medicine, Atlanta, GA, USA
e-mail: jevelaz@emory.edu; mschniederjan@emory.edu

L. Y. Ballester
Department of Pathology and Laboratory Medicine, McGovern Medical School, Houston, TX, USA
e-mail: leomar.y.ballester@uth.tmc.edu

Y. Ding, L. Zhang (eds.), *Practical Oncologic Molecular Pathology*, Practical Anatomic Pathology,
https://doi.org/10.1007/978-3-030-73227-1_6

25. What are some of the most common genetic alterations that characterize meningiomas?
26. The finding of strong nuclear immunoreaction with STAT6 immunostain in a dural-based tumor is supportive of what diagnosis?
27. What molecular genetic alterations can be used to differentiate between primary CNS melanocytic neoplasms and metastatic melanomas?
28. What are the most common mutations of papillary craniopharyngioma and adamantinomatous craniopharyngioma, respectively?

Frequently Asked Questions

1. **How has an accelerated understanding of molecular genetics impacted the diagnosis of central nervous system (CNS) tumors?**
   - The incorporation of molecular-genetic findings into brain tumor pathology has led to major reclassification of CNS tumor entities and has reshaped the standard of care for brain tumor diagnostics [1].
   - For the first time, the revised fourth edition of the World Health Organization (WHO) Classification of Tumours of the CNS [2] incorporated molecular parameters with histologic criteria to define many tumor entities [3]. In the past, previously recognized molecular-genetic alterations were regarded as associations that informed prognostic or predictive expectations.
   - The histologic diagnostic impression is now integrated with the results of molecular-genetic testing to allow better distinction amongst histologically overlapping entities [4, 5].
   - Major changes in the classification of diffuse gliomas, ependymal tumors, and CNS embryonal neoplasms followed rapidly evolving and increasing availability of high-throughput molecular platforms and, more recently, DNA methylation-based classification [6, 7]. Less common CNS tumor entities have also seen significant advances [8].
   - The integration of molecular parameters into the classification of CNS tumors has improved the interobserver variability in the diagnosis of diffuse gliomas [9, 10]. Importantly, there is no molecular signature for so-called "mixed gliomas," "oligoastrocytomas," and "glioblastoma (GBM) with oligodendroglioma component" as current diagnostic algorithms resolve these tumors into IDH-mutant astrocytomas, oligodendrogliomas, or IDH-wildtype diffuse gliomas at the molecular level [11, 12].
   - The **C**onsortium to **I**nform **M**olecular and **P**ractical **A**pproaches to **CNS** **T**umor **T**axonomy – **N**ot **O**fficial **W**HO (cIMPACT-NOW) was established in 2016 and constituted three separate working committees to address practice gaps in classification, grading questions and challenges in neuropathology, allow for more rapid integration of molecular advances into routine clinical care, provide practice guidelines to practicing neuropathologists, and offer suggestions for future WHO classification updates [13, 14].
2. **What are some of the most common molecular methods utilized in brain tumor diagnostics?**
   - A variety of methods are available and routinely used in clinical practice to evaluate protein expression and genomic alterations in brain tumors.
   - Immunohistochemistry is a widely available surrogate to detect the presence of mutant proteins like BRAF V600E, H3.3 K27M, and IDH1 R132H.
   - Immunohistochemistry to identify loss of protein expression, by deletion and/or mutational loss of epitopes, is also an important part of brain tumor diagnosis. Examples include loss of ATRX expression in IDH-mutant diffuse astrocytomas and loss of SMARCB1/INI1 expression in atypical teratoid/rhabdoid tumor (AT/RT).
   - Single gene sequencing (e.g., Sanger sequencing) can be used to identify mutations in specific genes of interest although this is being replaced by next-generation sequencing (NGS) assays that allow the evaluation of multiple genes simultaneously.
   - Pyrosequencing can be used to assess specific codons (e.g., codon 132 of the *IDH1* gene or codon 27 of the *H3F3A* gene). This technique is amenable to evaluation of multiple samples in a multi-well format. However, it is limited to the assessment of one codon at time.
   - NGS is a preferred method to evaluate brain tumors because it allows the detection of mutations, gene fusions, and copy number alterations (CNAs). Hundreds of genes can be evaluated at once in a single assay.
   - Fluorescence in situ hybridization (FISH) is routinely used for evaluation of 1p/19q codeletion in oligodendrogliomas. It can also be used to detect deletions, duplications, rearrangements, fusions, and amplifications in pieces of tissue too small for other molecular methods.
   - Single-nucleotide polymorphism (SNP) arrays perform genome-wide assessment for CNAs in brain tumors including the combined gain of chromosome 7/loss of chromosome 10 and *EGFR* amplification that characterize IDH-wildtype GBM. Similarly, whole arm 1p/19q codeletion can be assessed by SNP arrays.
   - DNA methylation profiles of tumors are a combination of somatically acquired DNA methylation changes superimposed on the background methyl-

ation pattern of the cell of origin. These profiles are reproducible in clinical pathology settings and can be used to subclassify CNS tumors. Methylation arrays are increasingly being used to classify CNS tumors, especially when histologic and sequence-based findings are inconclusive. The main limitation of this technique is that the instrumentation and informatic tools required are not readily available.

- Gene expression analysis (transcriptomics) can be used to identify some tumor subtypes. For example, nanostring technology has been used to determine the four molecular subgroups of medulloblastoma. RNA sequencing by NGS can also be used for global gene expression analysis.
- See Table 6.1.

3. **What is the significance of identifying an *IDH1* or *IDH2* mutation by immunohistochemistry or sequencing analysis in a glial proliferation?**
   - Identifying an IDH mutation in a glial proliferation essentially rules out the possibility of reactive gliosis and supports the diagnosis of a diffuse glioma [15].
   - Parsons et al. [16] and Yan et al. [17] first established IDH-mutant diffuse gliomas as a form of disease that could not be differentiated histologically from their IDH-wildtype counterparts but exhibited distinct clinical behavior.
   - Somatic heterozygous *IDH1* mutations are regarded as initiating events in gliomagenesis [18].
   - Mutations within the enzymatic active sites of *IDH1* and *IDH2* lead to a gain-of-function resulting in the accumulation of the oncometabolite 2-hydroxyglutarate [19–22]. This oncometabolite results in global DNA hypermethylation and other genome-wide epigenetic alterations [23–25]. IDH mutations are not exclusive to gliomas as they have also been detected in subsets of acute myeloid leukemia, cholangiocarcinomas, chondrosarcomas, and melanomas [22].
   - Within the current diagnostic algorithms, more than 80% of diffuse astrocytomas (WHO grades 2–3) and all oligodendrogliomas are IDH-mutant [2, 16, 17, 26, 27].
   - *IDH1* and *IDH2* mutations result in a substitution of a key arginine within the enzymatic active sites at codons R132 and R172, respectively [28, 29]. The *IDH1* R132H variant is the most common mutation, accounting for 92.7% of all IDH mutations. Non-

Table 6.1 Common techniques for evaluation of genomic alterations in CNS tumors

Technique	Common application in CNS tumor diagnosis	Advantages	Limitations
Immunohistochemistry	Detection of lineage-specific proteins Detection of mutant protein expression Identifying loss of expression of mutant proteins	Relatively inexpensive Relatively quick and easy to analyze Readily available in clinical laboratories Requires minimal tumor tissue	Limited to one mutant allele per antibody and will not detect others Staining pattern may not always correlate with presence or absence of a genomic alteration Subjective interpretation
Fluorescence in situ hybridization	Copy number, e.g., 1p/19q codeletion, *EGFR* amplification Gene fusions and rearrangements via break-apart and fusion probes	Requires minimal tumor tissue Simple to perform and interpret	False-positive 1p19q codeletion due to partial deletions Break-apart probes not specific for fusion partner Limited to individual genes/loci
Next-generation sequencing	Evaluation of mutations (SNV), copy number alterations, and gene fusions	Ability to evaluate numerous genes simultaneously	Assessment of copy alterations may have limited sensitivity RNA needed for fusion detection
Methylation-specific PCR	Evaluation of MGMT promoter methylation	Relatively inexpensive Fast turn-around time	Requires large amounts of nucleic acid Bisulfite conversion can damage DNA and the assay can be technically challenging
Single-nucleotide polymorphism (SNP) array	Evaluation of copy number alterations and/or chromosomal defects	Allows genome-wide evaluation of copy number in detail Less expensive than NGS	Limited ability to detect mutations as SNPs Limited to alterations that impact copy number or LOH
Methylation array	Classification of CNS tumor type based on genome-wide methylation pattern Evaluation of MGMT promoter methylation	Reliable tumor classification Not sensitive to tissue quality, can use necrotic, over-fixed, old tissue	Analysis infrastructure and algorithms are not readily available Requires large amounts of nucleic acid
Pyrosequencing	Evaluation of single-nucleotide variants (SNV)	Inexpensive, sensitive, fast turn-around time	Use restricted to detection of SNVs in a single gene

canonical *IDH1* mutations include the R132C (4.1%), R132S (1.5%), R132G (1.4%), and R132L (0.2%) variants [29]. *IDH2* mutations account for approximately 3% of IDH mutations but are overrepresented in oligodendrogliomas, IDH-mutant and 1p/19q codeleted. The R172 codon of the *IDH2* gene is homologous to the R132 codon of the *IDH1* gene, and the most common variant mutations include R172K (65%), R172M (19%), and R172W (16%) [29].

- A highly sensitive and specific monoclonal antibody (IDH1R132H) that recognizes the mutant protein is widely available and routinely utilized in the diagnostic neuropathology setting [30]. Gene sequencing is necessary to detect non-R132H variant mutations.
- Recently, a distinct subset of cerebellar IDH-mutant diffuse astrocytic tumors has recently been characterized. Most of these tumors harbor non-canonical IDH mutations and the frequency of *ATRX* alterations is lower than in hemispheric IDH-mutant diffuse astrocytomas [31].

4. **Is *IDH1* and *IDH2* gene sequencing necessary in GBMs arising in patients aged 55 years and older that are negative for the IDH1 R132H immunostain?**
   - It has been suggested that *IDH1* and *IDH2* gene sequencing may not be warranted in the setting of a negative R132H immunostain in GBMs arising in patients older than 55 years due to the rarity of non-R132H *IDH1* mutations in patients in this age group [3, 32–34].
   - In a study of cost effectiveness that addressed IDH testing in diffuse gliomas, a negligible prevalence of noncanonical IDH mutations was seen in GBM patients over the age of 55 years suggesting that there is limited value in testing for variant *IDH1/2* mutations by sequencing in this population and supporting this age-based cutoff to improve test utilization and balance cost effectiveness in clinical practice [33].
5. **What is the utility of *ATRX* and *TP53* mutations in the classification of an IDH-mutant infiltrating glioma?**
   - Approximately two-thirds of IDH-mutant lower-grade diffuse gliomas had intact 1p/19q and of these 94% had *TP53* mutations and 86% had a functional loss of ATRX [26].
   - The finding of an IDH mutation by IDH1 R132H immunohistochemistry (IHC) or sequencing is evaluated in conjunction with p53 and ATRX immunostains. In the setting of a confirmed IDH mutation, strong p53 immunoreactivity and loss of nuclear expression with ATRX IHC are excellent surrogates of *TP53* mutation and ATRX loss at the genetic level and supportive of an integrated diagnosis of an IDH-mutant astrocytoma.
6. **What is the current consensus on grading of IDH-mutant astrocytomas and what is the clinical significance of incorporation of molecular genetic parameters into grading algorithms?**
   - The incorporation of IDH mutational status into the classification of diffuse astrocytomas resulted in challenges to the time-honored histologic grading criteria established decades before the discovery of *IDH1* and *IDH2* mutations [35–37].
   - Previously, the distinction between diffuse astrocytoma (WHO grade 2) and anaplastic astrocytoma (WHO grade 3) rested in the identification of mitotic activity. However, it was shown that conspicuous mitotic activity was not highly informative of clinical outcomes in IDH-mutant infiltrating astrocytomas [35]. IDH-mutant diffuse and anaplastic astrocytomas were found to arise at a similar age and showed little survival differences [36].
   - Efforts during the past several years focused in optimizing risk-stratification within IDH-mutant astrocytomas and identifying molecular parameters that may help in grading algorithms ("molecular grading") [38–40]. Homozygous *CDKN2A/B* deletion has been associated with shorter survival in IDH-mutant astrocytomas and has prognostic power superior to microvascular proliferation and necrosis [39, 40].
   - The cIMPACT-NOW update 5 addressed grading criteria and terminology of IDH-mutant astrocytomas [41]. Furthermore, the cIMPACT-NOW update 6 addressed new entities and diagnostic principle recommendations for future CNS tumor classification and grading [42]. Given the well-established survival advantage of IDH-mutant astrocytomas when compared to their wildtype counterparts, it has been recommended to discontinue the term "glioblastoma, IDH-mutant" [42]. The introduction of *CDKN2A/B* homozygous deletion to complement histologic grading algorithms and to complement histologic features was suggested. The presence of *CDKN2A/B* homozygous deletion denotes grade 4 behavior and outcomes [42].
7. **What is the molecular signature of oligodendrogliomas?**
   - The molecular signature of oligodendroglioma is defined by an *IDH1* or *IDH2* mutation *and* whole-arm codeletion of chromosomes 1p and 19q. By definition, the combination of both alterations is required for the now codified diagnosis of "oligodendroglioma, IDH-mutant and 1p/19q-codeleted." [2]
   - *IDH2* mutations are more common in oligodendrogliomas than in IDH-mutant astrocytomas.

- The oligodendroglial phenotype was tightly associated with the loss of 1p/19q by Reifenberger et al. [43] and the correlation to enhanced treatment response quickly followed in a study by Cairncross et al. [44]
- Now considered as a diagnostic signature, the codeletion is known to be mediated through an unbalanced translocation t(1;19)(q10;p10) followed by the loss of the derivative chromosome, resulting in whole-arm losses of 1p and 19q [45, 46].
- *CIC*, *FUBP1*, *NOTCH1*, and *TERT* promoter mutations are common in oligodendroglioma, IDH-mutant and 1p/19q-codeleted [26].
- Loss of chromosome 4 is seen in approximately 25% of cases with very few other recurring copy number alterations [26, 38].
- Oligodendrogliomas are graded on the basis of mitotic activity, microvascular proliferation, and necrosis; however, some genetic events including *NOTCH1* mutations, PI3K pathway alterations, and certain CNAs have been associated with disease progression and worse outcomes [47–50].

8. **What is a disadvantage of FISH test for 1p/19q codeletion in infiltrating gliomas?**
   - Whole-arm loss of chromosome 1p and 19q are invariably associated with *IDH1* and *IDH2* mutations. As stated above, whole-arm 1p/19q codeletion is essential to define an oligodendroglioma.
   - FISH for 1p/19q remains a popular method for assessing codeletions. However, FISH recognizes probe-specific focal losses that in the setting of genomic instability in high-grade astrocytomas may lead to a false positive result and possible misclassification [51, 52]. Hence, partial 1p/19q codeletion called positive by FISH is diagnostically a false-positive result because it is not indicative of the translocation that results in complete loss of 1p and 19q.
   - A small percentage of GBMs can show 1p/19q codeletion when tested by FISH. In a large cohort of GBMs (n = 491), Clark et al. [52] found that 5.7% had 1p/19q codeletion by either FISH or polymerase chain reaction (PCR)-based loss of heterozygosity; however, the vast majority of these showed other IDH-wildtype GBM signatures such as chromosome 10q loss of heterozygosity or *EGFR* amplifications. More recently, Ball et al. [53] studied a cohort of 223 diffuse astrocytic gliomas WHO grades 2–4 and estimated the overall false-positive FISH 1p/19q codeletion rate was 3.6%.
   - Testing platforms that are able to discriminate partial from whole-arm 1p/19q codeletion, such as molecular inversion probe arrays and NGS are becoming increasingly available and reduce the risk of a false positive result.
9. **What is the significance of identifying a concurrent gain of chromosome 7 and loss of chromosome 10, an *EGFR* amplification, and/or *TERT* promoter mutation in a diffuse astrocytic glioma without microvascular proliferation and necrosis?**
   - Diffuse astrocytomas lacking histologic criteria for a diagnosis of GBM but harboring genetic alterations classic of IDH-wildtype GBM behave aggressively [26, 27, 54, 55].
   - Stichel et al. [56] found that the combination of any two of *EGFR* amplification, the combined +7/−10 copy number signature, or *TERT* promoter mutation is highly specific for IDH-wildtype GBM and that the combination of all three events is exclusively seen in IDH-wildtype GBM.
   - The cIMPACT-NOW update 3 recognized high-level *EGFR* amplification, or combined +7/−10 copy number signature, or *TERT*-p mutation as markers highly specific of aggressive behavior and incorporated them as a requirement for a diagnosis of "diffuse astrocytic glioma, IDH-wildtype, with molecular features of GBM, WHO grade 4" [57].
   - Further survival analysis by Tesileanu et al. [58] showed similar behavior and outcomes of diffuse astrocytic glioma, IDH-wildtype, with molecular features of GBM, WHO grade 4, and IDH-wildtype GBM and proposed they be also classified as IDH-wildtype GBMs.
   - The cIMPACT-NOW update 6 recognizes these alterations as sufficient for a diagnosis of IDH-wildtype GBM. Hence, an IDH-wildtype diffuse astrocytoma can be diagnosed as "glioblastoma, IDH-wildtype, WHO grade 4" if (a) there is microvascular proliferation and/or necrosis or (b) if there is one or more of these three genetic signatures: *EGFR* amplification, combined +7/−10 CNA, or *TERT* promoter mutation [42]. This change reflects the need to simplify nomenclature and facilitate clinical trial entry.
10. **What is the significance of finding an H3 K27M mutation in a diffuse midline glioma?**
   - The entity of "diffuse midline glioma, H3 K27M-mutant, WHO grade 4" was first codified in 2016 to highlight the tight relationship of a form of high-grade glioma arising in a midline anatomic compartment [2]. Diffuse midline glioma H3 K27M-mutant is genetically distinct from other IDH-wildtype diffuse astrocytic gliomas.
   - Following the identification of the H3 K27M mutation in circumscribed and lower-grade glial/glioneuronal tumors, the cIMPACT-NOW issued a clarification on the entity to emphasize that the diag-

nostic criteria must be that of (a) an infiltrating glioma that (b) arises in a midline location [59]. "Diffuse midline glioma, H3 K27M-mutant, WHO grade 4" entity is reserved for tumors meeting the above stated criteria and should not be applied to other tumors that are H3 K27M –mutant [59].

- Mutations within the N-terminal tail of the histone variants H3.3 (encoded by the *H3F3A* and *H3F3B* genes) or H3.1 (encoded by the *HIST1H3B* and *HIST1H3C* genes) were first identified in the pediatric population and noted to be highly prevalent in diffuse intrinsic pontine gliomas. Tumors harboring these mutations have been increasingly recognized in other midline locations of adolescents and adults [60–65].
- Many studies have confirmed dismal prognosis in diffuse midline gliomas with H3 K27M mutations; hence, the entity was codified as a WHO grade 4 disease [62, 63, 66, 67]. Several studies that included adult patients have reinforced bad outcomes in this population [54, 68, 69]. There may be some differences in outcome depending on the anatomic site involved [70].
- H3 K27M mutations can be detected by immunohistochemistry with a sensitivity and specificity approaching 100% [61]. Loss of nuclear expression of H3K27 trimethylation by immunohistochemistry is often seen in H3 K27M-mutant tumors, although subjectivity in interpreting this immunostain has been documented [71].

11. **What is the significance of finding H3.3 G34 mutation in a hemispheric diffuse glioma and what are some of the clinicopathologic features of this tumor?**
    - The cIMPACT-NOW update 6 recommends the inclusion of "Diffuse glioma, H3.3 G34-mutant" in the upcoming WHO classification, corresponding to a WHO grade 4 disease [42]. These tumors have poor outcomes but have better prognosis than H3 K27M-mutant diffuse midline gliomas [72, 73].
    - Diffuse glioma, H3.3 G34-mutant preferentially occurs in the hemispheres of adolescents [60]. The driving mutation occurs in the gene encoding histone H3.3 at amino acid 34 and results in a substitution of glycine for either arginine or valine (G34R/V) [60].
    - These tumors exhibit histologic heterogeneity and can exhibit primitive neuroectodermal tumor or embryonal-like histomorphologic features [72, 74–76].
    - A new H3 G34R antibody has been developed to aid in the detection of such mutations [77]. These tumors have high rates of *TP53* mutations and *ATRX* alterations and immunohistochemistry for p53 and ATRX may be contributory when considering this entity in the differential diagnosis [72].
12. **What is the clinical utility of *MGMT* methylation analysis and what are the recommended methods to assess it?**
    - One of the most important prognostic and predictive biomarkers used in the clinical management of patients with GBM is the methylation status of the promoter for *O6-methylguanine-DNA methyltransferase* (*MGMT*). MGMT is a DNA repair enzyme with the ability to restore guanine from O6-methylguanine loss induced by alkylating agents such as Temozolomide [78–82]. Hence, low levels of MGMT would be expected to correlate with an improved treatment response to alkylating agents.
    - The expression level of MGMT is determined in large part by the methylation status of the gene's promoter.
    - Most investigations have shown that epigenetic gene silencing of *MGMT* by promoter methylation is a strong predictor of prolonged survival, independent of other clinical factors or treatment [83]. It has also been demonstrated that *MGMT* promoter methylation is associated with prolonged progression-free survival (PFS) and overall survival(OS) in patients with GBM treated with chemotherapy and radiation therapy [82–88].
    - In the clinical setting, *MGMT* promoter methylation is typically assessed by methylation-specific PCR or pyrosequencing [80, 81, 83, 89–91]. Some laboratories report the promoter methylation status as "low level" and "high level," or indicate that "partial methylation" is present, yet the clinical implications of this distinction are not fully understood. MGMT IHC is currently not recommended for clinical practice [80, 92, 93].
13. **What is the frequency and distribution of the *KIAA1549-BRAF* fusion and other MAPK pathway alterations in pilocytic astrocytomas?**
    - Pilocytic astrocytomas (WHO grade 1) are the most common brain tumors of childhood and are often found in the cerebellum with the classic radiologic presentation of a cyst with a mural enhancing nodule, however it can arise throughout the neuraxis. The most classic histomorphology is that of a biphasic low grade glioma with Rosenthal fibers and microcysts. Pilocytic astrocytomas generally have favorable prognosis [2].
    - Mitogen-activated protein kinase (MAPK) pathway alterations are characteristic of pilocytic astrocytomas and other pediatric type low-grade glial/glioneuronal tumors [often considered together as low-grade neuroepithelial tumors (LGNTs)]. These include

BRAF mutation or fusion, *FGFR1* mutation or structural rearrangement, *NF1* mutation, NTRK-family receptor kinase gene fusions, and other less frequent alterations such as *KRAS* mutations and *RAF1* fusions [94–98]. The elucidation of these genetic events within the past decade has led to parallel development of drugs targeting them [97, 98].
- The *KIAA1549-BRAF* fusion resulting from tandem duplication in the chromosome 7q34 region is a defining genetic event that is present in more than 70% of pilocytic astrocytomas across all anatomic compartments [96, 99, 100]. Approximately 90% of pilocytic astrocytomas arising in the cerebellum harbor this characteristic fusion [96]. Although the *KIAA1549-BRAF* is also the most frequent alteration elsewhere (approximately 50% of supratentorial cases), the frequency of alternate MAPK pathway alterations is comparatively increased [96].
- BRAF V600E mutations occur in a small subset of pilocytic astrocytomas [95].

14. **What are some of the most common genetic alterations in pediatric low-grade neuroepithelial tumors?**
    - Pediatric tumors are biologically and genetically dissimilar to their adult counterparts [94, 101, 102]. As an example, IDH-mutations and *TERT*-p mutations are very rare in childhood tumors [103, 104].
    - Alterations of the MAPK pathway are the most common drivers of LGNTs [94, 105]. For instance, the *KIAA1549-BRAF* fusion is characteristic of pilocytic astrocytomas, as stated above.
    - The most common pediatric brain tumors are low-grade gliomas, typically characterized by a mutually exclusive, single dominant somatic genetic event that affects genes such as *NF1*, *RAF1*, *BRAF*, *FGFR1*, or *MYB* (or its homolog, *MYBL1*) [94, 106]. Zhang et al. [94] found mutually exclusive *FGFR1* and *MYB* or *MYBL1* aberrations were present in 56% of diffuse gliomas.
    - Qaddoumi et al. [107] also found that most LGNTs (84%) analyzed by whole-genome sequencing were characterized by a single driver genetic alteration. They also found that the most common pathogenic alterations in LGNTs were in *FGFR1/FGFR2/FGFR3*, *BRAF*, or *MYB/MBL1*, occurring in 78% of the cohort cases. *FGFR1* alterations aligned with LGNTs that showed a predominant "oligodendroglioma-like" morphology while *MYB* fusion genes were the most common genetic alteration in diffuse astrocytomas (41%) [107].
    - In a recent analysis of 1,000 pediatric low-grade gliomas, Ryall et al. [102] found that 84% harbored a driver alteration, while those without an identified alteration also often exhibited upregulation of the RAS/MAPK pathway, demonstrating nearly universal activation of this key pathway in pediatric low-grade glioma. *KIAA1549-BRAF* fusion, *BRAF* V600E, and *NF1* mutations account for 2/3 of alterations in pediatric low-grade glioma [102].
    - The cIMPACT-NOW update 6 recommends that the diagnosis of "pediatric-type" IDH-wildtype and H3-wildtype diffuse gliomas be rendered in an integrated, tiered approach where both the histopathology and the genetic alterations are combined [42].
    - Pleomorphic xanthoastrocytomas (PXAs) exhibit the highest frequency of *BRAF* V600E mutations; however, they also occur in gangliogliomas (~30%), dysembryoplastic neuroepithelial tumors (~30%), pilocytic astrocytomas (~5%), and diffuse astrocytomas (17–43%) [2, 102, 103, 105, 107, 108].
    - Diffuse leptomeningeal glioneuronal tumor preferentially occurs in children and is characterized by widespread leptomeningeal growth, an oligodendroglial-like phenotype and high frequency of *KIAA1549-BRAF* fusion with either chromosome 1p deletion or 1p/19q codeletion without concurrent IDH mutations [109, 110].
    - Polymorphous low-grade neuroepithelial tumor of the young predominantly occurs in children and young adults and is associated with epilepsy. The tumor exhibits a diffuse pattern of growth, an oligodendroglial-like phenotype, calcifications and characteristic CD34 immunoreaction along with frequent alterations of *FGFR2*, *FGFR3*, or *BRAF* genes [111, 112].

15. **What is the best diagnosis for an infiltrative appearing glioma with perivascular affinity and a *MYB-QKI* fusion?**
    - Angiocentric glioma (WHO grade 1) is an uncommon glioma that primarily affects children and young adults. As one of the low-grade developmental and epilepsy-associated brain tumors (LEATs), angiocentric gliomas are often associated with epilepsy [113]. Histologically, the tumor exhibits ependymal differentiation, characteristically shows an angiocentric growth pattern and has an infiltrative appearance [2].
    - The *MYB-QKI* fusion is the prototypic rearrangement that characterizes angiocentric gliomas and represents a good example of phenotype-genotype correlation [107, 114].
    - Angiocentric gliomas are typically classified as "low-grade glioma, MYB/MYBL1" methylation class together with others tumors that lack an angiocentric growth pattern and/or the classic *MYB-QKI* fusion [6]. One such example is isomorphic diffuse glioma that also shows recurrent *MYB* and *MYBL1* alterations and exhibits a DNA-methylation profile closely

related to angiocentric glioma albeit forming distinct groups in t-SNE analyses [115].

16. **What is the frequency of *BRAF* mutation and *CDKN2A/B* homozygous deletion in PXA and what is the significance of these findings in the differential diagnosis?**
    - PXA (WHO grade 2) is a rare, well-circumscribed/poorly infiltrative glioma that commonly arises in children and young adults particularly in the temporal lobe. The tumor is characterized by a combination of spindle-shaped cells, xanthomatous change, eosinophilic granular bodies, and large pleomorphic multinucleated tumor cells [116].
    - PXAs exhibit the highest frequency of *BRAF* V600E mutations among CNS tumors, being present in approximately 60–78% of cases [2, 108, 116].
    - Loss of chromosome 9 and homozygous *CDKN2A/B* deletions are recognized as hallmark alterations of PXA and were initially estimated to occur in about 50–60% of cases when studied by comparative genomic hybridization [117]. More recently, Vaubel et al. [118] identified that 87% of PXAs showed homozygous deletion of *CDKN2A/B* using molecular inversion probe chromosomal microarray.
    - Anaplastic PXA (WHO grade 3) was codified in the 2016 revised fourth edition of the WHO classification and is associated with shorter OS and recurrence free survival. These tumors show more than 5 mitoses per 10 high-power fields [2]. *BRAF* V600E mutations and *CDKN2A/B* often occur in anaplastic PXAs but several recent studies have highlighted additional molecular-genetic features such as *TERT* alterations [116, 118–120]. Epithelioid GBM exhibits overlapping features both at the histologic and genomic levels and needs to be carefully excluded from a differential diagnosis that includes anaplastic PXA [121, 122]. Methylation profiling may be helpful in classifying difficult cases [123].
17. **What are some of the most common genetic alterations in pediatric high-grade gliomas?**
    - Although relatively rare, malignant gliomas in children represent the greatest cause of cancer-related deaths under the age of 19 years [101, 124]. In one recent study addressing causes of deaths in the pediatric neuro-oncology population, high-grade gliomas and diffuse intrinsic pontine gliomas accounted for 6.3% and 7.1% of the studied brain tumor cohort yet accounted for 49.3% of total deaths [125].
    - Diffuse intrinsic pontine gliomas often harbor mutations in the genes encoding histones H3.3 and H3.1 and exhibit WHO grade 4 behavior, as described above. *ACVR1* mutations can occur in up to a third of diffuse intrinsic pontine gliomas [64, 126].
    - In an integrated, large-scale genomic and epigenetic analyses of 202 pediatric GBMs Korshunov et al. [73] unexpectedly showed that 20% displayed methylation profiles similar to either low-grade gliomas or PXAs, had a better OS and were enriched for PXA-associated molecular alterations including *BRAF* V600E mutations and homozygous *CDKN2A* deletions. The remaining 162 pediatric GBMs stratified into the following 4 subgroups: IDH1-mutant (6%), H3.3 G34-mutant (15%), H3.3/H3.1 K27-mutant (43%), and those GBMs that were wild type for H3 and IDH (36%) [73]. In a subsequent study of the H3-/IDH-wildtype subset pediatric GBMs, 3 biologically and clinically distinct molecular subtypes with different genomic and epigenetic signatures were identified and classified as "pedGBM_MYCN," "pedGBM_RTK1," and "pedGBM_RTK2," which were respectively enriched for *MYCN*, *PDGFRA*, and *EGFR* amplifications [127].
    - Mackay et al. [101] performed an integrated molecular analysis in over a 1000 cases of pediatric high-grade gliomas which, among many important findings, confirmed the rarity of IDH-mutations in this population (6.25%), highlighted the rarity of common adult IDH-wildtype GBM alterations (*EGFR* amplification identified in less than 5% of cases) and further accentuated the high frequency of histone H3 variant mutations in the pediatric population (50.3% in this cohort).
    - Recent advances have been made regarding the biology and genetic underpinnings of congenital and infantile diffuse gliomas, which appear clinically distinct than their counterparts in older children despite similar histologies [128–131]. In infancy the association between tumor grade and outcome is less predictable and may exhibit paradoxical survival and better response to treatment when compared to older children [128]. Of potential clinical relevance, a subset of congenital/infant high-grade gliomas harbor *ALK*/*ROS1*/*MET*/NTRK-family fusions for which targeted therapies exist [128–131].
18. **What are recent advances in the molecular classification of ependymal tumors?**
    - The cIMPACT-NOW updates 6 and 7 recognize the biologic heterogeneity of ependymomas across CNS anatomic compartments and favors categorizing them by anatomic site and subgrouping them by genetic and epigenetic signature [42, 132].
    - The principle of separation of ependymomas by anatomic site follows methylome profiling that showed the largest differences were between anatomic compartments, despite similar histomorphologic appearance [132, 133]. The cIMPACT-NOW

update 7 proposed considering methylation profiling as a front-line diagnostic test when ependymoma is a consideration in the differential diagnosis [132].

- Pajtler et al. [134] recognized nine molecular subgroups of ependymoma across anatomic compartments by genome-wide methylation and gene expression profiling as follows:
  - Supratentorial compartment
    1. *C11orf95-RELA* fusion positive
    2. *YAP1-MAMLD1* or *YAP1-FAM118B* fusion positive
    3. Subependymoma
  - Posterior fossa compartment
    1. Group A
    2. Group B
    3. Subependymoma
  - Spinal cord compartment
    1. Ependymoma (classic)
    2. Myxopapillary ependymoma
    3. Subependymoma
- More recently, a subset of aggressive spinal cord ependymoma with its own methylation class has been described [135–137]. These tumors tend to occur in young adults in an intradural/extramedullary localization and are characterized by *MYCN* amplification, anaplastic histology, early dissemination, and absence of *NF2* mutations.
- The majority of classic spinal cord ependymoma is characterized by loss of chromosome 22q (including *NF2*). *NF2* mutations also occur in a subset [134].

19. **What is the clinical significance of detecting a *C11orf95-RELA* fusion in a pediatric supratentorial ependymoma?**
    - Ependymoma, RELA fusion-positive was codified in the revised fourth edition of the WHO CNS classification [2]. Approximately 75% of this subset of supratentorial ependymoma arises in children with a median age of 8 years [134].
    - More than 70% of supratentorial ependymomas harbor the *C11orf95-RELA* fusion, the most common recurrent genetic alteration in ependymomas [134, 138]. This oncogenic driver is mediated through chromothripsis of chromosome 11q13.1 and results in nuclear translocation of p65-RelA protein and NF-kB signaling activation [138].
    - Immunohistochemistry for p65-RelA is a sensible and reproducible method for detection of NF-kB pathway signaling activation, which could be used as a surrogate marker for the fusion event. The concordance between IHC for p65-RelA and RELA FISH was 100% in one study [139]. Pages et al. [139] demonstrated that concordance between p65-RelA IHC and DNA methylome analysis for the detection of the *RELA* fusion-positive ependymomas was high, with 96.4% agreement ($\kappa = 0.916$; CI95[0.754–1]). The concordance between RELA FISH and DNA methylation assay for the detection of these tumors was also high, with an overall agreement of 95.2% ($\kappa = 0.859$; CI95[0.592–1]) [139].
    - L1CAM immunoreaction by IHC also correlates well with the *C11orf95-RELA* fusion [138]. The fusion may also be detected by RT-PCR although alternate fusions may render a false negative result [139, 140].
    - Homozygous *CDKN2A* deletions were frequently detected in supratentorial *RELA* fusion-positive ependymomas and not in *YAP1* fusion-positive tumors [134].
    - In a large retrospective cohort, Pajtler et al. [134] found that supratentorial *RELA* fusion-positive ependymomas show dismal outcome with 10-year OS rates of approximately 50% and PFS rates of 20%.
20. **What CNAs differentially characterize posterior fossa ependymomas groups A and B and how can they be diagnosed in daily practice?**
    - Several studies have revealed the existence of two demographically, transcriptionally, genetically, and clinically distinct groups of posterior fossa ependymomas that have been termed "group A" and "group B." Posterior fossa group A patients are younger, have laterally located tumors with a balanced genome, and are much more likely to experience recurrence, metastasis at recurrence, and death when compared with the posterior fossa group B patients. Nearly all cases of posterior fossa group A arises in children aged below 8 years (median age: 3 years), whereas posterior fossa group B patients are older children and young adults [134, 141].
    - Although posterior fossa group A ependymomas have a tendency for balanced genomes, they are enriched for chromosome 1q gain, a known independent factor of poor prognosis [134, 141–143]. Posterior fossa group B ependymomas usually exhibit numerous CNAs involving whole chromosomes or chromosomal arms, including loss of 1, 2, 3, 6, 8, 10, 14q, 17q, and 22q, and gain of 4, 5q, 7, 9, 11, 12, 15q, 18, 20, and 21q [141].
    - Several studies have shown marked reductions of H3 K27 trimethylation immunostaining in posterior fossa group A ependymomas compared to group B tumors and have supported its use as an independent biomarker of poor prognosis and as a diagnostic aid to segregate these posterior fossa ependymomas with 99% sensitivity and 100% specificity [144, 145]. Of note, between 0.6 and 4.2% of group A ependymomas have been observed to harbor H3 K27M muta-

tions, the significance of which is currently unknown [146, 147].

- Witt et al. [141] reported 5-year PFS and OS of 47% and 69%, for group A ependymomas and 79% and 95% for group B ependymomas, respectively. Furthermore, Pajtler et al. [134] found that posterior fossa group A ependymomas show dismal outcome with 10-year OS rates of approximately 50% and PFS rates of 20%.

21. **What are some of the hallmark genomic alterations most commonly utilized in medulloblastoma diagnostics?**
    - The genetic classification for medulloblastoma (WHO grade 4) was introduced to the WHO Classification of CNS Tumors for the first time on 2016 [2]. The current consensus criteria for genetically defined medulloblastoma include four main subgroups termed WNT-activated, SHH-activated, group 3 and group 4 [148–151]. The recognition of these molecular subtypes has aided in algorithms for risk stratification in the clinical setting [150, 152].
    - WNT-activated medulloblastomas account for approximately 10% of all medulloblastomas, and up to 90% have exon 3 *CTNNB1* somatic mutations [148, 153–155].
    - SHH-activated tumors account for approximately 30% of all medulloblastomas and are further stratified on the basis of *TP53* mutations with those that are *TP53*-mutant having a grim prognosis [148, 154–156]. In this subset, *TP53* mutations correlate with anaplastic histology, a high rate of chromothripsis and tetraploidy, chromosome 17p loss, and *MYCN* amplification [156–158]. *PTCH1*, *SUFU*, and *SMO* mutations as well as other SHH-signaling pathway gene alterations are characteristic of SHH-activated medulloblastomas [154, 159]. Losses of *PTCH1* (chromosome 9q.22) are present in up to two thirds of SHH-activated medulloblastomas [155, 160, 161]. *TERT*-p mutations are overrepresented in SHH-activated medulloblastomas [162].
    - Group 3 and group 4 medulloblastomas are often considered together as a "non-WNT/non-SHH" group since they are not easily separated by readily available biomarker approaches. Together they account for the majority of all medulloblastomas (approximately 60%). MYC amplifications are almost exclusive to group 3 medulloblastomas and chromosome 17 alterations are found in approximately 80% of group 4 medulloblastomas [160, 163]. Both groups 3 and 4 medulloblastomas can exhibit an isochromosome 17q (approximately 60% in group 3 and 80% in group 4), making it the most common genetic abnormality in all medulloblastomas [7]. Group 3 medulloblastoma tend to have more CNAs, most frequently gain of 1q and 7, and loss of 10q. Besides isochromosome 17q, most abundant in group 4 medulloblastomas is gain of 7p and loss of 8 [7]. Among group 3 medulloblastomas, chromosome 1q gain, 17p loss, 17q gain, isochromosome 17q, and MYC amplification are associated with worse outcomes. In contrast, gains of chromosome 17 and loss of chromosome 11 have been associated with better outcomes in group 4 medulloblastomas [164].
    - Molecular subclassification of medulloblastomas was originally established by sequencing, gene expression, and transcriptomic analysis, but, more recently, DNA methylation profiling has superseded these other methodologies to become the "gold standard" [7, 165–167]. In one practical immunohistochemical approach, IHC for beta-catenin, GAB1, and YAP1 are performed to stratify medulloblastomas into molecular subgroups [160, 168]. Nuclear immunoreactivity of beta-catenin IHC is a surrogate for beta-catenin mutations in WNT pathway tumors, but it can be hard to interpret. WNT-driven medulloblastomas also express cytoplasmic and nuclear YAP1. GAB1 immunoreactivity is only observed in SHH-activated medulloblastomas alongside expression of YAP1. Non-WNT/non-SHH medulloblastomas are GAB1 and YAP1 negative [160, 163, 168].
    - In a study that included 1022 medulloblastoma patients, germline mutations were present in 6% of all medulloblastomas with the highest prevalence in the SHH-activated group. The consensus medulloblastoma predisposition genes include *APC*, *BRCA2*, *PALB2*, *PTCH1*, *SUFU*, and *TP53* [169].

22. **The finding of loss of nuclear expression of INI1 (SMARCB1) immunostain in an embryonal appearing neoplasm arising in a young child is diagnostic of what entity?**
    - Atypical teratoid/rhabdoid tumors (AT/RTs), WHO grade 4, are highly aggressive brain tumors that typically occur in early childhood. The vast majority of tumors show inactivation of *SMARCB1* (INI1, hSNF5, BAF47; chromosome 22q11.2), a core member of the adenosine triphosphate (ATP)-dependent SWI/SNF chromatin- remodeling complex. To a lesser extent, a subset of AT/RTs shows loss-of-function mutations of *SMARCA4* (BRG1) at chromosome 19p13.2 [170–173]. The genome of AT/RTs is not complex and exhibits a low mutational load [174]. Johann et al. [174] recently described three epigenetically distinct subgroups of AT/RTs exhibiting clinicopathologic differences.
    - Despite marked histologic heterogeneity, tumor cells in AT/RTs exhibit eccentric nuclei, vesicular chroma-

tin, conspicuous nucleoli, and cytoplasmic globular inclusions.

- Screening for germline mutations in AT/RTs should be a consideration particularly when arising in the very young, as roughly one third of cases arise in the setting of rhabdoid tumor predisposition syndrome [175, 176].
- AT/RTs can be identified by loss of INI1 immunostain nuclear expression in tumor cells. Internal normal tissue structures serve as a positive control, as INI1 expression is retained in normal cells. For example, endothelial cells within a *SMARCB1*-deficient tumor will be positive for INI1 immunostain.
- Loss of INI1 expression can be found in AT/RTs, epithelioid malignant peripheral nerve sheath tumors, epithelioid sarcomas, extraskeletal myxoid chondrosarcomas, myoepithelial carcinomas, renal medullary carcinomas, and renal rhabdoid tumors [177–184]. The spectrum of *SMARCB1*-deficient tumors continues to expand [184, 185].

23. **What emerging CNS tumor entities are characterized by *BCOR*, *MN1*, *FOXR2*, and *CIC* gene alterations?**
    - In 2016, Sturm et al. [186] described four new uncommon CNS tumor entities derived from DNA methylation, and transcriptomic and copy number profiling of CNS primitive neuroectodermal tumors. These were defined by recurrent genetic alterations and distinct clinical and histomorphologic features and designated as (I) CNS neuroblastoma with *FOXR2* activation, (II) CNS Ewing sarcoma family tumor with *CIC* alteration, (III) CNS high-grade neuroepithelial tumor with *MN1* alteration, and (IV) CNS high-grade neuroepithelial tumor with *BCOR* alteration. Following emerging evidence, the cIMPACT-now update 6 recommends further refinement with the codification of the following tumors in the next WHO classification as "CNS neuroblastoma, *FOXR2*-activated," *CIC* sarcoma (aligned with the WHO classification of tumors of soft tissue and bone), "astroblastoma, *MN1*-altered," and "CNS tumor with *BCOR* internal tandem duplication." [42]
    - The *BCOR* exon 15 internal tandem duplication is often the solitary pathogenic alteration of "CNS tumors with *BCOR* internal tandem duplication" but in a subset also co-occurs with other genetic events such as *CDKN2A/B* homozygous deletion, *TERT* alterations, and mutations in *TP53*, *BCORL1*, *EP300*, *SMARCA2*, and *STAG2* genes [187]. This tumor arises in the cerebral or cerebellar hemispheres of younger children and exhibits ependymoma-like perivascular pseudorosettes and glioma-like fibrillarity [186, 187].
    - The diagnosis of astroblastoma has well-recognized inter-observer variation and they do not exhibit a distinct methylation class [7]. In their study, Sturm et al. [186] recognized that a proportion of histologically diagnosed astroblastomas classified as high-grade neuroepithelial tumors with *MN1* alteration but not all tumors within this class exhibited the histomorphology of astroblastomas. The CNS high-grade neuroepithelial tumor with *MN1* alteration methylation class can harbor *MN1-BEND2* fusions and, to a lesser extent, *MN1-CXXC5* fusions, and can show losses of chromosomes 16q and 22q and chromothripsis of chromosome X [7, 186, 188]. Recent publications have highlighted the molecular heterogeneity of histologically diagnosed astroblastomas and have emphasized the need for molecular-genetic testing to exclude alternate diagnoses including PXA, ependymomas, and IDH-wildtype GBM [188–190].
    - CNS Ewing sarcoma family of tumors with CIC alterations as described by Sturm et al. [186] are likely to be termed "CIC sarcomas" as they occur in the bone and soft tissue counterparts [191–193]. These tumors often exhibit a small round cell phenotype but can show areas of spindling. Tumors arising within the CNS can harbor *CIC-NUTM1* fusions; however, the most common fusion in the bone and soft tissues is *CIC-DUX4* [186, 193, 194]. Rare CNS cases have been described to harbor the *CIC-DUX4* fusion [195, 196].
    - CNS neuroblastomas with *FOXR2* activation show embryonal architecture and a small cell phenotype along with neuropil and neuronal differentiation with scattered ganglion cells. These tumors reveal genomic alterations and structural alterations involving the *FOXR2* gene locus including fusions, tandem duplications, deletion, or chromothripsis [186, 197]. These tumors show gains of chromosome 1 and 8 and losses on chromosome 16 [7, 197].

24. **The finding of a focal amplification or fusion at chromosome 19q13.42 is characteristic of which family of CNS tumors?**
    - 'Embryonal tumor with multilayered rosettes, C19MC-altered' represents the consolidation of three previously codified entities (embryonal tumor with abundant neuropil with true rosettes, ependymoblastoma, and medulloepithelioma) into a single entity defined by a highly specific focal amplification and fusion of chromosome 19q13.42 that encodes the largest human microRNA cluster (C19MC) [198–201].

- These tumors are characterized by pseudostratified/multilayered rosettes and exhibit aggressive behavior, therapy resistance, and poor survival; hence, they represent a WHO grade 4 disease [202]. The focal amplification of chromosome 19q13 is definitional, although there is a subset of tumors that histomorphologically fit this entity but lack the amplification and also fall within this methylation class family [7]. Chromosome 2 gain is present in 60% of these tumors [7].
- Despite their highly heterogeneous histology these tumors are characterized by specific high expression of the RNA-binding protein LIN28A. Immunohistochemistry for LIN28A is often used as a diagnostic marker for these tumors [202, 203].

25. **What are some of the most common genetic alterations that characterize meningiomas?**
    - Meningiomas are tumors that originate from the meninges, the membrane that covers the brain and spinal cord, and they represent approximately 30% of all primary brain tumors, the vast majority of which are benign WHO grade I tumors (more than 80%) [204, 205]. Multiple histologic variants across WHO grades 1–3 are recognized and codified in the WHO classification of CNS tumors [2].
    - Neurofibromatosis type 2 (NF2) is a genetic disorder that predisposes patients to the development of certain tumors such as the hallmark bilateral acoustic schwannomas and multiple meningiomas (the second most common tumor in the syndrome). Meningiomas occur in more than half of NF2 patients and always have chromosome 22 abnormalities [205–208]. Meningiomas can also arise in the context of other germline syndromes including some with alterations in the SWI/SNF chromatin-related pathway [205].
    - The most common genomic alteration in sporadic meningiomas is loss of chromosome 22 in the vast majority of meningiomas (up to 70%), which includes the *NF2* gene [204, 205, 208]. Inactivating *NF2* mutations can occur in up to 50% of tumors with loss of chromosome 22 [208]. The majority of chromosomal changes are whole chromosomal arm losses with a tendency to increase in frequency in correlation to grade and risk of recurrence/progression such as loss of chromosome 1p [204, 208].
    - Differences among sporadic, NF2-associated, pediatric, and radiation-induced meningiomas have been documented, and non-sporadic meningiomas have a higher incidence of multiple chromosomal abnormalities at presentation [208–210]. Recently, a subgroup of NF2-wildtype pediatric and young adult meningiomas were found to harbor *YAP1-FAM118B* fusions previously described in an important molecular subset of supratentorial ependymomas, therefore expanding the genomic spectrum of meningiomas [211].
    - Several phenotype-genotype correlations are recognized in meningiomas as delineated below:
      i. Recurrent mutations in *TRAF7, AKT1, KLF4*, and *SMO* are present in up to 40% of sporadic meningiomas, preferentially in skull base tumors and almost always occurring without associated *NF2* mutation or chromosome 22 loss [205, 212, 213]. Mutations in *TRAF7* are the second most common genomic alteration in meningiomas. Mutations in *TRAF7* frequently co-occur with mutations in *KLF4* (p.K09Q) or *AKT1* (p.E17K) [213].
      ii. In the skull base, mutations correlate with different sites of origin. The majority of meningiomas in the lateral or posterior regions have *NF2* loss, while meningiomas in the anterior and medial regions have mutations in *TRAF7*, and *AKT1*, *TRAF7*, and *KLF4* or *SMO* [213].
      iii. The BRCA1-associated protein (BAP1) is a tumor suppressor gene inactivated in a subset of high-grade rhabdoid meningiomas. Meningiomas with BAP1 loss are clinically aggressive and have shorter time to recurrence. In a subset of patients, the BAP1-inactivating mutations are of germline origin (BAP1 tumor predisposition syndrome) [214, 215].
      iv. Angiomatous meningiomas have a tendency to harbor multiple polysomies across the genome, most commonly of chromosome 5 [216]. More recently, microcystic meningiomas have been shown to harbor a similar genetic profile as angiomatous meningiomas, including a hyperdiploid genome and chromosome 5 polysomy [217].
      v. Nearly all cases of secretory meningioma harbor mutations in both KLF4(K409Q) and TRAF7 but lack mutations in *NF2* [218].
      vi. In the context of familial, hereditary multiple spinal meningioma syndrome, clear cell meningiomas are associated with *SMARCE1* loss-of-function mutations [219].
    - Recent epigenetic analyses revealed robust DNA methylation signatures that correlated with previously described risk-associated chromosomal CNAs and stratified patients by recurrence risk [220, 221]. Losses of chromosome 1p, 6q, 14q, and 18q and gain of 1p were identified as indicators of poor outcome [220]. A methylome-based prediction model of early recurrence risk has been developed for meningiomas which was found to offer important prognostic information [222].

26. **The finding of strong nuclear immunoreaction with STAT6 immunostain in a dural-based tumor is supportive of what diagnosis?**
    - Solitary fibrous tumors (SFTs) are rare soft tissue tumors that can form nearly anywhere in the body. Solitary fibrous tumors most often occur in the lining around the outside of the lungs (pleural solitary fibrous tumors) but have also been found in other sites, including the neuraxis as meningeal tumors. SFTs are composed of spindled to ovoid cells in a patternless architecture with prominent stromal collagen and branching (staghorn-like) vessels. It can sometimes be difficult to distinguish SFTs from other intracranial mesenchymal tumors including meningiomas and sarcomas.
    - A *NAB2–STAT6* gene fusion, resulting in a chimeric protein in which a repressor domain of NGFI-A binding protein 2 (EGR1 binding protein 2) (NAB2) is replaced with the carboxy-terminal transactivation domain from signal transducer and activator of transcription 6, interleukin-4-induced (STAT6), has been identified as a consistent finding in SFTs [223, 224]. This gene fusion results in nuclear localization of the chimeric protein, which can be visualized with an antibody against the STAT6 protein [225–227].
    - The revised fourth edition of the WHO classification of CNS tumors restructured solitary fibrous tumor and hemangiopericytomas (SFT/HPC) as one entity and introduced a grading system to accommodate this change [2].
    - A number of studies, including CNS tumor series, have reported phenotype-genotype correlations based in differences of histopathology and type of *NAB2-STAT6* fusion [228–230].
27. **What molecular genetic alterations can be used to differentiate between primary CNS melanocytic neoplasms and metastatic melanomas?**
    - The most common genetic alterations that drive melanocytic proliferations vary by anatomic location. Knowledge of the oncogenic drivers of melanocytic neoplasms can help identify the primary site of origin and help distinguish metastatic from primary CNS lesions [231–233]. Some of the most important genetic correlations include the following:
    - The *BRAF* V600E mutation is the most common genetic alteration in cutaneous melanomas.
    - Melanomas from acral skin and mucosal regions frequently have alterations in *KIT*.
    - Melanocytic proliferations in the CNS of adult patients (including ocular melanomas) frequently have alterations in *GNAQ* and *GNA11*.
    - *NRAS* mutations occur in primary CNS melanocytic tumors of children and underlie the pathogenesis of neurocutaneous melanosis.
28. **What are the most common mutations of papillary craniopharyngioma and adamantinomatous craniopharyngioma, respectively?**
    - Craniopharyngiomas are tumors that originate in the sellar region. Two types of craniopharyngiomas are recognized based on histologic characteristics: papillary and adamantinomatous. Papillary craniopharyngiomas occur almost exclusively in adults while adamantinomatous craniopharyngiomas can occur in children or adults.
    - Adamantinomatous craniopharyngioma consists of a proliferation of squamous cells with peripheral palisading, stellate reticulum, and wet keratin. Mutations in *CTNNB1* (beta-catenin) have been identified in approximately 95% of adamantinomatous craniopharyngiomas [234, 235].
    - Beta-catenin is involved in the Wnt-signaling pathway. Beta-catenin moves into the nucleus and regulates gene expression. Mutations in *CTNNB1* can interfere with the degradation of beta-catenin, resulting in increased protein levels and aberrant nuclear localization. Nuclear expression of beta-catenin (which can be assessed by immunohistochemistry) is a good surrogate marker for *CTNNB1* mutations in adamantinomatous craniopharyngiomas.

Papillary craniopharyngiomas are characterized by the presence of fibrovascular cores with non-keratinizing squamous epithelium. The *BRAF* V600E mutation is present in approximately 95% of papillary craniopharyngiomas [235].

Case Presentations

Case 1

Learning Objective

Highlight the diagnostic algorithm of IDH-mutant gliomas and the practical workup utilized to differentiate between IDH-mutant astrocytomas and oligodendrogliomas, IDH-mutant and 1p/19q codeleted.

Case History

A 49-year-old female presented with a seizure and a history of previously diagnosed "oligoastrocytoma, WHO grade 2" 8 years earlier. At that time, she also presented with seizures and MRI revealed a partially cystic, T2-hyperintense, non-enhancing right temporal lobe tumor which was resected and followed by imaging surveillance. No chemotherapy or radiotherapy was given prior to the resection of progressive disease.

Histologic Features

- H&E sections (Fig. 6.1a) revealed a moderately cellular infiltrating glioma composed of cells with variable nuclear contours ranging from round to elongate, irregular forms. Conspicuous mitotic activity was identified. There was no necrosis or microvascular proliferation.
- By immunohistochemistry, IDH R132H immunostain diffusely highlighted tumor cells (Fig. 6.1b). Immunohistochemistry for p53 showed strong and diffuse overexpression in tumor nuclei (Fig. 6.1c). ATRX immunostain highlighted loss of nuclear expression in tumor nuclei (Fig. 6.1d). Of note, ATRX expression is retained in neurons, endothelial cells, and lymphocytes (internal positive control).

Genetic Study

SNP-array revealed multiple copy number alterations including partial gains and losses. Importantly, whole-arm codeletion of 1p/19q was not present. Homozygous deletion of *CDKN2A/B* was absent. There were no amplification events. Sequencing analysis confirmed the *IDH1* c.395G>A(pArg132His, R132H) sequence variation. MGMT promoter methylation was detected.

Final Diagnosis

Astrocytoma, IDH-mutant, WHO grade 3

Discussion

The molecular signature of IDH-mutant astrocytomas include *IDH1*/*IDH2*, *ATRX*, and *TP53* mutations. The immunoprofile is strongly supportive of the diagnosis as it confirmed the IDH1 R132H variant mutation; there was strong p53 overexpression and there was loss of ATRX nuclear expression. A diagnosis of oligoastrocytoma or mixed glioma is no longer supported since molecular-genetic alterations now stratify lower-grade infiltrating gliomas into IDH-mutant astrocytomas, oligodendrogliomas, or IDH-wildtype astrocytomas. In the context of an IDH-mutant glioma, the absence of whole-arm 1p/19q codeletion is inconsistent with the now molecularly defined oligodendroglioma. IDH-mutant astrocytomas have improved OS when compared to their IDH-wildtype counterparts.

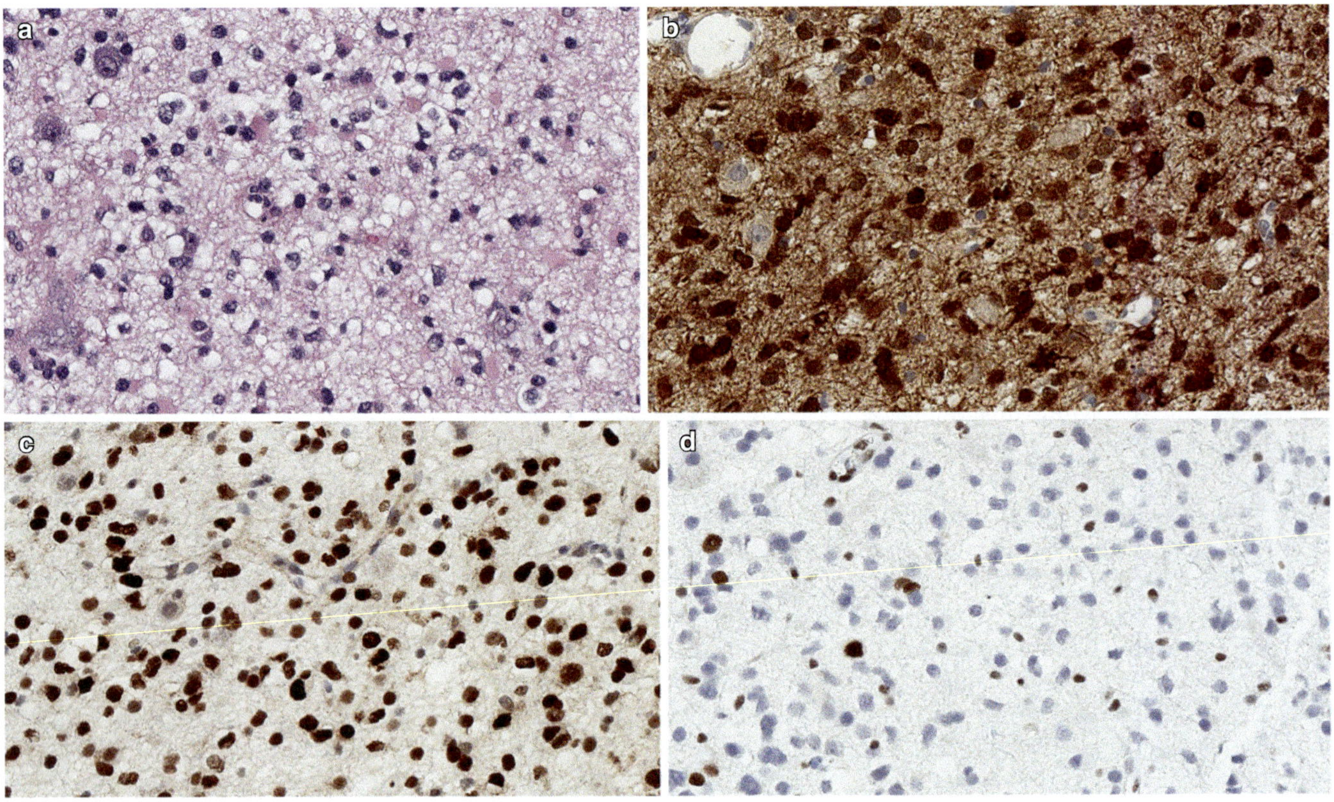

Fig. 6.1 Histomorphologic and immunostaining features of case 1. (**a**) H&E stain. (**b-d**) Immunohistochemical stains. (**b**) IDH R132H, (**c**) p53, (**d**) ATRX. (Original magnification: 400X)

Case 2

Learning Objective

Highlight the current classification of ependymomas and recognize an important subset of genetically defined supratentorial ependymoma.

Case History

A 13-year-old male that presented with generalized tonic clonic seizures. MRI revealed a 4 cm right frontal tumor in the precentral area that was heterogeneously hyperintense on T2-weighted images and showed heterogeneous solid and "ring-like" areas of enhancement. The tumor has recurred on multiple occasions requiring several modalities of adjuvant treatment, including chemotherapy and radiotherapy.

Histologic Features

- H&E sections (Fig. 6.2a) showed a well-circumscribed glioma with areas showing classic histologic features of ependymoma, including perivascular pseudorosettes. The tumor, however, exhibited heterogeneous features including areas of clearing, vacuolation, and prominent calcifications (not shown). Conspicuous mitotic activity was identified (Fig. 6.2b). Focal microvascular proliferation was present but there was no necrosis.
- Immunohistochemistry for GFAP was positive and EMA showed "dot-like" immunoreactivity as commonly seen in ependymomas. L1CAM immunostain was positive.
- The Ki-67 proliferation index was high.

Genetic Study

SNP-array detected a polyploid genome with multiple copy number alterations including complex abnormalities of chromosome 11 consistent with chromothripsis and suggestive of *C11orf95-RELA* fusion. FISH confirmed rearrangement of *RELA* and *C11orf95*.

Final Diagnosis

Supratentorial ependymoma, RELA-fusion positive (WHO grade 3)

Discussion

C11orf95-RELA fusion-positive ependymomas occur in the supratentorial compartment of children with a median age of 8 years. They exhibit aggressive behavior and poor outcomes. The diagnosis of ependymomas now integrates the anatomic compartment and molecular-genetic information. This case met histomorphologic criteria for an anaplastic designation (WHO grade 3).

Case 3

Learning Objective

Highlight the phenotype-genotype correlation of a tumor that may mimic a high-grade astrocytoma and comment on the utility of biomarkers in resolving the differential diagnosis.

Case History

A 21-year-old female presented with new onset seizures. MRI revealed a 1.4 cm area of abnormal T2/FLAIR signal with incomplete rim of enhancement in the right temporal lobe.

Histologic Features

- H&E sections (Fig. 6.3a, b) revealed a glial hypercellular tumor composed of numerous atypical pleomorphic astrocytes with abundant eosinophilic cytoplasm. In areas the tumor was remarkable for spindled and fascicular arrangements (Fig. 6.3a). Numerous eosinophilic granular bodies were identified (Fig. 6.3b), and perivascular lymphocytic cuffing was noted. Mitotic figures were inconspicuous. There was no necrosis or microvascular proliferation.

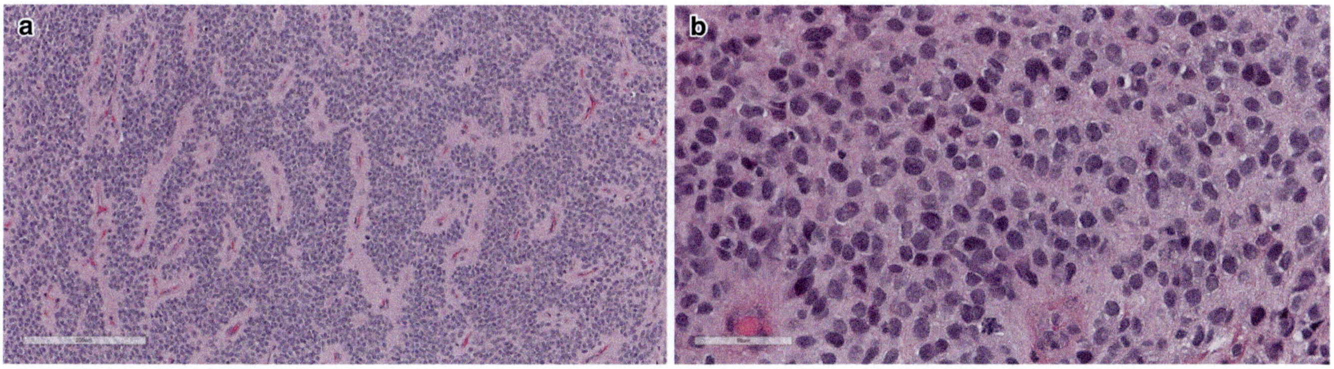

Fig. 6.2 Histomorphologic features of case 2. H&E stain, (**a**) (100X) shows classic histologic features of ependymoma, including perivascular pseudorosettes. (**b**) (400X) shows conspicuous mitotic activity

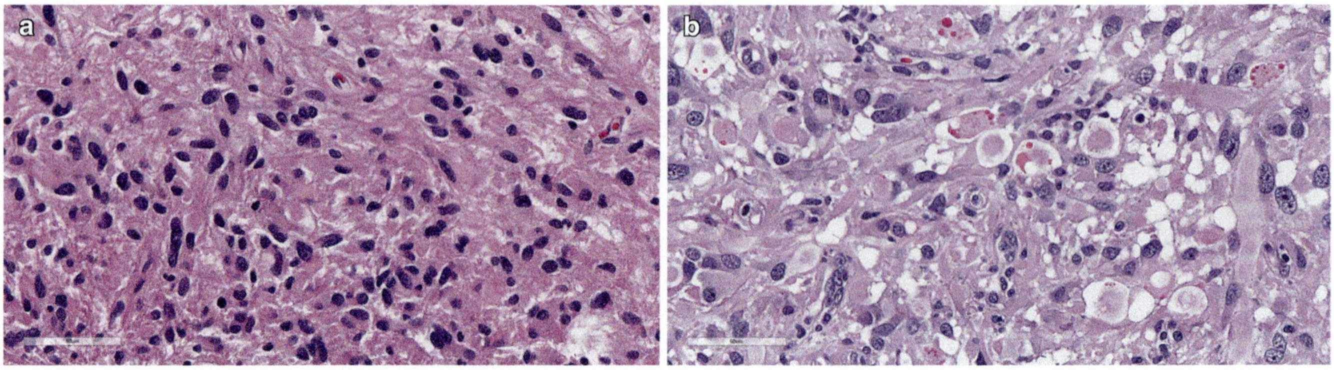

Fig. 6.3 Histomorphologic features of case 3. In areas the tumor was remarkable for spindled and fascicular arrangements (**a**). Numerous eosinophilic granular bodies were identified (**b**). H&E stain, (**a, b**) 400X

- Immunohistochemistry was negative for IDH1 R132H immunohistochemistry. ATRX immunostain highlighted intact nuclear expression, and p53 was just focally positive.
- The ki-67 proliferation index was very low.

Genetic Study

An SNP array detected a near tetraploid genome with predominantly whole chromosomal losses. Copy number alterations typical of IDH-wildtype GBM were absent (no combined +7/−10 CNA and no *EGFR* amplification). Homozygous loss of *CDKN2A/B* was present. Sequencing analysis confirmed the BRAF c. 1799T>A (p. Val600Glu, V600E) sequence variation.

Final Diagnosis

Pleomorphic xanthoastrocytoma, WHO grade 2

Discussion

Pleomorphic xanthoastrocytomas (PXAs) exhibit the highest frequency of *BRAF* V600E mutations among CNS tumors but they are not specific. These tumors typically arise in the temporal lobes of children or young adults and are characterized by a combination of spindle-shaped cells, xanthomatous change, eosinophilic granular bodies, and large pleomorphic multinucleated tumor cells that may elicit a differential that includes other high-grade astrocytomas. *BRAF* V600E mutations and homozygous deletion of *CDKN2A/B* are characteristic genetic abnormalities of PXA. The lack of mitoses in this case argues against an anaplastic PXA designation.

Case 4

Learning Objective

Highlight an aggressive embryonal neoplasm predominantly arising in childhood and the molecular signature that characterizes it.

Case History

A 7-month-old female presented with vomiting episodes, facial droop for 1 week, and subjective right sided extremity weakness. MRI revealed a 5 cm heterogeneous, right cerebellar mass with marked mass effect on the brainstem and fourth ventricle effacement. Heterogeneous and nodular enhancement was present. MR spectroscopy showed markedly elevated choline and decreased NAA, consistent with a high-grade neoplasm.

Histologic Features

- H&E sections showed sheets of malignant embryonal appearing cells with variable amounts of cytoplasm and vacuolation (Fig. 6.4a). In areas, a rhabdoid morphology with eccentric "inclusion-like" cytoplasm was appreciated in conjunction with prominent nucleoli. Conspicuous mitotic activity, necrosis, and microvascular proliferation were all present.
- Immunohistochemistry for INI1 showed loss of nuclear expression (Fig. 6.4b). Endothelial cells serve as internal positive control.

Genetic Study

No additional genetic studies were necessary after confirmation of loss of INI1/SMARCB1 by immunohistochemistry.

Final Diagnosis

Atypical teratoid/rhabdoid tumor, WHO grade 4

Discussion

Atypical teratoid/rhabdoid tumors are highly aggressive brain tumors that typically occur in early childhood. The vast majority of tumors show inactivation of *SMARCB1* (INI1, hSNF5, BAF47; chromosome 22q11.2) and can be identified by loss of INI1 immunohistochemistry. A small subset of these tumors will have intact INI1 but show loss-of-function mutations of *SMARCA4* (BRG1) at chromosome 19p13.2, which can be identified with BRG1 immunohistochemistry.

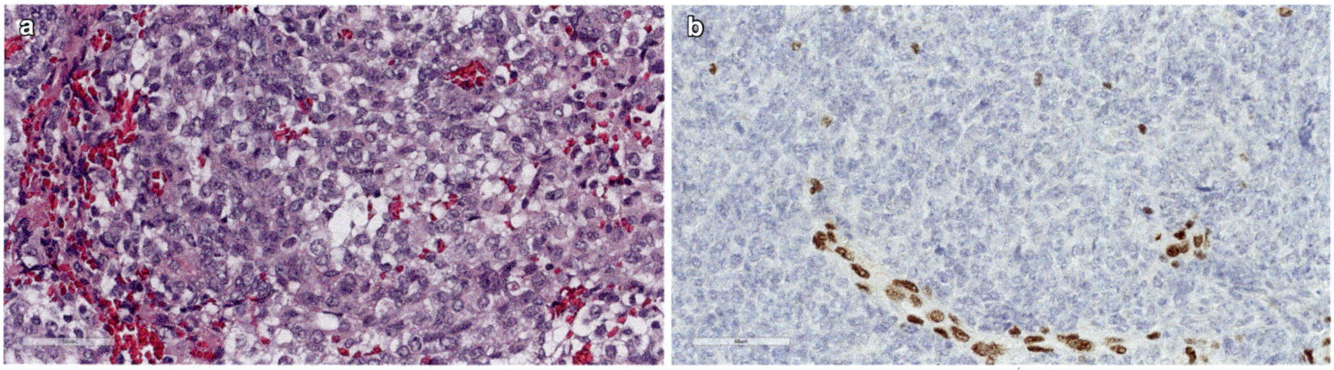

Fig. 6.4 **Histomorphologic and immunostaining features of case 4.** (**a**) H&E stained section shows sheets of malignant embryonal appearing cells with variable amounts of cytoplasm and vacuolation. (**b**) INI1 immunostain. (Original magnification 400X)

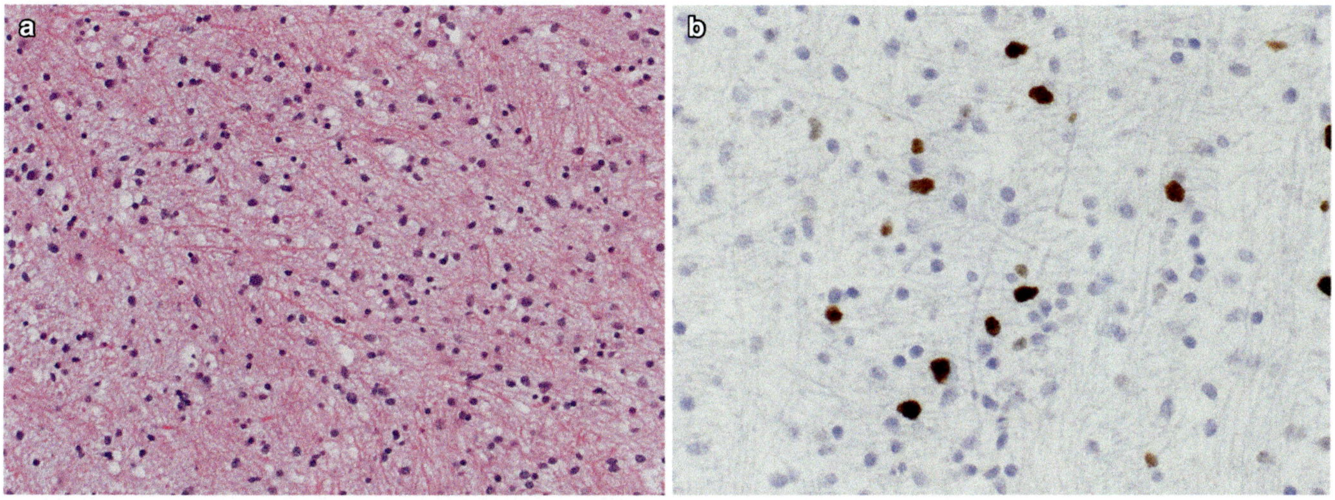

Fig. 6.5 **Histomorphologic and immunostaining features of case 5.** (**a**) H&E section (200X) shows mildly hypercellular white matter infiltrated by a sparse population of cells with irregular nuclear contours and mild cytologic atypia. (**b**) Ki-67 immunostain (400X)

These immunostains are highly contributory in ruling out other diagnosis in the differential, including medulloblastoma and other embryonal neoplasms.

Case 5

Learning Objective

Highlight the classification of pediatric-type diffuse gliomas and one of the common genetic drivers in tumors arising in this population.

Case History

A 2-year-old male presented with episodes of staring and non-responsiveness and was found to have focal seizures. MRI revealed a poorly circumscribed T2-hyperintense lesion in the deep white matter of the right frontal lobe. A needle core biopsy was obtained from the lesion.

Histologic Features

- H&E sections (Fig. 6.5a) showed mildly hypercellular white matter infiltrated by a sparse population of cells with irregular nuclear contours and mild cytologic atypia. There was no necrosis or microvascular proliferation, and mitotic activity was not identified.
- By immunohistochemistry, the tumor cells retained ATRX expression, had weak and variable p53 staining (wild-type), and were negative for H3 K27M mutant protein.
- Ki-67 proliferation index was low (Fig. 6.5b).

Genetic Study

An NGS panel identified a truncating rearrangement in the *MYBL1* gene at a low allele frequency commensurate with the sparse infiltrate of tumor cells.

Final Diagnosis

Diffuse glioma, *MYBL1* altered

Discussion

Diffuse gliomas in children can have clinical behavior that does not match the histologic grading and generally require molecular characterization to more reliably predict outcomes. In this case, a bland, somewhat astrocytic diffuse glioma was shown to have a *MYBL1* gene alteration that is strongly associated with an indolent course. On the other hand, an equally bland tumor with an H3 K27M mutation would be expected to be aggressive and fatal within a couple of years. Regardless of histology, all diffuse gliomas in children should have a genetic driver identified in order to deliver the best care.

Case 6

Learning Objective

Highlight one of the recently described uncommon CNS tumor and its molecular signature.

Case History

A 13-year-old male presents with back pain and bilateral lower extremity weakness with difficulty walking. Spine MRI revealed an enhancing 2.4 cm intramedullary mass around T7–T8 with syrinx extending above and below the lesion. Following gross total resection and chemoradiation, there was rapid recurrence of disease with diffuse leptomeningeal dissemination.

Histologic Features

- H&E sections (Fig. 6.6a) showed a hypercellular tumor composed of relatively monotonous tumor nuclei with round to elongate contours and inconspicuous nucleoli. The background was mildly vacuolated. Scattered mitotic figures were identified.
- By immunohistochemistry, the tumor cells were positive for CD56, WT1 (nuclear – both N- and Carboxy-terminus) and focally positive for CD99 (membranous pattern). Immunohistochemistry for WT1 (N-terminus) is shown below (Fig. 6.6b). INI1 immunostain highlighted intact nuclear expression. Immunohistochemistry for GFAP, EMA, NeuN, and synaptophysin was negative.
- The Ki-67 proliferation index was high and focally approximated 50%.

Genetic Study

An NGS panel confirmed the *CIC-DUX4* gene fusion.

Final Diagnosis

CIC-DUX4 sarcoma

Discussion

Initially described as CNS Ewing sarcoma family of tumor with CIC alterations, tumors harboring CIC alterations will be recognized as "CIC sarcomas" as there is insufficient evidence to separate them from the bone and soft tissue counterparts. While the morphology may be that of a round cell sarcoma, areas of spindling and myxoid changes are not uncommon. Most tumors arising in the CNS have demonstrated *CIC-NUTM1* fusions with rare cases harboring the *CIC-DUX4* fusion most characteristic of tumors arising elsewhere. Nuclear WT1 is a common immunohistochemical finding. These tumors behave aggressively and have poor outcomes.

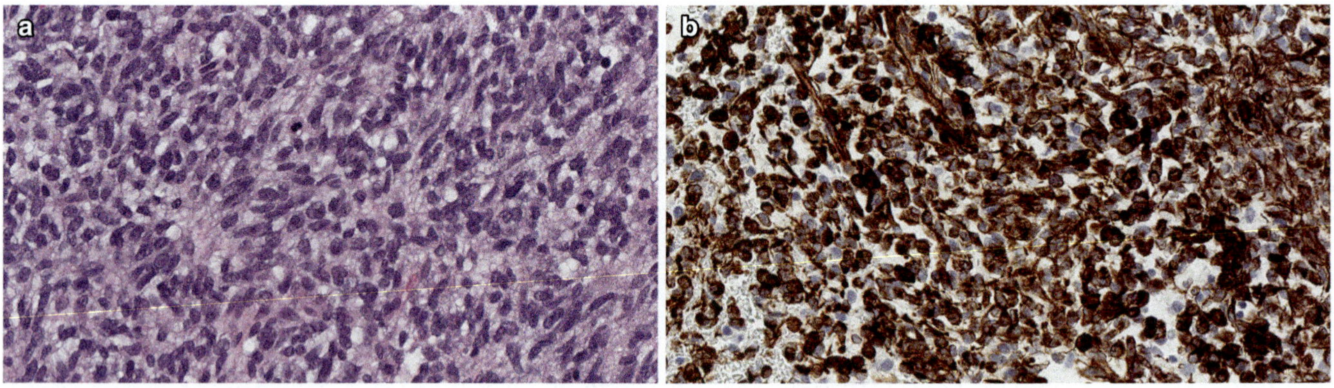

Fig. 6.6 Histomorphologic and immunostaining features of case 6. (**a**). H&E section (400X) shows hypercellular tumor composed of relatively monotonous tumor nuclei with round to elongate contours and inconspicuous nucleoli; the background is mildly vacuolated. (**b**). WT1 (N-terminus) immunostain.

References

1. Louis DN, Perry A, Burger P, et al. International society of neuropathology – Haarlem consensus guidelines for nervous system tumor classification and grading. Brain Pathol. 2014;24(5):429–35.
2. Louis DN, Ohgaki H, Wiestler OD, Cavenee WKE. WHO classification of tumours of the central nervous system. Revised 4th ed. Lyon: International Agency for Research on Cancer (IARC); 2016.
3. Louis DN, Perry A, Reifenberger G, et al. The 2016 World Health Organization classification of tumors of the central nervous system: a summary. Acta Neuropathol. 2016;131(6):803–20.
4. Velazquez Vega JE, Brat DJ. Incorporating advances in molecular pathology into brain tumor diagnostics. Adv Anat Pathol. 2018;25(3):143–71.
5. Spino M, Snuderl M. Genomic molecular classification of CNS malignancies. Adv Anat Pathol. 2020;27(1):44–50.
6. Capper D, Jones DTW, Sill M, et al. DNA methylation-based classification of central nervous system tumours. Nature. 2018;555(7697):469–74.
7. Capper D, Stichel D, Sahm F, et al. Practical implementation of DNA methylation and copy-number-based CNS tumor diagnostics: the Heidelberg experience. Acta Neuropathol. 2018;136(2):181–210.
8. Sahm F, Reuss DE, Giannini C, WHO 2016 Classification: changes and advancements in the diagnosis of miscellaneous primary CNS tumours. Neuropathol Appl Neurobiol . 2018;44(2):163–71.
9. van den Bent MJ. Interobserver variation of the histopathological diagnosis in clinical trials on glioma: a clinician's perspective. Acta Neuropathol. 2010;120(3):297–304.
10. Iorgulescu JB, Torre M, Harary M, et al. The misclassification of diffuse gliomas: rates and outcomes. Clin Cancer Res. 2019;25:2656.
11. Sahm F, Reuss D, Koelsche C, et al. Farewell to oligoastrocytoma: in situ molecular genetics favor classification as either oligodendroglioma or astrocytoma. Acta Neuropathol. 2014;128(4):551–9.
12. Hinrichs BH, Newman S, Appin CL, et al. Farewell to GBM-O: genomic and transcriptomic profiling of glioblastoma with oligodendroglioma component reveals distinct molecular subgroups. Acta Neuropathol Commun. 2016;4:4.
13. Louis DN, Aldape K, Brat DJ, et al. Announcing cIMPACT-NOW: the consortium to inform molecular and practical approaches to CNS tumor taxonomy. Acta Neuropathol. 2017;133(1):1–3.
14. Louis DN, Aldape K, Brat DJ, et al. cIMPACT-NOW (the consortium to inform molecular and practical approaches to CNS tumor taxonomy): a new initiative in advancing nervous system tumor classification. Brain Pathol. 2017;27(6):851–2.
15. Camelo-Piragua S, Jansen M, Ganguly A, Kim JC, Louis DN, Nutt CL. Mutant IDH1-specific immunohistochemistry distinguishes diffuse astrocytoma from astrocytosis. Acta Neuropathol. 2010;119(4):509–11.
16. Parsons DW, Jones S, Zhang X, et al. An integrated genomic analysis of human glioblastoma multiforme. Science. 2008;321(5897):1807–12.
17. Yan H, Parsons DW, Jin G, et al. IDH1 and IDH2 mutations in gliomas. N Engl J Med. 2009;360(8):765–73.
18. Watanabe T, Nobusawa S, Kleihues P, Ohgaki H. IDH1 mutations are early events in the development of astrocytomas and oligodendrogliomas. Am J Pathol. 2009;174(4):1149–53.
19. Dang L, White DW, Gross S, et al. Cancer-associated IDH1 mutations produce 2-hydroxyglutarate. Nature. 2009;462(7274):739–44.
20. Dang L, Yen K, Attar EC. IDH mutations in cancer and progress toward development of targeted therapeutics. Ann Oncol. 2016;27(4):599–608.
21. Xu W, Yang H, Liu Y, et al. Oncometabolite 2-hydroxyglutarate is a competitive inhibitor of alpha-ketoglutarate-dependent dioxygenases. Cancer Cell. 2011;19(1):17–30.
22. Wang HY, Tang K, Liang TY, et al. The comparison of clinical and biological characteristics between IDH1 and IDH2 mutations in gliomas. J Exp Clin Cancer Res. 2016;35:86.
23. Lu C, Ward PS, Kapoor GS, et al. IDH mutation impairs histone demethylation and results in a block to cell differentiation. Nature. 2012;483(7390):474–8.
24. Noushmehr H, Weisenberger DJ, Diefes K, et al. Identification of a CpG island methylator phenotype that defines a distinct subgroup of glioma. Cancer Cell. 2010;17(5):510–22.
25. Turcan S, Rohle D, Goenka A, et al. IDH1 mutation is sufficient to establish the glioma hypermethylator phenotype. Nature. 2012;483(7390):479–83.
26. Cancer Genome Atlas Research N, Brat DJ, Verhaak RG, et al. Comprehensive, integrative genomic analysis of diffuse lower-grade gliomas. N Engl J Med. 2015;372(26):2481–98.
27. Eckel-Passow JE, Lachance DH, Molinaro AM, et al. Glioma groups based on 1p/19q, IDH, and TERT promoter mutations in tumors. N Engl J Med. 2015;372(26):2499–508.
28. Balss J, Meyer J, Mueller W, Korshunov A, Hartmann C, von Deimling A. Analysis of the IDH1 codon 132 mutation in brain tumors. Acta Neuropathol. 2008;116(6):597–602.
29. Hartmann C, Meyer J, Balss J, et al. Type and frequency of IDH1 and IDH2 mutations are related to astrocytic and oligodendroglial differentiation and age: a study of 1,010 diffuse gliomas. Acta Neuropathol. 2009;118(4):469–74.
30. Capper D, Zentgraf H, Balss J, Hartmann C, von Deimling A. Monoclonal antibody specific for IDH1 R132H mutation. Acta Neuropathol. 2009;118(5):599–601.
31. Banan R, Stichel D, Bleck A, et al. Infratentorial IDH-mutant astrocytoma is a distinct subtype. Acta Neuropathol. 2020;140(4):569–81.
32. Chen L, Voronovich Z, Clark K, et al. Predicting the likelihood of an isocitrate dehydrogenase 1 or 2 mutation in diagnoses of infiltrative glioma. Neuro-Oncology. 2014;16(11):1478–83.
33. DeWitt JC, Jordan JT, Frosch MP, et al. Cost-effectiveness of IDH testing in diffuse gliomas according to the 2016 WHO classification of tumors of the central nervous system recommendations. Neuro-Oncology. 2017;19(12):1640–50.
34. Robinson C, Kleinschmidt-DeMasters BK. IDH1-mutation in diffuse gliomas in persons age 55 years and over. J Neuropathol Exp Neurol. 2017;76(2):151–4.
35. Olar A, Wani KM, Alfaro-Munoz KD, et al. IDH mutation status and role of WHO grade and mitotic index in overall survival in grade II-III diffuse gliomas. Acta Neuropathol. 2015;129(4):585–96.
36. Reuss DE, Mamatjan Y, Schrimpf D, et al. IDH mutant diffuse and anaplastic astrocytomas have similar age at presentation and little difference in survival: a grading problem for WHO. Acta Neuropathol. 2015;129(6):867–73.
37. Hartmann C, Hentschel B, Wick W, et al. Patients with IDH1 wild type anaplastic astrocytomas exhibit worse prognosis than IDH1-mutated glioblastomas, and IDH1 mutation status accounts for the unfavorable prognostic effect of higher age: implications for classification of gliomas. Acta Neuropathol. 2010;120(6):707–18.
38. Cimino PJ, Zager M, McFerrin L, et al. Multidimensional scaling of diffuse gliomas: application to the 2016 World Health Organization classification system with prognostically relevant molecular subtype discovery. Acta Neuropathol Commun. 2017;5(1):39.

39. Korshunov A, Casalini B, Chavez L, et al. Integrated molecular characterization of IDH-mutant glioblastomas. Neuropathol Appl Neurobiol. 2018;45:108.
40. Shirahata M, Ono T, Stichel D, et al. Novel, improved grading system(s) for IDH-mutant astrocytic gliomas. Acta Neuropathol. 2018;136(1):153–66.
41. Brat DJ, Aldape K, Colman H, et al. cIMPACT-NOW update 5: recommended grading criteria and terminologies for IDH-mutant astrocytomas. Acta Neuropathol. 2020;139(3):603–8.
42. Louis DN, Wesseling P, Aldape K, et al. cIMPACT-NOW update 6: new entity and diagnostic principle recommendations of the cIMPACT-Utrecht meeting on future CNS tumor classification and grading. Brain Pathol. 2020;30(4):844–56.
43. Reifenberger J, Reifenberger G, Liu L, James CD, Wechsler W, Collins VP. Molecular genetic analysis of oligodendroglial tumors shows preferential allelic deletions on 19q and 1p. Am J Pathol. 1994;145(5):1175–90.
44. Cairncross JG, Ueki K, Zlatescu MC, et al. Specific genetic predictors of chemotherapeutic response and survival in patients with anaplastic oligodendrogliomas. J Natl Cancer Inst. 1998;90(19):1473–9.
45. Griffin CA, Burger P, Morsberger L, et al. Identification of der(1;19)(q10;p10) in five oligodendrogliomas suggests mechanism of concurrent 1p and 19q loss. J Neuropathol Exp Neurol. 2006;65(10):988–94.
46. Jenkins RB, Blair H, Ballman KV, et al. A t(1;19)(q10;p10) mediates the combined deletions of 1p and 19q and predicts a better prognosis of patients with oligodendroglioma. Cancer Res. 2006;66(20):9852–61.
47. Wesseling P, van den Bent M, Perry A. Oligodendroglioma: pathology, molecular mechanisms and markers. Acta Neuropathol. 2015;129(6):809–27.
48. Giannini C, Scheithauer BW, Weaver AL, et al. Oligodendrogliomas: reproducibility and prognostic value of histologic diagnosis and grading. J Neuropathol Exp Neurol. 2001;60(3):248–62.
49. Aoki K, Nakamura H, Suzuki H, et al. Prognostic relevance of genetic alterations in diffuse lower-grade gliomas. Neuro-Oncology. 2018;20(1):66–77.
50. Halani SH, Yousefi S, Velazquez Vega J, et al. Multi-faceted computational assessment of risk and progression in oligodendroglioma implicates NOTCH and PI3K pathways. NPJ Precis Oncol. 2018;2:24.
51. Brat DJ, Seiferheld WF, Perry A, et al. Analysis of 1p, 19q, 9p, and 10q as prognostic markers for high-grade astrocytomas using fluorescence in situ hybridization on tissue microarrays from radiation therapy oncology group trials. Neuro-Oncology. 2004;6(2):96–103.
52. Clark KH, Villano JL, Nikiforova MN, Hamilton RL, Horbinski C. 1p/19q testing has no significance in the workup of glioblastomas. Neuropathol Appl Neurobiol. 2013;39(6):706–17.
53. Ball MK, Kollmeyer TM, Praska CE, et al. Frequency of false-positive FISH 1p/19q codeletion in adult diffuse astrocytic gliomas. Neurooncol Adv. 2020;2(1):vdaa109.
54. Reuss DE, Kratz A, Sahm F, et al. Adult IDH wild type astrocytomas biologically and clinically resolve into other tumor entities. Acta Neuropathol. 2015;130(3):407–17.
55. Reuss DE, Sahm F, Schrimpf D, et al. ATRX and IDH1-R132H immunohistochemistry with subsequent copy number analysis and IDH sequencing as a basis for an "integrated" diagnostic approach for adult astrocytoma, oligodendroglioma and glioblastoma. Acta Neuropathol. 2015;129(1):133–46.
56. Stichel D, Ebrahimi A, Reuss D, et al. Distribution of EGFR amplification, combined chromosome 7 gain and chromosome 10 loss, and TERT promoter mutation in brain tumors and their potential for the reclassification of IDHwt astrocytoma to glioblastoma. Acta Neuropathol. 2018;136(5):793–803.
57. Brat DJ, Aldape K, Colman H, et al. cIMPACT-NOW update 3: recommended diagnostic criteria for "diffuse astrocytic glioma, IDH-wildtype, with molecular features of glioblastoma, WHO grade IV". Acta Neuropathol. 2018;136(5):805–10.
58. Tesileanu CMS, Dirven L, Wijnenga MMJ, et al. Survival of diffuse astrocytic glioma, IDH1/2 wildtype, with molecular features of glioblastoma, WHO grade IV: a confirmation of the cIMPACT-NOW criteria. Neuro-Oncology. 2020;22(4):515–23.
59. Louis DN, Giannini C, Capper D, et al. cIMPACT-NOW update 2: diagnostic clarifications for diffuse midline glioma, H3 K27M-mutant and diffuse astrocytoma/anaplastic astrocytoma, IDH-mutant. Acta Neuropathol. 2018;135(4):639–42.
60. Lee J, Solomon DA, Tihan T. The role of histone modifications and telomere alterations in the pathogenesis of diffuse gliomas in adults and children. J Neuro-Oncol. 2017;132(1):1–11.
61. Solomon DA, Wood MD, Tihan T, et al. Diffuse midline gliomas with histone H3-K27M mutation: a series of 47 cases assessing the Spectrum of morphologic variation and associated genetic alterations. Brain Pathol. 2016;26(5):569–80.
62. Khuong-Quang DA, Buczkowicz P, Rakopoulos P, et al. K27M mutation in histone H3.3 defines clinically and biologically distinct subgroups of pediatric diffuse intrinsic pontine gliomas. Acta Neuropathol. 2012;124(3):439–47.
63. Schwartzentruber J, Korshunov A, Liu XY, et al. Driver mutations in histone H3.3 and chromatin remodelling genes in paediatric glioblastoma. Nature. 2012;482(7384):226–31.
64. Wu G, Diaz AK, Paugh BS, et al. The genomic landscape of diffuse intrinsic pontine glioma and pediatric non-brainstem high-grade glioma. Nat Genet. 2014;46(5):444–50.
65. Schreck KC, Ranjan S, Skorupan N, et al. Incidence and clinicopathologic features of H3 K27M mutations in adults with radiographically-determined midline gliomas. J Neuro-Oncol. 2019;143(1):87–93.
66. Karremann M, Gielen GH, Hoffmann M, et al. Diffuse high-grade gliomas with H3 K27M mutations carry a dismal prognosis independent of tumor location. Neuro-Oncology. 2018;20(1):123–31.
67. Sturm D, Witt H, Hovestadt V, et al. Hotspot mutations in H3F3A and IDH1 define distinct epigenetic and biological subgroups of glioblastoma. Cancer Cell. 2012;22(4):425–37.
68. Meyronet D, Esteban-Mader M, Bonnet C, et al. Characteristics of H3 K27M-mutant gliomas in adults. Neuro-Oncology. 2017;19(8):1127–34.
69. Kleinschmidt-DeMasters BK, Mulcahy Levy JM. H3 K27M-mutant gliomas in adults vs. children share similar histological features and adverse prognosis. Clin Neuropathol. 2018;37(2):53–63.
70. Wang L, Li Z, Zhang M, et al. H3 K27M-mutant diffuse midline gliomas in different anatomical locations. Hum Pathol. 2018;78:89–96.
71. Venneti S, Santi M, Felicella MM, et al. A sensitive and specific histopathologic prognostic marker for H3F3A K27M mutant pediatric glioblastomas. Acta Neuropathol. 2014;128(5):743–53.
72. Korshunov A, Capper D, Reuss D, et al. Histologically distinct neuroepithelial tumors with histone 3 G34 mutation are molecularly similar and comprise a single nosologic entity. Acta Neuropathol. 2016;131(1):137–46.
73. Korshunov A, Ryzhova M, Hovestadt V, et al. Integrated analysis of pediatric glioblastoma reveals a subset of biologically favorable tumors with associated molecular prognostic markers. Acta Neuropathol. 2015;129(5):669–78.
74. Gessi M, Gielen GH, Hammes J, et al. H3.3 G34R mutations in pediatric primitive neuroectodermal tumors of central nervous system (CNS-PNET) and pediatric glioblastomas: possible diagnostic and therapeutic implications? J Neuro-Oncol. 2013;112(1):67–72.

75. Neumann JE, Dorostkar MM, Korshunov A, et al. Distinct histomorphology in molecular subgroups of glioblastomas in young patients. J Neuropathol Exp Neurol. 2016;75(5):408–14.
76. Yoshimoto K, Hatae R, Sangatsuda Y, et al. Prevalence and clinicopathological features of H3.3 G34-mutant high-grade gliomas: a retrospective study of 411 consecutive glioma cases in a single institution. Brain Tumor Pathol. 2017;34(3):103–12.
77. Haque F, Varlet P, Puntonet J, et al. Evaluation of a novel antibody to define histone 3.3 G34R mutant brain tumours. Acta Neuropathol Commun. 2017;5(1):45.
78. Aldape K, Zadeh G, Mansouri S, Reifenberger G, von Deimling A. Glioblastoma: pathology, molecular mechanisms and markers. Acta Neuropathol. 2015;129(6):829–48.
79. Brandner S, von Deimling A. Diagnostic, prognostic and predictive relevance of molecular markers in gliomas. Neuropathol Appl Neurobiol. 2015;41(6):694–720.
80. Mansouri A, Hachem LD, Mansouri S, et al. MGMT promoter methylation status testing to guide therapy for glioblastoma: refining the approach based on emerging evidence and current challenges. Neuro Oncol. 2018;21:167.
81. Quillien V, Lavenu A, Ducray F, et al. Validation of the high-performance of pyrosequencing for clinical MGMT testing on a cohort of glioblastoma patients from a prospective dedicated multicentric trial. Oncotarget. 2016;7(38):61916–29.
82. Yang P, Zhang W, Wang Y, et al. IDH mutation and MGMT promoter methylation in glioblastoma: results of a prospective registry. Oncotarget. 2015;6(38):40896–906.
83. Hegi ME, Diserens AC, Gorlia T, et al. MGMT gene silencing and benefit from temozolomide in glioblastoma. N Engl J Med. 2005;352(10):997–1003.
84. Rivera AL, Pelloski CE, Gilbert MR, et al. MGMT promoter methylation is predictive of response to radiotherapy and prognostic in the absence of adjuvant alkylating chemotherapy for glioblastoma. Neuro-Oncology. 2010;12(2):116–21.
85. Wick W, Platten M, Meisner C, et al. Temozolomide chemotherapy alone versus radiotherapy alone for malignant astrocytoma in the elderly: the NOA-08 randomised, phase 3 trial. Lancet Oncol. 2012;13(7):707–15.
86. Weller M, Felsberg J, Hartmann C, et al. Molecular predictors of progression-free and overall survival in patients with newly diagnosed glioblastoma: a prospective translational study of the German glioma network. J Clin Oncol. 2009;27(34):5743–50.
87. Stupp R, Hegi ME, Mason WP, et al. Effects of radiotherapy with concomitant and adjuvant temozolomide versus radiotherapy alone on survival in glioblastoma in a randomised phase III study: 5-year analysis of the EORTC-NCIC trial. Lancet Oncol. 2009;10(5):459–66.
88. Hegi ME, Diserens AC, Godard S, et al. Clinical trial substantiates the predictive value of O-6-methylguanine-DNA methyltransferase promoter methylation in glioblastoma patients treated with temozolomide. Clin Cancer Res. 2004;10(6):1871–4.
89. Weller M, Stupp R, Reifenberger G, et al. MGMT promoter methylation in malignant gliomas: ready for personalized medicine? Nat Rev Neurol. 2010;6(1):39–51.
90. Appin CL, Brat DJ. Biomarker-driven diagnosis of diffuse gliomas. Mol Asp Med. 2015;45:87–96.
91. Christians A, Hartmann C, Benner A, et al. Prognostic value of three different methods of MGMT promoter methylation analysis in a prospective trial on newly diagnosed glioblastoma. PLoS One. 2012;7(3):e33449.
92. Tanboon J, Williams EA, Louis DN. The diagnostic use of immunohistochemical surrogates for signature molecular genetic alterations in gliomas. J Neuropathol Exp Neurol. 2016;75(1):4–18.
93. Preusser M, Charles Janzer R, Felsberg J, et al. Anti-O6-methylguanine-methyltransferase (MGMT) immunohistochemistry in glioblastoma multiforme: observer variability and lack of association with patient survival impede its use as clinical biomarker. Brain Pathol. 2008;18(4):520–32.
94. Zhang J, Wu G, Miller CP, et al. Whole-genome sequencing identifies genetic alterations in pediatric low-grade gliomas. Nat Genet. 2013;45(6):602–12.
95. Jones DT, Hutter B, Jager N, et al. Recurrent somatic alterations of FGFR1 and NTRK2 in pilocytic astrocytoma. Nat Genet. 2013;45(8):927–32.
96. Collins VP, Jones DT, Giannini C. Pilocytic astrocytoma: pathology, molecular mechanisms and markers. Acta Neuropathol. 2015;129(6):775–88.
97. Packer RJ, Pfister S, Bouffet E, et al. Pediatric low-grade gliomas: implications of the biologic era. Neuro-Oncology. 2017;19(6):750–61.
98. Jones DTW, Kieran MW, Bouffet E, et al. Pediatric low-grade gliomas: next biologically driven steps. Neuro-Oncology. 2017;20:160.
99. Jones DT, Kocialkowski S, Liu L, et al. Tandem duplication producing a novel oncogenic BRAF fusion gene defines the majority of pilocytic astrocytomas. Cancer Res. 2008;68(21):8673–7.
100. Pfister S, Janzarik WG, Remke M, et al. BRAF gene duplication constitutes a mechanism of MAPK pathway activation in low-grade astrocytomas. J Clin Invest. 2008;118(5):1739–49.
101. Mackay A, Burford A, Carvalho D, et al. Integrated molecular meta-analysis of 1,000 pediatric high-grade and diffuse intrinsic Pontine glioma. Cancer Cell. 2017;32(4):520–537 e525.
102. Ryall S, Zapotocky M, Fukuoka K, et al. Integrated molecular and clinical analysis of 1,000 pediatric low-grade gliomas. Cancer Cell. 2020;37(4):569–583 e565.
103. Gierke M, Sperveslage J, Schwab D, et al. Analysis of IDH1-R132 mutation, BRAF V600 mutation and KIAA1549-BRAF fusion transcript status in central nervous system tumors supports pediatric tumor classification. J Cancer Res Clin Oncol. 2016;142(1):89–100.
104. Koelsche C, Sahm F, Capper D, et al. Distribution of TERT promoter mutations in pediatric and adult tumors of the nervous system. Acta Neuropathol. 2013;126(6):907–15.
105. Ryall S, Tabori U, Hawkins C. A comprehensive review of paediatric low-grade diffuse glioma: pathology, molecular genetics and treatment. Brain Tumor Pathol. 2017;34(2):51–61.
106. Ellison DW, Hawkins C, Jones DTW, et al. cIMPACT-NOW update 4: diffuse gliomas characterized by MYB, MYBL1, or FGFR1 alterations or BRAF(V600E) mutation. Acta Neuropathol. 2019;137(4):683–7.
107. Qaddoumi I, Orisme W, Wen J, et al. Genetic alterations in uncommon low-grade neuroepithelial tumors: BRAF, FGFR1, and MYB mutations occur at high frequency and align with morphology. Acta Neuropathol. 2016;131(6):833–45.
108. Schindler G, Capper D, Meyer J, et al. Analysis of BRAF V600E mutation in 1,320 nervous system tumors reveals high mutation frequencies in pleomorphic xanthoastrocytoma, ganglioglioma and extra-cerebellar pilocytic astrocytoma. Acta Neuropathol. 2011;121(3):397–405.
109. Rodriguez FJ, Perry A, Rosenblum MK, et al. Disseminated oligodendroglial-like leptomeningeal tumor of childhood: a distinctive clinicopathologic entity. Acta Neuropathol. 2012;124(5):627–41.
110. Schniederjan MJ, Alghamdi S, Castellano-Sanchez A, et al. Diffuse leptomeningeal neuroepithelial tumor: 9 pediatric cases with chromosome 1p/19q deletion status and IDH1 (R132H) immunohistochemistry. Am J Surg Pathol. 2013;37(5):763–71.
111. Huse JT, Snuderl M, Jones DT, et al. Polymorphous low-grade neuroepithelial tumor of the young (PLNTY): an epileptogenic neoplasm with oligodendroglioma-like components, aberrant

CD34 expression, and genetic alterations involving the MAP kinase pathway. Acta Neuropathol. 2017;133(3):417–29.
112. Johnson DR, Giannini C, Jenkins RB, Kim DK, Kaufmann TJ. Plenty of calcification: imaging characterization of polymorphous low-grade neuroepithelial tumor of the young. Neuroradiology. 2019;61(11):1327–32.
113. Slegers RJ, Blumcke I. Low-grade developmental and epilepsy associated brain tumors: a critical update 2020. Acta Neuropathol Commun. 2020;8(1):27.
114. Bandopadhayay P, Ramkissoon LA, Jain P, et al. MYB-QKI rearrangements in angiocentric glioma drive tumorigenicity through a tripartite mechanism. Nat Genet. 2016;48(3):273–82.
115. Wefers AK, Stichel D, Schrimpf D, et al. Isomorphic diffuse glioma is a morphologically and molecularly distinct tumour entity with recurrent gene fusions of MYBL1 or MYB and a benign disease course. Acta Neuropathol. 2020;139(1):193–209.
116. Ida CM, Rodriguez FJ, Burger PC, et al. Pleomorphic Xanthoastrocytoma: natural history and long-term follow-up. Brain Pathol. 2015;25(5):575–86.
117. Weber RG, Hoischen A, Ehrler M, et al. Frequent loss of chromosome 9, homozygous CDKN2A/p14(ARF)/CDKN2B deletion and low TSC1 mRNA expression in pleomorphic xanthoastrocytomas. Oncogene. 2007;26(7):1088–97.
118. Vaubel R, Zschernack V, Tran QT, et al. Biology and grading of pleomorphic xanthoastrocytoma-what have we learned about it? Brain Pathol. 2020;31:20.
119. Vaubel RA, Caron AA, Yamada S, et al. Recurrent copy number alterations in low-grade and anaplastic pleomorphic xanthoastrocytoma with and without BRAF V600E mutation. Brain Pathol. 2018;28(2):172–82.
120. Phillips JJ, Gong H, Chen K, et al. The genetic landscape of anaplastic pleomorphic xanthoastrocytoma. Brain Pathol. 2019;29(1):85–96.
121. Alexandrescu S, Korshunov A, Lai SH, et al. Epithelioid glioblastomas and anaplastic epithelioid pleomorphic xanthoastrocytomas – same entity or first cousins? Brain Pathol. 2016;26(2):215–23.
122. Kleinschmidt-DeMasters BK, Aisner DL, Birks DK, Foreman NK. Epithelioid GBMs show a high percentage of BRAF V600E mutation. Am J Surg Pathol. 2013;37(5):685–98.
123. Korshunov A, Chavez L, Sharma T, et al. Epithelioid glioblastomas stratify into established diagnostic subsets upon integrated molecular analysis. Brain Pathol. 2018;28(5):656–62.
124. Ostrom QT, Gittleman H, Xu J, et al. CBTRUS statistical report: primary brain and other central nervous system tumors diagnosed in the United States in 2009–2013. Neuro-Oncology. 2016;18(suppl_5):v1–v75.
125. Renzi S, Michaeli O, Ramaswamy V, et al. Causes of death in pediatric neuro-oncology: the sickkids experience from 2000 to 2017. J Neuro-Oncol. 2020;149(1):181–9.
126. Fontebasso AM, Papillon-Cavanagh S, Schwartzentruber J, et al. Recurrent somatic mutations in ACVR1 in pediatric midline high-grade astrocytoma. Nat Genet. 2014;46(5):462–6.
127. Korshunov A, Schrimpf D, Ryzhova M, et al. H3-/IDH-wild type pediatric glioblastoma is comprised of molecularly and prognostically distinct subtypes with associated oncogenic drivers. Acta Neuropathol. 2017;134(3):507–16.
128. Guerreiro Stucklin AS, Ryall S, Fukuoka K, et al. Alterations in ALK/ROS1/NTRK/MET drive a group of infantile hemispheric gliomas. Nat Commun. 2019;10(1):4343.
129. Gilani A, Donson A, Davies KD, et al. Targetable molecular alterations in congenital glioblastoma. J Neuro-Oncol. 2020;146(2):247–52.
130. Viaene AN, Pu C, Perry A, Li MM, Luo M, Santi M. Congenital tumors of the central nervous system: an institutional review of 64 cases with emphasis on tumors with unique histologic and molecular characteristics. Brain Pathol. 2020;31:45.
131. Clarke M, Mackay A, Ismer B, et al. Infant high-grade gliomas comprise multiple subgroups characterized by novel targetable gene fusions and favorable outcomes. Cancer Discov. 2020;10(7):942–63.
132. Ellison DW, Aldape KD, Capper D, et al. cIMPACT-NOW update 7: advancing the molecular classification of ependymal tumors. Brain Pathol. 2020;30(5):863–6.
133. Pajtler KW, Mack SC, Ramaswamy V, et al. The current consensus on the clinical management of intracranial ependymoma and its distinct molecular variants. Acta Neuropathol. 2017;133(1):5–12.
134. Pajtler KW, Witt H, Sill M, et al. Molecular classification of ependymal tumors across all CNS compartments, histopathological grades, and age groups. Cancer Cell. 2015;27(5):728–43.
135. Swanson AA, Raghunathan A, Jenkins RB, et al. Spinal cord ependymomas with MYCN amplification show aggressive clinical behavior. J Neuropathol Exp Neurol. 2019;78(9):791–7.
136. Ghasemi DR, Sill M, Okonechnikov K, et al. MYCN amplification drives an aggressive form of spinal ependymoma. Acta Neuropathol. 2019;138(6):1075–89.
137. Raffeld M, Abdullaev Z, Pack SD, et al. High level MYCN amplification and distinct methylation signature define an aggressive subtype of spinal cord ependymoma. Acta Neuropathol Commun. 2020;8(1):101.
138. Parker M, Mohankumar KM, Punchihewa C, et al. C11orf95-RELA fusions drive oncogenic NF-kappaB signalling in ependymoma. Nature. 2014;506(7489):451–5.
139. Pages M, Pajtler KW, Puget S, et al. Diagnostics of pediatric supratentorial RELA ependymomas: integration of information from histopathology, genetics, DNA methylation and imaging. Brain Pathol. 2019;29(3):325–35.
140. Figarella-Branger D, Lechapt-Zalcman E, Tabouret E, et al. Supratentorial clear cell ependymomas with branching capillaries demonstrate characteristic clinicopathological features and pathological activation of nuclear factor-kappaB signaling. Neuro-Oncology. 2016;18(7):919–27.
141. Witt H, Mack SC, Ryzhova M, et al. Delineation of two clinically and molecularly distinct subgroups of posterior fossa ependymoma. Cancer Cell. 2011;20(2):143–57.
142. Korshunov A, Witt H, Hielscher T, et al. Molecular staging of intracranial ependymoma in children and adults. J Clin Oncol. 2010;28(19):3182–90.
143. Araki A, Chocholous M, Gojo J, et al. Chromosome 1q gain and tenascin-C expression are candidate markers to define different risk groups in pediatric posterior fossa ependymoma. Acta Neuropathol Commun. 2016;4(1):88.
144. Bayliss J, Mukherjee P, Lu C, et al. Lowered H3K27me3 and DNA hypomethylation define poorly prognostic pediatric posterior fossa ependymomas. Sci Transl Med. 2016;8(366):366ra161.
145. Panwalkar P, Clark J, Ramaswamy V, et al. Immunohistochemical analysis of H3K27me3 demonstrates global reduction in group-a childhood posterior fossa ependymoma and is a powerful predictor of outcome. Acta Neuropathol. 2017;134(5):705–14.
146. Ryall S, Guzman M, Elbabaa SK, et al. H3 K27M mutations are extremely rare in posterior fossa group a ependymoma. Childs Nerv Syst. 2017;33(7):1047–51.
147. Pajtler KW, Wen J, Sill M, et al. Molecular heterogeneity and CXorf67 alterations in posterior fossa group a (PFA) ependymomas. Acta Neuropathol. 2018;136(2):211–26.
148. Ramaswamy V, Remke M, Bouffet E, et al. Risk stratification of childhood medulloblastoma in the molecular era: the current consensus. Acta Neuropathol. 2016;131(6):821–31.
149. Northcott PA, Korshunov A, Witt H, et al. Medulloblastoma comprises four distinct molecular variants. J Clin Oncol. 2011;29(11):1408–14.
150. Northcott PA, Robinson GW, Kratz CP, et al. Medulloblastoma. Nat Rev Dis Primers. 2019;5(1):11.

151. Orr BA. Pathology, diagnostics, and classification of medulloblastoma. Brain Pathol. 2020;30(3):664–78.
152. Ellison DW, Kocak M, Dalton J, et al. Definition of disease-risk stratification groups in childhood medulloblastoma using combined clinical, pathologic, and molecular variables. J Clin Oncol. 2011;29(11):1400–7.
153. Clifford SC, Lusher ME, Lindsey JC, et al. Wnt/wingless pathway activation and chromosome 6 loss characterize a distinct molecular sub-group of medulloblastomas associated with a favorable prognosis. Cell Cycle. 2006;5(22):2666–70.
154. Northcott PA, Jones DT, Kool M, et al. Medulloblastomics: the end of the beginning. Nat Rev Cancer. 2012;12(12):818–34.
155. Northcott PA, Shih DJ, Peacock J, et al. Subgroup-specific structural variation across 1,000 medulloblastoma genomes. Nature. 2012;488(7409):49–56.
156. Zhukova N, Ramaswamy V, Remke M, et al. Subgroup-specific prognostic implications of TP53 mutation in medulloblastoma. J Clin Oncol. 2013;31(23):2927–35.
157. Jones DT, Jager N, Kool M, et al. Dissecting the genomic complexity underlying medulloblastoma. Nature. 2012;488(7409):100–5.
158. Kool M, Jones DT, Jager N, et al. Genome sequencing of SHH medulloblastoma predicts genotype-related response to smoothened inhibition. Cancer Cell. 2014;25(3):393–405.
159. Northcott PA, Buchhalter I, Morrissy AS, et al. The whole-genome landscape of medulloblastoma subtypes. Nature. 2017;547(7663):311–7.
160. Ellison DW, Dalton J, Kocak M, et al. Medulloblastoma: clinicopathological correlates of SHH, WNT, and non-SHH/WNT molecular subgroups. Acta Neuropathol. 2011;121(3):381–96.
161. Kool M, Korshunov A, Remke M, et al. Molecular subgroups of medulloblastoma: an international meta-analysis of transcriptome, genetic aberrations, and clinical data of WNT, SHH, group 3, and group 4 medulloblastomas. Acta Neuropathol. 2012;123(4):473–84.
162. Remke M, Ramaswamy V, Peacock J, et al. TERT promoter mutations are highly recurrent in SHH subgroup medulloblastoma. Acta Neuropathol. 2013;126(6):917–29.
163. Kaur K, Kakkar A, Kumar A, et al. Integrating molecular subclassification of medulloblastomas into routine clinical practice: a simplified approach. Brain Pathol. 2016;26(3):334–43.
164. Shih DJ, Northcott PA, Remke M, et al. Cytogenetic prognostication within medulloblastoma subgroups. J Clin Oncol. 2014;32(9):886–96.
165. Northcott PA, Shih DJ, Remke M, et al. Rapid, reliable, and reproducible molecular sub-grouping of clinical medulloblastoma samples. Acta Neuropathol. 2012;123(4):615–26.
166. Hovestadt V, Remke M, Kool M, et al. Robust molecular subgrouping and copy-number profiling of medulloblastoma from small amounts of archival tumour material using high-density DNA methylation arrays. Acta Neuropathol. 2013;125(6):913–6.
167. Schwalbe EC, Williamson D, Lindsey JC, et al. DNA methylation profiling of medulloblastoma allows robust subclassification and improved outcome prediction using formalin-fixed biopsies. Acta Neuropathol. 2013;125(3):359–71.
168. Pietsch T, Haberler C. Update on the integrated histopathological and genetic classification of medulloblastoma - a practical diagnostic guideline. Clin Neuropathol. 2016;35(6):344–52.
169. Waszak SM, Northcott PA, Buchhalter I, et al. Spectrum and prevalence of genetic predisposition in medulloblastoma: a retrospective genetic study and prospective validation in a clinical trial cohort. Lancet Oncol. 2018;19(6):785–98.
170. Biegel JA, Rorke LB, Emanuel BS. Monosomy 22 in rhabdoid or atypical teratoid tumors of the brain. N Engl J Med. 1989;321(13):906.
171. Biegel JA, Rorke LB, Packer RJ, Emanuel BS. Monosomy 22 in rhabdoid or atypical tumors of the brain. J Neurosurg. 1990;73(5):710–4.
172. Rorke LB, Packer RJ, Biegel JA. Central nervous system atypical teratoid/rhabdoid tumors of infancy and childhood: definition of an entity. J Neurosurg. 1996;85(1):56–65.
173. Biegel JA. Molecular genetics of atypical teratoid/rhabdoid tumor. Neurosurg Focus. 2006;20(1):E11.
174. Johann PD, Erkek S, Zapatka M, et al. Atypical teratoid/Rhabdoid tumors are comprised of three epigenetic subgroups with distinct enhancer landscapes. Cancer Cell. 2016;29(3):379–93.
175. Fossey M, Li H, Afzal S, et al. Atypical teratoid rhabdoid tumor in the first year of life: the Canadian ATRT registry experience and review of the literature. J Neuro-Oncol. 2017;132(1):155–62.
176. Lafay-Cousin L, Hawkins C, Carret AS, et al. Central nervous system atypical teratoid rhabdoid tumours: the Canadian paediatric brain tumour consortium experience. Eur J Cancer. 2012;48(3):353–9.
177. Chbani L, Guillou L, Terrier P, et al. Epithelioid sarcoma: a clinicopathologic and immunohistochemical analysis of 106 cases from the French sarcoma group. Am J Clin Pathol. 2009;131(2):222–7.
178. Judkins AR, Mauger J, Ht A, Rorke LB, Biegel JA. Immunohistochemical analysis of hSNF5/INI1 in pediatric CNS neoplasms. Am J Surg Pathol. 2004;28(5):644–50.
179. Hornick JL, Dal Cin P, Fletcher CD. Loss of INI1 expression is characteristic of both conventional and proximal-type epithelioid sarcoma. Am J Surg Pathol. 2009;33(4):542–50.
180. Hollmann TJ, Hornick JL. INI1-deficient tumors: diagnostic features and molecular genetics. Am J Surg Pathol. 2011;35(10):e47–63.
181. Kohashi K, Oda Y, Yamamoto H, et al. SMARCB1/INI1 protein expression in round cell soft tissue sarcomas associated with chromosomal translocations involving EWS: a special reference to SMARCB1/INI1 negative variant extraskeletal myxoid chondrosarcoma. Am J Surg Pathol. 2008;32(8):1168–74.
182. Cheng JX, Tretiakova M, Gong C, Mandal S, Krausz T, Taxy JB. Renal medullary carcinoma: rhabdoid features and the absence of INI1 expression as markers of aggressive behavior. Mod Pathol. 2008;21(6):647–52.
183. Biegel JA, Tan L, Zhang F, Wainwright L, Russo P, Rorke LB. Alterations of the hSNF5/INI1 gene in central nervous system atypical teratoid/rhabdoid tumors and renal and extrarenal rhabdoid tumors. Clin Cancer Res. 2002;8(11):3461–7.
184. Kohashi K, Oda Y. Oncogenic roles of SMARCB1/INI1 and its deficient tumors. Cancer Sci. 2017;108(4):547–52.
185. Fuller CE. All things rhabdoid and SMARC: an enigmatic exploration with Dr. Louis P. Dehner. Semin Diagn Pathol. 2016;33(6):427–40.
186. Sturm D, Orr BA, Toprak UH, et al. New brain tumor entities emerge from molecular classification of CNS-PNETs. Cell. 2016;164(5):1060–72.
187. Ferris SP, Velazquez Vega J, Aboian M, et al. High-grade neuroepithelial tumor with BCOR exon 15 internal tandem duplication-a comprehensive clinical, radiographic, pathologic, and genomic analysis. Brain Pathol. 2020;30(1):46–62.
188. Lehman NL, Usubalieva A, Lin T, et al. Genomic analysis demonstrates that histologically-defined astroblastomas are molecularly heterogeneous and that tumors with MN1 rearrangement exhibit the most favorable prognosis. Acta Neuropathol Commun. 2019;7(1):42.
189. Lehman NL, Hattab EM, Mobley BC, et al. Morphological and molecular features of astroblastoma, including BRAFV600E mutations, suggest an ontological relationship to other cortical-based gliomas of children and young adults. Neuro-Oncology. 2017;19(1):31–42.

190. Wood MD, Tihan T, Perry A, et al. Multimodal molecular analysis of astroblastoma enables reclassification of most cases into more specific molecular entities. Brain Pathol. 2017;28:192.
191. Specht K, Sung YS, Zhang L, Richter GH, Fletcher CD, Antonescu CR. Distinct transcriptional signature and immunoprofile of CIC-DUX4 fusion-positive round cell tumors compared to EWSR1-rearranged Ewing sarcomas: further evidence toward distinct pathologic entities. Genes Chromosomes Cancer. 2014;53(7):622–33.
192. Yoshimoto T, Tanaka M, Homme M, et al. CIC-DUX4 induces small round cell sarcomas distinct from Ewing sarcoma. Cancer Res. 2017;77(11):2927–37.
193. Antonescu CR, Owosho AA, Zhang L, et al. Sarcomas with CIC-rearrangements are a distinct pathologic entity with aggressive outcome: a clinicopathologic and molecular study of 115 cases. Am J Surg Pathol. 2017;41(7):941–9.
194. Le Loarer F, Pissaloux D, Watson S, et al. Clinicopathologic features of CIC-NUTM1 sarcomas, a new molecular variant of the family of CIC-fused sarcomas. Am J Surg Pathol. 2019;43(2):268–76.
195. Yamada S, Muto J, De Leon JCA, et al. Primary spinal intramedullary Ewing-like sarcoma harboring CIC-DUX4 translocation: a similar cytological appearance as its soft tissue counterpart but no lobulation in association with desmoplastic stroma. Brain Tumor Pathol. 2020;37(3):111–7.
196. Bielle F, Zanello M, Guillemot D, et al. Unusual primary cerebral localization of a CIC-DUX4 translocation tumor of the Ewing sarcoma family. Acta Neuropathol. 2014;128(2):309–11.
197. Holsten T, Lubieniecki F, Spohn M, et al. Detailed clinical and histopathological description of 8 cases of molecularly defined CNS neuroblastomas. J Neuropathol Exp Neurol. 2021;80(1):52–9.
198. Korshunov A, Remke M, Gessi M, et al. Focal genomic amplification at 19q13.42 comprises a powerful diagnostic marker for embryonal tumors with ependymoblastic rosettes. Acta Neuropathol. 2010;120(2):253–60.
199. Korshunov A, Sturm D, Ryzhova M, et al. Embryonal tumor with abundant neuropil and true rosettes (ETANTR), ependymoblastoma, and medulloepithelioma share molecular similarity and comprise a single clinicopathological entity. Acta Neuropathol. 2014;128(2):279–89.
200. Spence T, Sin-Chan P, Picard D, et al. CNS-PNETs with C19MC amplification and/or LIN28 expression comprise a distinct histogenetic diagnostic and therapeutic entity. Acta Neuropathol. 2014;128(2):291–303.
201. Pfister S, Remke M, Castoldi M, et al. Novel genomic amplification targeting the microRNA cluster at 19q13.42 in a pediatric embryonal tumor with abundant neuropil and true rosettes. Acta Neuropathol. 2009;117(4):457–64.
202. Lambo S, von Hoff K, Korshunov A, Pfister SM, Kool M. ETMR: a tumor entity in its infancy. Acta Neuropathol. 2020;140(3):249–66.
203. Korshunov A, Ryzhova M, Jones DT, et al. LIN28A immunoreactivity is a potent diagnostic marker of embryonal tumor with multilayered rosettes (ETMR). Acta Neuropathol. 2012;124(6):875–81.
204. Lee Y, Liu J, Patel S, et al. Genomic landscape of meningiomas. Brain Pathol. 2010;20(4):751–62.
205. Bi WL, Abedalthagafi M, Horowitz P, et al. Genomic landscape of intracranial meningiomas. J Neurosurg. 2016;125(3):525–35.
206. Evans DG, Sainio M, Baser ME. Neurofibromatosis type 2. J Med Genet. 2000;37(12):897–904.
207. Evans DG. Neurofibromatosis 2 [bilateral acoustic neurofibromatosis, central neurofibromatosis, NF2, neurofibromatosis type II]. Genet Med. 2009;11(9):599–610.
208. Ragel BT, Jensen RL. Molecular genetics of meningiomas. Neurosurg Focus. 2005;19(5):E9.
209. Suppiah S, Nassiri F, Bi WL, et al. Molecular and translational advances in meningiomas. Neuro-Oncology. 2019;21(Suppl 1):i4–i17.
210. Toland A, McNulty SN, Pekmezci M, et al. Pediatric meningioma: a clinicopathologic and molecular study with potential grading implications. Brain Pathol. 2020;30(6):1134–43.
211. Schieffer KM, Agarwal V, LaHaye S, et al. YAP1-FAM118B fusion defines a rare subset of childhood and young adulthood Meningiomas. Am J Surg Pathol. 2020;45:329.
212. Brastianos PK, Horowitz PM, Santagata S, et al. Genomic sequencing of meningiomas identifies oncogenic SMO and AKT1 mutations. Nat Genet. 2013;45(3):285–9.
213. Clark VE, Erson-Omay EZ, Serin A, et al. Genomic analysis of non-NF2 meningiomas reveals mutations in TRAF7, KLF4, AKT1, and SMO. Science. 2013;339(6123):1077–80.
214. Shankar GM, Abedalthagafi M, Vaubel RA, et al. Germline and somatic BAP1 mutations in high-grade rhabdoid meningiomas. Neuro-Oncology. 2017;19(4):535–45.
215. Shankar GM, Santagata S. BAP1 mutations in high-grade meningioma: implications for patient care. Neuro-Oncology. 2017;19(11):1447–56.
216. Abedalthagafi MS, Merrill PH, Bi WL, et al. Angiomatous meningiomas have a distinct genetic profile with multiple chromosomal polysomies including polysomy of chromosome 5. Oncotarget. 2014;5(21):10596–606.
217. Kuroi Y, Akagawa H, Shibuya M, Onda H, Maegawa T, Kasuya H. Identification of shared genomic aberrations between angiomatous and microcystic meningiomas. Neurooncol Adv. 2019;1(1):vdz028.
218. Reuss DE, Piro RM, Jones DT, et al. Secretory meningiomas are defined by combined KLF4 K409Q and TRAF7 mutations. Acta Neuropathol. 2013;125(3):351–8.
219. Smith MJ, O'Sullivan J, Bhaskar SS, et al. Loss-of-function mutations in SMARCE1 cause an inherited disorder of multiple spinal meningiomas. Nat Genet. 2013;45(3):295–8.
220. Olar A, Wani KM, Wilson CD, et al. Global epigenetic profiling identifies methylation subgroups associated with recurrence-free survival in meningioma. Acta Neuropathol. 2017;133(3):431–44.
221. Sahm F, Schrimpf D, Stichel D, et al. DNA methylation-based classification and grading system for meningioma: a multicentre, retrospective analysis. Lancet Oncol. 2017;18(5):682–94.
222. Nassiri F, Mamatjan Y, Suppiah S, et al. DNA methylation profiling to predict recurrence risk in meningioma: development and validation of a nomogram to optimize clinical management. Neuro-Oncology. 2019;21(7):901–10.
223. Chmielecki J, Crago AM, Rosenberg M, et al. Whole-exome sequencing identifies a recurrent NAB2-STAT6 fusion in solitary fibrous tumors. Nat Genet. 2013;45(2):131–2.
224. Robinson DR, Wu YM, Kalyana-Sundaram S, et al. Identification of recurrent NAB2-STAT6 gene fusions in solitary fibrous tumor by integrative sequencing. Nat Genet. 2013;45(2):180–5.
225. Schweizer L, Koelsche C, Sahm F, et al. Meningeal hemangiopericytoma and solitary fibrous tumors carry the NAB2-STAT6 fusion and can be diagnosed by nuclear expression of STAT6 protein. Acta Neuropathol. 2013;125(5):651–8.
226. Demicco EG, Harms PW, Patel RM, et al. Extensive survey of STAT6 expression in a large series of mesenchymal tumors. Am J Clin Pathol. 2015;143(5):672–82.
227. Fritchie KJ, Jin L, Rubin BP, et al. NAB2-STAT6 gene fusion in meningeal hemangiopericytoma and solitary fibrous tumor. J Neuropathol Exp Neurol. 2016;75(3):263–71.
228. Barthelmess S, Geddert H, Boltze C, et al. Solitary fibrous tumors/hemangiopericytomas with different variants of the NAB2-STAT6 gene fusion are characterized by specific histomorphology and distinct clinicopathological features. Am J Pathol. 2014;184(4):1209–18.

229. Tai HC, Chuang IC, Chen TC, et al. NAB2-STAT6 fusion types account for clinicopathological variations in solitary fibrous tumors. Mod Pathol. 2015;28(10):1324–35.
230. Fritchie K, Jensch K, Moskalev EA, et al. The impact of histopathology and NAB2-STAT6 fusion subtype in classification and grading of meningeal solitary fibrous tumor/hemangiopericytoma. Acta Neuropathol. 2019;137(2):307–19.
231. Kusters-Vandevelde HV, Kusters B, van Engen-van Grunsven AC, Groenen PJ, Wesseling P, Blokx WA. Primary melanocytic tumors of the central nervous system: a review with focus on molecular aspects. Brain Pathol. 2015;25(2):209–26.
232. van de Nes J, Gessi M, Sucker A, et al. Targeted next generation sequencing reveals unique mutation profile of primary melanocytic tumors of the central nervous system. J Neuro-Oncol. 2016;127(3):435–44.
233. van Engen-van Grunsven AC, Kusters-Vandevelde H, Groenen PJ, Blokx WA. Update on molecular pathology of cutaneous melanocytic lesions: what is new in diagnosis and molecular testing for treatment? Front Med (Lausanne). 2014;1:39.
234. Sekine S, Shibata T, Kokubu A, et al. Craniopharyngiomas of adamantinomatous type harbor beta-catenin gene mutations. Am J Pathol. 2002;161(6):1997–2001.
235. Brastianos PK, Taylor-Weiner A, Manley PE, et al. Exome sequencing identifies BRAF mutations in papillary craniopharyngiomas. Nat Genet. 2014;46(2):161–5.

7 Lung Cancer

Ruifang Zheng and Linsheng Zhang

List of Frequently Asked Questions

1. What are the major types of lung cancer and how are they different in the molecular mechanisms of tumorigenesis?
2. What are the clinically significant genetic abnormalities seen in lung adenocarcinoma?
3. What is the mutation landscape of squamous cell carcinoma of the lung?
4. When is mutation testing for squamous cell carcinoma indicated?
5. What is the mutation landscape of small cell lung cancer?
6. Are there any clinically significant genetic alterations associated with other relatively uncommon lung cancer types?
7. What is the purpose of molecular genetic testing for lung cancer?
8. What genes/mutations should be tested for non-small-cell lung cancer?
9. When should a lung cancer sample be tested for mutation profile?
10. When multiple lung cancer lesions and/or multiple metastatic tumors are identified and excised/biopsied in one patient, should each of them be tested for mutation profile separately?
11. How are different types of genetic aberrations of lung cancer tested in the clinical diagnostic laboratories?
12. What are the benefits and challenges of using next generation sequencing-based tests for non-small-cell lung cancer?
13. What are the specimen types acceptable for mutation profiling of lung cancer?
14. What is the role of cell-free DNA testing (liquid biopsy) for lung cancer?
15. What is the clinical significance of tumor mutation burden (TMB) in lung cancer and how is it tested?
16. What other tests can be considered to provide guidance for immunotherapy of lung cancer?

R. Zheng · L. Zhang (✉)
Department of Pathology and Laboratory Medicine, Emory University School of Medicine, Atlanta, GA, USA
e-mail: ruifangzhengnj@gmail.com; linsheng.zhang@emory.edu

Frequently Asked Questions

1. **What are the major types of lung cancers and how are they different in the molecular mechanisms of tumorigenesis?**
   - Lung cancer is a common cancer and the leading cause of cancer deaths in the Western world. Although the incidence and death rate have been declining since 1990 per statistics published by the American Cancer Society in 2020 [1], lung cancer is still ranked #2 of all new cancer cases (excluding basal cell and squamous cell skin cancers and in situ carcinoma except urinary bladder) in both males and females (estimated over 110,000 cases in each sex in 2020) and #1 in all cancer deaths (72,500 males and 63,220 females, both >20% of all cancer deaths) in the United States.
   - In clinical practice, the major lung cancer types are non-small-cell lung cancer (NSCLC), including adenocarcinoma, squamous cell carcinoma, and other relatively less common types and small cell lung cancer (SCLC) [2]. Adenocarcinoma and squamous cell carcinoma comprise approximately 70%, SCLC 15–20% of all lung cancers [3].
   - Tobacco smoking has been recognized as the major cause of lung cancer, responsible for over 85% of all lung cancer cases [4]. The percentage of cigarette-smoking-caused lung cancers has declined thanks to the mass media campaigns and tobacco control policies [5, 6]. There are significant differences in the

Y. Ding, L. Zhang (eds.), *Practical Oncologic Molecular Pathology*, Practical Anatomic Pathology,
https://doi.org/10.1007/978-3-030-73227-1_7

molecular tumorigenesis between cigarette-smoking-related and unrelated lung cancers. The tobacco smoke carcinogen-induced mutations are frequently G to T transversions, such as *RAS* codon 12 GGT (glycine) mutated to TGT (cysteine) or GTT (valine), and loss of function mutations of the tumor suppressor gene *TP53*.

- Overall, activating mutations of oncogenes are frequently seen in adenocarcinoma not related to cigarette smoking, resulting in self-sufficiency in growth signals, insensitivity to antigrowth signals, and evasion of apoptosis. The clinically significant alterations in this category include activating mutations in genes encoding the epidermal growth factor receptor (ERBB receptor tyrosine kinases) and related elements in the cell proliferation and survival signal pathways, and rearrangement involving *ALK1* or *ROS1*. Loss of function mutations of tumor suppressor genes are more common in tobacco-related SCLC and SCC. These mutations also occur in adenocarcinoma of nonsmokers but are usually not the driver mutations [3].
- It is much more difficult to target a loss of function (tumor suppressor genes) than an activating alteration. Currently available targeted therapies, therefore, mostly apply to adenocarcinoma in non-smokers, whose tumors show so-called oncogene addiction. Small molecules inhibiting the protein kinases overactive due to genetic alterations represent the major breakthrough in the treatment of NSCLC. On the other hand, loss of tumor suppressor functions frequently results in accumulation of secondary mutations and higher mutation load in the tumor. These tumors are more likely to have neoantigens and, therefore, may respond better to immunotherapies, which is the second breakthrough of lung cancer treatment, clinically effective for the non-oncogene-addicted tumors.

2. **What are the clinically significant genetic abnormalities seen in lung adenocarcinoma?**
   - Multiple genetic abnormalities are associated with lung adenocarcinoma. According to the data archived at cBioportal.com, the most commonly mutated genes in lung adenocarcinoma are (in the order of highest to lowest) *TP53* (52.4%), *KRAS* (30.5%), *EGFR* (24.2%), *STK11* (16.8%), and *KEAP1* (15.8%); the genes most commonly involved in translocation/fusion are *ALK* (2.2%), *EML4* (2.0%), *ROS1* (1.5%), *CD74* (1.0%), and *RET* (1.0%). They can either be grouped into driver mutations versus non-driver mutations based on their roles in tumorigenesis, or into actionable mutations versus non-actionable mutations based on whether there are drugs targeting the specific mutation.
   - Currently, the actionable mutations/alterations in adenocarcinoma with approved drugs include [7, 8]:
     - ***EGFR* mutations**: Mutations occur throughout the *EGFR* (*ERBB1*) gene, resulting in abnormal activation of the EGFR kinase activity. Majority of the mutations occur in exon 18–21, encoding the protein kinase domain [9].
     - ***ALK* rearrangements**: *ELM4-ALK1* is the most common *ALK* fusion gene [10].
     - ***ROS1* rearrangements**: *ROS1* has various partner genes with *CD74* being the most common one [11].
     - ***MET* abnormalities** include exon 14 skipping and *MET* amplification, both leading to increased MET protein level and kinase activity [12].
     - ***BRAF* mutations**: *BRAF* mutations in lung adenocarcinoma have a different spectrum from that seen in melanoma; *BRAF* c.1799T > A; p.V600E only comprises approximately 50% of all *BRAF* mutations [13].
     - ***RET* rearrangements** are rare, present in only 1–2% of lung adenocarcinoma [14].
     - **Neurotrophic tyrosine receptor kinase (*NTRK*)** fusions: NTRK1 fusion proteins are relatively common in lung adenocarcinoma; NTRK2 and NTRK3 fusions are present at low frequencies [15].
     - ***HER2*:** Mutations in the kinase domain of *ERBB2* (*HER2/neu*), one of the epidermal growth factor receptor or ErbB family tyrosine kinases, are found in approximately 1–4% of lung adenocarcinomas [16–18]. They are seen in tumors with a similar phenotype to those harboring *EGFR* mutations.
   - *EGFR* mutations are the most common targetable mutations in lung adenocarcinoma and have a high prevalence in younger, female, Asian non-smoker patients. The inframe deletion in exon 19 (see case 1 as an example) and c.2573T > G; p.Leu858Arg (L858R) mutation in exon 21 together comprise approximately 90% of all *EGFR* mutations, with the prevalence of exon 19 deletion slightly higher than that of L858R [9]. These two mutations are sensitive to the tyrosine kinase inhibitors (TKIs). The responsiveness to TKIs varies for the other less commonly seen mutations, such as *EGFR* c.2155G > A; p.G719S, c.2582T > A; p.L861Q, and c.2303G > T; p.S768I, etc.
   - In addition to the targetable *EGFR* mutations, there are also mutations associated with drug resistance. Identifying them helps to predict the responsiveness to targeted therapy. Two well-defined *EGFR* mutations are associated with resistance to first- and second-generation EGFR TKIs. Patients carrying these two mutations usually respond to therapy with a third generation TKI.
     - The *EGFR* c.2369C > T; p.Thr790Met (T790M) mutation is the most common mutation in *EGFR* that is responsible for acquired resistance to the first- and second-generation TKIs. The incidence of

  T790M in treatment-naïve patients is less than 1%, whereas in first- and second-generation TKI-treated patients, it can be as high as ~50% [19, 20] (see case 2 as an example).
  - *EGFR* exon 20 insertion is considered the major mechanism of refractoriness to the first- and second-generation TKIs in treatment-naïve patients [21].
- *ALK1* or *ROS1* rearrangement creates a fusion protein with constitutive tyrosine kinase activity. They occur in lung adenocarcinoma at low frequency, with *ALK1* rearrangements in 1–3% and *ROS1* rearrangements in 0.7–3.4% of Caucasian patients [22] [23]. In NSCLC, *ELM4* is the most common fusion partner of *ALK1*; other partner genes, such as *TGF*, *KLC1*, and *KIKF5B*, are rare [24]. The partner gene provides the dimerization domain required for the constitutive activation of *ALK1* kinase [24, 25]. More than 20 variants of *ELM4-ALK1* fusion proteins have been identified, all containing the intracellular kinase domain of ALK1, but variable length of ELM4 due to different breakpoints. The trimerization domain (TD) of ELM4 is required for the constitutive activity of ELM4-ALK1 fusion protein. The presence and the length of the tandem atypical propeller (TAPE) domain of ELM4 affect protein localization and sensitivity to ALK1 inhibitors [10, 25, 26]. *CD74*, *SDC4*, *EZR*, and *SLC34A2* are well-documented *ROS1* fusion partners, among which *CD74* is the most common one, comprising approximately 38% of all *ROS1* fusions [11]. *ROS1* can also be rearranged to partner with *TPM3*, *MYH9*, *CCDC6*, *FIG*, *LRIG3*, *KDELR2*, *MSN*, *TMEM106B*, *TPD52L1*, *CLTC*, and *LIMA1* [27]. Unlike *ALK1* and *ROS1* rearrangements that have multiple breakpoints, *ROS1* fusions with *CD74* and *EZR* often occur at intron 33, whereas breakpoints at intron 31 are more frequently seen in fusions with *SDC4* and *SLC34A2* [11]. The underlying mechanisms of how the fusions lead to ROS1 kinase activation is currently unknown. The presence of *ALK1* or *ROS1* rearrangement predicts sensitivity to ALK1 or ROS1 kinase inhibitors. Due to a high degree of homology between the kinase domains of ALK1 and ROS1 [28], most of the currently available ALK inhibitors including crizotinib, ceritinib, lorlatinib, etc., also show cross inhibitory effect on ROS1 fusion proteins [29].
- *MET* exon 14 skipping refers to the loss of exon 14 due to mutations at the splice site or nearby introns. Exon 14 skipping and mutation of codon Y1003 prevent Casitas B-lineage lymphoma proto-oncogene (c-CBL) E3 ligase binding, resulting in decreased protein degradation and increased MET protein level, enhanced MET phosphorylation, and prolonged MET activation [12]. *MET* amplification is frequently seen in acquired resistance to *EGFR* inhibitors but also occurs in treatment-naïve patients. The increased MET activity due to exon 14 skipping and *MET* amplification are both sensitive to MET inhibitors [12, 30].
- *RET* rearrangement is rare in NSCLC with a frequency of 1–2% [14]. The *RET* fusion genes consist of the RET kinase domain and a dimerization domain provided by its partner gene. The dimerization confers constitutive RET kinase activity of the fusion protein [31]. Patients carrying *RET* fusion genes respond to multi-target tyrosine kinase inhibition; however, their clinical outcome is inferior to those with other oncogene-addicted NSCLC receiving selective TKIs [32].
- *BRAF* mutations in lung adenocarcinoma include c.1799T > A; p.Val600Glu (V600E), and non-V600E mutations, with an approximate ratio of 1:1. V600E mutation occurs in 1.5–3.5% of lung adenocarcinoma; non-V600E mutations can either be activating or inactivating [13]. *BRAF* rearrangements in lung adenocarcinoma are rare [33]. A novel fusion *SND1-BRAF* has been reported in lung adenocarcinoma in non-smokers with increased phosphorylation levels of MEK/ERK and cell proliferation by in vitro study [34].
- *NTRK* fusions in lung adenocarcinoma involve all three isoforms of *NTRK*s. *NTRK1* rearrangements are present in approximately 3%; *NTRK2* and *NTRK3* rearrangements in less than 1% of lung adenocarcinomas [15, 35]. There is a great diversity of *NTRK* gene partners, which render constitutive kinase activity to the fusion proteins and sensitivity to TKIs [36]. *MPRIP-NTRK1*, *CD74-NTRK1*, and *TMP53-NTRK2* are the relatively frequent fusions in lung adenocarcinoma [37].
- *HER2* mutations occur in exon 20 (insertion), the kinase, transmembrane, and extracellular domains; some of them may have concurrent *HER2* amplification [18]. *HER2*-mutated lung cancers are sensitive to kinase inhibitors like dacomitinib [38] and afatinib [17], HER2 monoclonal antibody trastuzumab [16] and ado-trastuzumab emtansine, a HER2-targeted antibody-drug conjugate [18].

3. **What is the mutation landscape of squamous cell carcinoma of the lung?**
   - Squamous cell carcinoma (SCC) has a strong association with tobacco smoking. Despite the relatively higher mutation burden, the typical tyrosine kinase gene mutations/aberrations seen in adenocarcinoma are rare in squamous cell carcinoma [39–41]. Mutations/aberrations detected in squamous cell lung carcinoma are similar to the squamous cell carcinoma from other organs, referred to as "squamousness" gene signatures [42, 43].
   - The most common genetic alterations in lung SCC occur in the cell cycle regulator genes, including

deletion and loss of function mutations in *TP53* (>75%) and *CDKN2A/B* (~70%) [39, 41]. *TP53* mutation-associated signature is a significant prognostic biomarker and potentially predictive of response to immunotherapies [44].

- Receptor tyrosine kinase (RTK) gene amplifications are present in >30% of lung SCC, with *EGFR* and *FGFR1* being most common; however, mutations/fusions are rare [40, 45]. *FGFR1* amplification is associated with better prognosis [46]. *ERBB* family mutations are seen in >20% of lung SCC; however, clinical responses to TKIs were not promising in the patients harboring these mutations, suggesting they are unlikely driver mutations [43].
- RAS, MAPK, and PI3K signaling pathway dysregulation is another feature of SCC, most commonly loss of *NF1*, amplification or mutation of *PIK3CA,* and loss of *PTEN.* The potential value for targeted therapy of these alterations is under investigation [40].
- Squamous cell carcinoma has been shown to have a higher tumor mutation burden (TMB) than adenocarcinoma [47]. In recent years, TMB has evolved as a novel biomarker to predict the sensitivity to immune-checkpoint inhibitors (see answers to question 15).

4. **When is mutation testing for squamous cell carcinoma indicated?**
   - Given that there is no effective targeted therapy for lung SCC in routine clinical practice, mutation profiling is not recommended for well-defined squamous cell carcinoma by the current practice guidelines [48].
   - Approximately 0.4–4% of all lung carcinomas contain both adeno and squamous components under the light microscope, and the frequency is even higher based on the ultrastructural appearance [49, 50]. These tumors may be sensitive to targeted therapies if related mutations are present [48]. Therefore, if the specimens from lung cancer, such as a small biopsy or needle aspiration, are not representative of the whole tumor, or the morphologic and immunophenotypic features are not entirely characteristic of SCC and a definitive classification is challenging, pathologists should consider mutation testing of the sample (see example case 4).
   - The current expert consensus opinion is that oncologists or pathologists may consider molecular testing in tumors other than adenocarcinoma when the probability of a targetable oncogenic driver is high based on the clinical features of the patient, including young age (<50 years) and absence of tobacco exposure history [28, 48, 51].
   - Although routine clinical testing of TMB has not been standardized, TMB assessment together with mutation profiling with targeted panel next generation sequencing (NGS) is a hot topic for molecular testing of NSCLC, including SCC [52–54].

5. **What is the mutation landscape of small cell lung cancer?**
   - Small cell carcinoma of the lung (SCLC) is a high-grade neuroendocrine tumor, possessing the worst prognosis among all lung carcinomas. There has not been any targeted therapy for SCLC so far. Recent genomic studies of SCLC reveal a complex genomic profile [55].
   - Both copy number gains and losses involving multiple chromosomes have been identified using array-based genomic analysis. Recurrent loss of 3p (*FHIT* and *RASSF1*), 17p (*TP53*), 13q (*RB1*), and 10q (*PTEN*) have been reported in multiple studies. The other commonly seen copy number gains/amplifications include 1p, 2p, and 8q harboring the *MYC* family genes [56–63].
   - SCLC has a high mutation rate partly attributed to exposure to tobacco carcinogens. Several pathways are involved in the mutations associated with SCLC. Deletion and/or loss of function mutations in *RB1* and *TP53* occur in >90% of the SCLC [63].
   - Alteration of telomere length is frequently detected in neuroendocrine carcinomas of the lung, greater in high grade forms (large cell neuroendocrine carcinoma and SCLC) [64]. *TERT* copy gain, together with *RB1* deletion, was an independent predictor of poor prognosis in a study by Simbolo et al. [65].
   - Large cell neuroendocrine carcinoma (LCNEC) is another form of high-grade carcinoma of neuroendocrine origin. There are similarities in the gene expression profiles suggesting a common origin of LCNEC and SCLC [66], and their molecular profiles are significantly different from that of low grade neuroendocrine tumors [67]. Molecular genetic distinction between LCNEC and SCLC has also been reported [68, 69]. However, the inconsistency of these findings and the clinical significance of the differences warrant further study.

6. **Are there any clinically significant genetic alterations associated with other relatively uncommon lung cancer types?**
   - Some of the other relatively uncommon lung cancer types included in the fourth edition of WHO Classification [2] are carcinosarcoma, pulmonary blastoma, NUT carcinoma, primary pulmonary lymphoepithelioma-like carcinoma (PLELC), and salivary-gland-type lung carcinomas.
   - Carcinosarcoma is an aggressive NSCLC that frequently contains a variety of components, with phenotypes ranging from adenocarcinoma, SCC, to different sarcomas. The mutation profiles corresponding to

different components may be present in one tumor. Multiple studies have reported that *TP53* mutations are frequently present, followed by *KRAS* mutation. Targetable mutations associated with adenocarcinoma, such as *EGFR* mutations and *ALK* rearrangement, are rarely detected, but *ALK* and *EGFR* amplification and overexpression are not uncommon [70–77]. One study found a high frequency of actionable *MET* mutations (8 of 36 cases tested) [78].

- Pulmonary blastomas are frequently associated with missense mutations of *CTNNB1* [79, 80], resulting in aberrant nuclear/cytoplasmic localization of beta-catenin protein and activation of the Wnt signaling pathway [81].
- No clinically significant mutation profile has been discovered in PLELC so far. One study found low TMB in PLELC despite relatively high frequency of *TP53* mutations [82].
- Salivary-gland-type lung carcinomas arise from the submucosal glands of the airway, accounting for <1% of all lung tumors [83]. Histologically, they resemble their salivary gland counterpart, and most of them also share the same genetic alterations. Table 7.1 lists the major types of pulmonary salivary gland tumors and their associated genetic signatures.
- NUT carcinomas carry the characteristic *NUT* rearrangement. The fusion partners are most commonly (70%) *BRD4* resulting from t(15;19) [84, 85]. *BRD3*, *BRD4*, and *NSD3* are other common gene partners of *NUT* [86]. The fusion protein causes epigenetic deregulation, resulting in loss of cell differentiation [87]. Detection of the *NUT* rearrangement in challenging cases provides evidence for a definitive diagnosis.

7. **What is the purpose of molecular genetic testing for lung cancer?**
    - As a standard of care, the purpose of performing mutation profiling for lung cancer in routine clinical practice is to select patients for mutation-based targeted therapy. In patients who developed resistance to a targeted therapy, mutation profiling is an important approach to search for resistance mechanisms.
    - When multiple lesions are present, mutation profiling may provide useful information to evaluate the origin of the different lesions, the clonal diversity, and clonal evolution (see questions 10 and 11 below).
    - Detecting characteristic genetic alterations provide definitive or additional supporting evidence for the diagnosis and classification of some special types of carcinomas (see answers to question 6 above).
    - Beyond the standard of care recommended by the practice guidelines, molecular tests should also be considered when there is compelling evidence from clinical trial results that investigational targeted therapies are effective. TMB is considered a promising biomarker independent of PD-L1 immunostaining to select lung cancer patients for immunotherapies.

8. **What genes/mutations should be tested for non-small-cell lung cancer?**
    - Genes with targetable mutations associated with non-squamous NSCLC are recommended by several published guidelines to be tested as the current standard of care [8, 48, 88]:
        - *EGFR* mutations, and *ALK1* and *ROS1* rearrangements must be tested as a separate single gene or panel test, for all lung adenocarcinoma patients. *BRAF, MET, RET, KRAS*, and *HER2* testing should be included in a larger panel whenever appropriate, if there is sufficient sample available [48].
        - *KRAS* mutation single gene test can be performed separately because of the high prevalence and the mutual exclusivity of *KRAS* mutation with *EGFR* mutations and *ALK* fusions in NSCLC. If *KRAS* mutation is detected, larger panel testing for other mutations is not necessary. Currently, there is no compelling evidence to support single gene tests for *BRAF, MET, RET,* and *HER2* [48].
        - The first-generation *NTRK* inhibitors, larotrectinib and entrectinib, were approved by the US Food and Drug Administration (US FDA) in 2017 for the treatment of any *NTRK*-fusion-positive cancers, including NSCLC [89]. When clinically indicated, testing for *NTRK* fusions in the absence of other driver alterations is recommended in the newer guidelines [8].
        - TMB testing to help selecting patients for immunotherapy [90], although not included in the guideline published in 2018 [48], may be considered for some patients with metastatic NSCLC [91].
        - Given the high prevalence of *EGFR* T790M mutation in acquired resistance to first- and second-generation EGFR TKIs, *EGFR* T790M must be tested in the setting of disease progression while on targeted therapy to select patients for third-generation TKIs [48].
        - Although mutations in the *ALK1* gene may be associated with drug resistance, current evidence is not sufficient to support routine testing for *ALK1* mutations.

Table 7.1 Pulmonary salivary-gland-type carcinomas and their genetic signatures

Tumor type	Genetic alteration
Mucoepidermoid carcinoma	*MECT1-MAML2* fusion
Adenoid cystic carcinoma	*MYB-NFIB* fusion
Pleomorphic adenoma and carcinoma ex pleomorphic adenoma	*PLAG1* rearrangement, *HMGA* amplification
Myoepithelial carcinoma	*EWSR1* rearrangement
Hyalinizing clear cell carcinoma	*EWSR1-ATF1* fusion

- *TP53* is altered in >40% of NSCLC and >80% of lung SCC [92]. Most clinical studies suggest that NSCLC with *TP53* alterations carry a worse prognosis and may be relatively more resistant to chemo- and radiation therapies [93]. Recently, *TP53* co-mutations in *EGFR*- mutated NSCLC have also been associated with poor outcome of TKI therapy [94]. *TP53* is usually included in the NGS panel for lung cancer mutation profiling to provide prognostic and predictive information.
- There are many genes/mutations associated with NSCLC for which targeted or specific therapies are in development. Testing these genes/mutations may be considered in specific patient groups to provide information for clinical trial recruitment.

9. **When should a lung cancer sample be tested for mutation profile?**
   - Lung cancer mutation testing/profiling is only required in patients presenting with advanced-stage (stage IV) or metastatic disease who are suitable for therapy, either at initial diagnosis or recurrent disease with progression, if not previously tested [8, 48, 88].
   - Molecular testing is encouraged for early-stage lung cancer [48]. Testing lung cancer samples from early-stage patients allows for obtaining molecular profiling results from high-quality resection specimen when it is readily available. These results are saved for the future in case the lung cancer progresses and it becomes necessary to have mutation profile results but it is difficult or unnecessary to obtain more sample. However, with the improvement of clinical management, a subset of early stage patients will be cured by surgical resection and/or chemoradiation therapy, thus, never needing the mutation profile. Each institution should set its own policy on testing patients with early-stage diseases.
   - Repeat testing on recurrent tumor or a blood sample (for circulating cell free tumor DNA) can be considered for patients who developed resistant or refractory disease to investigate the molecular basis of resistance and search for potential mutation targets to enroll the patients in clinical trials.
   - When a diagnosis is established and it is determined that molecular testing is necessary, tissue samples should be prioritized for molecular testing before exhaustion for other studies, especially when only cytology or limited biopsy samples are available. When the specimen size is small and additional studies are anticipated, it could be very helpful to cut multiple additional unstained sections upfront to avoid later refacing the tissue block for additional sections, which could result in significant loss of the limited tissue.
10. **When multiple lung cancer lesions and/or multiple metastatic tumors are identified and excised/biopsied in one patient, should each of them be tested for mutation profile separately?**
    - There is no significant clonal diversity in a tumor that would cause sampling bias in the molecular testing of NSCLC [95, 96]. Furthermore, the mutation patterns remain quite stable in metastatic and recurrent tumors [95]. Therefore, primary or metastatic tumors are equally suitable for molecular testing [97]. It is not necessary to test different regions of one tumor for mutation profiles, and routine testing of metastatic or recurrent lesions of a known primary NSCLC is not recommended.
    - In patients with synchronous multifocal lung cancers, these lesions can be metastatic from one primary or concurrent multiple primary lung cancers [98, 99]. Distinguishing multiple synchronous primary from metastatic malignant masses is important for lung cancer staging and has significant treatment implications because the treatment protocols for metastatic late-stage lung cancer is substantially different from early-stage disease (see case 3 as an example).
    - Comparing the histomorphologic features of multiple tumors can be a powerful tool to determine whether they are metastatic late-stage cancer or multiple primaries. However, histologic features are not always reliable [100]. Furthermore, when a metastatic cancer is identified in a patient with a history of more than one cancer of the same histologic type (i.e., adenocarcinoma of different organ origin), it could be more challenging to determine the origin of the metastatic cancer based on histologic and even immunophenotypic features.
    - Molecular profile as definitive clonal evidence for a tumor sample has been used to study clonal diversity, clonal evolution, and intra-tumor heterogeneity [95–97, 101]. Combining histomorphologic and genotypic assessments is the ultimate approach to the accurate staging of lung cancer and defining the origin and evolution of a metastatic cancer [102, 103].
    - The decision of whether to test each of the tumors should be based on the clinical context of the patients, and the communications between pathologists and clinicians [88]. Recurrent tumors are recommended to be re-tested only when there are clinical indications, such as progression under targeted therapy suggesting acquired resistance, pathologic evidences suggesting clonal evolution, or a different tissue/organ origin.
11. **How are different types of genetic aberrations of lung cancer tested in the clinical diagnostic laboratories?**
    - Many different molecular methods can be used to detect mutations and/or other genetic alterations in

NSCLC. Because only a few genes/alterations (*EGFR* mutations, *ALK1* and *ROS1* translocations) are mandatory to be tested, single-gene or small panel tests are still widely performed in clinical diagnostic laboratories. After the first practice guideline published in 2013, some manufacturers have made commercial test kits focused on NSCLC mutations. The characteristics, advantages, and disadvantages of different methods used in molecular tests of NSCLC are summarized in Table 7.2.

- Point mutations, either as single- or multi-nucleotide variants, frequently occur in *EGFR, KRAS, BRAF, HER2*, and many other genes and are detectable by almost any molecular testing methods, if designed appropriately. Mutant-allele-specific polymerase chain reaction (PCR) needs special primer design to detect multinucleotide variants (MNVs); the commercially available allele-specific primers or probes are usually not designed for the multinucleotide changes. For example, allele-specific PCR designed for BRAF c.1799T > A; p.V600E would not accurately detect less commonly seen c.1798_1799delinsAA; p.V600K or c.1798_1799delinsAG; p.V600R mutations. Droplet digital PCR method is a variant form of PCR that markedly increases the analytic sensitivity and quantitation accuracy. It is particularly useful when the sample contains a low percentage of tumor or mutant DNA, such as circulating cell-free DNA (cfDNA) extracted from blood (liquid biopsy).
- Small insertions and deletions (indels) frequently occur in mutant *EGFR* (exon 19 deletion, exon 20 insertion) and *HER2* (exon 20 insertion). Although a well-designed PCR method may detect most of the indels, relatively uncommon ones that have the same pathologic effect are usually not covered. A fragment size analysis or sequencing based method is preferred; the latter could provide detailed information of the nucleotide changes.
- Fusions genes resulting from chromosome rearrangements (*ALK1, ROS1, RET, NTRK*, rarely *BRAF* and *FGFR*) are detectable by fluorescence in situ hybridization (FISH) with excellent sensitivity and specificity, if the probes are designed appropriately (see case 5 as an example). Because these fusion genes are all transcribed to mRNA with fusion protein expression, mRNA-based reverse transcription (RT) PCR is also an excellent detection method, providing better analytic sensitivity than FISH. However, RT-PCR may not cover all the translocation variants because rare or novel variants are usually not included in the primer design.

Table 7.2 Molecular genetic methods used in pathologic characterization of NSCLC

Method	Major features	Examples
FISH	Specific probes to detect translocations and amplifications; usually 200 cells scored Relatively labor intensive and not easily automated	*ALK1* and *ROS1* rearrangements, *MET* amplification
Polymerase chain reaction (PCR)		
RT-PCR	Identify abnormalities in mRNA, testing for fusion RNA and aberrant splicing	*EML4-ALK1* fusion, *MET* exon 14 skipping
Mutant allele specific PCR	Excellent in detecting SNVs, MNVs and small indels Need specific primer/probe design for each mutation	*EGFR* point mutations (L858R, T790M), and some indels such as exon 19 deletions
Droplet digital PCR	Same as allele-specific PCR, excellent analytic sensitivity, best for low tumor/mutant percentage	cfDNA test (liquid biopsy)
Fragment size analysis	Identify indels only Analytic sensitivity ~5%	*EGFR* exon 19 deletion *HER2* exon 20 insertion
SNaPshot	PCR-based, multiplex with variable probe lengths Only detects SNVs	*EGFR* (SNVs), *BRAF* V600E *KRAS* codon 12 and 13 mutations
Sequencing		
Sanger sequencing	Read the nucleotide sequence of a fragment up to 1000 bp; analytic sensitivity (~20%) not optimal for specimens with low tumor content Low throughput	Confirmation of germline variants and novel fusions, or other abnormalities when tumor content is sufficient
Pyrosequencing	Similar to Sanger sequencing; better analytic sensitivity (~5%), shorter sequencing length. Not optimal for regions with homopolymers	*EGFR* (SNVs and indels) *BRAF* V600E *KRAS* codon 12 and 13 mutations
NGS	High throughput, covering many genes/mutations in one test. Potentially detects a wide range of alterations. See discussion in question 12	DNA + RNA panel for tissue cfDNA testing (liquid biopsy)

Abbreviations: *FISH* fluorescence in situ hybridization, *SNV* single-nucleotide variant, *MNV* multinucleotide variant, *RT-PCR* reverse transcription PCR, *cfDNA* cell-free DNA, *NGS* next-generation sequencing

- Targetable gene amplifications in lung cancer occur in *MET*, *HER2*, and *FGFR*. The detection of gene amplification is challenging by PCR or sequencing methods. FISH with a chromosome enumeration probe (CEP) as internal control is a sensitive and specific method to detect gene amplification. For example, *MET* amplification is defined as a *MET/CEP7* (chromosome 7 enumeration probe) ratio >2.2. The probe design for specific genes is required, and a standardized cutoff threshold is critical to define an amplification. A copy number array analysis can sensitively detect gene amplification at the whole-genome level, but it is too costly to be routinely performed; only selected patients may be indicated.
- More frequent than amplification, targetable alterations of *MET* include mutations at the RNA splice site or intronic region resulting in exon 14 skipping. Although many mutations have been confirmed resulting in exon 14 skipping, testing at the DNA level is challenging to recognize all the mutations to that effect [104]. Only an mRNA-based test (RT-PCR or RNA sequencing) could provide definitive evidence by amplifying the abnormally spliced mRNA with shorter length [105] (see case 6).
- Although it is easier to implement FDA-approved in vitro diagnostic (IVD) tests [106], the laboratory directors need to have a full understanding of the detection range of the PCR-based tests to know whether additional testing would be required if the results from the IVD tests are negative.
- Given the complexity and variable prevalence of the targetable genetic changes associated with NSCLC, there are different ways to approach the molecular testing in a clinical diagnostic laboratory [107]. It might be worthwhile for molecular diagnostic laboratories to establish a cost-effective test triaging an algorithm based on local resources and clinical requirements. Potentially practical algorithms include (1) test *KRAS* first, if any mutation identified, no other tests are indicated; (2) test *EGFR* first, if no mutation detected, reflex to *ALK1*, *ROS1* translocation, and/or *KRAS* mutation test, or a panel test to include more alterations. (3) start with a small panel to cover the most relevant genes, such as *EGFR* mutation and *ALK1* and *ROS1* translocations; if the results are all negative, then consider testing uncommon and investigational mutations with an expanded panel in a subgroup of patients as clinically indicated. In the future, most clinical laboratories will likely implement extensive large-panel NGS to cover all the mutations associated with NSCLC.
- Laboratories performing mutation tests for NSCLC should have a plan for reflex testing in case any sample fails the first test or the quality/quantity not sufficient to complete the routine tests. In our institution, we perform a small panel (26 genes) NGS for SNVs/MNVs and small indels, together with a FISH panel including *ALK1*, *ROS1*, *RET* translocations, and *MET* amplification. If a sample fails to qualify for the NGS test, it is reflexed to a SNaPshot panel for the hotspot mutations of 10 genes including *EGFR, KRAS,* and *BRAF*, together with a fragment size analysis for *EGFR* exon 19 deletion, exon 20 insertion, as well as *HER2* exon 20 insertion. This approach allows us to obtain the mutation profile of all the clinically significant alterations from almost any sample, small or large.
- In addition to molecular tests, immunohistochemical staining (IHC) for *ALK1* is considered as equivalent to FISH for ALK fusions; however, only the D5F3 antibody from Ventana has been approved by the FDA for patient selection for crizotinib treatment [106]. IHC can be used as a screening test for *ROS1* translocation; positive results must be confirmed by FISH [48]. *BRAF* V600E mutation can be screened by IHC with VE1 antibody; however, the performance characteristics need to be determined by the individual laboratory; and this antibody cannot detect *BRAF* non-V600E mutations. Due to the low prevalence of *HER2* amplification, the immunohistochemical stain of HER2 is not useful in predicting the treatment response of inhibitors or antibodies. IHC has no value in detecting *EGFR* mutations.

12. **What are the benefits and challenges of using next-generation sequencing (NGS)-based tests for non-small-cell lung cancer?**
    - If designed appropriately, one NGS test can cover multiple genes, various types of mutations/aberrations, including point mutations, deletions, insertions, and copy number variants. Sequencing libraries built from tumor RNA can be loaded together with that from DNA to identify fusion genes and assess gene expression levels. TMB, a potential biomarker for immunotherapy, can also be calculated based on the data from a large-panel NGS (see question 15).
    - Other advantages of NGS include low input of genetic materials, high sensitivity, and low cost per gene. When multiple gene targets are tested for lung cancer, an NGS panel is more cost effective over multiple single-gene tests [107]. The high analytic sensitivity of deep sequencing coupled with molecular barcoding (unique molecular identifier, UMI) provides an ideal method to detect low-frequency mutant alleles, making it suitable for circulating tumor DNA (ctDNA) testing using blood samples (see answers to question 14 below).

- Because detecting *ALK1* and *ROS1* fusions are clinically required, designing a cost effective small NGS panel to cover all the clinically significant NSCLC alterations is challenging. The targeted panel NGS test can also be challenging in detecting large indels and copy number changes due to problematic alignment algorithms of bioinformatic pipelines for large indels, and the limited, sometimes biased, data available to calculate a normalized diploid level.
- NGS panels, especially the large ones, generate a large amount of data. The post-sequencing analysis, variant interpretation, and data storage are current challenges for NGS tests. Furthermore, reporting many variants of uncertain significance (VUS) from a large panel may dilute the significance of clinically relevant mutations. Therefore, for the clinical mutation profiling of lung cancer, despite the increasing demand for larger panels from oncologists and patients, each molecular diagnostic laboratory needs to balance the panel size with the cost, turnaround time, and clinical relevance.

13. **What are the specimen types acceptable for mutation profiling of lung cancer?**
    - Formalin-fixed, paraffin-embedded (FFPE) tissues or cell blocks are widely validated for FISH and molecular testing of NSCLC. The unstained FFPE sections for molecular tests should be unbaked. The routine 5- to 10-μm thick sections are used, and the number of sections depends on the size of the tumor and the test to be performed. In general, five 5-μm thick sections should be enough for non-sequencing assays, and ten 5-μm sections may be preferable for NGS.
    - Fresh, frozen, or alcohol-fixed specimens are all acceptable for molecular tests; fresh or frozen specimens producing high-quality RNA are particularly good for RNA-based tests. However, each tissue type needs to be validated separately. Tissue samples treated with other methods such as acidic or heavy metal fixatives, or decalcifying solutions, should be avoided due to high false-negative rate [108–110].
    - Cytologic specimens including liquid-based cytology and fresh cell suspension, direct smear, and stained cytology slides can also be used for FISH and molecular tests. For cytology slides, Quick-diff is preferred than the Papanicolaou stain because DNA in the latter degrades faster [111].
    - Cellular fluids sampled from body cavities involved by metastatic tumors are usually sufficient for diagnostic evaluation, including molecular genetic testing. Peripheral blood, spinal fluid, and urine may be used to extract cfDNA for the assessment of therapy response and drug resistance in certain clinical circumstances.
    - Regardless which tissue/sample type is used for FISH or molecular tests, the tumor content (the percentage of malignant cell nuclei) should be determined by a pathologist examining the corresponding cytology smear or H&E slides. A training and feedback program for pathologists evaluating the tumor cell content can significantly improve the skill and accuracy of estimation [112]. The analytic sensitivity (lower limit of detection, LLOD) of each test is method dependent. The current guidelines strongly encourage laboratories to implement tests that can detect mutations in specimens with as low as 10% cancer cells (5% mutant allele frequency) [48]. Circling the tumor-rich area on an H&E slide for macrodissection should be routinely performed to increase the tumor cell percentage and improve test accuracy, especially when the overall tumor cell percentage is low [113].
14. **What is the role of cell-free DNA testing (liquid biopsy) for lung cancer?**
    - Detecting cancer-related mutations from the circulating tumor DNA (ctDNA) shed into blood by apoptotic or necrotic tumor cells is referred to as "liquid biopsy." Testing cfDNA from other body fluids can also be performed with the same methods [114]. As a minimally invasive procedure, liquid biopsy has quickly gained popularity among oncologists for NSCLC and other solid tumors.
    - Given the low concentration of cfDNA and variable fraction of ctDNA, a method with high analytic sensitivity is required for cfDNA-based cancer mutation detection. Currently most laboratories use droplet digital PCR or deep sequencing (NGS with high read depth) for cfDNA tests. The test protocols are challenging to validate and costly for each sample.
    - Studies have found excellent concordance and specificity (83.3–99.0%) of the mutation profiles detected from plasma compared with that from tissue samples. The clinical sensitivity of liquid biopsy ranges from 50% to 80% for guideline-recommended NSCLC biomarkers [48, 115–118].
    - It is assumed that mutations detected in ctDNA better reflect the heterogeneity of the tumors; therefore, mutation profiling with liquid biopsy could provide a more complete picture than testing tissue sampled from a single tumor region. On the other hand, the heterogeneous origin of ctDNA can complicate the result interpretation. A patient with lung cancer may have concurrent primary cancers in another organs; assigning a cfDNA mutation profile to lung cancer requires a complete evaluation of the patient to rule out other potential primary lesions.
    - Currently, there is not enough evidence to support the use of cfDNA molecular tests for the screening

and diagnosis of primary lung adenocarcinoma. When there is already a diagnosis of NSCLC but the tissue sample is insufficient for molecular testing, cfDNA assay is an option to identify targetable mutations [48].

- When there is a need to identify the acquired resistant mutations, especially when it is clinically unfeasible to perform invasive procedures for tissue sampling due to comorbidities and/or other contraindications, a rebiopsy can be avoided if the cfDNA test is positive. Otherwise tumor sample testing should still be pursued due to the lower clinical sensitivity of cfDNA testing [48].
- Serial sampling to monitor the mutation evolution using cfDNA, which is much easier than repeat tissue biopsies, could reveal critical information to recognize the heterogeneous molecular basis of EGFR TKI [119, 120] or ALK inhibitor resistance [121, 122], especially when acquired *EGFR* T790M mutation decreases with the expanded use of third-generation EGFR TKIs [123].

15. **What is the clinical significance of tumor mutation burden (TMB) in lung cancer and how is it tested?**
    - Tumor mutational burden (TMB) is a measurement of the total number of somatic mutations in the genome of tumor cells. It was originally defined as the number of nonsynonymous mutations per genome or per million base pairs (mut/Mb) calculated from the whole-genome (WGS) or whole-exon sequencing (WES) data [124]. The level of TMB is significantly variable across tumor types. NSCLC (both adenocarcinoma and squamous cell carcinoma) and SCLC have high average mutation burdens following melanoma [125, 126]. It is reasonably assumed that TMB can be a proxy for the number of neoantigens that is associated with the strength of immune response triggered by tumor cells.
    - Multiple studies have shown that high TMB is associated with better responses to immune checkpoint inhibitors (ICIs) in NSCLC, independent of the expression levels of PD-L1 [47, 90, 127, 128]. TMB is, thereby, recognized as a powerful biomarker to select patients for ICI therapy although there are still some controversial results by other studies [129, 130].
    - The gold standard for TMB was established from the data analysis of simultaneous WES of tumor and matched blood or normal tissue, in which only somatic nonsynonymous variants were included in the calculation. Recent studies demonstrated that data from NGS of a targeted panel with >300 genes could generate TMB results comparable to those calculated from WES [131–133].
    - Multiple factors can affect the accurate assessment and interpretation of TMB [134]:

      Preanalytical factors:
      - FFPE tissue is most frequently used for NGS testing. Tissue quality and processing can significantly affect the level of artifacts, especially false-positive variants from nucleotide modifications.
      - Tumor cell content and background tumor environment also affect the test results. Because a targeted panel sequencing can achieve higher sequencing depth than a WES, it is presumably more suitable for samples with lower tumor content that cannot be enriched (e.g., cytology cell block with relatively scattered tumor cells/clusters). However, this assumption has yet to be confirmed in clinical studies.
      - Multiple studies have confirmed that TMB from plasma ctDNA correlates well with that from tissue samples (bTMB vs. tTMB [115, 135, 136]). If the value of bTMB is confirmed by correlating with clinical outcomes of immunotherapy, the utility of liquid biopsy could be largely expanded (see more discussion in question 14).

      Analytical factors:
      - The methods to calculate TMB and the cutoff value of high TMB need to be adjusted and validated based on the sequencing data from different platforms.
      - To increase the accuracy of TMB measurement from targeted panel sequencing that generates less nonsynonymous variants, it is proposed to include synonymous variants and indels, which may render a better correlation with the TMB calculated from WES results.
      - When a tumor sample is sequenced without paired normal tissue or blood sample, the germline variants can only be filtered through bioinformatic analysis using germline variant databases. Not all germline variants can be recognized this way; therefore, the TMB is likely overestimated.

      Postanalytical factors:
      - The procedure of interpreting and reporting TMB results have not been standardized, especially when the data from a targeted panel NGS is used.
      - Currently there is no consensus cutoff value to define a high TMB. Although 10 mut/Mb is used as the threshold in the FDA approval of pembrolizumab for adults and children with TMB-H solid tumors [137], many WES-based studies reported TMB as total mutations per tumor. It is yet to be determined whether lung adenocarcinoma, SCC,

and SCLC need different TMB cutoff values to guide immunotherapy decisions.

– Before a consensus guideline is available for TMB reporting, the TMB Harmonization Consortium recommended that TMB be reported as mut/Mb [138]. The types of mutations included in the TMB calculation, the cutoff value, and the rationale to establish the cutoff should also be included in the report [139].

16. **What other tests can be considered to provide guidance for immunotherapy of lung cancer?**
    - Assessment of PD-L1 expression by IHC is widely accepted as a useful marker to select NSCLC patients for immunotherapy with ICIs [140], although there are no standardized method and interpretation guideline, and the predictive value is questioned in some studies [141]. In addition to the TMB test discussed above, a combination of multiple biomarkers may provide a better prediction of ICI response in NSCLC patients.
    - The mutation profiling routinely performed in most clinical laboratories for lung cancer has predictive value for ICI therapy. *EGFR* mutation, *ALK1*, or *ROS1* translocation-positive NSCLC usually responds poorly to ICIs even when the tumor expresses a high level of PD-L1 [142]. *TP53*-mutated, but *STK11* and *EGFR* wild-type NSCLCs are associated with longer disease-free survival (DFS) in ICI-treated patients [143].
    - The evolution of ctDNA level in plasma defined by changes of the mutant allele frequency, regardless of specific mutations, may predict ICI response. Low ctDNA at the first evaluation after nivolumab treatment was associated with better clinical response, progression-free survival (PFS), and overall survival in a recent study [144]. The ctDNA level may become an early predictor of a durable good response to nivolumab [145].

While most studies on the efficacy of immunotherapy focus on the potential neoantigens created from genetic alterations of the malignant cells (the target), investigating the T-cells (the effector) mediating the killing of tumor cells have also provided information potentially valuable to independently predict responses to immunotherapy [146–148]. More clinical studies are required to confirm the validity of these results.

Case Presentations

The clinical histories of these cases are slightly modified to simplify the presentation and avoid the potential association of any protected patient information.

Case 1

Learning Objectives

- To understand the NGS test result of *EGFR* exon 19 deletion
- To discuss the nomenclature of complex variants detected by NGS

Case History

A 60-year-old female with a smoking history 30 years ago has a right upper lobe lung mass found at a routine clinic visit. A computerized tomography (CT) scan confirms a 3.7 × 2.4 cm single lesion. A core biopsy is performed and reveals lung adenocarcinoma. The mass is excised by a robotic right upper lobectomy with additional lymphadenectomy. Figure 7.1a, b show the histomorphologic findings are characteristic of invasive adenocarcinoma, acinar predominant; there is also in situ nonmucinous adenocarcinoma with a lepidic component shown in (b). Metastasis tumor is found in one ipsilateral lymph node.

Pathological Diagnosis

Adenocarcinoma, acinar predominant (acinar 55%, micropapillary 40%, papillary 5%), moderately to poorly differentiated

Maximum tumor diameter: 3.6 cm. The adenocarcinoma is staged IIB (T2a N1 M0)

Molecular Genetic Study

A 26-gene NGS test is performed on the lobectomy specimen. Tumor content is enriched by macrodissection. The only clinically significant alteration detected is shown in Fig. 7.1c. This is a complex sequence variant in exon 19 of *EGFR*, with a 15-base-pair deletion (codon 746 glutamic acid to 750 alanine) and a C to T variant at codon 751 Threonine. Based on the original data displayed in the image, the inframe deletion is on the same allele with the single nucleotide variant (*cis* mutations). It would not be entirely wrong to report the two variants separately as "*EGFR* E746_A750del (c.2236_2250del)" and "*EGFR* T751I (c.2252C > T)"; in fact, if the original alignment reveals the two variants are on different alleles (*trans* mutations), they must be reported separately. However, it is more appropriate to combine them as one mutation in the nomenclature to reflect that the complex variants are on the same allele:

- *EGFR* (NM_005228.3) c.2236_2252delinsAT (p.E746_T751delinsI) in approximately 9% of alleles

Chromosome coordinates: chr7:55242466-55242482: GAATTAAGAGAAGCAAC > AT

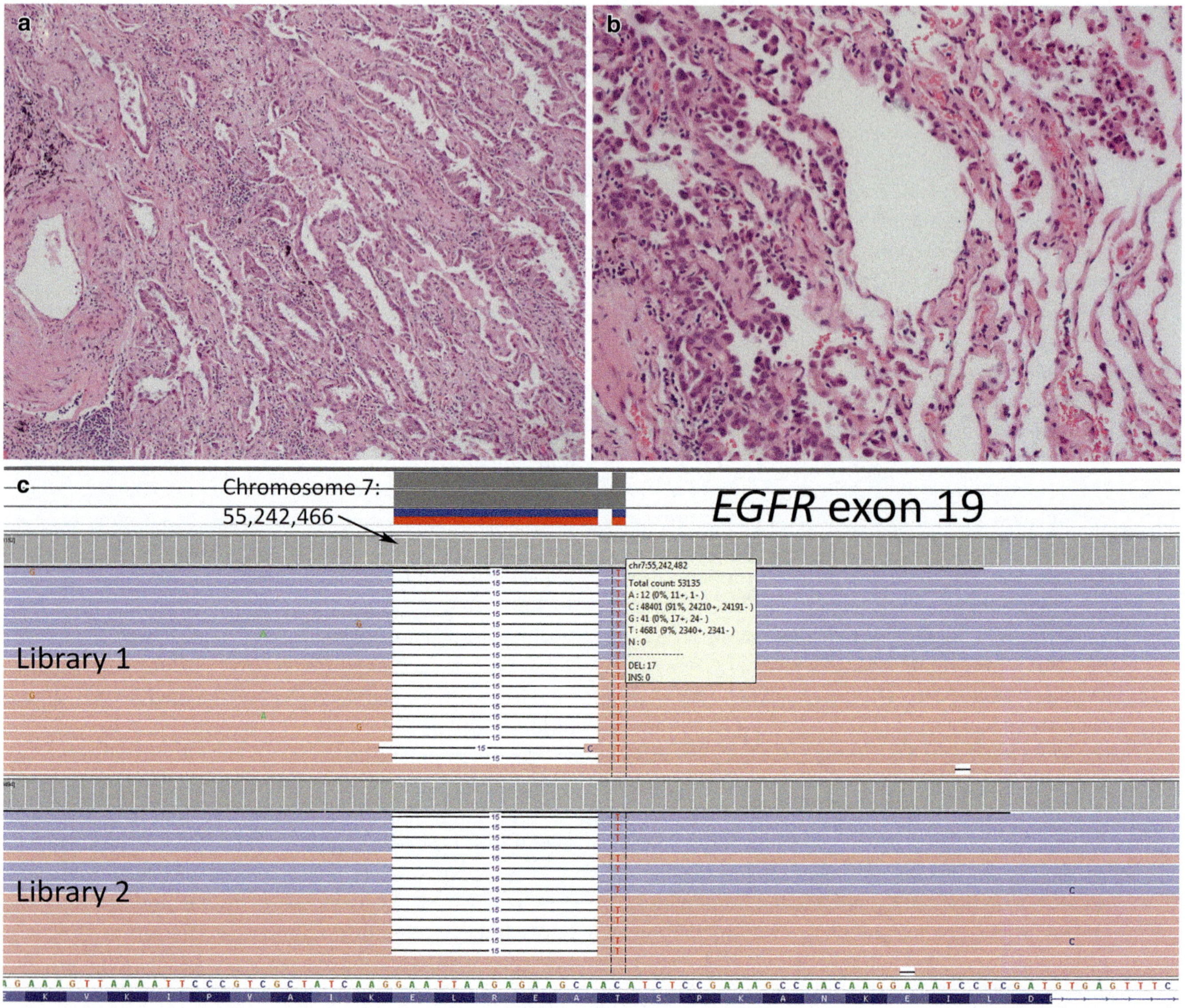

Fig. 7.1 Adenocarcinoma with *EGFR* exon 19 deletion. (**a**) and (**b**) Representative histomorphology images of the lobectomy specimen (H&E stain, A. 100X, B. 200X). (**c**) Screenshot of the NGS result displayed in the Integrative Genomics Viewer (IGV, Broad Institute) showing the *EGFR* exon 19 region. The NGS protocol leverages two separate libraries built from either strand of a DNA fragment (displayed on the upper and lower panel of image C, Library 1 and 2). The horizontal bars represent the sequencing reads, with purple and pink colors indicating read directions. The chromosome coordinates indicated in the image are based on the reference assembly hg19, GRCh37. The reference DNA sequence and corresponding amino acids are displayed on the bottom. A 15-base-pair deletion and a C > T single nucleotide variant (SNV) are seen on the same sequencing reads in both libraries and both read directions. As displayed on the yellow box, the total variant frequency is 9% in this result with a total read depth of 53,135

Clinical Follow-Up

The patient receives adjuvant chemotherapy after surgery. No new or enlarging suspicious pulmonary nodules detected by follow-up CT scan 9 months later.

Discussion

Approximately half of the *EGFR* mutations in NSCLC are inframe exon 19 deletions, such as the mutation detected in this patient. These deletions result in increased kinase activity of EGFR, lead to hyperactivation of downstream proliferation and pro-survival signaling pathways, and conferred increased sensitivity to EGFR tyrosine kinase inhibitor treatment.

As discussed above, the *EGFR* exon 19 inframe deletion in this case is complicated by an additional single-nucleotide variant. This specific variant is a known oncogenic variant described in TKI-responsive lung adenocarcinomas [149] and appears to be very similar to the well-characterized EGFR p. E746_A750del variant that confers TKI sensitivity in NSCLC.

The NGS result of this case signifies the importance for the molecular pathologists to review the original alignment data to generate an accurate mutation report.

Case 2

Learning Objective

The *EGFR* T790M mutation is the most common mechanism of acquired resistance after EGRF TKI-targeted therapy.

Case History

A 69-year-old male was diagnosed with bilateral metastatic adenocarcinoma of the lung with activating *EGFR* L858R mutation. He received targeted therapy using the first-generation TKI, erlotinib. Although he has no symptoms, based on imaging study results, the disease has slowly progressed in 2 years. A blood cfDNA test (liquid biopsy, performed by Guardant360® CDx) reported negative results; the original *EGFR* L858R mutation was not detected either. A biopsy of the right upper lobe lung lesion is performed.

Pathological Diagnosis

Before treatment (right lung transbronchial biopsy):

- Adenocarcinoma, non-mucinous with predominantly a lepidic growth pattern, intermediate nuclear grade

After 2 years of erlotinib treatment (right upper lobe, transbronchial biopsy):

- Adenocarcinoma, acinar-type growth pattern

Representative histomorphologic images of the two biopsies are shown in Fig. 7.2.

Molecular Genetic Studies

A 26-gene NGS test is performed on both biopsies.

Before treatment, two mutations detected:

- *EGFR* (NM_005228.3) c.2573T > G (p.Leu858Arg), 15% of alleles
- *TP53* (NM_000546.5) c.742C > T (p.Arg248Trp), 22% of alleles

After treatment, two new mutations detected:

- *CTNNB1* (NM_001098210.1) c.95A > C (p.Asp32Ala) 10% of alleles
- *EGFR* (NM_005228.3) c.2369C > T (p.Thr790Met), 9% of alleles; and c.2573T > G (p.Leu858Arg), 26% of alleles
- *TP53* (NM_000546.5) c.742C > T (p.Arg248Trp) 19% of alleles

Clinical Follow-Up

Erlotinib is discontinued after the second biopsy reported T790M mutation; treatment with third-generation EGFR inhibitor, osimertinib starts. Eight-weeks later, restaging CT scan shows about 50% size reduction in right upper lobe tumor and size reduction in scattered lung nodules. However, follow-up imaging scans 3 years later show the disease is still slowly progressing.

Discussion

Resistance to first- and second-generation EGFR TKIs can be either on-target that includes acquired EGFR resistance mutations or *EGFR* amplification or off-target that includes activation of non-EGFR pathways, lineage transformation, etc. *EGFR* T790M mutation is the most common on-target mechanism for the resistance of first- and second-generation EGFR TKIs. Molecular testing of T790M mutation is recommended for patients with disease progression while on EGFR TKI therapy, like in this case. Although liquid biopsy provides a minimally invasive way to detect additional mutations in these patients, the clinical sensitivity is relatively low. When a liquid biopsy result is negative, lesional tissue biopsy should be attempted. In this case, because the *EGFR* L858R mutation reported in the original biopsy sample was not detected by liquid biopsy, the negative result is problematic, and additional mutations are confirmed by follow-up tissue biopsy.

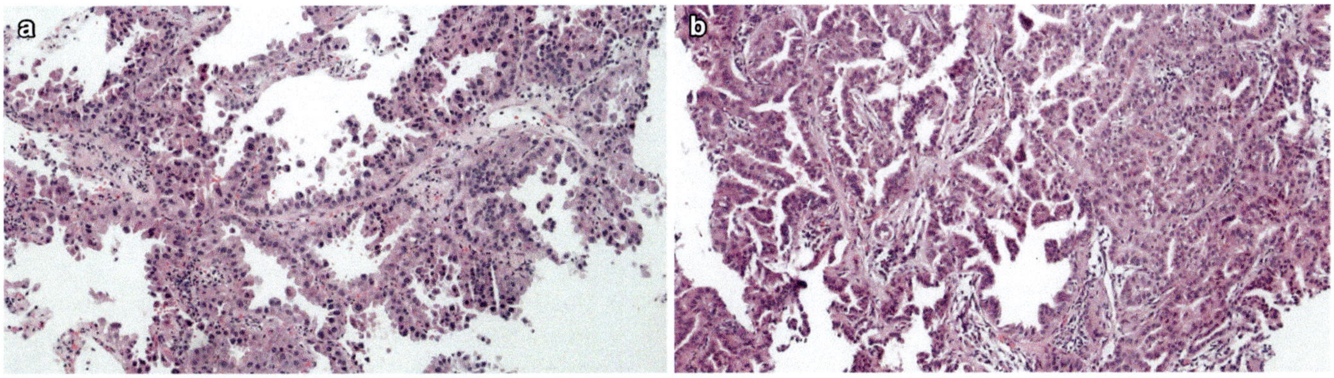

Fig. 7.2 Histomorphology of the adenocarcinoma biopsied before and after erlotinib treatment (H&E stain, 100X). (**a**) Before treatment: adenocarcinoma, primarily lepidic pattern; (**b**) After treatment: adenocarcinoma with a predominant acinar pattern

An additional *CTNNB1* p.Asp32Ala mutation is detected at the same allele frequency as *EGFR* T790M, further confirming the clonal evolution. It is not clear whether the *CTNNB1* and *TP53* mutations are associated with the patient's unsatisfactory response to the third-generation TKI therapy.

Case 3

Learning Objectives

- Synchronous multifocal lung cancers can be metastatic from one primary, or concurrent multiple primary lung cancers.
- Molecular profiling provides definitive clonal information for tumor samples. Combining histomorphologic and genotypic assessment is the ultimate approach to an accurate staging of lung cancer with multiple masses.

Case History

A 73-year-old female had a history of left breast cancer 20 years ago. A CT scan shows bilateral lung nodules. Three nodules located in the right lower lobe, middle lobe, and upper lobe are resected.

Pathologic Diagnosis

Right lower lobe (A):

- Adenocarcinoma, acinar type with lepidic pattern, maximum diameter 1.7 cm
- A separate nodule is consistent with metastatic carcinoma from breast (positively for GATA3 and mammaglobin; negative for TTF-1 and napsin)

Right middle lobe (B): Metastatic carcinoma from breast (based on morphology and IHC stains)

Right upper lobe (C):

- Adenocarcinoma, lepidic type (tumor size: 3.2 cm based on a CT scan report)

The histomorphologic features of the lung adenocarcinoma from block A2 and C1 are displayed in Fig. 7.3.

Molecular Genetic Studies

Only the lung cancer components (A2 and C1) are submitted for the 26-gene NGS test. The sequence variants detected are:

Right lower lobe (A2):

- *KRAS* (NM_033360) c.34G > T (p.G12C), 28% of alleles
- *APC* (NM_000038) c.3386T > C (p.L1129S), 46% of alleles

Right upper lobe (C1):

- *MET* (NM_001127500) c.3081_3082 + 2delAGGT (p. E1027fs), 14% of alleles; this deletion spans both exons and introns, most likely resulting in exon 14 skipping
- *APC* c.3386T > C (p.L1129S), 49% of alleles.

The two lesions are staged as separate primary tumors based on the molecular profiling results:

- Lower lobe stage: pT1b (1–2 cm)
- Upper lobe stage: pT2a: (3–4 cm)

Discussion

Multiple synchronous lung nodules are present in approximately 20% of the lung cancer cases [98, 99]. Determining whether they are independent primary tumors or intrapulmonary metastasis is crucial for the correct pathological staging and prognosis evaluation. Historically, the determination solely relied on histomorphologic features. Genetic studies can provide definitive evidence to determine the clonal relationship of different nodules. This patient presents with two separate lung adenocarcinomas at different lobes of the right lung, and the two tumor nodules share similar morphology. If one is primary and the other is metastasis, the stage will be pT4. In this case, the different driver mutations indicate they are two independent primary tumors; thus they are staged separately as pT1b and pT2a. Of note, the patient also has metastatic breast cancer nodules in the lung that are easily recognized by the different immunostaining patterns. If a metastatic cancer shows similar morphologic and immunostaining features with the primary lung cancer, it will be even more challenging to determine their origin without clonal evidence. A same *APC* sequence variant is detected in different primary lesions with an allele frequency close to 50%, suggesting this is most likely a germline variant. The *APC* p.L1129S is found in 0.10–0.24% of the general population (rs143638171). As a germline variant, it is considered benign or likely benign by contributors to NCBI's ClinVar database (https://www.ncbi.nlm.nih.gov/clinvar/RCV000077988/). However, this variant is usually not filtered out as a benign germline variant due to its low prevalence in the general population. This kind of variant of uncertain clinical significance (VUS) is frequently encountered in cancer mutation profiling.

Case 4

Learning Objectives

- A small subset of lung carcinomas contains both adeno and squamous components. Not all the different components can be sampled in a small biopsy.

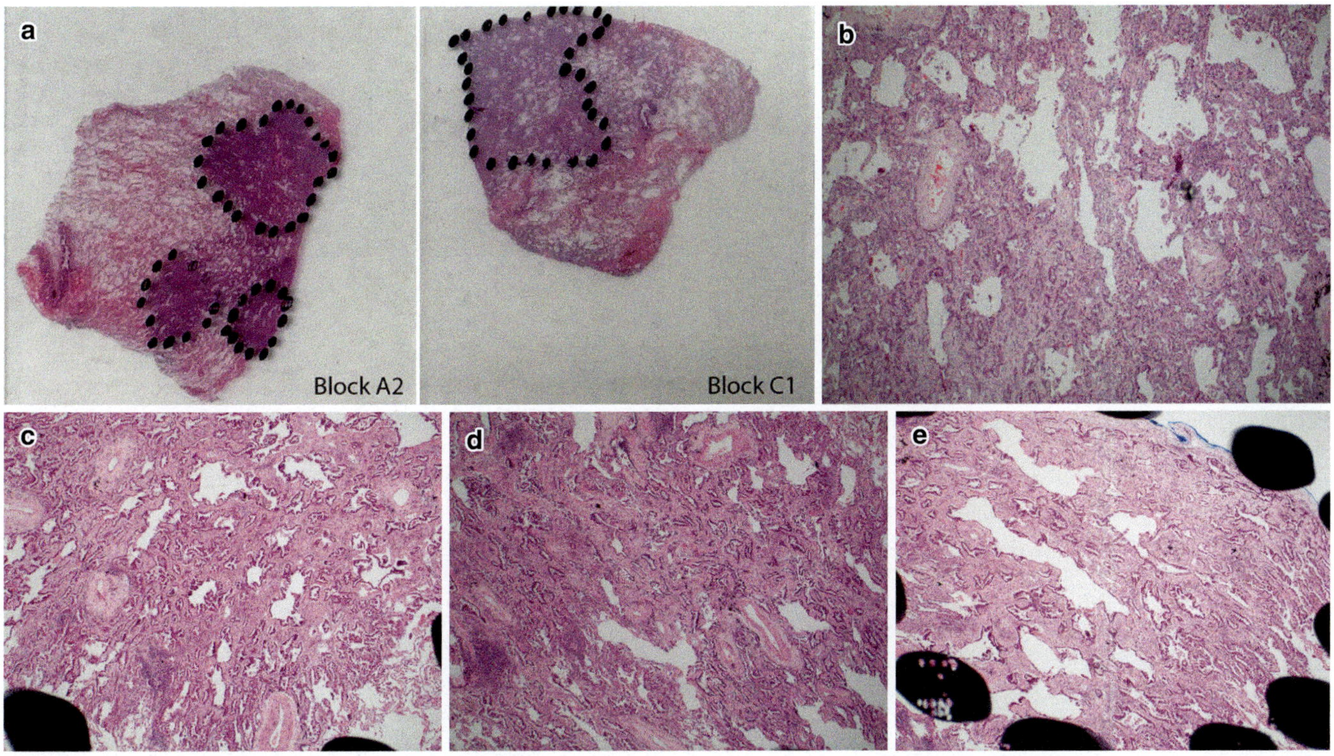

Fig. 7.3 Histomorphology of the adenocarcinomas from two different locations. (**a**) Photo taken directly on the glass slide of A2 (right lower lobe) and C1 (right upper lobe). These nodules have all been confirmed to be lung origin, not metastatic breast cancer, by IHC stains. Although three nodules are seen on slide A2, they partially merge with each other under microscopic observation. These nodules were not separated when preparing for the NGS test. (**b–e**) Microscopic images, H&E stain, 40X. (**b**) Lesion from C1; (**c**, **d**, **e**) Three nodules from A2. These lesions show similar histomorphologic features of adenocarcinoma. It is unable to determine whether they are independent primary adenocarcinomas or metastasis from one primary

- Even if only squamous cell carcinoma is present in a core biopsy, it may be considered for molecular testing when there is a possibility of unsampled adenocarcinoma based on the clinical history or clues from histomorphologic features.

Case History

A 55-year-old female has a left femoral pathologic fracture. She was diagnosed with lung adenocarcinoma 2 years ago and treated with osimertinib based on the molecular test findings. A total hip arthroplasty is performed, and the bone specimen is received for pathology examination.

Pathological Diagnosis

Right lower lobe lung biopsy (from 2 years ago):

- Adenocarcinoma, lung primary

Left femoral neck resection:

- Metastatic keratinizing squamous cell carcinoma

The histomorphology images of both the lung and bone lesions are shown in Fig. 7.4.

Molecular Genetic Studies

A 26-gene panel NGS test performed on both specimens identifies the same mutation profiles (displayed in Figs. 7.5 and 7.6).

Lung mass:

- *EGFR* (NM_005228.3) c.2235_2249del (p.E746_A750del), 53% of alleles
- *APC* (NM_000038.5) c.3479C > A (p.T1160K), 58% of alleles

Bone (left femoral neck):

- *EGFR* (NM_005228.3) c.2235_2249del (p.E746_A750del), 48% of alleles
- *APC* (NM_000038.5) c.3479C > A (p.T1160K), 63% of alleles

Discussion

The histologic feature of the metastatic bone lesion is diagnostic of keratinizing squamous cell carcinoma, making it difficult to determine its primary origin. Mutation profiling with NGS identifies the lung and bone lesions share the same mutations, including the driver mutation

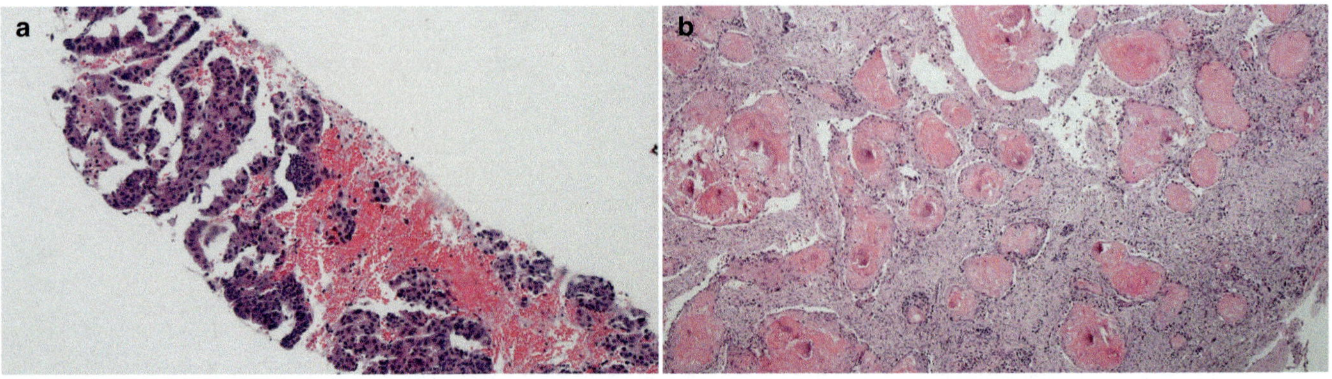

Fig. 7.4 Histomorphology of the primary and metastatic cancers. (**a**) Primary lung adenocarcinoma and (**b**) metastatic squamous cell carcinoma in the bone. (H&E stain, 100X)

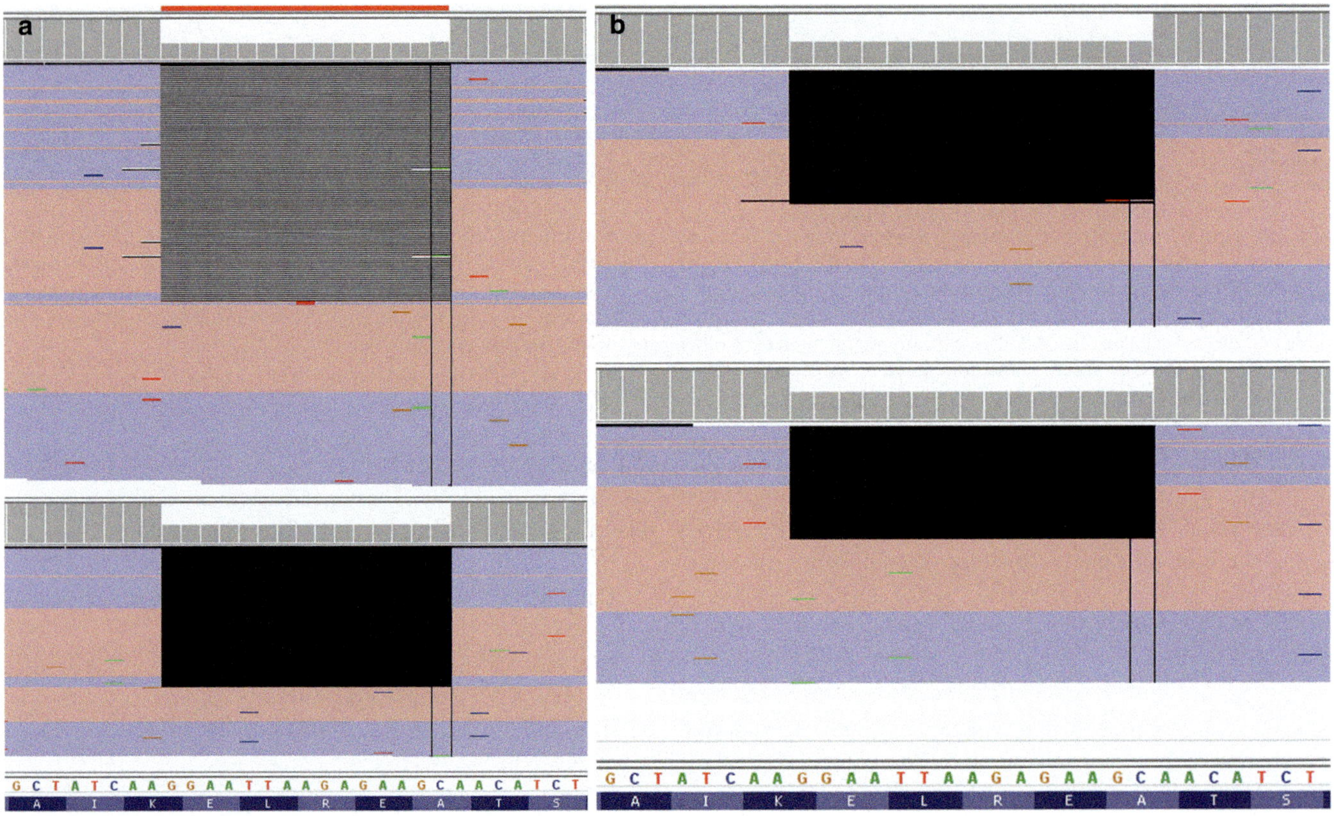

Figs. 7.5 and 7.6 Screenshots of the NGS results displayed in IGV. The screenshots demonstrate that the same sequence variants are present in both (**a**) primary lung cancer and (**b**) metastatic bone lesion. The NGS protocol is the same as described in Fig. 7.1. Figure 7.5 *EGFR* exon 19 deletion; Fig. 7.6 *APC* c.3479 C > A (p.T1160K). More detailed information about the variant reads is displayed in the yellow box

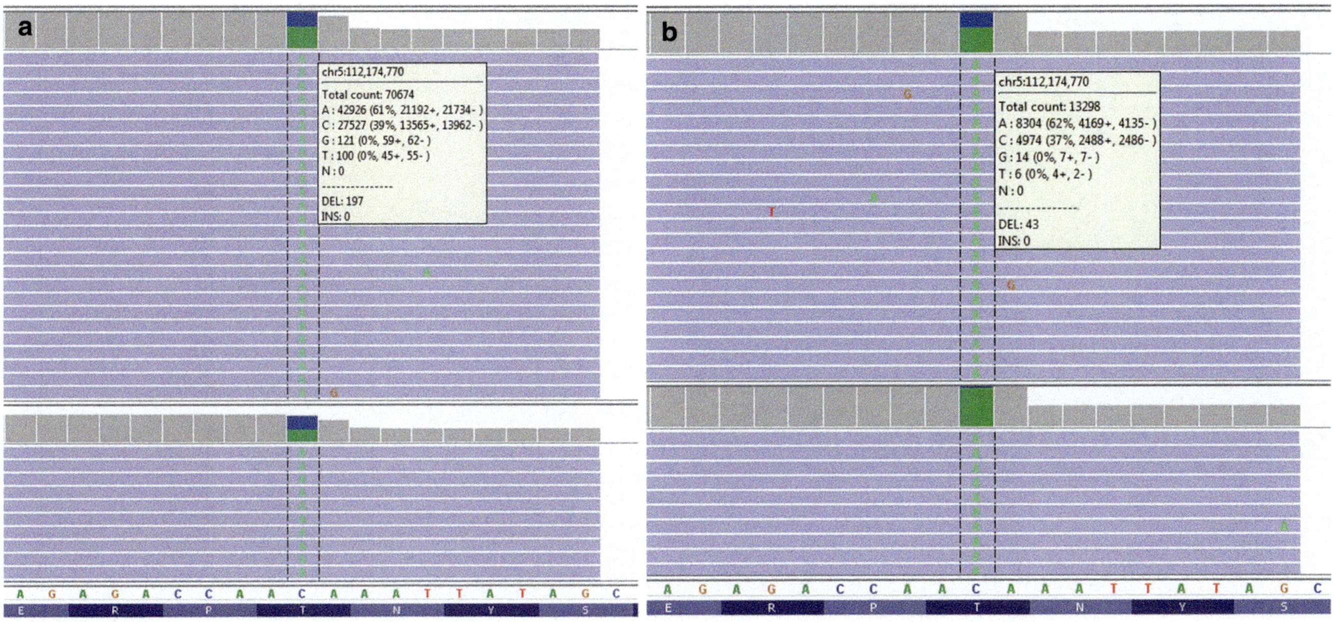

Figs. 7.5 and 7.6 (continued)

EGFR exon 19 deletion, indicating the bone lesion is a metastasis of the NSCLC. In that regard, the results of molecular testing are useful in determining the origin of the metastatic tumor, especially when the morphologic features are different.

More importantly, this case demonstrates that various components may be present or derived from an NSCLC. We can reasonably hypothesize that a squamous cell carcinoma component was present in the primary lung cancer but not sampled in the biopsy.

Re-biopsy sampling for molecular test is indicated in patients whose lung cancer progresses or metastasizes to other locations while on targeted therapy to identify possible loss of actionable *EGFR* mutations or acquisition of resistant mutations, such as *EGFR* C797S, L718Q, G724S, and S768I. In this case, no other *EGFR* mutations were detected in the metastatic carcinoma in the bone.

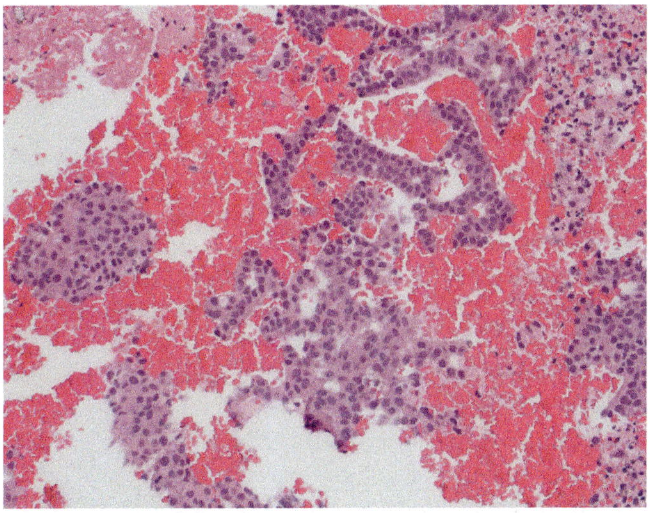

Fig. 7.7 Morphologic features of the tumor sample. Sections of the cell block made from the sub-carina lymph node fine needle aspiration sample showing malignant cells forming glandular architecture, consistent with lung adenocarcinoma. H&E stain, 200X

Case 5

Learning Objectives

- To understand the FISH method detecting chromosome rearrangements that result in fusion genes
- To recognize the variant signal pattern of *ALK1* break apart FISH result

Case History

A 69-year-old male, non-smoker, is referred to ophthalmology for two right choroidal lesions. He is treated with steroids, but the lesions grew. Metastatic cancer is suspected, and a positron emission tomography (PET) scan shows a non-FDG avid nodule in the right lower lung lobe measuring 2.6 × 2.4 cm and a subcarinal lymph node measuring 1.9 × 2.0 cm with FDG 3.8. Fine needle aspiration of the subcarinal lymph node is performed.

Pathologic Diagnosis

The cytology smear and cell block show malignant cells (Fig. 7.7); immunostains performed on the cell block sections reveal the malignant cells are positive for TTF1 and napsin, consistent with metastatic adenocarcinoma from lung primary.

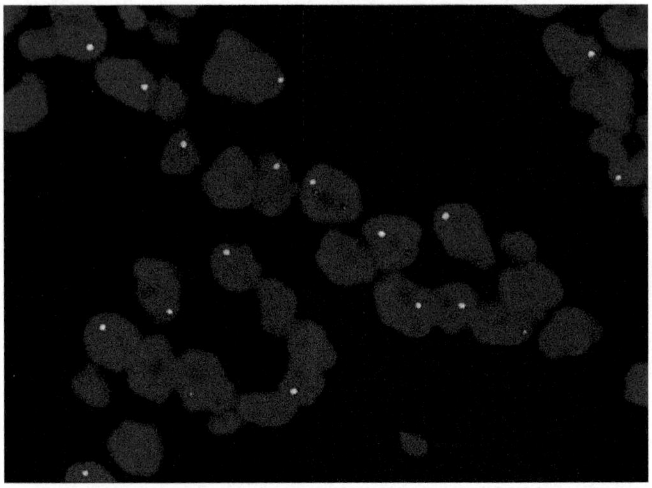

Fig. 7.8 Fluorescence in situ hybridization (FISH) of *ALK1* rearrangement. Dual-color break-apart probes show 1 fusion (red + green/yellow, the red part is smaller in many cells) and 1–2 red signals, indicating loss of 5′ (green) signal. Although rearrangement typically shows split of green and red signals, loss of 5′ green signal is a variant pattern indicating rearranged *ALK1* gene

FISH Analysis

- POSITIVE for variant *ALK1* gene rearrangement with loss of 5′ *ALK* in 81% of the 200 cells scored (Fig. 7.8)

Discussion

Although *ALK1* rearrangements are present only infrequently in NSCLC, they are targetable alterations required to be tested per current practice guidelines. FISH is a sensitive and specific method to detect *ALK* rearrangements (and other rearrangements such as *ROS1* and *RET*). To cover variable partners of *ALK1* fusion, a break apart-probe design is preferred in the clinical FISH laboratory because the specific partner does not affect the therapy response. In the fusion protein, only the ALK kinase portion is functionally relevant; therefore a variant rearrangement with loss of 5′ signal and retention of the 3′ kinase portion, like in this case, is considered positive for *ALK1* fusion.

EML4 is the most common gene partner of *ALK1*; both genes are located in the short (p) arm of chromosome 2. Segment inversion of chromosome 2p results in the constitutively active *ALK-EML4* fusion protein. *AlK1* can also fuse with other genes, such as *TFG, KIF5B, KLC1*, etc. In this case, an *ALK-EML4* fusion gene has been confirmed in a later liquid biopsy test.

Case 6

Learning Objective

- Splice site mutation caused *MET* exon 14 skipping can be recognized at the DNA level in many cases.
- Definitive diagnosis of *MET* exon 14 skipping may require confirmatory tests at the RNA level.

Case History

A 70-year-old male is found to have a right upper lobe lung nodule (1.1 × 1.0 cm) and a subpleural left lung nodule (0.7 × 0.7 cm) in the CT scan during the work-up for his bladder cancer. A right upper lobe wedge resection is performed.

Pathologic Diagnosis

- Pulmonary adeno-squamous carcinoma (1.1 × 1.0 × 1.0 cm)

The histomorphology of this case and a control case is shown in Fig. 7.9a, d.

Molecular Genetic Studies

The 26-gene panel NGS test is performed on the sample after enrichment of tumor cells by macrodissection. A right upper lobe nodule biopsied from an 88-year-old female is used as a control for this case; the same molecular test is also performed on the control case.

The following mutation is detected in the patient sample:

- *MET* (NM_001127500) c.3082 + 1G > C, 16% of alleles, at chromosome 7: 116412044

The splice site mutation is likely to cause exon 14 skipping. A different single-nucleotide mutation is detected in the control case: *MET* c.3061T > C (p.Y1021H), 28.39% at Chromosome 7: 116412022. This variant should not affect RNA splicing, and the mRNA length should be the same as wild-type mRNA.

The NGS results are displayed in Fig. 7.9b, e.

RT-PCR amplification of the *MET* region flanking exon 14 is performed. *ABL1* Transcript serves as the amplification internal control. The results are deployed in Fig. 7.9c, f. The amplicon size from this patient (166 bp) is shorter than that from the control patient (281 bp, expected normal mRNA length).

Discussion

MET exon 14 skipping is a driver mutation in NSCLCs, and the absence of exon 14 leads to decreased MET protein degradation and increased kinase activity. RNA splicing requires a donor site (5′ end of the intron), a branch site (near the 3′ end of the intron), and an acceptor site (3′ end of the intron). Mutations in these regions result in splicing error, leading to loss of exons or retraining of intron sequence. In this case, a G > C mutated splice donor site causes exon 14 skipping.

Although most mutations affecting RNA splicing can be identified by DNA sequencing and many have been confirmed by testing the mRNA, not all mutations causing *MET* exon 14 skipping are recognizable at the DNA level. A confirmatory RNA testing may be required if targeting MET active mutation is clinically indicated.

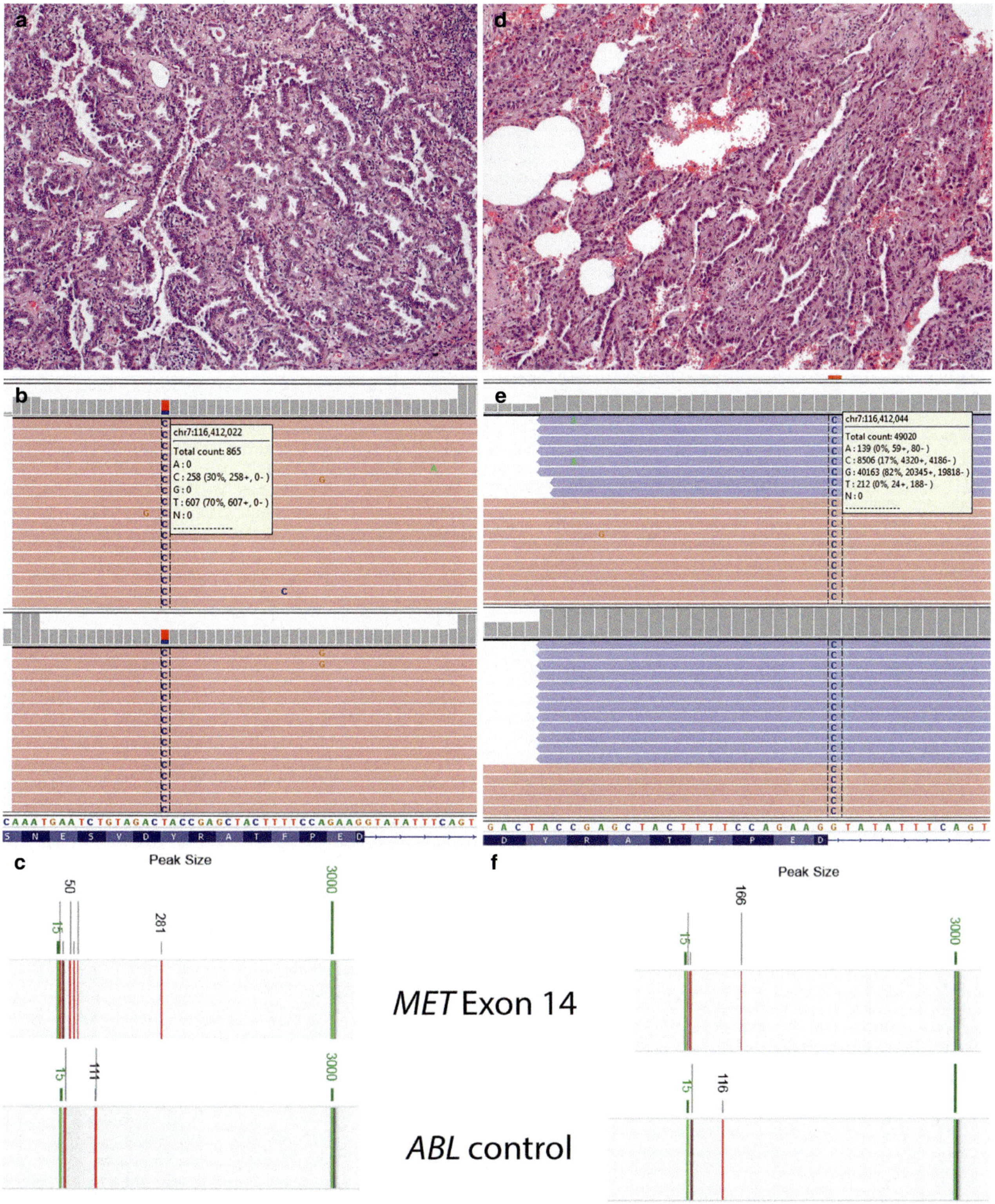

Fig. 7.9 Adenocarcinoma with *MET* exon 14 skipping mutation. This case (**d–f**) is illustrated in comparison to an adenocarcinoma with *MET* missense mutation (**a–c**). (**a**) and (**d**) Representative microscopic images, H&E stain, 100X. (**b**) and (**e**) IGV screenshots of NGS result. The NGS protocol is the same as described in Fig. 7.1. Displayed are the 3′ region of *MET* exon 14 and the 5′-region of intron 14–15. Of note, the *MET* c.3061 T > C (p.Y1021H) in the control case has only one read direction due to the limited read length, but both libraries 1 and 2 reveal the same variant (**b**). The *MET* exon 14 skipping is confirmed by a reverse transcription polymerase chain reaction (RT-PCR); *ABL* gene is used as the internal control for RT-PCR amplification. (**c** and **f**) PCR amplicons revealed by Qiaxcel® (Qiagen) capillary gel electrophoresis. A shorter amplicon is detected in the exon 14 skipping sample (166 bp in **f** vs. 281 bp in **c**). The expected *ABL* control amplicons (111/116 bp) are present in both cases

References

1. Siegel RL, Miller KD, Jemal A. Cancer statistics, 2020. CA Cancer J Clin. 2020;70(1):7–30.
2. Travis WD, et al. World Health Organization classification of tumours. In: Bosman FT, et al., editors. WHO classification of tumours of the lung, pleura, thymus and heart. 4th ed. Lyon: International Agency for Research on Cancer (IARC); 2015. p. 412.
3. Fong KM, et al. Molecular basis of lung carcinogenesis. In: Coleman WB, Tsongalis GJ, editors. The molecular basis of human cancer. New York: Springer; 2017. p. 447–96.
4. Gazdar AF, Minna JD. Cigarettes, sex, and lung adenocarcinoma. J Natl Cancer Inst. 1997;89(21):1563–5.
5. American Cancer Society®. *Cancer Facts & Figures 2020*. 2020 [cited October 28, 2020]; Available from: https://www.cancer.org/content/dam/cancer-org/research/cancer-facts-and-statistics/annual-cancer-facts-and-figures/2020/cancer-facts-and-figures-2020.pdf
6. Wakefield MA, et al. Impact of tobacco control policies and mass media campaigns on monthly adult smoking prevalence. Am J Public Health. 2008;98(8):1443–50.
7. Reckamp KL. Targeted therapy for patients with metastatic non-small cell lung cancer. J Natl Compr Cancer Netw. 2018;16(5s):601–4.
8. Ettinger DS, et al. NCCN guidelines insights: non-small cell lung cancer, version 1.2020. J Natl Compr Cancer Netw. 2019;17(12):1464–72.
9. da Cunha Santos G, Shepherd FA, Tsao MS. EGFR mutations and lung cancer. Annu Rev Pathol. 2011;6:49–69.
10. Sabir SR, et al. EML4-ALK variants: biological and molecular properties, and the implications for patients. Cancers (Basel). 2017;9(9):118.
11. Cui M, et al. Molecular and clinicopathological characteristics of ROS1-rearranged non-small-cell lung cancers identified by next-generation sequencing. Mol Oncol. 2020;14(11):2787–95.
12. Reungwetwattana T, et al. The race to target MET exon 14 skipping alterations in non-small cell lung cancer: the why, the how, the who, the unknown, and the inevitable. Lung Cancer. 2017;103:27–37.
13. Leonetti A, et al. BRAF in non-small cell lung cancer (NSCLC): pickaxing another brick in the wall. Cancer Treat Rev. 2018;66:82–94.
14. Cancer Genome Atlas Research N. Comprehensive molecular profiling of lung adenocarcinoma. Nature. 2014;511(7511):543–50.
15. Vaishnavi A, et al. Oncogenic and drug-sensitive NTRK1 rearrangements in lung cancer. Nat Med. 2013;19(11):1469–72.
16. Cappuzzo F, Bemis L, Varella-Garcia M. HER2 mutation and response to trastuzumab therapy in non-small-cell lung cancer. N Engl J Med. 2006;354(24):2619–21.
17. De Grève J, et al. Clinical activity of afatinib (BIBW 2992) in patients with lung adenocarcinoma with mutations in the kinase domain of HER2/neu. Lung Cancer. 2012;76(1):123–7.
18. Li BT, et al. Ado-trastuzumab emtansine for patients with HER2-mutant lung cancers: results from a phase II basket trial. J Clin Oncol. 2018;36(24):2532–7.
19. Li W, et al. Primary and acquired EGFR T790M-mutant NSCLC patients identified by routine mutation testing show different characteristics but may both respond to osimertinib treatment. Cancer Lett. 2018;423:9–15.
20. Assi H, et al. Prevalence of T790M mutation among TKI-therapy resistant Lebanese lung cancer patients based on liquid biopsy analysis: a first report from a major tertiary care center. Mol Biol Rep. 2019;46(4):3671–6.
21. Fang W, et al. EGFR exon 20 insertion mutations and response to osimertinib in non-small-cell lung cancer. BMC Cancer. 2019;19(1):595.
22. Cress WD, et al. Lung cancer mutations and use of targeted agents in Hispanics. Rev Recent Clin Trials. 2014;9(4):225–32.
23. Bubendorf L, et al. Testing for ROS1 in non-small cell lung cancer: a review with recommendations. Virchows Arch. 2016;469(5):489–503.
24. Shackelford RE, et al. ALK-rearrangements and testing methods in non-small cell lung cancer: a review. Genes Cancer. 2014;5(1–2):1–14.
25. Choi YL, et al. Identification of novel isoforms of the EML4-ALK transforming gene in non-small cell lung cancer. Cancer Res. 2008;68(13):4971–6.
26. Soda M, et al. Identification of the transforming EML4-ALK fusion gene in non-small-cell lung cancer. Nature. 2007;448(7153):561–6.
27. Lin JJ, Shaw AT. Recent advances in targeting ROS1 in lung cancer. J Thorac Oncol. 2017;12(11):1611–25.
28. Bergethon K, et al. ROS1 rearrangements define a unique molecular class of lung cancers. J Clin Oncol. 2012;30(8):863–70.
29. Le T, Gerber DE. ALK alterations and inhibition in lung cancer. Semin Cancer Biol. 2017;42:81–8.
30. Kawakami H, et al. Targeting MET amplification as a new oncogenic driver. Cancers (Basel). 2014;6(3):1540–52.
31. Bronte G, et al. Targeting RET-rearranged non-small-cell lung cancer: future prospects. Lung Cancer (Auckl). 2019;10:27–36.
32. Ackermann CJ, et al. Targeted therapy for RET-rearranged non-small cell lung cancer: clinical development and future directions. Onco Targets and Therapy. 2019;12:7857–64.
33. Reddy VP, Laurie MG, Elvin JA, Vergilio J-A, Suh J, Ramkissoon S, et al. BRAF fusions in clinically advanced non-small cell lung cancer: an emerging target for anti-BRAF therapies. J Clin Oncol. 2017;35:9072.
34. Jang JS, et al. Common oncogene mutations and novel SND1-BRAF transcript fusion in lung adenocarcinoma from never smokers. Sci Rep. 2015;5:9755.
35. Vaishnavi A, Le AT, Doebele RC. TRKing down an old oncogene in a new era of targeted therapy. Cancer Discov. 2015;5(1):25–34.
36. Russell JP, et al. The TRK-T1 fusion protein induces neoplastic transformation of thyroid epithelium. Oncogene. 2000;19(50):5729–35.
37. Ricciuti B, et al. Targeting NTRK fusion in non-small cell lung cancer: rationale and clinical evidence. Med Oncol. 2017;34(6):105.
38. Kris MG, et al. Targeting HER2 aberrations as actionable drivers in lung cancers: phase II trial of the pan-HER tyrosine kinase inhibitor dacomitinib in patients with HER2-mutant or amplified tumors. Ann Oncol. 2015;26(7):1421–7.
39. Okamoto T, et al. Clinical and genetic implications of mutation burden in squamous cell carcinoma of the lung. Ann Surg Oncol. 2018;25(6):1564–71.
40. Gandara DR, et al. Squamous cell lung cancer: from tumor genomics to cancer therapeutics. Clin Cancer Res. 2015;21(10):2236–43.
41. TCGA. Comprehensive genomic characterization of squamous cell lung cancers. Nature. 2012;489(7417):519–25.
42. Schwaederle M, et al. Squamousness: next-generation sequencing reveals shared molecular features across squamous tumor types. Cell Cycle. 2015;14(14):2355–61.
43. Friedlaender A, et al. Next generation sequencing and genetic alterations in squamous cell lung carcinoma: where are we today? Front Oncol. 2019;9:166.
44. Xu F, et al. A TP53-associated gene signature for prediction of prognosis and therapeutic responses in lung squamous cell carcinoma. Onco Targets Ther. 2020;9(1):1731943.

45. Kashima J, Kitadai R, Okuma Y. Molecular and morphological profiling of lung cancer: a foundation for "next-generation" pathologists and oncologists. Cancers (Basel). 2019;11(5):599.
46. Paik PK, et al. Next-generation sequencing of stage IV squamous cell lung cancers reveals an association of PI3K aberrations and evidence of clonal heterogeneity in patients with brain metastases. Cancer Discov. 2015;5(6):610–21.
47. Berland L, et al. Current views on tumor mutational burden in patients with non-small cell lung cancer treated by immune checkpoint inhibitors. J Thorac Dis. 2019;11(Suppl 1):S71–80.
48. Lindeman NI, et al. Updated molecular testing guideline for the selection of lung cancer patients for treatment with targeted tyrosine kinase inhibitors: guideline from the College of American Pathologists, the International Association for the Study of Lung Cancer, and the Association for Molecular Pathology. J Mol Diagn. 2018;20(2):129–59.
49. McDowell EM, et al. The respiratory epithelium. V. Histogenesis of lung carcinomas in the human. J Natl Cancer Inst. 1978;61(2):587–606.
50. Travis WD, et al. Introduction to the 2015 World Health Organization classification of tumors of the lung, pleura, thymus, and heart. J Thorac Oncol. 2015;10(9):1240–2.
51. Inamura K, et al. EML4-ALK lung cancers are characterized by rare other mutations, a TTF-1 cell lineage, an acinar histology, and young onset. Mod Pathol. 2009;22(4):508–15.
52. Heeke S, Hofman P. Tumor mutational burden assessment as a predictive biomarker for immunotherapy in lung cancer patients: getting ready for prime-time or not? Transl Lung Cancer Res. 2018;7(6):631–8.
53. Greillier L, Tomasini P, Barlesi F. The clinical utility of tumor mutational burden in non-small cell lung cancer. Transl Lung Cancer Res. 2018;7(6):639–46.
54. Alborelli I, et al. Tumor mutational burden assessed by targeted NGS predicts clinical benefit from immune checkpoint inhibitors in non-small cell lung cancer. J Pathol. 2020;250(1):19–29.
55. Umemura S, Tsuchihara K, Goto K. Genomic profiling of small-cell lung cancer: the era of targeted therapies. Jpn J Clin Oncol. 2015;45(6):513–9.
56. Kim YH, et al. Combined microarray analysis of small cell lung cancer reveals altered apoptotic balance and distinct expression signatures of MYC family gene amplification. Oncogene. 2006;25(1):130–8.
57. Rudin CM, et al. Comprehensive genomic analysis identifies SOX2 as a frequently amplified gene in small-cell lung cancer. Nat Genet. 2012;44(10):1111–6.
58. Semenova EA, et al. Transcription factor NFIB is a driver of small cell lung cancer progression in mice and marks metastatic disease in patients. Cell Rep. 2016;16(3):631–43.
59. D'Amico D, et al. High frequency of somatically acquired p53 mutations in small-cell lung cancer cell lines and tumors. Oncogene. 1992;7(2):339–46.
60. Yokomizo A, et al. PTEN/MMAC1 mutations identified in small cell, but not in non-small cell lung cancers. Oncogene. 1998;17(4):475–9.
61. Yuan J, et al. Expression of p16 and lack of pRB in primary small cell lung cancer. J Pathol. 1999;189(3):358–62.
62. Balsara BR, Testa JR. Chromosomal imbalances in human lung cancer. Oncogene. 2002;21(45):6877–83.
63. Kim KB, Dunn CT, Park KS. Recent progress in mapping the emerging landscape of the small-cell lung cancer genome. Exp Mol Med. 2019;51(12):1–13.
64. Nishio Y, et al. Telomere length, telomerase activity, and expressions of human telomerase mRNA component (hTERC) and human telomerase reverse transcriptase (hTERT) mRNA in pulmonary neuroendocrine tumors. Jpn J Clin Oncol. 2007;37(1):16–22.
65. Simbolo M, et al. Lung neuroendocrine tumours: deep sequencing of the four World Health Organization histotypes reveals chromatin-remodelling genes as major players and a prognostic role for TERT, RB1, MEN1 and KMT2D. J Pathol. 2017;241(4):488–500.
66. Jones MH, et al. Two prognostically significant subtypes of high-grade lung neuroendocrine tumours independent of small-cell and large-cell neuroendocrine carcinomas identified by gene expression profiles. Lancet. 2004;363(9411):775–81.
67. Swarts DR, Ramaekers FC, Speel EJ. Molecular and cellular biology of neuroendocrine lung tumors: evidence for separate biological entities. Biochim Biophys Acta. 2012;1826(2):255–71.
68. Hiroshima K, et al. Distinction of pulmonary large cell neuroendocrine carcinoma from small cell lung carcinoma: a morphological, immunohistochemical, and molecular analysis. Mod Pathol. 2006;19(10):1358–68.
69. Peng WX, et al. Array-based comparative genomic hybridization analysis of high-grade neuroendocrine tumors of the lung. Cancer Sci. 2005;96(10):661–7.
70. Terra SB, et al. Molecular characterization of pulmonary sarcomatoid carcinoma: analysis of 33 cases. Mod Pathol. 2016;29(8):824–31.
71. Ushiki A, et al. Genetic heterogeneity of EGFR mutation in pleomorphic carcinoma of the lung: response to gefitinib and clinical outcome. Jpn J Clin Oncol. 2009;39(4):267–70.
72. Toyokawa G, et al. The first case of lung carcinosarcoma harboring in-frame deletions at exon19 in the EGFR gene. Lung Cancer. 2013;81(3):491–4.
73. Fallet V, et al. High-throughput somatic mutation profiling in pulmonary sarcomatoid carcinomas using the LungCarta™ Panel: exploring therapeutic targets. Ann Oncol. 2015;26(8):1748–53.
74. Liang X, et al. Mutation landscape and tumor mutation burden analysis of Chinese patients with pulmonary sarcomatoid carcinomas. Int J Clin Oncol. 2019;24(9):1061–8.
75. Manabe S, et al. Analysis of targeted somatic mutations in pleomorphic carcinoma of the lung using next-generation sequencing technique. Thorac Cancer. 2020;11(8):2262–9.
76. Italiano A, et al. EGFR and KRAS status of primary sarcomatoid carcinomas of the lung: implications for anti-EGFR treatment of a rare lung malignancy. Int J Cancer. 2009;125(10):2479–82.
77. Pelosi G, et al. Multiparametric molecular characterization of pulmonary sarcomatoid carcinoma reveals a nonrandom amplification of anaplastic lymphoma kinase (ALK) gene. Lung Cancer. 2012;77(3):507–14.
78. Liu X, et al. Next-generation sequencing of pulmonary sarcomatoid carcinoma reveals high frequency of actionable MET gene mutations. J Clin Oncol. 2016;34(8):794–802.
79. Zhao J, et al. Clinicopathologic features and genomic analysis of pulmonary blastomatoid carcinosarcoma. BMC Cancer. 2020;20(1):248.
80. Macher-Goeppinger S, et al. Expression and mutation analysis of EGFR, c-KIT, and β-catenin in pulmonary blastoma. J Clin Pathol. 2011;64(4):349–53.
81. Nakatani Y, et al. Aberrant nuclear localization and gene mutation of beta-catenin in low-grade adenocarcinoma of fetal lung type: up-regulation of the Wnt signaling pathway may be a common denominator for the development of tumors that form morules. Mod Pathol. 2002;15(6):617–24.
82. Wu Q, et al. Primary pulmonary lymphoepithelioma-like carcinoma is characterized by high PD-L1 expression, but low tumor mutation burden. Pathol Res Pract. 2020;216(8):153043.
83. Falk N, et al. Primary pulmonary salivary gland-type tumors: a review and update. Adv Anat Pathol. 2016;23(1):13–23.
84. Xie XH, et al. Clinical features, treatment, and survival outcome of primary pulmonary NUT midline carcinoma. Orphanet J Rare Dis. 2020;15(1):183.

85. Sholl LM, et al. Primary pulmonary NUT midline carcinoma: clinical, radiographic, and pathologic characterizations. J Thorac Oncol. 2015;10(6):951–9.
86. French CA, et al. BRD-NUT oncoproteins: a family of closely related nuclear proteins that block epithelial differentiation and maintain the growth of carcinoma cells. Oncogene. 2008;27(15):2237–42.
87. Schwartz BE, et al. Differentiation of NUT midline carcinoma by epigenomic reprogramming. Cancer Res. 2011;71(7):2686–96.
88. Lindeman NI, et al. Molecular testing guideline for selection of lung cancer patients for EGFR and ALK tyrosine kinase inhibitors: guideline from the College of American Pathologists, International Association for the Study of Lung Cancer, and Association for Molecular Pathology. J Mol Diagn. 2013;15(4):415–53.
89. Drilon A. TRK inhibitors in TRK fusion-positive cancers. Ann Oncol. 2019;30(Suppl 8):viii23–30.
90. Hellmann MD, et al. Nivolumab plus Ipilimumab in lung cancer with a high tumor mutational burden. N Engl J Med. 2018;378(22):2093–104.
91. National Comprehensive Cancer Network (N.C.C.N®). *Non-Small Cell Lung Cancer (Version 8.2020)*. September 15, 2020 [Accessed: October 20, 2020]; Available from: https://www.nccn.org/professionals/physician_gls/pdf/nscl.pdf
92. Consortium TAPG. AACR project GENIE: powering precision medicine through an international consortium. Cancer Discov. 2017;7(8):818–31.
93. Mogi A, Kuwano H. TP53 mutations in nonsmall cell lung cancer. J Biomed Biotechnol. 2011;2011:583929.
94. Roeper J, et al. TP53 co-mutations in EGFR mutated patients in NSCLC stage IV: a strong predictive factor of ORR, PFS and OS in EGFR mt+ NSCLC. Oncotarget. 2020;11(3):250–64.
95. Yatabe Y, Matsuo K, Mitsudomi T. Heterogeneous distribution of EGFR mutations is extremely rare in lung adenocarcinoma. J Clin Oncol. 2011;29(22):2972–7.
96. Zhang J, et al. Intratumor heterogeneity in localized lung adenocarcinomas delineated by multiregion sequencing. Science. 2014;346(6206):256–9.
97. Sherwood J, et al. Mutation status concordance between primary lesions and metastatic sites of advanced non-small-cell lung cancer and the impact of mutation testing methodologies: a literature review. J Exp Clin Cancer Res. 2015;34:92.
98. Chang YL, Wu CT, Lee YC. Surgical treatment of synchronous multiple primary lung cancers: experience of 92 patients. J Thorac Cardiovasc Surg. 2007;134(3):630–7.
99. Arai J, et al. Clinical and molecular analysis of synchronous double lung cancers. Lung Cancer. 2012;77(2):281–7.
100. Girard N, et al. Comprehensive histologic assessment helps to differentiate multiple lung primary nonsmall cell carcinomas from metastases. Am J Surg Pathol. 2009;33(12):1752–64.
101. Gerlinger M, et al. Genomic architecture and evolution of clear cell renal cell carcinomas defined by multiregion sequencing. Nat Genet. 2014;46(3):225–33.
102. Chang JC, et al. Comprehensive next-generation sequencing unambiguously distinguishes separate primary lung carcinomas from intrapulmonary metastases: comparison with standard histopathologic approach. Clin Cancer Res. 2019;25(23):7113–25.
103. Schneider F, et al. Morphological and molecular approach to synchronous non-small cell lung carcinomas: impact on staging. Mod Pathol. 2016;29(7):735–42.
104. Awad MM, et al. MET exon 14 mutations in non-small-cell lung cancer are associated with advanced age and stage-dependent MET genomic amplification and c-met overexpression. J Clin Oncol. 2016;34(7):721–30.
105. Li Y, et al. Identification of MET exon14 skipping by targeted DNA- and RNA-based next-generation sequencing in pulmonary sarcomatoid carcinomas. Lung Cancer. 2018;122:113–9.
106. U.S. Food & Drug Administration (FDA). *List of Cleared or Approved Companion Diagnostic Devices (In Vitro and Imaging Tools)*. 2020 [cited October 27, 2020]; Available from: https://www.fda.gov/medical-devices/vitro-diagnostics/list-cleared-or-approved-companion-diagnostic-devices-vitro-and-imaging-tools
107. Layfield LJ, et al. Molecular testing strategies for pulmonary adenocarcinoma: an optimal approach with cost analysis. Arch Pathol Lab Med. 2019;143(5):628–33.
108. Nam SK, et al. Effects of fixation and storage of human tissue samples on nucleic acid preservation. Korean J Pathol. 2014;48(1):36–42.
109. Kim L, Tsao MS. Tumour tissue sampling for lung cancer management in the era of personalised therapy: what is good enough for molecular testing? Eur Respir J. 2014;44(4):1011–22.
110. Baloglu G, et al. The effects of tissue fixation alternatives on DNA content: a study on normal colon tissue. Appl Immunohistochem Mol Morphol. 2008;16(5):485–92.
111. Bellevicine C, et al. How to prepare cytological samples for molecular testing. J Clin Pathol. 2017;70(10):819–26.
112. Mikubo M, et al. Calculating the tumor nuclei content for comprehensive cancer panel testing. J Thorac Oncol. 2020;15(1):130–7.
113. Burghel GJ, et al. The importance of neoplastic cell content assessment and enrichment by macrodissection in cancer pharmacogenetic testing. J Clin Pathol. 2019;72(10):721–2.
114. Villatoro S, et al. Prospective detection of mutations in cerebrospinal fluid, pleural effusion, and ascites of advanced cancer patients to guide treatment decisions. Mol Oncol. 2019;13(12):2633–45.
115. Gandara DR, et al. Blood-based tumor mutational burden as a predictor of clinical benefit in non-small-cell lung cancer patients treated with atezolizumab. Nat Med. 2018;24(9):1441–8.
116. Leighl NB, et al. Clinical utility of comprehensive cell-free DNA analysis to identify genomic biomarkers in patients with newly diagnosed metastatic non–small cell lung cancer. Clin Cancer Res. 2019;25(15):4691–700.
117. Rijavec E, et al. Liquid biopsy in non-small cell lung cancer: highlights and challenges. Cancers (Basel). 2019;12(1):17.
118. Revelo AE, et al. Liquid biopsy for lung cancers: an update on recent developments. Ann Transl Med. 2019;7(15):349.
119. Chabon JJ, et al. Circulating tumour DNA profiling reveals heterogeneity of EGFR inhibitor resistance mechanisms in lung cancer patients. Nat Commun. 2016;7:11815.
120. Thress KS, et al. Acquired EGFR C797S mutation mediates resistance to AZD9291 in non-small cell lung cancer harboring EGFR T790M. Nat Med. 2015;21(6):560–2.
121. Dagogo-Jack I, et al. Tracking the evolution of resistance to ALK tyrosine kinase inhibitors through longitudinal analysis of circulating tumor DNA. JCO Precis Oncol. 2018;2:1–14.
122. McCoach CE, et al. Clinical utility of cell-free DNA for the detection of ALK fusions and genomic mechanisms of ALK inhibitor resistance in non–small cell lung cancer. Clin Cancer Res. 2018;24(12):2758–70.
123. Soria JC, et al. Osimertinib in untreated EGFR-mutated advanced non-small-cell lung cancer. N Engl J Med. 2018;378(2):113–25.
124. Chan TA, et al. Development of tumor mutation burden as an immunotherapy biomarker: utility for the oncology clinic. Ann Oncol. 2019;30(1):44–56.
125. Chalmers ZR, et al. Analysis of 100,000 human cancer genomes reveals the landscape of tumor mutational burden. Genome Med. 2017;9(1):34.
126. Alexandrov LB, et al. Signatures of mutational processes in human cancer. Nature. 2013;500(7463):415–21.
127. Carbone DP, et al. First-line nivolumab in stage IV or recurrent non-small-cell lung cancer. N Engl J Med. 2017;376(25):2415–26.
128. Socinski MA, et al. Atezolizumab for first-line treatment of metastatic nonsquamous NSCLC. N Engl J Med. 2018;378(24):2288–301.

129. Langer C, et al. OA04.05 KEYNOTE-021: TMB and outcomes for carboplatin and pemetrexed with or without pembrolizumab for nonsquamous NSCLC. J Thorac Oncol. 2019;14(10, Supplement):S216.
130. Garassino M, et al. OA04.06 evaluation of TMB in KEYNOTE-189: pembrolizumab plus chemotherapy vs placebo plus chemotherapy for nonsquamous NSCLC. J Thorac Oncol. 2019;14(10, Supplement):S216–7.
131. Bevins N, et al. Comparison of commonly used solid tumor targeted gene sequencing panels for estimating tumor mutation burden shows analytical and prognostic concordance within the cancer genome atlas cohort. J Immunother Cancer. 2020;8(1):e000613.
132. Chaudhary R, et al. A scalable solution for tumor mutational burden from formalin-fixed, paraffin-embedded samples using the Oncomine Tumor Mutation Load Assay. Transl Lung Cancer Res. 2018;7(6):616–30.
133. Rizvi H, et al. Molecular determinants of response to anti-programmed cell death (PD)-1 and anti-programmed death-ligand 1 (PD-L1) blockade in patients with non-small-cell lung cancer profiled with targeted next-generation sequencing. J Clin Oncol. 2018;36(7):633–41.
134. Li R, et al. Choosing tumor mutational burden wisely for immunotherapy: a hard road to explore. Biochim Biophys Acta Rev Cancer. 1874;2020(2):188420.
135. Wang Z, et al. Assessment of blood tumor mutational burden as a potential biomarker for immunotherapy in patients with non-small cell lung cancer with use of a next-generation sequencing cancer gene panel. JAMA Oncol. 2019;5(5):696–702.
136. Imperial R, et al. Matched whole-genome sequencing (WGS) and whole-exome sequencing (WES) of tumor tissue with circulating tumor DNA (ctDNA) analysis: complementary modalities in clinical practice. Cancers (Basel). 2019;11(9):1399.
137. U.S. Food & Drug Administration (FDA). *FDA approves pembrolizumab for adults and children with TMB-H solid tumors*. June 17, 2020; Available from: https://www.fda.gov/drugs/drug--approvals-and-databases/fda-approves-pembrolizumab-adults-and-children-tmb-h-solid-tumors
138. Merino DM, et al. Establishing guidelines to harmonize tumor mutational burden (TMB): in silico assessment of variation in TMB quantification across diagnostic platforms: phase I of the Friends of Cancer Research TMB Harmonization Project. J Immunother Cancer. 2020;8(1):e000147.
139. Büttner R, et al. Implementing TMB measurement in clinical practice: considerations on assay requirements. ESMO Open. 2019;4(1):e000442.
140. Brahmer J, et al. Nivolumab versus docetaxel in advanced squamous-cell non-small-cell lung cancer. N Engl J Med. 2015;373(2):123–35.
141. Rittmeyer A, et al. Atezolizumab versus docetaxel in patients with previously treated non-small-cell lung cancer (OAK): a phase 3, open-label, multicentre randomised controlled trial. Lancet. 2017;389(10066):255–65.
142. Miura Y, Sunaga N. Role of immunotherapy for oncogene-driven non-small cell lung cancer. Cancers (Basel). 2018;10(8):245.
143. Biton J, et al. TP53, STK11, and EGFR mutations predict tumor immune profile and the response to anti-PD-1 in lung adenocarcinoma. Clin Cancer Res. 2018;24(22):5710–23.
144. Giroux Leprieur E, et al. Circulating tumor DNA evaluated by Next-Generation Sequencing is predictive of tumor response and prolonged clinical benefit with nivolumab in advanced non-small cell lung cancer. Onco Targets Ther. 2018;7(5):e1424675.
145. Iijima Y, et al. Very early response of circulating tumour-derived DNA in plasma predicts efficacy of nivolumab treatment in patients with non-small cell lung cancer. Eur J Cancer. 2017;86:349–57.
146. Looney T, et al. TCR beta chain convergence defines the tumor infiltrating T cell repertoire of melanoma and non-small cell lung carcinoma. Ann Oncol. 2018;29:viii19–20.
147. Jermann P, et al. TCR-beta repertoire convergence and evenness are associated with response to immune checkpoint inhibitors. Ann Oncol. 2019;30:v851.
148. Han J, et al. TCR repertoire diversity of peripheral PD-1(+) CD8(+) T cells predicts clinical outcomes after immunotherapy in patients with non-small cell lung cancer. Cancer Immunol Res. 2020;8(1):146–54.
149. Pao W, et al. EGF receptor gene mutations are common in lung cancers from "never smokers" and are associated with sensitivity of tumors to gefitinib and erlotinib. Proc Natl Acad Sci U S A. 2004;101(36):13306–11.

Gastrointestinal, Hepatobiliary, and Pancreatic Tumors

8

Mohammad K. Mohammad and Guoli Chen

List of Frequently Asked Questions

1. What is the clinical significance of evaluating HER2 expression/amplification in gastric adenocarcinoma, and how to evaluate it?
2. What are the major molecular classification systems of gastric carcinoma and the differences among them?
3. What are the molecular mechanisms underlying development of gastrointestinal stromal tumor (GIST) and their clinical significance for targeted therapy?
4. What are the routinely tested molecular genetic biomarkers for clinical management of colorectal cancer (CRC) and their clinical significance?
5. What is the role of mismatch repair (MMR) protein deficiency in tumorigenesis of Lynch syndrome, and what are the recommended steps for Lynch syndrome screening in patients with CRC?
6. What are the commonly used methods for microsatellite instability (MSI) analysis?
7. What is the role of MMR/MSI testing in the prediction of immune checkpoint inhibitor treatment in CRC?
8. What are the common clinical syndromes associated with GI tract polyposis and their typical genetic alterations?
9. What are the emerging molecular targeted therapies for hepatocellular carcinoma (HCC)? What is the role of next-generation sequencing (NGS) technology in clinical management of HCC?
10. What is the morpho-molecular classification of liver cancer in correlation to clinicohistologic features?
11. What is the genetic landscape of pancreatic cancer and its potential clinical significance?
12. What is the significance of molecular diagnostics in cytologic samples of pancreatobiliary lesions? What is the role of NGS technology?

M. K. Mohammad
Department of Pathology and Laboratory Medicine, Geisinger Medical Center, Geisinger Commonwealth School of Medicine, Danville, PA, USA
e-mail: dr.mohammad.mohammad@aol.com

G. Chen (✉)
Department of Pathology and Laboratory Medicine, Geisinger Medical Center, Danville, PA, USA
e-mail: gchen1@geisinger.edu

Frequently Asked Questions

1. **What is the clinical significance of evaluating HER2 expression/amplification in gastric adenocarcinoma, and how to evaluate it?**
   - The World Health Organization (WHO) classifies gastric carcinoma (GC) into two main histological types, diffuse and intestinal. Diffuse gastric cancer type is more common in young patients with a multifocal potential and not often accompanied by intestinal metaplasia, while the intestinal cancer type is more frequently observed in older patients and follows multifocal atrophic gastritis [1].
   - Human epidermal growth factor receptor 2 (*HER2*) gene is a proto-oncogene located on chromosome 17q21 and encodes a transmembrane protein with tyrosine kinase activity and is more commonly overexpressed in intestinal-type (21.5%) than in diffuse-type (2%) gastric adenocarcinoma [2, 3]. HER2 protein overexpression is associated with decreased survival rates and clinicopathological progression characteristics, including serosal invasion, metastases, and higher disease stage [3].
   - Given the introduction of a targeting therapy, e.g., trastuzumab (a monoclonal antibody which binds to and inhibits HER2 signaling) for the treatment of patients with advanced gastric cancer, HER2 status assessment is now necessary for selecting patients eligible for this treatment. Testing for HER2 is recommended for any patient with gastric adenocarcinoma

Y. Ding, L. Zhang (eds.), *Practical Oncologic Molecular Pathology*, Practical Anatomic Pathology,
https://doi.org/10.1007/978-3-030-73227-1_8

(locally advanced, recurrent, or metastatic) based on the guidelines of the American Society of Clinical Oncology (ASCO), the College of American Pathologists (CAP), and the American Society for Clinical Pathology (ASCP) [2].

- HER2 studies in gastric adenocarcinoma, like those in breast cancers, include an initial evaluation of the protein expression levels by immunohistochemistry (IHC). Positive (IHC 3+) or negative (IHC 0 or 1+) HER2 IHC results do not mandate further in situ hybridization testing. Fluorescent in situ hybridization (FISH) is the gold standard but commonly performed whenever it is indicated by IHC results due to its higher cost and time consumption, as well as the need for a fluorescence microscope [3]. In particular, it is usually recommended for the equivocal cases of HER2 with a score of 2+ on IHC according to the currently recommended testing algorithms [4]. In situ hybridization cutoffs using either the HER2/CEP17 (centromeric region of chromosome 17) ratio or copy number-based assessment is applied to delineate the final HER2 status. Particularly, the in situ hybridization test results of HER2/CEP17 ratio ≥2 or an average HER2 copy number ≥6.0 signals/cell are considered positive.
- According to the guideline, pathologists should ensure that tissue specimens used for HER2 testing are rapidly placed in fixative, ideally within 1 hour (cold ischemic time) and are fixed in 10% neutral buffered formalin for 6–72 hours.
- According to the guideline, pathologists should select the tissue block with areas of lowest-grade tumor morphology for IHC and mark the areas of strongest intensity of IHC HER2 staining for subsequent FISH study if required.
- Currently, the analysis of HER2 expression/amplification is recommended in both gastric and gastroesophageal junction (GEJ) adenocarcinomas.

2. **What are the major molecular classification systems of gastric carcinoma and the differences among them?**
   - The Cancer Genome Atlas (TCGA) research network reported a comprehensive classification of the genetic alterations associated with gastric carcinoma, combining data from six different platforms: array-based somatic copy number analysis, whole-exome and genome sequencing, messenger RNA sequencing, microRNA sequencing, and reverse-phase protein array profiling, plus evaluation of microsatellite instability [5]. They proposed to classify GC into four subtypes: EBV-positive (EBV), microsatellite-unstable (MSI), genomically stable (GS), and chromosomal instability (CIN).
   - The Asian Cancer Research Group (ACRG) categorizes GC into four subtypes based on gene expression data [6]: microsatellite instability (MSI), epithelial-to-mesenchymal transition (EMT), and microsatellite stable (MSS)/TP53+ and MSS/TP53-. The MSI group was characterized by loss of MLH1 and was enriched by mutations in several oncogenic genes. The MSS and EMT (MSS/EMT) group was characterized by the loss of CDH1 and a gene expression signature that correlated with that of EMT.
   - The Singapore-Duke group was the first to describe GC molecular subtypes. Initially, they divided GC into two intrinsic genomic subtypes that had distinct patterns of gene expression: G-INT (genomic intestinal) and G-DIF (genomic diffuse). Subsequently, the Singapore-Duke group classified GC into three different subtypes: proliferative, metabolic, and mesenchymal.
   - Clinical application of the molecular classification systems is pending on more comprehensive and conclusive examination of their clinical correlation and significance [6].
3. **What are the molecular mechanisms underlying development of gastrointestinal stromal tumor (GIST) and their clinical significance for targeted therapy?**
   - Gastrointestinal stromal tumors (GISTs) are one of the two most common mesenchymal tumors in addition to leiomyoma of the GI tract with approximately 5000 new cases diagnosed annually. Approximately 10% of patients present with synchronous liver metastases at the time of diagnosis [7, 8].
   - Due to similarities between GIST cells and interstitial cells of Cajal (ICCs) in expressing cKIT/CD117, GIST is hypothesized to originate from the ICCs [9].
   - While GISTs can arise anywhere from the esophagus to rectum, the majority are sporadic in the stomach, arising with somatic gain-of-function mutations in the tyrosine kinase gene *KIT* [9]. A report from the National Institutes of Health Gastrointestinal Stromal Tumor Clinic documented that 85% of GISTs harbor a mutation in *KIT* or *PDGFRA* (platelet derived growth factor receptor alpha), leaving 10–15% of GISTs in adults and 85% of GISTs in children free of a mutation in either of these genes (wild-type GISTs) [9–11].
   - Recent studies have revealed genetic alterations in *EGFR* (epidermal growth factor receptor) in 0.93% (3/323) of primary GISTs, with no overlap with mutations in *KIT*, *PDGFRA*, *KRAS*, or *BRAF* [8]. *EGFR* mutations are associated with a gastric location and a female gender predominance with a low recurrence rate. *BRAF* mutation is associated with small-sized GISTs (4 mm in average) and is one of the earliest events in the GIST development. NF1-associated GISTs are also of small size with a dominant small intestine location and indolent clinical course [8]. *PIK3CA* mutation (p.H1047L) has also been reported in a GIST case with *KIT* exon 11 deletion [12].

Table 8.1 A brief summary of therapeutic response to various mutations in GIST

Mutation	Therapeutic response
KIT exon 11	Imatinib sensitive and regorafenib sensitive
KIT exon 9	Imatinib sensitive to higher dose and sunitinib sensitive
KIT exons 13, 14, 17, 18	Sunitinib sensitive
PDGFRA D842V (exon 18) *PDGFRA* exons 12, 14, and 18 (except for D842V)	Imatinib resistant while dasatinib sensitive Imatinib sensitive
KIT/PDGFRA wild-type (children)	Imatinib resistant, regorafenib sensitive, and dasatinib sensitive

PDGFRA platelet-derived growth factor receptor A

The therapeutic implications of the genetic alterations in GIST drivers are among the best documented of all solid tumors. GISTs respond to targeted therapy with imatinib [13]. However, the sequencing of *KIT* and *PDGFRA* genes should be considered a standard practice for the treatment of GIST patients regardless of whether the tumor overexpresses KIT (CD117) protein or not because different mutations predict different responses to the drug [14, 15] as briefly summarized in Table 8.1. For example, a decent study demonstrated that patients with *KIT* mutations have better clinical benefit rates and response to sunitinib compared to those with *PDGFRA* mutations [14], particularly those with *KIT* exon 9 or 11 mutations [12]. Moreover, GIST patients with *KIT* exon 9 mutations have higher clinical benefit rates over those with *KIT* exon 11 mutations. Recent guidelines recommend imatinib therapy for advanced GIST patients harboring a sensitive *KIT* mutation, while an increased dose of imatinib (800 mg daily) is suggested in patients with exon 9 mutations owing to an inferior outcome [7]. Imatinib 800 mg was associated with improved PFS compared with conventional dosing (400 mg daily) in this subset of patients.

4. **What are the routinely tested molecular genetic biomarkers for clinical management of colorectal cancer and their clinical significance?**
   - Primary colorectal carcinoma (CRC) is the second leading cause of death in the United States [16]. In 2020, the American Cancer Society expects approximately 147,950 individuals to be diagnosed with CRC with an estimate of 53,200 to die from the disease [17].
   - A variety of genetic alterations have been found in CRC (Table 8.2). The promise of personalized medicine has become a clinical reality with CRC treatment being at the forefront of this major evolution in medical field [18]. Alterations in EGFR and associated cell signaling transduction pathways are important in the carcinogenesis of CRC and other cancers; thus, tremendous effort has been put on developing agents targeting those pathways as shown in Fig. 8.1 [19]. For example, monoclonal antibody therapies including cetuximab and panitumumab targeting EGFR require molecular testing of specific molecular genes for proper patient selection and accurate CRC treatment; thus, a guideline has been published with the combined efforts of CAP, ASCP, AMP, and ASCO [20].
   - EGFR-targeted treatment is efficient only if there are no mutations found in *KRAS* and *NRAS* genes. Currently assays for the molecular mutational analysis of *KRAS* and *NRAS* genes should include at least codons 12, 13, 59, 61, 117, and 146.
   - Patients with mutant *BRAF* also seem to have a poor response to the treatment, although *BRAF* testing for this predictive purpose has not officially been recommended. *BRAF* p.V600 (c.1799) mutational analysis should be performed in patients with CRC, however, rather for the purposes of prognostic stratification and others that will be discussed below.
   - Other molecular markers that are potentially with clinical significance in EGFR signaling transduction pathways such as PI3K catalytic subunit (PIK3CA) and PTEN have been suggested to harbor aberrations in 30–40% of all sporadic CRC cases. A recent study suggested *PIK3CA* mutations may have clinical prognostic information in tumor stages I–III and that PIK3CA/PTEN deregulation, in addition to *RAS* and *BRAF* mutations, are considered a biomarker of the drug resistance [21]. Molecular analysis of these genes for the predictive purpose has not officially been recom-

Table 8.2 Common genetic mutations and incidences in colorectal cancer

Gene	Mutation	%
KRAS	Activating mutations at codon 12/13 and other codons	40%
BRAF	Activating mutation V600E	10%
CTNNB1 (β-catenin)	Activating mutations	2%
TGFBR2	Inactivating mutations	30%
TP53 mutations	Inactivating mutations	50%
APC mutations	Inactivating mutations	70%
CpG island methylator phenotype (CIMP)	Inactivating mutations methylation of at least three loci from a selected panel of five markers	15%
Mismatch repair genes	Inactivating mutations methylation	1–15%
18qLOH	Deletion in chromosome 18	50%
PIK3CA	Helical and kinase domain mutations	20%
PTEN	Loss of protein expression	30%

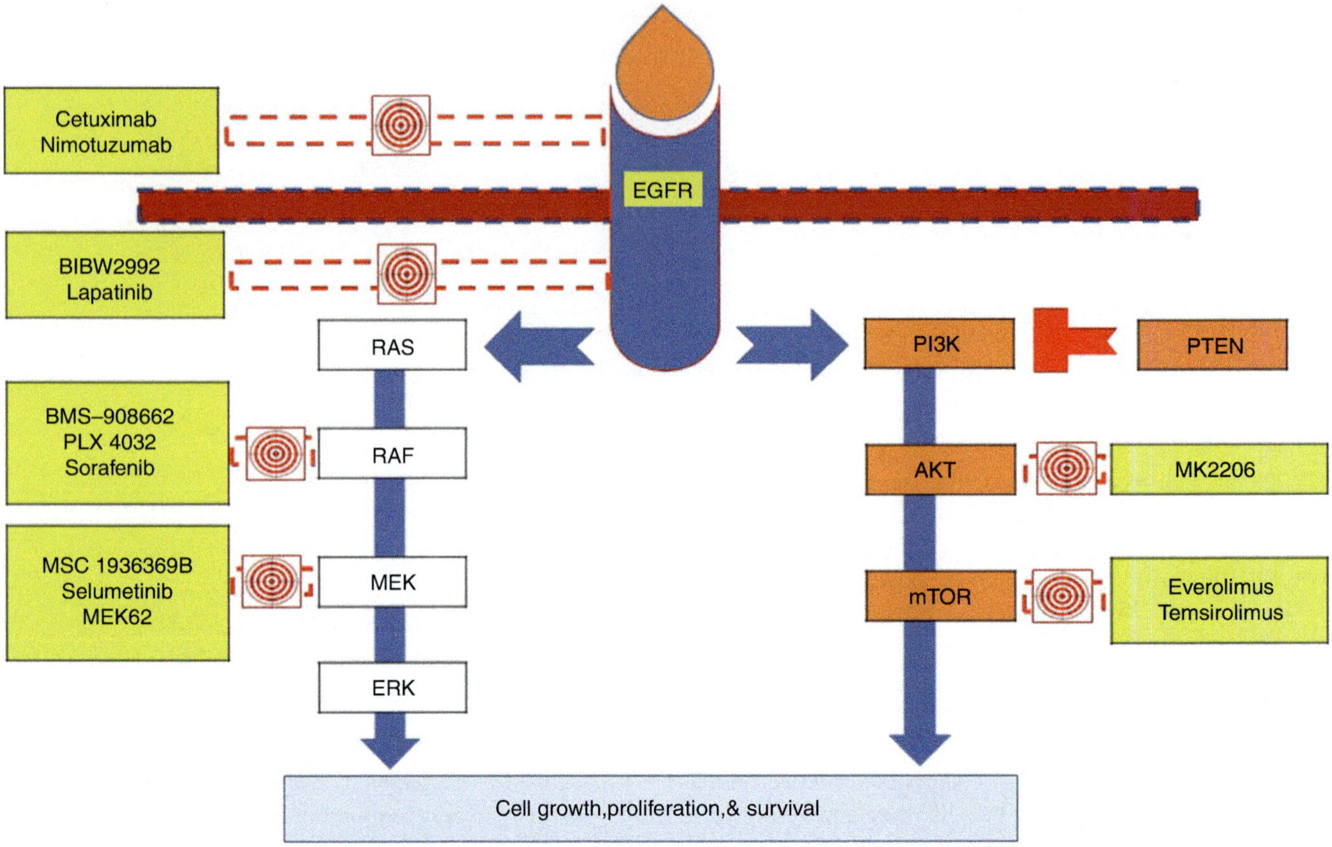

Fig. 8.1 Major EGFR signaling transduction pathways associated with tumorigenesis, and examplary drugs targeting EGFR and its downstream molecules. MEK: MAPK (mitogen-activated protein kinase) kinases/extracellular-signal-regulated kinases, ERK: extracellular-signal-related kinase, PTEN: phosphatase and tensin homolog

mended in this current guideline but is indicated and often included in a testing panel.

- Recently, *ERBB2* (*HER2*) amplification, *NTRK* fusions and other biomarkers have also been routinely tested in more and more institutes due to the availability/approval of targeting therapies for CRC patients [22].

5. **What is the role of mismatch repair (MMR) protein deficiency in tumorigenesis of Lynch syndrome, and what are the recommended steps for Lynch syndrome screening in patients with CRC?**
   - Approximately 3% of all patients with CRC have Lynch syndrome which is an autosomal-dominant inherent disease associated with germline mutations in MMR genes. To date, there are four key genes identified: mutL homologue 1 (*MLH1*), mutS homologue 2 (*MSH2*), mutS homologue 6 (*MSH6*), and postmeiotic segregation increased 2 (*PMS2*), so named because of their homology to the *E. coli* MMR genes [23, 24].
   - The MSH2 and MSH6 proteins form a heterodimeric complex (mutSα) which plays a role in the initial identification of mismatched bases and DNA repair. Similarly, MLH1 and PMS2 proteins always pair to function.
   - Overall, the MMR complex is one of the mechanisms correcting molecular genetic errors that frequently occur in the cells. When the MMR system develops a functional error or defect, namely, deficient mismatch repair (dMMR), this results in accumulation of genetic mutations in cancer-related genes and eventually tumorigenesis. A phenotype called microsatellite instability (MSI) is also a result of dMMR and may work as a surrogate test reflecting the dMMR status [25].
   - The occurrence of dMMR could be sporadic in origin which is commonly associated with the hypermethylation of *MLH1* promotor region or result from germline changes in a autosomal-dominant inherited predisposition condition, Lynch syndrome [23, 25]. Patients with Lynch syndrome are vulnerable to the development of different types of cancers earlier in their lives than normal population. CRC is the most common tumor associated with Lynch syndrome.
   - A testing algorithm combining clinical presentation, MMR IHC studies, and molecular tests on CRC tumor tissue has been developed to assess the MMR status and identify patients with a high risk of Lynch syn-

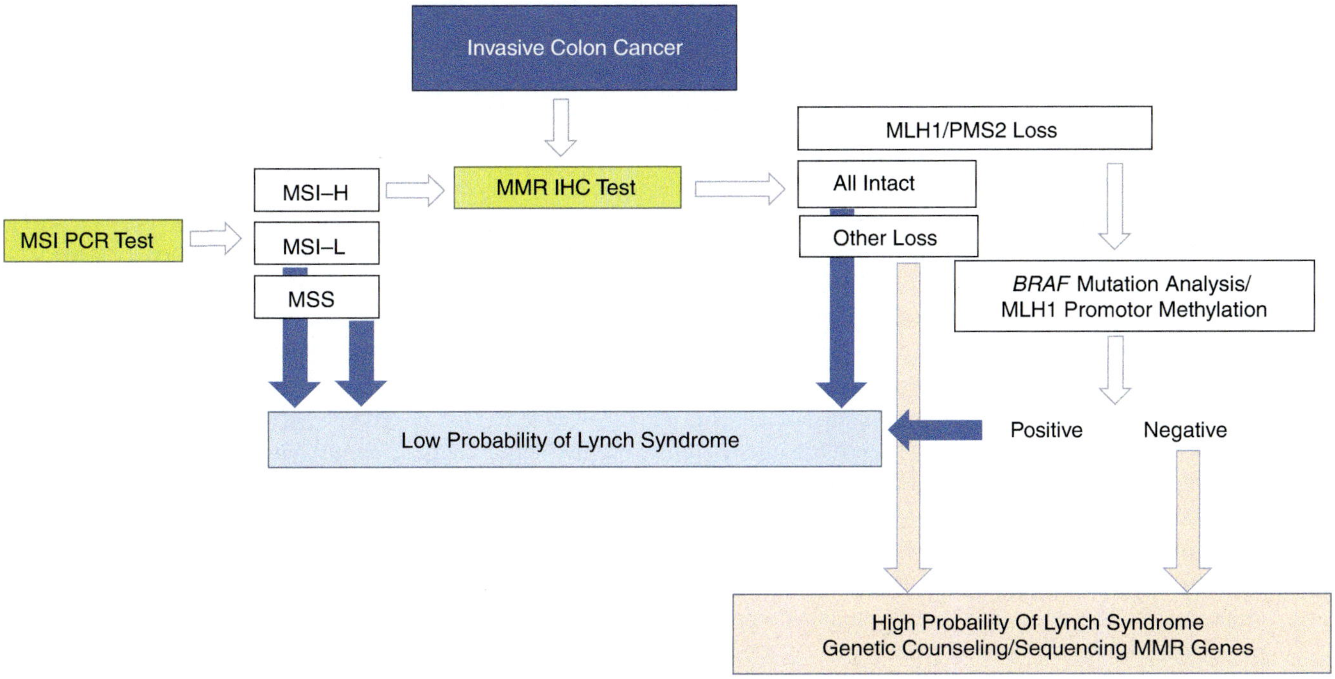

Fig. 8.2 An algorithm showing how to screen for Lynch Syndrome with CRC tissue, which is commonly initiated with IHC for MMR proteins, or alternatively, with a PCR-based molecular assay of microsatellite stability

drome from those with a sporadic origin (Fig. 8.2). Of note, neither clinical presentation, MMR IHC studies, nor MSI molecular tests are 100% accurate in the detection of dMMR/MSI-H tumors [23, 26]. IHC staining of the four MMR proteins is the widely adopted initial step, although it can alternatively be started with a molecular MSI testing. If IHC demonstrates MLH1 and PMS2 loss of nuclear expression in tumor cells with a *BRAF* (V600F) mutation and/or hypermethylation of *MLH1* promotor area present, the CRC is likely of sporadic dMMR. If neither a *BRAF* mutation nor hypermethylation is detected, or IHC demonstrates another protein loss pattern (e.g., PMS2 loss with intact MLH1, MSH6 and/or MSH2 loss), the CRC is then in an increased likelihood of Lynch syndrome with a strong indication for MMR gene sequencing. Under this circumstance, a genetic counselling should be first recommended. The likelihood of Lynch syndrome associated versus sporadic CRC may vary based on the clinical scenario even if there is a dMMR status detected. The IHCs of the four MMR proteins, *BRAF* mutation/MLH1 promotor methylation analysis, with or without MSI molecular testing in a screening algorithm should allow primary MMR subgroup stratification to the risk of Lynch syndrome for most cases.

- A guideline from the American College of Gastroenterology requires that all newly diagnosed colorectal cancers (CRCs) have to be evaluated for mismatch repair deficiency. Patients with personal history of a tumor showing evidence of mismatch repair deficiency with no demonstrated *BRAF* mutation or hypermethylation of *MLH1*, a known family mutation associated with Lynch syndrome, or a risk of ≥5% chance of Lynch syndrome (based on risk prediction models) should undergo genetic evaluation. Genetic testing of the suspected patients should include germline mutation testing for *MLH1*, *MSH2*, *MSH6*, *PMS2*, and/or *EPCAM* genes or the altered gene(s) indicated by immunohistochemistry [27]. For individuals at risk for Lynch syndrome, screening for colorectal cancer by colonoscopy should be performed at least every 2 years, beginning between ages 20 and 25 years. Annual colonoscopy should be considered in confirmed mutation carriers [17].

6. **What are the commonly used molecular methods for microsatellite instability analysis?**
   - Microsatellites are ubiquitous short repetitive DNA sequences with a length ranging from one to six core nucleotide repetitions (usually between 10 and 60 times). These DNA motifs are scattered throughout the coding and noncoding regions of the genome, often highly polymorphic among population while stable in individuals [28].
   - Microsatellite instability occurs when novel-sized alleles are detected in microsatellite loci in tumor DNA while are absent in normal constitutional DNA from the same person.

- The loss of nuclear expression of a single protein or a heterodimeric couple of the MMR complex suggests the presence of dMMR, as discussed. In rare cases of missense mutations *MLH1* or *MSH6* genes, however, IHC provides misleading information resulting from translated proteins with normal antibody affinity but missing functional activity. In these cases, PCR-based MSI analysis helps to determine whether there are true functional MMR proteins through the mutations [28, 29].
- For PCR-based MSI diagnostic assay, DNA is extracted from both tumor and normal tissue using fresh tissue or formalin-fixed, paraffin-embedded blocks. The size of PCR products obtained from normal tissue DNA is considered the normal (germline) size of the microsatellites that will be then compared to the PCR products obtained from the tumor. Therefore, microsatellite instability demonstrates changed lengths of PCR products due to either the insertion or deletion of repeating units in a microsatellite locus of the tumor compared to normal tissue. A validated panel of microsatellites by a National Cancer Institute (NCI) workshop, known as the Bethesda panel, is considered the reference panel for clinical and research testing [30, 31]. It consists of five mononucleotide repeats generally including *BAT25*, *BAT26*, *NR21*, *NR24*, and *Mono27*. More "alternative loci" are also provided.
- The NCI also defined the diagnostic criteria for microsatellite-high (MSI-H), microsatellite-low (MSI-L), and microsatellite-stable (MSS) phenotypes. When analyzing five loci, MSI-H is defined as instability at two loci or more and MSI-L as instability at one locus [32]. MSI-H colorectal tumors most often arise from the epigenetic silencing of *MLH1*, which is commonly a sporadic alteration. In contrast to MSI-H tumors, MSI-L tumors arise through the chromosomal instability carcinogenesis pathway, like MSS tumors [28, 32].
- In addition to a conventional PCR-based assay, the MSI testing can be performed in a panel employing the technology of next-generation sequencing (NGS). Some laboratories started applying NGS for microsatellite status evaluations. Like PCR, in most cases, NGS-based MSI determination needs paired tumor and normal tissue. Recently, an MSI assay that uses data from a commercially available NGS panel has been established. One advantage of this NGS-based assay is that it does not require matched normal tissue samples. Furthermore, NGS-based methods cover a broader range of microsatellite loci and are not limited to the five microsatellite sites used in the PCR-based method. The disadvantages include higher costs per sample for NGS technology in addition to a longer turnaround time in comparison to PCR- and IHC-based MSI analysis methods [29].
- MSI-H and dMMR are often used as exchangeable terms by a lot of colleagues in literature and practice.

7. **What is the role of MMR/MSI testing in prediction of immune checkpoint inhibitor treatment in CRC?**
   - Two programmed cell death 1 (PD1)-blocking antibodies, nivolumab and pembrolizumab, have demonstrated efficacy in patients with metastatic CRC of MSI-H/dMMR, with a granted FDA approval [33]. In the current practice, MSI-H/dMMR CRC patients typically require the use of immune checkpoint inhibitors in the third-line setting after progression with conventional treatments. However, the National Comprehensive Cancer Network (NCCN) guidelines for colon cancer and rectal cancer recommend nivolumab, with or without low-dose ipilimumab or pembrolizumab for patients with MSI-H/dMMR tumors immediately after first-line treatment and as first-line treatment for patients for whom intensive therapy is not appropriate.
   - MSI-H/dMMR status is thus a predictive biomarker for response to immune checkpoint inhibitors in CRC and other solid tumors. Patients with MSI-H/dMMR mCRC demonstrate improved responses to checkpoint inhibitor therapy versus those with MSS/pMMR mCRC. The NCCN guidelines for colon cancer and rectal cancer recommend that all patients with CRC, regardless of stage, receive MSI or MMR testing at the time of initial diagnosis.
   - Due to poor antigenicity, microsatellite-stable tumors are more likely to be immunotherapy resistant. Strategies to improve tumor antigenicity including increasing tumor antigen and major histocompatibility complex class I molecule expression, together with the ones altering the tumor microenvironment by increasing T-cell infiltration and activation, and shifting the cytokine milieu toward interferon-γ production are under investigation [34, 35].
8. **What are the common clinical syndromes associated with GI tract polyposis and their genetic alterations?**
   - Since the first description of the GI tract polyposis in 1939, a group of syndromes have been described with the propensity to develop polyps in the upper and lower GI tracts with a potential to develop cancers. These syndromes are usually autosomal-dominantly inherited [36].
   - Familial adenomatous polyposis (FAP) is caused by a germline mutation in one of the *APC* (adenomatous polyposis coli) alleles on chromosome 5q21 and characterized by multiple adenomatous polyps in the large bowel with 100% lifetime risk of colorectal cancer. Germline mutations are mainly found in the 5′ half of the *APC* gene, particularly in codons 1061 and 1309 with majority of mutations being frameshifts or nonsense mutations, leading to truncated APC proteins. Meanwhile, somatic *APC* mutations are more fre-

quently found in the mutation cluster region of exon 15, between codons 1286 and 1513. In classic FAP, patients have innumerable (>100 to thousands) adenomatous polyps located at the colorectum. A milder disease variant, termed attenuated FAP (AFAP), is characterized by the presence of less than 100 polyps (oligo polyposis) at the presentation and later onset of CRC (on average 12 years later than in classic FAP). FAP patients also develop duodenal and gastric polyps, and extraintestinal malignancies [37]. Without prophylactic proctocolectomy, invasive carcinoma usually develops before the fifth decade of life.

- Juvenile polyposis syndrome (JPS) carries mutations in the *BMPR1A* and *SMAD4* genes leading to multiple noncancerous growths called juvenile polyps before age 20. However, "juvenile" refers to the characteristics of the tissue that makes up the polyps, not the ages of the patients. Another form of JPS is juvenile polyposis/hereditary hemorrhagic telangiectasia syndrome which is a condition that involves both arteriovenous malformations and a tendency to develop polyps in the GI tract. The American College of Gastroenterology recommends that individuals with five or more juvenile polyps in the colorectum or any numbers of juvenile polyps in other parts of the GI tract should undergo evaluation for JPS [27, 38].
- Peutz-Jeghers syndrome (PJS) is inherited in an autosomal-dominant pattern. In about half of all cases, an affected person inherits a mutation in the *STK11* gene from one affected parent [36, 38]. The remaining cases occur in people with no history of PJS in their family. The extracolonic anomalies described in PJS include bladder, renal pelvis, bronchial, and nasal polyps. Skeletal anomalies and bony tumors, as well as ovarian lesions, such as cysts, cystadenomas, and malignant tumors, may also be associated. The American College of Gastroenterology recommends that patients with perioral or buccal pigmentation and/or two or more histologically characteristic gastrointestinal hamartomatous polyps or a family history of PJS should be evaluated for PJS [27, 38].
- Hereditary mixed polyposis syndrome (HMPS) is inherited in an autosomal-dominant pattern that predisposes to an increased risk of developing cancer and polyps with no specific gene mutation identified so far [36]. However, some families have an inherited mutation in the *GREM1* gene, with a majority of Ashkenazi Jewish ancestry. Polyps show evidence of mixed elements, such as tubular, villous and sessile adenomas, and atypical juvenile polyps with adenomatous and/or hyperplastic features.
- PTEN hamartoma tumor syndromes (Cowden and Bannayan-Riley-Ruvalcaba syndromes): both conditions can be caused by mutations in the *PTEN* gene with about half of all people with Bannayan-Riley-Ruvalcaba syndrome developing hamartomas in their intestines, known as hamartomatous polyps [36]. At least half of the affected infants have macrocephaly, and many also have a high birth weight and macrosomia. Other noncancerous growths often associated with Bannayan-Riley-Ruvalcaba syndrome include lipomas and angiolipomas. The American College of Gastroenterology recommends that individuals with multiple gastrointestinal hamartomas or ganglioneuromas should be evaluated for Cowden syndrome and related conditions [27].
- Cronkhite-Canada syndrome (CCS) has been described in 1955, by Cronkhite and Canada. CCS still has an obscure etiopathogenesis. Given the increased IgG4 mononuclear cell staining in CCS polyps, an autoimmune mechanism may be involved [39]. Malignant transformation of CCS polyps may occur, and the risk of CRC may warrant aggressive screening in CCS patients.

9. **What are the emerging molecular targeted therapies for hepatocellular carcinoma (HCC)? What is the role of NGS technology in the clinical management of HCC?**
   - Hepatocellular carcinoma (HCC) exhibits a diversity of molecular phenotypes that challenge the clinical management [40–42]. The integration of NGS technology into molecular characterization of HCC has provided a genetic landscape with multiple potential genetic targets to aid drug development of targeted therapy for advanced HCC [42].
   - Multiple studies have now identified common driver mutations among HCC tumors from patients with different ethnicities and etiologies. These most prevalent driver mutations are *TERT*, *CTNNB1*, *TP53*, *AXIN1*, *ARID1A*, and *ARID1B*, which unfortunately are commonly seen as "non-druggable."
   - Recent advances in the molecular field have managed to take NGS a step closer to directly affecting clinical care in HCC. Using MSK-IMPACT, an FDA-approved panel of 468 genes, is able to identify mutations that portend worse outcomes both with sorafenib and immune checkpoint inhibitors. Patients with oncogenic PI3K-mTOR alterations had significantly worse outcomes than those without when treated with sorafenib. Similarly, patients with an activating mutation of WNT/β-catenin were resistant to checkpoint inhibitor therapy [43]. In the last several years, successful novel types of drugs have emerged for clinical use [44]. As recommended by the updated Barcelona Clinic Liver Cancer (BCLC) treatment algorithms [45], the drugs can be categorized into the first-line

Table 8.3 Molecular targeted, immune, and combination therapies in HCC

Drug	Molecular target/Biomarker	Combination therapy	Molecular target/Biomarker
Sorafenib	VEGFR1/2/3; PDGFR; Ras/Raf/Mek/Erk	Atezolizumab + bevacizumab	PD-L1/VEGFA
Lenvatinib	VEGFR1/2/3; FGFR1/2/3/4; FGF; PDGFR2; RET	Durvalumab +/− tremelimumab	PD-L1/CTLA-4
Regorafenib	VEGFR1; RETRAF1; TIE-2; BRAF; PDGFR; FGFR	Nivolumab +/− ipilimumab	PD-1/CTLA-4
Cabozantinib	c-Met; VEGFR1/2/3	Galunisertib + sorafenib	TGF-βR1/VEGFRs, C-KIT, PDGFRB, RAF
Ramucirumab	VEGFR2	Mogamulizumab + nivolumab	CCR4/PD-1
Bevacizumab	VEGF	Pembrolizumab + epacadostat	PD-1/IDO1
Brivanib	VEGF; FGFR	Galunisertib + nivolumab	TGF-βR1/PD-1
Linifanib	VEGF; PDGFR	Apatinib + SHR1210	VEGFR2/PD-1
Sunitinib	VEGFR; PDGFRa/b; c-Kit	Spartalizumab +/− capmatinib	PD-1/MET
Erlotinib	EGFR	FGF401 +/− spartalizumab	FGFR4/PD-1
Cetuximab	EGFR	Pembrolizumab + sorafenib	PD-1/VEGFRs, C-KIT, PDGFRB, RAF
Lapatinib	EGFR	Pembrolizumab + lenvatinib	PD-1/VEGFR2, VEGFR3
Sirolimus	PI3K/Akt/mTOR	Spartalizumab + sorafenib	PD-1/VEGFRs, C-KIT, PDGFRB, RAF
Everolimus	PI3K/Akt/mTOR	Regorafenib + pembrolizumab	VEGFRs, FGFRs, C-KIT, PDGFRs, RAF/PD-1
Tivantinib	C-Met	Cabozantinib + nivolumab	MET, VEGFRs/PD-1
Tremelimumab	CTLA-4	Avelumab + axitinib	PD-L1/VEGFRs, C-KIT, PDGFRs
Nivolumab	PD-1	Ramucirumab + durvalumab	VEGFR2/PD-L1
Pembrolizumab	PD-1	XL888 + pembrolizumab	Hsp90/PD-1

and second-line ones, with targets including varied growth factors (Table 8.3). Other molecules, such as the selective CDK4/6inhibitors, are in the earlier stages of clinical development [46].

10. **What is the morpho-molecular classification of HCC in correlation to clinicohistologic features?**
    - HCC could be divided into two types based on proliferation: proliferative and non-proliferative. The latter has the characteristics of chromosomal stability and maintenance of expression of hepatocytic markers. They generally display a well-differentiated phenotype and constitute a homogeneous subtype with cholestasis and microtrabecular and pseudoglandular architectural patterns [47]. On the other hand, the proliferative HCC is associated with chromosomal instability and *TP53* mutations. They are usually poorly differentiated and include tumors with progenitor features. A morphological variant of proliferative HCC, for example, macro trabecular-massive (MTM-HCC) subtype, is associated with angiogenesis activation, *TP53* mutations, and *FGF19* amplifications [47]. Given the distinct molecular and histological features, the proposed subtypes of HCC are briefly summarized as follows and Table 8.4. In addition to these, morphological subtypes including lympoepithelioma-like HCC, combined hepatocellular-cholangiocarcinoma, sarcomatoid HCC and more are rare and with unclear molecular genetic changes.
    - Macro trabecular-massive HCC occurs in HBV-infected patients with high alpha-fetoprotein serum levels. It exhibits a very aggressive phenotype, with frequent satellite nodules and macrovascular and/or microvascular invasion. Angiogenesis activation associated gene expression is a hallmark feature.
    - Scirrhous HCC has abundant, dense fibrous stroma with the expression of various progenitor or cancer stem cell genes, including *CK7* (*KRT7*), *CK19* (*KRT19*), *THY1*, or *CD133* (*PROM1*). It also often show activation of transforming growth factor beta (TGF-β) pathway/epithelial-to-mesenchymal transition, with overexpression of *VIM, SNAIL (SNAI1), SMAD4* and *TWIST*.
    - Steatohepatitis HCC with morphological features of alcoholic or nonalcoholic steatohepatitis, with ballooned cells, Mallory bodies, and steatosis. It may be associated with overexpression of C-reactive protein – a target gene of JAK/STAT signalling pathway. Also this variant very rarely harbors Wnt/β-catenin pathway activation.
    - *CTNNB1*-mutated HCC shows retained expression of various genes involved in hepatocellular differentia-

Table 8.4 Morpho-molecular classification of HCC

Subtypes	Phenotypical features	Molecular mechanisms	Genetic alterations
Macro tubular-massive	CK19 expression; satellite nodules; Vascular invasion	Angiogenesis cell proliferation Lack of immune infiltration	*TP53/FGF19*
Progenitor	CK19 + PDL1 expression	TGFB, NOTCH, IGF2 pathways	*TP53*, CIN
CTNNB1	Glutamine synthase	Bile salt transporter dysregulation	*CTNNB1*
Steatohepatitis	Loss of CPR expression; Loss of satellite nodules/vascular invasion	JAK/STAT pathway Infiltration by T cells and neutrophils	*CTNNB1*, *TP53*, *TERT*
Scirrhous	CK19 expression	EMT activation	*CTNNB1*, *TSC1/TSC2*

tion and function, such as *APOB*, *ALB*, *HNF1A*, or *HNF4A*. HCCs with mutations in *CTNNB1* display a particular phenotype with well-differentiated morphology, microtrabecular and pseudoglandular architectural patterns, intratumour cholestasis and lack of immune infiltration.

- Progenitor HCC may be the result of a dedifferentiation of neoplastic hepatocytes or reflect the malignant transformation of hepatic progenitor cells. Neoplastic cells of progenitor HCC are characterized by CK19 expression.
- Fibrolamellar HCC is a well-established and rare (<1%) subtype of HCC with microscopic examination showing compact clusters of cells embedded in a lamellar, hyaline, and fibrotic stroma. Pure ones harbor a unique gene expression profile, with overexpression of *ERBB2*, and various neuroendocrine genes including *PCSK1*, *NTS*, *CALCA*, and *DNAJB1-PRKACA* fusion.

11. **What is the genetic landscape of pancreatic cancer and its potential clinical significance?**
    - Pancreatic carcinogenesis is a stepwise successive accumulation of gene mutations during the transformation of a pre-invasive pancreatic lesion to pancreatic cancer, particularly, pancreatic ductal adenocarcinoma (PDAC) [48, 49]. In addition to activating mutations in *KRAS*, the most common genetic alterations, mutations in other driver genes such as *CDKN2A*, *TP53*, or *SMAD4* are randomly associated to *KRAS* mutations, generating a heterogeneous genetic landscape between patients [50–52]. The pivotal molecular alterations that define the development of pancreatic tumors could be classified into three categories: oncogenes, tumor-suppressor genes, and genome-maintenance genes as shown in Table 8.5 [53, 54].
    - PDAC, recently, has been classified into clinical subgroups based on the predominant genomic profiles including basal-like, stroma-activated, desmoplastic, pure classical, and immune classical types [55]. The Cancer Genome Atlas has identified *KRAS*, *TP53*, *SMAD4*, and *CDKN2A* as the most commonly mutated genes in the mutational landscape of pancreatic adenocarcinomas [56]. Integrated whole-genome analysis identified ongoing genomic instability due to aberrations in mutant genes *KRAS* and *GATA6* [57].

Table 8.5 Genetic landscape of pancreatic tumors

Genetic mutations (%)	Tumor type
KRAS (95%) *TP53* (35–40%) *CDKN2A/p16* (95–100%) *SMAD4* (45–60%)	PDAC
KRAS (45–50%) *GNAS* (30–50%)	IPMN
KRAS (20–50%) *GNAS* (25–50%)	MCNs
KRAS (70%) *TP53* (20%) *GNAS* (5%)	PanIN
CTNNB1 (90–100%)	SPN
APC (50–60%) *CTNNB1* (30–40%) *TP53* (30–40%)	PAAC
VHL (40–50%)	SCA
MEN1 (10–30%)	P-NETs

Abbreviations: *PDAC* pancreatic ductal adenocarcinoma, *IPMN* intraductal papillary-mucinous neoplasm, *MCNs* mucinous cystic neoplasms, *PanIN* pancreatic intraepithelial neoplasia, *SPN* solid-pseudopapillary neoplasm, *PACC* pancreatic acinar cell carcinoma, *SCA* serous cystadenoma of the pancreas, *p-NETs* pancreatic neuroendocrine tumors

- In addition to the above genetic mutations, chromosomal abnormalities are involved in pancreatic carcinogenesis including allelic loss mainly in chromosomes 17p, 18q, 9p, 12q and less often in 1p, 6p, 6q, 8p, 10p, 10q, 12p, 21q, and 22q. Cases with chromosomal additions have been documented as well, such as in chromosomes 7 and 20.11. Many tumor suppressor genes are positioned in these locations, e.g., *TP53* at chromosome 17p, *SMAD4* at chromosome 18q, and *p16INK4a* (*MTS1*) gene at chromosome 9p [53, 58].
- Although over 90% of PDACs harbor activating mutations in *KRAS*, the inhibition of RAS activation or its downstream signaling with inhibitors has not demonstrated a significant benefit yet. More than six signaling pathways stem from RAS; if one is impaired, the others can pick up the slack or circumvent it. PI3K pathway inhibition when combined

with RAF-MEK- ERK inhibition is currently under investigation [59, 60].

- According to the current NCCN Guidelines of Oncology for Pancreatic Adenocarcinoma, version 1.2020, all patients with pancreatic cancer should undergo genetic testing including *BRCA1*, *BRCA2*, *CDH1*, *PALB2*, *PTEN*, and *TP53* genes.

12. **What is the significance of molecular diagnostics in cytologic samples of pancreatobiliary lesions? What is the role of NGS technology?**
   - The cytopathologic evaluation of pancreatic lesions is an extremely valuable technique widely used to diagnose and characterize pancreatic lesions with a minimal risk to patients. The increased use of endoscopic ultrasound-guided fine-needle aspiration (EUS-FNA) has further improved the procurement of cellular samples of targeted lesions [52, 61]. The collected cytologic samples are used for morphological, chemical, and molecular analysis for diagnosis and presurgical risk stratification. For example, the combination of endoscopic ultrasound-guided cytopathology and *RAS* mutation assay has been proved to improve the diagnosis of pancreatic cancer with reducing false-negative results compared to cytopathology alone [61–63].
   - Pancreatic cysts are a heterogeneous group of lesions that include injury and inflammation-related nonneoplastic conditions and neoplasms. Most neoplastic cysts are of ductal mucinous lineage mainly as intraductal papillary-mucinous neoplasms (IPMN) and mucinous cystic neoplasm (MCN), in addition to serous lineage (serous cystadenoma and rarely cystadenocarcinoma). The addition of molecular testing could be particularly helpful in cases where cytology and CEA are noncontributory and thus significantly improve the sensitivity of pancreatic cyst fluid analysis. One of the proposed working algorithms in this regard is shown in Fig. 8.3, although none has been

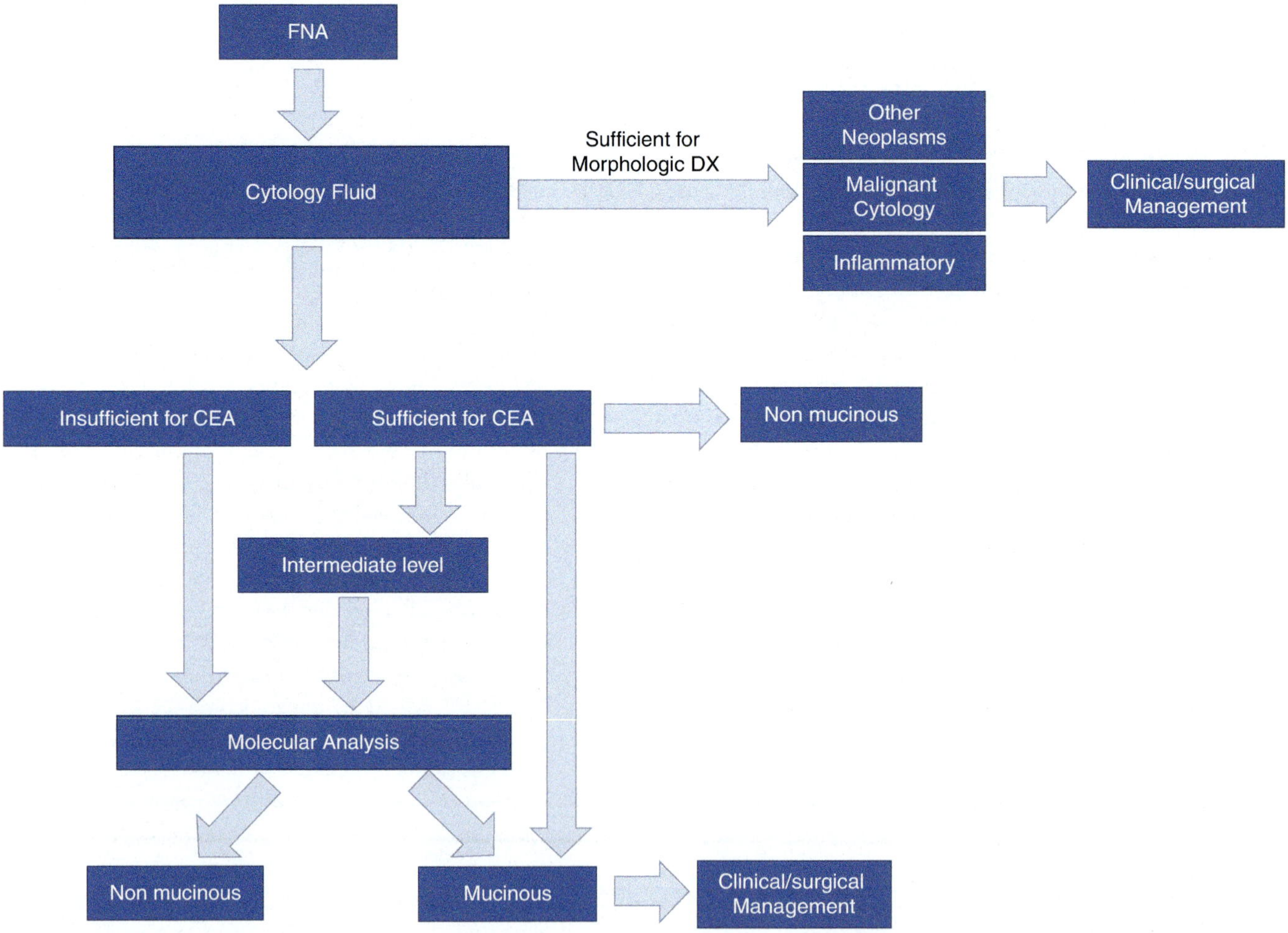

Fig. 8.3 A proposed algorithm for the role of molecular diagnostics in preoperative cytological workup of pancreatic cystic lesions and risk stratification

formally recommended by a major organization guideline.

- A recent study has shown that analysis of *KRAS* and loss of heterozygosity significantly help in the differential diagnosis of cystic mucinous pancreatic lesions (IPMN and MCN) when preoperative cytology is not sufficient or carcinoembryonic antigen (CEA) levels in cyst fluid are indeterminate [61]. Studies showed that 91% of the IPMNs had a mutation in either *KRAS* or *GNAS*, and almost half had a mutation in both genes [61, 62]. The biomarkers were able to detect serous cystadenomas and MCNs with 91% and 75% specificity, respectively, and 100% sensitivity, and IPMNs with 97% specificity and 76% sensitivity.
- NGS, given its high throughput and sensitive nature, is a favorable molecular assay platform particularly when only a limited amount of cyst fluid could be aspirated [61]. Several studies have proved increased sensitivity and specificity using NGS analysis of EUS-FNA samples for the diagnosis of pancreatic lesions of malignant potential. Similarly, studies have also demonstrated increased sensitivity and specificity using NGS analysis of EUS-FNA samples than other conventional mutation analysis for the diagnosis of pancreatic solid tumors. In pancreatic FNA specimens, NGS analysis of *KRAS* mutations have increased clinical sensitivity up to 74%, which is far superior to the values obtained by both allele-specific real-time PCR (52.8%) and Sanger sequencing (42.1%), with maintaining clinical specificity at 100% [52].
- With bile duct brushings, the addition of fluorescence in situ hybridization (FISH) to cytology is an established ancillary test for the diagnosis of bile duct carcinoma. Meanwhile, NGS is as sensitive as the analysis of aneuploidy by FISH for identifying pancreatobiliary duct malignancies in preoperative settings [61].

Case Presentations

Case 1

Learning Objective

Current routine molecular testing algorithm and interpretation for CRC patients

Case History

A 65-year-old gentleman with a history of colorectal cancer status post colectomy and chemo-adjuvant therapy 2 years ago is now presenting with multiple lesions in the liver and lung by radiographic imaging. A biopsy of the liver lesions was performed and sent to pathology laboratory for evaluation.

Surgical Pathology Findings

Metastatic colorectal adenocarcinoma; IHCs show loss of nuclear expression of MLH1 and PMS2 in tumor cells, while MSH2 and MSH6 expressions are intact (Fig. 8.4).

Molecular Genetic Findings

KRAS and *NRAS* mutational analysis is negative, while *BRAF* mutational testing reveal the presence of V600E mutation.

Final Diagnosis/Summary

Metastatic colorectal adenocarcinoma; dMMR, low probability of Lynch syndrome

Follow-Up

The patient received checkpoint immunotherapy and shows improvement.

Discussion

Selecting CRC patients particularly those with end-stage or metastatic tumors for monoclonal antibody therapies targeting EGFR requires the molecular mutational analysis of *KRAS* and *NRAS* gene codons 12, 13, 59, 61, 117, and 146. The presence of a mutation excludes patients from this treatment. In general, *BRAF* mutational analysis is also included in an initial testing panel. Patients with mutant *BRAF* typically seem to have a poor response to the treatment as well, although *BRAF* testing for this predictive purpose has not officially been recommended. *BRAF* p.V600 mutational analysis should be performed in patients with CRC indeed for the purposes of prognostic stratification. Other molecular markers that are potentially with clinical significance in EGFR signaling transduction pathways such as *PIK3CA* and *PTEN* have been suggested. A recent study suggested *PIK3CA* mutations may have clinical prognostic information in tumor stages I–III and that PIK3CA/PTEN deregulation, in addition to *KRAS* and *BRAF* mutations, are considered a biomarker of the drug resistance.

In addition to the role in screening for Lynch syndrome and some prognostic significance, the MSI-H/dMMR status is a predictive biomarker for response to immune checkpoint inhibitors in CRC and other solid tumors. Patients with MSI-H/dMMR mCRC demonstrate improved responses with checkpoint inhibitor therapy versus those with MSS/pMMR mCRC. The NCCN guidelines for colon cancer and rectal cancer recommend that all patients with CRC, regardless of stage, receive MSI or MMR testing at the time of initial diagnosis. Of note, *ERBB2* (*HER2*) amplification and *NTRK* fusions have also become a part of routinely tested

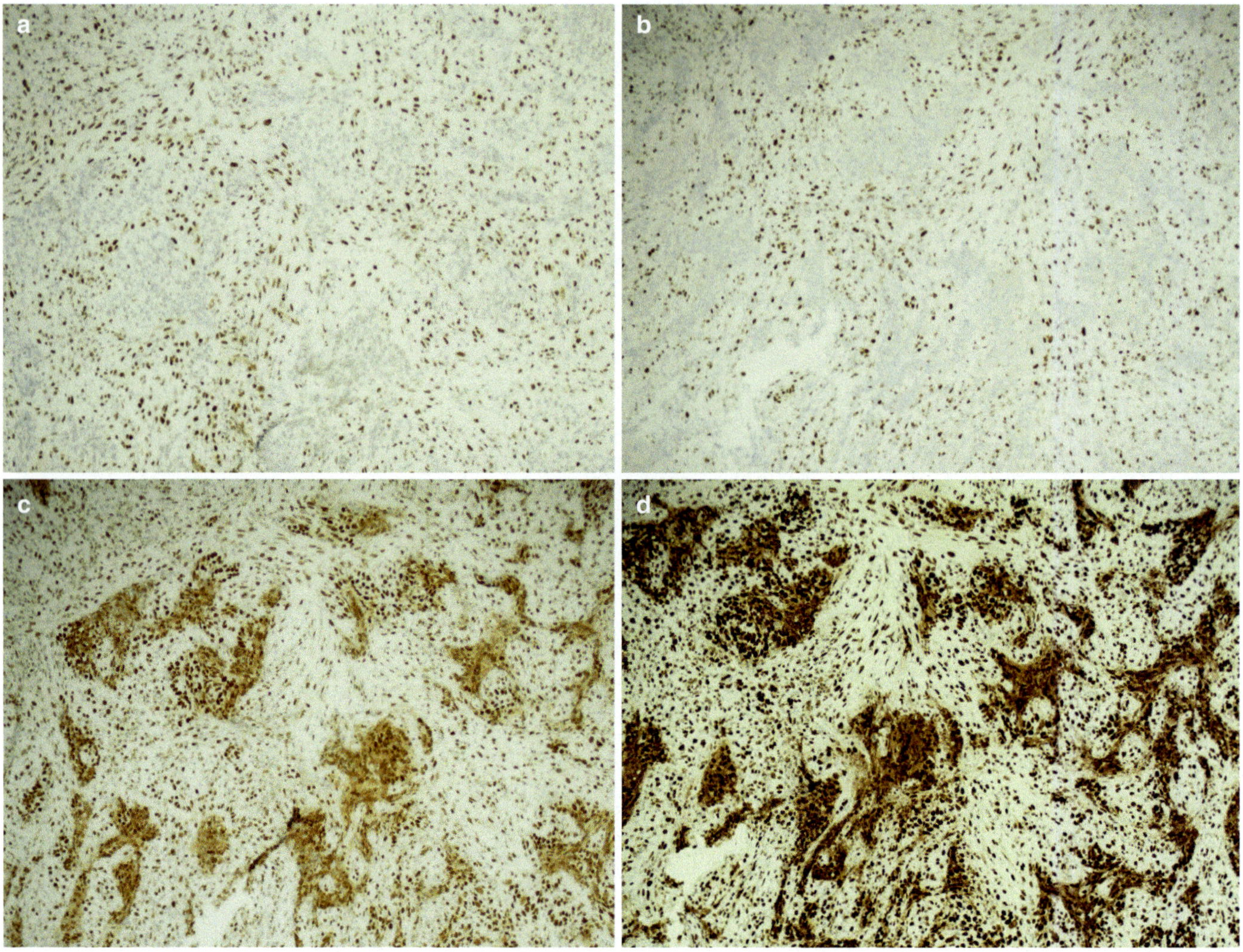

Fig. 8.4 Immunostains of MMR proteins for case 1 show loss of nuclear expression of MLH1 (**a**) and PMS2 (**b**) proteins in tumor cells while intact expression of MSH2 (**c**) and MSH6 (**d**) proteins. Tumor surrounding stromal and inflammatory cells are used as an internal positive control

biomarkers due to the availability/approval of targeting therapies for CRC patients.

Case 2

Learning Objective

Current screening algorithm for Lynch syndrome in CRC patients and unusual result interpretation

Case History

A 53-year-old woman recently developed bowel habit changes but with no substantial change in her weight, diet, or appetite. Colonoscopy revealed a large mass in the mid-colon, and following staging CT scans confirmed a circumferential mass without evidence for distant metastatic diseases. She has a strong family history of breast cancer with her mother and aunt.

Surgical Pathology Findings

Invasive moderately differentiated colorectal adenocarcinoma; IHCs show complete loss of MLH1 and PMS2, partial loss of MSH2 and MSH6 nuclear expression in tumor cells (Fig. 8.5).

Molecular Genetic Findings

KRAS, *NRAS* and *BRAF* mutational analysis is negative.

Final Diagnosis/Summary

Invasive moderately differentiated colorectal adenocarcinoma; high probability of Lynch syndrome; genetic counselling and/or MMR gene sequencing is recommended.

Follow-Up

Extended right hemicolectomy was conducted and revealed a 9.4-cm pT3N2b adenocarcinoma. The patient was also seen by a genetic counselor. A specimen was sent to an out-

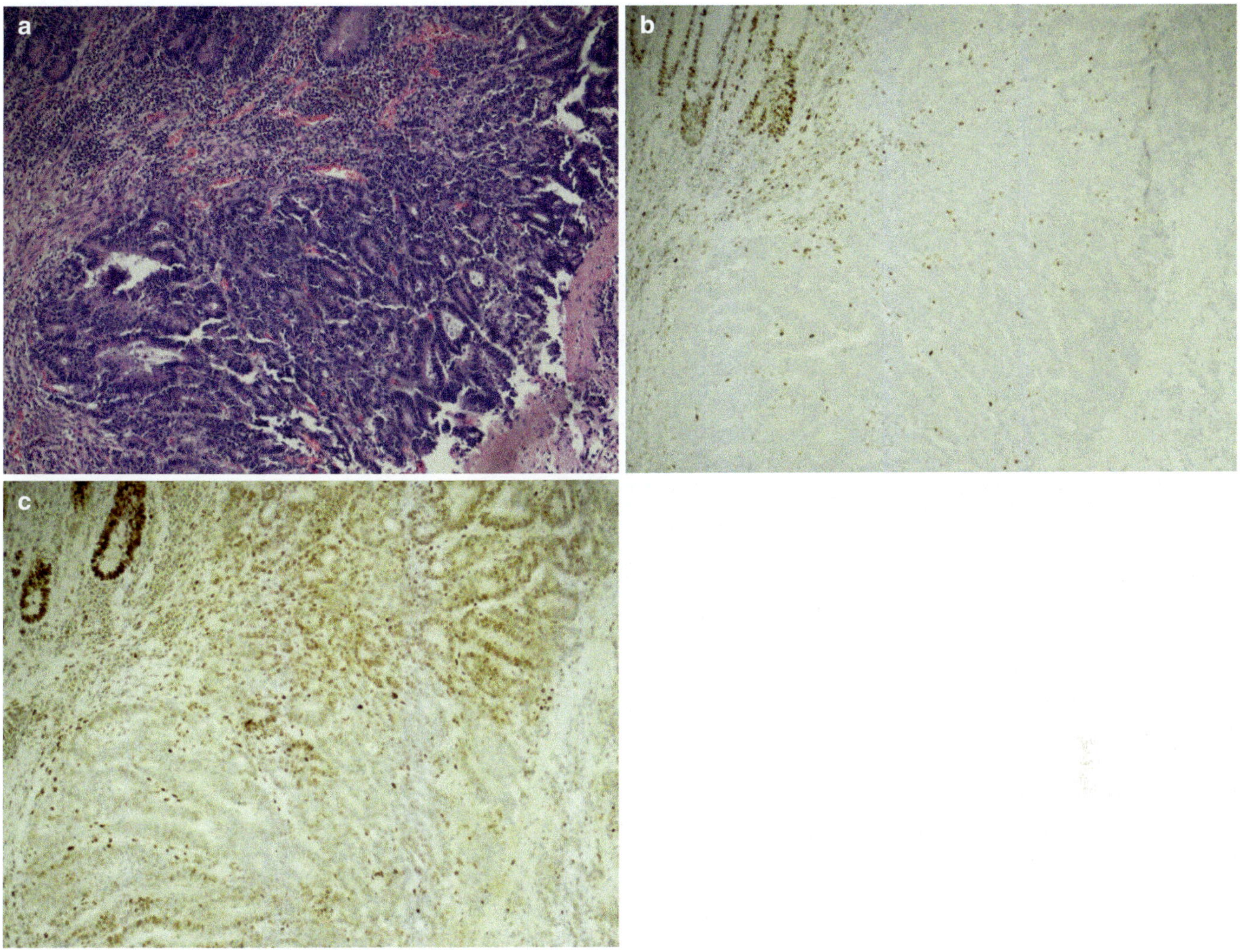

Fig. 8.5 (**a**) H&E stain shows benign colonic epithelium (on the left) and CRC (on the right) for case 2. Immunostains of MMR proteins show complete loss of nuclear expression of MLH1/PMS2 in tumor cells (**b**), while partial loss of MSH2/MSH6 (**c**). Surrounding stromal and inflammatory cells are used as an internal positive control

side lab with the patient's consent for genetic sequencing of MMR genes which reveal a germline mutation in the *MLH1* gene.

Discussion

dMMR results in the accumulation of genetic mutations in cancer-related genes and eventually tumorigenesis. The occurrence of dMMR could be sporadic in origin, or result from germline changes in an autosomal-dominant-inherited predisposition condition, such as Lynch syndrome [23]. Patients with Lynch syndrome are vulnerable to the development of different types of cancers earlier in their lives than normal population. CRC is the most common one. The American College of Gastroenterology requires that all newly diagnosed colorectal cancers (CRCs) should be evaluated for mismatch repair deficiency.

A testing algorithm combining clinical presentation, MMR IHCs, and MSI and other molecular tests on CRC tumor tissue has been developed to assess the MMR status and furtherly the risk of patients for Lynch syndrome (Fig. 8.2). Evaluation may be initiated by immunohistochemical stains for the MLH1/MSH2/MSH6/PMS2 proteins or molecular testing for microsatellite instability. IHC staining is the widely adopted initial step due to its better feasibility and cost efficiency. The most common dMMR pattern demonstrated with IHC is MLH1 and PMS2 loss of nuclear expression in tumor cells. As to this scenario, if with a *BRAF* (V600F) mutation and/or hypermethylation of *MLH1* promotor area present, the CRC is likely of sporadic dMMR. Otherwise and other common protein loss patterns include PMS2 loss with intact MLH1, MSH6 and/or MSH2 loss are all considered with an increased likelihood of Lynch syndrome with a strong indication for further evaluation, e.g., MMR gene sequencing. Under this circumstance, a genetic counselling should be first recommended.

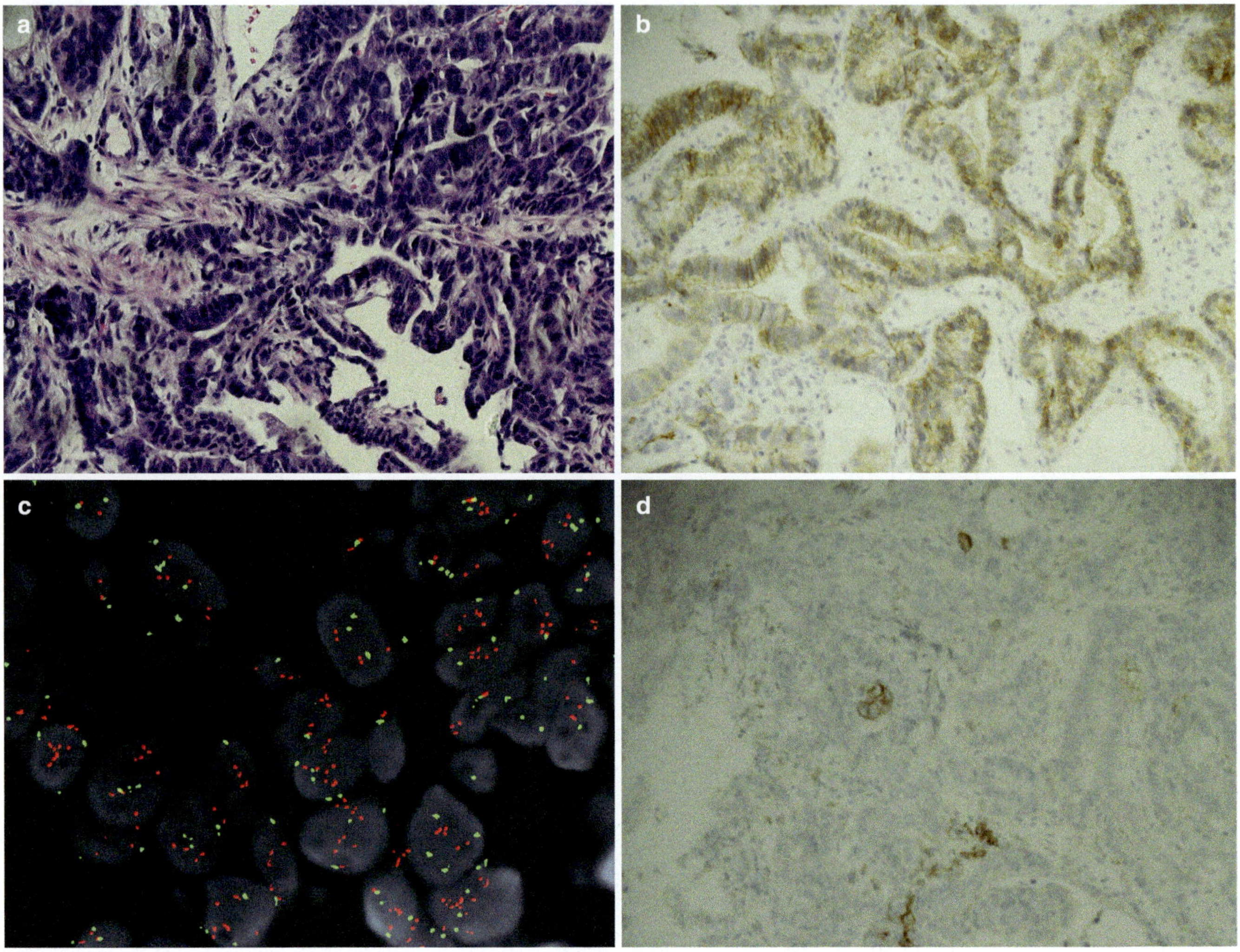

Fig. 8.6 (**a**) H&E stain shows gastric adenocarcinoma for case 3. (**b**) Immunostains of HER2 proteins show equivocal staining score (2+); a subsequent FISH study is negative for *HER2* amplification (**c**). PD-L1 IHC shows a CPS >1% (**d**)

Rarely, unusual IHC patterns can be seen. For example, in the case presented above, it is still unclear why there is partial loss of MSH2/MSH6 in addition to MLH1/PMS2 loss. Overall, they may represent a real dMMR status or are due to artifacts. To accurately interpret an unusual IHC pattern of MMR proteins, a few suggestions may be considered: (1) verify internal and external controls, particularly take advantage of tumor surrounding non-tumor cells (e.g., stromal cells and inflammatory cells) as an internal positive staining control; (2) be aware of unusual but real dMMR staining patterns and manifestations of common staining artifacts; (3) consider another methodology such as MSI molecular testing when IHCs result are undeterminable. In general, PCR based MSI testing generates less ambiguous cases than IHCs, although it is more costly and cannot tell which protein is lost when a MSI-high status is identified; and (4) repeat the IHCs if a staining artifact is suspected. Of note, clinical presentation, MMR IHC studies, or MSI tests are not 100% accurate in the detection of dMMR/MSI-H tumors [23, 26]. Combining them together with or without other molecular tests should allow MMR status clarification for most cases.

Case 3

Learning Objective

Current HER2 testing algorithm for gastric adenocarcinoma and the role of PD-L1 IHC in prediction of immune checkpoint inhibitor therapy

Case History

A 57-year-old man with past medical histories of hyperlipidemia, hypertension, and known severe CAD is now presenting with complaints of centrally located chest pain, associated shortness of breath, diaphoresis, nausea, and recent weight loss. Upper GI endoscopy reveals a malignant appearing gastric mass near the gastroesophageal junction, and a biopsy was performed. Imaging studies shows multiple small lung and liver lesions highly suspicious for metastases.

Surgical Pathology Findings

Invasive moderately differentiated gastric adenocarcinoma (Fig. 8.6a). By IHC, Her-2/neu expression is equivocal (score 2+) (Fig. 8.6b).

Molecular Genetic Findings

FISH shows "not amplified": HER2/CEN-17 ratio 1.8 (Reference range: <2) (Fig. 8.6c).

Final Diagnosis/Summary

Invasive moderately differentiated gastric adenocarcinoma; negative for HER2 amplification

Follow-Up

Due to the patients' existing medical morbidities and clinical evidence of liver and lung metastases, the clinical team excluded him as a surgical candidate; immune checkpoint inhibitor therapy was brought up. Per request, an IHC stain of PD-L1 was performed, and a CPS score of >1 was reported (Fig. 8.6d).

Discussion

With the approval of HER2 targeting therapy for patients with advanced gastric cancer, an assessment of HER2 overexpression/amplification to select patients eligible for this treatment is recommended for any patient with gastric and GEJ adenocarcinomas (locally advanced, recurrent, or metastatic) based on the guidelines of ASCO, CAP, and ASCP [2]. A HER2 testing algorithm (Fig. 8.7) in gastric adenocarcinoma, like the one in breast cancers, include an initial evaluation of the protein expression levels by IHC. Positive (IHC 3+) or negative (IHC 0 or 1+) HER2 IHC results will be reported, respectively, without further studies. However, the equivocal cases of HER2 with a score of 2+ on IHC will warrant a FISH assay according to the currently recommended testing algorithms [4].

In addition to MSI-H/dMMR status in CRC and other solid tumors as discussed above, predictive biomarkers that have been extensively studied and used in clinical and/or scientific settings for checkpoint immune therapy predominantly include the expression of PD-1 and PD-L1, tumor inflammatory microenvironment, and tumor mutational burden [64]. The FDA has approved companion PD-L1 diagnostic tests in a variety of tumor types. However, each companion test uses its own reagents, working conditions, and interpretation criteria. To predict the response to immune checkpoint inhibitors in patients with gastric/GEJ adenocarcinomas by PD-L1 IHC, a concept of the combined positive score (CPS) was proposed. It was employed as part of a companion diagnostics package approved by the FDA in 2017 for the treatment of gastric adenocarcinoma with pembrolizumab [65]. To calculate a CPS, the pathologist must count the number of PD-L1-positive cells including tumor cells, lymphocytes, and

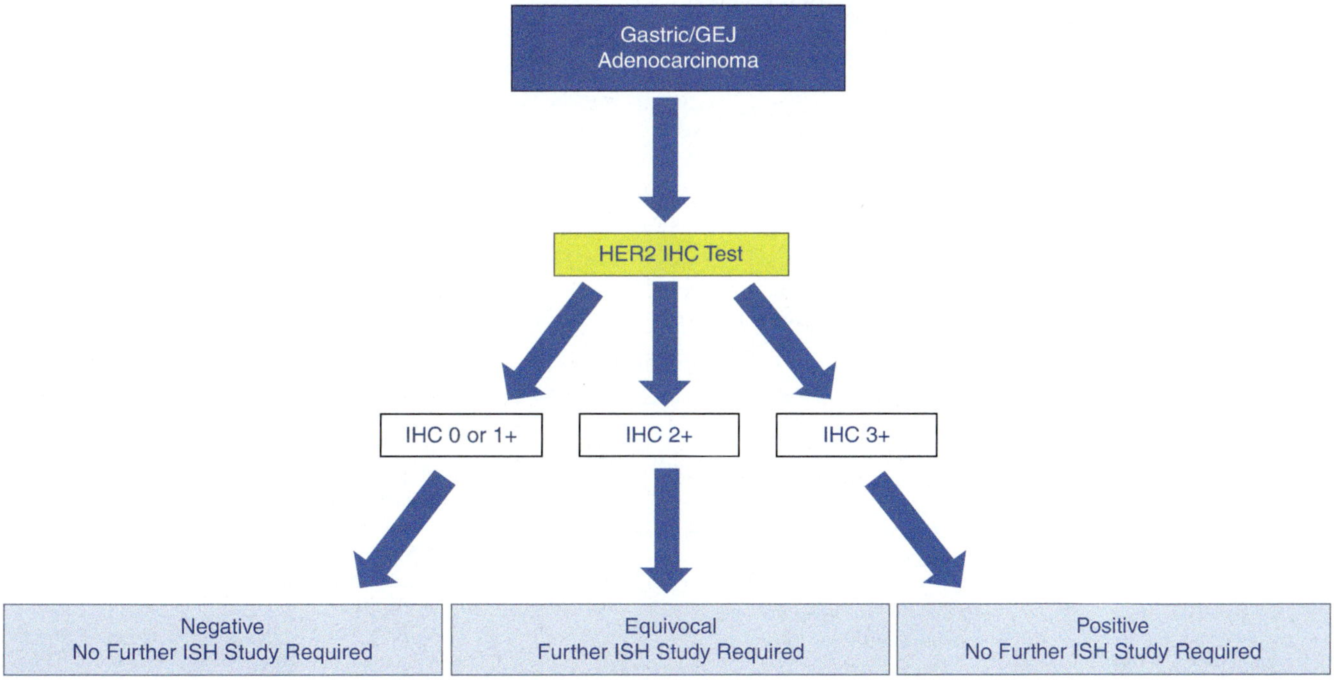

Fig. 8.7 An algorithm of HER2 amplification testing in gastric/GEJ adenocarcinoma, which is commonly initiated with IHC for HER2 protein and subsequently followed by a FISH assay if the IHC score is equivocal

macrophages; divide that total by the number of viable tumor cells; and multiply by 100. For gastric or GEJ adenocarcinoma, a CPS score ≥1 recognizes responders who are eligible for treatment with pembrolizumab. CPS ≥1 is the minimum PD-L1 expression threshold for patients to qualify for treatment with pembrolizumab; however, studies have suggested that patients with higher CPS scores may gain greater benefit [66]. The PD-L1 antibody used in the approved companion diagnostic panel is 22C3 primary antibody from Dako; therefore, another interesting issue is whether different PD-L1 antibodies from different vendors may have similar predictive values with similar interpretation criteria. This currently remains unclear until large-scale studies are conducted.

References

1. Milne AN, et al. Nature meets nurture: molecular genetics of gastric cancer. Hum Genet. 2009;126(5):615–28.
2. Azarhoosh R, Ebneghasem R, Besharat S. HER-2/neu gene amplification in gastric adenocarcinoma and its relationship with clinical and pathological findings. J Gastrointest Oncol. 2017;8(6):1046–50.
3. Abrahao-Machado LF, Scapulatempo-Neto C. HER2 testing in gastric cancer: an update. World J Gastroenterol. 2016;22(19):4619–25.
4. Zhao D, Klempner SJ, Chao J. Progress and challenges in HER2-positive gastroesophageal adenocarcinoma. J Hematol Oncol. 2019;12(1):50.
5. Cancer Genome Atlas Research N. Comprehensive molecular characterization of gastric adenocarcinoma. Nature. 2014;513(7517):202–9.
6. Serra O, et al. Comparison and applicability of molecular classifications for gastric cancer. Cancer Treat Rev. 2019;77:29–34.
7. Casali PG, et al. Gastrointestinal stromal tumours: ESMO-EURACAN Clinical Practice Guidelines for diagnosis, treatment and follow-up. Ann Oncol. 2018;29(Suppl 4):iv267.
8. Niinuma T, Suzuki H, Sugai T. Molecular characterization and pathogenesis of gastrointestinal stromal tumor. Transl Gastroenterol Hepatol. 2018;3:2.
9. Oppelt PJ, Hirbe AC, Van Tine BA. Gastrointestinal stromal tumors (GISTs): point mutations matter in management, a review. J Gastrointest Oncol. 2017;8(3):466–73.
10. Heinrich MC, et al. PDGFRA activating mutations in gastrointestinal stromal tumors. Science. 2003;299(5607):708–10.
11. Boikos SA, et al. Molecular subtypes of KIT/PDGFRA wild-type gastrointestinal stromal tumors: a report from the National Institutes of Health Gastrointestinal Stromal Tumor Clinic. JAMA Oncol. 2016;2(7):922–8.
12. Serrano C, George S. Gastrointestinal stromal tumor: challenges and opportunities for a new decade. Clin Cancer Res. 2020;26(19):5078–85.
13. Li GZ, Raut CP. Targeted therapy and personalized medicine in gastrointestinal stromal tumors: drug resistance, mechanisms, and treatment strategies. Onco Targets Ther. 2019;12:5123–33.
14. Tan S, et al. Genomic subtypes of GISTs for stratifying patient response to sunitinib following imatinib resistance: a pooled analysis and systematic review. Dis Markers. 2018;2018:1368617.
15. Demetri GD, et al. Efficacy and safety of imatinib mesylate in advanced gastrointestinal stromal tumors. N Engl J Med. 2002;347(7):472–80.
16. Siegel RL, Miller KD, Jemal A. Cancer statistics, 2020. CA Cancer J Clin. 2020;70(1):7–30.
17. Siegel RL, et al. Colorectal cancer statistics, 2020. CA Cancer J Clin. 2020;70:145.
18. Pritchard CC, Grady WM. Colorectal cancer molecular biology moves into clinical practice. Gut. 2011;60(1):116–29.
19. Merla A, Goel S. Novel drugs targeting the epidermal growth factor receptor and its downstream pathways in the treatment of colorectal cancer: a systematic review. Chemother Res Pract. 2012;2012:387172.
20. Sepulveda AR, et al. Molecular biomarkers for the evaluation of colorectal cancer: guideline from the American Society for Clinical Pathology, College of American Pathologists, Association for Molecular Pathology, and American Society of Clinical Oncology. Arch Pathol Lab Med. 2017;141(5):625–57.
21. Eklof V, et al. The prognostic role of KRAS, BRAF, PIK3CA and PTEN in colorectal cancer. Br J Cancer. 2013;108(10):2153–63.
22. Lee MKC, Loree JM. Current and emerging biomarkers in metastatic colorectal cancer. Curr Oncol. 2019;26(Suppl 1):S7–S15.
23. Richman S. Deficient mismatch repair: read all about it (review). Int J Oncol. 2015;47(4):1189–202.
24. Engel C, et al. Associations of pathogenic variants in MLH1, MSH2, and MSH6 with risk of colorectal adenomas and tumors and with somatic mutations in patients with lynch syndrome. Gastroenterology. 2020;158(5):1326–33.
25. Olkinuora A, et al. Molecular basis of mismatch repair protein deficiency in tumors from lynch suspected cases with negative germline test results. Cancers (Basel). 2020;12(7):1.
26. Funkhouser WK Jr, et al. Relevance, pathogenesis, and testing algorithm for mismatch repair-defective colorectal carcinomas: a report of the association for molecular pathology. J Mol Diagn. 2012;14(2):91–103.
27. Syngal S, et al. ACG clinical guideline: genetic testing and management of hereditary gastrointestinal cancer syndromes. Am J Gastroenterol. 2015;110(2):223–62; quiz 263.
28. Gilson P, et al. Evaluation of 3 molecular-based assays for microsatellite instability detection in formalin-fixed tissues of patients with endometrial and colorectal cancers. Sci Rep. 2020;10(1):16386.
29. Ratti M, et al. Microsatellite instability in gastric cancer: molecular bases, clinical perspectives, and new treatment approaches. Cell Mol Life Sci. 2018;75(22):4151–62.
30. Murphy KM, et al. Comparison of the microsatellite instability analysis system and the Bethesda panel for the determination of microsatellite instability in colorectal cancers. J Mol Diagn. 2006;8(3):305–11.
31. Perucho M. Correspondence re: C.R. Boland et al., A National Cancer Institute workshop on microsatellite instability for cancer detection and familial predisposition: development of international criteria for the determination of microsatellite instability in colorectal cancer. Cancer Res., 58:5248–5257. Cancer Res, 1999. 1998;59(1):249–56.
32. Pawlik TM, Raut CP, Rodriguez-Bigas MA. Colorectal carcinogenesis: MSI-H versus MSI-L. Dis Markers. 2004;20(4–5):199–206.
33. Ganesh K, et al. Immunotherapy in colorectal cancer: rationale, challenges and potential. Nat Rev Gastroenterol Hepatol. 2019;16(6):361–75.
34. Morse MA, Hochster H, Benson A. Perspectives on treatment of metastatic colorectal cancer with immune checkpoint inhibitor therapy. Oncologist. 2020;25(1):33–45.
35. Dai D, et al. Association between the microsatellite instability status and the efficacy of postoperative adjuvant chemoradiotherapy in patients with gastric cancer. Front Oncol. 2019;9:1452.
36. Calva D, Howe JR. Hamartomatous polyposis syndromes. Surg Clin North Am. 2008;88(4):779–817, vii.
37. Brosens LA, et al. Gastrointestinal polyposis syndromes. Curr Mol Med. 2007;7(1):29–46.
38. Kanth P, et al. Hereditary colorectal polyposis and cancer syndromes: a primer on diagnosis and management. Am J Gastroenterol. 2017;112(10):1509–25.
39. Bettington M, et al. The challenging diagnosis of Cronkhite-Canada syndrome in the upper gastrointestinal tract: a series of 7 cases with clinical follow-up. Am J Surg Pathol. 2014;38(2):215–23.

40. Jain S, et al. Molecular genetics of hepatocellular neoplasia. Am J Transl Res. 2010;2(1):105–18.
41. Desert R, et al. Human hepatocellular carcinomas with a periportal phenotype have the lowest potential for early recurrence after curative resection. Hepatology. 2017;66(5):1502–18.
42. Thillai K, Ross P, Sarker D. Molecularly targeted therapy for advanced hepatocellular carcinoma – a drug development crisis? World J Gastrointest Oncol. 2016;8(2):173–85.
43. Dominguez DA, Wang XW. Impact of next-generation sequencing on outcomes in hepatocellular carcinoma: how precise are we really? J Hepatocell Carcinoma. 2020;7:33–7.
44. Montironi C, Montal R, Llovet JM. New drugs effective in the systemic treatment of hepatocellular carcinoma. Clin Liver Dis (Hoboken). 2019;14(2):56–61.
45. Liu Z, et al. Molecular targeted and immune checkpoint therapy for advanced hepatocellular carcinoma. J Exp Clin Cancer Res. 2019;38(1):447.
46. De Mattia E, et al. Pharmacogenetics of the systemic treatment in advanced hepatocellular carcinoma. World J Gastroenterol. 2019;25(29):3870–96.
47. Calderaro J, et al. Molecular and histological correlations in liver cancer. J Hepatol. 2019;71(3):616–30.
48. Hidalgo M. Pancreatic cancer. N Engl J Med. 2010;362(17):1605–17.
49. Sakorafas GH, Smyrniotis V. Molecular biology of pancreatic cancer: how useful is it in clinical practice? JOP. 2012;13(4):332–7.
50. Waddell N, et al. Whole genomes redefine the mutational landscape of pancreatic cancer. Nature. 2015;518(7540):495–501.
51. Nicolle R, et al. Establishment of a pancreatic adenocarcinoma molecular gradient (PAMG) that predicts the clinical outcome of pancreatic cancer. EBioMedicine. 2020;57:102858.
52. de Biase D, et al. The role of next-generation sequencing in the cytologic diagnosis of pancreatic lesions. Arch Pathol Lab Med. 2018;142(4):458–64.
53. Strimpakos AS, Syrigos KN, Saif MW. The molecular targets for the diagnosis and treatment of pancreatic cancer. Gut Liver. 2010;4(4):433–49.
54. Yachida S, et al. Clinical significance of the genetic landscape of pancreatic cancer and implications for identification of potential long-term survivors. Clin Cancer Res. 2012;18(22):6339–47.
55. Puleo F, et al. Stratification of pancreatic ductal adenocarcinomas based on tumor and microenvironment features. Gastroenterology. 2018;155(6):1999–2013. e3
56. Zarkavelis G, et al. Genetic mapping of pancreatic cancer by targeted next-generation sequencing in a cohort of patients managed with nab-paclitaxel-based chemotherapy or agents targeting the EGFR axis: a retrospective analysis of the Hellenic Cooperative Oncology Group (HeCOG). ESMO Open. 2019;4(5):e000525.
57. Chan-Seng-Yue M, et al. Transcription phenotypes of pancreatic cancer are driven by genomic events during tumor evolution. Nat Genet. 2020;52(2):231–40.
58. Chang DK, Grimmond SM, Biankin AV. Pancreatic cancer genomics. Curr Opin Genet Dev. 2014;24:74–81.
59. Amanam I, Chung V. Targeted therapies for pancreatic cancer. Cancers (Basel). 2018;10(2):36.
60. Sato-Dahlman M, Wirth K, Yamamoto M. Role of gene therapy in pancreatic cancer-a review. Cancers (Basel). 2018;10(4):103.
61. Al-Haddad M. Role of emerging molecular markers in pancreatic cyst fluid. Endosc Ultrasound. 2015;4(4):276–83.
62. de la Fuente J, Majumder S. Molecular diagnostics and testing for pancreatic cysts. Curr Treat Options Gastroenterol. 2020 Jan 27. Online ahead of print.
63. Bournet B, et al. KRAS G12D mutation subtype is a prognostic factor for advanced pancreatic adenocarcinoma. Clin Transl Gastroenterol. 2016;7:e157.
64. Gibney GT, Weiner LM, Atkins MB. Predictive biomarkers for checkpoint inhibitor-based immunotherapy. Lancet Oncol. 2016;17(12):e542–51.
65. Fashoyin-Aje L, et al. FDA approval summary: pembrolizumab for recurrent locally advanced or metastatic gastric or gastroesophageal junction adenocarcinoma expressing PD-L1. Oncologist. 2019;24(1):103–9.
66. Das S, et al.: All in the levels-programmed death-ligand 1 expression as a biomarker for immune checkpoint inhibitor response in patients with gastrointestinal cancer. Oncologist. 2021;26(1):e186-e188.

Skin Tumors

9

Cynthia Reyes Barron and Bruce R. Smoller

List of Frequently Asked Questions

1. Cutaneous melanoma is a skin cancer with variable presentations and outcomes. Does molecular genetics help classify melanoma into subtypes and explain clinical behavior of malignancies?
2. How can molecular testing serve as a tool in the diagnosis of melanoma?
3. What molecular tests may be used to differentiate between nevoid malignant melanoma and benign melanocytic nevi?
4. What molecular studies help define and classify Spitz tumors and predict clinical behavior?
5. What are proliferative nodules and what molecular findings help distinguish them from malignant melanoma?
6. How can molecular studies help stage malignant melanoma?
7. What are the clinical implications of *BRAF* mutations in cutaneous melanoma?
8. What methods are commonly used clinically to determine *BRAF* mutation status and what are the limitations of each?
9. Is testing for *BRAF* mutation status indicated for all cases of cutaneous melanoma?
10. What other targetable mutations are commonly seen in cutaneous melanoma?
11. Does molecular testing help predict prognosis for melanoma patients?
12. Is gene expression profiling available for other cutaneous malignancies?
13. How does molecular testing aid in the diagnosis of Muir-Torre syndrome (MTS) in patients presenting with cutaneous sebaceous tumors?
14. How do T-cell gene rearrangements help in the diagnosis of mycosis fungoides?
15. Are cytogenetic studies necessary for the unequivocal diagnosis of dermatofibrosarcoma protuberans (DFSP)?

Frequently Asked Questions

1. **Cutaneous melanoma is a skin cancer with variable presentations and outcomes. Does molecular genetics help classify melanoma into subtypes and explain clinical behavior of malignancies?**
   - There are multiple schemes of melanoma classification with biologic and clinical implications. Sequencing results of the Cancer Genome Atlas Network provided the framework to classify cutaneous melanoma based on genomic alterations. Genomic subtypes were defined according to the most prevalent mutated genes into four categories: *BRAF* mutated, *RAS* mutated, *NF1* mutated, and triple wild-type [1]. Mutations in three genes (*BRAF*, *NRAS*, and *NF1*) may be responsible for the initiation of melanoma tumorigenesis. *BRAF* mutations may occur in childhood or young adulthood and lead to melanoma development 20–30 years later. Other genes such as *TERT*, *CDKN2A*, and *ARID1A* are commonly mutated in melanomas and may represent later events contributing to malignancy progression. Mutations in *PTEN* and *TP53* likely occur late in melanomagenesis and are indicative of more aggressive disease [2].
   - The 2018 WHO Classification of Skin Tumours placed melanomas into three principal categories: tumors associated with cumulative solar damage, tumors not consistently associated with cumulative solar damage, and nodular melanoma [3]. Recent discoveries in molecular genetics has revealed that distinct biological pathways exist corresponding to distinct molecular

C. Reyes Barron · B. R. Smoller (✉)
Department of Pathology and Laboratory Medicine, University of Rochester Medical Center, Rochester, NY, USA
e-mail: creyesba711@gmail.com; bruce_smoller@urmc.rochester.edu

Y. Ding, L. Zhang (eds.), *Practical Oncologic Molecular Pathology*, Practical Anatomic Pathology,
https://doi.org/10.1007/978-3-030-73227-1_9

alterations commonly seen in lesions of the various WHO categories [2, 4].

- Mutational signatures, tracked in the Catalogue of Somatic Mutations in Cancer (COSMIC), are patterns of somatic mutations that help categorize malignancies. Instead of focusing on driver or passenger mutations of specific genes, mutational signatures depict patterns of genetic insults, both exogenous and endogenous, throughout a person's lifetime. The patterns are determined by assessing substitutions of base pairs and the bases immediately 5′ and 3′ to the base substitutions. Over 30 signatures have been defined using whole exome and whole genome sequencing [5]. Signature 7 is associated with ultraviolet light exposure and the resulting DNA damage which consists predominantly of cytosine to thymine substitutions at dipyrimidines. Melanomas can be categorized into low and high cumulative solar damage lesions that also correspond to those that are non-signature 7 and signature 7, respectively. Studies have shown that melanomas with signature 7 have better overall survival [6].

2. **How can molecular testing serve as a tool in the diagnosis of melanoma?**
   - While the vast majority of melanomas are diagnosed on histologic criteria alone with or without the use of immunohistochemical stains (IHC), there are cases that pose a diagnostic challenge (see Chart 9.1).
   - Certain benign melanocytic lesions can mimic malignant melanoma, and making a distinction is challenging histologically, even for experienced dermatopathologists. These include differentiating between nevoid melanoma and benign melanocytic nevi, Spitz melanoma from Spitz nevi, and infiltrative melanoma within congenital nevi from proliferative nodules [8].
   - Diagnostically indeterminate lesions may be treated with conservative complete excision and close follow-up. However, an unequivocal diagnosis of melanoma would result in more appropriate treatment, possibly with wider margins on excision and sentinel lymph node dissection, in some cases.
   - Molecular studies are emerging as valuable ancillary tests to aid in the diagnosis of malignancy for challenging lesions. Taken in conjunction with histopathologic features, results of molecular tests may help distinguish benign from malignant lesions.
   - Although most pathology laboratories do not have the technical capabilities to perform ancillary molecular testing themselves, dermatopathologists may send samples to outside laboratories or consultants to obtain results. A survey of dermatopathologists attending the American Society of Dermatopathology Annual Meeting, 2016, revealed that approximately 31% of those surveyed perform molecular testing at their insti-

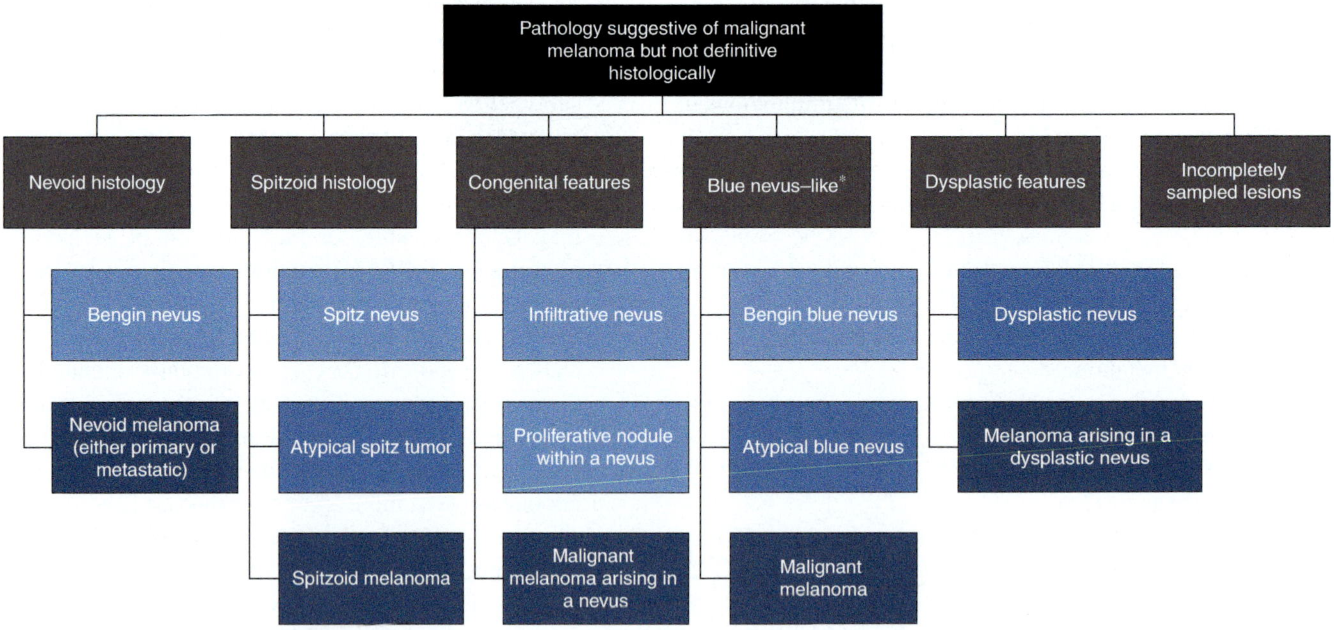

Chart 9.1 Summary of histologic features that may be seen in equivocal melanocytic lesions and the corresponding differential diagnoses. CGH and FISH studies have been deemed usually appropriate as ancillary studies to aid in diagnosis in such cases by the American Society of Dermatopathology (*Only CGH and not FISH is considered appropriate in this scenario) [7]

Table 9.1 Overview of copy number variants (CNVs) frequently seen in melanocytic lesions

Copy number variants overview					
Diagnosis	Losses	Gains	Other	Notes	References
Melanoma (general)	3p, 9p, 9q, 10p, 10q, 11q	1q, 4q, 6p, 7p, 7q, 8q, 11q, 17q, 20q		6p gain indicates an unfavorable prognosis	[9, 12]
Melanoma in blue nevus	1p and 4q	1q, 4p, 6p, 8q	Gains and losses of entire arms		[3, 13]
Melanoma at acral site	6q, 15q	4q, 5p, 11q, 12q			[9]
Melanoma, lentigo maligna type	13q, 17p				[9]
Melanoma arising in congenital nevus	Homozygous loss of 9p21	High gains at 6p25			[3, 14]
Proliferative nodule			Gains and losses of whole chromosomes		[14]
Spitz nevus		11p (~20%)		Most have no CNVs	[3]
Atypical Spitz tumor	Homozygous loss of 9p21			Loss associated with the risk of metastatic/ aggressive disease	[15]

tutions and 54% either use molecular testing in their practice or expect consultants to use molecular testing when indicated [9].

- Evidence exists for the utility of comparative genomic hybridization (CGH) and fluorescence in situ hybridization (FISH) for the analysis of melanocytic lesions. Single nucleotide polymorphism array comparative genomic hybridization (SNP-aCGH) is a platform used in many molecular laboratories that has the capability of providing data on copy number variants as well as loss of heterozygosity.
- Copy number variants (CNVs), as determined by CGH, are indicative of malignant behavior in melanocytic lesions (see Table 9.1). In particular, one study showed that melanocytic neoplasms with adverse clinical behavior had more than three CNVs [10]. Therefore, performing SNP-CGH on lesions with atypical features but indefinite for malignancy may be an adequate ancillary study for determining malignancy. Benign melanocytic nevi, with few exceptions, do not harbor CNVs [11].
- FISH studies may be used to confirm specific variants identified by CGH and may also provide sufficient evidence of malignancy independently. Multiple FISH panels have shown adequate specificity and sensitivity in identifying malignant melanoma [9].
- The American Society of Dermatopathology (ASDP) has developed appropriate use criteria for molecular testing in cutaneous lesions including melanocytic neoplasms. They enumerated 30 specific clinical scenarios involving melanocytic lesions and their expert panel concluded that FISH or CGH are "usually appropriate" to diagnose melanoma in both pediatric and adult cases of uncertain malignancy by histopathologic assessment. The use of qRT-PCR panels was rated rarely appropriate or of uncertain appropriateness in these same scenarios [7]. Specific diagnostic dilemmas are further discussed.

3. **What molecular tests may be used to differentiate between nevoid malignant melanoma and benign melanocytic nevi?**
   - Nevoid melanoma histologically looks deceptively benign. The melanocytes appear to grow in well-circumscribed nests and cytologic atypia is absent to subtle, mimicking benign nevi. Mitotic figures may be difficult to identify [8].
   - The ASDP appropriate use criteria rates both FISH and CGH as appropriate for distinguishing these entities [7].
   - Assays using various combinations of FISH probes have been tested to assess utility in the diagnosis of malignant melanoma and in distinguishing malignancy from benign nevi. A FISH assay consisting of four probes which target 9p21 (*CDKN2A*), 6p25 (*RREB1*), 11q13 (*CCND1*), and 8q24 (*MYC*) has a sensitivity of 94% and specificity of 96% [16]. Gains and losses at these loci are seen much more commonly in melanomas than nevi. However, most studies have been conducted comparing histologically definitively malignant and definitively benign lesions. One study showed that the sensitivity of FISH for detecting malignancy in borderline lesions was 61% [17].
   - Array-CGH may be better suited to discriminate between benign nevi and malignant melanoma than FISH in cases that are borderline histologically [17]. The loss of entire chromosomes is one potential pitfall leading to false positives using FISH that is avoided with CGH. Such losses are indicative of benign lesions and can be seen in nevi while more focal copy number alterations are consistent with malignant behavior. The targeted nature of FISH testing fails to discriminate between a whole chromo-

some loss and focal copy number losses involving one or a few genes. CGH provides a broad view of copy number alterations across the genome which is advantageous, particularly in malignancies such as melanoma which can be very variable at the histologic as well as molecular level.

- Procuring fresh tissue from biopsied or resected skin lesions for molecular testing is not practical in the standard surgical pathology workflow. Obtaining sufficient good quality DNA for CGH testing from FFPE may be challenging, particularly when the lesion is small or there is low tumor percentage in a specimen. Microdissection of FFPE is often necessary to separate lesional cells from surrounding cells including lymphocytes and uninvolved epidermal keratinocytes, to obtain sufficient tumor DNA [18].
- FISH has the advantage of requiring less tissue. Once a slide is prepared from FFPE, counting only 30 cells from the lesion in question may be sufficient to assess abnormalities. This requires pathologists or technicians trained in the use of fluorescent microscopy and reading FISH studies.
- The choice of appropriate probes for FISH testing allows detection of balanced translocations which are missed by CGH. However, FISH is limited by the number of probes. Typically, a maximum of four probes are used in a set which means that four regions of the genome can be targeted per test [18]. Although research has revealed high sensitivity and specificity for the detection of melanoma using 4-probe sets, aberrations will be missed if they are not specifically targeted.
- FISH may be less expensive, have a shorter turnaround time, and be available in more laboratories than CGH [18].

4. **What molecular studies help define and classify Spitz tumors and predict clinical behavior?**
   - Spitz tumors are a distinct class of melanocytic lesions consisting of spindle and epithelioid cells that are frequently seen in pediatric patients and young adults although they may occur at any age [8]. Histologically and molecularly, Spitz tumors occur on a spectrum ranging from benign nevi to highly aggressive malignant melanoma with a diagnosis of atypical Spitz tumor falling between these two diagnostic poles. An atypical Spitz tumor, also referred to as a Spitz tumor of uncertain malignant potential (STUMP), may be particularly challenging diagnostically. Criteria including clinical features, histologic architecture, cellular morphology, and mitotic activity are helpful in distinguishing Spitz nevi from atypical Spitz tumors and Spitz melanoma but distinguishing between the latter two may remain difficult [19].
   - While Spitz nevi may display characteristically benign features such as symmetry and maturation of melanocytes, atypical features such as cellular pleomorphism, and increased mitoses may lead to a diagnosis of atypical Spitz nevus or Spitz melanoma [4]. Atypical Spitz tumors have clinical behavior intermediate between nevi and melanoma and may metastasize, most often to regional lymph nodes. Lymph node involvement does not necessarily portend a worse outcome as in cases of definitive melanoma [20].
   - Spitz tumors have molecular characteristics that distinguish them from other melanocytic lesions, but are heterogeneous as a category, as well. Molecular findings correspond with histologic features, prognosis, and treatment response [21].
   - Activating *HRAS* mutations are rarely seen in other melanocytic lesions but are present in approximately 15% of Spitz nevi and are often accompanied by copy number gains at 11p [20, 22]. Importantly, *HRAS* mutations have not been identified in Spitz melanomas, making this molecular finding highly predictive of benign behavior [22]. Isolated loss of 6p23 in atypical Spitz tumors may also indicate a benign course [22].
   - *BAP1* inactivated Spitzoid tumors, also known as BAP1-inactivated melanocytic tumors (BIMT), harbor inactivating mutations of *BAP1,* as the name implies. These lesions characteristically also carry the *BRAFV600E* mutation. They generally follow an indolent course according to multiple studies [4, 20, 22]. Nevertheless, this entity has recently been recognized as separate from Spitz tumors and additional outcome studies are necessary to better understand their biologic behavior [23]. Although histologically, they share many features with Spitz tumors, they are considered lesions in the low cumulative solar damage pathway, separate from Spitz tumors, in the 2018 WHO classification [3].
   - Approximately 50% of Spitz tumors harbor a translocation or fusion involving *ALK*, *ROS1*, *NTRK1*, *RET*, *MET*, or *BRAF*. These translocations span the spectrum of tumors from Spitz nevi to Spitz melanoma, and their presence is not helpful in distinguishing between benign and malignant tumors [22]. Most tumors with *ALK* translocations are classified as atypical Spitz tumors and very rarely Spitz melanoma [22]. In cases where lymph nodes are involved or there is clinical concern for spread or recurrence of disease, Spitz tumors with *ALK*, *ROS1*, or *RET* fusions may be treated with kinase inhibitors such as crizotinib [20].
   - Other mutations may be associated with an aggressive clinical course and molecular testing may help

guide clinical decisions in cases of atypical Spitz tumors. Mutations in the *TERT* promoter are associated with the spread of disease and poor outcomes [24]. In one study, homozygous loss of 9p21 had a strong association with death due to Spitz melanoma [25]; however, others have not supported these findings and additional studies are warranted in larger cohorts with longer follow-up [22].

- CGH and FISH are both considered appropriate studies to aid in diagnosis and classification of Spitz tumors for pediatric and adult patients according to the ASDP criteria [7]. As with other melanocytic lesions, identification of multiple copy number variants by CGH is more likely to be seen in Spitz melanoma than in Spitz nevi [26]. Additional studies are necessary to further clarify the molecular findings in atypical Spitz tumors lying in the middle of the malignancy spectrum and determining the best diagnostic markers.

5. **What are proliferative nodules and what molecular findings help distinguish them from malignant melanoma?**
   - One of the most challenging distinctions to make histologically is between a proliferative nodule and malignant melanoma in a congenital nevus. By definition, proliferative nodules are mitotically active nests of melanocytes within the dermis. They are concerning for melanoma because they may have features seen in malignancies including increased mitotic activity, high cellularity, and nuclear atypia [8]. Proliferative nodules may arise in giant congenital nevi in pediatric patients, and are much more common than melanoma in this population; however, the risk of melanoma also exists [14].
   - CGH studies have shown that proliferative nodules may have whole chromosome gains or losses. As previously discussed, melanomas are likely to have partial chromosome gains and losses across the genome. This difference in copy number variant patterns may help differentiate between benign and malignant lesions [14, 27].
   - CGH and FISH are both considered appropriate studies to aid in the distinction of malignant melanoma from proliferative nodules for pediatric and adult patients according to the ASDP criteria [7].
6. **How can molecular studies help stage malignant melanoma?**
   - Maximum tumor depth, also known as Breslow thickness, is measured from the granular layer to the deepest invasive tumor cell and is the most important parameter for staging melanoma. The challenge comes with the realization that not all melanocytes found in the dermis are necessarily malignant. Compound nevi and intradermal nevi are benign lesions with populations of melanocytes in the dermis. The depth of these benign melanocytes is not indicative of risk and has no staging significance. Not uncommonly, melanoma develops within or in association with a benign nevus. Differentiating between the two populations of melanocytes, benign nevus cells and the malignant melanoma cells intermixed within the dermis, may be very challenging. Melanoma is stage T1 if the Breslow depth is under 1.0 mm, T2 if greater than 1.0 and up to 2.0 mm, T3 if greater than 2.0 mm and up to 4.0 mm and T4 if greater than 4.0 mm according to the eighth edition of the AJCC staging manual [28].
   - Because FISH studies are performed directly on tissue sections and are evaluated on the glass slide, they may be used to highlight malignant cells in the dermis and differentiate them from benign melanocytes [29]. IHC is generally not useful for this purpose because the stains commonly used for melanocytic lesions, including S100, SOX10, and Melan-A, will highlight melanocytes whether they are benign or malignant. FISH will show cytogenetic abnormalities in the malignant cells that are not present in the benign nevus cells allowing pathologists to measure Breslow depth more accurately and properly stage a lesion.
7. **What are the clinical implications of *BRAF* mutations in cutaneous melanoma?**
   - Approximately 40–60% of primary cutaneous melanomas harbor a somatic *BRAF* mutation [30]. The *BRAF* V600E amino acid substitution of glutamic acid for valine is the most common mutation occurring in approximately 90% of *BRAF* mutated melanomas, with *V600K* and others occurring infrequently [1, 30, 31].
   - *BRAF* mutations can be divided into three classes with varying sensitivities to targeted therapy. Mutations at amino acid position 600 (V600E/K/D/R or M) are in class 1 and are sensitive to *BRAF* inhibitors such as vemurafenib. Tumors with class 2 or class 3 mutations, which include amino acid substitutions at other regions of the protein and fusions that affect kinase activity, are generally insensitive to vemurafenib and other targeted therapies in this family [32].
   - Tumors with a *BRAF* mutation are found in younger patients, are more commonly located on the trunk, and develop on skin with low cumulative solar damage [2, 31, 33]. Histologically, cumulative solar damage is identified by the presence of solar elastosis which consists of degenerated elastic fibers in the superficial dermis. Skin of the head and neck and distal extremities is more likely to have solar elastosis

and melanomas with higher cumulative solar damage.
- Because over 80% of benign melanocytic nevi may also harbor a *BRAF* mutation, particularly *BRAF* V600E, it is not helpful in distinguishing benign from malignant lesions [34]. However, nevi have few additional pathogenic mutations and overall low mutational burden in contrast to melanoma [2].
- Targeted therapy with *BRAF* inhibitors, often in combination with *MEK* inhibitors, has become standard of care for patients with metastatic *BRAF*-mutated melanoma. The use of *BRAF* inhibitors alone results in the eventual development of resistance and disease progression in virtually all cases and cutaneous toxicities including promotion of secondary tumors such as squamous cell carcinomas. Combination therapy with a *MEK* inhibitor may reduce toxicity and deter the development of resistance [35]. Multiple studies have shown that targeted therapy with combination *BRAF* and *MEK* inhibitors has greatly improved overall survival in melanoma patients with advanced disease [36–38]. One-year survival for patients with a *BRAF* mutation was 83% for those treated with targeted therapy versus 29% for those not treated, in one study [33].

8. **What methods are commonly used clinically to determine *BRAF* mutation status and what are the limitations of each?**
   - Although it is possible to assess *BRAF* mutation status from circulating tumor DNA in blood samples, the sensitivity is approximately 76% for *BRAF* V600E and this method is not commonly used clinically [39].
   - Testing is typically conducted on tumor tissue obtained either from the biopsy at the time of diagnosis or resection specimen. Since complete surgical excision of the primary tumor and/or metastasis is usually part of the treatment plan, tissue samples are generally available and provide the opportunity to assess histologic characteristics as well as conduct tissue molecular testing. Multiple assays exist to evaluate *BRAF* status using formalin fixed paraffin embedded tissue (FFPE) [40].
   - Immunohistochemistry (IHC) may be used as a screening tool for the *BRAF* V600E mutation using monoclonal antibody VE1. This method detects the mutant protein in the cytoplasm of tumor cells using a commercially available kit. The relatively quick turn-around time allows patients to begin targeted therapy soon after diagnosis. Moreover, the cost is low and most pathology labs are already equipped to perform IHC tests. The sensitivity and specificity may be as high as 97% and 98%, respectively [41]. Only the V600E mutation is detected; therefore, a negative result does not exclude other *BRAF* mutations and additional testing is recommended. Confirmation of positive results with a molecular method is also standard practice [42].
   - There are many techniques based on real-time PCR available for *BRAF* mutation testing. Several commercial platforms are FDA approved and offer the benefit of automation with the capability of extracting DNA directly from FFPE without the need for manual extraction, decreasing technical time and effort required to obtain *BRAF* status. Results may be ready in approximately 2 hours from the time the FFPE tissue sample is loaded. They are not limited to the detection of the V600E mutant and can detect the other common variants at this location including V600K/R/M. One such platform demonstrated a sensitivity of 100% and specificity of 94% [43]. Although it is a practical option and may be more rapid and automated than next generation sequencing (NGS) panels, it does require initial investment on the platform and the cost of disposable cartridges. Also, the test is limited to one gene, *BRAF*, and only specific targets within the gene, commonly at the site of amino acid 600. If the results are negative, genetic testing for mutations on other genes associated with melanoma may be desirable for patient care.
   - Pyrosequencing is an excellent option for *BRAF* mutation testing and validated assays have been used for many years. Because the majority of *BRAF* mutations in melanocytic lesions occur at a hotspot location, pyrosequencing is an efficient and effective method of detection and it can be used to identify multiple variants [44]. Pyrosequencing can be performed directly from FFPE tissue samples on commercially available automated platforms, with high concordance to conventional dideoxy sequencing methods. The analytic sensitivity may be as low as 2%, much lower than what is seen in dideoxy sequencing [45]. As with other automated systems, the availability and initial investment in instrumentation is a limiting factor.
   - NGS sequencing platforms that simultaneously sequence multiple genes have the advantage of providing a broader assessment of mutation status [46]. The ability to detect *BRAF* mutations across the gene and identify mutations in genes such as *NRAS* and *KIT* using a single assay is a valuable feature. It allows for the evaluation of multiple therapeutic targets in one step as well as generating data with potential to be significant as knowledge of the genetic landscape of cancer increases and new treatments are developed. However, the analysis of the data gener-

ated is not trivial and must be accurate to determine significance. The sensitivity and specificity for detecting *BRAF* mutations may be as high as 98% and 100%, respectively [40]. Sequencing platforms require a substantial initial investment although various commercially available solid tumor panels have clinical utility across cancer types and may be a more efficient use of resources than performing multiple individual tests when the initial targeted gene results are negative.

9. **Is testing for *BRAF* mutation status indicated for all cases of cutaneous melanoma?**
   - According to the National Comprehensive Cancer Network, genetic testing for *BRAF* mutations is indicated for all patients with Stage III disease [42]. Targeted therapy with *BRAF* inhibitors has been shown to improve outcomes in patients with certain *BRAF* mutations as discussed above and results of genetic testing will guide patient treatment decisions.
   - Patients with Stage IV disease or clinical recurrence should be tested for *BRAF* mutations if not previously tested [42]. As with Stage III disease, *BRAF* status will guide treatment.
   - Testing for patients with Stage I and II disease is not recommended unless the patient is being considered for a clinical trial and the results will determine eligibility [42]. Otherwise, *BRAF* status will not affect management. Melanoma at early stages is treated with surgical resection with clear margins and systemic therapy is generally not necessary [36].
   - Because tissue from the metastasis represents the most advanced disease, it is preferred for *BRAF* testing, when available. Although *BRAF* mutation is usually an early event in the development of melanoma [2], studies have shown that tumor heterogeneity exists and selective pressures may favor one clone over another and the metastasis may not harbor the same mutation. Patients whose primary tumors were *BRAF* wild-type may have metastatic disease that is *BRAF* mutated [30].
   - In any case, if single gene testing is used and *BRAF* is wild-type, molecular testing with a larger panel may be warranted to assess for the presence of other possibly targetable driver mutations and qualification for clinical trial enrollment [42].
10. **What other targetable mutations are commonly seen in cutaneous melanoma?**
    - Melanomas harbor more somatic mutations than other cancer types, likely due to the damaging influence of ultraviolet radiation and its role in tumorigenesis [5]. The high mutational burden of these tumors may explain why they are so susceptible to immunotherapy; however, finding adequate targeted therapies has proved challenging [47, 48]. Clinical trials are underway for multiple therapies targeting various driver mutations. Molecular studies may allow clinicians to determine if patients with specific mutations qualify for these trials.
    - *KIT* mutations are seen in melanomas occurring at mucosal sites and acral sites, such as palms and soles, more commonly than chronically sun-exposed skin (10–15% versus less than 2%) and even less frequently in skin without significant cumulative solar damage [35]. *KIT* mutation testing is warranted in mucosal and acral melanomas. Approximately 30–50% of melanomas with activating mutations in *KIT* will respond to targeted therapy with *KIT* inhibitors such as imatinib, although the response is not significant in tumors with *KIT* amplifications [49]. In particular, melanomas with *KIT* mutations in exons 11 and 13 may have significant response to *KIT* inhibitors [50].
    - *NRAS* mutations are present in approximately 15–30% of melanomas and are more common in melanomas occurring in skin with high cumulative solar damage [2, 48]. Clinical trials with new *MEK* inhibitors have shown promising results in progression-free survival for *NRAS* mutated melanoma [51, 52]. *MEK* inhibitor treatment is currently only available as part of a clinical trial.
    - Approximately 21% of cutaneous melanomas harbor genetic alterations in *CDKN2A* including copy number variants and mutations. IHC testing showing loss of p16 is a screening tool for mutations of the *CDKN2A* gene [3]. Several trials are underway targeting the *CDKN2A/CDK4* pathway of tumorigenesis with results pending [48].
11. **Does molecular testing help predict prognosis for melanoma patients?** (See Chart 9.2.)
    - CNV burden, an indication of chromosome instability, may correlate with prognosis in melanoma with greater CNV burden seen in patients with worse outcomes [53]. Array CGH, which determines CNVs across the genome, may be suitable for determining prognosis.
    - CNVs detected by FISH may have prognostic value, as well. Gains at 11q13 and 8q24 were significantly associated with poor prognosis and disease progression in one study [54].
    - Several commercial gene expression profiling (GEP) panels are available to place melanomas into prognostic categories. These panels assess DNA expression by determining levels of mRNA of carefully selected genes that may be differentially expressed in tumors with greater metastatic potential [55]. FFPE

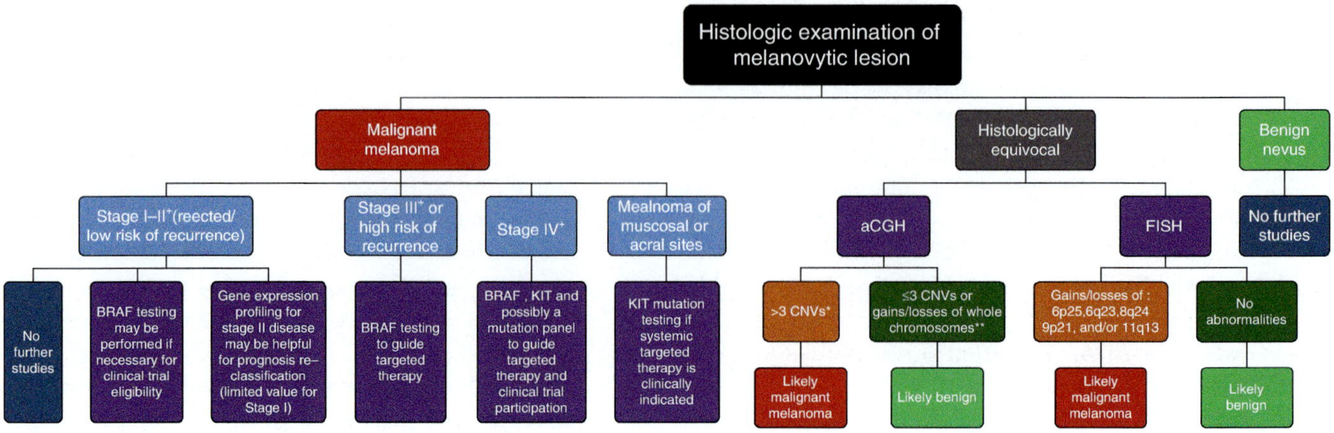

Chart 9.2 Approach to molecular testing for melanocytic lesions +Staging based on the American Joint Committee on Cancer (AJCC) melanoma staging system
* Excluding CNVs thought to be inconsequential: 3p21 loss, 11p gain (may be seen in Spitz nevi), 1q22-q23.1 loss and whole chromosome losses and gains [10]
** Excluding homozygous loss of CDKN2A, or gains of 11q13, 8q24, or 6p25 [10]

from either a biopsy or resection specimen is adequate for testing.

- GEP panels have not replaced TNM staging, but may provide supplementary information to guide clinical management in certain cases and in conjunction with histopathologic features.
- Patients placed in high-risk categories by GEP may undergo sentinel lymph node biopsy or have closer follow-up and imaging studies.
- Although the use of GEP is becoming increasingly popular, limited outcome data exists. A recent meta-analysis reports that GEP tests may have particularly limited utility in Stage I disease with poor concordance of high- and low-risk categories with tumor recurrence and disease progression [56]. However, most patients with Stage II disease that had disease progression were correctly classified as high risk by GEP [56].
- Selecting the appropriate patients to undergo GEP testing will decrease the burden of false-positive results that may lead to over-treatment and false-negative results that provide misplaced reassurance. A multidisciplinary approach with collaboration including dermatologists, oncologists, surgeons, and pathologists reviewing each case is beneficial.

12. **Is gene expression profiling available for other cutaneous malignancies?**
    - Commercial GEP panels have recently become available for cutaneous squamous cell carcinoma. Like those developed for melanoma, they categorize tumors into low and high risk for metastasis and may guide decisions on patient follow-up, surveillance, and adjuvant therapies. Initial studies show promising results with a positive predictive value of 60% for the highest category and negative predictive value of 90% for a validated test [57]. Additional studies are underway.
13. **How does molecular testing aid in the diagnosis of Muir-Torre syndrome (MTS) in patients presenting with cutaneous sebaceous tumors?**
    - MTS, a subtype of hereditary non-polyposis colorectal cancer syndrome (Lynch syndrome), is an autosomal-dominant disorder leading to DNA microsatellite instability and the development of multiple sebaceous tumors on the skin as well as colorectal, endometrial, ovarian, and urothelial malignancies [58].
    - The sebaceous tumors associated with MTS range from benign sebaceous adenomas and sebaceomas to sebaceous carcinoma. Presence of multiple keratoacanthomas or reticulated acanthomas with sebaceous differentiation is also associated with MTS [58].
    - Muir-Torre syndrome is usually caused by mutations in the DNA mismatch repair genes, *MLH1*, *PMS2*, *MSH2*, or *MSH6* leading to microsatellite instability. A variant of MTS is associated with biallelic inactivation of *MYH* [59].
    - IHC is an important screening tool that can be applied to either the sebaceous tumors or visceral malignancies. Loss of staining with antibodies against *MLH1*, *PMS2*, *MSH2*, and/or *MSH6* may be indicative of a mismatch repair deficiency (MMR). Approximately 67% of sebaceous tumors will show loss of at least one MMR protein by IHC and 60% of those have loss of *MSH2* and/or associated loss of its partner *MSH6* [60].
    - Patients with MTS often present with cutaneous complaints first although sebaceous tumors may develop concurrently or after visceral malignancies. The diag-

nosis of multiple sebaceous tumors, particularly in patients 60 years of age or older, warrants additional testing for MMR [7]. However, age at presentation and other clinical features such as site of the lesion may not be predictive of MMR and some recommend screening all sebaceous tumors by IHC [60].

- Loss of mismatch repair proteins may be a sporadic and is not diagnostic of MTS. Approximately 33% of cases with the loss of a MMR protein by IHC will have germline deficiencies [58]. Germline testing for mutations in the MMR proteins is appropriate, particularly if there is high clinical suspicion of MTS, to guide patient care and adequate screening for visceral malignancies [59]. Genetic counseling is also important to help families understand their risks.
- Microsatellite instability testing is conducted using PCR and comparing the presence of microsatellite repeats in patient samples to normal tissue at standardized sites. In addition, targeted NGS panels have been developed that provide accurate assessment of MSI in small samples [61].

14. **How do T-cell gene rearrangements help in the diagnosis of mycosis fungoides?**
    - Mycosis fungoides (MF) is the most common cutaneous T-cell lymphoma (CTCL) and is characterized by clonal proliferation of malignant epidermotropic T-cells [62]. MF usually affects adults, presenting as erythematous patches and plaques in skin that is sun-protected such as the trunk [63].
    - There are multiple classes of MF with varying clinical and histologic features. MF is known as the "great imitator" because the initial clinical presentation is often non-specific and can simulate many benign inflammatory skin conditions ranging from psoriasis to infectious entities [64]. Both clinical presentation and histopathology are necessary for definitive diagnosis and should be evaluated in conjunction due to the non-specific nature of findings [63].
    - Ancillary molecular studies play a critical role in the analysis of the skin biopsy because the identification of a malignant T-cell clone supports a definitive diagnosis. The most widely used assay is PCR-based amplification of the T-cell receptor (TCR) gamma gene and gel electrophoresis to identify a clonal band [62].
    - Sufficient T-cells must be present in the tissue sample in order to obtain a valid result and avoid a false negative. Also, a small fraction of the T-cells may have the same rearrangement, leading to a false impression of clonality. Diagnosis may be particularly challenging in early lesions.
    - The identification of a clonal population of T-cells does not automatically render a diagnosis of MF because a clone may be present in various non-cancerous diseases including infection [65]. Nevertheless, in the appropriate clinical context and with the appropriate histologic findings, a clonal TCR does support the diagnosis and may be the definitive evidence of malignancy.
    - The clinical-pathologic correlation is so important in the diagnosis of MF that the ASDP appropriate use criteria incorporate specific clinical presentations in their recommendations. For example, in patients presenting with at least one scaly patch or plaque clinically concerning for MF and histology that is concerning, suspicious or suggestive of MF, TCR testing is appropriate [7].
    - NGS shows promise in improving sensitivity for the detection of T-cell clonality compared to other methods [66, 67]. One benefit of this method is the ability to characterize the specific sequence of the clone, providing the opportunity to follow the clone through treatment and disease progression.
    - Clonality tests using high throughput sequencing (NGS) can detect the malignant T-cell clone from peripheral blood samples even when flow cytometry studies fail to detect peripheral blood involvement in patients with MF/CTCL. The identification of a malignant clone in the peripheral blood with the same rearrangement as that seen in a skin biopsy, even when present in low numbers, provides valuable evidence of disease [68]. Peripheral blood testing is less invasive than skin biopsy and often adequate to follow disease progression, recurrence, and response to therapy.
    - MF may be clinically indolent, slowly progressive, or aggressive. Molecular findings may help determine prognosis. Tumor clone frequency determined by high throughput sequencing of the T-cell receptor beta gene may be a marker for aggressive disease [69], although such testing is not routinely performed.
15. **Are molecular genetic studies necessary for the unequivocal diagnosis of dermatofibrosarcoma protuberans (DFSP)?**
    - DFSP is a malignant spindle cell tumor often diagnosed in young to middle-aged adults that is low-grade and generally has a good prognosis. Although it rarely metastasizes, the tumor may be locally destructive with high risk of recurrence. Tumors may undergo fibrosarcomatous transformation and proper treatment is imperative to prevent complications [70].
    - Typically, the tumor exhibits spindle cells that are monomorphic and grow in an infiltrative pattern from the dermis into the subcutis. Unlike benign dermatofibromas, DFSPs usually stain diffusely with CD34. However, CD34 is not specific and can stain other spindle cell tumors of varying malignant potential that occur in the skin [71].
    - DFSPs are characterized by the cytogenetic aberration, t(17;22)(q22;q13) or a supernumerary ring

chromosome that result in a *COL1A1* and *PDGFB* fusion. In cases where the tumor cells stain positive for CD34 but the histology is not typical or appears high-grade, the ASDP considers cytogenetic testing appropriate for diagnosis [7].

- FISH using separate probes for the *COL1A1* gene and *PDGFB* gene may be used to detect the translocation. In one study, FISH detected the translocation in 96% of tumors with diagnoses of DFSP considered certain by histopathologic criteria [72].
- Metastatic cases or cases with fibrosarcomatous change may be more aggressive clinically and are more likely to have atypical histology and loss of CD34 staining, making cytogenetic studies more critical for diagnosis [73].
- The tyrosine kinase inhibitor, imatinib, may be effective in treating DFSPs and is used in cases with extensive or metastatic disease that are not amenable to surgery [74]. When this targeted therapy is being considered, cytogenetic testing is appropriate to confirm the translocation [7].

Case Presentations

Case 1

Learning Objective

Comparative genomic hybridization (CGH) provides a view of copy number variants (CNVs) across the whole genome. Benign melanocytic lesions have few to no copy number variants while malignant melanomas harbor many. CGH is a valuable diagnostic tool for differentiating between benign and malignant melanocytic lesions, particularly if the histology is indefinite.

Case History

A 45-year-old female saw a dermatologist to ask about removing a dark mole on the bridge of her nose for cosmetic reasons (see Fig. 9.1a). She had first noticed the mole 4 years prior and thought it was growing. The lesion was a 3 mm papule that was darkly pigmented and well circumscribed. She had no personal or family history of cancer. A shave biopsy was performed and sent to pathology to confirm the benign nature of what appeared to be a nevus, clinically.

Histologic Findings

The biopsy showed an atypical melanocytic neoplasm within the dermis. The melanocytes were epithelioid with ample cytoplasm, large and hyperchromatic nuclei, and scattered nucleoli, characteristic of a Spitzoid tumor (see Fig. 9.1b). Although the melanocytes did not appear to mature, a full assessment of maturation was not possible since they extended to the base of the biopsy. Mitotic figures were identified and a Ki-67 IHC stain showed a proliferation rate of approximately 10%. A severely atypical Spitz tumor and Spitz melanoma were in the differential diagnosis.

Genetic Study

SNP-aCGH was performed from the FFPE biopsy tissue specimen showing a gain at 5p15.33 (TERT), loss at 6q22.33-q27 (MYB), amplification of 7q31.33-q34 (BRAF), and loss at 7q36.1-q36.3 (see Fig. 9.1c).

Final Diagnosis

Favor malignant melanoma (Spitz melanoma).

Follow-Up

The patient underwent a wide local excision, sentinel lymph node biopsy, and reconstruction with facial plastics. On full excision, the Breslow thickness was 2.1 mm. A sentinel lymph node in the parotid gland was negative for melanoma. The tumor stage was pT3N0 (Stage IIa). The patient is healing well after the surgery and will be followed by oncology and dermatology.

Discussion

Although melanoma is generally diagnosed by histologic examination of the tissue specimen, certain cases are particularly challenging. A correct diagnosis was critically important in this case because of the sensitive site of the lesion. A wide excision of melanoma of the nasal bridge can be disfiguring and cause significant morbidity. Sentinel lymph node biopsy in the parotid must be performed with the least damage to surrounding structures including the facial nerve. The patient obtained a superficial biopsy initially, with little clinical concern that pathology would return a diagnosis of malignancy. The biopsy was superficial, yet there was enough evidence to consider malignant melanoma in the differential diagnosis. However, it was difficult to call the lesion malignant with certainty. The difference in treatment between an atypical and malignant diagnosis could potentially be critical at this site. A superficial, though complete excision with slow Mohs would have been appropriate for an atypical Spitz tumor. Since molecular studies provided additional evidence of malignancy, a deeper surgical excision with wide margins and sentinel lymph node biopsy was indicated. The patient received appropriate treatment and will have closer follow-up because SNP-aCGH was performed.

This case also illustrates the need for molecular studies to provide sensitive and specific results from small tissue samples that are formalin fixed and paraffin embedded. The initial biopsy was a superficial shave biopsy about 2 mm in depth. Less than 50% of the nucleated cells in the specimen were malignant melanocytes. Furthermore, the tissue was processed as a standard biopsy with no foresight of the need for molecular testing. The biopsy was

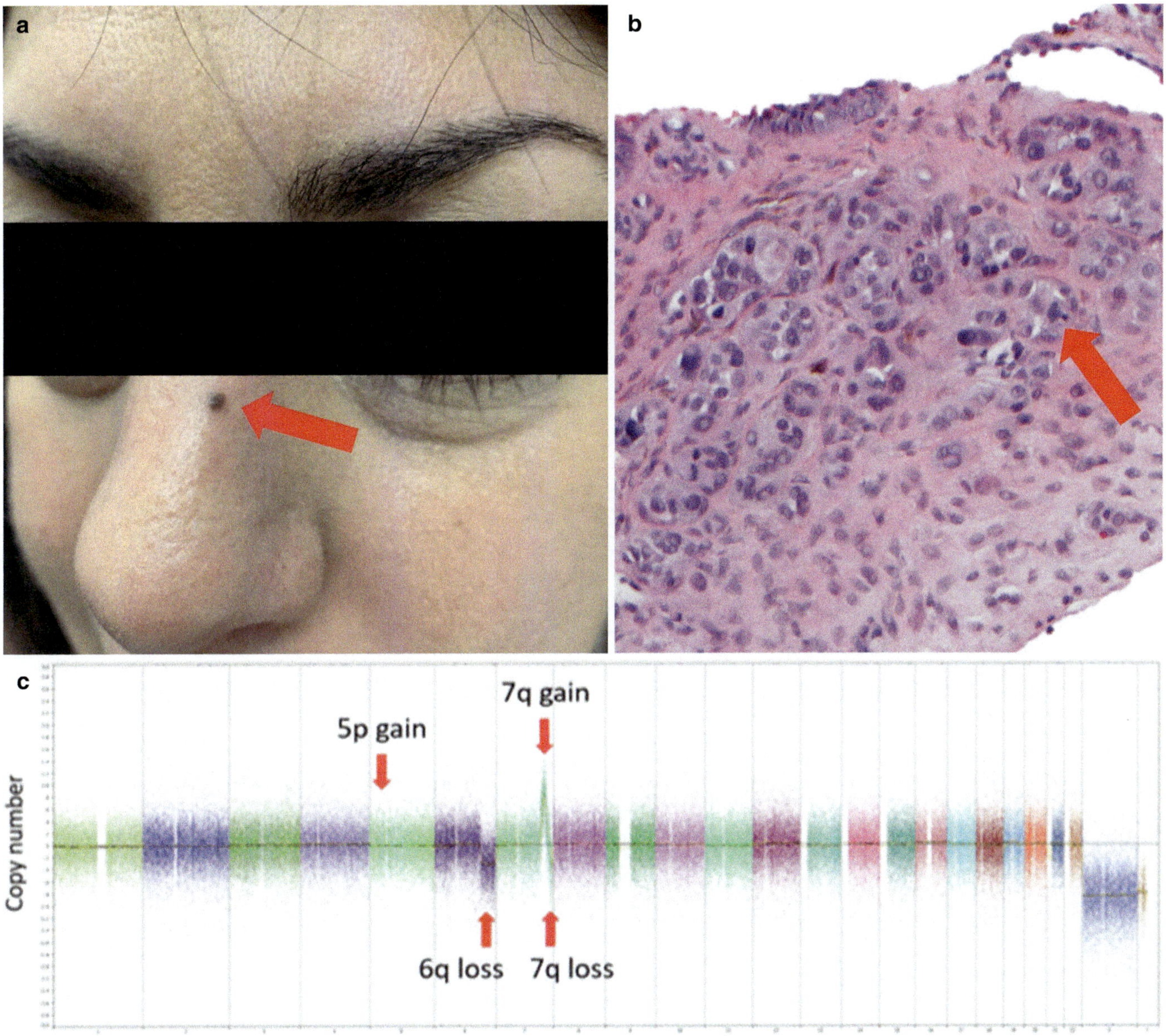

Fig. 9.1 (**a**) Patient with concerning papule on the bridge of her nose (indicated by a red arrow). (**b**) Biopsy showing an atypical Spitzoid melanocytic proliferation in the dermis. (The red arrow indicates a mitotic figure. H&E stain, original amplification 200 X). (**c**) Results of SNP-aCGH showing multiple copy number variants. (Photo courtesy of Dr. May P. Chang, University of Michigan Medical School)

placed directly into formalin at the bedside as soon as it was taken from the patient. After appropriate fixation, it was grossed and embedded in paraffin. In order to conduct molecular testing, an adequate method for collecting sufficient good quality DNA from the FFPE tissue must be part of the protocol. In this case, SNP-aCGH provided clear results from limited tissue.

Case 2

Learning Objective

Targeted therapy is available for patients with advanced melanoma that carry a *BRAF* mutation. Molecular testing for this mutation is imperative in order to identify patients that may benefit.

Case History

A 54-year-old female with a past medical history of obesity, depression, and hypothyroidism presented to her primary care physician for a routine medical exam. A 2 × 2 cm irregular patch was identified in her mid-lower back (see Fig. 9.2a). The lesion had variegated color and asymmetry. The patient reported that it had been present for several years and was not certain if there had been any changes. Her physician biopsied the lesion and sent it for pathologic evaluation. After the biopsy diagnosis, the patient proceeded to have a full excision of the lesion with sentinel lymph node biopsy.

Histologic Findings

The biopsy showed atypical melanocytes extending from the dermal-epidermal junction and invading into the dermis to a depth of 1.1 mm (see Fig. 9.2b). A diagnosis of malignant melanoma was rendered. Pagetoid melanocytes were present focally. No ulceration, no lymphovascular or perineural invasion, and no mitotic figures were identified. Residual melanoma with similar histologic features was seen on the

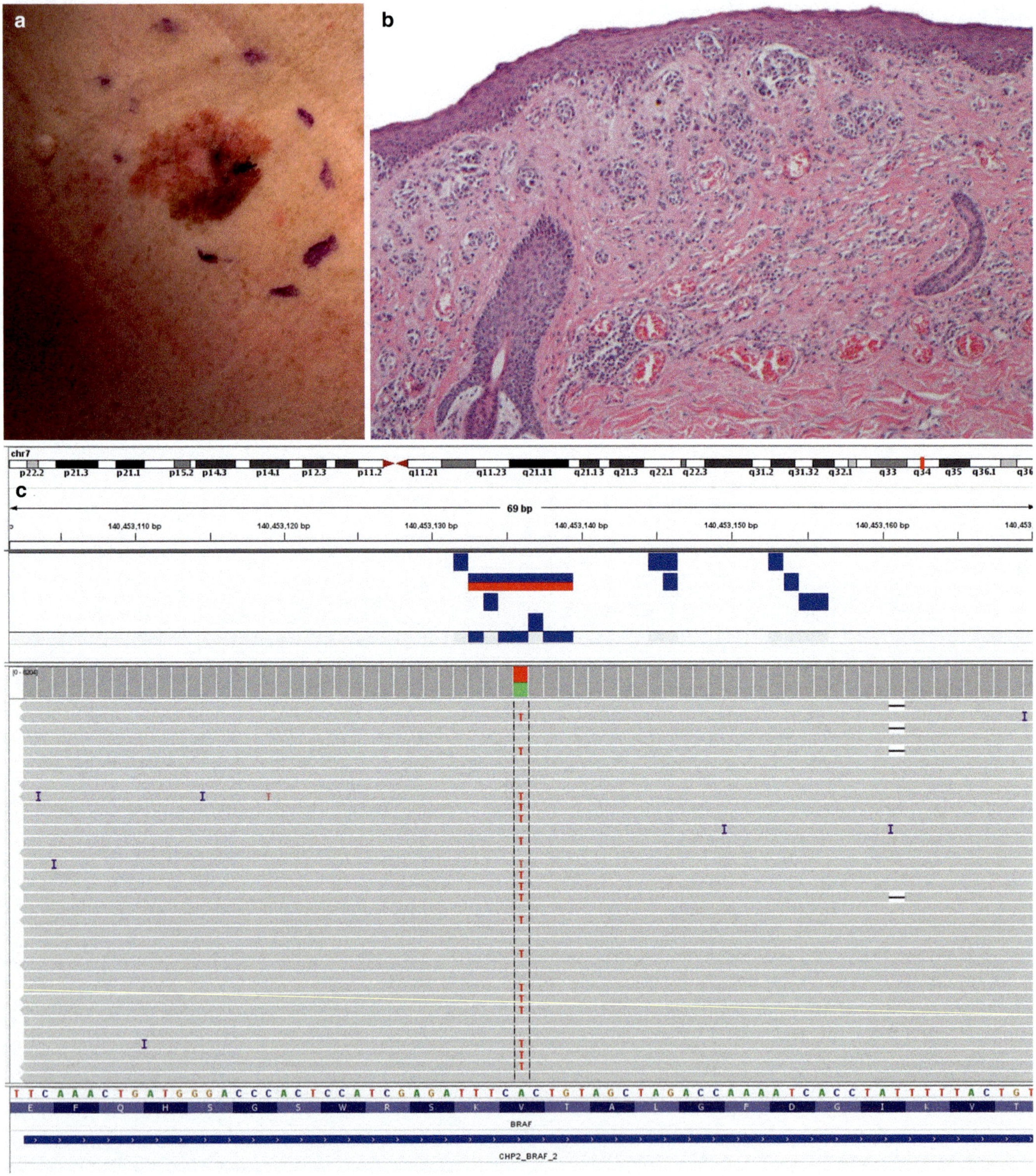

Fig. 9.2 (**a**) Lesion on mid-lower back with variegated pigment, asymmetry, and irregular borders, clinically concerning for melanoma. (**b**) Invasive malignant melanoma seen in the biopsy specimen (H&E stain, original amplification 100 X). (**c**) Sequencing results showing the *BRAF* V600E mutation

excision specimen and metastatic melanoma was identified in one sentinel lymph node. The final pathologic stage was pT2aN1Mx, corresponding to Clinical Stage III.

Genetic Study

A molecular next-generation sequencing solid tumor mutation panel, which included sequencing of the *BRAF* gene, was used to identify the *BRAF* V600E mutation in the patient's excisional specimen (see Fig. 9.2c). No other pathogenic mutations were seen.

Final Diagnosis

Malignant melanoma positive for pathogenic mutation in *BRAF* V600E.

Follow-Up

The patient is receiving treatment with combination *BRAF* and *MEK* inhibitors (vemurafenib plus cobimetinib). She is tolerating the treatment well and recent imaging studies have been negative for disease progression.

Discussion

Testing for BRAF mutations is indicated in all patients with Stage III disease because systemic targeted therapy is considered. This patient's positive lymph node classified her disease as Stage III. *BRAF* mutations are found in 40–60% of malignant melanoma cases and the most common mutation is V600E. Melanomas that carry this mutation respond to *BRAF* inhibitors. Studies have shown that combination treatment with a *MEK* inhibitor improves outcomes and decreases toxicity. Unfortunately, most cases will develop resistance to *BRAF* inhibitors and eventually progress. The addition of *MEK* inhibitors to the treatment regimen prolongs the benefit and improves survival. The NGS panel that was used to sequence this patient's tumor also included sequencing data on other cancer related genes. Although in this case, the results were normal for all genes on the panel other than *BRAF*, mutations in other genes including *KIT* and *CDKN2A* may allow patients to qualify for clinical trials with targeted treatments in development.

Case 3

Learning Objective

The diagnosis of a sebaceous neoplasm, whether benign or malignant, may be the first indication that a patient has Muir-Torre syndrome. Testing for mismatch repair deficiency and identifying microsatellite instability helps render the diagnosis and guide genetic counseling and cancer surveillance.

Case History

A 47-year-old male with a past medical history of hypercholesterolemia and asthma presented to his dermatologist for an annual skin check. He was concerned about multiple pink papules on his face that seemed to be growing. Several papules were deemed to be seborrheic keratoses, clinically. A 0.4 × 0.5 cm papule on the right jawline was biopsied and sent to surgical pathology for evaluation (see Fig. 9.3a).

Histologic Findings

The biopsy showed lobules of basaloid squamous epithelium with interspersed sebaceous cells with downward growth into the dermis. The cells displayed cytologic atypia and there were readily identifiable mitotic figures (see Fig. 9.3b). Immunohistochemistry for mismatch repair proteins showed that the neoplastic cells had complete loss of MSH2 and MSH6 while MLH1 and PMS2 were retained.

Genetic Study

A fluorescent PCR-based assay with capillary electrophoresis was used to compare alleles at five marker sites in normal and patient samples to assess microsatellite instability. The patient's sample was abnormal at all five marker sites for a diagnosis of microsatellite instability - high (see Fig. 9.3c).

Additional Clinical History

The diagnosis of sebaceous carcinoma and MSI-high prompted screening colonoscopy. Several tubular adenomas were resected, one of which showed invasive colonic adenocarcinoma. He underwent sigmoid colon resection and lymph node dissection revealed metastatic colon cancer to one lymph node.

Final Diagnosis

Muir-Torre syndrome with microsatellite instability.

Follow-Up

The patient has had multiple sebaceous adenomas, sebaceomas, and sebaceous carcinomas treated since his original diagnosis. He continues to have close surveillance of his remaining colon for colorectal adenocarcinoma. He was recently diagnosed with urothelial cancer. His younger brother is undergoing heightened cancer screening with colonoscopies and skin checks.

Discussion

Muir-Torre syndrome is a rare autosomal dominant disease that is a variant of hereditary nonpolyposis colorectal cancer syndrome (Lynch syndrome). In Muir-Torre, patients have at least one sebaceous skin tumor along with a visceral cancer including endometrial, urothelial, ovarian, or colorectal cancer. Sebaceous tumors may develop after malignancy at other sites; however, the skin lesions are often noted by patients before symptoms of other tumors are apparent. Therefore, the diagnosis of sebaceous adenoma, sebaceoma, or sebaceous carcinoma in the skin should prompt consideration of additional testing, if clinically indicated. Although

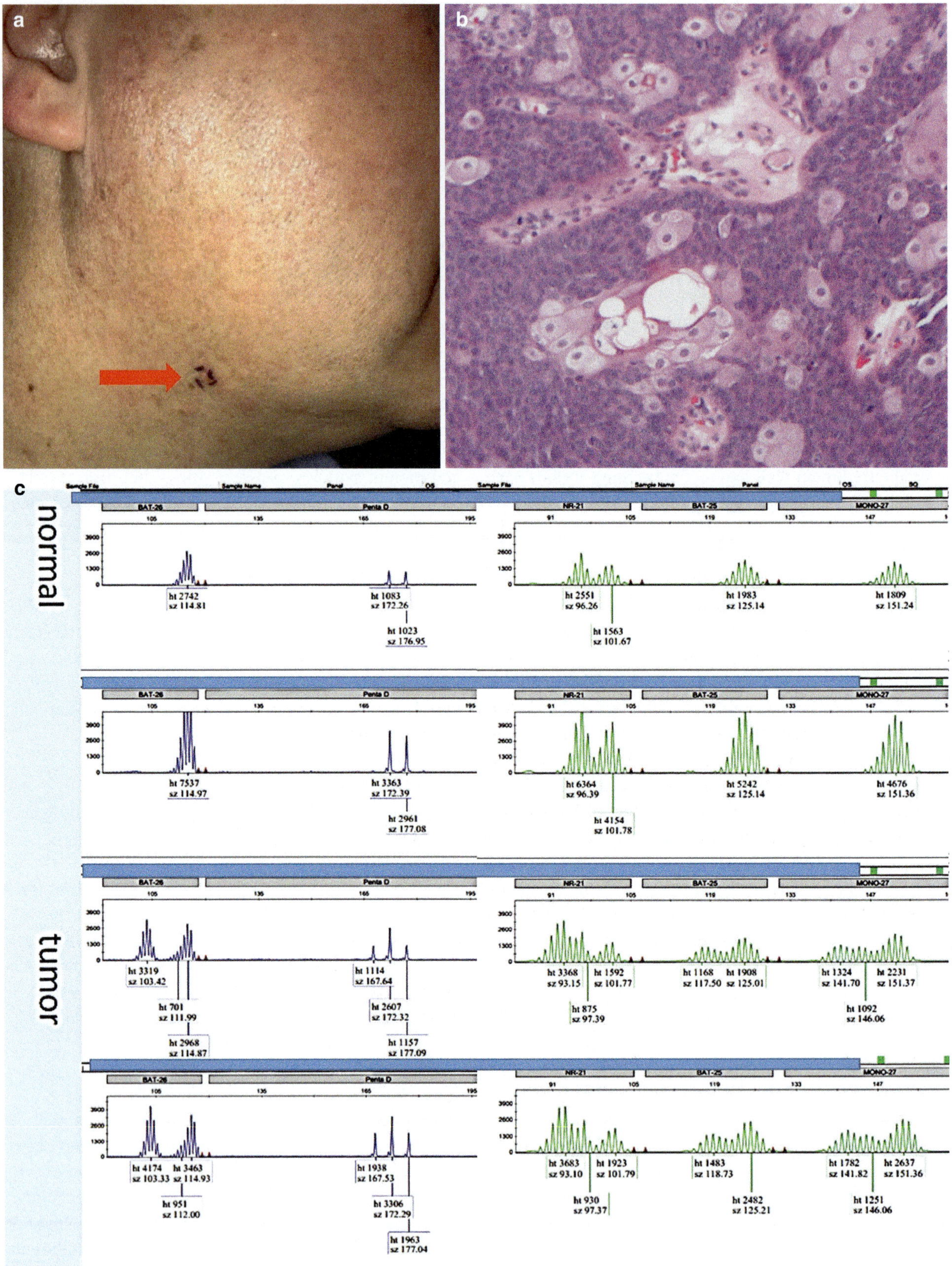

Fig. 9.3 (**a**) Pink papule on right jawline that was biopsied. (**b**) Biopsy showing basaloid proliferation of atypical cells with sebaceous differentiation and mitoses (H&E stain, original amplification 200 X). (**c**) Electropherogram results of microsatellite instability molecular testing illustrating allelic profiles, generated by PCR amplification, at five marker sites in both a normal control and the patient sample. The five marker sites were selected for their sensitivity and specificity in the detection of microsatellite instability (MSI). Samples in which at least two markers are abnormal are considered MSI-high. The patient sample contains alleles that are not present in the normal control at all five marker sites indicating MSI-high status due to mismatch-repair deficiency

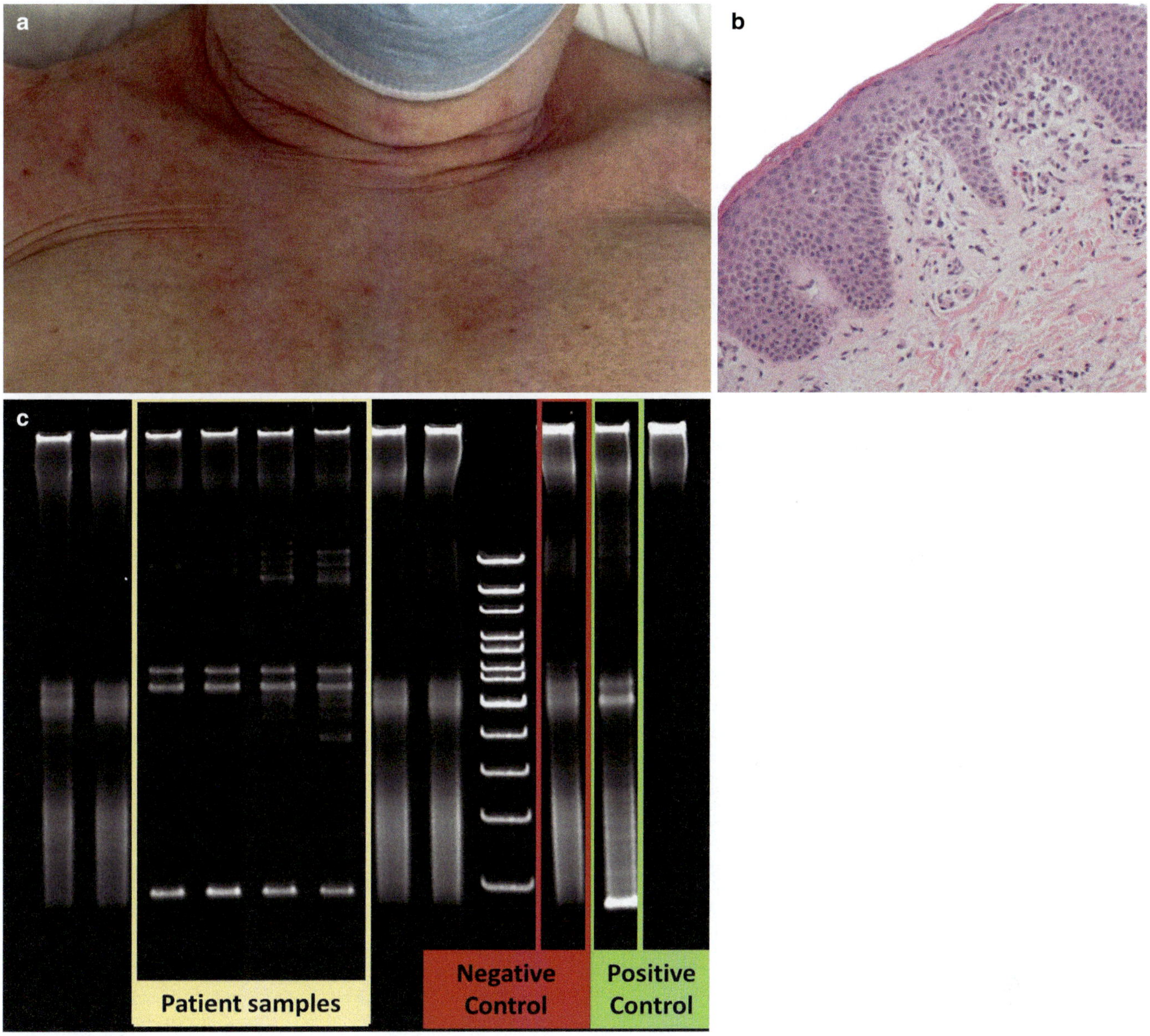

Fig. 9.4 (**a**) Erythematous, pruritic rash involving the chest. (**b**) Biopsy showing mild dermal lymphocytic infiltrate with focal epidermotropism (H&E stain, original amplification 200 X). (**c**) Polyacrylamide gel showing distinct bands in repeat patient samples, indicating a positive T-cell receptor gene rearrangement. The positive control is labeled in green and the polyclonal (negative control) is labeled in red

sebaceous adenomas and sebaceomas are benign tumors, their presence may herald the presence of visceral malignancies in patients with Muir-Torre. IHC is an excellent screening test for deficiency in mismatch repair proteins. Abnormal loss of expression may warrant molecular studies for microsatellite instability.

Case 4

Learning Objective

The presence of a clonal T-cell receptor gene rearrangement provides evidence for mycosis fungoides, and taken together with the clinical presentation and histologic findings, is important in making the diagnosis.

Case History

A 57-year-old female presented to her dermatologist with a complaint of erythematous, pruritic patches focally involving her face, neck, chest, abdomen, and bilateral thighs to encompass less than 10% of her body surface area (see Fig. 9.4a). The pruritic rash had been present for approximately 4 months. She did not recall any recent changes in soaps or lotions, there were no aggravating factors, and over-the-counter anti-itch medications were not helpful. She was otherwise healthy and had no history of malignancy. Biopsies were taken from lesions on the thigh and chest.

Histologic Findings

Both biopsies showed similar findings. The epidermis was mildly acanthotic with no spongiosis. There was a sparse lymphocytic infiltrate in the papillary dermis and lymphocytes at the dermal-epidermal junction as well as few scattered lymphocytes in the epidermis (see Fig. 9.4b). Immunohistochemical stains showed that the epidermotropic lymphocytes were positive for CD3 and CD4 and most had lost mature T-cell marker, CD7.

Genetic Study

T-cell receptor gamma gene rearrangement studies conducted by PCR and polyacrylamide gel electrophoresis were strongly positive (see Fig. 9.4c).

Final Diagnosis

Mycosis fungoides, patch stage.

Follow-Up

The patient is being treated with topical steroid creams and was counseled on the appropriate use of moisturizers to relieve discomfort. Since she is at the patch stage of mycosis fungoides and has limited body surface involvement, her disease may follow an indolent course for many years. She is being seen by her dermatologist every 6 months to monitor disease.

Discussion

This lesion was difficult to classify because the lymphocytic infiltrate was very sparse. There were several concerning features such as epidermotropism of the lymphocytes and loss of the mature T-cell marker, CD7 by IHC. Although the histologic findings were suspicious for MF, they were not diagnostic on their own. In early stages of MF, the population of malignant T-cells is often sparse and T-cell gene rearrangements may show a weak positive or false negative. Multiple repeat biopsies may be necessary for definitive diagnosis if the clinical suspicion is high. A validated molecular test with good sensitivity is imperative to identify a clonal population in such samples. The T-cell gene rearrangement for this patient was determined by a PCR, heteroduplex formation and polyacrylamide gel electrophoresis assay developed and validated in the laboratory. The strong TCR rearrangement supported the diagnosis of MF and was sufficient evidence to render the diagnosis when taken together with the clinical and histologic findings in this case.

References

1. Cancer Genome Atlas N. Genomic classification of cutaneous melanoma. Cell. 2015;161(7):1681–96.
2. Shain AH, Bastian BC. From melanocytes to melanomas. Nat Rev Cancer. 2016;16(6):345–58.
3. Elder DE, Bastian BC, Cree IA, Massi D, Scolyer RA. The 2018 World Health Organization classification of cutaneous, mucosal, and uveal melanoma: detailed analysis of 9 distinct subtypes defined by their evolutionary pathway. Arch Pathol Lab Med. 2020;144(4):500–22.
4. Bastian BC. The molecular pathology of melanoma: an integrated taxonomy of melanocytic neoplasia. Annu Rev Pathol. 2014;9:239–71.
5. Alexandrov LB, Nik-Zainal S, Wedge DC, Aparicio SAJR, Behjati S, Biankin AV, et al. Signatures of mutational processes in human cancer. Nature. 2013;500(7463):415–21.
6. Trucco LD, Mundra PA, Hogan K, Garcia-Martinez P, Viros A, Mandal AK, et al. Ultraviolet radiation-induced DNA damage is prognostic for outcome in melanoma. Nat Med. 2019;25(2):221–4.
7. Vidal CI, Armbrect EA, Andea AA, Bohlke AK, Comfere NI, Hughes SR, et al. Appropriate use criteria in dermatopathology: initial recommendations from the American Society of Dermatopathology. J Cutan Pathol. 2018;45(8):563–80.
8. Harvey NT, Wood BA. A practical approach to the diagnosis of melanocytic lesions. Arch Pathol Lab Med. 2019;143(7): 789–810.
9. Emanuel PO, Andea AA, Vidal CI, Missall TA, Novoa RA, Bohlke AK, et al. Evidence behind the use of molecular tests in melanocytic lesions and practice patterns of these tests by dermatopathologists. J Cutan Pathol. 2018;45(11):839–46.
10. Alomari AK, Miedema JR, Carter MD, Harms PW, Lowe L, Durham AB, et al. DNA copy number changes correlate with clinical behavior in melanocytic neoplasms: proposal of an algorithmic approach. Mod Pathol. 2020;33(7):1307–17.
11. Wang L, Rao M, Fang Y, Hameed M, Viale A, Busam K, et al. A genome-wide high-resolution array-CGH analysis of cutaneous melanoma and comparison of array-CGH to FISH in diagnostic evaluation. J Mol Diagn. 2013;15(5):581–91.
12. Mesbah Ardakani N, Thomas C, Robinson C, Mina K, Harvey NT, Amanuel B, et al. Detection of copy number variations in melanocytic lesions utilising array based comparative genomic hybridisation. Pathology. 2017;49(3):285–91.
13. Chan MP, Andea AA, Harms PW, Durham AB, Patel RM, Wang M, et al. Genomic copy number analysis of a spectrum of blue nevi identifies recurrent aberrations of entire chromosomal arms in melanoma ex blue nevus. Mod Pathol. 2016;29(3):227–39.
14. Yelamos O, Arva NC, Obregon R, Yazdan P, Wagner A, Guitart J, et al. A comparative study of proliferative nodules and lethal melanomas in congenital nevi from children. Am J Surg Pathol. 2015;39(3):405–15.
15. Lee JJ, Lian CG. Molecular testing for cutaneous melanoma: an update and review. Arch Pathol Lab Med. 2019;143(7):811–20.
16. Gerami P, Li G, Pouryazdanparast P, Blondin B, Beilfuss B, Slenk C, et al. A highly specific and discriminatory FISH assay for distinguishing between benign and malignant melanocytic neoplasms. Am J Surg Pathol. 2012;36(6):808–17.
17. Carter MD, Durham AB, Miedema JR, Harms PW, Chan MP, Patel RM, et al. Molecular testing of borderline cutaneous melanocytic lesions: SNP array is more sensitive and specific than FISH. Hum Pathol. 2019;86:115–23.
18. March J, Hand M, Truong A, Grossman D. Practical application of new technologies for melanoma diagnosis: part II. Molecular approaches. J Am Acad Dermatol. 2015;72(6):943–58; quiz 59-60
19. Hillen LM, Van den Oord J, Geybels MS, Becker JC, Zur Hausen A, Winnepenninckx V. Genomic landscape of Spitzoid neoplasms impacting patient management. Front Med. 2018;5:344.
20. Wiesner T, Kutzner H, Cerroni L, Mihm MC Jr, Busam KJ, Murali R. Genomic aberrations in spitzoid melanocytic tumours and their implications for diagnosis, prognosis and therapy. Pathology. 2016;48(2):113–31.
21. Amin SM, Haugh AM, Lee CY, Zhang B, Bubley JA, Merkel EA, et al. A comparison of morphologic and molecular features of

BRAF, ALK, and NTRK1 fusion Spitzoid neoplasms. Am J Surg Pathol. 2017;41(4):491–8.
22. Tetzlaff MT, Reuben A, Billings SD, Prieto VG, Curry JL. Toward a molecular-genetic classification of Spitzoid neoplasms. Clin Lab Med. 2017;37(3):431–48.
23. Zhang AJ, Rush PS, Tsao H, Duncan LM. BRCA1-associated protein (BAP1)-inactivated melanocytic tumors. J Cutan Pathol. 2019;46(12):965–72.
24. Lee S, Barnhill RL, Dummer R, Dalton J, Wu J, Pappo A, et al. TERT promoter mutations are predictive of aggressive clinical behavior in patients with Spitzoid melanocytic neoplasms. Sci Rep. 2015;5:11200.
25. Gerami P, Scolyer RA, Xu X, Elder DE, Abraham RM, Fullen D, et al. Risk assessment for atypical spitzoid melanocytic neoplasms using FISH to identify chromosomal copy number aberrations. Am J Surg Pathol. 2013;37(5):676–84.
26. Ali L, Helm T, Cheney R, Conroy J, Sait S, Guitart J, et al. Correlating array comparative genomic hybridization findings with histology and outcome in spitzoid melanocytic neoplasms. Int J Clin Exp Pathol. 2010;3(6):593–9.
27. Bastian BC, Xiong J, Frieden IJ, Williams ML, Chou P, Busam K, et al. Genetic changes in neoplasms arising in congenital melanocytic nevi: differences between nodular proliferations and melanomas. Am J Pathol. 2002;161(4):1163–9.
28. AJCC Cancer Staging Manual. 8th ed. New York: Springer International Publishing; 2017.
29. Newman MD, Lertsburapa T, Mirzabeigi M, Mafee M, Guitart J, Gerami P. Fluorescence in situ hybridization as a tool for microstaging in malignant melanoma. Mod Pathol. 2009;22(8): 989–95.
30. Cheng L, Lopez-Beltran A, Massari F, MacLennan GT, Montironi R. Molecular testing for BRAF mutations to inform melanoma treatment decisions: a move toward precision medicine. Mod Pathol. 2018;31(1):24–38.
31. Kim SY, Kim SN, Hahn HJ, Lee YW, Choe YB, Ahn KJ. Metaanalysis of BRAF mutations and clinicopathologic characteristics in primary melanoma. J Am Acad Dermatol. 2015;72(6):1036–46 e2.
32. Yao Z, Yaeger R, Rodrik-Outmezguine VS, Tao A, Torres NM, Chang MT, et al. Tumours with class 3 BRAF mutants are sensitive to the inhibition of activated RAS. Nature. 2017;548(7666):234–8.
33. Menzies AM, Haydu LE, Visintin L, Carlino MS, Howle JR, Thompson JF, et al. Distinguishing clinicopathologic features of patients with V600E and V600K BRAF-mutant metastatic melanoma. Clin Cancer Res. 2012;18(12):3242–9.
34. Pollock PM, Harper UL, Hansen KS, Yudt LM, Stark M, Robbins CM, et al. High frequency of BRAF mutations in nevi. Nat Genet. 2003;33(1):19–20.
35. McArthur GA, Ribas A. Targeting oncogenic drivers and the immune system in melanoma. J Clin Oncol. 2013;31(4):499–506.
36. Devji T, Levine O, Neupane B, Beyene J, Xie F. Systemic therapy for previously untreated advanced BRAF-mutated melanoma: a systematic review and network meta-analysis of randomized clinical trials. JAMA Oncol. 2017;3(3):366–73.
37. Robert C, Grob JJ, Stroyakovskiy D, Karaszewska B, Hauschild A, Levchenko E, et al. Five-year outcomes with dabrafenib plus trametinib in metastatic melanoma. N Engl J Med. 2019;381(7):626–36.
38. Robert C, Karaszewska B, Schachter J, Rutkowski P, Mackiewicz A, Stroiakovski D, et al. Improved overall survival in melanoma with combined dabrafenib and trametinib. N Engl J Med. 2015;372(1):30–9.
39. Santiago-Walker A, Gagnon R, Mazumdar J, Casey M, Long GV, Schadendorf D, et al. Correlation of BRAF mutation status in circulating-free DNA and tumor and association with clinical outcome across four BRAFi and MEKi clinical trials. Clin Cancer Res. 2016;22(3):567–74.
40. Vanni I, Tanda ET, Spagnolo F, Andreotti V, Bruno W, Ghiorzo P. The current state of molecular testing in the BRAF-mutated melanoma landscape. Front Mol Biosci. 2020;7:113.
41. Long GV, Wilmott JS, Capper D, Preusser M, Zhang YE, Thompson JF, et al. Immunohistochemistry is highly sensitive and specific for the detection of V600E BRAF mutation in melanoma. Am J Surg Pathol. 2013;37(1):61–5.
42. Network NCC. Cutaneous Melanoma (Version 3.2020) 2020 [Available from: https://www.nccn.org/professionals/physician_gls/default.aspx#melanoma
43. Bisschop C, Ter Elst A, Bosman LJ, Platteel I, Jalving M, van den Berg A, et al. Rapid BRAF mutation tests in patients with advanced melanoma: comparison of immunohistochemistry, droplet digital PCR, and the Idylla mutation platform. Melanoma Res. 2018;28(2):96–104.
44. Spittle C, Ward MR, Nathanson KL, Gimotty PA, Rappaport E, Brose MS, et al. Application of a BRAF pyrosequencing assay for mutation detection and copy number analysis in malignant melanoma. J Mol Diagn. 2007;9(4):464–71.
45. Tan YH, Liu Y, Eu KW, Ang PW, Li WQ, Salto-Tellez M, et al. Detection of BRAF V600E mutation by pyrosequencing. Pathology. 2008;40(3):295–8.
46. Mancini I, Simi L, Salvianti F, Castiglione F, Sonnati G, Pinzani P. Analytical evaluation of an NGS testing method for routine molecular diagnostics on melanoma formalin-fixed, paraffin-embedded tumor-derived DNA. Diagnostics. 2019;9(3):1–14.
47. Davis EJ, Johnson DB, Sosman JA, Chandra S. Melanoma: what do all the mutations mean? Cancer. 2018;124(17):3490–9.
48. Vanni I, Tanda ET, Dalmasso B, Pastorino L, Andreotti V, Bruno W, et al. Non-BRAF mutant melanoma: molecular features and therapeutical implications. Front Mol Biosci. 2020;7:172.
49. Hodi FS, Corless CL, Giobbie-Hurder A, Fletcher JA, Zhu M, Marino-Enriquez A, et al. Imatinib for melanomas harboring mutationally activated or amplified KIT arising on mucosal, acral, and chronically sun-damaged skin. J Clin Oncol. 2013;31(26):3182–90.
50. Carvajal RD, Antonescu CR, Wolchok JD, Chapman PB, Roman RA, Teitcher J, et al. KIT as a therapeutic target in metastatic melanoma. JAMA. 2011;305(22):2327–34.
51. Queirolo P, Spagnolo F. Binimetinib for the treatment of NRAS-mutant melanoma. Expert Rev Anticancer Ther. 2017;17(11):985–90.
52. Dummer R, Schadendorf D, Ascierto PA, Arance A, Dutriaux C, Di Giacomo AM, et al. Binimetinib versus dacarbazine in patients with advanced NRAS-mutant melanoma (NEMO): a multicentre, open-label, randomised, phase 3 trial. Lancet Oncol. 2017;18(4):435–45.
53. Hirsch D, Kemmerling R, Davis S, Camps J, Meltzer PS, Ried T, et al. Chromothripsis and focal copy number alterations determine poor outcome in malignant melanoma. Cancer Res. 2013;73(5):1454–60.
54. Gerami P, Jewell SS, Pouryazdanparast P, Wayne JD, Haghighat Z, Busam KJ, et al. Copy number gains in 11q13 and 8q24 [corrected] are highly linked to prognosis in cutaneous malignant melanoma. J Mol Diagn. 2011;13(3):352–8.
55. Gerami P, Cook RW, Wilkinson J, Russell MC, Dhillon N, Amaria RN, et al. Development of a prognostic genetic signature to predict the metastatic risk associated with cutaneous melanoma. Clin Cancer Res. 2015;21(1):175–83.
56. Marchetti MA, Coit DG, Dusza SW, Yu A, McLean L, Hu Y, et al. Performance of gene expression profile tests for prognosis in patients with localized cutaneous melanoma: a systematic review and meta-analysis. JAMA Dermatol. 2020;
57. Farberg AS, Hall MA, Douglas L, Covington KR, Kurley SJ, Cook RW, et al. Integrating gene expression profiling into NCCN high-risk cutaneous squamous cell carcinoma management recommendations: impact on patient management. Curr Med Res Opin. 2020;36(8):1301–7.

58. Iacobelli J, Harvey NT, Wood BA. Sebaceous lesions of the skin. Pathology. 2017;49(7):688–97.
59. John AM, Schwartz RA. Muir-Torre syndrome (MTS): an update and approach to diagnosis and management. J Am Acad Dermatol. 2016;74(3):558–66.
60. Jessup CJ, Redston M, Tilton E, Reimann JD. Importance of universal mismatch repair protein immunohistochemistry in patients with sebaceous neoplasia as an initial screening tool for Muir-Torre syndrome. Hum Pathol. 2016;49:1–9.
61. Li K, Luo H, Huang L, Luo H, Zhu X. Microsatellite instability: a review of what the oncologist should know. Cancer Cell Int. 2020;20:16.
62. Smoller BR. Mycosis fungoides: what do/do not we know? J Cutan Pathol. 2008;35(Suppl 2):35–9.
63. Bagherani N, Smoller BR. An overview of cutaneous T cell lymphomas. F1000Res. 2016;5.
64. Hodak E, Amitay-Laish I. Mycosis fungoides: a great imitator. Clin Dermatol. 2019;37(3):255–67.
65. Hristov AC, Tejasvi T, Wilcox RA. Mycosis fungoides and Sezary syndrome: 2019 update on diagnosis, risk-stratification, and management. Am J Hematol. 2019;94(9):1027–41.
66. Sufficool KE, Lockwood CM, Abel HJ, Hagemann IS, Schumacher JA, Kelley TW, et al. T-cell clonality assessment by next-generation sequencing improves detection sensitivity in mycosis fungoides. J Am Acad Dermatol. 2015;73(2):228–36. e2
67. Fujii K, Kanekura T. Next-generation sequencing Technologies for Early-Stage Cutaneous T-cell lymphoma. Front Med. 2019;6:181.
68. Kirsch IR, Watanabe R, O'Malley JT, Williamson DW, Scott LL, Elco CP, et al. TCR sequencing facilitates diagnosis and identifies mature T cells as the cell of origin in CTCL. Sci Transl Med. 2015;7(308):308ra158.
69. de Masson A, O'Malley JT, Elco CP, Garcia SS, Divito SJ, Lowry EL, et al. High-throughput sequencing of the T cell receptor beta gene identifies aggressive early-stage mycosis fungoides. Sci Transl Med. 2018;10(440):1–28.
70. Allen A, Ahn C, Sangueza OP. Dermatofibrosarcoma Protuberans. Dermatol Clin. 2019;37(4):483–8.
71. Carter JM, Weiss SW, Linos K, DiCaudo DJ, Folpe AL. Superficial CD34-positive fibroblastic tumor: report of 18 cases of a distinctive low-grade mesenchymal neoplasm of intermediate (borderline) malignancy. Mod Pathol. 2014;27(2):294–302.
72. Karanian M, Perot G, Coindre JM, Chibon F, Pedeutour F, Neuville A. Fluorescence in situ hybridization analysis is a helpful test for the diagnosis of dermatofibrosarcoma protuberans. Mod Pathol. 2015;28(2):230–7.
73. Ha SY, Lee SE, Kwon MJ, Kim YJ, Lee EH, Seo J, et al. PDGFB rearrangement in dermatofibrosarcoma protuberans: correlation with clinicopathologic characteristics and clinical implications. Hum Pathol. 2013;44(7):1300–9.
74. Navarrete-Dechent C, Mori S, Barker CA, Dickson MA, Nehal KS. Imatinib treatment for locally advanced or metastatic dermatofibrosarcoma protuberans: a systematic review. JAMA Dermatol. 2019;155(3):361–9.

Soft Tissue Tumors

10

Anthony P. Martinez

List of Frequently Asked Questions

1. What is the role of molecular testing in round cell sarcomas?
2. How are undifferentiated round cell sarcomas classified? What are the most common fusions?
3. Is FISH testing for Ewing sarcoma and other undifferentiated round cell sarcomas enough? What is the role of next-generation sequencing (NGS) in Ewing sarcoma and other undifferentiated small round cell sarcomas?
4. What are some of the limitations for using NGS on undifferentiated round cell sarcomas?
5. What is the role of molecular testing in adipocytic tumors?
6. What is the sensitivity of *MDM2* FISH for the diagnosis of ALT/WDL? What is the benefit of using FISH testing in problematic lipomatous tumors?
7. When is it appropriate to use *MDM2* FISH testing in dedifferentiated liposarcoma? Are there any potential pitfalls?
8. What molecular fusion is seen in myxoid liposarcoma? What other molecular alterations can be seen?
9. What is the role of molecular testing in vascular tumors?
10. Are there any benign vascular tumors that may benefit from ancillary molecular testing?
11. What intermediate or low-grade vascular neoplasms are often confirmed with the use of molecular testing?
12. What is the role of molecular testing in angiosarcoma?
13. What is the role of molecular testing in skeletal muscle tumors?
14. What fusions are seen in alveolar rhabdomyosarcoma? What other alterations can be seen? How sensitive and specific is FISH testing and what are possible reasons for a negative result?
15. What entities are encompassed under the umbrella term "sindle cell/sclerosing rhabdomyosarcoma"? What rearrangements and/or mutations are seen? How does this impact prognosis?
16. What is the role of molecular testing in tumors of uncertain differentiation? What are the common fusions found in these tumors? What testing modalities are commonly employed and are there any limitations?
17. What is the role of molecular testing in fibroblastic/myofibroblastic tumors? What are the common fusions found in these tumors? What testing modalities are commonly employed and are there any limitations?

Frequently Asked Questions

1. **What is the role of molecular testing in undifferentiated round cell sarcomas?**
   - The differential for undifferentiated round cell sarcomas is broad. In fact, there are so many that the use of mnemonics is often employed just to remember the differential (Table 10.1). The role of molecular is to provide a definitive diagnosis on limited tissue samples to ensure appropriate treatment (e.g., neoadjuvant chemotherapy) and prognostic data when applicable.
   - Molecular testing is often considered an ancillary technique after an initial round of sorting with immunohistochemical stains (lymphoma/leukemia versus Ewing versus Rhabdomyosarcoma); however, many tumors can have overlapping histologic and immunohistochemical features, and in these cases the use of molecular testing is invaluable.
2. **How are undifferentiated round cell sarcomas classified? What are the most common fusions?**
   - Undifferentiated round cell sarcomas are classified as Ewing sarcoma, round cell sarcoma with *EWSR1*-

A. P. Martinez (✉)
Department of Pathology and Laboratory Medicine, Department of Dermatology, Emory University School of Medicine, Atlanta, GA, USA
e-mail: anthonymartinezmd@gmail.com

Y. Ding, L. Zhang (eds.), *Practical Oncologic Molecular Pathology*, Practical Anatomic Pathology, https://doi.org/10.1007/978-3-030-73227-1_10

non-ETS fusions, *CIC*-rearranged sarcoma, and sarcoma with *BCOR* genetic alterations [1] (Table 10.2).

- Ewing sarcoma (EWS) is the prototypical small round cell sarcoma that involves *EWSR1* on 22q12 with members of the ETS (E-26 transformation specific) transcription factors creating *EWSR1-ETS* fusions.
  - Most commonly involved fusion involves *FLI1* [2] on 11q24 in ~85% of cases followed by *ERG* on 21q22 in ~10% of cases [3].
  - Other less common fusions involved *ETV1* (ETS-variant gene 1) on 7p22 [4], *ETV4* (*ETS*-variant gene 4) on 17q12 [5], and *FEV* (fifth Ewing sarcoma variant) on 2q33 [6].
- Because *EWSR1* is a member of FET family, other members including *FUS* (Fused in Sarcoma) can rarely substitute for *EWSR1* creating FET/ETS fusions.
  - Known fusions include *FUS-ERG* and *FUS-FEV* [7, 8].
  - *TAF15* other member of FET family could, in theory, substitute for *FUS* or *EWSR1*.
- Round cell sarcoma with EWSR1-non-ETS fusions.
  - *EWSR1-NFATC2* and *EWSR1-PATZ1* tend to be not respond as well to neoadjuvant chemotherapy [9].
  - DNA methylations studies confirm distinct profiling from *EWSR1*-ETS and *CIC* or *BCOR* rearranged sarcomas [10, 11].
- *CIC*-rearranged sarcomas account for the vast majority of "Ewing-like" sarcomas.
  - Most commonly involve *CIC-DUX4* but other partners include *FOXO4* [12, 13], *NUTM1* [14], and *NUTM2A* [15].
  - Can also show trisomy 8 and *MYC* amplifications [16].
  - *CIC-LEUTX* can be seen as a subset of angiosarcomas [17].
  - Not chemosensitive like EWS and have a worse overall survival [18].
    Tend to affect the deep soft tissue of the trunk and lower extremities of young adults (third to fourth decade).
    Exception are the *CIC-NUTM1* fusion which involves the bones of young children [14].
  - Potential pitfall.
    A subset of angiosarcomas can show *CIC* gene abnormalities, most often mutations, but rearrangements have also been reported [17].

Table 10.1 Differential of small round cell tumors

Mnemonic	Tumor
M	Melanoma
R	Rhabdomyosarcoma (alveolar subtype)
S	Synovial sarcoma
L	Lymphoma/leukemia
E	Ewing sarcoma and other undifferentiated round cell tumors (BCOR, CIC, etc.)
M	Merkel cell carcinoma
O	Olfactory neuroblastoma
N	Neuroblastoma
S	Small cell carcinoma

Table 10.2 Undifferentiated round cell sarcomas

WHO terminology	Age	Sex	Location	Fusion(s)	IHC	Other
Ewing sarcoma	Peak incidence in second decade Older patients tend to be extraskeletal	M > F	Bones (long bones, pelvis, ribs) >> > soft tissue	*EWSR1-FLI* (~85%) *EWSR1-ERG* (~10%)	CD99 (strong, membranous), NKX2.2, FLI1 and ERG depending on fusion	Small % involves *FUS* from FET family) to other ETS genes (*ETV1*, *ETV4*, *FEV*)
Round cell sarcoma with *EWSR1*-non-ETS-fusions	Median age = fourth decade (*NFATC2*) Mean age = fifth decade (*PATZ1*)	M >> > F (*NFATC2*) M = F (*PATZ1*)	Long bones (*NFATC2*) Soft tissue (*PATZ1*)	*EWSR1-NFATC2* *FUS-NFATC2* *EWSR1-PATZ1*	CD99 (50%), NKX2.2 and focal AE1/AE3 (*NFATC2*) Co-expression of myogenic and neural markers (*PATZ1*)	*EWSR1-NFATC2* often shows concurrent amplification of 5′ probe by break-apart FISH
CIC-rearranged sarcoma	Median = third and fourth decades	M > F	Trunk and lower extremities deep soft tissue	CIC-DUX4 (95%)	CD99, ETV4, DUX4, WT1	Small % involves fusion to *FOXO4*, *LEUTX*, *NUTM1*, and *NUTM2* Trisomy 8 with *MYC* amplifications
Sarcoma with *BCOR* genetic alterations	Most common in first-second decade (>90%)	M >> > F	Bone > soft tissue	*BCOR-CCNB3* *BCOR*-ITD	CD99 (50%), BCOR, cyclin D1, SATB2, TLE1	Rare fusions include *BCOR-MAML3* and *BCOR-ZC3H7B*

IHC immunohistochemistry, *M* male, *F* female

- *BCOR*-rearranged sarcoma.
  - Most frequent is *BCOR-CCNB3*; but others include internal tandem duplication (*BCOR*-ITD), *KMT2D-BCOR*, *BCOR-ZC3H7B*, and *BCOR-MAML3* [19, 20].
  - Tend to affect the bones of child/adolescents (80% in first two decades) [21, 22].
  - More common in males and have a similar overall survival compared to EWS [19].

3. **Is FISH testing for Ewing sarcoma and other undifferentiated round cell sarcomas enough? What is the role of next-generation sequencing (NGS) in Ewing sarcoma and other undifferentiated small round cell sarcomas?**
   - FISH testing, primarily through break-apart assays, is no longer considered enough by most soft tissue pathologists. This is in part due to some overlapping histology and immunohistochemistry with non-ETS fusions and other round cell sarcomas with specific gene rearrangements that can have a different prognosis (see below). The role of NGS is to identify specific gene fusions that may dictate treatment and prognosis.
   - *EWSR1* break-apart FISH testing can sometimes create false positives in non-EWS tumors [23].
     - Often with tumors showing concurrent *SMARCB1* deletions since genes are located only 5.5 Mb from each other.
   - Around 50% of previously diagnosed undifferentiated round cell sarcomas, most commonly defined as negative for *EWSR1* rearrangement by FISH, have disease defining fusions [24–26], most commonly *CIC* and *BCOR*.
   - Because both *EWSR1* and *PATZ1* are located on the same chromosome and are ~2 mb away from each other, a FISH break-apart probe may result in a false negative due to the short distance between the inversion of the involved genes.
   - A subset of *CIC*-rearranged sarcomas may be missed using FISH as opposed to NGS testing [27–29].
     - Exact reason for false negatives is unknown, but it may be due to cryptic insertions beyond the resolution of the FISH assay.
4. **What are some of the limitations for using NGS on undifferentiated round cell sarcomas?**
   - Occasionally, *CIC*-rearranged sarcomas can be missed on RNA-based sequencing and this may be related to a failure of algorithmic analysis [29].
     - This may be in part due to repetitive sequences that can be seen with *DUX4* on chromosomes 4q35.2 and 10q26.3 and are filtered out by algorithms.
     - Use of "Grep" command may help detect fusion when missed by other programs such as FusionMap, FusionFinder, and ChimeraScan programs [30].
   - There is still a small subset of undifferentiated round cell sarcomas that lack an identifiable fusion. These cases may benefit from array-based DNA-methylation profiling to determine if they cluster with a known group (e.g., *CIC*, *BCOR*) or if it will change management (i.e., use of neoadjuvant chemotherapy).
5. **What is the role of molecular testing in adipocytic tumors?**
   - Many adipocytic neoplasms have specific molecular mutations or rearrangements (Table 10.3). The primary role for molecular testing is to confirm or establish the diagnosis in problematic situations (see below).
6. **What is the sensitivity of *MDM2* FISH for the diagnosis of ALT/WDL? What is the benefit of using FISH testing in problematic lipomatous tumors?**
   - Atypical lipomatous tumor/well-differentiated liposarcoma (ALT/WDL) is defined by the amplification

Table 10.3 Alterations in lipomatous neoplasms

Neoplasm	Alteration	Molecular testing usually needed?	Role of testing if used
Lipoma	*HMGA2* rearrangements	No	Exclude WDL
Angiolipoma	*PRKD2* mutations	No	None
Hibernoma	Translocations and interstitial deletions of 11q that localize to *MEN1* and *AIP*	No	Exclude WDL
Lipoblastoma	*PLAG1* rearrangements	No	Exclude MLS and WDL
Spindle cell/ pleomorphic lipoma	*RB1* deletions	No	Exclude WDL
Chondroid lipoma	*MRTFB* rearrangement (previously called *MKL2*)	No	Exclude WDL and MLS
MLS	*DDIT3* rearrangements	Yes	For confirmation and exclude DDLS and other round cell sarcomas
WDL/DDLS	*MDM2* amplification	Yes	Exclude benign lipomatous neoplasms or confirm DDLS
Pleomorphic liposarcoma	Complex chromosomal aberrations	Yes	Exclude DDLS

WDL well-differentiated liposarcoma, *MLS*, myxoid liposarcoma, *DDLS* dedifferentiated liposarcoma

of *MDM2* originating from the region of 12q14-q15, and because of its relative increased sensitivity and specificity compared to other methods such as Q-PCR and immunohistochemistry, FISH is now considered the gold standard for diagnosis [31–33].
  - Sensitivity in literature is considered to be greater than 90% [31, 32]; however, many studies were done on non-problematic tumors.
  - Cytogenetic analysis often shows supernumerary ring and giant chromosomes that originate from the 12q14-q15 region [34].
- In problematic tumors, using the following criteria for *MDM2* FISH testing may identify up to 1/3 of cases that would otherwise be classified as lipoma [35, 36]:
  - Recurrent lipomas.
  - Tumors with equivocal cytologic atypia.
  - Retroperitoneal, intra-abdominal, and pelvic tumors.
  - Deep extremity tumors larger than 10 cm in patients over 50.

7. **When is it appropriate to use *MDM2* FISH testing in dedifferentiated liposarcoma (DDLPS)? Are there any potential pitfalls?**
   - Similar to ALT/WDLs, DDLPS are usually straightforward and do not need molecular testing if background WDL is present along with the high-grade component.
   - There are certain situations when testing is helpful, and these include:
     - When the differential includes primary retroperitoneal myxoid liposarcoma.
     - When then dedifferentiated component looks like another tumor such as myxoid liposarcoma or pleomorphic liposarcoma.
   - Potential pitfalls in dedifferentiated liposarcomas; the following situations might be misinterpreted as MDM2 amplification:
     - *STAT6*, which is associated with solitary fibrous tumors (*NAB2-STAT6* fusions) [37], is located in 12q13 and can show amplification by FISH [38] and can also show nuclear immunohistochemical staining for STAT6.
     - *DDIT3*, which is associated with myxoid liposarcoma (*FUS-DDIT3*) is located on 12q13.2, and DDLPS can show amplification of *DDIT3* in tumors that often have myxoid liposarcoma-like morphology [39].
   - Both ALTs and DDLPS can occasionally demonstrate multiple faint alphoid signals that represent satellite DNA of chromosome 12 [31].
     - This could be misinterpreted as gain of copy number.
8. **What molecular fusion is seen in myxoid liposarcoma (MLPS)? What other molecular alterations can be seen?**
   - Translocations of *FUS-DDIT3* [40] in >95% and *EWSR1-DDIT3* [41] in less than 5% are considered pathognomonic for MLPS.
     - Break-apart FISH for *DDIT3* is considered sensitive and specific [42].
   - Approximately 50% have *TERT* promoter mutations [43].
   - ~25% of PI3K/mTOR mutations, most often gain of function mutations [44].
   - Diagnosis of high-grade MLPS when >5% round cell change.
     - High-grade MLPS have higher rate of metastasis and death [45].
     - Presence of necrosis is also associated with adverse prognosis [45].
9. **What is the role of molecular testing in vascular tumors?**
   - Many vascular tumors have known mutations or rearrangements; however, molecular testing is really only performed in a handful of vascular tumors (Table 10.4),

Table 10.4 Commonly assessed molecular alterations in vascular lesions

WHO terminology	Common locations	Primary molecular alteration	Routine testing needed?	Role of testing if used
Epithelioid hemangioma	Head and neck, distal extremities, trunk	*FOS* or *FOSB* rearrangement	No but may be helpful in difficult cases	Exclude epithelioid angiosarcoma
Pseudomyogenic hemangioendothelioma	Lower and upper extremities, trunk	*SERPINE1-FOSB* and *ACTB-FOSB* rearrangements	No	Exclude epithelioid hemangioendothelioma and epithelioid sarcoma
Epithelioid hemangioendothelioma	Soft tissue, lung, liver	*WWTR1-CAMTA1* and *YAP-TFE3*	Yes and no	Exclude epithelioid angiosarcoma and also helpful if surrogate IHC for CAMTA1 not available
Secondary (radiation-induced) AS	Breast, other irradiated sites	*MYC* amplification	No	Equivocal cases where IHC may be considered false positive to exclude AVL

IHC immunohistochemistry, *AS* angiosarcoma, *AVL* atypical vascular lesion and these are usually problematic or equivocal, borderline cases where the diagnosis is between benign and malignant and/or it will affect treatment/management.

10. **Are there any benign vascular tumors that may benefit from ancillary molecular testing?**
    - Epithelioid hemangioma is traditionally considered on spectrum and synonymous with the term angiolymphoid hyperplasia with eosinophilia (ALHE).
      - WHO no longer recommends the use of this terminology.
      - Interestingly, many cases of ALHE lack *FOS* or *FOSB* rearrangements [46].
    - Epithelioid hemangioma is characterized by recurrent fusion of *FOS* or *FOSB* genes in ~50% of cases [46].
      - FOS partners include *LMNA*, *MBNL1*, *VIM*, and l*incRNA* [47, 48].
      - FOSB partners include *ZFP36*, *WWTR1*, or *ACTB* [47, 49].
    - Molecular testing may be beneficial in cases that are referred to as atypical epithelioid hemangiomas [50], which can show some features such as solid growth and necrosis that would raise the differential of epithelioid angiosarcoma.
11. **What intermediate or low-grade vascular neoplasms are often confirmed with the use of molecular testing?**
    - Pseudomyogenic hemangioendothelioma (PMHE).
      - When originally described, it was called epithelioid sarcoma-like hemangioendothelioma [51].
      - Molecular testing can be helpful because the tumor is often confused for other entities such as carcinoma or an epithelioid sarcoma.

        Showing diffuse keratin (AE1/AE3) and vascular markers expression (ERG, FLI). About 50% express CD31 [52].
      - Characterized by *SERPINE1-FOSB* and *ACTB-FOSB* fusions [49, 53].
    - Epithelioid hemangioendothelioma (EHE).
      - Malignant vascular tumor that most commonly involves the somatic soft tissue but also visceral organs such as the lung and liver [54].
      - In classic cases, molecular testing is likely not needed; however, if surrogate IHC is not available or if there is a need to exclude epithelioid angiosarcoma, then molecular testing is helpful.
      - Characterized by *WWTR1-CAMTA1* fusion in >90% of cases [55] and *YAP1-TFE3* in approximately 10% of cases [56].

        CAMTA1 and TFE3 immunohistochemistry are often used as a surrogate for molecular testing [56, 57].
12. **What is the role of molecular testing in radiation-associated angiosarcoma?**
    - High-level *MYC* gene amplifications are characteristic of post-irradiation and chronic lymphedema-associated (Stewart-Treves) angiosarcoma [58].
    - Primary role of FISH testing is rule-in/-out angiosarcoma in difficult cases or when IHC is felt to represent a false positive [59].
      - ~25% of cases can show co-amplification of *FLT4* [58].
      - *FLT4* amplified lesion lack *KDR* and *PLCG1* mutations that can be seen in both secondary and primary angiosarcomas [17].
    - Potential pitfall is that a small subset of primary angiosarcomas can show both MYC overexpression by IHC and *MYC* amplification, so clinical context is needed [60].
13. **What is the role of molecular testing in skeletal muscle tumors?**
    - Molecular testing for sarcomas showing skeletal muscle differentiation (rhabdomyoblastic) is continuing to evolve. The main role of molecular testing is for confirmation of alveolar rhabdomyosarcoma and to exclude other sarcomas with specific rearrangements or in specific situations where there may be a clinical need for mutational status (e.g., *MYOD1* status in pediatric spindle cell rhabdomyosarcoma) or prognosis (e.g., congenital spindle cell rhabdomyosarcoma).
14. **What fusions are seen in alveolar rhabdomyosarcoma? What other alterations can be seen? How sensitive and specific is FISH testing and what are possible reasons for a negative result?**
    - Alveolar rhabdomyosarcoma (ARMS).
      - Second most common type of rhabdomyosarcoma [61].
      - Primitive round cell sarcoma characterized by *PAX3-FOXO1*, most commonly or *PAX7-FOXO1* fusions [62].

        Amplifications of *MYCN* and *CDK4* can often be seen in *PAX3-FOXO1* fusions [63, 64].

        Amplification of 1p36 which encompasses *PAX7* can be seen in *PAX7-FOXO1* fusions [65].

        Break-apart FISH for *FOXO1* is generally considered to be 100% specific [66] but still a subset (~15%) of ARMS that are negative.

        (a) Likely a combination of low-level fusions, cryptic fusions, and true fusion-negative cases [67].
      - *ALK* copy number gains can be seen but has not played a role in therapy [68, 69].
      - Prognosis worse than fusion-negative rhabdomyosarcoma and ERMS [70].

15. **What entities are encompassed under the umbrella term "sindle cell/sclerosing rhabdomyosarcoma"? What rearrangements and/or mutations are seen? How does this impact prognosis?**
    - Congenital spindle cell rhabdomyosarcoma.
      - Characterized by *VGLL2/NCOA2/CITED2* rearrangements.
        Fusions involve *VGLL2-CITED2, VGLL2-NCOA2, SRF-NCOA2, TEAD1-NCOA2* [71, 72].
      - Tend to present within first year and commonly involve the trunk and have a favorable prognosis.
        Exceptions are those with *MYOD1* mutations that tend to have a poor prognosis [72].
    - Spindle cell rhabdomyosarcoma with *FUS-TFCP2* and *EWSR1-TFCP2* fusions [11].
      - Can involve both bone and soft tissue, involve both children and adults, tend to be confused for an Ewing-like sarcoma, and behave aggressively.
    - Adult spindle cell/sclerosing rhabdomyosarcoma.
      - A subset shows *MYOD1* mutations [73, 74].
        Usually homozygous mutation in exon 1 (pL122R) but can also have heterozygous mutations.
        More commonly seen in sclerosing subtype and can also harbor coexistent *PIK3CA* mutations [74].
    - Histiocyte-rich rhabdomyoblastic tumor.
      - Provisional entity most often confused with spindle cell rhabdomyosarcoma [75].
      - Does not have *MYOD1* mutations, is usually encapsulated with surrounding lymphoid aggregates and a prominent histiocytic inflammatory infiltrate.
      - Good prognosis with no recurrences or metastasis [76].
      - Mentioned because angiomatoid fibrous histiocytoma would be on the histologic differential and molecular testing may be needed to exclude.
16. **What is the role of molecular testing in tumor of uncertain differentiation? What are the common fusions found in these tumors? What testing modalities are commonly employed and are there any limitations?**
    - Many soft tissue tumors of uncertain differentiation have unique molecular rearrangements that routinely primarily to confirm a diagnosis. See below for specifics on the individual tumors that are commonly tested.
    - Angiomatoid fibrous histiocytoma (AFH).
      - Primarily occurs in children and young adults (<40 years) primarily in the dermis/subcutis of the extremities, although can occur anywhere where normal lymph nodes are found [77].
      - Most frequent fusion is *EWSR1-CREB1* seen in >90% of cases [78].
        Less commonly *EWSR1-ATF1* and less commonly *FUS-ATF1*.
        FISH break-apart probes are generally sensitive for detecting either the *EWSR1* or the *FUS* rearrangement in AFH but up to 25% cases can be missed [79].
        (a) May possibly represent cryptic rearrangements not detectable through FISH probes or represent other fusion(s).
      Immunohistochemistry.
        (a) Most show co-expression of EMA and desmin [77].
        (b) Recently, many have been shown to variably express ALK although this does not correlate with molecular alteration [80].
    - Synovial sarcoma (SS).
      - Primarily occurs in the deep soft tissue of the extremities of adolescents or young adults and vast majority occur before age 50 [81].
      - Monophasic subtype more common than biphasic.
      - Because synovial sarcomas express EMA and cyokeratins [82], molecular testing can help exclude sarcomatoid carcinoma, in cases with treatment effect where the original material is not available for review and in more poorly differentiated cases.
      - Most common fusion is *SS18-SSX1* between exon 10 of *SS18* and exon 6 of *SSX* and less commonly involves *SSX2*, *SSX4* or *SS18L-SSX1* [83, 84].
        Many centers employ the use of break-apart FISH which in some studies shows sensitivity of around 85% versus 95% when compared to PCR [83].
    - Alveolar soft part sarcoma.
      - Mainly affects young adults, most commonly involves the deep soft tissue of the extremities followed by the trunk [85].
        More commonly affects head and neck in children.
      - Characterized by *ASPSCR1-TFE3* fusion [86].
      - Molecular testing either by FISH or NGS only necessary in difficult or selected cases.
        Strong and diffuse TFE3 by IHC and classic morphology is considered sufficient for the diagnosis [87].
    - Clear cell sarcoma.
      - Mainly affects young adults, most commonly as deep-seated locations of the distal extremities, with the majority arising near the foot/ankle [88].
      - Because of the expression of melanocytic markers [89], immunohistochemical distinction from melanoma not possible and molecular has become the mainstay for definitive distinction.

  - Most common fusion involves *EWSR1-ATF1* most commonly between exon 8 of *EWSR1* and exon 4 of *ATF1* [90].
    - Other variant translocations involve fusion of *EWSR1-CREB1* [89].
    - Rare cases can also show concurrent BRAF mutations [91], further blurring the differential with melanoma.
- Extraskeletal myxoid chondrosarcoma.
  - Most commonly affects adults (median age 50 years) in the deep soft tissue of the proximal extremities and limb girdles [92].
  - Most commonly involves rearrangements of *NR4A3* with either *EWSR1* or *TAF15* [93].
    - Rare fusions involving *TCF12-NR4A3* and *TFG-NR4A3* have also been identified [94, 95].
    - More recently, a *HSPA8-NR4A3* fusion has been identified [96].
  - No other sarcoma has been found to have *NR4A3* fusions, so its detection is considered pathognomonic.
- Desmoplastic small round cell tumor (DSRCT).
  - Most commonly affects children and young adults in the abdomen/peritoneal cavity [97].
    - Striking male predominance.
  - Because of its histologic overlap with other small round cell tumors (e.g., Ewing, alveolar rhabdomyosarcoma), the use of ancillary immunohistochemical stains, and molecular testing is often employed.
    - Most cases show expression for keratins, desmin, and WT1 (C-terminus) [97].
    - On molecular level, characterized by recurrent fusion most commonly involving first seven exons of *EWSR1* and exons 8–10 of *WT1* [98].
- Intimal sarcoma.
  - Malignant sarcoma involving the great vessels of the heart and is now considered the most common [99].
  - FISH for MD*M2* amplification is often necessary as these tumors can have non-distinctive histology.
  - The use of array-CGH can often also show amplification of *KIT* and *PDGFRA*, gain of *EGFR*, and loss of *CDKN2A* [99].

17. **What is the role of molecular testing in fibroblastic/myofibroblastic tumors? What are the common molecular alterations found in these tumors? What testing modalities are commonly employed and are there any limitations?**
    - Many fibroblastic/myofibroblastic tumors have distinct molecular mutations or fusions that are characteristics, but because ancillary testing methods such as immunohistochemistry are so cheap and have a faster turn-around-time, molecular testing is generally not needed. In addition, some of these tumors are benign and the cost of performing the molecular testing cannot be generally justified (Table 10.5). See below for specifics on the individual tumors for potential scenarios where ancillary molecular techniques may be employed.
    - Nodular fasciitis
      - Self-limited mesenchymal neoplasm that most commonly affects young adults of the subcutis of the upper extremities, trunk, head, and neck [100].
      - Most cases show classic histology and show myofibroblastic differentiation with actin positivity [101] in a "tram-track" pattern, so there is no need for molecular confirmation.
      - Difficult or unusual cases may benefit from molecular testing in order to exclude a more worrisome lesion.
        - Most often characterized by rearrangements between *USP6* and *MYH9* [102].
        - An exceptional case associated with multiple recurrences and metastatic disease has been associated with *PPP6R3-USP6* [103].
      - A subset of cellular fibromas of tendon sheath have been found to have *USP6* rearrangements [104].
    - *EWSR1-SMAD3*-positive fibroblastic tumor
      - Benign fibroblastic tumor that often involves the dermis/subcutis of acral sites [105].
      - Typically are positive for ERG but negative for SMA, CD34, CD31, and S100 [105].
        - It is unclear if these tumors represent a spectrum of similar pediatric fibroblastic neoplasms, and indeed, some cases classified initially as one entity are sometimes re-classified as another based on molecular testing [106].
    - Soft tissue angiofibroma
      - Benign fibroblastic neoplasm affecting middle-aged adults in the extremities, most commonly the leg [107].
      - Characterized by *NCOA2* rearrangements most often to *AHRR* [108].
        - Other fusion partners include *GTF2I-NCOA2* and *GAB1-ABL1* [109, 110].
      - In most cases, molecular testing is not needed to confirm the rearrangements.
        - The main role of molecular testing is to exclude lesions that can have some histologic overlap and can behave more aggressively or have metastatic potential such as solitary

Table 10.5 Fibroblastic and myofibroblastic tumors with characteristic molecular findings that are not routinely tested

WHO classification	Age	Common location	Molecular	Routine molecular testing needed?
Nodular fasciitis	Young adults	Subcutis of upper extremities, trunk, head, and neck	*USP6* rearrangement	No
Fibrous hamartoma of infancy	Children	Axilla, trunk, extremities	*EGFR* mutations	No
Myofibroblastoma	Adults	Inguinal/groin area	Loss of *RB1*	No
Calcifying aponeurotic fibroma	Children, teenagers	Palmar surface of hands and fingers	*FN1-EGF* fusion	No
EWSR1-SMAD3-positive tumor	Wide age range	Hands and feet	*EWSR1-SMAD3*	Yes
Angiofibroma of soft tissue	Middle-aged adults	Extremities, most commonly the leg	*NCOA2* rearrangements	No
Cellular angiofibroma	Adults	Inguinal region	Loss of *RB1*	No
Acral fibromyxoma	Adults	Fingers and toes	Loss of *RB1*	No
Gardner fibroma	Children	Back, paraspinal, head, and neck	Germline *APC* mutation	No
Desmoid fibromatosis	Young adults	Extremities, abdominal wall, chest wall	*CTNNB1* mutations; germline *APC* in Gardner syndrome	No
Giant cell fibroblastoma/ dermatofibrosarcoma protuberans	Children/adults	Trunk, groin, extremities	*COL1A1-PDGFB*	No
Solitary fibrous tumor	Adults	Anywhere but more common in deep soft tissue	*NAB2-STAT6*	No
Inflammatory myofibroblastic tumor	Children, young adults	Abdominal viscera and soft tissue	*ALK*, *ROS*, *NTRK3* gene rearrangements	No
Infantile fibrosarcoma	Children <2 years	Extremities, trunk, head, and neck	*NTRK3* fusions	Yes
Low-grade fibromyxoid sarcoma	Young to middle aged adults	Extremities and trunk	*FUS-CREB3L2* or *FUS-CREB3L1*	No
Sclerosing epithelioid fibrosarcoma	Middle-aged to elderly adults	Extremities and trunk	*EWSR1-CREBL1*	No

fibrous tumor, low-grade fibromyxoid sarcoma, and a low-grade myxofibrosarcoma.

- Desmoid-type fibromatosis
  - Locally aggressive fibroblastic neoplasm with a propensity for local recurrence that primarily affects young adults and most commonly involves the extremities, trunk, and abdominal cavity [111].
  - Point mutations involved two codon of exon 3 of *CTNNB1* are found in the majority of sporadic tumors [112].
    Immunostain for beta-catenin often used as a surrogate marker.
  - Smaller percentage is associated with Gardner syndrome and show germline mutations in *APC* gene but can also show sporadic mutations [113].
- Giant cell fibroblastoma/dermatofibrosarcoma protuberans
  - Although listed separately in WHO, they are thought to be spectrums of the same neoplasm with the former arising primarily in children.
  - Lesions defined by *COL1A1-PDGFB* fusion.
    ~2% of cases may be cryptic, and another small percentage may show alternate fusions involving *PDGFB* including *COL6A3-PDGFD* and *EMILIN2-PDGFD* [114].
  - Reasons to perform break-apart FISH or NGS.
    Extensively myxoid lesion where classic architecture is not present.
    Metastatic/recurrent disease where original material is not available.
    Small samples where only "herringbone" pattern is present and the differential would include synovial sarcoma, MPNST, and fibrosarcomatous DFSP.
- Solitary fibrous tumor
  - Commonly affects adults and can occur at any site but more common in deep soft tissue and extrapleural locations [115].
  - NAB2-STAT6 fusion is pathognomonic [37].
  - Molecular testing not generally needed as STAT6 IHC is generally considered sensitive and specific [38].
    Dedifferentiated liposarcomas can occasionally show STAT6 expression, so this may be an instance where molecular testing is indicated.
- Infantile fibrosarcoma
  - Commonly affects children less than 2 years and involves the extremities, trunk, head and neck.

   - Most cases harbor an *ETV6-NTRK3* fusion [116]. Other cases have *NTRK1*, *NTRK2*, *BRAF*, and *MET* fusions [117–119].
   - Cases with *NTRK* rearrangements often show pan-TRK IHC expression [120].
- Low-grade fibromyxoid sarcoma (LGFMS)
   - Malignant fibroblastic neoplasm that most commonly affects young to middle-aged adults of the deep extremities and trunk [121].
   - Characterized by fusions most commonly involving *FUS-CREB3L2* or *FUS CREB3L1* [122].
     Less commonly can involve *EWSR1* [123].
   - MUC4 IHC is generally considered sensitive and specific for the diagnosis, so routine molecular testing is not needed [124].
     Selected cases tested when MUC4 IHC is negative or not available.
- Sclerosing epithelioid fibrosarcoma
   - Malignant fibroblastic neoplasm with subset that is related to LGFMS both histologically and molecularly and can have a similar age and site distribution [125].
   - Most common fusion is *EWSR1-CREB3L1* [126].
     Other fusions show *FUS* or *PAX5* with *CREB3L2*, *CREB3L3*, or *CREM* [127, 128].
   - Similarly to LGFMS, MUC4 IHC is considered sensitive and specific and is present in ~90% of cases [129], so routine molecular testing is not often needed.

Case 1

Case History

30-year-old previously healthy male presents with progressively worsening double vision for 1 month with associated vertigo and balance difficulties. This has been compounded by neuropathic back pain that radiates to the abdomen. An imaging CT shows a 9 cm chest wall mass that encases the eighth and ninth rib with a mild periosteal reaction without frank osseous invasion. The radiologic differential would be a malignant solitary fibrous tumor versus lymphoma versus, less likely metastatic disease.

Histologic Features

A CT-guided biopsy demonstrates a basaloid population of epithelioid cells with crush artifact and scattered admixed spindle cells (Fig. 10.1). Immunostains are positive for AE1/AE3 (focal), EMA (rare), and the spindled cells are positive for SOX10. The cells are negative for CD3, CD20, CK7, CK20, TTF1, desmin, chromogranin A, and SALL4.

Choice of Molecular Testing

Given the presence of admixed spindled cells that are SOX10 positive, the preliminary differential was a round cell sarcoma with an *EWSR1-PATZ1* fusion (*EWSR1*-non-ETS fusion). As this particular fusion is not responsive to traditional chemotherapy, a decision was made to perform RNA sequencing to confirm or rule out the fusion as opposed to simply using an *EWSR1* break-apart FISH probe which has a faster turn-around time.

Molecular Study

An Archer® NGS fusion study revealed an *ESWR1* (Exon 7)-*FLI1* (Exon 5) fusion. (The NGS fusion study was performed using 26 gene FusionPlex Sarcoma panel, ArcherDx, Boulder, CO; validated in the molecular diagnostic laboratory for clinical testing.)

Final Diagnosis

Ewing Sarcoma with *EWSR1-FLI1* fusion.

Case Discussion

This case demonstrates that although break-apart FISH would have detected the *EWSR1* rearrangement, RNA sequencing provided the correct information for the diagnosis and also provided the treating clinicians with the correct clinical information to begin EWS chemotherapy regimen that would not have been started if this case truly demonstrated a *PATZ1* fusion.

Case 2

Case History

A 13-year-old female noticed a lump in her groin for 2 weeks. She had a history of a neoplasm removed from her right knee 5 years ago. Ultrasound showed a 4 cm lymph node concerning for malignancy. Upon further investigation, the patient had been diagnosed with an angiomatoid fibrous histiocytoma. Given that lesion was removed years ago without recurrence, the current lesion is suspicious for metastasis.

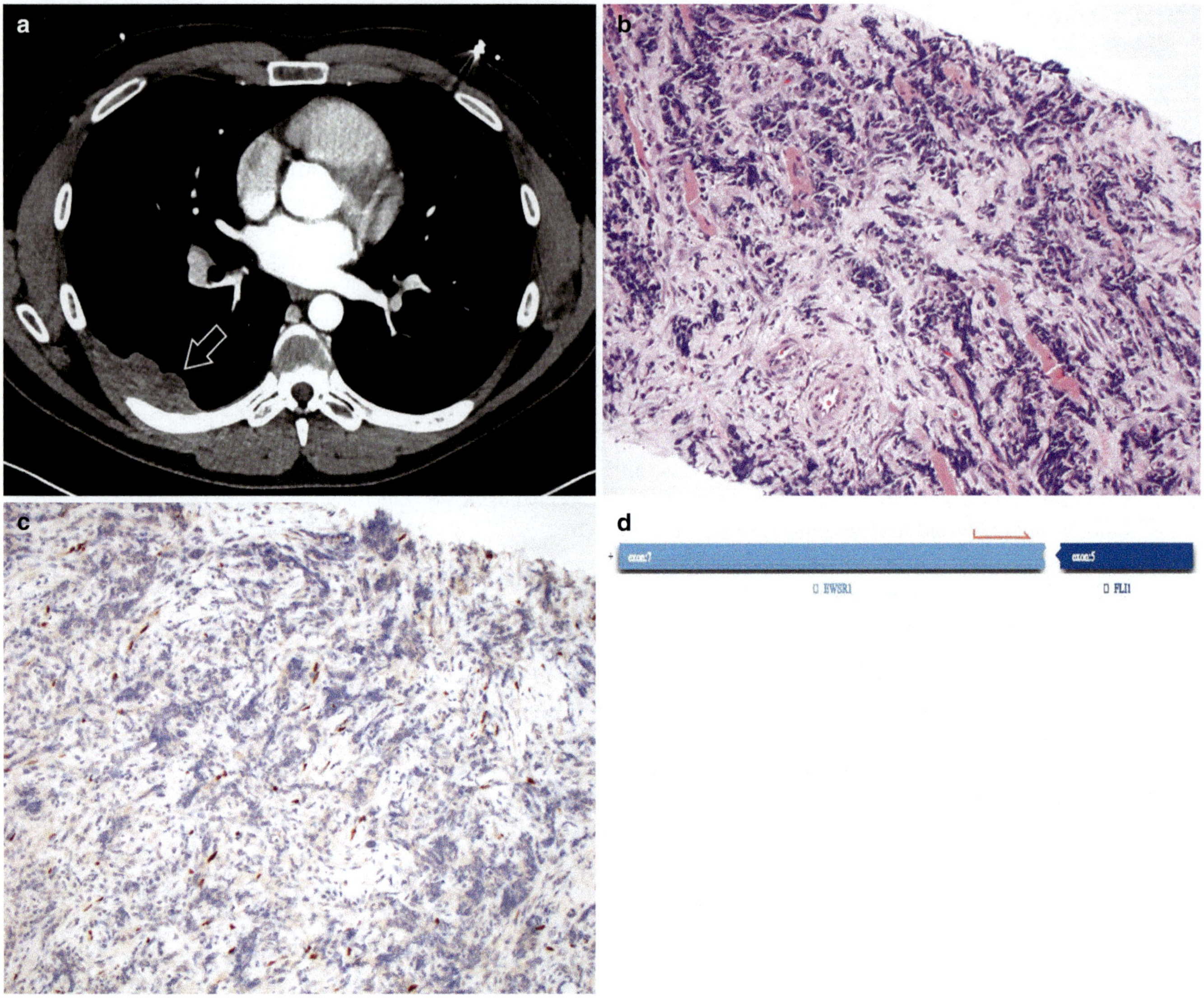

Fig. 10.1 Axial CT shows a posterior chest wall mass (**a**) that is composed of small round blue cells admixed with spindle cells (**b**) that are positive for SOX10 (**c**) that can of be seen in *EWSR1-PATZ1* fusion. Interestingly, however, NGS revealed an *EWSR1-FLI1* fusion (**d**)

Histologic Features

Sections show a tumor composed of spindled to epithelioid cells arranged in a syncytial pattern that is involving a lymph node (Fig. 10.2). Immunostains are positive for EMA and desmin.

Molecular Study

An Archer® NGS fusion study found an *EWSR1-ATF1* gene fusion.

Final Diagnosis

Metastatic angiomatoid fibrous histiocytoma.

Case Discussion

While angiomatoid fibrous histiocytomas can have surrounding lymphoid aggregates, the current case illustrates a rare metastasis to the locoregional lymph nodes that happens in <5% of cases. *EWSR1-CREB1* fusions are the most common fusions in angiomatoid fibrous histiocytoma, but *ATF1* fusions are more frequently associated with extrasomatic soft tissue cases. In the current case, FISH break-apart would have been an option. However, one potential limitation is that FISH testing cannot always discriminate between a simple terminal deletion of the 3' *EWSR1* and translocation involving the remaining 5′ portion of *EWSR1* with another gene. In addition, rare fusions involving *FUS* can happen and would be missed by that assay.

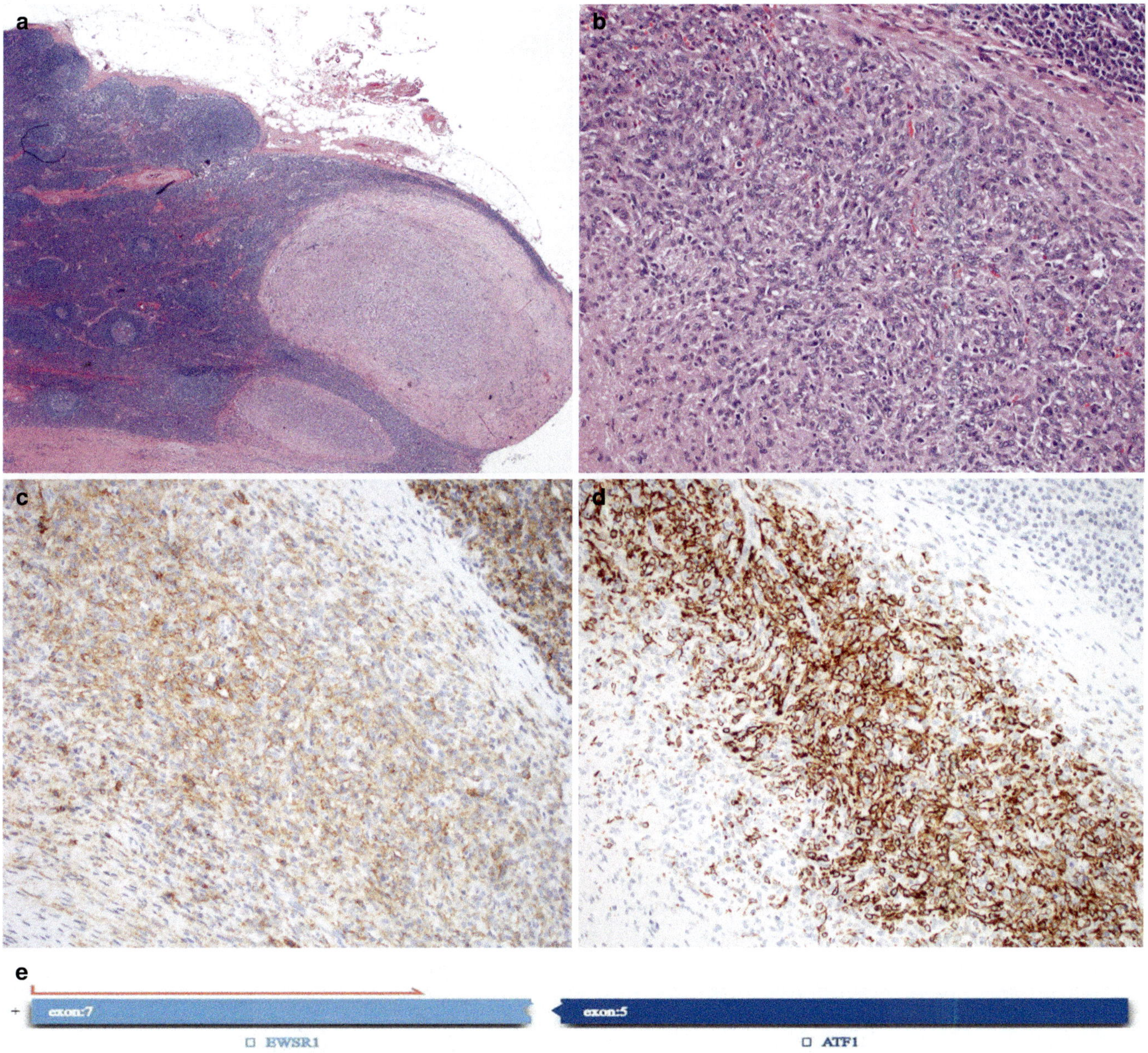

Fig. 10.2 Low power shows a metastatic deposit in a lymph node (**a**). Higher power shows uniform histiocytoid cells (**b**) that are positive for both EMA (**c**) and desmin (**d**). NGS reveal an *EWSR1-ATF1* fusion (**e**)

Case 3

Case History

A 25-year-old male presented with several week history of pleuritic chest pain. He was treated by his PCP with a trial of steroids and Z-Pak which failed to improve his symptoms. On initial examination, a right upper quadrant ultrasound demonstrated two hepatic masses. A follow-up MRI showed innumerable masses along the liver that appear external to liver parenchyma. There was also a large confluent mass anteriorly between the liver and the diaphragm that measured 10 cm.

Histologic Features

Core biopsy shows a malignant small round cell tumor arranged in nest and sheets with intervening fibrous stroma (Fig. 10.3). Immunostains are positive for AE1/AE3, Desmin, and CD99 (patchy) and are negative for WT1, CK5/6, MYOD1, CD45, Melan-A, and TTF1.

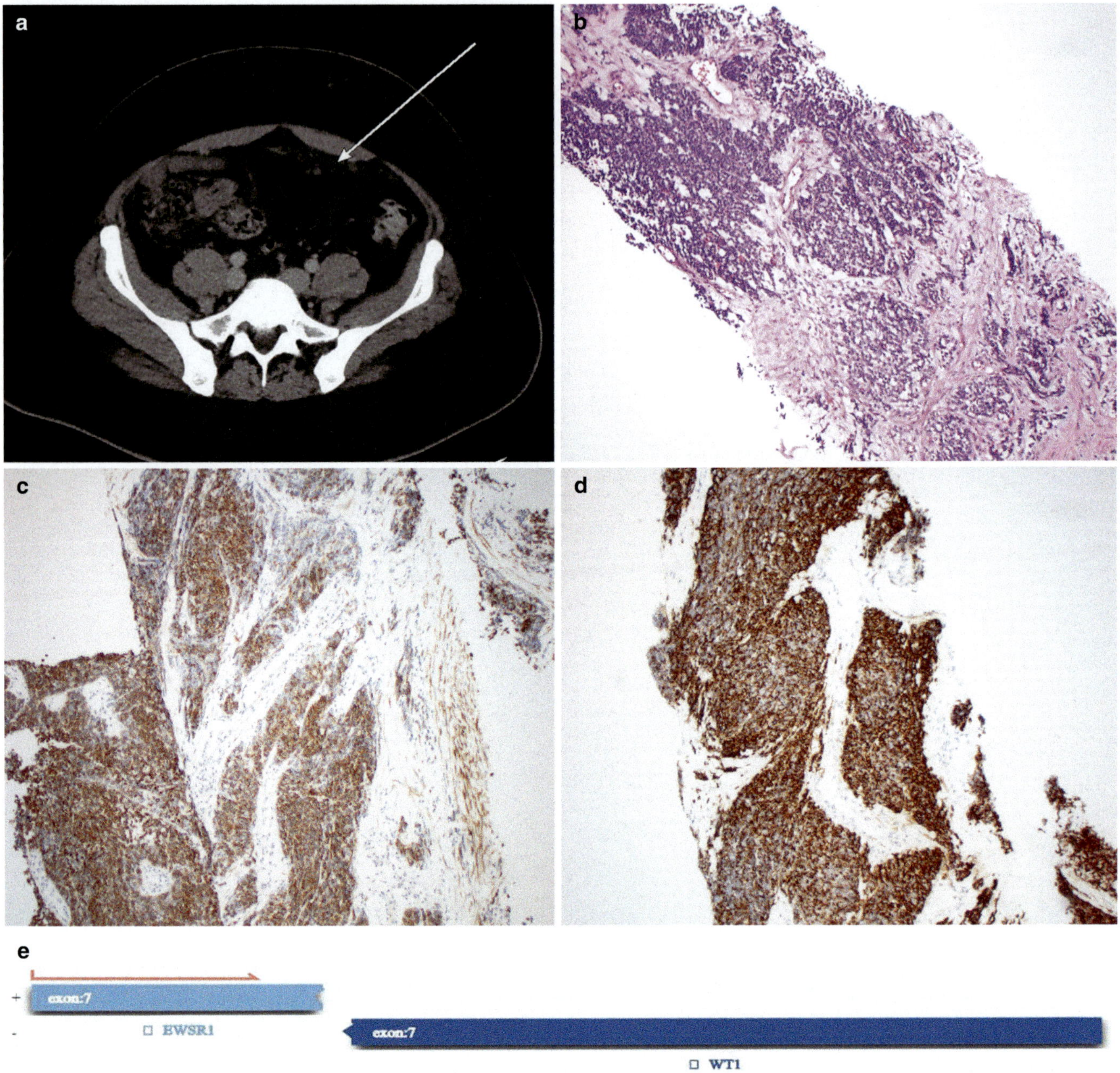

Fig. 10.3 Axial MRI shows multiple peritoneal surface masses throughout the abdomen (**a**). Biopsy shows a small round cell tumor growing in sheets with intervening fibrous stroma (**b**) that is strongly positive for AE1/AE3 (**c**) and desmin (**d**). NGS revealed an *EWSR1-WT1* fusion (**e**)

Molecular Study

An Archer® NGS fusion study revealed an *EWSR1-WT1* fusion.

Final Diagnosis

Desmoplastic small round cell tumor.

Case Discussion

The most common transcript for DSRCT involves the first 7 exons of *EWSR1* fusing to exons 8–10 of *WT1*; however variant translocations exist. This patient underwent 8 cycles of chemotherapy and repeat imaging revealed persistent abdominal lesions with persistent mediastinal lymphadenopathy. The patient is currently scheduled for resection of the mediastinal lesions with a plan for subsequent abdominal

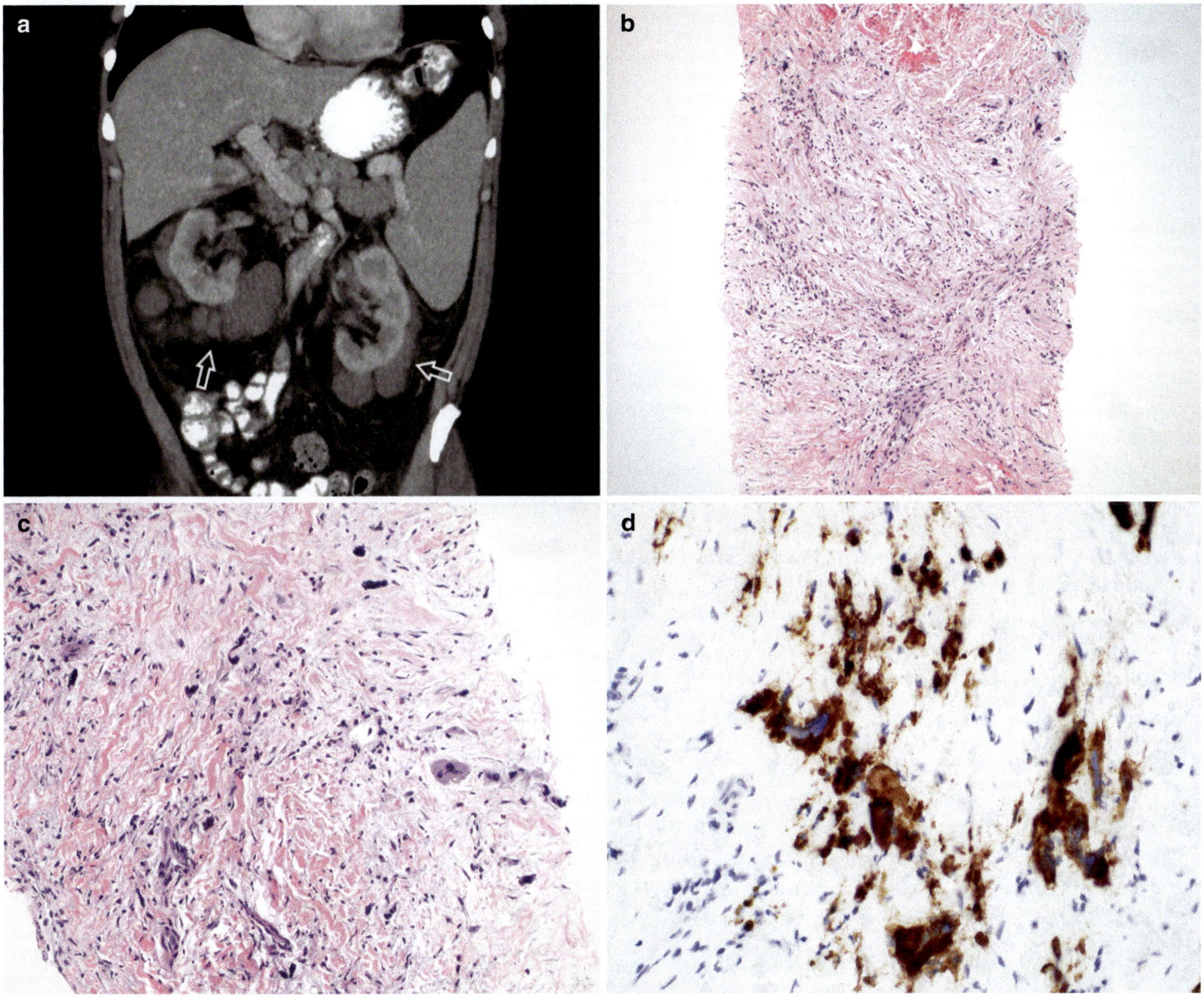

Fig. 10.4 Coronal CT shows multiple soft tissue masses bilaterally included around the kidneys (**a**). Biopsy of retroperitoneum at low power shows a fibrous spindle cell lesion with scattered enlarged and hyperchromatic cells (**b**). Higher power reveals the pleomorphic cells show smudgy chromatin and multinucleate forms (**c**) that are positive for CD61 (**d**)

exploration and cytoreductive surgery. Despite multimodality therapy, the 5-year overall survival rate is low.

Case 4

Case History

A 50-year-old male had a history of essential thrombocytosis diagnosed 20 years ago. His most recent blood cell counts revealed the following: WBC 3.3 K/μL, Hb 9.3 g/dL, Hct 38%, Plt 331 K/μL. He had had worsening anemia of the past year with increasing splenomegaly. A CT of the abdomen and pelvis revealed a 19.5 cm spleen as well as numerous soft tissue masses encompassing the right and left kidney but clinically the patient has been asymptomatic.

Histologic Features

Core biopsy shows a variably cellular lesion composed of small, bland spindled cells arranged in vague fascicles set in a myxo-collagenous stroma with scattered hyperchromatic pleomorphic cells with smudgy chromatin (Fig. 10.4). An immunostain is positive for CD61 and negative for MDM2.

FISH Results

Negative for *MDM2* amplification.

Final Diagnosis

Sclerosing extramedullary hematopoietic tumor.

Case Discussion

Sclerosing extramedullary hematopoietic tumor is an extramedullary complication associated with myeloproliferative neoplasms. The presence of atypical megakaryocytes in the retroperitoneum raises the differential of a well-differentiated liposarcoma; however, they stain appropriately with CD61 and FISH for *MDM2* is negative to help exclude a liposarcoma. In this case, the diagnosis would have been extremely difficult if the clinical history was not available.

Case 5

Case History

A 35-year-old female with no significant past medical history presented with a back mass that was clinically felt to be a lipoma or a cyst. Nothing was done at that time on initial presentation, and she returned to clinic a couple months later because the mass increased in size and it was excised by a surgeon.

Histologic Features

Sections show a cellular lesion composed of spindled and epithelioid cells arranged in sheets and nests with areas of peritheliomatous growth with associated necrosis, brisk mitotic activity and areas of clear cell and myxoid change. In addition, there are nodular areas of fascicular growth with intervening dense fibrous septa (Fig. 10.5). Immunostains are positive for CD99, FLI1 and WT1 and are negative for CD45, AE1/AE3, Cam5.2, PAX8, desmin, hmb-45, SOX10, and BCOR.

Molecular Study

An Archer® NGS fusion study revealed a fusion transcript of *CIC* (exon 20) and *FOXO4* (exon 2).

Final Diagnosis

CIC-rearranged sarcoma.

Case Discussion

CIC-rearranged sarcoma is an undifferentiated round cell sarcoma that most commonly involves a *CIC-DUX4* fusion. The nodular growth pattern in the current case along with the zone of necrosis and strong nuclear expression of WT1 is suggestive of a *CIC*-rearranged sarcoma. Interestingly the presence of clear cell change can sometimes be associated with *EWSR1-FEV*; however, because response to chemotherapy is dependent on the specific fusion transcript detected NGS testing is becoming the gold standard in the diagnosis of round cell sarcomas.

Case 6

Case History

An 80-year-old female with a left chest wall mass that was felt to be recurrent myxoid liposarcoma. She was originally diagnosed at an outside facility with a retroperitoneal primary myxoid liposarcoma 5 years ago and is status post two resections. The current lesion measures up to 16 cm. No history of molecular/FISH testing is found.

Histologic Features

Sections show a predominant low-grade myxoid adipocytic lesion with a plexiform vasculature and signet-type lipoblasts. A few sections demonstrate more increased cellularity and atypia with spindled cells arranged in fascicles with scattered pleomorphic forms and conspicuous mitotic activity. Within the cellular areas, focal osteoid formation is present (Fig. 10.6). An immunostain for MDM2 is focally positive.

FISH Results

Positive for *MDM2* amplification with a ratio of *MDM2* fluorescent signal to chromosome 12 centromere signal of 15.

Final Diagnosis

Dedifferentiated liposarcoma.

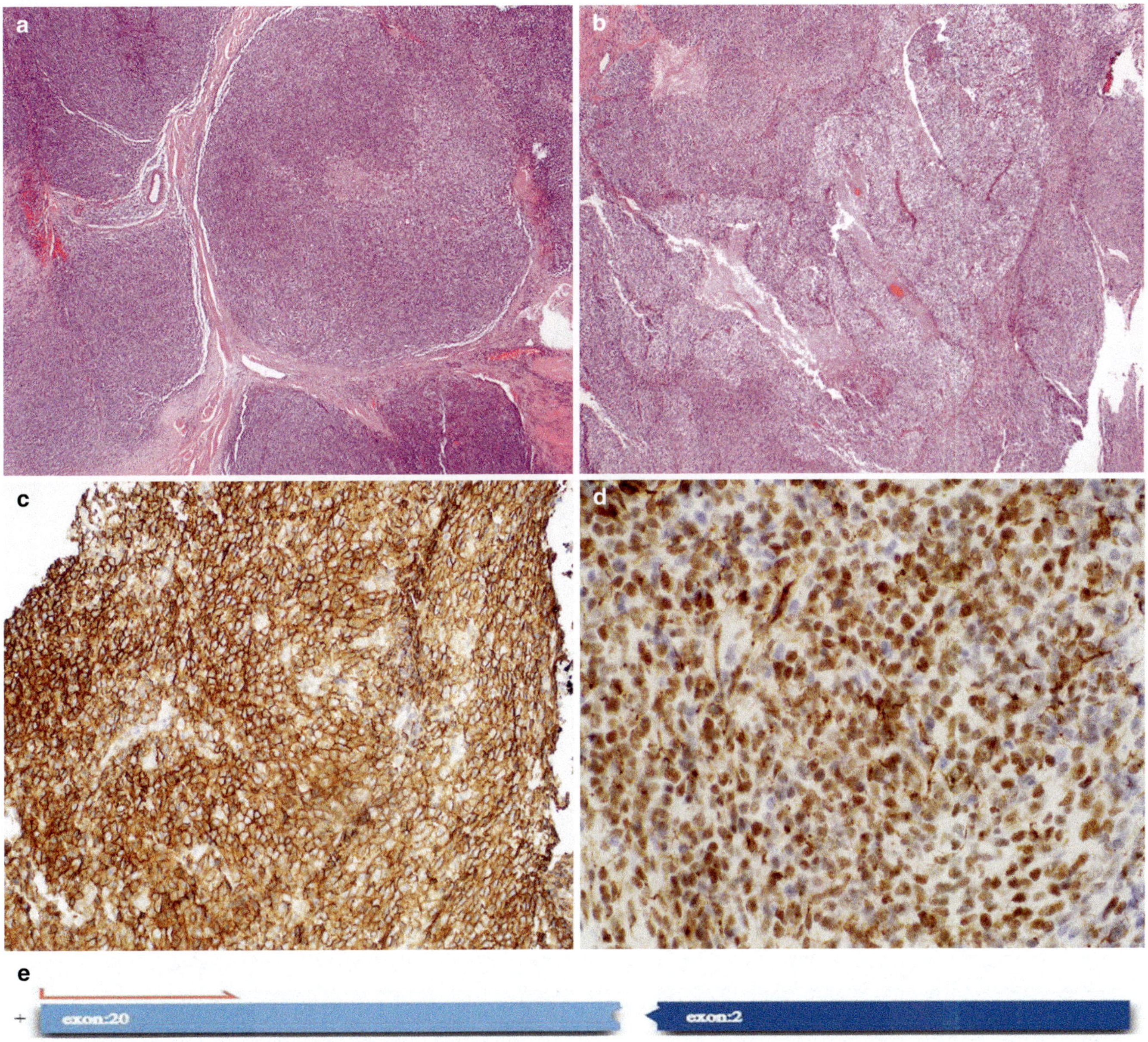

Fig. 10.5 Low power shows nodular growth pattern with intervening fibrous septa (**a**) and areas of clear cell change with zones of necrosis (**b**). Medium power shows strong, membranous CD99 (**c**) and nuclear WT1 (**d**). NGS revealed a fusion transcript of *CIC* (exon 20) and *FOXO4* (exon 2) (**e**)

Case Discussion

The patient's history of a retroperitoneal primary myxoid liposarcoma is noted. Although primary retroperitoneal myxoid liposarcomas do exist, they are rare and a retroperitoneal dedifferentiated liposarcoma with areas reminiscent of myxoid liposarcoma would be much more likely. As the current specimen showed a high-grade spindle cell component which would be unusual for a high-grade myxoid liposarcoma, FISH testing was employed and is amplified.

Case 7

Case History

A 25-year-old female presented with a complaint of swelling and a slowly enlarging mass of the lower lip. Clinical exam demonstrated a mobile and well-circumscribed lesion suggestive of a benign process.

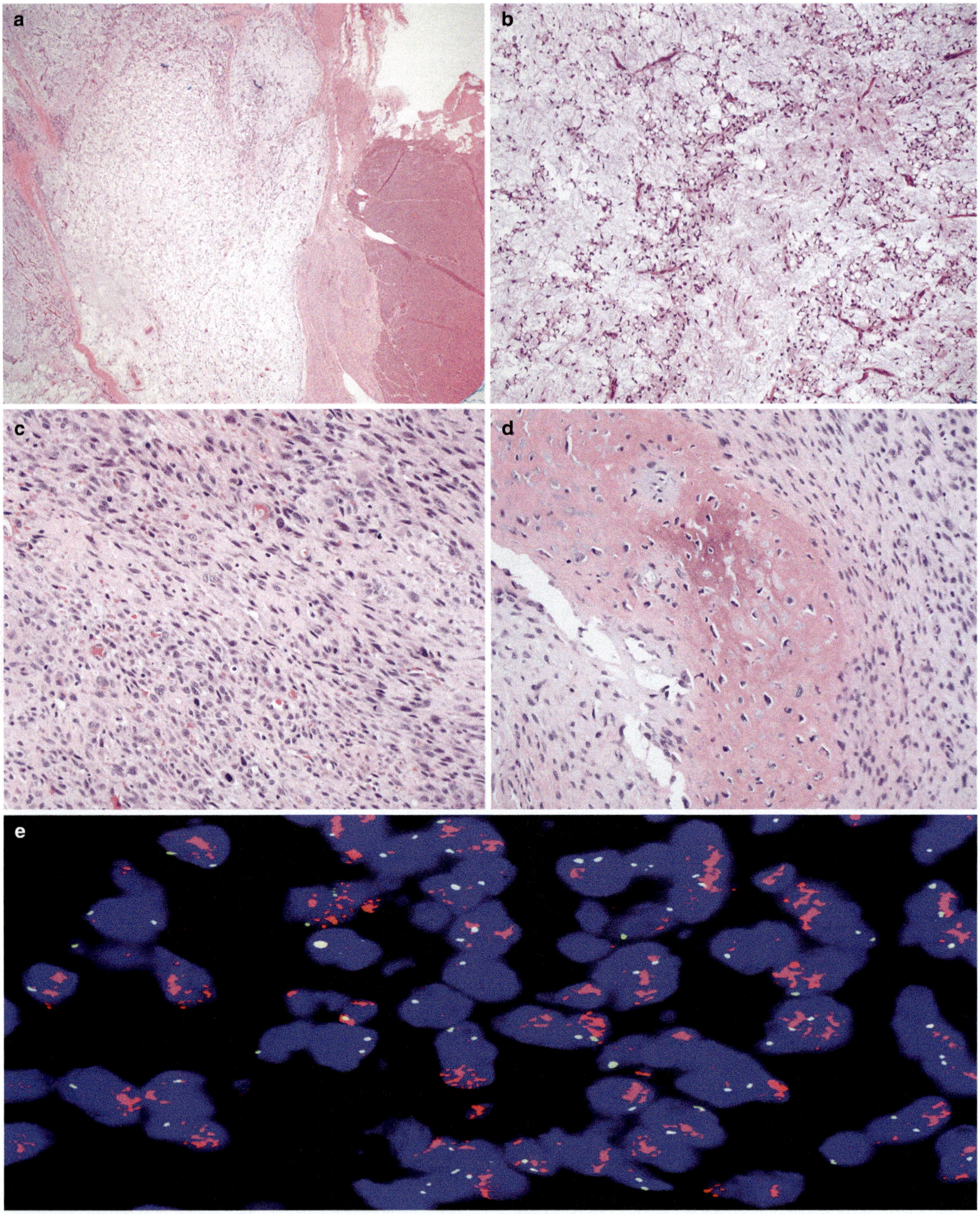

Fig. 10.6 Low power shows a nodular myxoid lesion (**a**) with plexiform vasculature and scattered signet-type lipoblasts (**b**). Higher power demonstrates spindled fascicular growth with conspicuous mitoses with pleomorphic forms (**c**) and osteoid formation (**d**). FISH testing demonstrates amplification of *MDM2* (**e**)

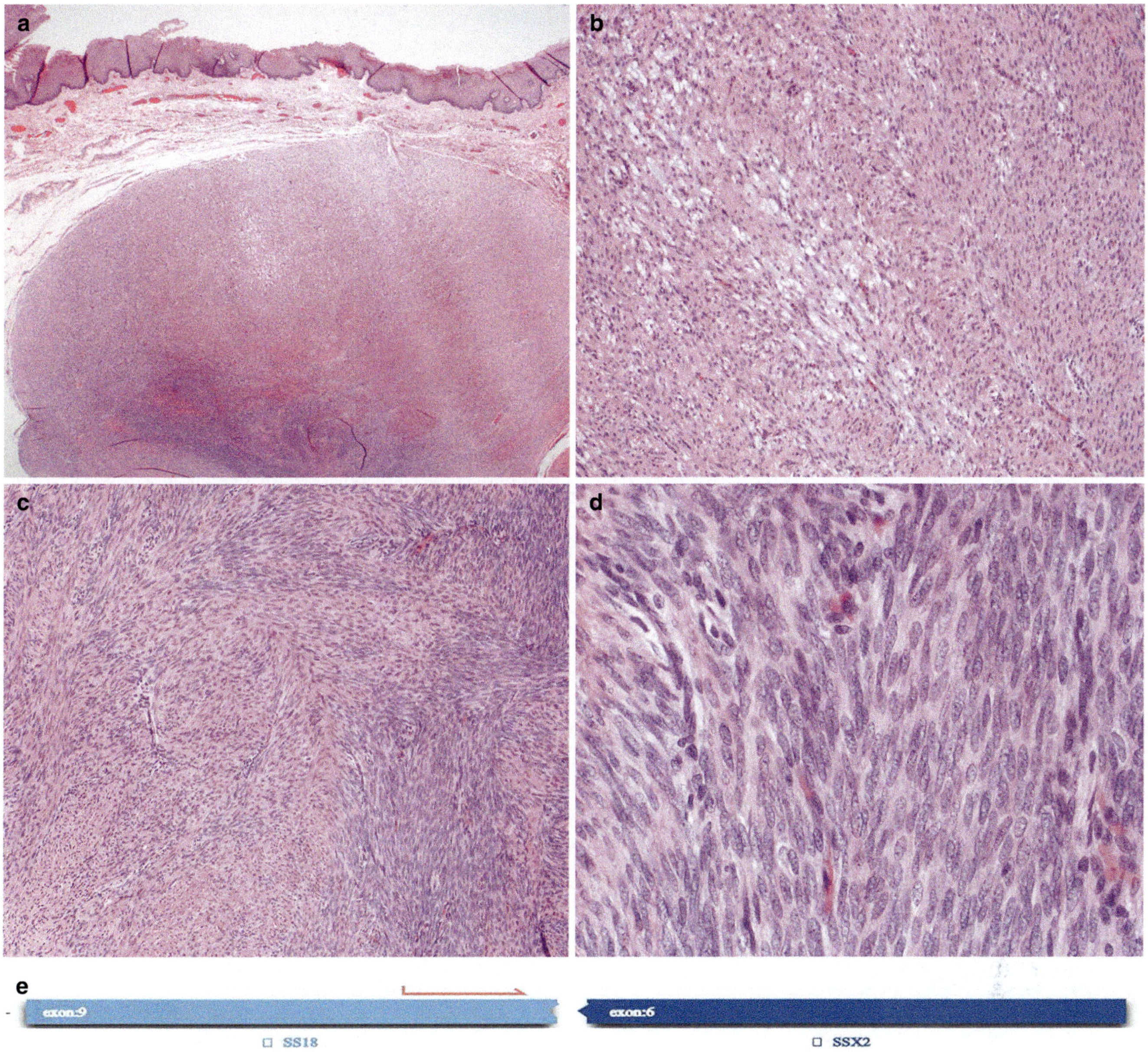

Fig. 10.7 Low power shows a well-circumscribed submucosal mass (**a**) that is composed of loose fibrous spindle cell areas (**b**) admixed with more cellular basophilic areas (**c**). Higher power shows the monotonous spindle cell population with overlapping nuclei (**d**). NGS revealed a *SS18-SSX2* fusion (**e**)

Histologic Features

Sections show a relatively well-circumscribed submucosal spindle cell lesion. The spindle cells show fascicular growth and are monomorphic with relatively bland elongated to wavy nuclei with finely granular chromatin, inconspicuous nucleoli, and minimal cytoplasm (Fig. 10.7). Immunostains are positive for EMA (patchy) and are negative for CD34, desmin, S100 protein, and STAT6.

Molecular Study

An Archer® NGS fusion study revealed a *SS18-SSX2* fusion transcript.

Final Diagnosis

Monophasic synovial sarcoma.

Case Discussion

The most common fusion in synovial sarcoma is *SS18-SSX1*, but a majority of *SS18-SSX2* are the monophasic subtype and they are more common in females. Less than 10% of synovial sarcomas involve the head and neck region and a well-circumscribed growth can give a false impression of a benign process. Although NGS was performed, break-apart FISH for *SS18* would have been a reasonable ancillary testing method choice.

Case 8

Case History

A 40-year-old female presented to her dermatologist with a left lower leg nodule. The clinical differential was broad and included lymphoma, a granulomatous process, a deep fungal infection versus a metastasis of unknown primary.

Histologic Features

A punch biopsy shows a cellular dermal-based mesenchymal neoplasm composed of basaloid cells growing in nests and sheets. The cells have scant cytoplasm and mitotic activity is conspicuous (Fig. 10.8). Immunostains are positive for desmin, myogenin, and myoD1 and are negative for AE1/AE3, S100, chromogranin, CK20, TTF1, TdT, and CD45.

Molecular Study

An Archer® NGS fusion study revealed a fusion transcript of *PAX3* (exon 7) and *FOXO4* (exon 2).

Final Diagnosis

Alveolar rhabdomyosarcoma.

Case Discussion

The patient underwent chemotherapy, and at the time of resection, the tumor was approximately 10% viable with negative margins and one lymph node positive for metastatic disease. Approximately 8 months later, she had a recurrence at the original site that was resection and most recent imaging studies have been negative.

Case 9

Case History

A 60-year-old female with a history of clear cell sarcoma that was diagnosed at an outside facility with break-apart FISH for *EWSR1*. She had lung metastases but had been on 4 cycles of pembrolizumab but developed a possible recurrence in the groin.

Histologic Features

Biopsy showed a subcutaneous clear cell neoplasm composed of relatively uniform cells arranged in pseudo-alveolar nests with surrounding fibrous septa (Fig. 10.9). Immunostains were positive for Melan-A and SOX10 and negative for AE1/AE3.

Molecular Study

An Archer® NGS fusion study revealed no database fusions.

Reflective FISH Results

Positive for *EWSR1* gene rearrangement in 33% of cells.

Final Diagnosis

Recurrent clear cell sarcoma.

Case Discussion

This is a challenging case that was discussed at length at the multidisciplinary tumor boards. It was suggested that perhaps there is potentially a DNA only fusion without an RNA transcript secondary to the immunotherapy that may account for the NGS testing being negative. Conversely, it is possible that the *EWSR1* FISH is a false positive. The FISH probe used in the most recent cytogenetic test is actually proximal to the 5′ portion of *EWSR1* and not a part of the gene itself. So, it is possible that the break is next to but not within the actual gene. That being said, the mutational burden was also low and other mutations commonly seen in melanoma (the main histologic differential) were not seen. Taken together, it was felt clinically that the lesion most likely represents clear cell sarcoma and the patient is currently continuing immunotherapy treatment.

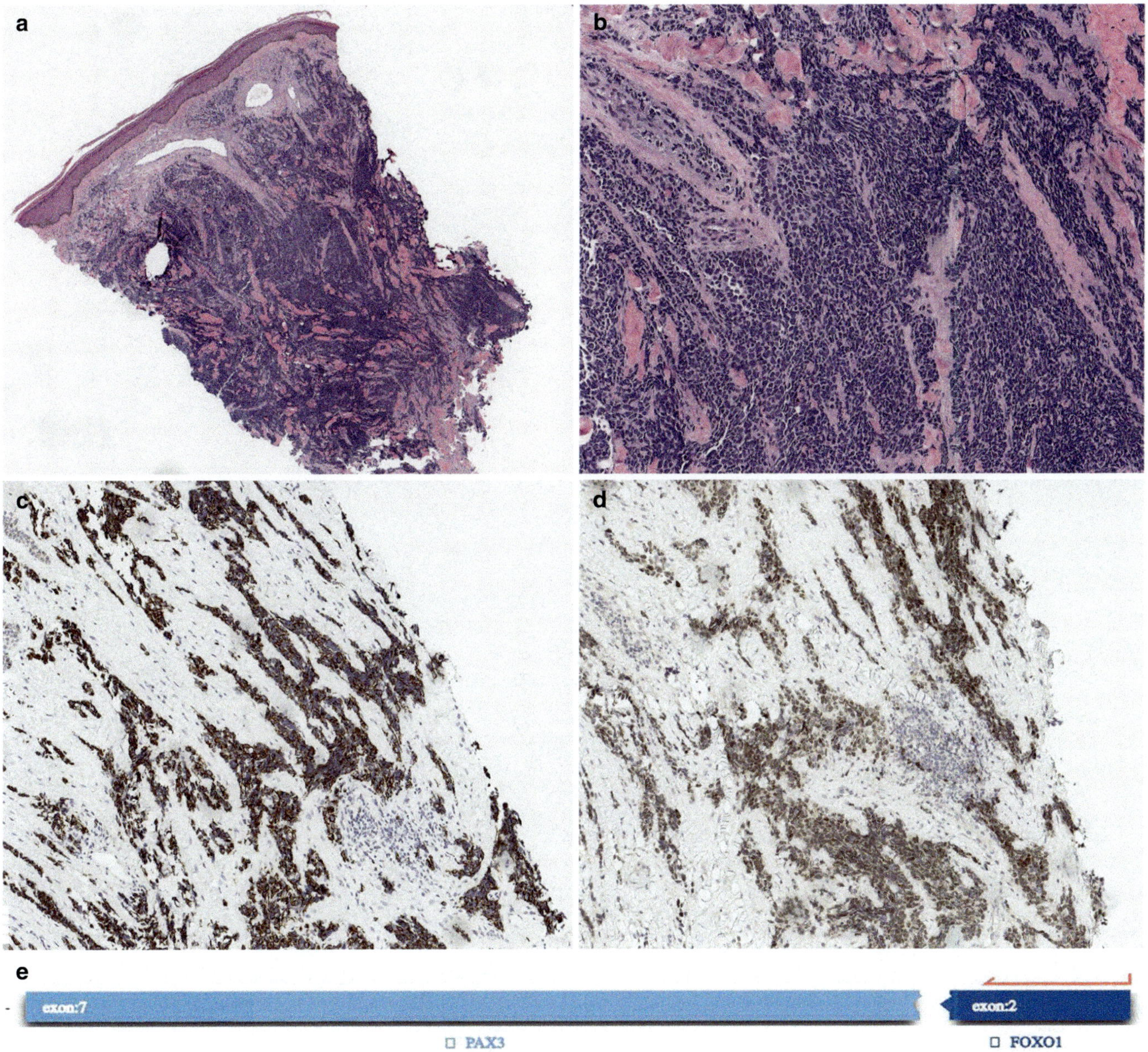

Fig. 10.8 Low power shows a cellular dermal basaloid neoplasm (**a**). Higher power shows a small round cell tumor growing in sheets and nests (**b**). The tumor cells are positive for desmin (**c**) and myo-D1 (**d**). NGS revealed a *PAX3-FOXO1* fusion (**e**)

Case 10

Case History

A 75-year-old male presented with a right posterior thigh mass. A CT exam showed a solid enhancing intramuscular mass that measured 5.2 cm. A CT biopsy was performed for diagnosis given the concern for a soft tissue sarcoma.

Histologic Features

A biopsy shows a myxoid mesenchymal neoplasm composed of monotonous spindled cells with admixed more epithelioid cells growing in reticular cords (Fig. 10.10). Immunostains show patchy EMA and are negative for AE1/AE3, S100 and synaptophysin.

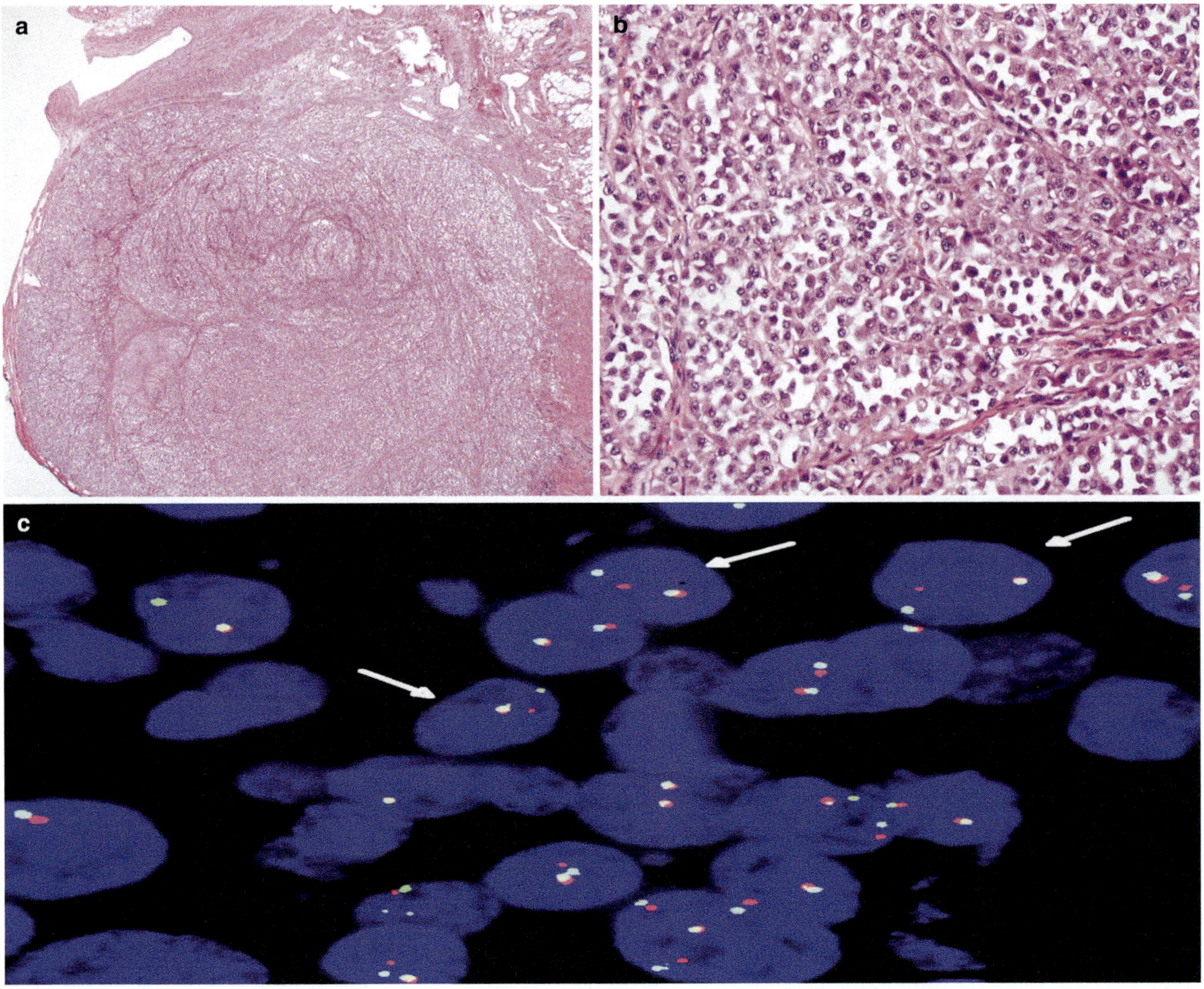

Fig. 10.9 Low power shows a subcutaneous clear cell neoplasm with intervening fibrous septa (**a**). Higher power shows a relatively monotonous population of epithelioid cells arranged in pseudo-alveolar nests (**b**). FISH testing demonstrates an *EWSR1* rearrangement (**c**)

Molecular Study

An Archer® NGS fusion study revealed an *EWSR1-NR4A3* fusion.

Final Diagnosis

Extraskeletal myxoid chondrosarcoma.

Case Discussion

The growth pattern of the cells is highly suggestive of an extraskeletal myxoid chondrosarcoma and the absence keratin and myoepithelial markers would make myoepithelioma less likely. However, because the immunophenotype of EMC is often non-distinct, routine molecular testing is performed when this diagnosis is entertained and the finding of a *NR4A3* rearrangement is pathognomonic.

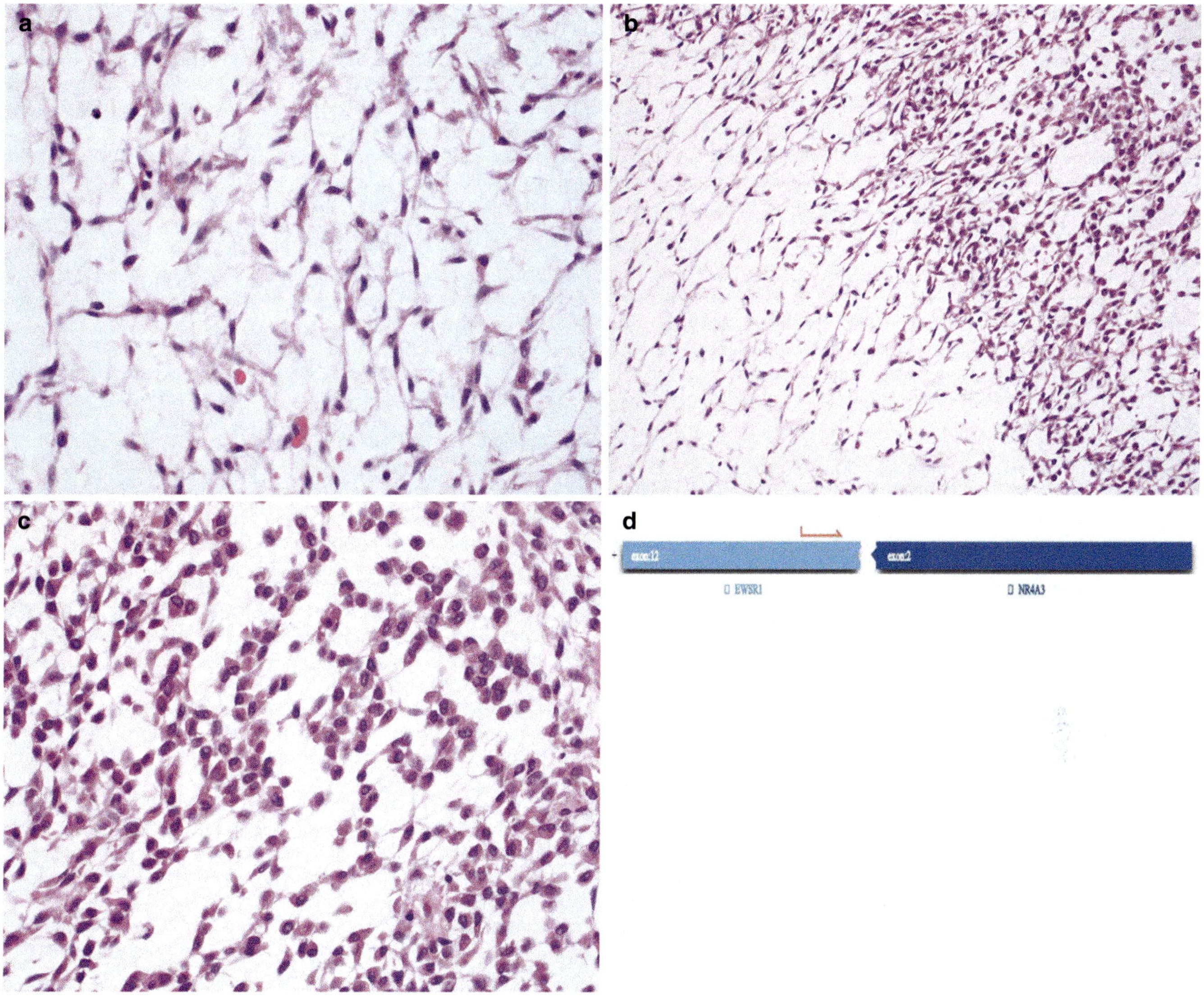

Fig. 10.10 Sections show a myxoid spindle lesion with eosinophilic cytoplasm growing in cords (**a**) with a transition to more cellular areas (**b**) with the cells becoming more epithelioid (**c**). NGS revealed an *EWSR1-NR4A3* fusion (**d**)

References

1. Board WCoTE. Soft tissue and bone tumours: international agency for research on cancer; 2020.
2. Delattre O, Zucman J, Plougastel B, Desmaze C, Melot T, Peter M, et al. Gene fusion with an ETS DNA-binding domain caused by chromosome translocation in human tumours. Nature. 1992;359(6391):162–5.
3. Delattre O, Zucman J, Melot T, Garau XS, Zucker JM, Lenoir GM, et al. The Ewing family of tumors – a subgroup of small-round-cell tumors defined by specific chimeric transcripts. N Engl J Med. 1994;331(5):294–9.
4. Jeon IS, Davis JN, Braun BS, Sublett JE, Roussel MF, Denny CT, et al. A variant Ewing's sarcoma translocation (7;22) fuses the EWS gene to the ETS gene ETV1. Oncogene. 1995;10(6):1229–34.
5. Kaneko Y, Yoshida K, Handa M, Toyoda Y, Nishihira H, Tanaka Y, et al. Fusion of an ETS-family gene, EIAF, to EWS by t(17;22)(q12;q12) chromosome translocation in an undifferentiated sarcoma of infancy. Genes Chromosomes Cancer. 1996;15(2):115–21.
6. Peter M, Couturier J, Pacquement H, Michon J, Thomas G, Magdelenat H, et al. A new member of the ETS family fused to EWS in Ewing tumors. Oncogene. 1997;14(10):1159–64.
7. Shing DC, McMullan DJ, Roberts P, Smith K, Chin SF, Nicholson J, et al. FUS/ERG gene fusions in Ewing's tumors. Cancer Res. 2003;63(15):4568–76.
8. Ng TL, O'Sullivan MJ, Pallen CJ, Hayes M, Clarkson PW, Winstanley M, et al. Ewing sarcoma with novel translocation t(2;16) producing an in-frame fusion of FUS and FEV. J Mol Diagn. 2007;9(4):459–63.
9. Bridge JA, Sumegi J, Druta M, Bui MM, Henderson-Jackson E, Linos K, et al. Clinical, pathological, and genomic features of EWSR1-PATZ1 fusion sarcoma. Mod Pathol. 2019;32(11):1593–604.
10. Koelsche C, Kriegsmann M, Kommoss FKF, Stichel D, Kriegsmann K, Vokuhl C, et al. DNA methylation profiling distinguishes Ewing-like sarcoma with EWSR1-NFATc2 fusion from Ewing sarcoma. J Cancer Res Clin Oncol. 2019;145(5):1273–81.

11. Watson S, Perrin V, Guillemot D, Reynaud S, Coindre JM, Karanian M, et al. Transcriptomic definition of molecular subgroups of small round cell sarcomas. J Pathol. 2018;245(1):29–40.
12. Solomon DA, Brohl AS, Khan J, Miettinen M. Clinicopathologic features of a second patient with Ewing-like sarcoma harboring CIC-FOXO4 gene fusion. Am J Surg Pathol. 2014;38(12):1724–5.
13. Sugita S, Arai Y, Tonooka A, Hama N, Totoki Y, Fujii T, et al. A novel CIC-FOXO4 gene fusion in undifferentiated small round cell sarcoma: a genetically distinct variant of Ewing-like sarcoma. Am J Surg Pathol. 2014;38(11):1571–6.
14. Le Loarer F, Pissaloux D, Watson S, Godfraind C, Galmiche-Rolland L, Silva K, et al. Clinicopathologic features of CIC-NUTM1 sarcomas, a new molecular variant of the family of CIC-fused sarcomas. Am J Surg Pathol. 2019;43(2):268–76.
15. Sugita S, Arai Y, Aoyama T, Asanuma H, Mukai W, Hama N, et al. NUTM2A-CIC fusion small round cell sarcoma: a genetically distinct variant of CIC-rearranged sarcoma. Hum Pathol. 2017;65:225–30.
16. Smith SC, Buehler D, Choi EY, McHugh JB, Rubin BP, Billings SD, et al. CIC-DUX sarcomas demonstrate frequent MYC amplification and ETS-family transcription factor expression. Mod Pathol. 2015;28(1):57–68.
17. Huang SC, Zhang L, Sung YS, Chen CL, Kao YC, Agaram NP, et al. Recurrent CIC gene abnormalities in Angiosarcomas: a molecular study of 120 cases with concurrent investigation of PLCG1, KDR, MYC, and FLT4 gene alterations. Am J Surg Pathol. 2016;40(5):645–55.
18. Antonescu CR, Owosho AA, Zhang L, Chen S, Deniz K, Huryn JM, et al. Sarcomas with CIC-rearrangements are a distinct pathologic entity with aggressive outcome: a clinicopathologic and molecular study of 115 cases. Am J Surg Pathol. 2017;41(7):941–9.
19. Kao YC, Owosho AA, Sung YS, Zhang L, Fujisawa Y, Lee JC, et al. BCOR-CCNB3 fusion positive sarcomas: a clinicopathologic and molecular analysis of 36 cases with comparison to morphologic spectrum and clinical behavior of other round cell sarcomas. Am J Surg Pathol. 2018;42(5):604–15.
20. Specht K, Zhang L, Sung YS, Nucci M, Dry S, Vaiyapuri S, et al. Novel BCOR-MAML3 and ZC3H7B-BCOR gene fusions in undifferentiated small blue round cell sarcomas. Am J Surg Pathol. 2016;40(4):433–42.
21. Krskova L, Kabickova E, Drahokoupilova E, Kopeckova K, Plank L, Vitkova P, et al. An undifferentiated sarcoma with BCOR-CCNB3 fusion transcript – pathological and clinical retrospective study. Neoplasma. 2018;65(4):630–6.
22. Yamada Y, Kuda M, Kohashi K, Yamamoto H, Takemoto J, Ishii T, et al. Histological and immunohistochemical characteristics of undifferentiated small round cell sarcomas associated with CIC-DUX4 and BCOR-CCNB3 fusion genes. Virchows Arch. 2017;470(4):373–80.
23. Huang SC, Zhang L, Sung YS, Chen CL, Kao YC, Agaram NP, et al. Secondary EWSR1 gene abnormalities in SMARCB1-deficient tumors with 22q11-12 regional deletions: potential pitfalls in interpreting EWSR1 FISH results. Genes Chromosomes Cancer. 2016;55(10):767–76.
24. Mantilla JG, Ricciotti RW, Chen E, Hoch BL, Liu YJ. Detecting disease-defining gene fusions in unclassified round cell sarcomas using anchored multiplex PCR/targeted RNA next-generation sequencing-molecular and clinicopathological characterization of 16 cases. Genes Chromosomes Cancer. 2019;58(10):713–22.
25. Rekhi B, Kembhavi P, Mishra SN, Shetty O, Bajpai J, Puri A. Clinicopathologic features of undifferentiated round cell sarcomas of bone & soft tissues: an attempt to unravel the BCOR-CCNB3- & CIC-DUX4-positive sarcomas. Indian J Med Res. 2019;150(6):557–74.
26. Italiano A, Chen CL, Thomas R, Breen M, Bonnet F, Sevenet N, et al. Alterations of the p53 and PIK3CA/AKT/mTOR pathways in angiosarcomas: a pattern distinct from other sarcomas with complex genomics. Cancer. 2012;118(23):5878–87.
27. Yoshida A, Arai Y, Kobayashi E, Yonemori K, Ogura K, Hama N, et al. CIC break-apart fluorescence in-situ hybridization misses a subset of CIC-DUX4 sarcomas: a clinicopathological and molecular study. Histopathology. 2017;71(3):461–9.
28. Hung YP, Fletcher CD, Hornick JL. Evaluation of ETV4 and WT1 expression in CIC-rearranged sarcomas and histologic mimics. Mod Pathol. 2016;29(11):1324–34.
29. Kao YC, Sung YS, Chen CL, Zhang L, Dickson BC, Swanson D, et al. ETV transcriptional upregulation is more reliable than RNA sequencing algorithms and FISH in diagnosing round cell sarcomas with CIC gene rearrangements. Genes Chromosomes Cancer. 2017;56(6):501–10.
30. Panagopoulos I, Gorunova L, Bjerkehagen B, Heim S. The "grep" command but not FusionMap, FusionFinder or ChimeraScan captures the CIC-DUX4 fusion gene from whole transcriptome sequencing data on a small round cell tumor with t(4;19)(q35;q13). PLoS One. 2014;9(6):e99439.
31. Kashima T, Halai D, Ye H, Hing SN, Delaney D, Pollock R, et al. Sensitivity of MDM2 amplification and unexpected multiple faint alphoid 12 (alpha 12 satellite sequences) signals in atypical lipomatous tumor. Mod Pathol. 2012;25(10):1384–96.
32. Sirvent N, Coindre JM, Maire G, Hostein I, Keslair F, Guillou L, et al. Detection of MDM2-CDK4 amplification by fluorescence in situ hybridization in 200 paraffin-embedded tumor samples: utility in diagnosing adipocytic lesions and comparison with immunohistochemistry and real-time PCR. Am J Surg Pathol. 2007;31(10):1476–89.
33. Clay MR, Martinez AP, Weiss SW, Edgar MA. MDM2 and CDK4 immunohistochemistry: should it be used in problematic differentiated lipomatous tumors?: a new perspective. Am J Surg Pathol. 2016;40(12):1647–52.
34. Dal Cin P, Kools P, Sciot R, De Wever I, Van Damme B, Van de Ven W, et al. Cytogenetic and fluorescence in situ hybridization investigation of ring chromosomes characterizing a specific pathologic subgroup of adipose tissue tumors. Cancer Genet Cytogenet. 1993;68(2):85–90.
35. Clay MR, Martinez AP, Weiss SW, Edgar MA. MDM2 amplification in problematic lipomatous tumors: analysis of FISH testing criteria. Am J Surg Pathol. 2015;39(10):1433–9.
36. Zhang H, Erickson-Johnson M, Wang X, Oliveira JL, Nascimento AG, Sim FH, et al. Molecular testing for lipomatous tumors: critical analysis and test recommendations based on the analysis of 405 extremity-based tumors. Am J Surg Pathol. 2010;34(9):1304–11.
37. Robinson DR, Wu YM, Kalyana-Sundaram S, Cao X, Lonigro RJ, Sung YS, et al. Identification of recurrent NAB2-STAT6 gene fusions in solitary fibrous tumor by integrative sequencing. Nat Genet. 2013;45(2):180–5.
38. Doyle LA, Tao D, Marino-Enriquez A. STAT6 is amplified in a subset of dedifferentiated liposarcoma. Mod Pathol. 2014;27(9):1231–7.
39. Mantilla JG, Ricciotti RW, Chen EY, Liu YJ, Hoch BL. Amplification of DNA damage-inducible transcript 3 (DDIT3) is associated with myxoid liposarcoma-like morphology and homologous lipoblastic differentiation in dedifferentiated liposarcoma. Mod Pathol. 2019;32(4):585–92.
40. Crozat A, Aman P, Mandahl N, Ron D. Fusion of CHOP to a novel RNA-binding protein in human myxoid liposarcoma. Nature. 1993;363(6430):640–4.
41. Panagopoulos I, Lassen C, Isaksson M, Mitelman F, Mandahl N, Aman P. Characteristic sequence motifs at the breakpoints of the hybrid genes FUS/CHOP, EWS/CHOP and FUS/ERG in myxoid liposarcoma and acute myeloid leukemia. Oncogene. 1997;15(11):1357–62.

42. Narendra S, Valente A, Tull J, Zhang S. DDIT3 gene break-apart as a molecular marker for diagnosis of myxoid liposarcoma – assay validation and clinical experience. Diagn Mol Pathol. 2011;20(4):218–24.
43. Koelsche C, Renner M, Hartmann W, Brandt R, Lehner B, Waldburger N, et al. TERT promoter hotspot mutations are recurrent in myxoid liposarcomas but rare in other soft tissue sarcoma entities. J Exp Clin Cancer Res. 2014;33:33.
44. Trautmann M, Cyra M, Isfort I, Jeiler B, Kruger A, Grunewald I, et al. Phosphatidylinositol-3-kinase (PI3K)/Akt signaling is functionally essential in myxoid liposarcoma. Mol Cancer Ther. 2019;18(4):834–44.
45. Antonescu CR, Tschernyavsky SJ, Decuseara R, Leung DH, Woodruff JM, Brennan MF, et al. Prognostic impact of P53 status, TLS-CHOP fusion transcript structure, and histological grade in myxoid liposarcoma: a molecular and clinicopathologic study of 82 cases. Clin Cancer Res. 2001;7(12):3977–87.
46. Huang SC, Zhang L, Sung YS, Chen CL, Krausz T, Dickson BC, et al. Frequent FOS gene rearrangements in epithelioid hemangioma: a molecular study of 58 cases with morphologic reappraisal. Am J Surg Pathol. 2015;39(10):1313–21.
47. Adam J, Adamova D, Aggarwal MM, Rinella GA, Agnello M, Agrawal N, et al. Measurement of pion, kaon and proton production in proton-proton collisions at [formula: see text] TeV. Eur Phys J C Part Fields. 2015;75(5):226.
48. van IDG, de Jong D, Romagosa C, Picci P, Benassi MS, Gambarotti M, et al. Fusion events lead to truncation of FOS in epithelioid hemangioma of bone. Genes Chromosomes Cancer. 2015;54(9):565–74.
49. Agaram NP, Zhang L, Cotzia P, Antonescu CR. Expanding the Spectrum of genetic alterations in pseudomyogenic hemangioendothelioma with recurrent novel ACTB-FOSB gene fusions. Am J Surg Pathol. 2018;42(12):1653–61.
50. Antonescu CR, Chen HW, Zhang L, Sung YS, Panicek D, Agaram NP, et al. ZFP36-FOSB fusion defines a subset of epithelioid hemangioma with atypical features. Genes Chromosomes Cancer. 2014;53(11):951–9.
51. Billings SD, Folpe AL, Weiss SW. Epithelioid sarcoma-like hemangioendothelioma. Am J Surg Pathol. 2003;27(1):48–57.
52. Hornick JL, Fletcher CD. Pseudomyogenic hemangioendothelioma: a distinctive, often multicentric tumor with indolent behavior. Am J Surg Pathol. 2011;35(2):190–201.
53. Walther C, Tayebwa J, Lilljebjorn H, Magnusson L, Nilsson J, von Steyern FV, et al. A novel SERPINE1-FOSB fusion gene results in transcriptional up-regulation of FOSB in pseudomyogenic haemangioendothelioma. J Pathol. 2014;232(5):534–40.
54. Weiss SW, Enzinger FM. Epithelioid hemangioendothelioma: a vascular tumor often mistaken for a carcinoma. Cancer. 1982;50(5):970–81.
55. Errani C, Zhang L, Sung YS, Hajdu M, Singer S, Maki RG, et al. A novel WWTR1-CAMTA1 gene fusion is a consistent abnormality in epithelioid hemangioendothelioma of different anatomic sites. Genes Chromosomes Cancer. 2011;50(8):644–53.
56. Antonescu CR, Le Loarer F, Mosquera JM, Sboner A, Zhang L, Chen CL, et al. Novel YAP1-TFE3 fusion defines a distinct subset of epithelioid hemangioendothelioma. Genes Chromosomes Cancer. 2013;52(8):775–84.
57. Doyle LA, Fletcher CD, Hornick JL. Nuclear expression of CAMTA1 distinguishes epithelioid hemangioendothelioma from histologic mimics. Am J Surg Pathol. 2016;40(1):94–102.
58. Guo T, Zhang L, Chang NE, Singer S, Maki RG, Antonescu CR. Consistent MYC and FLT4 gene amplification in radiation-induced angiosarcoma but not in other radiation-associated atypical vascular lesions. Genes Chromosomes Cancer. 2011;50(1):25–33.
59. Ginter PS, Mosquera JM, MacDonald TY, D'Alfonso TM, Rubin MA, Shin SJ. Diagnostic utility of MYC amplification and anti-MYC immunohistochemistry in atypical vascular lesions, primary or radiation-induced mammary angiosarcomas, and primary angiosarcomas of other sites. Hum Pathol. 2014;45(4):709–16.
60. Shon W, Sukov WR, Jenkins SM, Folpe AL. MYC amplification and overexpression in primary cutaneous angiosarcoma: a fluorescence in-situ hybridization and immunohistochemical study. Mod Pathol. 2014;27(4):509–15.
61. Newton WA Jr, Gehan EA, Webber BL, Marsden HB, van Unnik AJ, Hamoudi AB, et al. Classification of rhabdomyosarcomas and related sarcomas. Pathologic aspects and proposal for a new classification – an intergroup rhabdomyosarcoma study. Cancer. 1995;76(6):1073–85.
62. Rudzinski ER, Anderson JR, Chi YY, et al. Histology, fusion status, and outcome in metastatic rhabdomyosarcoma: A report from the Children's Oncology Group. Pediatr Blood Cancer. 2017;64(12):10.1002/pbc.26645. https://doi.org/10.1002/pbc.26645.
63. Hachitanda Y, Toyoshima S, Akazawa K, Tsuneyoshi M. N-myc gene amplification in rhabdomyosarcoma detected by fluorescence in situ hybridization: its correlation with histologic features. Mod Pathol. 1998;11(12):1222–7.
64. Ragazzini P, Gamberi G, Pazzaglia L, Serra M, Magagnoli G, Ponticelli F, et al. Amplification of CDK4, MDM2, SAS and GLI genes in leiomyosarcoma, alveolar and embryonal rhabdomyosarcoma. Histol Histopathol. 2004;19(2):401–11.
65. Duan F, Smith LM, Gustafson DM, Zhang C, Dunlevy MJ, Gastier-Foster JM, et al. Genomic and clinical analysis of fusion gene amplification in rhabdomyosarcoma: a report from the children's oncology group. Genes Chromosomes Cancer. 2012;51(7):662–74.
66. Downs-Kelly E, Shehata BM, Lopez-Terrada D, Weaver J, Patel RM, Hartke M, et al. The utility of FOXO1 fluorescence in situ hybridization (FISH) in formalin-fixed paraffin-embedded specimens in the diagnosis of alveolar rhabdomyosarcoma. Diagn Mol Pathol. 2009;18(3):138–43.
67. Barr FG, Qualman SJ, Macris MH, Melnyk N, Lawlor ER, Strzelecki DM, et al. Genetic heterogeneity in the alveolar rhabdomyosarcoma subset without typical gene fusions. Cancer Res. 2002;62(16):4704–10.
68. van Gaal JC, Flucke UE, Roeffen MH, de Bont ES, Sleijfer S, Mavinkurve-Groothuis AM, et al. Anaplastic lymphoma kinase aberrations in rhabdomyosarcoma: clinical and prognostic implications. J Clin Oncol. 2012;30(3):308–15.
69. Wierdl M, Tsurkan L, Chi L, Hatfield MJ, Tollemar V, Bradley C, et al. Targeting ALK in pediatric RMS does not induce antitumor activity in vivo. Cancer Chemother Pharmacol. 2018;82(2):251–63.
70. Rudzinski ER. Histology and fusion status in rhabdomyosarcoma. Am Soc Clin Oncol Educ Book. 2013:425–8.
71. Mosquera JM, Sboner A, Zhang L, Kitabayashi N, Chen CL, Sung YS, et al. Recurrent NCOA2 gene rearrangements in congenital/infantile spindle cell rhabdomyosarcoma. Genes Chromosomes Cancer. 2013;52(6):538–50.
72. Alaggio R, Zhang L, Sung YS, Huang SC, Chen CL, Bisogno G, et al. A molecular study of pediatric spindle and sclerosing rhabdomyosarcoma: identification of novel and recurrent VGLL2-related fusions in infantile cases. Am J Surg Pathol. 2016;40(2):224–35.
73. Szuhai K, de Jong D, Leung WY, Fletcher CD, Hogendoorn PC. Transactivating mutation of the MYOD1 gene is a frequent event in adult spindle cell rhabdomyosarcoma. J Pathol. 2014;232(3):300–7.
74. Agaram NP, Chen CL, Zhang L, LaQuaglia MP, Wexler L, Antonescu CR. Recurrent MYOD1 mutations in pediatric and adult sclerosing and spindle cell rhabdomyosarcomas: evidence for a common pathogenesis. Genes Chromosomes Cancer. 2014;53(9):779–87.

75. Martinez AP, Fritchie KJ, Weiss SW, Agaimy A, Haller F, Huang HY, et al. Histiocyte-rich rhabdomyoblastic tumor: rhabdomyosarcoma, rhabdomyoma, or rhabdomyoblastic tumor of uncertain malignant potential? A histologically distinctive rhabdomyoblastic tumor in search of a place in the classification of skeletal muscle neoplasms. Mod Pathol. 2019;32(3):446–57.
76. Bourgeau M, Martinez AP. Histiocyte-rich rhabdomyoblastic tumor: a report of two cases and a review of the differential diagnoses. Virchows Arch. 2021;478(2):367–73.
77. Fanburg-Smith JC, Miettinen M. Angiomatoid "malignant" fibrous histiocytoma: a clinicopathologic study of 158 cases and further exploration of the myoid phenotype. Hum Pathol. 1999;30(11):1336–43.
78. Antonescu CR, Dal Cin P, Nafa K, Teot LA, Surti U, Fletcher CD, et al. EWSR1-CREB1 is the predominant gene fusion in angiomatoid fibrous histiocytoma. Genes Chromosomes Cancer. 2007;46(12):1051–60.
79. Tanas MR, Rubin BP, Montgomery EA, Turner SL, Cook JR, Tubbs RR, et al. Utility of FISH in the diagnosis of angiomatoid fibrous histiocytoma: a series of 18 cases. Mod Pathol. 2010;23(1):93–7.
80. Cheah AL, Zou Y, Lanigan C, Billings SD, Rubin BP, Hornick JL, et al. ALK expression in angiomatoid fibrous histiocytoma: a potential diagnostic pitfall. Am J Surg Pathol. 2019;43(1):93–101.
81. Ladanyi M, Antonescu CR, Leung DH, Woodruff JM, Kawai A, Healey JH, et al. Impact of SYT-SSX fusion type on the clinical behavior of synovial sarcoma: a multi-institutional retrospective study of 243 patients. Cancer Res. 2002;62(1):135–40.
82. Pelmus M, Guillou L, Hostein I, Sierankowski G, Lussan C, Coindre JM. Monophasic fibrous and poorly differentiated synovial sarcoma: immunohistochemical reassessment of 60 t(X;18)(SYT-SSX)-positive cases. Am J Surg Pathol. 2002;26(11):1434–40.
83. Amary MF, Berisha F, Bernardi Fdel C, Herbert A, James M, Reis-Filho JS, et al. Detection of SS18-SSX fusion transcripts in formalin-fixed paraffin-embedded neoplasms: analysis of conventional RT-PCR, qRT-PCR and dual color FISH as diagnostic tools for synovial sarcoma. Mod Pathol. 2007;20(4):482–96.
84. Storlazzi CT, Mertens F, Mandahl N, Gisselsson D, Isaksson M, Gustafson P, et al. A novel fusion gene, SS18L1/SSX1, in synovial sarcoma. Genes Chromosomes Cancer. 2003;37(2):195–200.
85. Wang H, Jacobson A, Harmon DC, Choy E, Hornicek FJ, Raskin KA, et al. Prognostic factors in alveolar soft part sarcoma: a SEER analysis. J Surg Oncol. 2016;113(5):581–6.
86. Ladanyi M, Lui MY, Antonescu CR, Krause-Boehm A, Meindl A, Argani P, et al. The der(17)t(X;17)(p11;q25) of human alveolar soft part sarcoma fuses the TFE3 transcription factor gene to ASPL, a novel gene at 17q25. Oncogene. 2001;20(1):48–57.
87. Argani P, Lal P, Hutchinson B, Lui MY, Reuter VE, Ladanyi M. Aberrant nuclear immunoreactivity for TFE3 in neoplasms with TFE3 gene fusions: a sensitive and specific immunohistochemical assay. Am J Surg Pathol. 2003;27(6):750–61.
88. Enzinger FM. Clear-cell sarcoma of tendons and aponeuroses. An analysis of 21 cases. Cancer. 1965;18:1163–74.
89. Hisaoka M, Ishida T, Kuo TT, Matsuyama A, Imamura T, Nishida K, et al. Clear cell sarcoma of soft tissue: a clinicopathologic, immunohistochemical, and molecular analysis of 33 cases. Am J Surg Pathol. 2008;32(3):452–60.
90. Panagopoulos I, Mertens F, Debiec-Rychter M, Isaksson M, Limon J, Kardas I, et al. Molecular genetic characterization of the EWS/ATF1 fusion gene in clear cell sarcoma of tendons and aponeuroses. Int J Cancer. 2002;99(4):560–7.
91. Park BM, Jin SA, Choi YD, Shin SH, Jung ST, Lee JB, et al. Two cases of clear cell sarcoma with different clinical and genetic features: cutaneous type with BRAF mutation and subcutaneous type with KIT mutation. Br J Dermatol. 2013;169(6):1346–52.
92. Enzinger FM, Shiraki M. Extraskeletal myxoid chondrosarcoma. An analysis of 34 cases. Hum Pathol. 1972;3(3):421–35.
93. Panagopoulos I, Mertens F, Isaksson M, Domanski HA, Brosjo O, Heim S, et al. Molecular genetic characterization of the EWS/CHN and RBP56/CHN fusion genes in extraskeletal myxoid chondrosarcoma. Genes Chromosomes Cancer. 2002;35(4):340–52.
94. Agaram NP, Zhang L, Sung YS, Singer S, Antonescu CR. Extraskeletal myxoid chondrosarcoma with non-EWSR1-NR4A3 variant fusions correlate with rhabdoid phenotype and high-grade morphology. Hum Pathol. 2014;45(5):1084–91.
95. Hisaoka M, Ishida T, Imamura T, Hashimoto H. TFG is a novel fusion partner of NOR1 in extraskeletal myxoid chondrosarcoma. Genes Chromosomes Cancer. 2004;40(4):325–8.
96. Urbini M, Astolfi A, Pantaleo MA, Serravalle S, Dei Tos AP, Picci P, et al. HSPA8 as a novel fusion partner of NR4A3 in extraskeletal myxoid chondrosarcoma. Genes Chromosomes Cancer. 2017;56(7):582–6.
97. Lae ME, Roche PC, Jin L, Lloyd RV, Nascimento AG. Desmoplastic small round cell tumor: a clinicopathologic, immunohistochemical, and molecular study of 32 tumors. Am J Surg Pathol. 2002;26(7):823–35.
98. Ladanyi M, Gerald W. Fusion of the EWS and WT1 genes in the desmoplastic small round cell tumor. Cancer Res. 1994;54(11):2837–40.
99. Neuville A, Collin F, Bruneval P, Parrens M, Thivolet F, Gomez-Brouchet A, et al. Intimal sarcoma is the most frequent primary cardiac sarcoma: clinicopathologic and molecular retrospective analysis of 100 primary cardiac sarcomas. Am J Surg Pathol. 2014;38(4):461–9.
100. Meister P, Buckmann FW, Konrad E. Extent and level of fascial involvement in 100 cases with nodular fasciitis. Virchows Arch A Pathol Anat Histol. 1978;380(2):177–85.
101. Montgomery EA, Meis JM. Nodular fasciitis. Its morphologic spectrum and immunohistochemical profile. Am J Surg Pathol. 1991;15(10):942–8.
102. Erickson-Johnson MR, Chou MM, Evers BR, Roth CW, Seys AR, Jin L, et al. Nodular fasciitis: a novel model of transient neoplasia induced by MYH9-USP6 gene fusion. Lab Investig. 2011;91(10):1427–33.
103. Guo R, Wang X, Chou MM, Asmann Y, Wenger DE, Al-Ibraheemi A, et al. PPP6R3-USP6 amplification: novel oncogenic mechanism in malignant nodular fasciitis. Genes Chromosomes Cancer. 2016;55(8):640–9.
104. Carter JM, Wang X, Dong J, Westendorf J, Chou MM, Oliveira AM. USP6 genetic rearrangements in cellular fibroma of tendon sheath. Mod Pathol. 2016;29(8):865–9.
105. Kao YC, Flucke U, Eijkelenboom A, Zhang L, Sung YS, Suurmeijer AJH, et al. Novel EWSR1-SMAD3 gene fusions in a group of acral fibroblastic spindle cell neoplasms. Am J Surg Pathol. 2018;42(4):522–8.
106. Al-Ibraheemi A, Folpe AL, Perez-Atayde AR, Perry K, Hofvander J, Arbajian E, et al. Aberrant receptor tyrosine kinase signaling in lipofibromatosis: a clinicopathological and molecular genetic study of 20 cases. Mod Pathol. 2019;32(3):423–34.
107. Marino-Enriquez A, Fletcher CD. Angiofibroma of soft tissue: clinicopathologic characterization of a distinctive benign fibrovascular neoplasm in a series of 37 cases. Am J Surg Pathol. 2012;36(4):500–8.
108. Jin Y, Moller E, Nord KH, Mandahl N, Von Steyern FV, Domanski HA, et al. Fusion of the AHRR and NCOA2 genes through a recurrent translocation t(5;8)(p15;q13) in soft tissue angiofibroma results in upregulation of aryl hydrocarbon receptor target genes. Genes Chromosomes Cancer. 2012;51(5):510–20.
109. Arbajian E, Magnusson L, Mertens F, Domanski HA, Vult von Steyern F, Nord KH. A novel GTF2I/NCOA2 fusion gene empha-

sizes the role of NCOA2 in soft tissue angiofibroma development. Genes Chromosomes Cancer. 2013;52(3):330–1.
110. Bekers EM, Groenen P, Verdijk MAJ, Raaijmakers-van Geloof WL, Roepman P, Vink R, et al. Soft tissue angiofibroma: Clinicopathologic, immunohistochemical and molecular analysis of 14 cases. Genes Chromosomes Cancer. 2017;56(10):750–7.
111. Crago AM, Denton B, Salas S, Dufresne A, Mezhir JJ, Hameed M, et al. A prognostic nomogram for prediction of recurrence in desmoid fibromatosis. Ann Surg. 2013;258(2):347–53.
112. Lazar AJ, Tuvin D, Hajibashi S, Habeeb S, Bolshakov S, Mayordomo-Aranda E, et al. Specific mutations in the beta-catenin gene (CTNNB1) correlate with local recurrence in sporadic desmoid tumors. Am J Pathol. 2008;173(5):1518–27.
113. Miyaki M, Konishi M, Kikuchi-Yanoshita R, Enomoto M, Tanaka K, Takahashi H, et al. Coexistence of somatic and germ-line mutations of APC gene in desmoid tumors from patients with familial adenomatous polyposis. Cancer Res. 1993;53(21):5079–82.
114. Dadone-Montaudie B, Alberti L, Duc A, Delespaul L, Lesluyes T, Perot G, et al. Alternative PDGFD rearrangements in dermatofibrosarcomas protuberans without PDGFB fusions. Mod Pathol. 2018;31(11):1683–93.
115. Enzinger FM, Smith BH. Hemangiopericytoma. An analysis of 106 cases. Hum Pathol. 1976;7(1):61–82.
116. Knezevich SR, McFadden DE, Tao W, Lim JF, Sorensen PH. A novel ETV6-NTRK3 gene fusion in congenital fibrosarcoma. Nat Genet. 1998;18(2):184–7.
117. Flucke U, van Noesel MM, Wijnen M, Zhang L, Chen CL, Sung YS, et al. TFG-MET fusion in an infantile spindle cell sarcoma with neural features. Genes Chromosomes Cancer. 2017;56(9):663–7.
118. Kao YC, Fletcher CDM, Alaggio R, Wexler L, Zhang L, Sung YS, et al. Recurrent BRAF gene fusions in a subset of pediatric spindle cell sarcomas: expanding the genetic spectrum of tumors with overlapping features with infantile fibrosarcoma. Am J Surg Pathol. 2018;42(1):28–38.
119. Suurmeijer AJH, Dickson BC, Swanson D, Zhang L, Sung YS, Cotzia P, et al. A novel group of spindle cell tumors defined by S100 and CD34 co-expression shows recurrent fusions involving RAF1, BRAF, and NTRK1/2 genes. Genes Chromosomes Cancer. 2018;57(12):611–21.
120. Rudzinski ER, Lockwood CM, Stohr BA, Vargas SO, Sheridan R, Black JO, et al. Pan-Trk immunohistochemistry identifies NTRK rearrangements in pediatric mesenchymal tumors. Am J Surg Pathol. 2018;42(7):927–35.
121. Folpe AL, Lane KL, Paull G, Weiss SW. Low-grade fibromyxoid sarcoma and hyalinizing spindle cell tumor with giant rosettes: a clinicopathologic study of 73 cases supporting their identity and assessing the impact of high-grade areas. Am J Surg Pathol. 2000;24(10):1353–60.
122. Mertens F, Fletcher CD, Antonescu CR, Coindre JM, Colecchia M, Domanski HA, et al. Clinicopathologic and molecular genetic characterization of low-grade fibromyxoid sarcoma, and cloning of a novel FUS/CREB3L1 fusion gene. Lab Investig. 2005;85(3):408–15.
123. Lau PP, Lui PC, Lau GT, Yau DT, Cheung ET, Chan JK. EWSR1-CREB3L1 gene fusion: a novel alternative molecular aberration of low-grade fibromyxoid sarcoma. Am J Surg Pathol. 2013;37(5):734–8.
124. Doyle LA, Moller E, Dal Cin P, Fletcher CD, Mertens F, Hornick JL. MUC4 is a highly sensitive and specific marker for low-grade fibromyxoid sarcoma. Am J Surg Pathol. 2011;35(5):733–41.
125. Meis-Kindblom JM, Kindblom LG, Enzinger FM. Sclerosing epithelioid fibrosarcoma. A variant of fibrosarcoma simulating carcinoma. Am J Surg Pathol. 1995;19(9):979–93.
126. Arbajian E, Puls F, Magnusson L, Thway K, Fisher C, Sumathi VP, et al. Recurrent EWSR1-CREB3L1 gene fusions in sclerosing epithelioid fibrosarcoma. Am J Surg Pathol. 2014;38(6):801–8.
127. Dewaele B, Libbrecht L, Levy G, Brichard B, Vanspauwen V, Sciot R, et al. A novel EWS-CREB3L3 gene fusion in a mesenteric sclerosing epithelioid fibrosarcoma. Genes Chromosomes Cancer. 2017;56(9):695–9.
128. Arbajian E, Puls F, Antonescu CR, Amary F, Sciot R, Debiec-Rychter M, et al. In-depth genetic analysis of sclerosing epithelioid fibrosarcoma reveals recurrent genomic alterations and potential treatment targets. Clin Cancer Res. 2017;23(23):7426–34.
129. Doyle LA, Wang WL, Dal Cin P, Lopez-Terrada D, Mertens F, Lazar AJ, et al. MUC4 is a sensitive and extremely useful marker for sclerosing epithelioid fibrosarcoma: association with FUS gene rearrangement. Am J Surg Pathol. 2012;36(10):1444–51.

Genitourinary Neoplasms

11

Yi Ding, Khaleel I. Al-Obaidy, and Liang Cheng

List of Frequently Asked Questions

1. What are the most common molecular assays currently available in the sporadic genitourinary (GU) system neoplasia?
2. When should a molecular assay for *VHL* mutations or 3p deletions be considered in working up a renal cell carcinoma?
3. What are the commonly seen genetic alterations in chromophobe renal cell carcinoma?
4. What molecular assays can be used to aid the subtyping of papillary renal cell carcinoma (PRCC)?
5. What molecular assays should be considered to help differentiate translocation-associated renal cell carcinoma (tRCC) from other subtypes of renal cell carcinoma (RCC)?
6. What molecular assays are available when a hereditary RCC syndrome is considered?
7. What are the commonly seen genetic alterations in Wilms tumor?
8. What is the most used molecular test in urothelial carcinoma (UC) screening?
9. Besides UroVysion assay, what are other molecular assays available for UC and their indications?
10. What is the clinical utility of ETS gene fusions in diagnosis of prostate adenocarcinoma?
11. Besides the ETS gene family, what are other commonly observed molecular genetic abnormalities in prostatic cancer and their prognostic significance?
12. For prostatic cancer, what is the current utilization of gene expression profiling (GEP) assay?
13. Is there a prostate cancer screening algorithm available?
14. What are the commonly seen molecular changes in testicular germ cell tumors (GCTs)?

Y. Ding (✉)
Department of Laboratory Medicine, Geisinger Health, Danville, PA, USA
e-mail: yding1@geisinger.edu

K. I. Al-Obaidy · L. Cheng
Department of Pathology and Laboratory Medicine, Indiana University School of Medicine, Indianapolis, IN, USA
e-mail: lcheng@iupui.edu

Frequently Asked Questions

1. **What are the most common molecular assays currently available in the sporadic genitourinary (GU) system neoplasia?**
   - With increasing understanding of the genetic landscape of the tumors of the genitourinary system, it is proved that many types of GU tumors are associated with, and even defined by, recurrent genomic abnormalities.
   - Table 11.1 reviews the majority of the clinically relevant molecular assays currently available that may aid in the diagnosis, prognosis, and treatment of neoplasia in the genitourinary system.
   - It should be noted that there remain significant practice gaps for the implementation of this increasing knowledge into clinical practice.
2. **When should a molecular assay for *VHL* mutations or 3p deletions be considered in working up a renal cell carcinoma?**
   - More than 90% of sporadic clear cell renal cell carcinoma (CCRCC) harbors genomic alterations, most commonly copy number loss, on chromosome arm 3p, on which the tumor suppressor genes, such as *VHL*, *PBRM1*, *BAP1*, and *SETD2*, are located [1–3].
   - Most diagnostic pathology practice in a routine setting is based on histologic evaluation, possibly combined with immunohistochemistry (IHC). In rare challenging cases or in cases with a small biopsy or scant material, a molecular assay, including mutation analysis, FISH assay, and methylation studies, for 3p loss or *VHL* mutation can certainly provide supporting evidence for diagnosis [2].

Y. Ding, L. Zhang (eds.), *Practical Oncologic Molecular Pathology*, Practical Anatomic Pathology,
https://doi.org/10.1007/978-3-030-73227-1_11

Table 11.1 Main molecular assays in the genitourinary neoplasms

Organ	Target	Diagnosis	Method	Specimen
Kidney	*VHL* gene and chromosome 3	Clear cell RCC	FISH, sequencing	Fresh or FFPE tissue
	Chromosome 7 and 17 trisomy Chromosome Y deletion in male patients	Papillary RCC	FISH	Fresh or FFPE tissue
	TFE3 and *TFEB*	Translocation-associated RCC	IHC, FISH	Fresh or FFPE tissue
	ALK	ALK-rearranged RCC	Gene sequencing, FISH	Fresh or FFPE tissue
	Chromosome 7 and 17 trisomy Chromosome Y deletion in male patients *KRAS* mutation	Papillary renal neoplasm with reverse polarity	Gene sequencing, FISH	Fresh or FFPE tissue
	NTRK	Cellular congenital mesoblastic nephroma	IHC, FISH, sequencing	Fresh or FFPE tissue,
Bladder	Chromosome 3, 7, 9p, and 17; *TERT* promoter mutations; *FGFR* gene alterations	Urothelial carcinoma	FISH, molecular techniques	Urine, fresh or FFPE tissue, cytology smear, urine
Prostate	*ERG*	Prostatic adenocarcinoma and small cell carcinoma	IHC, FISH	Fresh or FFPE tissue
	TMPRSS2: *ERG* and *PCA3*	Screening for prostatic adenocarcinoma	TMA	Urine
	BRAF, *RAF1*	ETS-negative prostate cancer	FISH, sequencing	Fresh or FFPE tissue
	AR signaling status, AR-V7	Castration-resistant prostatic adenocarcinoma	Molecular techniques	Fresh or FFPE tissue, blood
	BRCA1, *BRCA2*, *HOXB13*	Pathogenic germline mutations increasing risk of prostate cancer	Molecular techniques	Fresh or FFPE tissue, blood
Testis	Isochromosome 12p	Germ cell tumor	FISH	FFPE tissue, semen

RCC renal cell carcinoma; *FISH* fluorescence in situ hybridization; *IHC* immunohistochemistry

- Notably, FISH analysis is unable to detect some cases of *VHL* loss, and other copy number assessment should be considered to identify copy number deletion, missense, and truncating mutations in *VHL*, which commonly occur in CCRCC.
- Emerging biomarkers, such as *VHL*, *PBRM1*, *BAP1*, and *SETD2*, although not being used routinely, may have increasing roles in renal cancer management. For example, it has been demonstrated that tumors harboring *PBRM1* mutation have more favorable behavior, whereas tumors with *BAP1* or *SETD2* mutations likely to have more aggressive behavior [4, 5].

3. **What are the commonly seen genetic alterations in chromophobe renal cell carcinoma?**
   - Like other RCC, chromophobe RCC can be usually diagnosed by typical histologic evaluation, with IHC in some cases.
   - Conventional cytogenetics can be used to detect commonly seen cytogenetic changes in chromophobe RCC including:
     - Hypodiploidy
     - Loss of chromosomes 1,2,6,10,13,17,21 and Y [6]
   - Commonly seen gene mutations include [7]:
     - Mutations in tumor suppressor genes: *TP53* (20–30%), *PTEN* (5–10%)
     - Rearrangements in *TERT* promoter region (~10%)
   - For tumors with hybrid chromophobe and oncocytic morphology and Birt-Hogg-Dube syndrome is suspected; genetic counseling and analysis of the *FLCN* (folliculin) gene should be considered [8, 9].
4. **What molecular assays can be used to aid the subtyping of papillary renal cell carcinoma (PRCC)?**
   - Papillary RCC (PRCC) is the second most common type of RCC and accounts for 15–20% of RCCs.
   - Papillary RCC is further subdivided into type 1 and type 2 PRCC, in which type 1 is more uniform on morphologic, immunophenotypic, and molecular features than type 2.
   - The difference between type 1 and type 2 PRCC is not only histologic but also prognostic and genomic, as patients with type 2 PRCC typically have worse outcomes than patients with type 1 PRCC.
   - Type 1 PRCC is frequently associated with trisomy of chromosomes 7 and 17 and loss of chromosome Y, whereas recent studies have shown that although these cytogenetic changes can also be observed in type 2 PRCC, it is more characterized by other genetic alterations. Indeed, type 2 PRCC is now considered likely more than one diagnostic entity (Table 11.2) [10, 11].
   - Nonetheless, there is currently no clinically available molecular assay to aid in the diagnosis of type 2 PRCC,

Table 11.2 Comparison of type 1 and type 2 PRCC

	Type 1 PRCC	Type 2 PRCC
Histology and immunophenotype	More uniform	Likely a mixture of multiple entities
cytogenetic changes	Trisomy or polysomic chromosomes 7 and 17 Loss of chromosome Y Gain of chromosomes 3,12,16, and 20	Gain of chromosomes 12,16, and 20
Gene mutations	*MET* mutations in the hereditary papillary RCC syndrome and sporadic type I PRCC [12–18]	*CDKN2A* silencing, *SETD2* mutations [10]

but FISH for trisomy 7 and/or 17 could be used in cases in which type 1 PRCC is a consideration. Notably, type 1 PRCC can have considerable morphologic overlap with mucinous tubular and spindle cell carcinoma and clear cell papillary RCC, both of which lack trisomies 7 and 17; thus, FISH for trisomy 7 and/or 17 may be especially useful in this differential diagnosis.

- Papillary renal neoplasm with reverse polarity is a newly proposed entity. It shows architectural and immunohistochemical overlap with PRCC. However, it has distinctively a single layer of apically located nuclei with positive GATA3 and LICAM and negative vimentin immunostaining. This sets it apart from PRCC, clear cell PRCC, and Xp11 translocation RCC. Recurrent *KRAS* point mutation identified in this entity is distinctly different from other renal cell neoplasms.

5. **What molecular assays should be considered to help differentiate translocation-associated TCC (tRCC) from other subtypes of RCC?**
   - Translocation-associated RCC (tRCC) is a subtype of RCC defined by a translocation involving the microphthalmia (MiT) subfamily of transcription factors includes the most common *TFE3* located at Xp11.2 and less common *TFEB*, *TFC*, and *MITF* [19].
   - The diagnosis of tRCC is mainly based on typical morphologic features such as nested and papillary growth pattern, mixture of clear and eosinophilic cells with unusually voluminous cytoplasm, psammomatous calcifications, and hyalinized stroma.
   - In the difficult cases with considerable morphologic overlap between tRCC and other RCC subtypes, such as CCRCC and PRCC.
     - Immunohistochemistry, such as melanocytic markers, TFE3 or TFEB, is often useful but not sensitive or specific for tRCC.
     - Break-apart FISH analysis for *TFE3* and *TFEB* gene rearrangements is highly sensitive and specific for tRCC and should be used to aid the diagnosis of tRCC [20, 21].
     - Other molecular techniques including sequencing can be used to detect gene rearrangement in cases with suspected false-negative FISH results and uncommon fusions not covered by FISH.
6. **What molecular assays are available when a hereditary RCC syndrome is considered?**
   - Hereditary RCC syndromes mainly include:
     - Hereditary leiomyomatosis and RCC (HLRCC) syndrome
     - Succinate dehydrogenase (SDH)-deficient RCC
     - von Hippel-Lindau syndrome
     - Hereditary papillary RCC
     - Birt-Hogg-Dube syndrome
     - Tuberous sclerosis
   - When encountering one or multiple renal tumors in a young patient, communication with clinicians, genetic counseling, and molecular assays for germline mutations should be considered to evaluate for a hereditary renal cancer syndrome (Table 11.3).
7. **What are the commonly seen genetic alterations in Wilms tumor?**
   - Wilms tumor is the most common childhood renal malignancy and could be associated with a variety of syndromes, which mainly include:
     - WAGR syndrome: **W**ilms tumor, **a**niridia, **g**enitourinary abnormalities, and mental **r**etardation
     - Denys-Drash and Frasier syndrome
     - Beckwith-Wiedemann syndrome
   - Genetic alteration has been identified in one-third of Wilms tumor-associated syndromes and is summarized in Table 11.4. In addition, mutations in *CTNNB1*, *WTX*, and *TP53* are identified in 10–15% of these syndromes [27].
8. **What is the most used molecular test in urothelial carcinoma (UC) screening?**
   - The most widely used molecular assay in UC screening is urine-based UroVysion (Vysis Inc) test.
   - UroVysion is a FISH assay performed on exfoliated cells in urine that assesses the aneuploidy of chromosomes 3, 7, and 17, as well as the loss of chromosome 9p21 locus, all of which are abnormalities characteristic of UC [28].
   - UroVysion test can be used as an aid for the initial diagnosis of bladder carcinoma in patients with hematuria. Because of its relatively high sensitivity and specificity for UC, this test has been implemented into many bladder cancer screening programs.
   - UroVysion can also be used to monitor tumor recurrence in patients with a history of UC or for stratification of patients with an abnormal cytology result and no clinical or cystoscopic evidence of a bladder tumor

Table 11.3 Major molecular genetic alterations in hereditary renal cell syndromes

Hereditary RCC syndromes	Associated neoplasms	Germline mutation	Mutation detection
Hereditary leiomyomatosis and RCC (HLRCC) syndrome [22, 23]	Leiomyomatosis of the skin and uterus **RCC** with type 2 papillary RCC-like morphology with prominent nucleoli Pheochromocytoma (rarely)	Fumarate hydratase (*FH*) gene with autosomal-dominant fashion	IHC for FH; IHC for 2SC (accumulates in the cytoplasm of HLRCC-associated RCC); Sequencing of *FH* gene
Succinate dehydrogenase (SDH)-deficient RCC [24, 25]	Paraganglioma/ pheochromocytoma Gastrointestinal stromal tumor **SDH-deficient RCC** Pituitary adenoma	One of the *SDH* genes (A–D), most commonly *SDHB* with autosomal-dominant fashion	SDHB IHC (loss of SDHB expression by IHC confirms inactivation of an *SDH* gene but is not necessarily diagnostic of inactivation of the *SDHB* gene) Sequencing of *SDH* genes
von Hippel-Lindau syndrome [26]	**Multiple CCRCC and renal cysts** Hemangioblastoma of the CNS and retina Pheochromocytoma Pancreatic cysts and neuroendocrine tumors Epididymal and broad ligament cystadenomas Endolymphatic sac tumors of the inner ear	*VHL* gene	Gene sequencing, FISH
Hereditary papillary RCC	Multiple, bilateral PRCCs	*MET* gene	Gene sequencing
Birt-Hogg-Dube syndrome	Multiple, bilateral kidney tumors, including a characteristic hybrid oncocytic tumor	*FCLN* gene	Gene sequencing
Tuberous sclerosis	A morphologically unique RCCs	*TSC1* and *TSC2* genes	Gene sequencing

CNS central nervous system; *2SC* 2-succinyl-cysteine

Table 11.4 Major genetic changes of Wilms tumor-associated syndromes

Congenital syndromes associated with Wilms tumor	Genetic changes
WAGR syndrome	Deletion mutations in *WT1* gene
Denys-Drash syndrome	Missense mutations in *WT1* gene
Beckwith-Wiedemann syndrome	Loss of imprinting or uniparental disomy of *IGF2* gene in chromosome 11p15.5

[29]. However, more recent studies demonstrate that the sensitivity and positive predictive value of UroVysion, particularly for low-grade urothelial carcinoma, may not be as optimal as initially thought [30].

9. **Besides UroVysion assay, what are other molecular assays available for UC and their indications?**
   - Besides cytogenetic alterations in UC, *TERT* promoter point mutations are commonly present in 60% to 80% of UC, and it appears to be early events in the oncogenesis of UC [31, 32].
   - Because *TERT* promoter mutations do not occur in reactive urothelial lesions [33], it has practical implications to test this mutation under at least three situations:
     1. In the differential diagnosis of UC versus non-neoplastic benign mimics (e.g., cystitis glandularis)
     2. In the differential diagnosis of UC versus other GU malignancy, such as prostatic cancer
     3. In urine cytology case suspicious for recurrent UC screening
   - Limitations of *TERT* promoter mutation test include the following:
     – It is not specific for UC. *TERT* promoter mutations are also present in benign urothelial neoplasms, such as urothelial papilloma, papillary urothelial neoplasm of low malignant potential, bladder squamous cell carcinoma, sarcomatoid carcinoma, and urachal carcinomas [34–37]. In addition, they are also reported to be present in neoplasms of other organs, such as glioblastoma and melanoma.
     – A negative *TERT* promoter mutation result does not exclude the possibility of a urothelial neoplasm.
   - *FGFR3* mutations, primarily point mutations and translocations, can be detected in nonmuscle-invasive bladder cancer as well as up to 10–15% of muscle-invasive bladder cancer cases [38, 39]. Because FGFR3 is a target of pan-FGFR inhibitors, the National Comprehensive Cancer Network (NCCN) has recently recommended that molecular tests for *FGFR3* mutations should be considered in patients with advanced stage bladder cancer.

10. **What is the clinical utility of ETS gene fusions in diagnosis of prostate adenocarcinoma?**
    - The ETS family of transcription factors is composed of approximately 27 members which are frequently involved in gene fusions. ETS fusion genes have been detected in a variety of malignancies such as *EWS* gene fusions in Ewing's sarcoma, *TEL(ETV6)* gene fusions in leukemia, and *ERG* gene fusions in prostate cancer [40–42].
    - More than 20 *ERG* fusion partners have been reported in prostate cancer, and about 50% is fusion of *TMPRSS2* to *ERG* [43, 44].
    - *ERG* fusion transcripts can be detected in up to 50% of prostate tumors. Although the diagnosis of most prostate tumors are based on histologic and immunohistochemistry evaluation, FISH or sequence for *ERG* may provide help in the difficult cases to aid the diagnosis of prostatic adenocarcinoma versus a benign process.
    - Most ETS rearrangements can be detected by FISH using a break-apart probe for *ERG* (chromosome 21q22). IHC using an anti-ERG antibody, which detects the *ERG* gene fusion product, can also detect *ERG* aberrations.
    - Limitations:
      - A negative *ERG* FISH or IHC result does not exclude the diagnosis of prostatic adenocarcinoma.
      - IHC for ERG may be positive in high-grade prostatic intraepithelial neoplasia (HGPIN).
      - Overexpression of *ERG* by itself is not a diagnostic criterion for malignancy.
11. **Besides the ETS gene family, what are other commonly observed molecular genetic abnormalities in prostatic cancer and their prognostic significance?**
    - *PTEN*, the tumor-suppressor gene, and proliferation index Ki67 are emerging biomarkers in localized prostate cancer and may be used to guide clinical management.
    - *PTEN* inactivation, either by gene deletion, rearrangement, or truncation mutations, have been described in about 20% of primary and up to 40% of metastatic prostate cancer. Depending on the mutation type, FISH or IHC assays are the commonly used methods to assess *PTEN* status [45–48].
    - Clinical significance of *PTEN* inactivation in prostate cancer include [46, 48–50]:
      - *PTEN* inactivation is associated with rising levels of prostate-specific antigen (PSA) in the serum.
      - Patients with heterogeneous or subclonal *PTEN* loss generally have worse outcomes than those with intact *PTEN* but better outcome than patients with homogenous or clonal *PTEN* loss.
      - Patients with compound *PTEN* inactivation and *ERG* rearrangement have better clinical outcomes compared with those with *PTEN* inactivation but wild-type *ERG* gene.
    - Because *PTEN* inactivation shows a strong positive correlation with pathologic stage in prostate cancer, the analysis of *PTEN* status and Ki67 level should be considered to facilitate the assessment of the pathologic grade of the tumor especially in the core biopsy settings [51].
12. **For prostatic cancer, what is the current utilization of gene expression profiling (GEP) assay?**
    - Gene expression profiling (GEP) is introduced to risk-stratify prostatic cancer patients and guide treatment decisions between therapeutic intervention and active surveillance.
    - Several commercially available clinical GEP assays have been developed, including Prolaris® assay (Myriad Genetics, Salt Lake City, UT), OncotypeDX® Prostate Cancer Assay (Genomic Health, Redwood City, CA), Decipher® Prostate Cancer Classifier (GenomeDx Biosciences, Vancouver, BC, Canada), and ProMark™ Protein Biomarker Test (Metamark Genetics, Cambridge, MA). The characteristic features of these assays are summarized in Table 11.5 [52–57].
    - Although with potential benefit in providing additional information in aiding treatment decisions and preventing unnecessary rebiopsy procedure and its related cost, GEP assay's clinical utility is still not well defined at current practice, and most of such tests are performed upon clinician's requests. Further evidence of GEP performance and patients' follow-up is desirable to evaluate its value to guide future utilization.
13. **Is there a prostate cancer screening algorithm available?**
    - A review of more than 60 studies of screening for prostate cancer including approximately 2 million people demonstrated that prostate-specific antigen (PSA) screening has been shown to substantially reduce prostate cancer mortality. It is also known to be associated with false-positive results, overdiagnosis, unnecessary biopsies with associated risks of morbidity, and increased risks associated with treatments that may not prolong life. A novel or modified screening algorithm is imperative to replace the PSA-alone prostate cancer screening practice.

Table 11.5 Representative gene expression profiling assays for prostate cancer

GEP	Sample type	Targets	Risk calculation
ConfirmMDx® Prostate Cancer Assay	Previously biopsied prostate cancer negative tissue	Detect the DNA methylation status of *GSTP1*, *APC*, and *RASSF1* genes using methylation-specific PCR (MSP)	The likelihood of GS ≤ 6 and GS ≥ 7 prostate cancer being detected on repeat biopsy is calculated by incorporating DNA methylation intensity with clinical risk factors, including PSA, DRE, age, and histopathology of the previous biopsy
Decipher® Prostate Cancer Classifier	Radical prostatectomy tissue in newly diagnosed patients with localized cancer	A GEP panel of 22 genes	A continuous risk score between 0 and 1 to predict the probability of clinical metastasis within 5 years of radical prostatectomy
OncotypeDX® Prostate Cancer Assay	Prostate biopsy	A GEP panel of 17 genes (12 cancer-related and 5 reference genes) to generate a GPS.	Combination of GPS (0–100) with PSA, Gleason score, and tumor stage
Prolaris® assay	Prostate biopsy or prostatectomy sample	A GEP panel of 46 genes (31 CCP genes and 15 housekeeper genes) to generate a CCP score	Combination of GS, PSA, clinical stage, and CCP score
ProMark™ Protein Biomarker Test	Prostate biopsy	A quantitative protein based multiplex immunofluorescence in situ imaging platform measuring eight protein biomarkers	An algorithmically derived risk score between 1 and 100

GS Gleason score; *PSA* prostate-specific antigen; *DRE* digital rectal exam; *CCP* cell cycle progression; *GPS* genomic prostate score [58]

- Several new screening tests, including serum or blood-based such as 4Kscore, prostate health index (PHI), and Stockholm3(STHLM3) test and urine-based such as prostate cancer antigen 3 (PCA3) and HOXC6/DLX1, have been shown to be more accurate and generally better than PSA-alone screening. Combinations of molecular tests with multiparametric magnetic resonance imaging (mpMRI) are also gaining popularity for its ability to determine clinically significant cancer.
- In summary, a shared decision-making approach is currently used for prostate cancer screening, and patients are encouraged to decide for themselves whether the benefits of screening outweigh the harms.

14. **What are the commonly seen molecular changes in testicular germ cell tumors (GCTs)?**
    - Germ cell tumors (GCTs) account for most testicular neoplasms, especially in young adult men.
    - Alteration of chromosome 12p is the hallmark biomarker of germ cell tumors. Isochromosome 12p is the most common alteration observed in about ~80% of cases seen in almost all invasive tumors, but not in isolated germ cell neoplasia in situ without an adjacent invasive component [58].
    - Most common genetic changes in GCTs are the copy number gain of chromosome 12p, which can be detected in ~80% of GCTs by FISH, microarray, or next-generation sequencing (NGS).
    - Driver mutations in *KIT*, *KRAS*, and *NRAS* genes have also been reported in 5–30% of seminoma and up to 15% of non-seminoma patients [59–62].

Case Presentations

Case 1

Learning Objective

Histological, immunophenotypic, and molecular features of papillary renal neoplasm with reverse polarity.

Case History

The patient is a 54-year-old female with a history of end-stage renal disease who was found to have an incidental 2-cm right renal mass during routine workup for consideration of renal transplantation. She underwent total nephrectomy.

Histologic Findings

Histologic examination showed an intracystic papillary tumor. The papillae were arborized and covered by a single layer of cuboidal cells with eosinophilic cytoplasm. The nuclei were monotonous and rounded and were characteristically apical in location. They had a low WHO/ISUP nuclear grade with no prominent nucleoli. The papillary cores were fibrotic and contained sparse inflammatory cells. No hemorrhage, necrosis, or mitotic figures were seen. The tumor was positive for GATA3 and L1CAM and negative for AMACR and vimentin by immunohistochemistry (Fig. 11.1a–d).

- *Question 1: After reviewing this preliminary information, what are the major differential diagnosis?*
- *Question 2: Which molecular studies could be ordered to help the diagnosis?*

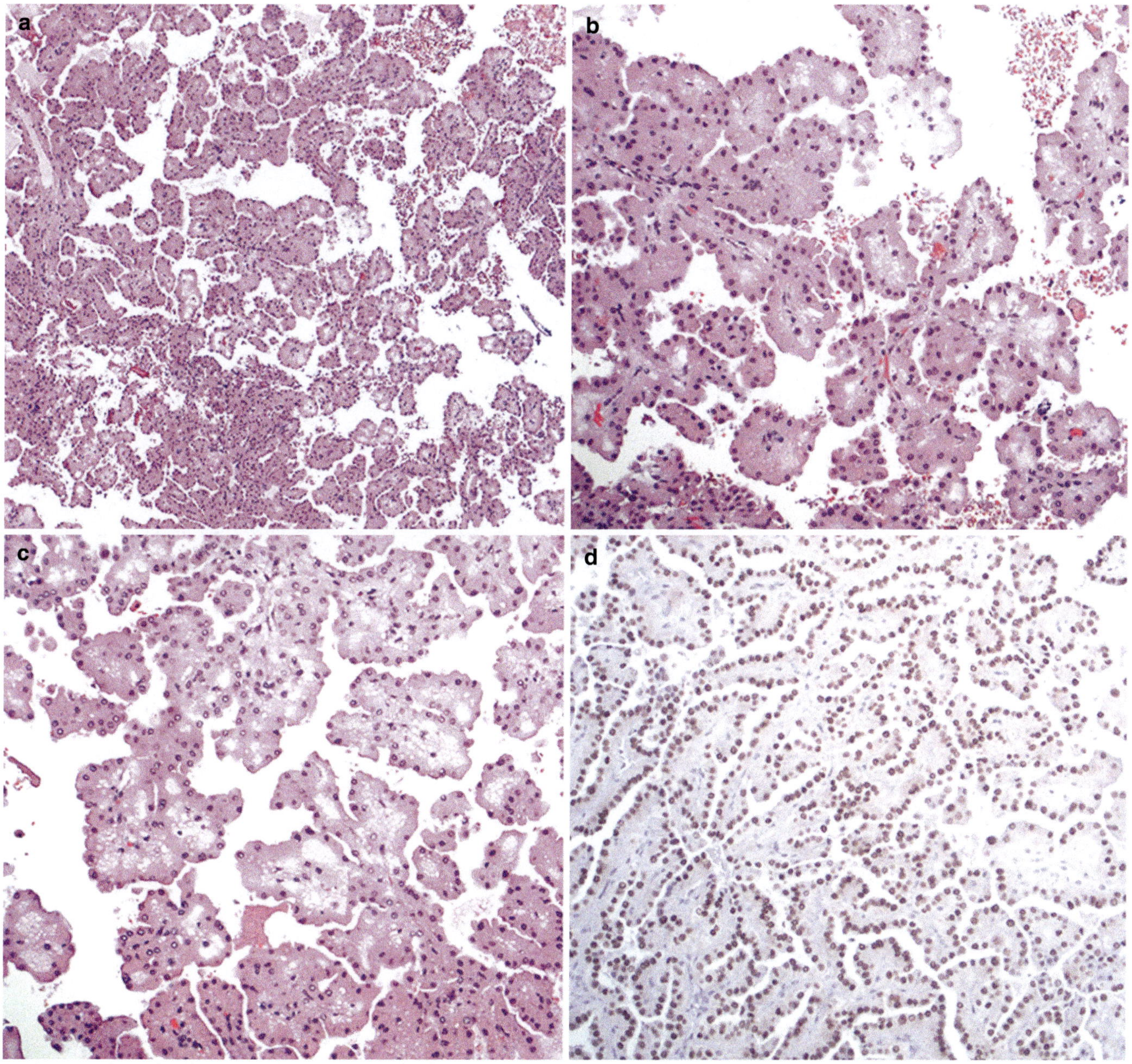

Fig. 11.1 Papillary renal neoplasm with reverse polarity. It is formed by arborizing papillary architecture with centrally hyalinized fibrovascular core (H&E stain, 100×) [53] (**a**). The papillae are covered by a single layer of cuboidal cells with eosinophilic cytoplasm and apically located nuclei (reversely polarized) (H&E stain, 200×) (**b**, **c**). Prominent intracytoplasmic vacuolization is present (**c**). GATA-3 immunostain is uniformly positive (H&E stain, 200×) (**d**)

Based on the described histologic findings, the major differential diagnosis includes papillary renal cell carcinoma, type 1 or type 2, and other papillary renal cell neoplasms. FISH analysis to identify the presence of chromosomal abnormalities including gains or losses of 3p, 7, 17, and Y would provide useful information to diagnose.

Molecular Genetic Study

FISH analysis showed the presence of trisomy of chromosome 7 and disomy of chromosome 17 (Fig. 11.2). Next-generation sequencing identified *KRAS* p.G12V (c.34G > T) mutation.

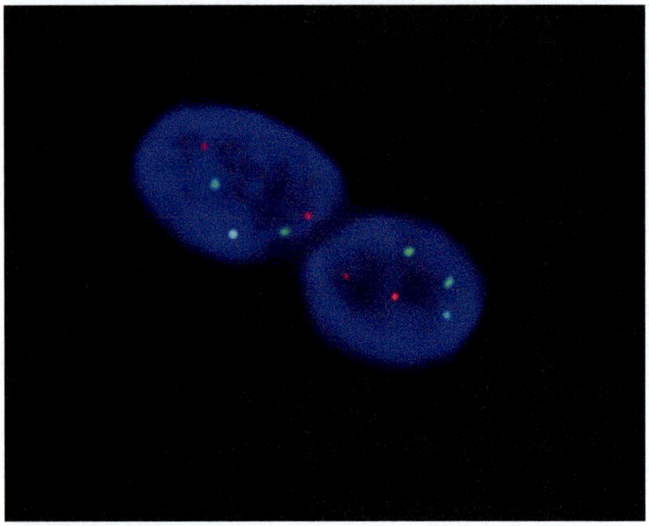

Fig. 11.2 FISH analysis showed the presence of trisomy 7 and disomy of chromosome 17

Final Diagnosis

Papillary renal neoplasm with reverse polarity

Follow-Up

The patient was followed up for 48 months and had no evidence of tumor recurrence or metastasis.

Discussion

Papillary renal neoplasm with reverse polarity is an epithelial renal tumor and a newly proposed entity [63]. Although papillary renal neoplasm with reverse polarity has papillary or tubulopapillary architecture, which overlaps with PRCC, it also has distinctively apically located nuclei away from the basement membrane. Together with other morphological findings, including the single layer of eosinophilic cells with finely granular cytoplasm, inconspicuous nucleoli, and lack of intracellular hemosiderin, mitotic figures or necrosis, these features set this entity apart from PRCC, clear cell PRCC, and Xp11 translocation RCC. Immunophenotypically, papillary renal neoplasm with reverse polarity are positive for GATA3 and LICAM and negative for vimentin and AMACR (except for blush-like positive in some cases).

Besides the well-known histologic heterogeneity in papillary renal cell carcinoma (PRCC), especially in type 2, type 1 PRCCs are associated with *MET* alterations, whereas a variety of gene alterations, such as *CDKN2A* inactivation and *SETD2* mutations, have been reported in type 2. *KRAS* point mutation is associated with papillary renal neoplasm with reverse polarity which is distinctly different from other renal cell neoplasms [64].

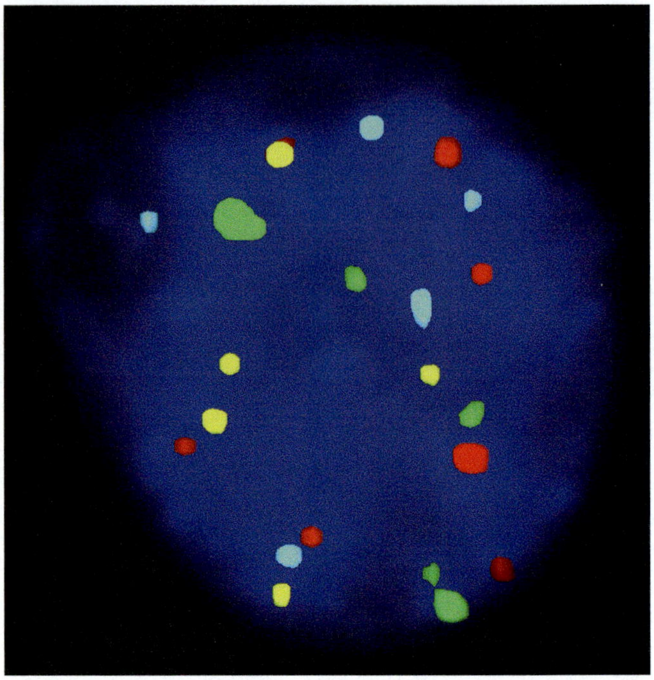

Fig. 11.3 UroVysion FISH analysis was positive for polysomy of chromosomes 3, 7, 17, and 9p21

Case 2

Learning Objective

Utilization of UroVysion FISH analysis for bladder cancer screening

Case History

The patient is an 84-year-old male with a history of prostatectomy for high-grade prostatic adenocarcinoma with salvage radiation and hormonal therapy. Fifteen years after his prostatectomy, he presented with gross hematuria, and cytology showed rare atypical urothelial cell suspicious for high-grade urothelial carcinoma. The urine specimen was sent for UroVysion analysis.

Molecular Genetic Study

UroVysion FISH analysis was positive for polysomy of chromosomes 3, 7, 17, and 9p21 (Fig. 11.3). The patient underwent a cystoscopy which was sent for pathology evaluation.

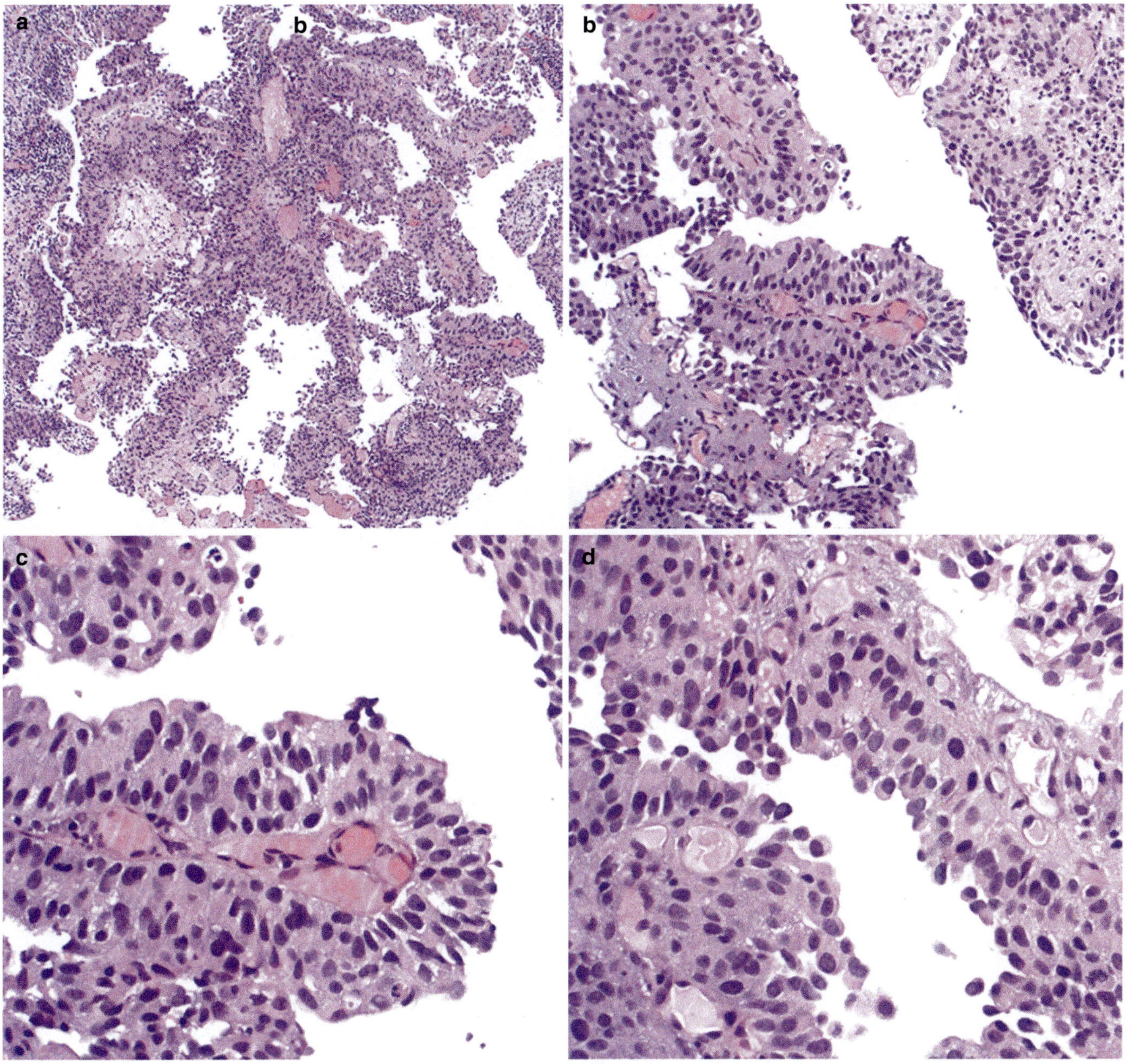

Fig. 11.4 High-grade papillary urothelial carcinoma. The papillae are covered by proliferating urothelial cells (H&E stain, 100×) (**a**), showing disorderly oriented nuclei, with marked cytologic atypia, nuclear hyperchromasia, and prominent nucleoli (H&E stain, 200×) (**b–d**)

Histologic Findings

Histologic examination shows neoplastic urothelial proliferation formed of multiple fibrovascular cores, covered by variably thickened urothelial cells. The cells show moderate to significant cytologic atypia, nuclear enlargement, and hyperchromasia. Loss of nuclear polarity and prominent nucleoli are also seen (Fig. 11.4a–d).

Final Diagnosis

Papillary urothelial carcinoma, noninvasion, high grade

Follow-Up

The patient had a tumor recurrence 2 years later which was cystoscopically resected and showed invasion into the lamina propria. He was followed up for 70 months with no evidence of recurrence.

Discussion

This case represents a typical situation when UroVysion FISH study is indicated for bladder cancer screening. Besides it can also be used to monitor tumor recurrence based on its high specificity for high-grade urothelial carcinoma.

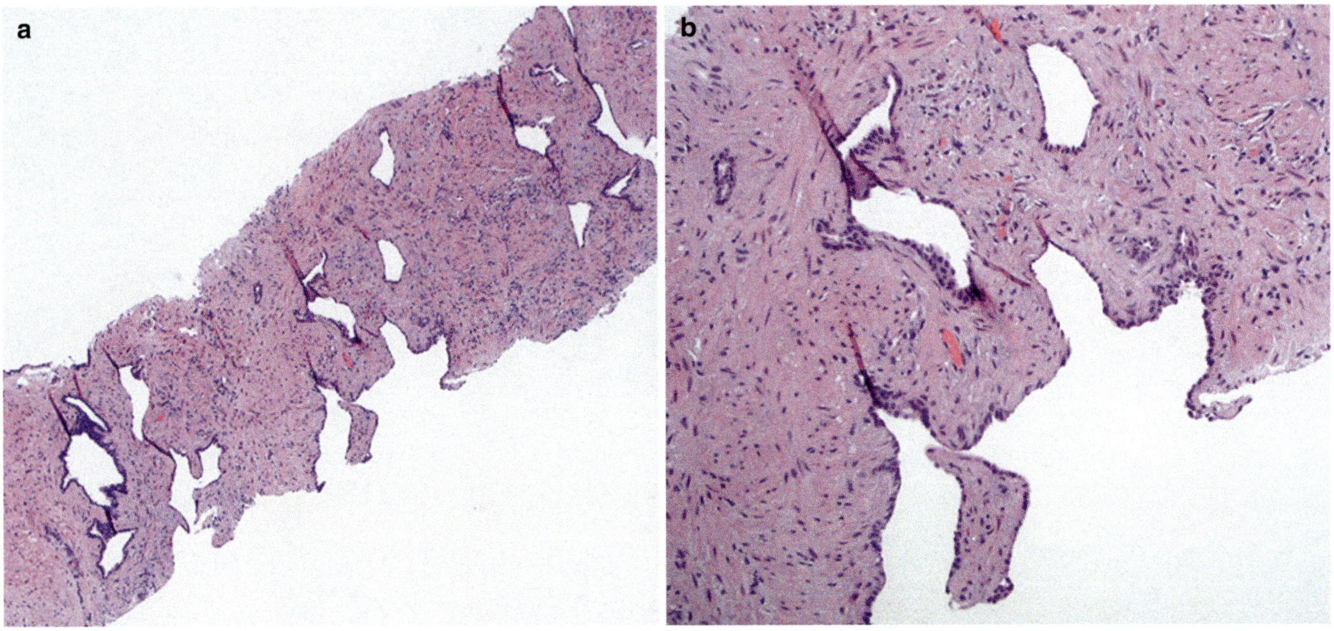

Fig. 11.5 Prostatic atrophy. The prostatic parenchyma shows widely spaced prostatic glands with dilated lumens and separated by prominent stromal elements (H&E stain, 40×) (**a**). The glands are lined by cells with minimal amount of cytoplasm and crowded nuclei (H&E stain, 200×) (**b**)

Case 3

Learning Objective

Emerging gene expression profiling (GEP) assay for risk-stratify patients with increased risk for prostate cancer

Case History

The patient is a 69-year-old male with no known significant medical history, who presented for evaluation of two episodes of elevated prostate specific antigen (PSA) of up to 6.25 ng/ml during surveillance examination within 6 months.

Histologic Findings

Histologic examination showed cores of prostatic tissue composed of glands with dilated lumens that are lined by cells with minimal amount of cytoplasm and crowded nuclei. Stromal fibrosis is also prominent (Fig. 11.5a–b).

Molecular Genetic Study

The case was sent to ConfirmMDx for prostate cancer DNA (*GSTP1*, *APC*, and *RASSF1*) methylation study and was negative.

Final Diagnosis

Benign prostatic tissue with atrophy

Follow-Up

Given the negative biopsy and ConfirmMDx findings, the patient elected to be followed up by serial PSA monitoring. The subsequent PSA levels fell below 4 ng/ml.

Discussion

The ConfirmMDx assay (MDxHealth, Irvine, CA) is a commercially available test designed to improve patient stratification, and it could be considered in men with an elevated PSA level (≥4.0 ng/ml) and/or abnormal digital rectal exam (DRE) but with cancer-negative prostate biopsy [65, 66]. The DNA methylation status of three genes, *GSTP1*, *APC*, and *RASSF1*, is evaluated on the core biopsy, and the result indicates the likelihood of Gleason score (GS) ≤ 6 and GS ≥7 prostate cancer being detected. Urologists should incorporate the ConfirmMDx result together with PSA, DRE, age, and histopathology findings to stratify patients for active monitoring or repeat biopsy/MRI examination.

References

1. Brugarolas J. Molecular genetics of clear-cell renal cell carcinoma. J Clin Oncol. 2014;32(18):1968–76.
2. Magers MJ, Cheng L. Practical molecular testing in a clinical genitourinary service. Arch Pathol Lab Med. 2020;144(3):277–89.
3. Klatte T, Said JW, Seligson DB, Rao PN, de Martino M, Shuch B, et al. Pathological, immunohistochemical and cytogenetic features of papillary renal cell carcinoma with clear cell features. J Urol. 2011;185(1):30–5.
4. Chen YB, Xu J, Skanderup AJ, Dong Y, Brannon AR, Wang L, et al. Molecular analysis of aggressive renal cell carcinoma with unclassified histology reveals distinct subsets. Nat Commun. 2016;7:13131.
5. Piva F, Santoni M, Matrana MR, Satti S, Giulietti M, Occhipinti G, et al. BAP1, PBRM1 and SETD2 in clear-cell renal cell carcinoma: molecular diagnostics and possible targets for personalized therapies. Expert Rev Mol Diagn. 2015;15(9):1201–10.

6. Speicher MR, Schoell B, du Manoir S, Schrock E, Ried T, Cremer T, et al. Specific loss of chromosomes 1, 2, 6, 10, 13, 17, and 21 in chromophobe renal cell carcinomas revealed by comparative genomic hybridization. Am J Pathol. 1994;145(2):356–64.
7. Davis CF, Ricketts CJ, Wang M, Yang L, Cherniack AD, Shen H, et al. The somatic genomic landscape of chromophobe renal cell carcinoma. Cancer Cell. 2014;26(3):319–30.
8. Delongchamps NB, Galmiche L, Eiss D, Rouach Y, Vogt B, Timsit MO, et al. Hybrid tumour 'oncocytoma-chromophobe renal cell carcinoma' of the kidney: a report of seven sporadic cases. BJU Int. 2009;103(10):1381–4.
9. Petersson F, Gatalica Z, Grossmann P, Perez Montiel MD, Alvarado Cabrero I, Bulimbasic S, et al. Sporadic hybrid oncocytic/chromophobe tumor of the kidney: a clinicopathologic, histomorphologic, immunohistochemical, ultrastructural, and molecular cytogenetic study of 14 cases. Virchows Arch. 2010;456(4):355–65.
10. Pitra T, Pivovarcikova K, Alaghehbandan R, Hes O. Chromosomal numerical aberration pattern in papillary renal cell carcinoma: review article. Ann Diagn Pathol. 2019;40:189–99.
11. Saleeb RM, Brimo F, Farag M, Rompre-Brodeur A, Rotondo F, Beharry V, et al. Toward biological subtyping of papillary renal cell carcinoma with clinical implications through histologic, immunohistochemical, and molecular analysis. Am J Surg Pathol. 2017;41(12):1618–29.
12. Schmidt L, Duh FM, Chen F, Kishida T, Glenn G, Choyke P, et al. Germline and somatic mutations in the tyrosine kinase domain of the MET proto-oncogene in papillary renal carcinomas. Nat Genet. 1997;16(1):68–73.
13. Zbar B, Tory K, Merino M, Schmidt L, Glenn G, Choyke P, et al. Hereditary papillary renal cell carcinoma. J Urol. 1994;151(3):561–6.
14. Dharmawardana PG, Giubellino A, Bottaro DP. Hereditary papillary renal carcinoma type I. Curr Mol Med. 2004;4(8):855–68.
15. Rhoades Smith KE, Bilen MA. A review of papillary renal cell carcinoma and MET inhibitors. Kidney Cancer. 2019;3(3):151–61.
16. Gilbert JA. Savolitinib for MET-driven papillary renal cell carcinoma. Lancet Oncol. 2017;18(8):e440.
17. Akhtar M, Al-Bozom IA, Al HT. Papillary Renal Cell Carcinoma (PRCC): an update. Adv Anat Pathol. 2019;26(2):124–32.
18. Lubensky IA, Schmidt L, Zhuang Z, Weirich G, Pack S, Zambrano N, et al. Hereditary and sporadic papillary renal carcinomas with c-met mutations share a distinct morphological phenotype. Am J Pathol. 1999;155(2):517–26.
19. Argani P. MiT family translocation renal cell carcinoma. Semin Diagn Pathol. 2015;32(2):103–13.
20. Green WM, Yonescu R, Morsberger L, Morris K, Netto GJ, Epstein JI, et al. Utilization of a TFE3 break-apart FISH assay in a renal tumor consultation service. Am J Surg Pathol. 2013;37(8): 1150–63.
21. Rao Q, Williamson SR, Zhang S, Eble JN, Grignon DJ, Wang M, et al. TFE3 break-apart FISH has a higher sensitivity for Xp11.2 translocation-associated renal cell carcinoma compared with TFE3 or cathepsin K immunohistochemical staining alone: expanding the morphologic spectrum. Am J Surg Pathol. 2013;37(6):804–15.
22. Harrison WJ, Andrici J, Maclean F, Madadi-Ghahan R, Farzin M, Sioson L, et al. Fumarate hydratase-deficient uterine leiomyomas occur in both the syndromic and sporadic settings. Am J Surg Pathol. 2016;40(5):599–607.
23. Trpkov K, Hes O, Agaimy A, Bonert M, Martinek P, Magi-Galluzzi C, et al. Fumarate hydratase-deficient renal cell carcinoma is strongly correlated with fumarate hydratase mutation and hereditary leiomyomatosis and renal cell carcinoma syndrome. Am J Surg Pathol. 2016;40(7):865–75.
24. Gill AJ. Succinate dehydrogenase (SDH) and mitochondrial driven neoplasia. Pathology. 2012;44(4):285–92.
25. Gill AJ. Succinate dehydrogenase (SDH)-deficient neoplasia. Histopathology. 2018;72(1):106–16.
26. Cheng L, Williamson SR, Zhang S, Maclennan GT, Montironi R, Lopez-Beltran A. Understanding the molecular genetics of renal cell neoplasia: implications for diagnosis, prognosis and therapy. Expert Rev Anticancer Ther. 2010;10(6):843–64.
27. Huppmann AR. Educational case: Wilms tumor. Acad Pathol. 2018;5:2374289518781582.
28. Halling KC, Kipp BR. Bladder cancer detection using FISH (UroVysion assay). Adv Anat Pathol. 2008;15(5):279–86.
29. Moonen PM, Merkx GF, Peelen P, Karthaus HF, Smeets DF, Witjes JA. UroVysion compared with cytology and quantitative cytology in the surveillance of non-muscle-invasive bladder cancer. Eur Urol. 2007;51(5):1275–80. discussion 80
30. Dimashkieh H, Wolff DJ, Smith TM, Houser PM, Nietert PJ, Yang J. Evaluation of urovysion and cytology for bladder cancer detection: a study of 1835 paired urine samples with clinical and histologic correlation. Cancer Cytopathol. 2013;121(10):591–7.
31. Giedl J, Rogler A, Wild A, Riener MO, Filbeck T, Burger M, et al. TERT core promotor mutations in early-onset bladder cancer. J Cancer. 2016;7(8):915–20.
32. Rachakonda PS, Hosen I, de Verdier PJ, Fallah M, Heidenreich B, Ryk C, et al. TERT promoter mutations in bladder cancer affect patient survival and disease recurrence through modification by a common polymorphism. Proc Natl Acad Sci U S A. 2013;110(43):17426–31.
33. Zhong M, Tian W, Zhuge J, Zheng X, Huang T, Cai D, et al. Distinguishing nested variants of urothelial carcinoma from benign mimickers by TERT promoter mutation. Am J Surg Pathol. 2015;39(1):127–31.
34. Wang CC, Huang CY, Jhuang YL, Chen CC, Jeng YM. Biological significance of TERT promoter mutation in papillary urothelial neoplasm of low malignant potential. Histopathology. 2018;72(5):795–803.
35. Isharwal S, Hu W, Sarungbam J, Chen YB, Gopalan A, Fine SW, et al. Genomic landscape of inverted urothelial papilloma and urothelial papilloma of the bladder. J Pathol. 2019;248(3):260–5.
36. Kurtis B, Zhuge J, Ojaimi C, Ye F, Cai D, Zhang D, et al. Recurrent TERT promoter mutations in urothelial carcinoma and potential clinical applications. Ann Diagn Pathol. 2016;21:7–11.
37. Cheng L, Davidson DD, Wang M, Lopez-Beltran A, Montironi R, Wang L, et al. Telomerase reverse transcriptase (TERT) promoter mutation analysis of benign, malignant and reactive urothelial lesions reveals a subpopulation of inverted papilloma with immortalizing genetic change. Histopathology. 2016;69(1):107–13.
38. Sjodahl G, Lauss M, Lovgren K, Chebil G, Gudjonsson S, Veerla S, et al. A molecular taxonomy for urothelial carcinoma. Clin Cancer Res. 2012;18(12):3377–86.
39. Robertson AG, Kim J, Al-Ahmadie H, Bellmunt J, Guo G, Cherniack AD, et al. Comprehensive molecular characterization of muscle-invasive bladder cancer. Cell. 2017;171(3):540–56. e25
40. Bohlander SK. ETV6: a versatile player in leukemogenesis. Semin Cancer Biol. 2005;15(3):162–74.
41. Khoury JD. Ewing sarcoma family of tumors. Adv Anat Pathol. 2005;12(4):212–20.
42. Hollenhorst PC, McIntosh LP, Graves BJ. Genomic and biochemical insights into the specificity of ETS transcription factors. Annu Rev Biochem. 2011;80:437–71.
43. Kumar-Sinha C, Tomlins SA, Chinnaiyan AM. Recurrent gene fusions in prostate cancer. Nat Rev Cancer. 2008;8(7):497–511.
44. Tomlins SA, Rhodes DR, Perner S, Dhanasekaran SM, Mehra R, Sun XW, et al. Recurrent fusion of TMPRSS2 and ETS transcription factor genes in prostate cancer. Science. 2005;310(5748): 644–8.
45. Jamaspishvili T, Berman DM, Ross AE, Scher HI, De Marzo AM, Squire JA, et al. Clinical implications of PTEN loss in prostate cancer. Nat Rev Urol. 2018;15(4):222–34.
46. Lotan TL, Wei W, Ludkovski O, Morais CL, Guedes LB, Jamaspishvili T, et al. Analytic validation of a clinical-grade PTEN

immunohistochemistry assay in prostate cancer by comparison with PTEN FISH. Mod Pathol. 2016;29(8):904–14.
47. Picanco-Albuquerque CG, Morais CL, Carvalho FL, Peskoe SB, Hicks JL, Ludkovski O, et al. In prostate cancer needle biopsies, detections of PTEN loss by fluorescence in situ hybridization (FISH) and by immunohistochemistry (IHC) are concordant and show consistent association with upgrading. Virchows Arch. 2016;468(5):607–17.
48. Lotan TL, Heumann A, Rico SD, Hicks J, Lecksell K, Koop C, et al. PTEN loss detection in prostate cancer: comparison of PTEN immunohistochemistry and PTEN FISH in a large retrospective prostatectomy cohort. Oncotarget. 2017;8(39):65566–76.
49. Bismar TA, Hegazy S, Feng Z, Yu D, Donnelly B, Palanisamy N, et al. Clinical utility of assessing PTEN and ERG protein expression in prostate cancer patients: a proposed method for risk stratification. J Cancer Res Clin Oncol. 2018;144(11):2117–25.
50. Reid AH, Attard G, Ambroisine L, Fisher G, Kovacs G, Brewer D, et al. Molecular characterisation of ERG, ETV1 and PTEN gene loci identifies patients at low and high risk of death from prostate cancer. Br J Cancer. 2010;102(4):678–84.
51. Lotan TL, Gurel B, Sutcliffe S, Esopi D, Liu W, Xu J, et al. PTEN protein loss by immunostaining: analytic validation and prognostic indicator for a high risk surgical cohort of prostate cancer patients. Clin Cancer Res. 2011;17(20):6563–73.
52. Cuzick J, Berney DM, Fisher G, Mesher D, Moller H, Reid JE, et al. Prognostic value of a cell cycle progression signature for prostate cancer death in a conservatively managed needle biopsy cohort. Br J Cancer. 2012;106(6):1095–9.
53. Klein EA, Cooperberg MR, Magi-Galluzzi C, Simko JP, Falzarano SM, Maddala T, et al. A 17-gene assay to predict prostate cancer aggressiveness in the context of Gleason grade heterogeneity, tumor multifocality, and biopsy undersampling. Eur Urol. 2014;66(3):550–60.
54. Erho N, Crisan A, Vergara IA, Mitra AP, Ghadessi M, Buerki C, et al. Discovery and validation of a prostate cancer genomic classifier that predicts early metastasis following radical prostatectomy. PLoS One. 2013;8(6):e66855.
55. Kornberg Z, Cooperberg MR, Cowan JE, Chan JM, Shinohara K, Simko JP, et al. A 17-gene genomic prostate score as a predictor of adverse pathology in men on active surveillance. J Urol. 2019;202(4):702–9.
56. Freedland SJ, Gerber L, Reid J, Welbourn W, Tikishvili E, Park J, et al. Prognostic utility of cell cycle progression score in men with prostate cancer after primary external beam radiation therapy. Int J Radiat Oncol Biol Phys. 2013;86(5):848–53.
57. Ross AE, Johnson MH, Yousefi K, Davicioni E, Netto GJ, Marchionni L, et al. Tissue-based genomics augments post-prostatectomy risk stratification in a natural history cohort of intermediate- and high-risk men. Eur Urol. 2016;69(1):157–65.
58. Al-Obaidy KI, Chovanec M, Cheng L. Molecular characteristics of testicular germ cell tumors: pathogenesis and mechanisms of therapy resistance. Expert Rev Anticancer Ther. 2020;20(2):75–9.
59. McIntyre A, Summersgill B, Grygalewicz B, Gillis AJ, Stoop J, van Gurp RJ, et al. Amplification and overexpression of the KIT gene is associated with progression in the seminoma subtype of testicular germ cell tumors of adolescents and adults. Cancer Res. 2005;65(18):8085–9.
60. Kemmer K, Corless CL, Fletcher JA, McGreevey L, Haley A, Griffith D, et al. KIT mutations are common in testicular seminomas. Am J Pathol. 2004;164(1):305–13.
61. Litchfield K, Summersgill B, Yost S, Sultana R, Labreche K, Dudakia D, et al. Whole-exome sequencing reveals the mutational spectrum of testicular germ cell tumours. Nat Commun. 2015;6:5973.
62. Cheng L, Lyu B, Roth LM. Perspectives on testicular germ cell neoplasms. Hum Pathol. 2017;59:10–25.
63. Al-Obaidy KI, Eble JN, Cheng L, Williamson SR, Sakr WA, Gupta N, et al. Papillary renal neoplasm with reverse polarity: a morphologic, immunohistochemical, and molecular study. Am J Surg Pathol. 2019;43(8):1099–111.
64. Al-Obaidy KI, Eble JN, Nassiri M, Cheng L, Eldomery MK, Williamson SR, et al. Recurrent KRAS mutations in papillary renal neoplasm with reverse polarity. Mod Pathol. 2020;33(6):1157–64.
65. Waterhouse RL Jr, Van Neste L, Moses KA, Barnswell C, Silberstein JL, Jalkut M, et al. Evaluation of an epigenetic assay for predicting repeat prostate biopsy outcome in African American men. Urology. 2019;128:62–5.
66. Van Neste L, Groskopf J, Grizzle WE, Adams GW, DeGuenther MS, Kolettis PN, et al. Epigenetic risk score improves prostate cancer risk assessment. Prostate. 2017;77(12):1259–64.

Hereditary Cancer Syndromes and Inherited Cancer Risks

12

Kristin K. Deeb, Mariana Kekis, and Tatiana Tvrdik

List of Frequently Asked Questions

1. What are hereditary cancer syndromes?
2. How have molecular events of critical cellular pathways further contributed to our understanding of hereditary and sporadic cancer development?
3. What are the general features suggesting the presence of hereditary cancer syndrome or inherited cancer risks?
4. What are genetic predispositions to hematologic malignancies syndromes?
5. What are the indications of a myeloid neoplasm (MDS, AML, or lymphoblastic leukemia) with germline predisposition?
6. Why is it important to pursue germline testing?
7. Who is involved in ordering, counseling, and interpreting germline testing?
8. What are the current techniques for germline cancer testing?
9. What are the common cancer predisposition genes detected by somatic testing?
10. What types of variants are detected and reported by germline genetic testing?
11. What types of variants are detected and reported by somatic testing?
12. What is variant allele frequency (VAF)? Can VAF on a somatic NGS assay be used to predict a variant with a germline origin?
13. What are the guidelines for variant interpretation and reporting for somatic and for germline findings?
14. How should a finding suggestive of a pathogenic variant in a hereditary cancer gene be confirmed when it is observed by somatic testing of a tumor biopsy?
15. What type of sample should be tested to determine if a pathogenic variant has a germline origin for non-hematological malignancies (solid tumors)?
16. What are molecular genetic testing considerations for germline predisposition for hematologic malignancies?
17. What other molecular possibilities can be considered when germline cancer predisposition is suspected, but no pathogenic variant was identified?
18. Do discrepancies in variant interpretation occur between laboratories when interpreting germline variants?

Frequently Asked Questions

1. **What are hereditary cancer syndromes?**
   - The causes of cancer are a mixture of environmental and genetic alterations. A hereditary cancer syndrome is a genetic predisposition to certain types of cancer, often with a significantly or moderately increased risks of cancer, and may account for 5% to 10% of all cancers in patients with early onset or family history of disease [1–3].
   - Hereditary cancer syndromes are characterized by germline pathogenic variants associated with high probability of cancer development.
   - Most hereditary cancer syndromes are autosomal dominant with relatively high penetrance, but there are also autosomal recessive conditions (Table 12.1).
   - In most cases, tumors of hereditary cancer syndromes typically develop at a younger age compared to sporadic tumors, and multiple primary tumors can arise.
   - Environmental factors contribute to the modulation of extent of cancer risk.

K. K. Deeb (✉) · T. Tvrdik
Department of Pathology and Laboratory Medicine, Emory University School of Medicine, Atlanta, GA, USA
e-mail: kristin.deeb@emory.edu; tatiana.tvrdik@emory.edu

M. Kekis
Laboratory Medicine and Genetics, Trillium Health Partners, Mississauga, ON, Canada
e-mail: mariana.kekis@thp.ca

Y. Ding, L. Zhang (eds.), *Practical Oncologic Molecular Pathology*, Practical Anatomic Pathology,
https://doi.org/10.1007/978-3-030-73227-1_12

Table 12.1 Selected examples of hereditary cancer syndromes

Syndromes	Inheritance patterns and gene(s)	Tumor types	Reference(s)
A. Hereditary breast cancer syndromes			
Hereditary breast cancer and ovarian cancer syndrome	**AD:** *BRCA1, BRCA2*	Breast cancer Ovarian cancer Prostate cancer Pancreatic cancer Fanconi anemia/medulloblastoma	[4]
Li-Fraumeni Syndrome	**AD:** *TP53*	Soft tissue sarcoma Breast cancer Osteosarcoma Leukemia Brain tumors Adrenocortical carcinoma	[5]
Cowden Syndrome	**AD:** *PTEN*	Breast cancer Thyroid cancer Endometrial and other cancers	[6]
Bannayan-Riley-Ruvalcaba syndrome	**AD:** *PTEN*	Breast cancer Meningioma Thyroid follicular cell tumors	[6]
Ataxia-telangiectasia	**AR:** *ATM*	Breast cancer Leukemia, lymphoma	[7]
B. Hereditary gastrointestinal malignancies			
HNPCC, including "Lynch II" Syndrome	**AD:** *MLH1, MSH2, MSH6*	Colon cancer Endometrial cancer Ovarian cancer Renal pelvis cancers Ureteral cancers Pancreatic cancer Stomach and small bowel cancers Hepatobiliary cancers	[8]
Familial polyposis, including attenuated phenotype	**AD:** *APC*	Colon cancer	[9]
Hereditary diffuse gastric cancer	**AD:** *CDH1*	Stomach cancers	[10]
Juvenile polyposis	**AD:** *SMAD4, BMPR1A*	Gastrointestinal cancers Pancreatic cancer	[11]
Peutz-Jeghers syndrome	**AD:** *STK11*	Colon cancer Small bowel cancer Breast cancer Ovarian cancer Pancreatic cancer	[12]
Melanoma pancreatic cancer syndrome	**AD:** *CDKN2A*	Pancreatic cancer Melanoma	[13, 14]
Hereditary pancreatitis	**AD:** *PRSS1*	Pancreatic cancer	[15, 16]
Turcot Syndrome	**AD:** *APC, MLH1, PMS2*	Colon cancer Basal cell carcinoma Ependymoma Medulloblastoma Glioblastoma	[17]
Familial gastrointestinal stromal tumor	**AD:** *KIT*	Gastrointestinal stromal tumors	[18–20]
C. Genitourinary cancer predisposition syndromes			
Hereditary prostate cancer	**AD:** *BRCA2, CHEK2, ATM, BRCA1, HOXB13*	Prostate cancer	[21, 22]
Simpson-Golabi-Behmel syndrome	**XLR:** *GPC3, GPC4*	Embryonal tumors Wilms tumor	[23]
von Hippel-Lindau syndrome	**AD:** *VHL*	Hemangioblastomas of retina and central nervous system Renal cell cancer Pheochromocytomas	[24]

Table 12.1 (continued)

Syndromes	Inheritance patterns and gene(s)	Tumor types	Reference(s)
Beckwith-Wiedemann syndrome	**AD:** *CDKN1C, NSD1*	Wilms tumor Hepatoblastoma Adrenal carcinoma Gonadoblastoma	[25]
Wilms tumor syndrome	**AD:** *WT1*	Wilms tumor WAGR: Wilms tumor, aniridia, genitourinary abnormalities, intellectual disability	[26]
Birt-Hogg-Dubé syndrome	**AD:** *FLCN*	Renal tumors	[27]
Renal cell carcinoma	**AD:** *RNF139* Constitutional t(3;8) translocation	Renal cell cancer	[28–30]
Rhabdoid tumor predisposition syndrome	**AD:** *SMARCA4, SMARCB1*	Rhabdoid tumors Medulloblastoma Choroid plexus tumors Primitive neuroectodermal tumors	[31]
D. Central nervous system/vascular cancer			
Hereditary paraganglioma	**AD:** *MAX, SDHA, SDHAF2, SDHD, SDHC, SDHB, TMEM127*	Paraganglioma Pheochromocytoma	[32]
Retinoblastoma	**AD:** *RB1*	Retinoblastoma Osteosarcoma	[33]
Rhabdoid tumor predisposition syndrome	**AD:** *SMARCA4, SMARCB1*	Rhabdoid tumors Medulloblastoma Choroid plexus tumors Primitive neuroectodermal tumors	[31]
E. Sarcoma/bone cancer predisposition syndromes			
Hereditary multiple osteochondromas	**AD:** *EXT1, EXT2*	Osteochondroma	[34]
Hereditary leiomyomatosis and renal cell cancer (HLRCC)	**AD:** *FH*	Papillary renal cell carcinoma Uterine leiomyosarcomas	[35–37]
Werner syndrome	**AD:** *WRN*	Sarcoma/osteosarcoma Meningioma	[38]
F. Endocrine cancer predisposition syndromes			
MEN1	**AD:** *MEN1*	Pancreatic islet cell tumors Pituitary adenomas Parathyroid adenomas	[39]
MEN2	**AD:** *RET*	Medullary thyroid cancers Pheochromocytoma Parathyroid hyperplasia	[40]
G. Genodermatoses with cancer predisposition			
Melanoma syndromes	**AD:** *CDKN2A, CDK4, MC1R, POT1*	Malignant melanoma	[41]
Basal cell cancers, Gorlin syndrome	**AD:** *PTCH1*	Basal cell cancers Brain tumors	[42, 43]
Cowden Syndrome	**AD:** *PTEN*	See above	[44]
Neurofibromatosis 1	**AD:** *NF1*	Neurofibrosarcomas Pheochromocytomas Optic gliomas Meningiomas	[45]
Neurofibromatosis 2	**AD:** *NF2*	Vestibular schwannomas	[46]
Tuberous sclerosis	**AD:** *TSC1, TSC2*	Myocardial rhabdomyoma Multiple bilateral renal angiomyolipoma Ependymoma Renal cancer Giant cell astrocytoma	[47]

(continued)

Table 12.1 (continued)

Syndromes	Inheritance patterns and gene(s)	Tumor types	Reference(s)
Carney complex	**AD:** *PRKAR1A*	Myxoid subcutaneous tumors Primary adrenocortical nodular hyperplasia Testicular Sertoli cell tumor Atrial myxoma Pituitary adenoma Mammary fibroadenoma Thyroid carcinoma Schwannoma	[48]
H. Germline predisposition associated with increased risk of hematological malignancies			
Familial AML with mutated *CEBPA*	**AD:** *CEBPA*	AML	[49, 50]
Familial MDS/AML with mutated *GATA2* (Emberger syndrome, MonoMac syndrome)	**AD:** *GATA2*	MDS, AML, CMML *Additional clinical findings* Warts Atypical mycobacteria Lymphedema Deafness Pulmonary alveolar proteinosis Arterio-venous malformations	[51, 52]
Familial MDS/AML with mutated *DDX41*	**AD:** *DDX41*	MDS	[53–55]
Familial platelet disorder with propensity to myeloid malignancy	**AD:** *RUNX1*	MDS, AML, ALL *Additional clinical findings* Thrombocytopenia Abnormal platelet function	[56, 57]
Thrombocytopenia 2	**AD:** *ANKRD26*	MDS, AML *Additional clinical findings* Thrombocytopenia Abnormal platelet function	[58, 59]
Thrombocytopenia 5	**AD:** *ETV6*	MDS, AML, ALL *Additional clinical findings* Thrombocytopenia Abnormal platelet function	[59–61]
Familial acute lymphoblastic leukemia	**AD:** *PAX5, ETV6, SH2B3, IKZF1*	ALL	[60, 62–65]
Susceptibility to ALL3	**AD:** *PAX5*	ALL	[64, 66, 67]
Li-Fraumeni syndrome	**AD:** *TP53*	ALL, MDS, AML *Nonhematological malignancies* Breast, soft tissue sarcoma, brain, adrenocortical carcinoma, lung, colon, pancreas, Wilms, prostate	[5]
Constitutional mismatch repair deficiency syndrome	**AR:** *MLH1, MSH2, MSH6, PMS2*	Lymphoma, ALL, AML *Nonhematological malignancies* CNS, GI tract, other (see above) *Additional clinical findings* Café-au-lait spots, axillary freckling, Lisch nodules, neurofibromas, intestinal adenomas	[68, 69]
MIRAGE syndrome	**AD:** *SAMD9*	MDS, AML Cytopenias *Additional clinical findings* Short stature, adrenal hypoplasia, infections; CNS, GI, GU, and skeletal abnormalities	[70]
Ataxia-pancytopenia syndrome	**AD:** *SAMD9L*	MDS, AML Bone marrow failure *Additional clinical findings* Ataxia (variable)	[71]

Table 12.1 (continued)

Syndromes	Inheritance patterns and gene(s)	Tumor types	Reference(s)
Bone marrow failure syndrome 1	**AD:** *SRP72*	MDS Bone marrow failure *Additional clinical findings* Sensorineural hearing loss	[55, 72, 73]
Bloom syndrome	**AR:** *BLM*	Lymphoma, MDS, ALL *Nonhematological malignancies* Colon, skin cancer, squamous cell carcinomas of head and neck, Wilms tumor, and others, at early age *Additional clinical findings* Facial rash with butterfly pattern, other dermatologic manifestations, chronic obstructive lung disease, endocrine abnormalities	[74]
Fanconi anemia	**AR:** *FANCA, FANCC, BRCA2, FANCD2, FANCDE, FANCF, FANCG, FANCI, BRIP1, FANCL, FANCM, PALB2, RAD51C, SLX4, ERCC4, RAD51, BRCA1, UBE2T, XRCC2, REV7* **XLR:** *FANCB*	MDS, AML (risk 7% and 9%, respectively) ALL with FANCD1 (*BRCA2*) *Nonhematological malignancies* Squamous cell carcinomas of the head and neck, vulva, GI tract; liver tumors; brain tumors; and Wilms tumor [FANCD1 (*BRCA2*)] *Additional clinical findings* Low birth weight; short stature; skin pigmentation (café-au-lait spots); radial anomalies; facial dysmorphism; renal, gonadal, cardiac, GI, and CNS abnormalities; deafness	[75]
Severe congenital neutropenia	**AD:** *ELANE, CSF3R, GFI1* **AR:** *HAX1, G6PC3* **XLR:** *WAS*	MDS, AML (risk 21–40%) *Additional clinical findings* Neurological abnormalities (*HAX1*) Cardiac abnormalities (*G6PC3*)	[76–78]
Shwachman-Diamond syndrome	**AR:** *SBDS*	AML, MDS (risk 5–24%) Preceding isolated neutropenia *Additional clinical findings* Pancreatic insufficiency; short stature; steatorrhea; thoracic dysplasia; skeletal abnormalities (metaphyseal dysostosis)	[79]
Diamond-Blackfan anemia	**AD:** *RPS19, RPS17, RPS24, RPL35A, RPL5, RPL11, RPS7, RPS26, RPS10* **XLR:** *GATA1, TSR2*	MDS, AML, ALL (risk 5%) *Nonhematological malignancies* Osteosarcoma, soft tissue sarcomas *Additional clinical findings* Small stature; congenital anomalies: craniofacial, Pierre Robin sequence, cardiac, skeletal, genitourinary	[80]
Nijmegen breakage syndrome	**AR:** *NBN*	Lymphoma *Nonhematological malignancies* Glioma, medulloblastoma, rhabdomyosarcoma *Additional clinical findings* Severe microcephaly, abnormal facies, other malformations	[81]
Autoimmune lymphoproliferative disorder	**AD:** *CASP10, FAS, FASLG*	Lymphoma	[82]
Immunodeficiency syndromes: Wiskott-Aldrich Common variable immune deficiency Severe combined immune deficiency	**XLR:** *WAS* **AR:** Unknown **XLR, AR:** *IL2RG, ADA, JAK3, RAG1, RAG2, IL7R, CD45, DCLRE1C*	Hematopoietic malignancies Lymphomas B-cell lymphoma *Additional clinical findings* Thrombocytopenia, neutropenia, eczema, infections, autoimmune disorders	[83–85]
Ataxia telangiectasia	**AR:** *ATM*	Leukemia Lymphoma *Nonhematological malignancies* Solid tumors	[7]

(continued)

Table 12.1 (continued)

Syndromes	Inheritance patterns and gene(s)	Tumor types	Reference(s)
Noonan syndrome	**AD:** *PTPN11, SOS1, RAF1, KRAS, NRAS, BRAF, MAP2K1*	Juvenile myelomonocytic leukemia (JMML) *Nonhematological malignancies* Rhabdomyosarcoma, neuroblastoma *Additional clinical findings* Short stature, macrocephaly, feeding difficulty, cardiac defects, other	[86, 87]
Telomere biology disorders, including dyskeratosis congenita and syndromes due to *TERC* or *TERT* mutations	**AD:** *TERT, TERC, TINF2, RTEL1, PARN* **XLR:** *DKC1* **AR:** *NOP10, NHP2, WRAP53, RTEL1, TERT, CTC1, STN1, PARN*	MDS, AML (2–30% risk) Bone marrow failure *Non-hematological malignancies* Squamous cell carcinoma of head and neck, GI tract *Additional clinical findings* Nail dystrophy, abnormal skin and pigmentation, rash, oral leukoplakia, pulmonary fibrosis, hepatic fibrosis, short stature, vascular anomalies, early graying of hair, hair loss, dental, CNS, GI and GU abnormalities	[88]

Abbreviations: *AD* autosomal dominant, *AR* autosomal recessive, *XLR* X-linked recessive, *OMIM* Online Mendelian Inheritance in Man, *ALL* acute lymphoblastic leukemia, *MDS* myelodysplastic syndrome, *AML* acute myeloid leukemia, *MEN* multiple endocrine neoplasia, *HNPCC* hereditary nonpolyposis colorectal cancer

- With increased genetic testing, new susceptibility genes continue to be identified, and while at a lower penetrance, they may expand the spectrum of cancer predisposition.

2. **How have molecular events of critical cellular pathways further contributed to our understanding of hereditary and sporadic cancer development?**
   - The hallmarks of cancer described by Hanahan and Weinberg were seminal to our understanding of cancer's most common traits [89, 90]:
     – Selective growth and proliferative advantage by sustaining self-sufficiency in growth signals/mitotic stimulation and evading anti-growth signals
     – Activating tissue invasion and metastasis
     – Enabling replicative immortality
     – Inducing and sustaining angiogenesis/vascularization
     – Resisting apoptosis
     – Deregulating cellular energy metabolism
     – Evading immune modulation and destruction
     – Enabling characteristics of tumor-promoting inflammation and promoting genomic instability and mutation
   - Knudson's "two-hit" theory of cancer causation, through the study of retinoblastoma, provided an early explanation correlating hereditary and non-hereditary incidences of similar cancers.
     – Retinoblastoma can be (a) sporadic, unilateral, with 30 month as the average age of onset, or (b) familial, bilateral, with 14 month as the average age of onset, and accompanied by other cancers.
     – Retinoblastoma develops only if **both** *RB1* alleles are inactive. Familial retinoblastoma is inherited as autosomal dominant (AD) of *RB1* gene, with 90% penetrance. In familial cases of retinoblastoma, one *RB1* pathogenic variant is inherited, and only one further mutation of the *RB1* gene in any retinal cells is therefore necessary for tumorigenesis.
     – Knudson's two-hit theory of carcinogenesis states that a cell can initiate tumor only with two damaged alleles. Carcinogenesis in retinoblastoma became a model to describe how inheritance of an altered gene predisposes the carrier to cancer.
   - The concept of multi-hit hypothesis [91], in which one particular gene that plays a critical role in maintaining a constant cell regulation (gatekeeper) in a certain tissue type, is dysregulated in cancer development.
   - The major classes of cancer genes are classified into those that normally inhibit cellular proliferation (tumor suppressors), those that activate proliferation (oncogenes), and those that involve DNA repair. Comparison of key features of tumor suppressor genes and oncogenes is shown in Table 12.2.
     – Tumor suppressor genes mediate progress through the cell cycle. Cancers are frequently initiated by failure of tumor suppressor genes.
       - Typically, the loss of function of one allele is recessive at cellular level (loss of one allele does not cause disease) and requires a second mutation ("second hit") of another normal allele for cancer development.
     – Oncogenes are mutated derivatives of proto-oncogenes involved in the deregulation of cell cycle control and signal transduction cascade.

Table 12.2 Comparison of features of tumor suppressor genes and oncogenes

Feature	Tumor suppressor genes	Oncogenes
Function	Regulation of cell growth, proliferation, and apoptosis	Promotes cell growth and proliferation
Mutation type	Both alleles affected for gene inactivation Deletion Loss of heterozygosity	Only one allele mutated Gene amplifications Hypomethylation Base-pair substitution (constitutive activation) Chromosome rearrangements (translocations)
Effect of mutation	Loss of function	Gain of function
Germline pathogenic variant that results in hereditary cancer syndrome	Seen in most tumor suppressor genes	Seen in only a few oncogenes

  - Unlike tumor suppressor genes, oncogenes are usually dominant at the cellular level: only a single copy of a mutated oncogene is required to contribute to the multistep process of tumor progression.
  - Oncogenes are typically activated by gain-of-function mutations, gene amplifications (i.e., increased number of gene copy through trisomy or other mechanism), hypomethylation of the 5′ region of an oncogene (which increases transcription), or chromosome rearrangement (upregulating the oncogene).
  - Abnormalities in oncogenes have broad tissue specificity and are rarely inherited.
- Cancer development is a multistage process in which a cell accumulates damage in several critical genes related to cell cycle regulation and/or differentiation. Genetic alterations of cell regulatory systems are the primary basis of carcinogenesis.
- A pathogenic variant, or deleterious mutation, in tumor suppressor genes or oncogenes associated with a hereditary cancer syndrome increases an individual's predisposition to certain types of non-hematologic cancers and hematologic malignancies (Table 12.1).
  - Most hereditary cancer syndromes exhibit autosomal-dominant (AD) inheritance, such as hereditary breast cancer and ovarian cancer syndrome, Lynch syndrome, Li-Fraumeni syndrome, Cowden syndrome, Peutz-Jeghers syndrome, familial adenomatous polyposis (FAP), hereditary leiomyomatosis and renal cancer syndrome, and hereditary diffuse gastric cancer (Table 12.1).
  - Inherited pathogenic variants are dominant alleles at the level of the individual (i.e., heterozygotes are predisposed to develop the disease) but recessive at the level of the cell (i.e., heterozygous cells do not form tumors; both alleles mutated for gene inactivation).

3. **What are the general features suggesting the presence of hereditary cancer syndrome or inherited cancer risks?**
   - Although familial disease clusters can be caused by shared environmental factors, there are several factors that allude to genetic causation of cancer. There are particular clinical appearances and genetic features of hereditary cancer that are present in the patient and/or in the patient's family history.
   - General features suggesting presence of a hereditary cancer syndrome include:
     - An early age of onset
     - Association with other clinical presentations or congenital defects
     - Presence of multiple neoplasms and/or rare morphological features
     - Multiple primary neoplasms within the same organ
     - Bilateral tumors in paired organ or lobes
     - Non-clonal tumors that are multifocal or in different organ systems and tissues in the same individual
     - Neoplasms occurring in gender that is not usually affected
   - Family history can help identify individuals at risk for developing cancer and typically involves several close relatives with the same or genetically associated cancers or family members with same rare cancer. Indicated family history includes:
     - One first-degree relative with the same or related tumor and one of individual features presented
     - ≥2 first-degree relatives with neoplasms in the same site, with neoplasms belonging to known familial cancer syndrome, or with rare tumors
     - ≥2 relatives in two generations with tumors of same site
4. **What are genetic predispositions to hematologic malignancies syndromes?**
   - Predisposition to hematological disorders have been observed in well-described inherited syndromes which also exhibit additional non-hematological findings and often present in childhood. These predisposing hematologic malignancies, listed in Table 12.1H, include bone marrow failure syndromes (e.g., Fanconi anemia) and telomere biology disorders (e.g., dyskeratosis congenita) [92–94].
   - With increasing use of molecular profiling and panel-based testing for hereditary cancers, it has become

apparent that some cases of myeloid neoplasms, particularly myelodysplastic syndrome (MDS), acute myeloid leukemia (AML), and aplastic anemia, occur in association with inherited genetic conditions or de novo germline pathogenic variants characterized by specific genetic and clinical findings [95–100].

- Familial B-lymphoblastic leukemia (B-ALL) is associated with germline pathogenic variants in *PAX5*, *ETV6*, *SH2B3*, and *IKZF1* genes [60, 62–65].
- Myeloid neoplasms associated with predisposing germline pathogenic variants are currently recognized as a new provisional entity within the World Health Organization (WHO) leukemia classification scheme [95, 101].
  - Myeloid neoplasms with germline predisposition without a preexisting disorder or organ dysfunction include:
    - Acute myeloid leukemia with germline *CEBPA* mutation
    - Myeloid neoplasms with germline *DDX41* mutation
  - Myeloid neoplasms with germline predisposition consisting of thrombocytopenia and preexisting platelet disorders include germline mutations in *RUNX1*, *ANKRD26*, and *ETV6* genes.
  - Myeloid neoplasms with germline predisposition and other organ dysfunction include (Table 12.1H) [51, 101–103]:
    - Myeloid neoplasms with germline *GATA2* mutation
    - Myeloid neoplasms associated with bone marrow failure syndromes
    - Myeloid neoplasms associated with telomere biology disorders
    - Juvenile myelomonocytic leukemia (JMML) associated with neurofibromatosis, Noonan syndrome, or Noonan syndrome-like disorders
    - Myeloid neoplasms associated with Down syndrome

5. **What are the indications of a myeloid neoplasm (MDS, AML, or lymphoblastic leukemia) with germline predisposition?**
   - Personal history of multiple cancers and family history (first- or second-degree relative) of a hematological neoplasm or solid tumor.
   - Patients presenting thrombocytopenia, bleeding propensity, or macrocytosis prior to a diagnosis of MDS/AML.
   - Patient or first- or second-degree relative presenting with well-defined inherited syndrome that exhibit additional non-hematological findings, such as abnormal nails or skin pigmentation, oral leukoplakia, idiopathic pulmonary fibrosis, unexplained liver disease, lymphedema, atypical infections, immune deficiencies, congenital limb anomalies, or short stature should also be given consideration for a germline predisposition [104].
6. **Why is it important to pursue germline testing?**
   - Identifying individuals who have a cancer predisposition syndrome has benefits for the patient and for at-risk relatives.
   - It is important to evaluate patients with cancer for clinical signs of a possible underlying hereditary cancer syndrome that may require germline testing and take family history of cancers to identify those who have a hereditary predisposition to develop malignancy or increased risk for additional primary cancers.
   - Finding a germline pathogenic variant in a patient with cancer is a starting point to personalized short- and long-term management and recommendations. These may include modified/increased cancer screening, consideration of risk-reducing interventions, tailored chemotherapy strategies, and determination of eligibility for cancer trials, providing prognosis for the current disease and for any additional primary and secondary malignancies.
   - Identifying the familial pathogenic variant by targeted genetic testing in at-risk relatives is an important initial step in guiding them for any appropriate screening and prevention strategies.
   - Allogeneic hematopoietic stem cell transplantation is an important treatment option and frequently the only potential cure for many hematopoietic and lymphoid neoplasms. It is critical to recognize a germline pathogenic variant associated with predispositions to hematologic malignancies in the proband patient, so that potential related donors can be tested and those carrying the variant be excluded.
7. **Who is involved in ordering, counseling, and interpreting germline testing?**
   - Before undergoing germline genetic testing, individuals benefit from referral to cancer genetic counselors. Genetic counseling is generally not required before germline genetic testing, the exception being insurance companies that necessitate a genetics professional to conduct a pretest counseling in order to authorize genetic testing. However, a number of professional organizations underscore the importance of genetic counseling in the cancer risk assessment and genetic testing process [105].
   - Session with a genetic counselor, in-person, telephone-based, or via telemedicine counseling services includes collecting information from three- to four-generation pedigree on relatives with cancer diagnoses, age of onset/cause of death, and any prior genetic testing.

- Genetic counselors provide pretest education and lead discussions to obtain informed consent. They review the purpose of genetic testing, possible outcome test results, management implications, benefits, risks, and limitations, as well as the voluntary nature of testing. They can prepare the patient for the conversation with the clinician, address psychosocial issues, and make referrals.
- Genetic counselors understand the limitations of various forms of genetic tests and can help guide providers and educate patients about the value and selection of tests, including gene selections to determine the best approach. Educational handouts, videos, presentations, online pedigree collection tools, and chatbots, such as Genetic Information Assistance, can serve as alternatives to pretest counseling [106].
- Genetic testing may be ordered by a cancer genetics professional, oncology provider, primary care provider, or other non-genetics professional healthcare providers in collaboration with healthcare professionals experienced in cancer genetics [107].
- Genetic counselors also provide post-test counseling, discuss and aid in test results interpretation, and document cancer risks associated with the identified pathogenic variant. They help patients understand and adapt to the medical, psychological, and familial implications of test results. Genetic counselors help coordinate genetic counseling and cascade testing of at-risk relatives or recommend further testing in the family based on family history.

8. **What are the current techniques for germline cancer testing?**
    - The majority of current germline genetic tests for hereditary cancer employ massively parallel sequencing (MPS)/next-generation sequencing (NGS) technology and include panels of genes. A number of genes on panels may range from a few, focusing on a specific type of cancer, to large comprehensive panels covering many cancer conditions. Careful selection of genes on NGS panels is important to ensure comprehensive testing. This may be especially important when family history includes several cancer types [108–110].
    - Broad multigene panels in appropriately ascertained individuals have the potential to detect more pathogenic germline variants in moderate- and high-penetrance cancer susceptibility genes. However, large gene panels also typically result in returning a considerable proportion of variants of uncertain significance. Here, gene-specific variant interpretation guidelines may help to lower the number of variants classified as uncertain [111, 112].
    - The massively parallel sequencing technology and bioinformatics pipelines routinely detect single-nucleotide variants and short (oftentimes less than 60-bp long) deletions and insertions, and typically yield high depth of sequencing reads.
    - Some tests detect large deletions, duplications, and insertions from massively parallel sequencing data using custom designed bioinformatic pipelines. The large pathogenic/likely pathogenic variants are typically confirmed by orthogonal methods such as targeted microarray, multiplex ligation-dependent probe amplification (MLPA), or quantitative polymerase chain reaction (qPCR). Other tests utilize MLPA or exonic oligonucleotide-based comparative genomic hybridization microarray to detect deletions and duplications.
    - Currently, only a few clinical tests include RNA sequencing of complementary DNA obtained by reverse transcription polymerase chain reaction (RT-PCR). This RNA methodology is helping to get functional evidence for classification of certain variants. The analysis in peripheral blood samples is limited to genes expressed in human lymphocytes.
    - Single gene testing is oftentimes performed by Sanger sequencing and MLPA technology to detect deletions and duplications. Sanger sequencing is also used to fill-in the gaps in targeted gene regions not fully covered by NGS.
    - Genes with known pseudogenes require the combination of NGS and specific custom-gene methods, such as long-range PCR [113].
    - Whole-genome DNA and RNA sequencing (WGS) and matched WGS of tumor and germline DNA in solid tumor cancers currently represent the most comprehensive approach to detect hereditary cancer susceptibility. However, these tests are mostly limited to academic research settings [114, 115].
    - The future in precision oncology belongs to long-read sequencing and optical mapping technologies that will help to identify large-scale genomic alterations and phase haplotypes [116] including pharmacogenomic variants known to modulate drug metabolism or mediate adverse effects in response to treatment [117].
9. **What are the common cancer predisposition genes detected by somatic testing?**
    - Germline variants are often detected in *ATM*, *BRCA1*, *BRCA2*, *CEBPA*, *CHEK2*, *DDX41*, *GATA2*, *MUTYH*, *RUNX1*, and *TP53* genes in solid tumors and hematopoietic malignancies panels [72, 109, 118, 119].
    - The number of germline pathogenic variants may vary in different genes. A study of germline testing following tumor sequencing in patients with cancer

found 39% of pathogenic variants in *BRCA1* and *BRCA2* and 28% in *MLH1*, *MSH2*, *MSH6*, and *PMS2* genes, but only 4% in *TP53* gene is of germline origin [120].

- Genotypic heterogeneity surrounding predisposition to cancers [109] means that pathogenic germline variants in genes such as *BRCA1* and *BRCA2* are being detected in patients with cancers not typically associated with these genes, such as in colorectal, thyroid, endometrial, and other cancer types [120].

10. **What types of variants are detected and reported by germline genetic testing?**
    - The gene content of germline testing panels is distinct from somatic panels.
    - Germline genetic testing involves NGS analysis of group of genes which have been associated with a particular hereditary cancer syndrome. An individual who meets the criteria of being at risk of a hereditary cancer syndrome would undergo testing for all of the genes implicated in that specific syndrome.
    - For example, in the case of hereditary breast and ovarian cancers, a gene panel involving 20–40 genes may be undertaken, depending on the genetic test (see Table 12.1 for a list of syndromes and their associated genes).
    - The entire coding sequence of most genes included on such panels is analyzed. These panels involve the analysis of the DNA sequence of these genes, as well as the copy number analysis of exons and the region within 10–20 bp of their boundaries.
    - Detection of pathogenic variants in regulatory regions, or large structural variants, such as the Bolland inversion in *MSH2* [121] or the *Alu* repeat insertions in *BRCA2* [122], may also be included in some tests.
    - The variants detected upon a sequencing run are automatically filtered based on a number of criteria, including their prevalence in population controls and if they represent known benign variants. The remaining variants are curated based on whether or not sufficient evidence exists to determine if they affect the function of the gene in which they were identified.
    - Identified DNA sequence alterations include missense and nonsense variants, small deletions or insertions of DNA sequence, and deletions involving single or multiple exons.
    - These are classified into one of the three categories in the final report: a variant of uncertain significance, a likely pathogenic variant, or a pathogenic variant. The criteria for the classification of variants are addressed in question #13.
11. **What types of variants are detected and reported by somatic testing?**
    - Somatic NGS analysis involves analyzing genes, or regions within genes, which may impact the clinical management of a tumor.
    - These analyses may involve the coding sequences of the entire genes or be limited to "hotspot" regions which encompass known clinically actionable variants.
    - Notably, this type of analysis often does not include the genes which predispose to hereditary cancer syndrome, since these genes are often the one of the first hits to occur in a tumor and may not drive its progression. An example of a current exception to this rule involves the detection of mutations in *BRCA1* and *BRCA2* in high-grade serious ovarian tumors, which is an eligibility criteria for treatment by poly ADP ribose polymerase (PARP) inhibition [123].
    - Somatic variants are classified by whether they affect the diagnosis, prognosis, or treatment of the tumor and are reported as Tier 1 (variants of strong clinical significance), Tier II (variants of potential clinical significance), and Tier III (variants of unknown clinical significance). The criteria for the classification of somatic variants is addressed in question #13.
    - Somatic variants will not be detected in normal tissue; therefore, the detection sensitivity is affected by the tumor cell content in the tested tissue.
12. **What is variant allele frequency (VAF)? Can VAF on a somatic NGS assay be used to predict a variant with a germline origin?**
    - VAF is the proportion of NGS reads which display a particular DNA sequence variant.
    - The VAF is a reflection of the abundance of the variant in the sample from which the respective DNA specimen was extracted.
    - In a germline NGS assay, a heterozygous variant, where one out of two alleles have undergone a sequence change, is expected to have a VAF of approximately 0.50, where 50% of the reads over a specific nucleotide position showed a sequence alteration. A homozygous variant, which arises when both copies of a gene undergo a change, may be expected to have a VAF approaching 1.0.
    - In a somatic NGS assay, DNA sequence variants may present with a range of VAF values [124], which may reflect the tumor cell percentage in the tissue and the genetic complexity of the tumor specimen.
    - Intratumor heterogeneity, chromosomal structural changes, clonality, and sample choice may affect the VAF values. As such, incidental pathogenic germline variants may also present at a range of VAF values [124] and should not be used as a sole criteria as to whether or not to recommend follow-up by germline NGS panel testing.

13. **What are the guidelines for variant interpretation and reporting for somatic and for germline findings?**
    - Variant interpretation guidelines for germline and somatic reporting are distinct.
    - As stated previously, somatic variants are classified based on whether they may impact the clinical management of the tumor.
    - The Association for Molecular Pathology (AMP), the American Society of Clinical Oncology (ASCO), and the College of American Pathologists (CAP) established guidelines for the interpretation of somatic findings from NGS analysis [125].
    - Variants detected in tumor specimens are annotated using the information available from the medical literature, online databases, and clinical trial repositories. Somatic variant interpretation focusses on whether or not a DNA variant can impact clinical care, and these variants are classified into four tiers, depending on its significance in the diagnosis, prognosis, or therapy of a tumor (discussed in Chap. 1, question #8 of this book; and more details in reference [125]).
    - Guidelines for germline variant interpretation were outlined by the American College of Medical Genetics and Genomics (ACMGG) and the Association for Molecular Pathology (AMP) [126].
    - Germline variant interpretation focusses on whether or not the respective change in a gene alters the function of the gene that, in the case of hereditary cancer testing, predisposes the individual to the development of a tumor.
    - This variant curation process includes searching databases and the medical literature for evidence pertaining to the population frequency of a variant, segregation with disease in multiple individuals and families, experimental studies which have examined the effect of the variant on the expression of the gene or the function of its encoded protein, and in silico predictions of the pathogenicity of the variant, among other criteria [126]. These criteria are weighed, with the strongest ones contributing more heavily toward meeting the scoring threshold for classification [126].
    - Pathogenic variants are those which meet the strongest criteria for causing a hereditary predisposition to cancer. In the context of hereditary cancer testing, these variants may include nonsense or splice variants, which may affect the expression of the mRNA or protein product; missense variants which lie in a critical domain or mutational hotspot and disrupt the function of the protein encoded by the gene; and variants with low frequency in population controls, but which are enriched in affected individuals and segregate in families with the cancer predisposition. Likely pathogenic variants are those which meet most, but not necessarily, all of these criteria.
    - Variants of uncertain significance lack evidence for being benign or causative. They may fulfill some of the criteria for each of these categories, but sufficient evidence is lacking to make a definitive classification.
    - Likely benign or benign variants are not typically reported.
    - While the somatic variant classification guidelines suggest likely pathogenic or pathogenic germline variants are classified as Tier 1 variants in the somatic framework [125], it is important to note that many of them do not affect the diagnosis, prognosis, or treatment of the tumor. Rather, these at-risk variants, upon confirmation in the germline, may influence preventative action, such as early and ongoing surveillance for cancer emergence.
14. **How should a finding suggestive of a pathogenic variant in a hereditary cancer gene be confirmed when it is observed by somatic testing of a tumor biopsy?**
    - Tumor tissue samples tested by NGS may contain somatic, germline, and clonal hematopoietic DNA changes (there are always some blood cells in the tumor tissue).
    - After a potentially germline pathogenic variant is detected by NGS testing (Fig. 12.1), the patient's provider facilitates genetic counseling and, when appropriate, testing to confirm germline status [119].
    - In the absence of concurrent analyses of matched normal and tumor samples from a patient, suspicion for a pathogenic germline variant should be followed by NGS testing by a germline assay of a normal tissue, after obtaining patient consent (Fig. 12.1).
    - When somatic or germline testing is performed on a peripheral blood sample, a pathogenic variant detected at a low variant frequency (less than 30%) may be due to somatic mosaicism, clonal hematopoiesis, sequencing artifact, or tumor pathogenic variant detected in the blood from a circulating hematologic malignancy or from solid tumors [127].
15. **What type of sample should be tested to determine if a pathogenic variant has a germline origin for non-hematological malignancies (solid tumors)?**
    - Confirmation of germline status can be achieved by identifying the *pathogenic variant* in a second tissue, such as peripheral blood, fibroblast cultures, or hair follicles such as eyebrow samples. Some testing laboratories also accept skin biopsies and buccal and saliva samples. Additionally, reactive, benign lymph nodes from matched tumor specimen that do not have epithelial cell components and

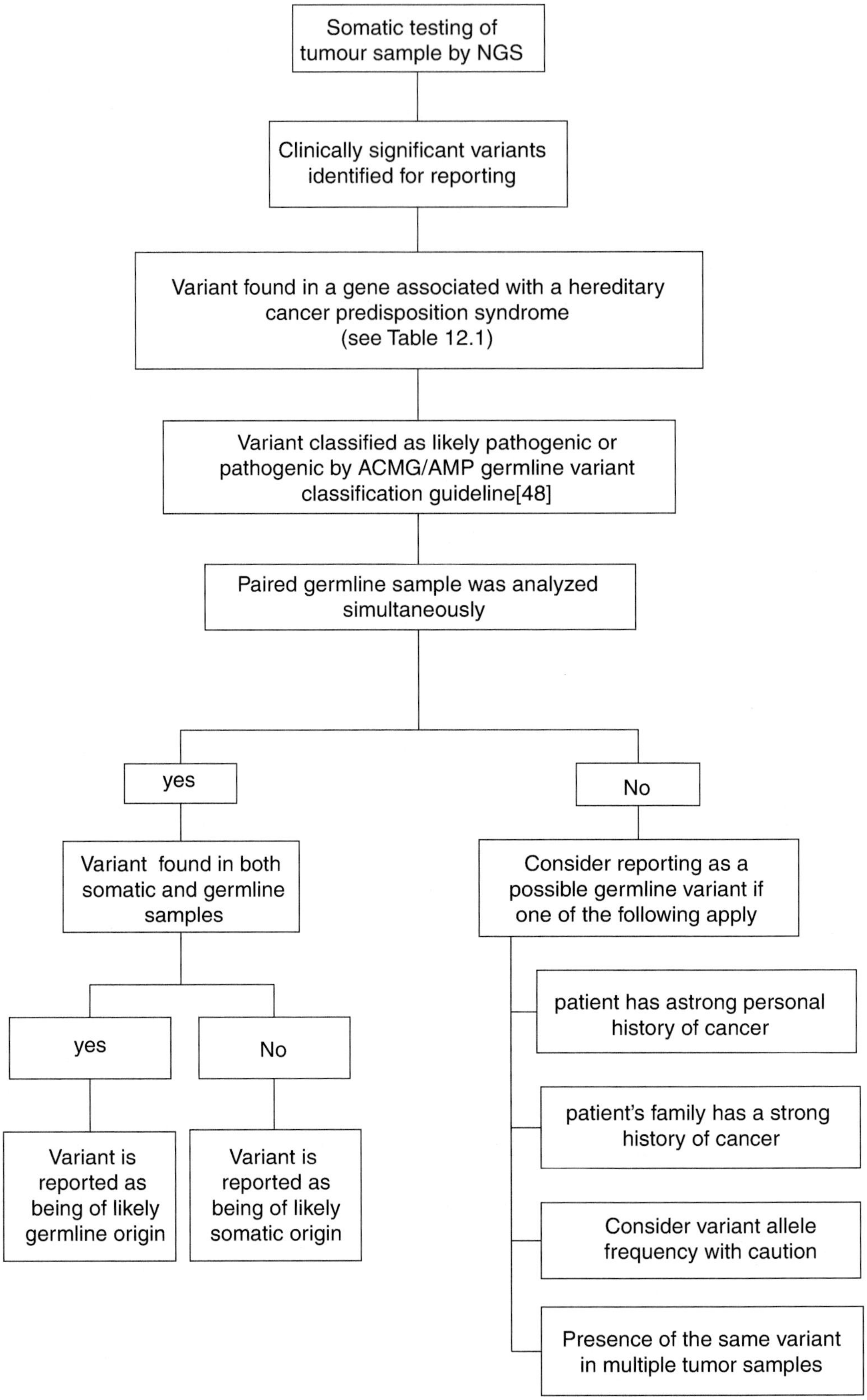

Fig. 12.1 Schematic diagram of differentiating between somatic and germline variants when variants are identified by tumor-based sequencing

morphohistochemically negative for metastatic tumor can be used for germline testing if consent is obtained from patient undergoing somatic testing (Case 6).

- As a rule, tissue samples for germline testing should not be contaminated with blood. However, failing to identify pathogenic variant in a different tissue type does not exclude a possibility of mosaicism.
- When germline origin of a pathogenic variant is confirmed, patient's provider discusses associated cancer risks, screening recommendations, referrals, possible implications for treatment, further genetic counseling, and testing at-risk relatives of individuals for the familial pathogenic variant.
- Access to the proband's test report with confirmed germline pathogenic test result is necessary for family members considering testing.

16. **What are molecular genetic testing considerations for germline predisposition for hematologic malignancies?**
    - Genes involved in germline predisposition for hematologic malignancies can also be mutated as acquired mutations in MDS/AML; therefore, it is important to perform germline testing on constitutional DNA.
    - Both the blood and bone marrow are affected in MDS/AML and should be used cautiously as a source for germline DNA. Although growth cultures of skin fibroblasts are usually the gold standard for germline studies, DNA from the hair and nail can be used as a source for germline DNA. Saliva and buccal swabs should be used with caution and should not be considered as pure germline material as they are often contaminated with blood cells that can confound germline analysis.
    - Healthy potential hematopoietic stem cell donor (family members) who is planning to donate to a family member with a hematologic malignancy with MDS, AML, or lymphoblastic leukemia should be tested for germline familial pathogenic variant.
    - Recommendations for an individual diagnosed with a hematologic predisposition syndrome include expert consultation or referral to specialized center, genetic counseling trained in inherited hematopoietic malignancies, updated personal/family history, physical examination and baseline CBC with differential and microscopy review for dysplasias, bone marrow evaluation with cytogenetic/FISH and molecular analysis, and HLA typing and referral to allogenic stem cell transplant center [128].
17. **What other molecular possibilities can be considered when germline cancer predisposition is suspected, but no pathogenic variant was identified?**
    - The gene of interest was not included on the panel test.
    - Variant is a deletion, duplication, insertion, or a structural variant that the test cannot detect.
    - Variant is in the pseudogene-associated region that the test cannot distinguish.
    - Variant is in the intronic or untranslated region that is not covered by the test.
    - Variant is in the homopolymer region not called by NGS pipeline.
    - Variant is in low-coverage region that was not filled-in by Sanger sequencing.
    - Variant was identified but misclassified or was omitted from the report.
    - Variant was not detected (when tested by a genotyping assay, Sanger sequencing, or during amplification-based target enrichment) due to single nucleotide polymorphism causing allelic dropout.
18. **Do discrepancies in variant interpretation occur between laboratories when interpreting germline variants?**
    - Discrepancies between laboratories in the interpretation of variants detected by germline sequencing have been reported.
    - An example of a discrepancy in variant interpretation is provided in case presentation #2.
    - While some laboratories use the ACMG/AMP guidelines as recommended, others have reportedly modified the criteria that they employ [129]. Some laboratories also modify the weight of certain criteria [130], which has been widely discussed in the community.
    - Despite this, the concordance of classifications of variants in hereditary breast, ovarian, colorectal, and related cancers approached 98.8% by one estimate [131].
    - Gene- or syndrome-specific variant interpretation criteria have been developed for some hereditary cancer predisposition genes [132, 133], and additional ones are currently under development. These may lead to an even higher rate of consistency in variant classification going forward.

Case Presentations

Case 1

Learning Objectives

Understand the clinical and family history risk factors of an inherited breast cancer syndrome; understand the molecular genetic testing that is performed when a suspicion of a hereditary breast cancer syndrome arises.

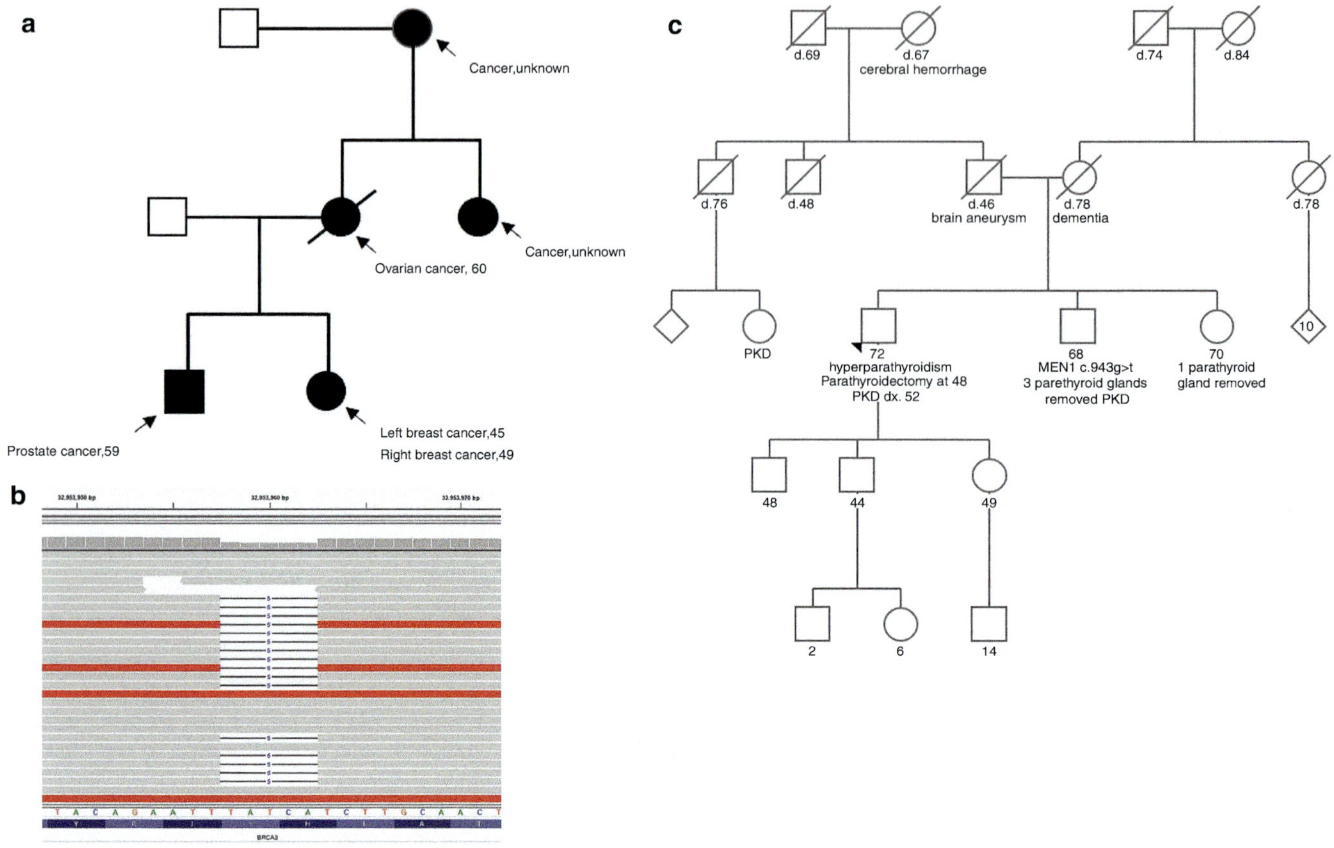

Fig. 12.2 (**a**) Pedigree of a family affected with breast, ovarian, and prostate cancers (Case 1). The proband, with bilateral breast cancer, has a *BRCA2* pathogenic variant, associated with hereditary breast and ovarian cancer syndrome. (**b**) An example of NGS reads showing the deletion of five base pairs in the BRCA2 gene, leading to a frameshift. (**c**) Pedigree for patient described in Case 2

Case History

A 51-year-old female diagnosed with breast cancer of the left side at 45 years of age (ER+/PR+/Her2-) and breast cancer of the right side (ER-/PR-/Her2-) at 49 years of age (Fig. 12.2a). One of her brothers was diagnosed with prostate cancer at 59 years of age, and her mother was diagnosed with ovarian cancer at 60 years of age. Her maternal grandmother and a maternal aunt also presented with cancer, although the type of cancer and the age of diagnosis were not known.

Genetic Study

Based on the personal and family history of breast, prostate, and ovarian cancers, the patient was deemed to be a candidate to undergo genetic testing for hereditary breast and ovarian cancers. DNA was extracted from a blood sample and analyzed by NGS for DNA sequence changes in 19 genes associated with hereditary breast and ovarian cancer.

A pathogenic variant was identified in *BRCA2*, c.9026_9030del p.(Tyr3009Serfs*7) (Fig. 12.2b). The allele frequency of this variant was ~45%, suggesting that this change is heterozygous. This variant resulted in an amino acid substitution of tyrosine at amino acid position 3009 with serine, followed by an alteration in the reading frame and introduction of a premature translation termination codon seven amino acids downstream. Using the ACMG/AMP guidelines [126], this variant was classified as pathogenic based on the following criteria:

- The variant is a null variant in the *BRCA2* gene, where the loss of function of one copy of the gene (haploinsufficiency) is the disease mechanism (ACMGG PVS1).
- The variant was present at very low frequency in population controls (0.00041% in the Genome Aggregation Database (gnomAD) (ACMGG PM2).
- The variant was catalogued in ClinVar (ID: 38204), where it was reported to be pathogenic by several submitting laboratories (ACMGG PP5).

Final Diagnosis

The pathogenic variant in *BRCA2* confirmed the diagnosis of a hereditary breast and ovarian cancer syndrome.

Follow-Up

The patient underwent a bilateral mastectomy and a bilateral salpingo-oophorectomy and was being monitored annually for melanoma. Genetic counselling and testing of family members for the c.9026_9030del p.(Tyr3009Serfs*7) variant in *BRCA2* was recommended.

Discussion

The cancer risks associated with pathogenic variants in *BRCA2* include fallopian tube cancer, peritoneal cancer, and increased risk of breast and prostate cancers in men. Increased risk of pancreatic cancer has also been reported in men and women.

Case 2

Learning Objective

Understand the clinical and family history of hyperparathyroidism; multiple endocrine neoplasia type 1 (MEN1) cancer syndrome; understand variant interpretation in the context of family history.

Case History

A 72-year-old male diagnosed with hyperparathyroidism (PHPT) at 36 years of age presents with hypercalcemia. Since the initial diagnosis, he has undergone four parathyroidectomies, implantation of parathyroid tissue, pulmonary embolism, and polycystic kidney disease (PKD) stage 3. His father died of a brain aneurysm at age 46. His brother had a notable history of PHPT and three surgeries, and his sister had a parathyroidectomy in her late 50s. No other MEN1-related tumors were reported in the personal or family history. His family history is shown in Fig. 12.2c.

Genetic Study

The patient's brother tested positive for a pathogenic variant, c.943G > T p.(Asp315Tyr), in the *MEN1* gene. His sister did not have genetic testing. The patient is likely to test positive for the *MEN1* pathogenic variant identified in his brother given his history of PHPT. His son tested negative for autosomal recessive form of PKD through carrier screening. Genetic testing of this patient resulted in the same heterozygous c.943G > T variant in *MEN1*, but classified as variant of uncertain significance (VUS) by a different laboratory.

There was a discrepancy in the interlaboratory classification of the *MEN1* variant occurred in this family.

Concordant interpretation from both laboratories:

- The *MEN1* p.(Asp315Tyr) variant is non-conservative amino acid substitution. The sequence change replaces aspartic acid with tyrosine at codon 315 of MEN1 protein.
- This variant was reported as a novel variant in a family with MEN1 [134] and in a family with MEN1 non-functioning microadenoma and non-functioning pancreatic cyst [135].

Discordant interpretation of both laboratories:

Laboratory A (tested brother)	Laboratory B (tested patient)
• Not reported in NHLBI Exome Sequencing Project. • Missense variants in nearby residues have been reported in association with MEN1.	• Present in population databases; ExAC 0.001%. • SIFT: Deleterious, PolyPhen-2: benign. • The algorithm to predict effect on RNA splicing suggests that the variant may create or strengthen splice site, but not confirmed by transcriptional studies.

Final Diagnosis

Reevaluation of the variant was requested of both laboratories given the family and clinical history.

Follow-Up

The patient's personal and family history of PHPT is consistent with multiple endocrine neoplasia type 1 (MEN1). Annual biochemical screening and periodic imaging (i.e., abdominal CT/MRI, pituitary MRI) is recommended for individuals with MEN1. Continue to manage patient as if he has MEN1 and recommend PTH/Ca screening for children and additional PKD testing. The patient's sister, who had undergone a parathyroidectomy, was tested.

Individuals with MEN1 have increased risks for pituitary tumors, parathyroid tumors, and pancreatic tumors (i.e., insulinoma, gastrinoma). Although more rare, carcinoid tumors (of the lung and thymus) and adrenocortical tumors can also be seen in individuals with MEN1. Annual biochemical screening and periodic imaging is recommended.

Discussion

Testing of patient's sister for VUS reclassification is recommended. If there is more supporting evidence of multiple co-segregation of multiple affected family members (in addition to brother and proband) according to the ACMG/AMP guidelines [126] along with pathogenic moderate (PM) evidence consisting of low frequency/absent in population, computational, and predictive data of novel missense change at an amino acid residue where different pathogenic missense change has been reported before and predicted change of RNA splicing and supporting evidence of publication from reputable sources, the evidence would support a "likely pathogenic" variant this family.

His first-degree relatives also have a 50% chance to carry the same variant and would be recommended to pursue genetic counseling/testing.

Case 3

Learning Objective

To review the role of epimutations as a cause of Lynch syndrome; to describe the inheritance patterns of *MLH1* epimutations and discuss implications of variant reclassification on patient care and management.

Case History

The patient was diagnosed with uterine cancer at 38 years of age, right-sided colon cancer at 47 years of age, and stage IIA sigmoid colon cancer at 65 years. Molecular testing demonstrated microsatellite instability (MSI) – high – and was positive for a *BRAF* p.(Val600Glu) mutation.

Genetic Study

Initial molecular testing was negative for genes on a colon cancer panel (*APC*, *AXIN2*, *BMPR1A*, *BRCA1*, *BRCA2*, *CDH1*, *CHEK2*, *EPCAM* (deletion/duplication testing only), *GREM1* (promoter region deletion/duplication testing only), *MLH1*, *MSH2*, *MSH6*, *MUTYH*, *PMS2*, *POLD1*, *POLE*, *PTEN*, *STK11*, *TP53*). Two years after the initial molecular results, an amended report showed a heterozygous likely pathogenic *MLH1* variant, c.27G > A p.(Arg9=) (silent). The sequence change affects codon 9 of *MLH1* mRNA and is a "silent" change that does not change amino acid sequence. This variant is not present in population databases (not listed in gnomAD) and has shown to segregate in families with Lynch syndrome-associated tumors [136, 137]. ClinVar contains an entry for this variant (Variation ID: 186982). This variant demonstrated low-level methylation and segregates in Lynch syndrome families [136, 137].

Final Diagnosis

Reevaluation of the variant colon cancer panel sequencing data resulted an amendment of a negative report. A likely pathogenic *MLH1* variant, c.27G > A, is a "silent" change that did not alter amino acid sequence, but instead a constitutional epigenetic aberration in the *MLH1* gene.

Follow-Up

There is a 50% risk for offspring. Continued screening for this patient was recommended: (1) annual urine microscopy, (2) colonoscopy very 1–2 years, (3) upper endoscopy every 3–5 years since the patient's paternal aunt had stomach cancer at 30 years of age, and (4) continue annual mammograms with family history of breast cancer. Genetic counseling and testing for family members were also encouraged.

Discussion

Constitutional *MLH1* epimutation refers to an epigenetic aberration that is present on one parental allele throughout normal tissues and represses or activates expression from the affected allele. There are two categories of epimutations: primary and secondary. Primary epimutation arises spontaneously and is established at an early stage of development before the differentiation of the three germ layers (endoderm, ectoderm, and mesoderm). Primary epimutation is liable in germline and is reversible between successive generations due to erasure in germline; hence, inheritance is unpredictable. On the other hand, secondary epimutation is caused by *cis*-acting DNA sequence alteration that is present in the germline and follows Mendelian autosomal-dominant inheritance pattern [138]. Epimutations at the *MLH1* locus preferentially arise on the maternal allele and constitute the first "hit" in Knudson's two-hit hypothesis that predisposes carriers to cancer. The heterozygous *MLH1* c.27G > A silent variant is a secondary epimutation and follows a Mendelian autosomal-dominant inheritance pattern. Therefore, there is a 50% risk for offspring in this family.

The screening algorithm for *MLH1* epimutation testing of Lynch syndrome is rather complex, lacks consensus, and does not account for family history [138]. Epimutation is only suspected in patients with a personal history of Lynch syndrome-type tumor at age under 60 years at first cancer presentation with or without a family history. The major difference in epimutation carriers is the lack of family history due to de novo epimutations. The overlapping pathology features of *MLH1* methylation and loss of MLH1 expression with sporadic MSI cancers further confound *MLH1* epimutation testing such that sporadic tumor cases can have *MLH1* methylation and *BRAF* p.(Val600Glu) mutation. Consideration for genetics referral is usually indicated when MLH1 protein loss and/or MSI-high are detected in histopathologic review of the tumor.

Testing for *MLH1* epimutation (constitutional methylation) is performed with paired normal tissue or blood DNA. Other factors contributory to rarity of reported *MLH1* epimutation cases are false-negative results due to potential for mosaicism, variable inheritance pattern, and cost-effectiveness of screening (both normal and tumor tissues need to be tested simultaneously). Therefore, *MLH1* epimutations are likely overlooked and underdiagnosed. However, testing should be considered in individuals with young diagnosis or when high suspicion for Lynch syndrome.

Case 4

Learning Objective

Recognize the possibility of mosaicism in genetic testing and explanations for detected mosaicism in peripheral blood.

Case History

The patient has a personal and family history of cancer (Fig. 12.3). She has a personal history of papillary thyroid

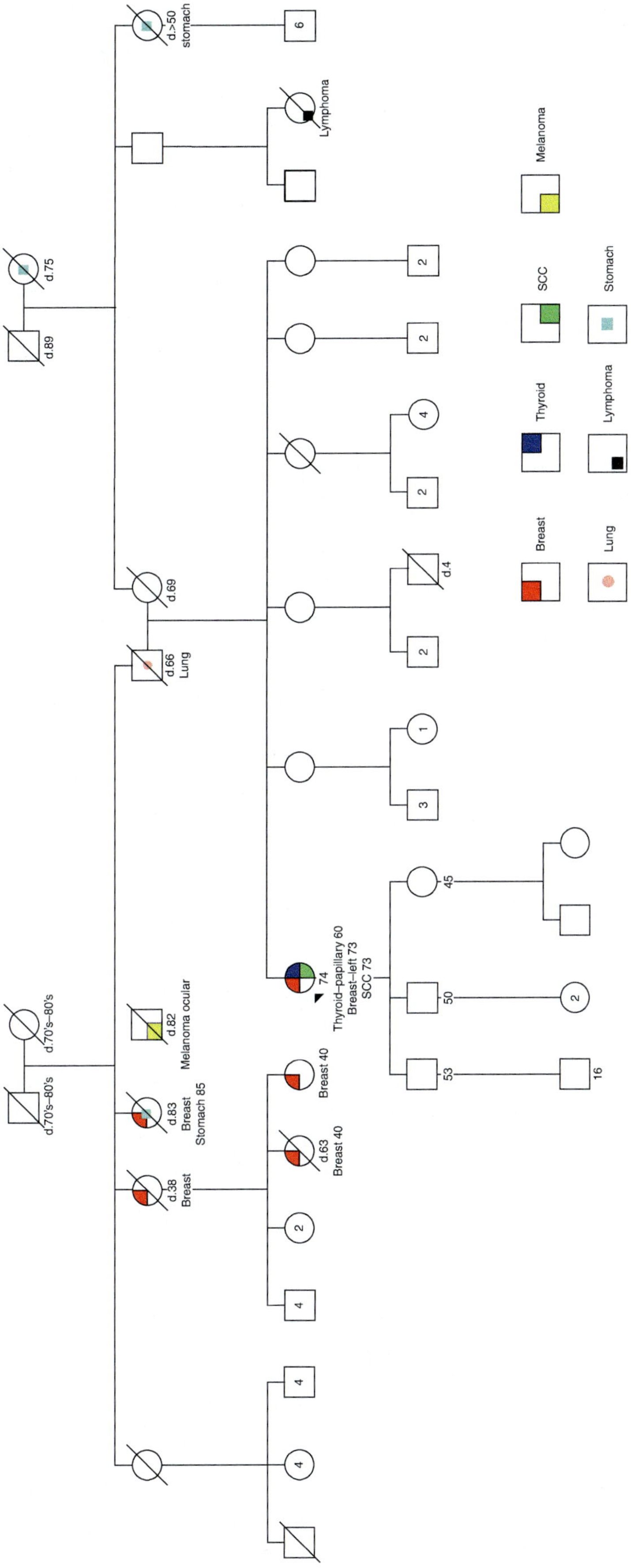

Fig. 12.3 Pedigree of a family with multiple family members affected with different tumor types suggestive of a hereditary cancer syndrome. The proband (noted with an *arrow*) harbors a mosaic germline *TP53* pathogenic variant

cancer at age 60 (treated with thyroidectomy), left breast cancer at age 73 treated with lumpectomy, and squamous cell carcinoma on her leg at age 73 treated with radiation and local chemotherapy. She also has a strong family history of cancer in her father (smoker), paternal aunt (breast cancer at age 40), and two paternal cousins (breast cancer in their 40s) among other family members with cancers, including lymphoma and ocular melanoma.

Genetic Study

Hereditary cancer panel testing was performed on a blood sample. Results indicated a variant of uncertain significance (VUS) in the *TP53* gene (possibly mosaic), c.700 T > C p.(Tyr234His), and a VUS in the *PDGFRA* gene, c.2164A > T p.(Ile722Phe). Given these variants were classified as VUS and no other family members were tested at the time, her surveillance for cancers did not change based on these results and was guided instead by her personal history.

Final Diagnosis

The patient has a *TP53* p.(Tyr234His) variant of uncertain significance, possibly mosaic with an estimated 11–15% allele frequency. Given the clinical history of the patient, testing of skin was recommended to determine whether the *TP53* variant is germline.

Follow-Up

Subsequent reanalysis of this patient's *TP53* variant p.(Tyr234His) years later reclassified the VUS to a likely pathogenic variant. Evaluation of the skin biopsy (fibroblast cells) was negative for the *TP53* variant. Since the variant was not detected in fibroblast cells, it is determined to be of somatic origin. Although constitutional mosaicism is a possibility, given the low allele frequency of 10–15% detected in a blood sample aging-related acquired clonal hematopoiesis is suspected [139]. The *TP53* likely pathogenic variant p.(Tyr234His), if constitutional mosaic, is associated with autosomal dominant Li-Fraumeni syndrome. Regardless, close surveillance for breast cancer by mammograms, colonoscopy, and periodic skin examination due to her history of skin cancer is part of the continued care due to the patient's history.

Discussion

TP53 is a cancer predisposition gene with autosomal-dominant inheritance for Li-Fraumeni syndrome, with an overall cancer risk for Li-Fraumeni syndrome (up to 100% in women) and NCCN guidelines for patients with germline pathogenic variants on the *TP53* gene. However, given the mosaic nature of the *TP53* likely pathogenic variant and the recognized possibility of aging-related clonal hematopoiesis, it is not known, although unlikely, whether there is mosaicism in other organs, such as ovarian tissues.

There are several possible explanations for a mosaic germline *TP53* variant detected in the blood of this patient's case:

- The mutation previously detected in the *TP53* gene may be somatic (developed over lifetime and not present in every cell of the patient's body) and may represent clonal hematopoiesis of indeterminate potential (CHIP) [140] – expanded the number of mutated stem cells that are different than normal blood cells, often as a result of aging.
- Mosaic Li-Fraumeni syndrome.
- Hematologic malignancy/pre-malignancy (i.e., leukemia).
- Circulating tumor cells.

Case 5

Learning Objective

Recognize that somatic findings may sometimes suggest a hereditary cancer syndrome.

Case History

A 37-year-old woman was diagnosed with high-grade serous ovarian cancer. Following resection and debulking, a tumor sample was analyzed for actionable variants in *BRCA1* and *BRCA2* to determine eligibility for treatment with poly-adenosine diphosphate-ribose polymerase (PARP) inhibitors.

Genetic Study

A sample of formalin-fixed paraffin-embedded resected tumor with 90% tumor cellularity was submitted for DNA extraction and NGS analysis of the *BRCA1* and *BRCA2* genes. A variant was detected in the *BRCA1* gene, c.2999delA p.(Glu1000Glyfs*24), at an allele frequency of 77%. This variant resulted in the deletion of one nucleotide, an adenine, at position 2999 of the *BRCA1* coding sequence, leading to premature translation termination. This variant was classified using the criteria recommended by the Association for Molecular Pathology [125] as Tier 1 (variant with strong clinical significance) since it had therapeutic implications with respect to PARP inhibitor therapy, as well the possibility that it may represent a pathogenic germline variant. Genetic counseling and germline testing were recommended.

Subsequent testing of DNA extracted from a blood sample from this patient also detected the c.2999delA p.(Glu1000Glyfs*24) variant in *BRCA1*. The allele frequency of the variant was 46%, consistent with a heterozygous germline change. The variant was classified as pathogenic using the criteria established by the ACMG and AMP for germline findings [126] using the following criteria:

- The variant is a null variant in the *BRCA1* gene, where the loss of function of one copy of the gene (haploinsufficiency) is the disease mechanism (ACMGG PVS1).
- The variant was not reported in population controls (ACMGG PM2).
- The variant was catalogued in ClinVar (ID: 54744), where it was reported to be pathogenic by several submitting laboratories (ACMGG PP5).

Final Diagnosis
The pathogenic variant in *BRCA1* confirmed the diagnosis of a hereditary breast and ovarian cancer syndrome.

Follow-Up
Genetic counselling and testing of family members for the c.2999delA p.(Glu1000Glyfs*24) variant in *BRCA1* was recommended.

Discussion
Mutations identified by somatic testing may represent ones which arose in the germline. If a germline variant is suspected, a referral for genetic counseling is recommended to facilitate additional testing on a normal tissue, such as the blood. Variant allele frequency of the somatic mutation should not alone be used to assess whether a variant arose in the germline, since a range of frequency values have been associated with germline findings [124]. Variant allele frequencies may be influenced by a number of factors, including tumor cellularity and heterogeneity and concomitant copy number changes in the sample.

Case 6

Learning Objective
Recognize the possibility of a germline pathogenic variant in somatic tumor testing and recommend appropriate testing of other tissue types when paired blood sample is not available. Acknowledge how different mutations in different tumor sites are critical for cancer staging or determining different primary tumors.

Case History
A 68-year-old-female has clinical history of early-stage breast cancer. She underwent a lumpectomy, radiation, and tamoxifen treatment. Adjuvant therapy was completed within treatment course. Approximately 12 years later, she developed intermittent febrile episodes, which was treated as Lyme disease with doxycycline. She denied tobacco use. Subsequent chest X-ray showed a right upper lobe (RUL) lung mass and multiple bilateral subcentimeter lung nodules that had significant uptake by PET scan. No uptake was seen in other lung nodules by PET, nor evidence of any regional or distant metastatic adenocarcinoma.

Histologic Features
Multiple lung nodules located on the right lower lobe (2×) and right upper lobe (1×) were assessed and were all reported as invasive adenocarcinomas with different morphohistological features (Fig. 12.4a–f).

- Tumor #1, right lower lobe (RLL; E2), had acinar and lepidic pattern with abundant lymphoid infiltrate.
- Tumor #2, right upper lobe (RUL; G3), was a 3.8-cm tumor with scar and had an acinar with minimal lepidic pattern and fibrotic stroma.
- Tumor #3, right lower lobe (RLL; H1), was a 0.8-cm tumor with an acinar pattern with loose connective tissue stroma.

Genetic Study
NGS mutation profiling using a 26-gene panel, when specimens were adequate, and allele-specific PCR-based lung cancer mutation panel (SNaPshot) testing were performed on the lung biopsies. An earlier sample of an RUL biopsy with limited tissue sample identified an *EGFR* p.(Thr790Met) mutation by SNaPshot. Subsequent SNaPshot molecular testing on tumors #1–3 identified the following molecular changes (Fig. 12.4g):

- Tumor #1 RLL (limited tissue, tumor cell content ~50%), tested by SNaPshot, had two *EGFR* variants, p.(Thr790Met) and p.(Gly719Ser), and was negative for *EGFR* and *ERBB2* (*HER2*) indel.
- Tumor #2 RUL (tumor cell content ~40%), tested by NGS mutation profiling using a 26-gene panel, identified two *EGFR* variants, p.(Thr790Met) and p.(Leu858Arg), at variant allele frequencies (VAF) of 52% and 17%, respectively, and a *TP53* p.(Arg273His) variant at a VAF of 23%.
- Tumor #3 RLL (tumor cell content ~40%), also tested by NGS mutation profiling using a 26-gene panel, identified the *EGFR* p.(Thr790Met) variant at a VAF of 46% and *EGFR* exon 19 deletion (15-bp) c.2238_2252del15 p.(Leu747_Thr751del) at a VAF of 19%.

Final Diagnosis
Non-small cell lung carcinoma with *EGFR* mutations. Different *EGFR* driver mutations in separate tumor nodules confirmed multiple *primary* tumors. Given the allele frequencies of *EGFR* p.(Thr790Met) variant in all three tumor nodules were close to 50%, it is possible that this mutation was germline. Additional germline testing was requested by the oncologist.

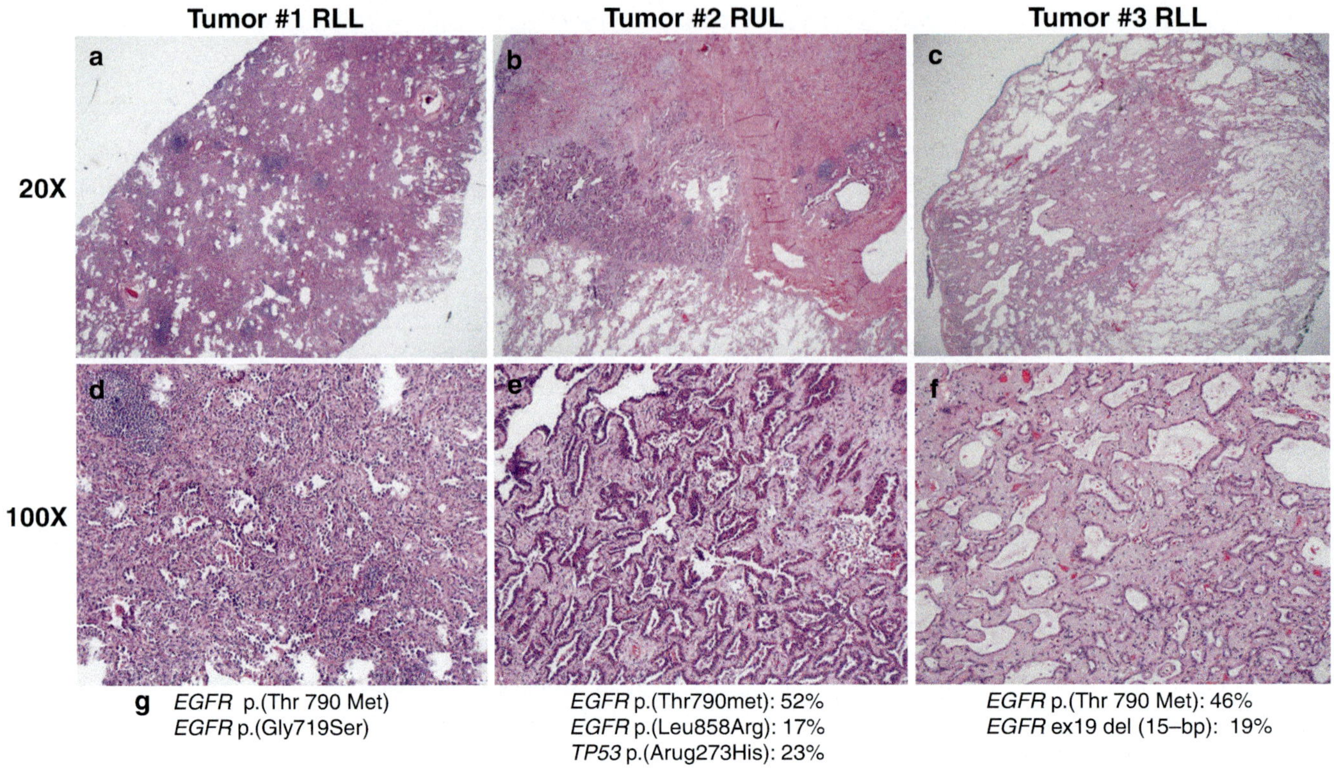

Fig. 12.4 H&E stain of multiple lung nodules at different locations. (**a**, **d**) Tumor #1 (block E2), located in the right lower lobe (RLL), has acinar and lepidic pattern with abundant lymphoid infiltrate. (**b**, **e**) Tumor #2 (block G3) situated in the right upper lobe (RUL) has an acinar with minimal lepidic pattern and fibrotic stroma. (**c**, **f**) Tumor #3 (block H1), located in the right lower lobe (RLL), has an acinar pattern with loose connective tissue stroma, and (**g**) tumor-associated sequencing results with gene mutations in *EGFR* and *TP53*. The variant allele frequency is shown next to the gene variant. Microscope objectives 20× (**a–c**) and 100× (**d–f**)

Follow-Up

Patient received adjuvant chemotherapy with carboplatin and pemetrexed and received periodic imaging and had stable subcentimeter pulmonary nodules. Paired peripheral blood was not available for germline testing. Consent had to be obtained from patient to proceed with additional testing of reactive benign lymph node, obtained during tumor resection, to determine whether the *EGFR* p.(Thr790Met) variant was germline. Morphologic and immunostain examination of reactive lymph node was negative for metastatic tumor and had no epithelial cell components. Target SNaPshot testing demonstrated a *EGFR* p.(Thr790Met).

Discussion

Different driver mutations observed in separate tumor nodules confirmed lung adenocarcinoma with multiple primary site tumors which had to be staged separately. Therefore, the three nodules were restaged as the following:

- Tumor #1, RLL: acinar predominant, 1.2 cm with 0.8 cm invasive component, pT1aN0
- Tumor #2, RUL: acinar predominant with mucinous features, 3.8 cm with scar, pT2aN0
- Tumor #3, RLL: acinar predominant, 0.8 cm with invasion, pT1aN0

Morphologic examination of reactive benign lymph node confirmed an *EGFR* p.(Thr790Met) germline variant. Somatic *EGFR* p.(Thr790Met) mutation is rare in untreated *EGFR*-mutated tumors (<5%) and is frequently detected (50%) in *EGFR*-mutated tumors with acquired resistance to first- and second-generation *EGFR* tyrosine kinase inhibitors (TKIs). Patients with the *EGFR* p.(Thr790Met) variant are treated with osimertinib, a third-generation TKI that irreversibly binds and inhibits p.(Thr790Met)-mutated *EGFR*.

Germline *EGFR* p.(Thr790Met) pathogenic variant has been reported in rare cases of lung cancer [141]. Germline carriers of *EGFR* p.(Thr790Met) have a unique autosomal-dominant hereditary lung cancer syndrome, with a preliminary estimate of 31% risk for lung cancer in never smoker carriers [142]. Of lung cancer tumors arising in germline *EGFR* p.(Thr790Met) carriers, approximately 73% of the cases contained a second activating *EGFR* gene mutation, as seen in this case [142].

Patients with germline pathogenic variant can develop multiple tumors with different somatic mutations, as in the case of this patient. In addition, recognizing different mutations is critical for cancer staging; in this case, there were three distinct primary tumors. In conclusion, it is not uncommon to detect potentially pathogenic germline variants in somatic cancer mutation profiling tests. Additional germline testing must be discussed with oncologists and consent, and counseling of patient should be obtained prior to testing.

Case 7

Learning Objective

Recognize a germline pathogenic variant in somatic tumor testing, apply evidence-based variant classification, recommend germline testing of different tissue type, and show the importance of further monitoring for secondary cancers.

Case History

A 55-year-old woman, with no prior history of tobacco use, had a lung nodule detected in the right middle lobe during a clinical visit. She did not experience weight loss, coughing, or pain. PET scan showed a 2-cm ^{18}Fluorodeoxyglucose uptake in the right middle lobe (RML) nodule and 8-mm non-FDG right upper lobe (RUL) nodule. The patient had a RML lobectomy, and two separate nodules were found at pathology examination, large (E2) and small (E6).

Histologic Features

Lung biopsy of the right middle lobe identified two distinct nodules with different morphological patterns (Fig. 12.5a–d). The final morphohistological diagnosis was pulmonary adenocarcinoma, acinar predominant with lesser components of micropapillary and lepidic growth. The two nodules identified were:

- Tumor #1, large nodule 4.4 × 3.0 × 1.4 cm (E2), was acinar and micropapillary pattern with a stage of pT2bN0.
- Tumor #2, small nodule 0.8 × 0.9 × 0.6 cm (E6), had a lepidic pattern with follicular lymphoid infiltrate and was minimally invasive.
- The RUL lesion was not biopsied.

Genetic Study

NGS mutation profiling using a 26-gene panel was performed on both lesions and identified the following molecular changes (Fig. 12.5e):

- Tumor #1, RML large nodule, had an *EGFR* 15-bp exon 19 deletion, c.2238_2252del p.(Leu747_Thr751del), and *TP53* c.455C > T p.(Pro152Leu) mutation at variant allele frequencies of 18% and 58%, respectively.
- Tumor #2, RML small nodule, had a different *EGFR* 15-bp exon 19 deletion, c.2236_2250del p.(Glu746_

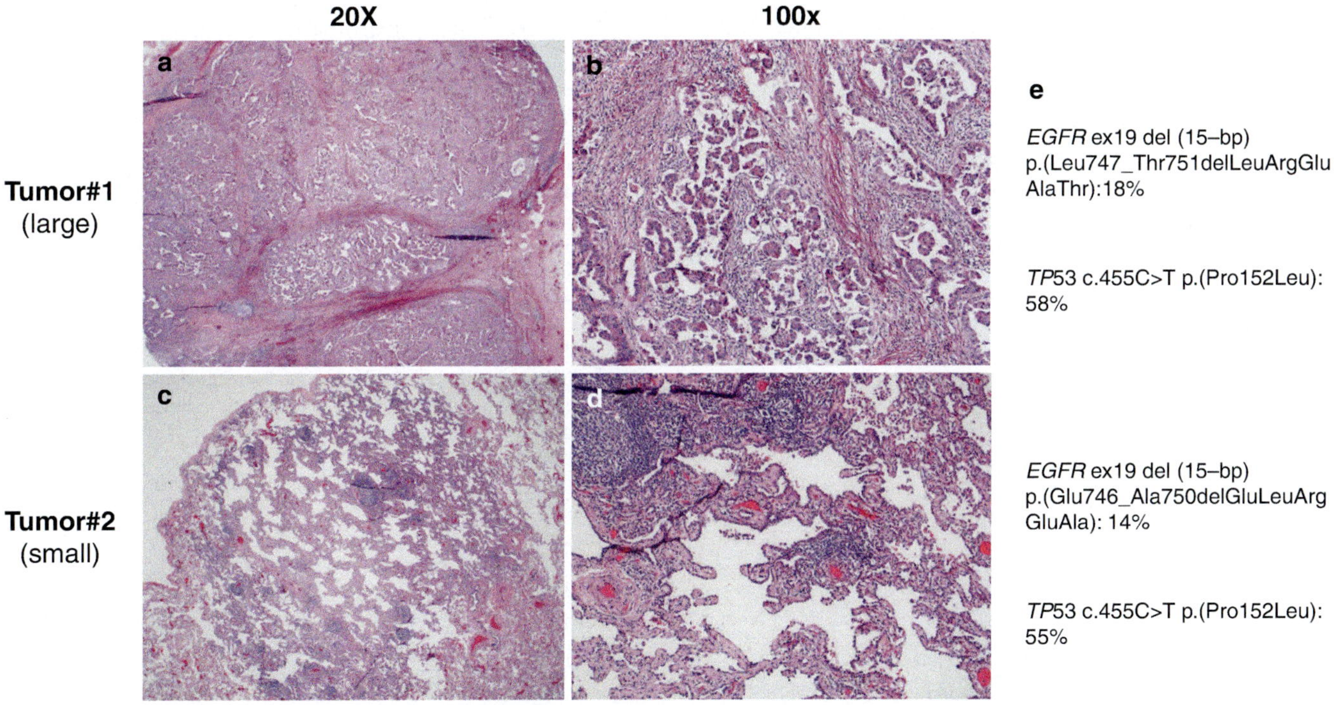

Fig. 12.5 H&E stain of two distinct lung nodules from the right middle lobe. (**a**, **c**) Tumor #1 (block E2), large nodule, has an acinar and micropapillary pattern with a stage of pT2bN0, and (**b**, **d**) Tumor #2 (block E6), small nodule, has a lepidic pattern with follicular lymphoid infiltrate and was minimally invasive. (**e**) Tumor-associated sequencing identified gene mutations in *EGFR* and *TP53*. The variant allele frequency is reported next to the gene variant. Microscope objectives 20× (**a**, **c**) and 100× (**b**, **d**)

Ala750del), and *TP53* c.455C > T p.(Pro152Leu) mutation at variant allele frequencies of 14% and 55%, respectively.

Given the variant allele frequencies of *TP53* c.455C > T p.(Pro152Leu) mutation in both nodules were close to 50%, the possibility of a *TP53* germline variant was suspected. After patient's consent, additional testing of peripheral blood confirmed a germline *TP53* p.(Pro152Leu) pathogenic variant in this patient.

Final Diagnosis

Non-small cell lung carcinoma with *EGFR* somatic mutations with germline *TP53* p.(Pro152Leu) pathogenic variant associated with Li-Fraumeni syndrome.

Follow-Up

The patient underwent adjuvant chemotherapy with cisplatin and pemetrexed. No lung nodules were detected in post-treatment CT scan. Due to the presence of the germline *TP53* pathogenic variant p.(Pro152Leu), the patient will need continual monitoring for secondary cancers by CT and MRI.

Discussion

The *TP53* gene is highly mutated in lung cancer (46% adenocarcinoma and 81% squamous cell carcinoma). Hotspot somatic mutations in *TP53* are typically related to smoking and associated with poor treatment response and unfavorable outcome. However, germline *TP53* pathogenic variants are not commonly detected in lung cancer [143]. *TP53* transactivation assay demonstrated a low-functioning allele and dominant negative effect and loss of function of TP53 protein (ACMGG PS3; [144, 145]). This particular *TP53* variant has been reported in multiple families with Li-Fraumeni-like (LFL) syndrome (ACMGG PP1; [146]) and in individuals affected with adrenocortical cancer, breast cancer, gastric cancer, or colorectal cancer and melanoma (ACMGG PS4; [147–150]). Additionally, this variant co-segregated with disease in multiple affected family members (ACMGG PP1; [151]).

This variant was catalogued in ClinVar (ID: 152480), where it was reported to be pathogenic by several submitting laboratories (ACMGG PP5). In summary, *TP53* c.455C > T p.(Pro152Leu) met the criteria to be classified as pathogenic for Li-Fraumeni syndrome in an autosomal-dominant manner based upon multiple reports in affected individuals, segregation studies, low frequency in controls, and functional evidence [126].

The authors acknowledge the gracious contributions of cases by genetic counselors Christine Tallo, MMSc, CGC and Christine Stanislaw, MMSc, CGC (Cases 2–4) from the Winship Cancer Institute of Emory University, and Dr. Linsheng Zhang (Cases 6 and 7) from the Department of Pathology and Laboratory Medicine of Emory University.

References

1. Hereditary Cancer Syndromes and Risk Assessment. ACOG Committee Opinion, Number 793. Obstet Gynecol. 2019;134(6):e143–e9. https://doi.org/10.1097/AOG.0000000000003562.
2. Rahman N. Realizing the promise of cancer predisposition genes. Nature. 2014;505(7483):302–8. https://doi.org/10.1038/nature12981.
3. Garber JE, Offit K. Hereditary cancer predisposition syndromes. J Clin Oncol. 2005;23(2):276–92. https://doi.org/10.1200/JCO.2005.10.042.
4. Petrucelli N, Daly MB, Pal T. BRCA1- and BRCA2-associated hereditary breast and ovarian cancer. In: Adam MP, Ardinger HH, Pagon RA, Wallace SE, Bean LJH, Mirzaa G, et al., editors. GeneReviews((R)). Seattle; 1993.
5. Schneider K, Zelley K, Nichols KE, Garber J. Li-Fraumeni syndrome. In: Adam MP, Ardinger HH, Pagon RA, Wallace SE, Bean LJH, Mirzaa G, et al., editors. GeneReviews((R)). Seattle; 1993.
6. Eng C. PTEN Hamartoma tumor syndrome. In: Adam MP, Ardinger HH, Pagon RA, Wallace SE, Bean LJH, Mirzaa G, et al., editors. GeneReviews((R)). Seattle; 1993.
7. Rothblum-Oviatt C, Wright J, Lefton-Greif MA, McGrath-Morrow SA, Crawford TO, Lederman HM. Ataxia telangiectasia: a review. Orphanet J Rare Dis. 2016;11(1):159. https://doi.org/10.1186/s13023-016-0543-7.
8. Duraturo F, Liccardo R, De Rosa M, Izzo P. Genetics, diagnosis and treatment of Lynch syndrome: old lessons and current challenges. Oncol Lett. 2019;17(3):3048–54. https://doi.org/10.3892/ol.2019.9945.
9. Jasperson KW, Patel SG, Ahnen DJ. APC-associated polyposis conditions. In: Adam MP, Ardinger HH, Pagon RA, Wallace SE, Bean LJH, Mirzaa G, et al., editors. GeneReviews((R)). Seattle; 1993.
10. Kaurah P, Huntsman DG. Hereditary diffuse gastric cancer. In: Adam MP, Ardinger HH, Pagon RA, Wallace SE, Bean LJH, Mirzaa G, et al., editors. GeneReviews((R)). Seattle; 1993.
11. Larsen Haidle J, Howe JR. Juvenile polyposis syndrome. In: Adam MP, Ardinger HH, Pagon RA, Wallace SE, Bean LJH, Mirzaa G, et al., editors. GeneReviews((R)). Seattle; 1993.
12. McGarrity TJ, Amos CI, Baker MJ. Peutz-Jeghers Syndrome. In: Adam MP, Ardinger HH, Pagon RA, Wallace SE, Bean LJH, Mirzaa G, et al., editors. GeneReviews((R)). Seattle; 1993.
13. Gironi LC, Colombo E, Farinelli P, Giorgione R, Bozzola C, Ogliara P, et al. Germline CDKN2A mutations in childhood melanoma: a case of melanoma-pancreatic cancer syndrome. Int J Dermatol. 2015;54(12):e553–5. https://doi.org/10.1111/ijd.12933.
14. Bottillo I, Valiante M, Menale L, Paiardini A, Papi L, Janson G, et al. A novel CDKN2A in-frame deletion associated with pancreatic cancer-melanoma syndrome. Dermatol Online J. 2020;26(8)
15. Shelton C, Solomon S, LaRusch J, Whitcomb DC. PRSS1-related hereditary pancreatitis. In: Adam MP, Ardinger HH, Pagon RA, Wallace SE, Bean LJH, Mirzaa G, et al., editors. GeneReviews((R)). Seattle; 1993.
16. Shelton C, LaRusch J, Whitcomb DC. Pancreatitis overview. In: Adam MP, Ardinger HH, Pagon RA, Wallace SE, Bean LJH, Mirzaa G, et al., editors. GeneReviews((R)). Seattle; 1993.
17. Khattab A, Monga DK. Turcot syndrome. Treasure Island: StatPearls; 2020.
18. Fornasarig M, Gasparotto D, Foltran L, Campigotto M, Lombardi S, Del Savio E, et al. A novel kindred with familial gastrointestinal stromal tumors caused by a rare KIT germline mutation (N655K): clinico-pathological presentation and TKI sensitivity. J Pers Med. 2020;10(4) https://doi.org/10.3390/jpm10040234.

19. Halpern AL, Torphy RJ, McCarter MD, Sciotto CG, Glode LM, Robinson WA. A familial germline mutation in KIT associated with achalasia, mastocytosis and gastrointestinal stromal tumors shows response to kinase inhibitors. Cancer Genet. 2019.;233–234:1–6. https://doi.org/10.1016/j.cancergen.2019.02.001.
20. Das S, Salami SS, Spratt DE, Kaffenberger SD, Jacobs MF, Morgan TM. Bringing prostate cancer germline genetics into clinical practice. J Urol. 2019;202(2):223–30. https://doi.org/10.1097/JU.0000000000000137.
21. Giri VN, Hegarty SE, Hyatt C, O'Leary E, Garcia J, Knudsen KE, et al. Germline genetic testing for inherited prostate cancer in practice: implications for genetic testing, precision therapy, and cascade testing. Prostate. 2019;79(4):333–9. https://doi.org/10.1002/pros.23739.
22. Heidegger I, Tsaur I, Borgmann H, Surcel C, Kretschmer A, Mathieu R, et al. Hereditary prostate cancer – primetime for genetic testing? Cancer Treat Rev. 2019;81:101927. https://doi.org/10.1016/j.ctrv.2019.101927.
23. Sajorda BJ, Gonzalez-Gandolfi CX, Hathaway ER, Kalish JM. Simpson-Golabi-Behmel syndrome Type 1. In: Adam MP, Ardinger HH, Pagon RA, Wallace SE, Bean LJH, Mirzaa G, et al., editors. GeneReviews((R)). Seattle; 1993.
24. van Leeuwaarde RS, Ahmad S, Links TP, Giles RH. Von Hippel-Lindau syndrome. In: Adam MP, Ardinger HH, Pagon RA, Wallace SE, Bean LJH, Mirzaa G, et al., editors. GeneReviews((R)). Seattle; 1993.
25. Brioude F, Kalish JM, Mussa A, Foster AC, Bliek J, Ferrero GB, et al. Expert consensus document: clinical and molecular diagnosis, screening and management of Beckwith-Wiedemann syndrome: an international consensus statement. Nat Rev Endocrinol. 2018;14(4):229–49. https://doi.org/10.1038/nrendo.2017.166.
26. Dome JS, Huff V. Wilms tumor predisposition. In: Adam MP, Ardinger HH, Pagon RA, Wallace SE, Bean LJH, Mirzaa G, et al., editors. GeneReviews((R)). Seattle; 1993.
27. Sattler EC, Steinlein OK. Birt-Hogg-Dube syndrome. In: Adam MP, Ardinger HH, Pagon RA, Wallace SE, Bean LJH, Mirzaa G, et al., editors. GeneReviews((R)). Seattle; 1993.
28. Smith PS, Whitworth J, West H, Cook J, Gardiner C, Lim DHK, et al. Characterization of renal cell carcinoma-associated constitutional chromosome abnormalities by genome sequencing. Genes Chromosomes Cancer. 2020;59(6):333–47. https://doi.org/10.1002/gcc.22833.
29. Kato T, Franconi CP, Sheridan MB, Hacker AM, Inagakai H, Glover TW, et al. Analysis of the t(3;8) of hereditary renal cell carcinoma: a palindrome-mediated translocation. Cancer Genet. 2014;207(4):133–40. https://doi.org/10.1016/j.cancergen.2014.03.004.
30. Poland KS, Azim M, Folsom M, Goldfarb R, Naeem R, Korch C, et al. A constitutional balanced t(3;8)(p14;q24.1) translocation results in disruption of the TRC8 gene and predisposition to clear cell renal cell carcinoma. Genes Chromosomes Cancer. 2007;46(9):805–12. https://doi.org/10.1002/gcc.20466.
31. Nemes K, Bens S, Bourdeaut F, Hasselblatt M, Kool M, Johann P, et al. Rhabdoid tumor predisposition syndrome. In: Adam MP, Ardinger HH, Pagon RA, Wallace SE, Bean LJH, Mirzaa G, et al., editors. GeneReviews((R)). Seattle; 1993.
32. Else T, Greenberg S, Fishbein L. Hereditary paraganglioma-pheochromocytoma syndromes. In: Adam MP, Ardinger HH, Pagon RA, Wallace SE, Bean LJH, Mirzaa G, et al., editors. GeneReviews((R)). Seattle; 1993.
33. Lohmann DR, Gallie BL. Retinoblastoma. In: Adam MP, Ardinger HH, Pagon RA, Wallace SE, Bean LJH, Mirzaa G, et al., editors. GeneReviews((R)). Seattle; 1993.
34. Wuyts W, Schmale GA, Chansky HA, Raskind WH. Hereditary multiple osteochondromas. In: Adam MP, Ardinger HH, Pagon RA, Wallace SE, Bean LJH, Mirzaa G, et al., editors. GeneReviews((R)). Seattle; 1993.
35. Ooi A. Advances in hereditary leiomyomatosis and renal cell carcinoma (HLRCC) research. Semin Cancer Biol. 2020;61:158–66. https://doi.org/10.1016/j.semcancer.2019.10.016.
36. Trpkov K, Hes O, Agaimy A, Bonert M, Martinek P, Magi-Galluzzi C, et al. Fumarate Hydratase-deficient renal cell carcinoma is strongly correlated with Fumarate Hydratase mutation and hereditary Leiomyomatosis and renal cell carcinoma syndrome. Am J Surg Pathol. 2016;40(7):865–75. https://doi.org/10.1097/PAS.0000000000000617.
37. Chayed Z, Kristensen LK, Ousager LB, Ronlund K, Bygum A. Hereditary leiomyomatosis and renal cell carcinoma: a case series and literature review. Orphanet J Rare Dis. 2021;16(1):34. https://doi.org/10.1186/s13023-020-01653-9.
38. Oshima J, Martin GM, Hisama FM. Werner syndrome. In: Adam MP, Ardinger HH, Pagon RA, Wallace SE, Bean LJH, Mirzaa G, et al., editors. GeneReviews((R)). Seattle; 1993.
39. Giusti F, Marini F, Brandi ML. Multiple Endocrine Neoplasia Type 1. In: Adam MP, Ardinger HH, Pagon RA, Wallace SE, Bean LJH, Mirzaa G, et al., editors. GeneReviews((R)). Seattle; 1993.
40. Eng C. Multiple Endocrine Neoplasia Type 2. In: Adam MP, Ardinger HH, Pagon RA, Wallace SE, Bean LJH, Mirzaa G, et al., editors. GeneReviews((R)). Seattle; 1993.
41. Leachman SA, Lucero OM, Sampson JE, Cassidy P, Bruno W, Queirolo P, et al. Identification, genetic testing, and management of hereditary melanoma. Cancer Metastasis Rev. 2017;36(1):77–90. https://doi.org/10.1007/s10555-017-9661-5.
42. Bresler SC, Padwa BL, Granter SR. Nevoid basal cell carcinoma syndrome (Gorlin syndrome). Head Neck Pathol. 2016;10(2):119–24. https://doi.org/10.1007/s12105-016-0706-9.
43. Soura E, Eliades PJ, Shannon K, Stratigos AJ, Tsao H. Hereditary melanoma: update on syndromes and management: genetics of familial atypical multiple mole melanoma syndrome. J Am Acad Dermatol. 2016;74(3):395–407.; quiz 8–10. https://doi.org/10.1016/j.jaad.2015.08.038.
44. Lopes S, Vide J, Moreira E, Azevedo F. Cowden syndrome: clinical case and a brief review. Dermatol Online J. 2017;23(8)
45. Friedman JM. Neurofibromatosis 1. In: Adam MP, Ardinger HH, Pagon RA, Wallace SE, Bean LJH, Mirzaa G, et al., editors. GeneReviews((R)). Seattle; 1993.
46. Evans DG. Neurofibromatosis 2. In: Adam MP, Ardinger HH, Pagon RA, Wallace SE, Bean LJH, Mirzaa G, et al., editors. GeneReviews((R)). Seattle; 1993.
47. Northrup H, Koenig MK, Pearson DA, Au KS. Tuberous sclerosis complex. In: Adam MP, Ardinger HH, Pagon RA, Wallace SE, Bean LJH, Mirzaa G, et al., editors. GeneReviews((R)). Seattle; 1993.
48. Stratakis CA, Raygada M. Carney complex. In: Adam MP, Ardinger HH, Pagon RA, Wallace SE, Bean LJH, Mirzaa G, et al., editors. GeneReviews((R)). Seattle; 1993.
49. Tawana K, Rio-Machin A, Preudhomme C, Fitzgibbon J. Familial CEBPA-mutated acute myeloid leukemia. Semin Hematol. 2017;54(2):87–93. https://doi.org/10.1053/j.seminhematol.2017.04.001.
50. Tawana K, Wang J, Renneville A, Bodor C, Hills R, Loveday C, et al. Disease evolution and outcomes in familial AML with germline CEBPA mutations. Blood. 2015;126(10):1214–23. https://doi.org/10.1182/blood-2015-05-647172.
51. West AH, Godley LA, Churpek JE. Familial myelodysplastic syndrome/acute leukemia syndromes: a review and utility for translational investigations. Ann N Y Acad Sci. 2014;1310:111–8. https://doi.org/10.1111/nyas.12346.
52. McReynolds LJ, Calvo KR, Holland SM. Germline GATA2 mutation and bone marrow failure. Hematol Oncol Clin North Am. 2018;32(4):713–28. https://doi.org/10.1016/j.hoc.2018.04.004.

53. Diness BR, Risom L, Frandsen TL, Hansen B, Andersen MK, Schmiegelow K, et al. Putative new childhood leukemia cancer predisposition syndrome caused by germline bi-allelic missense mutations in DDX41. Genes Chromosomes Cancer. 2018;57(12):670–4. https://doi.org/10.1002/gcc.22680.
54. Cheah JJC, Hahn CN, Hiwase DK, Scott HS, Brown AL. Myeloid neoplasms with germline DDX41 mutation. Int J Hematol. 2017;106(2):163–74. https://doi.org/10.1007/s12185-017-2260-y.
55. Babushok DV, Bessler M, Olson TS. Genetic predisposition to myelodysplastic syndrome and acute myeloid leukemia in children and young adults. Leuk Lymphoma. 2016;57(3):520–36. https://doi.org/10.3109/10428194.2015.1115041.
56. Sood R, Kamikubo Y, Liu P. Role of RUNX1 in hematological malignancies. Blood. 2017;129(15):2070–82. https://doi.org/10.1182/blood-2016-10-687830.
57. Yokota A, Huo L, Lan F, Wu J, Huang G. The clinical, molecular, and mechanistic basis of RUNX1 mutations identified in hematological malignancies. Mol Cells. 2020;43(2):145–52. https://doi.org/10.14348/molcells.2019.0252.
58. Kewan T, Noss R, Godley LA, Rogers HJ, Carraway HE. Inherited thrombocytopenia caused by germline ANKRD26 mutation should be considered in young patients with suspected myelodysplastic syndrome. J Investig Med High Impact Case Rep. 2020;8:2324709620938941. https://doi.org/10.1177/2324709620938941.
59. Perez Botero J, Dugan SN, Anderson MW. ANKRD26-related thrombocytopenia. In: Adam MP, Ardinger HH, Pagon RA, Wallace SE, Bean LJH, Mirzaa G, et al., editors. GeneReviews((R)). Seattle; 1993.
60. Rampersaud E, Ziegler DS, Iacobucci I, Payne-Turner D, Churchman ML, Schrader KA, et al. Germline deletion of ETV6 in familial acute lymphoblastic leukemia. Blood Adv. 2019;3(7):1039–46. https://doi.org/10.1182/bloodadvances.2018030635.
61. Noetzli L, Lo RW, Lee-Sherick AB, Callaghan M, Noris P, Savoia A, et al. Germline mutations in ETV6 are associated with thrombocytopenia, red cell macrocytosis and predisposition to lymphoblastic leukemia. Nat Genet. 2015;47(5):535–8. https://doi.org/10.1038/ng.3253.
62. Pui CH, Nichols KE, Yang JJ. Somatic and germline genomics in paediatric acute lymphoblastic leukaemia. Nat Rev Clin Oncol. 2019;16(4):227–40. https://doi.org/10.1038/s41571-018-0136-6.
63. Churchman ML, Qian M, Te Kronnie G, Zhang R, Yang W, Zhang H, et al. Germline genetic IKZF1 variation and predisposition to childhood acute lymphoblastic leukemia. Cancer Cell. 2018;33(5):937–48. e8. https://doi.org/10.1016/j.ccell.2018.03.021.
64. Auer F, Ruschendorf F, Gombert M, Husemann P, Ginzel S, Izraeli S, et al. Inherited susceptibility to pre B-ALL caused by germline transmission of PAX5 c.547G>A. Leukemia. 2014;28(5):1136–8. https://doi.org/10.1038/leu.2013.363.
65. Perez-Garcia A, Ambesi-Impiombato A, Hadler M, Rigo I, LeDuc CA, Kelly K, et al. Genetic loss of SH2B3 in acute lymphoblastic leukemia. Blood. 2013;122(14):2425–32. https://doi.org/10.1182/blood-2013-05-500850.
66. Gu Z, Churchman ML, Roberts KG, Moore I, Zhou X, Nakitandwe J, et al. PAX5-driven subtypes of B-progenitor acute lymphoblastic leukemia. Nat Genet. 2019;51(2):296–307. https://doi.org/10.1038/s41588-018-0315-5.
67. Shah S, Schrader KA, Waanders E, Timms AE, Vijai J, Miething C, et al. A recurrent germline PAX5 mutation confers susceptibility to pre-B cell acute lymphoblastic leukemia. Nat Genet. 2013;45(10):1226–31. https://doi.org/10.1038/ng.2754.
68. Abedalthagafi M. Constitutional mismatch repair-deficiency: current problems and emerging therapeutic strategies. Oncotarget. 2018;9(83):35458–69. https://doi.org/10.18632/oncotarget.26249.
69. Lavoine N, Colas C, Muleris M, Bodo S, Duval A, Entz-Werle N, et al. Constitutional mismatch repair deficiency syndrome: clinical description in a French cohort. J Med Genet. 2015;52(11):770–8. https://doi.org/10.1136/jmedgenet-2015-103299.
70. Tanase-Nakao K, Olson TS, Narumi S. MIRAGE syndrome. In: Adam MP, Ardinger HH, Pagon RA, Wallace SE, Bean LJH, Mirzaa G, et al., editors. GeneReviews((R)). Seattle; 1993.
71. Phowthongkum P, Chen DH, Raskind WH, Bird TD. SAMD9L-related ataxia-pancytopenia syndrome. In: Adam MP, Ardinger HH, Pagon RA, Wallace SE, Bean LJH, Mirzaa G, et al., editors. GeneReviews((R)). Seattle; 1993.
72. Bannon SA, DiNardo CD. Hereditary predispositions to myelodysplastic syndrome. Int J Mol Sci. 2016;17(6) https://doi.org/10.3390/ijms17060838.
73. Kirwan M, Walne AJ, Plagnol V, Velangi M, Ho A, Hossain U, et al. Exome sequencing identifies autosomal-dominant SRP72 mutations associated with familial aplasia and myelodysplasia. Am J Hum Genet. 2012;90(5):888–92. https://doi.org/10.1016/j.ajhg.2012.03.020.
74. Flanagan M, Cunniff CM. Bloom syndrome. In: Adam MP, Ardinger HH, Pagon RA, Wallace SE, Bean LJH, Mirzaa G, et al., editors. GeneReviews((R)). Seattle; 1993.
75. Mehta PA, Tolar J. Fanconi anemia. In: Adam MP, Ardinger HH, Pagon RA, Wallace SE, Bean LJH, Mirzaa G, et al., editors. GeneReviews((R)). Seattle; 1993.
76. Banka S. G6PC3 deficiency. In: Adam MP, Ardinger HH, Pagon RA, Wallace SE, Bean LJH, Mirzaa G, et al., editors. GeneReviews((R)). Seattle; 1993.
77. Chandra S, Bronicki L, Nagaraj CB, Zhang K. WAS-related disorders. In: Adam MP, Ardinger HH, Pagon RA, Wallace SE, Bean LJH, Mirzaa G, et al., editors. GeneReviews((R)). Seattle; 1993.
78. Skokowa J, Dale DC, Touw IP, Zeidler C, Welte K. Severe congenital neutropenias. Nat Rev Dis Primers. 2017;3:17032. https://doi.org/10.1038/nrdp.2017.32.
79. Nelson A, Myers K. Shwachman-Diamond syndrome. In: Adam MP, Ardinger HH, Pagon RA, Wallace SE, Bean LJH, Mirzaa G, et al., editors. GeneReviews((R)). Seattle; 1993.
80. Clinton C, Gazda HT. Diamond-Blackfan anemia. In: Adam MP, Ardinger HH, Pagon RA, Wallace SE, Bean LJH, Mirzaa G, et al., editors. GeneReviews((R)). Seattle; 1993.
81. Varon R, Demuth I, Chrzanowska KH. Nijmegen breakage syndrome. In: Adam MP, Ardinger HH, Pagon RA, Wallace SE, Bean LJH, Mirzaa G, et al., editors. GeneReviews((R)). Seattle; 1993.
82. Bleesing JJH, Nagaraj CB, Zhang K. Autoimmune lymphoproliferative syndrome. In: Adam MP, Ardinger HH, Pagon RA, Wallace SE, Bean LJH, Mirzaa G, et al., editors. GeneReviews((R)). Seattle; 1993.
83. Han SS, Wen KK, Vyas YM. Deficiency of Wiskott-Aldrich syndrome protein has opposing effect on the pro-oncogenic pathway activation in nonmalignant versus malignant lymphocytes. Oncogene. 2021;40(2):345–54. https://doi.org/10.1038/s41388-020-01533-3.
84. Mastio J, Saeed MB, Wurzer H, Krecke M, Westerberg LS, Thomas C. Higher incidence of B cell malignancies in primary immunodeficiencies: a combination of intrinsic genomic instability and exocytosis defects at the immunological synapse. Front Immunol. 2020;11:581119. https://doi.org/10.3389/fimmu.2020.581119.
85. Mayor PC, Eng KH, Singel KL, Abrams SI, Odunsi K, Moysich KB, et al. Cancer in primary immunodeficiency diseases: cancer incidence in the United States immune deficiency network registry. J Allergy Clin Immunol. 2018;141(3):1028–35. https://doi.org/10.1016/j.jaci.2017.05.024.
86. Smpokou P, Zand DJ, Rosenbaum KN, Summar ML. Malignancy in Noonan syndrome and related disorders. Clin Genet. 2015;88(6):516–22. https://doi.org/10.1111/cge.12568.

87. Strullu M, Caye A, Lachenaud J, Cassinat B, Gazal S, Fenneteau O, et al. Juvenile myelomonocytic leukaemia and Noonan syndrome. J Med Genet. 2014;51(10):689–97. https://doi.org/10.1136/jmedgenet-2014-102611.
88. Niewisch MR, Savage SA. An update on the biology and management of dyskeratosis congenita and related telomere biology disorders. Expert Rev Hematol. 2019;12(12):1037–52. https://doi.org/10.1080/17474086.2019.1662720.
89. Fouad YA, Aanei C. Revisiting the hallmarks of cancer. Am J Cancer Res. 2017;7(5):1016–36.
90. Hanahan D, Weinberg RA. The hallmarks of cancer. Cell. 2000;100(1):57–70. https://doi.org/10.1016/s0092-8674(00)81683-9.
91. Kinzler KW, Vogelstein B. Lessons from hereditary colorectal cancer. Cell. 1996;87(2):159–70. https://doi.org/10.1016/s0092-8674(00)81333-1.
92. Stieglitz E, Loh ML. Genetic predispositions to childhood leukemia. Ther Adv Hematol. 2013;4(4):270–90. https://doi.org/10.1177/2040620713498161.
93. Nickels EM, Soodalter J, Churpek JE, Godley LA. Recognizing familial myeloid leukemia in adults. Ther Adv Hematol. 2013;4(4):254–69. https://doi.org/10.1177/2040620713487399.
94. Seif AE. Pediatric leukemia predisposition syndromes: clues to understanding leukemogenesis. Cancer Genet. 2011;204(5):227–44. https://doi.org/10.1016/j.cancergen.2011.04.005.
95. Czuchlewski DR, Peterson LC. Myeloid neoplasms with germline predisposition: a new provisional entity within the World Health Organization classification. Surg Pathol Clin. 2016;9(1):165–76. https://doi.org/10.1016/j.path.2015.09.010.
96. Zhang MY, Keel SB, Walsh T, Lee MK, Gulsuner S, Watts AC, et al. Genomic analysis of bone marrow failure and myelodysplastic syndromes reveals phenotypic and diagnostic complexity. Haematologica. 2015;100(1):42–8. https://doi.org/10.3324/haematol.2014.113456.
97. Ghemlas I, Li H, Zlateska B, Klaassen R, Fernandez CV, Yanofsky RA, et al. Improving diagnostic precision, care and syndrome definitions using comprehensive next-generation sequencing for the inherited bone marrow failure syndromes. J Med Genet. 2015;52(9):575–84. https://doi.org/10.1136/jmedgenet-2015-103270.
98. Furutani E, Shimamura A. Germline genetic predisposition to hematologic malignancy. J Clin Oncol. 2017;35(9):1018–28. https://doi.org/10.1200/JCO.2016.70.8644.
99. Muramatsu H, Okuno Y, Yoshida K, Shiraishi Y, Doisaki S, Narita A, et al. Clinical utility of next-generation sequencing for inherited bone marrow failure syndromes. Genet Med. 2017;19(7):796–802. https://doi.org/10.1038/gim.2016.197.
100. Shimamura A. Aplastic anemia and clonal evolution: germ line and somatic genetics. Hematology Am Soc Hematol Educ Program. 2016;2016(1):74–82. https://doi.org/10.1182/asheducation-2016.1.74.
101. Arber DA, Orazi A, Hasserjian R, Thiele J, Borowitz MJ, Le Beau MM, et al. The 2016 revision to the World Health Organization classification of myeloid neoplasms and acute leukemia. Blood. 2016;127(20):2391–405. https://doi.org/10.1182/blood-2016-03-643544.
102. Godley LA. Inherited predisposition to acute myeloid leukemia. Semin Hematol. 2014;51(4):306–21. https://doi.org/10.1053/j.seminhematol.2014.08.001.
103. Owen C, Barnett M, Fitzgibbon J. Familial myelodysplasia and acute myeloid leukaemia – a review. Br J Haematol. 2008;140(2):123–32. https://doi.org/10.1111/j.1365-2141.2007.06909.x.
104. Churpek JE, Lorenz R, Nedumgottil S, Onel K, Olopade OI, Sorrell A, et al. Proposal for the clinical detection and management of patients and their family members with familial myelodysplastic syndrome/acute leukemia predisposition syndromes. Leuk Lymphoma. 2013;54(1):28–35. https://doi.org/10.3109/10428194.2012.701738.
105. Board PCGE: Cancer genetics risk assessment and counseling (PDQ®): Health Professional Version. 2020. https://www.ncbi.nlm.nih.gov/books/NBK65817/. Accessed 28 Jan 2021.
106. Szymaniak BM, Facchini LA, Giri VN, Antonarakis ES, Beer TM, Carlo MI, et al. Practical considerations and challenges for germline genetic testing in patients with prostate cancer: recommendations from the germline genetics working group of the PCCTC. JCO Oncol Pract. 2020;16(12):811–9. https://doi.org/10.1200/OP.20.00431.
107. Cohen SA, Bradbury A, Henderson V, Hoskins K, Bednar E, Arun BK. Genetic Counseling and testing in a community setting: quality, access, and efficiency. Am Soc Clin Oncol Educ Book. 2019;39:e34–44. https://doi.org/10.1200/EDBK_238937.
108. Samadder NJ, Riegert-Johnson D, Boardman L, Rhodes D, Wick M, Okuno S, et al. Comparison of universal genetic testing vs guideline-directed targeted testing for patients with hereditary cancer syndrome. JAMA Oncol. 2020; https://doi.org/10.1001/jamaoncol.2020.6252.
109. LaDuca H, Polley EC, Yussuf A, Hoang L, Gutierrez S, Hart SN, et al. A clinical guide to hereditary cancer panel testing: evaluation of gene-specific cancer associations and sensitivity of genetic testing criteria in a cohort of 165,000 high-risk patients. Genet Med. 2020;22(2):407–15. https://doi.org/10.1038/s41436-019-0633-8.
110. Mandelker D, Zhang L, Kemel Y, Stadler ZK, Joseph V, Zehir A, et al. Mutation detection in patients with advanced cancer by universal sequencing of cancer-related genes in tumor and normal DNA vs guideline-based germline testing. JAMA. 2017;318(9):825–35. https://doi.org/10.1001/jama.2017.11137.
111. Ritter DI, Rao S, Kulkarni S, Madhavan S, Offit K, Plon SE. A case for expert curation: an overview of cancer curation in the Clinical Genome Resource (ClinGen). Cold Spring Harb Mol Case Stud. 2019;5(5) https://doi.org/10.1101/mcs.a004739.
112. Fortuno C, Lee K, Olivier M, Pesaran T, Mai PL, de Andrade KC, et al. Specifications of the ACMG/AMP variant interpretation guidelines for germline TP53 variants. Hum Mutat. 2020; https://doi.org/10.1002/humu.24152.
113. Gould GM, Grauman PV, Theilmann MR, Spurka L, Wang IE, Melroy LM, et al. Detecting clinically actionable variants in the 3′ exons of PMS2 via a reflex workflow based on equivalent hybrid capture of the gene and its pseudogene. BMC Med Genet. 2018;19(1):176. https://doi.org/10.1186/s12881-018-0691-9.
114. Mandelker D, Zhang L. The emerging significance of secondary germline testing in cancer genomics. J Pathol. 2018;244(5):610–5. https://doi.org/10.1002/path.5031.
115. Rusch M, Nakitandwe J, Shurtleff S, Newman S, Zhang Z, Edmonson MN, et al. Clinical cancer genomic profiling by three-platform sequencing of whole genome, whole exome and transcriptome. Nat Commun. 2018;9(1):3962. https://doi.org/10.1038/s41467-018-06485-7.
116. Sakamoto Y, Sereewattanawoot S, Suzuki A. A new era of long-read sequencing for cancer genomics. J Hum Genet. 2020;65(1):3–10. https://doi.org/10.1038/s10038-019-0658-5.
117. van der Lee M, Kriek M, Guchelaar HJ, Swen JJ. Technologies for pharmacogenomics: a review. Genes (Basel). 2020;11(12) https://doi.org/10.3390/genes11121456.
118. Feurstein S, Zhang L, DiNardo CD. Accurate germline RUNX1 variant interpretation and its clinical significance. Blood Adv. 2020;4(24):6199–203. https://doi.org/10.1182/bloodadvances.2020003304.
119. Kraft IL, Godley LA. Identifying potential germline variants from sequencing hematopoietic malignancies. Hematology Am

Soc Hematol Educ Program. 2020;2020(1):219–27. https://doi.org/10.1182/hematology.2020006910.

120. Lincoln SE, Nussbaum RL, Kurian AW, Nielsen SM, Das K, Michalski S, et al. Yield and utility of germline testing following tumor sequencing in patients with cancer. JAMA Netw Open. 2020;3(10):e2019452. https://doi.org/10.1001/jamanetworkopen.2020.19452.
121. Rhees J, Arnold M, Boland CR. Inversion of exons 1-7 of the MSH2 gene is a frequent cause of unexplained Lynch syndrome in one local population. Familial Cancer. 2014;13(2):219–25. https://doi.org/10.1007/s10689-013-9688-x.
122. Peixoto A, Santos C, Rocha P, Pinheiro M, Principe S, Pereira D, et al. The c.156_157insAlu BRCA2 rearrangement accounts for more than one-fourth of deleterious BRCA mutations in northern/central Portugal. Breast Cancer Res Treat. 2009;114(1):31–8. https://doi.org/10.1007/s10549-008-9978-4.
123. George A, Kaye S, Banerjee S. Delivering widespread BRCA testing and PARP inhibition to patients with ovarian cancer. Nat Rev Clin Oncol. 2017;14(5):284–96. https://doi.org/10.1038/nrclinonc.2016.191.
124. Meric-Bernstam F, Brusco L, Daniels M, Wathoo C, Bailey AM, Strong L, et al. Incidental germline variants in 1000 advanced cancers on a prospective somatic genomic profiling protocol. Ann Oncol. 2016;27(5):795–800. https://doi.org/10.1093/annonc/mdw018.
125. Li MM, Datto M, Duncavage EJ, Kulkarni S, Lindeman NI, Roy S, et al. Standards and guidelines for the interpretation and reporting of sequence variants in cancer: a joint consensus recommendation of the Association for Molecular Pathology, American Society of Clinical Oncology, and College of American Pathologists. J Mol Diagn. 2017;19(1):4–23. https://doi.org/10.1016/j.jmoldx.2016.10.002.
126. Richards S, Aziz N, Bale S, Bick D, Das S, Gastier-Foster J, et al. Standards and guidelines for the interpretation of sequence variants: a joint consensus recommendation of the American College of Medical Genetics and Genomics and the Association for Molecular Pathology. Genet Med. 2015;17(5):405–24. https://doi.org/10.1038/gim.2015.30.
127. Batalini F, Peacock EG, Stobie L, Robertson A, Garber J, Weitzel JN, et al. Li-Fraumeni syndrome: not a straightforward diagnosis anymore-the interpretation of pathogenic variants of low allele frequency and the differences between germline PVs, mosaicism, and clonal hematopoiesis. Breast Cancer Res. 2019;21(1):107. https://doi.org/10.1186/s13058-019-1193-1.
128. Godley LA, Shimamura A. Genetic predisposition to hematologic malignancies: management and surveillance. Blood. 2017;130(4):424–32. https://doi.org/10.1182/blood-2017-02-735290.
129. Niehaus A, Azzariti DR, Harrison SM, DiStefano MT, Hemphill SE, Senol-Cosar O, et al. A survey assessing adoption of the ACMG-AMP guidelines for interpreting sequence variants and identification of areas for continued improvement. Genet Med. 2019;21(8):1699–701. https://doi.org/10.1038/s41436-018-0432-7.
130. Amendola LM, Jarvik GP, Leo MC, McLaughlin HM, Akkari Y, Amaral MD, et al. Performance of ACMG-AMP variant-interpretation guidelines among nine Laboratories in the Clinical Sequencing Exploratory Research Consortium. Am J Hum Genet. 2016;98(6):1067–76. https://doi.org/10.1016/j.ajhg.2016.03.024.
131. Yang S, Lincoln SE, Kobayashi Y, Nykamp K, Nussbaum RL, Topper S. Sources of discordance among germ-line variant classifications in ClinVar. Genet Med. 2017;19(10):1118–26. https://doi.org/10.1038/gim.2017.60.
132. Mester JL, Ghosh R, Pesaran T, Huether R, Karam R, Hruska KS, et al. Gene-specific criteria for PTEN variant curation: recommendations from the ClinGen PTEN Expert Panel. Hum Mutat. 2018;39(11):1581–92. https://doi.org/10.1002/humu.23636.
133. Lee K, Krempely K, Roberts ME, Anderson MJ, Carneiro F, Chao E, et al. Specifications of the ACMG/AMP variant curation guidelines for the analysis of germline CDH1 sequence variants. Hum Mutat. 2018;39(11):1553–68. https://doi.org/10.1002/humu.23650.
134. Ellard S, Hattersley AT, Brewer CM, Vaidya B. Detection of an MEN1 gene mutation depends on clinical features and supports current referral criteria for diagnostic molecular genetic testing. Clin Endocrinol. 2005;62(2):169–75. https://doi.org/10.1111/j.1365-2265.2005.02190.x.
135. White HD, Blair J, Pinkney J, Cuthbertson DJ, Day R, Weber A, et al. Improvement in the care of multiple endocrine neoplasia type 1 through a regional multidisciplinary clinic. QJM. 2010;103(5):337–45. https://doi.org/10.1093/qjmed/hcq020.
136. Leclerc J, Flament C, Lovecchio T, Delattre L, Ait Yahya E, Baert-Desurmont S, et al. Diversity of genetic events associated with MLH1 promoter methylation in Lynch syndrome families with heritable constitutional epimutation. Genet Med. 2018;20(12):1589–99. https://doi.org/10.1038/gim.2018.47.
137. Ward RL, Dobbins T, Lindor NM, Rapkins RW, Hitchins MP. Identification of constitutional MLH1 epimutations and promoter variants in colorectal cancer patients from the Colon Cancer Family Registry. Genet Med. 2013;15(1):25–35. https://doi.org/10.1038/gim.2012.91.
138. Hitchins MP. Finding the needle in a haystack: identification of cases of Lynch syndrome with MLH1 epimutation. Familial Cancer. 2016;15(3):413–22. https://doi.org/10.1007/s10689-016-9887-3.
139. Coffee B, Cox HC, Bernhisel R, Manley S, Bowles K, Roa BB, et al. A substantial proportion of apparently heterozygous TP53 pathogenic variants detected with a next-generation sequencing hereditary pan-cancer panel are acquired somatically. Hum Mutat. 2020;41(1):203–11. https://doi.org/10.1002/humu.23910.
140. Steensma DP, Bejar R, Jaiswal S, Lindsley RC, Sekeres MA, Hasserjian RP, et al. Clonal hematopoiesis of indeterminate potential and its distinction from myelodysplastic syndromes. Blood. 2015;126(1):9–16. https://doi.org/10.1182/blood-2015-03-631747.
141. Oxnard GR, Miller VA, Robson ME, Azzoli CG, Pao W, Ladanyi M, et al. Screening for germline EGFR T790M mutations through lung cancer genotyping. J Thorac Oncol. 2012;7(6):1049–52. https://doi.org/10.1097/JTO.0b013e318250ed9d.
142. Gazdar A, Robinson L, Oliver D, Xing C, Travis WD, Soh J, et al. Hereditary lung cancer syndrome targets never smokers with germline EGFR gene T790M mutations. J Thorac Oncol. 2014;9(4):456–63. https://doi.org/10.1097/JTO.0000000000000130.
143. Gibbons DL, Byers LA, Kurie JM. Smoking, p53 mutation, and lung cancer. Mol Cancer Res. 2014;12(1):3–13. https://doi.org/10.1158/1541-7786.MCR-13-0539.
144. Kato S, Han SY, Liu W, Otsuka K, Shibata H, Kanamaru R, et al. Understanding the function-structure and function-mutation relationships of p53 tumor suppressor protein by high-resolution missense mutation analysis. Proc Natl Acad Sci U S A. 2003;100(14):8424–9. https://doi.org/10.1073/pnas.1431692100.
145. Giacomelli AO, Yang X, Lintner RE, McFarland JM, Duby M, Kim J, et al. Mutational processes shape the landscape of TP53 mutations in human cancer. Nat Genet. 2018;50(10):1381–7. https://doi.org/10.1038/s41588-018-0204-y.
146. Monti P, Ciribilli Y, Jordan J, Menichini P, Umbach DM, Resnick MA, et al. Transcriptional functionality of germ line p53 mutants influences cancer phenotype. Clin Cancer Res. 2007;13(13):3789–95. https://doi.org/10.1158/1078-0432.CCR-06-2545.
147. Yurgelun MB, Masciari S, Joshi VA, Mercado RC, Lindor NM, Gallinger S, et al. Germline TP53 mutations in patients with early-

onset colorectal cancer in the Colon Cancer Family Registry. JAMA Oncol. 2015;1(2):214–21. https://doi.org/10.1001/jamaoncol.2015.0197.
148. Millar S, Bradley L, Donnelly DE, Carson D, Morrison PJ. Familial pediatric endocrine tumors. Oncologist. 2011;16(10):1388–96. https://doi.org/10.1634/theoncologist.2011-0120.
149. Masciari S, Dewanwala A, Stoffel EM, Lauwers GY, Zheng H, Achatz MI, et al. Gastric cancer in individuals with Li-Fraumeni syndrome. Genet Med. 2011;13(7):651–7. https://doi.org/10.1097/GIM.0b013e31821628b6.
150. Wagner J, Portwine C, Rabin K, Leclerc JM, Narod SA, Malkin D. High frequency of germline p53 mutations in childhood adrenocortical cancer. J Natl Cancer Inst. 1994;86(22):1707–10. https://doi.org/10.1093/jnci/86.22.1707.
151. Varley JM, McGown G, Thorncroft M, James LA, Margison GP, Forster G, et al. Are there low-penetrance TP53 alleles? Evidence from childhood adrenocortical tumors. Am J Hum Genet. 1999;65(4):995–1006. https://doi.org/10.1086/302575.

Part III

Molecular Hematopathology

Acute Myeloid Leukemia

13

Guang Yang and Linsheng Zhang

List of Frequently Asked Questions

1. What is the role of molecular genetics in the diagnosis and laboratory evaluation of acute myeloid leukemia (AML)?
2. What molecular genetic tests should be considered for the initial diagnostic workup of AML?
3. How do the sample types, sample quality, and sample processing affect the molecular genetic/cytogenetic tests for AML?
4. What are the significant molecular genetic abnormalities applied in the risk stratification of AML?
5. Which types of AML are defined by genetic abnormalities and do not require at least 20% blasts in the marrow or blood to make a diagnosis?
6. Which test should I choose when acute promyelocytic leukemia (APL) is suspected based on the morphologic characteristics observed on the blood or bone marrow smear?
7. How should we work up AML cases with morphologic and immunophenotypic features of APL but lacking *PML-RARA*?
8. What mutation tests should be expedited for AML to facilitate the early treatment decision?
9. What is the clinical significance of *BCR-ABL1* fusion in AML?
10. What are the clinical implications of *FLT3* mutations in AML, and how are *FLT3* mutations tested in the clinical laboratories?
11. What is the clinical significance of *NPM1* mutation in AML, and how do we test *NPM1* mutations?
12. What are the characteristics of *CEBPA* mutations in AML and how are *CEBPA* mutations detected in the clinical laboratories?
13. What is the clinical significance of *TP53* mutations in AML and how do we test *TP53* mutations?
14. What are the *RUNX1* mutations frequently seen in AML and their clinical significance?
15. What is the role of *GATA1* mutation in transient abnormal myelopoiesis (TAM) and myeloid leukemia associated with Down syndrome (MLADS)?
16. What ancillary tests should be considered toward a diagnosis of AML with myelodysplasia-related changes?
17. How frequently should molecular testing or mutation profiling be repeated in the clinical follow-up of the AML patients after treatment?
18. What is the role of molecular methods in the minimal/measurable residual disease (MRD) detection of AML and how are they performed in the clinical laboratories?

Frequently Asked Questions

1. **What is the role of molecular genetics in the diagnosis and laboratory evaluation of acute myeloid leukemia (AML)?**
   - Acute myeloid leukemia (AML) is characterized by the clonal expansion of myeloid blasts in the peripheral blood, bone marrow, or other tissues; it is a heterogeneous disease at the genetic level. In the 1970s, the French-American-British (FAB) classification of acute leukemia was introduced based largely on morphologic characteristics and cytochemical staining results [1]. Over the last few decades, our understanding of the cellular and molecular biology of AML has been significantly enhanced by the application of flow cytometric analysis and different molecular genetic

G. Yang
Department of Pathology and Laboratory Medicine, University of Pennsylvania, Philadelphia, PA, USA
e-mail: guang.yang@pennmedicine.upenn.edu

L. Zhang (✉)
Department of Pathology and Laboratory Medicine, Emory University School of Medicine, Atlanta, GA, USA
e-mail: linsheng.zhang@emory.edu

Y. Ding, L. Zhang (eds.), *Practical Oncologic Molecular Pathology*, Practical Anatomic Pathology,
https://doi.org/10.1007/978-3-030-73227-1_13

technologies. In 2008, the first complete DNA sequence of a human cancer genome was obtained from a cytogenetically normal AML patient [2]. The advances in sequencing technology have led to the discovery of many novel mutations in AML, providing deeper insights into its mutational landscape [3].

- Published in 2001, updated in 2008 and 2016, the World Health Organization (WHO) classification of tumors of hematopoietic and lymphoid tissues (abbreviated as WHO classification henceforth in this chapter) incorporates cytogenetics and molecular genetics together with the clinical features, the morphologic and immunophenotypic characteristics to define disease entities of clinical significance [4]. Of all the parameters that are integrated to yield a final diagnosis and appropriate classification of AML, the most clinically relevant are genetic abnormalities [5]. The revised WHO classification defines 25 subtypes of AML, including 11 entities in the category of "acute myeloid leukemia with recurrent genetic abnormalities" [6].
- Molecular genetic analysis of AML has become essential not only for diagnosis and classification but also for prognostic stratification, treatment guidance, and monitoring of minimal/measurable residual disease (MRD). Genetic testing of multiple genes relevant to the pathobiology of leukemogenesis and clinical management is already the standard of care in patients with AML.

2. **What molecular genetic tests should be considered for the initial diagnostic workup of AML?**
   - When the diagnosing criteria for acute myeloid leukemia are met, the accurate classification of AML requires multidisciplinary ancillary studies including immunophenotyping (flow cytometry and/or immunohistochemistry) and molecular genetic analysis. According to the National Comprehensive Cancer Network (NCCN) and College of American Pathologists and the American Society of Hematology guidelines [7], cytogenetic analyses, including karyotype and fluorescence in situ hybridization (FISH), are necessary for risk stratification and to guide the therapy of AML. All patients should be tested for mutations in *ASXL1*, *KIT*, *FLT3* (ITD and TKD), *NPM1*, *CEBPA*, *IDH1/IDH2*, *RUNX1*, and *TP53*. Multiplex gene panel tests or next-generation sequencing (NGS) can be performed to develop a more comprehensive prognostic assessment [7]. The revised 2017 European Leukemia Net (ELN) recommendations and the 2017 College of American Pathologists and the American Society of Hematology guidelines also recommend screening cytogenetic abnormalities, gene mutations, and gene rearrangements in the initial diagnostic workup of AML (summarized in Table 13.1) [8, 9].
   - Many molecular genetic methodologies are currently available for clinical workup of AML; they have distinct performance characteristics and different requirements for specimens (see Table 13.2). It is critical for pathologists and laboratory diagnosticians to understand their advantages and limitations, as well as some caveats that may arise in the interpretation of the results [10, 11].
   - It had been a common practice for clinical laboratories to perform selected or a panel of FISH tests in conjunction with conventional karyotyping to detect the cytogenetic abnormalities associated with AML, both at initial diagnosis and during follow-up monitoring. Recent studies have questioned the value and cost-effectiveness of this approach [12, 13]. When 20 well-displayed karyotypes are available for analysis, FISH adds mini-

Table 13.1 Recommendations of molecular genetic screening in the initial diagnostic workup of AML

Cytogenetics	1. Results from cytogenetics should be obtained preferably within 5–7 days 2. At least 20 bone marrow metaphases are needed to define a normal karyotype and recommended to describe an abnormal karyotype 3. Abnormal karyotypes may be obtained from blood specimens 4. Testing for t(9;22)(q34.1;q11.2); *BCR-ABL1* and *KMT2A* translocations should be performed in confirmed mixed phenotype acute leukemia
Gene mutations	1. *FLT3-ITD* (strongly recommended) 2. *IDH1*, *IDH2*, *TET2*, *WT1*, *DNMT3A*, *NPM1*, *CEBPA*, *RUNX1*, *FLT3*, *TP53*, *ASXL1* 3. Results of *NPM1* and *FLT3* mutational screening should be available within 48–72 h (at least in patients eligible for intensive chemotherapy)[a] and results from additional molecular genetics within the first treatment cycle 4. Mutational analysis of *KIT* should be performed in confirmed core-binding factor AML
Gene rearrangements	1. *PML-RARA*, *CBFB-MYH11*, *RUNX1-RUNX1T1*, *BCR-ABL1*, and other fusion genes (as indicated by pathologic and clinical features) 2. Screening for gene rearrangements should be performed by FISH or multiplex PCR if rapid information is needed for recommendation of suitable therapy, if chromosome morphology is of poor quality or if there is typical morphology but the suspected cytogenetic abnormality is not present

[a]The list of genes/mutations for which the tests should be expedited is determined by locally available treatment options (see more discussion in question 8)

Table 13.2 Different cytogenetic and molecular genetic methods used in the laboratory analysis of AML

Methodology	Characteristics, clinical utility, and advantages	Limitations and caveats
Conventional karyotyping	Global genomic view; identifies unknown/unexpected abnormalities Detects numerical and structural chromosome aberrations (i.e., translocation, inversion, large deletion, or gains)	Requires fresh, sterile live cells (in vitro culture) Low resolution (~5–10 Mb in routine practice) Long turnaround time (days) and labor intensive
Fluorescence in situ hybridization (FISH)	Targeted assessment of well-defined abnormalities Technically straightforward and shorter turnaround time Can be performed on interphase nuclei, suitable for fixed cells and FFPE tissue	Only detects alterations covered by the probe design Requires rigorous quality standards Low resolution (~100 kb)
Chromosomal microarray analysis (CMA)	Broad to whole-genome coverage Detecting small copy number variants (CNVs) such as microdeletion and microduplication Works for both fresh and FFPE tissue	Usually cannot detect balanced translocations Analytic sensitivity generally at ≥20% of alleles frequency Average resolution of ~30 kb throughout the genome Not routinely used in AML diagnosis
Endpoint and real-time polymerase chain reaction (PCR)	Assessment of genetic abnormalities and mutations of a small targeted region Excellent analytic sensitivity and specificity, suitable for minimal residual disease (MRD) monitoring Technically straightforward and fast turnaround time Can be multiplexed for a variety of targets Can be designed for quantitative test (real-time PCR) Suitable for a broad range of sample types, including FFPE tissue	Need to know the exact target sequence for primer design Mutation at the primer binding site may cause false-negative result (allele drop out) Can be potentially "too sensitive" for clinical significance
Digital PCR (dPCR)	Excellent sensitivity for minimal disease monitoring.	Requires special instruments and protocols
Sanger sequencing	Detecting single/multiple nucleotide variants (SNV, MNV) or small insertions/deletions (indels) Confirmation of novel fusions or other abnormalities	Single gene target Limited sequencing length (~300–1000 base pairs) Analytic sensitivity usually >15% allele frequency, not suitable for follow up studies
Next-generation sequencing (NGS)	Simultaneous screening of multiple genes in multiple samples Quantitative and sensitive detection of unknown/unexpected genomic alterations within the designed scope	Relatively expensive and longer turnaround time High complexity of workflow and result analysis Currently only for targeted genes/hotspots in clinical laboratories Detecting translocation (especially those without fusion RNA products) is challenging

mal value to identify AML-related cytogenetic abnormalities, especially for diagnostic samples where sufficient blasts are present to generate neoplastic karyotypes. Many hematologists and hematopathologists have started abandoning routine FISH tests and adding NGS-based mutation profiling for AML diagnostic workup. Given the quicker turnaround time and better sensitivity in some cases (e.g., cryptic *CBFB-MYH11* rearrangement not recognizable by karyotyping [14]), FISH tests still have diagnostic value in selected patients based on the clues from clinical presentations and pathologic features [15]. FISH for a cytogenetic abnormality known to be present in the leukemic cells is suitable for follow-up samples to reveal low-level leukemic clones [13].

3. **How do the sample types, sample quality and sample processing affect the molecular genetic/cytogenetic tests for AML?**
   - A successful molecular diagnostic test starts from the reliable and robust extraction of nucleic acids. Fresh specimens such as blood, bone marrow aspirate, and fresh tissue or fluids are the ideal sources of nucleic acids.
   - The most commonly used sample types for genetic testing of AML are whole blood and bone marrow (aspirate and biopsy core). Sometimes other types of samples, such as fine-needle aspirate and/or biopsy tissue, body fluids including cerebrospinal fluid (CSF), pleural fluid, and peritoneal fluid, might also be taken for pathologic evaluation, especially when blasts are not identified or present at low percentage in the blood and bone marrow.
   - To collect samples for molecular genetic testing, ethylenediaminetetraacetic acid (EDTA) is the preferred anticoagulant (lavender-top tube), but citrate (yellow-top tube) is also acceptable. Heparin (green-top tube) is the least preferred anticoagulant for molecular testing because of its inhibitory effects on key enzymes in the polymerase chain reaction (PCR) [16]. However, heparin is the preferred anticoagulant for FISH and chromosome analysis (conventional karyotyping).

- Chromosome analysis requires live cells to perform in vitro culture. In contrast, a variety of samples can be used for FISH, array, and molecular studies (see Table 13.2).
- As the most commonly used tissue fixative, neutral buffered formalin can cause cross-linking of nucleic acid with protein, nucleic acid fragmentation, and other artifacts [17]. Longer fixation time is associated with a decreased yield of nucleic acid. Long storage time of formalin-fixed paraffin-embedded (FFPE) tissue blocks is related to increased nucleic acid degradation. A method validated for fresh tissue samples therefore cannot be used to test FFPE unless the same clinical performances are also validated.
- Bone marrow trephine biopsy specimens need decalcification before being embedded in the tissue block for optimal histologic sectioning. The most commonly used decalcification agents usually contain strong acids (i.e., formic acid, acetic acid, picric acid, or nitric acid), resulting in the degradation of nucleic acids. The decalcified specimens, therefore, are not suitable for molecular analysis. Some studies showed that slow decalcification with EDTA results in the better preservation of nucleic acids [18–20]. However, validating test performance is required before EDTA-decalcified tissue samples can be used for molecular testing in the case fresh samples are not available.

4. **What are the significant molecular genetic abnormalities applied in the risk stratification of AML?**
   - Both conventional cytogenetics and the molecular genetic studies of various alterations are powerful prognostic factors of AML. The revised 2017 ELN recommendations for diagnosis and management of AML in adults integrate cytogenetic and molecular features to classify AML patients into three prognostic risk groups that differ based on the rates of complete remission, disease-free survival, and overall survival. These risk categories are "favorable," "intermediate," and "adverse" [8]. A recent study confirmed the critical importance of genomic abnormalities to the prognosis of AML and proposed a genomic-based classification of AML [3]. Generally, the chromosome copy number and structural abnormalities have more significant effects on the clinical outcomes than isolated gene mutations.
   - The abnormalities indicating adverse risks are as follows:

     Cytogenetic abnormalities:
     1. Balanced translocations including t(6,9)(p23;q34.1); *DEK-NUP214*, t(v;11q23.3); *KMT2A* rearranged, t(9,22)(q34.1;q11.2); *BCR-ABL1*, inv(3)(q21.3q26.2), or t(3,3)(q21.3;q26.2); *GATA2*, *MECOM* (*EVI1*)
     2. Monosomy 5 or del(5q), monosomy 7, monosomy 17, or abn(17p), which is defined as loss or disruption of 17p13 (*TP53* locus) [21]
     3. Complex karyotype: defined as three or more unrelated chromosome abnormalities, in the absence of one of the WHO-designated recurrent translocations or inversions, including t(8,21); inv(16) or t(16,16); t(9,11); t(v;11)(v;q23.3); t(6,9); inv(3) or t(3,3); and AML with *BCR-ABL1*
     4. Monosomal karyotype: the presence of one single monosomy (excluding the loss of X or Y) in association with at least one additional monosomy or structural chromosome abnormality (excluding core-binding factor AML) [8]

     Molecular abnormalities (gene mutations):
     1. Wild-type *NPM1* with *FLT3-ITD* high allele burden (≥ 0.5)
     2. *DNMT3A/NPM1/FLT3* triple mutations [22]
     3. Mutated *RUNX1* or *ASXL1* (exception: not as an adverse prognostic marker if they co-occur with favorable-risk AML subtypes)
     4. Mutated *TP53*, which is frequently associated with complex and monosomal karyotype
   - The abnormalities indicating favorable risks are:

     Cytogenetic abnormalities:
     1. Core-binding factor AML: t(8,21)(q22;q22.1); *RUNX1-RUNX1T1* and inv(16)(p13.1q22) or t(16,16)(p13.1;q22); *CBFB-MYH11*
     2. APL with *PML-RARA*

     Molecular abnormalities:
     1. Mutated *NPM1* without *FLT3*-ITD or with low *FLT3*-ITD allelic ratio (< 0.5, controversial [23])
     2. Double (biallelic) *CEBPA* mutation
     3. *IDH2* p.R172 mutations and no other class-defining lesions [3]
   - Cases with t(9;11)(p21.3;q23.3); *MLLT3-KMT2A* and other cytogenetic and molecular abnormalities (including various combinations of *NPM1/CEBPA/FLT3* mutations) not classified as adverse or favorable are in the "intermediate" risk group.
   - Besides the genetic abnormalities listed above, additional genetic abnormalities may coexist and influence the biologic and clinical behavior of AML, including response to therapy and overall survival. For instance,

KIT gene mutations are commonly seen in core-binding factor AML and are associated with relatively adverse prognosis [24].

- Given the complexity of molecular genetic changes associated with AML, recently there were efforts to build knowledge banks and computerized algorithms to integrate clinical, laboratory, and molecular genetic information to assist the best clinical decision-making [25, 26]. Free online tools based on these studies are available (http://www.amlcompositemodel.org/ and https://cancer.sanger.ac.uk/aml-multistage/, for research use only). We can expect this new trend in precision medicine for AML to progress and expand with the accumulation of big data, to establish robust models facilitated by artificial intelligence.

5. **Which types of AML are defined by genetic abnormalities and do not require at least 20% blasts in the marrow or blood to make a diagnosis?**
   - Traditionally, AML has been distinguished from other myeloid neoplasms based on a minimum blast cell percentage in the bone marrow or peripheral blood. The threshold of blast cell percentage required for a diagnosis of acute leukemia has been arbitrarily set at 30% by the French-American-British (FAB) cooperative group [1]. In 2008, the WHO classification reduced the blast threshold for the diagnosis of AML from 30% to 20% in the bone marrow or peripheral blood [27].
   - Several specific entities in the category "AML with recurrent genetic abnormalities" have been defined without regard to blast cell count in the 2008 WHO classification [24]. In the appropriate clinical settings, a diagnosis of AML can be rendered even when the blast percentage in the peripheral blood and/or bone marrow is less than 20%, when any one of the following three genetic abnormalities is present:
     1. t(8,21)(q22;q22.1);RUNX1-RUNX1T1
     2. inv(16)(p13.1q22) or t(16;16)(p13.1;q22);CBFB-MYH11
     3. PML-R*ARA* fusion
   - Of note, AML can also be diagnosed when there is only extramedullary involvement, such as myeloid sarcoma, or at least 20% blasts are identified in body fluids such as cerebral spinal fluids, without requiring at least 20% blasts in the blood and/or bone marrow.
6. **Which test should I choose when acute promyelocytic leukemia (APL) is suspected based on the morphologic characteristics observed on blood or bone marrow smear?**
   - Among all acute leukemias, acute promyelocytic leukemia (APL) is a distinct subtype with the most compelling genotype-phenotype (morphology and immunophenotype) correlation. The classic hypergranular APL often exhibits abundant cytoplasmic granules and bundles of Auer rods, while the hypogranular variant commonly shows indistinct granules and folded nuclei. When blasts with these features are seen in blood smear (see Case 1), APL should be highly suspected.
   - APL is considered a hematologic emergency because of the high early mortality rate related to disseminated intravascular coagulation (DIC). Rapid diagnosis and prompt treatment with differentiation agent all-trans retinoic acid (ATRA) is critical to prevent early mortality of APL patients [28]. Although flow cytometric immunophenotyping can provide further evidence to support the likelihood of APL, definitive diagnosis requires molecular genetic tests to demonstrate *PML-RARA* fusion gene. Emergency (STAT) testing for *PML-RARA* translocation to confirm the diagnosis of APL is critical for making the early treatment decision [28].
   - Several testing methods including karyotyping, FISH, and reverse transcription-polymerase chain reaction (RT-PCR) have been used to detect the *PML-RARA* fusion. Both rapid hybridization FISH and rapid RT-PCR can usually provide reasonable turnaround time for a STAT *PML-RARA* detection. FISH test may be more cost-effective since separate controls are needed for the PCR test; however, PCR test provides simpler workflow [29] and better sensitivity [30]. In addition, some clinical laboratories also utilized an immunofluorescent method using antibodies directed against the PML protein for the rapid diagnosis of APL [31].
   - Real-time (quantitative) reverse transcription PCR (RT-qPCR) for *PML-RARA* transcript level detection is the only method that can provide sufficient sensitivity to monitor the treatment response and MRD. It is also performed at initial diagnosis (in addition to the STAT test) to establish a baseline *PML-RARA* transcript level [28].
7. **How should we work up AML cases with morphologic and immunophenotypic features of APL but lacking *PML-RARA*?**
   - Although t(15;17)(q24.1;q21.2);*PML-RARA* is seen in approximately 99% of APLs, variant translocations of *RARA* with different fusion partners other than *PML* occur in approximately 1% of the remaining cases that show the same morphologic and immunophenotypic features as APL with *PML-RARA*. The variant partner genes include *BCOR*, *FIP1L1*, *FNDC3B*, *GTF2I*, *IRF2BP2*, *NABP1*, *NPM1*, *NUMA*, *OBFC2A*, *PRKAR1A*, *STAT3*, *STAT5B*, *TBLR*, *TFG*, and *ZBTB16* [32].
   - Per the current WHO classification, only APL with *PML-RARA* is considered as a distinct entity, because

other APL cases with variant *RARA* translocation partners are not as exquisitely responsive to ATRA and arsenic trioxide (ATO) treatment. Cases with variant translocations are diagnosed as APL with a variant *RARA* translocation [6].

- Variant *RARA* translocations with non-*PML* fusion partners are uncommon but create significant diagnostic and therapeutic challenges. These rare APL cases are important to be recognized because they often have morphologic features resembling typical APL, but some variants, such as those harboring *ZBTB16-RARA* and *STAT5B-RARA*, are resistant to ATRA and therefore have a poorer prognosis [33].
- When testing for t(15;17)(q24.1;q21.2);*PML-RARA* is negative, conventional karyotyping and FISH can provide complementary information suggesting the presence of a variant translocation involving *RARA*. Conventional karyotyping would identify the variant translocations except in cases with cryptic fusion genes. FISH analysis using *RARA* dual-color break-apart probes detects split *RARA* signals in interphase nuclei [34], indicating variant translocation in *PML-RARA* negative cases.
- RNA-based NGS (RNA-seq) can be designed to comprehensively interrogate the fusion genes related to AML, including APL with *PML-RARA* and variant *RARA* fusions. Transcriptome sequencing has the power to identify all the RNA fusions, including novel fusion transcripts. These methods have been used to detect novel *RARA* fusion partners [33]; however, its clinical utility is very limited due to the complexity of the workflow and analysis.

8. **What mutation tests should be expedited for AML to facilitate the early treatment decision?**
   - Over the past few years, several novel agents targeting specific proteins with altered activities have been approved by the US Food and Drug Administration (FDA) for the treatment of AML, providing additional options both in the frontline and relapsed or refractory settings [35]. In this era of new drugs, the timely identification of actionable mutations at diagnosis and at relapse is critical for the clinical management of AML patients [36].
   - These new targeted drugs include midostaurin and gilteritinib to target FLT3 (ITD or TKD mutations), ivosidenib and enasidenib to target mutant isocitrate dehydrogenase 1 and 2 (IDH1/2), and venetoclax to target B-cell lymphoma 2 (BCL2), respectively. Recent studies highlight the promising efficacy of venetoclax (BCL2 inhibitor)-based therapy in *NPM1*-mutated AML [37, 38].
   - NCCN guidelines recommend that molecular and cytogenetic analyses for immediately actionable mutations such as *CBF*, *FLT3* (ITD/TKD), *NPM1*, *IDH1*, and *IDH2* mutations should be expedited [7]. Each clinical laboratory may establish a protocol for fast turnaround time mutation testing for AML based on local resources, clinical indications, and treatment options.

9. **What is the clinical significance of *BCR-ABL1* fusion in AML?**
   - AML with *BCR-ABL1* is now listed as a provisional entity in the category of "AML with recurrent genetic abnormalities" in the 2016 revised WHO classification [6]. The incidence of Philadelphia chromosome in de novo AML ranges from 0.5% to 3%, with most cases demonstrating the p210 fusion [39–41].
   - Because FISH or molecular testing for *BCR-ABL1* is not routinely performed in cases meeting diagnostic criteria of AML, and there are no unique morphologic or immunophenotypic features to suggest AML with *BCR-ABL1*; currently most cases are identified by conventional karyotyping. In order to make this diagnosis, there should also be no evidence of co-occurring genetic aberrations used to define other entities in the category of AML with recurrent genetic abnormalities [6].
   - Due to the low incidence, our knowledge about the morphologic, immunophenotypic, and molecular genetic features of AML with *BCR-ABL1* is based on limited studies. In a patient with no history of CML, it is challenging to distinguish de novo AML from the myeloid blast phase (MBP) of CML. Compared to CML-MBP, the following features support AML with *BCR-ABL1* [6].
     1. No previous abnormal blood cell counts, less splenomegaly, lower basophilia [42]
     2. Less cellular bone marrow (average 80% versus >95%) and dwarf megakaryocytes [42]
     3. Additional cytogenetic abnormalities different from those present in CML-MBP [40]
     4. Co-occurring AML-associated mutations such as *NPM1* and *FLT3-ITD* [40]
     5. Loss of *IKZF1* and *CDKN2A* and cryptic deletions within *IGH* and T-Cell Receptor genes [43]
   - AML with *BCR-ABL1* is classified as a high-risk disease by the ELN [8, 42]. However, a study suggested that the aggressive nature of this entity is not because of *BCR-ABL1* itself but rather due to other high-risk cytogenetic/molecular features that are present in the vast majority of cases [44]. Some reports showed that the survival of AML with *BCR-ABL1* patients may be improved with tyrosine kinase inhibitor (TKI) therapy followed by allogeneic hematopoietic cell transplant [45, 46].

- Cases of AML developed subclonal population with *BCR-ABL1* have been reported [47–53]. These are not considered in the subtype of AML with *BCR-ABL1*. However, it is also recommended these cases be treated with BCR-ABL TKIs [6, 53, 54].

10. **What are the clinical implications of *FLT3* mutations in AML, and how are *FLT3* mutations tested in the clinical laboratories?**
    - FMS-like tyrosine kinase 3 (FLT3) is a member of the type III receptor tyrosine kinase family and consists of five immunoglobulin-like domains in the extracellular region, a juxtamembrane (JM) domain, a tyrosine kinase (TK) domain separated by a kinase insert domain, and a C-terminal domain in the intracellular region (Fig. 13.1a). Ligand binding to the FLT3 extracellular domain promotes receptor dimerization and subsequent tyrosine kinase domain activation. As such, a series of intracellular signaling molecules are activated through JAK/STAT, PI3K/AKT, and MAPK/ERK signal transduction. FLT3 protein plays an important role in the survival and proliferation of early hematopoietic progenitor cells [55, 56].
    - *FLT3* gene mutations occur in approximately one-third of all AML patients. *FLT3* mutation is not spe-

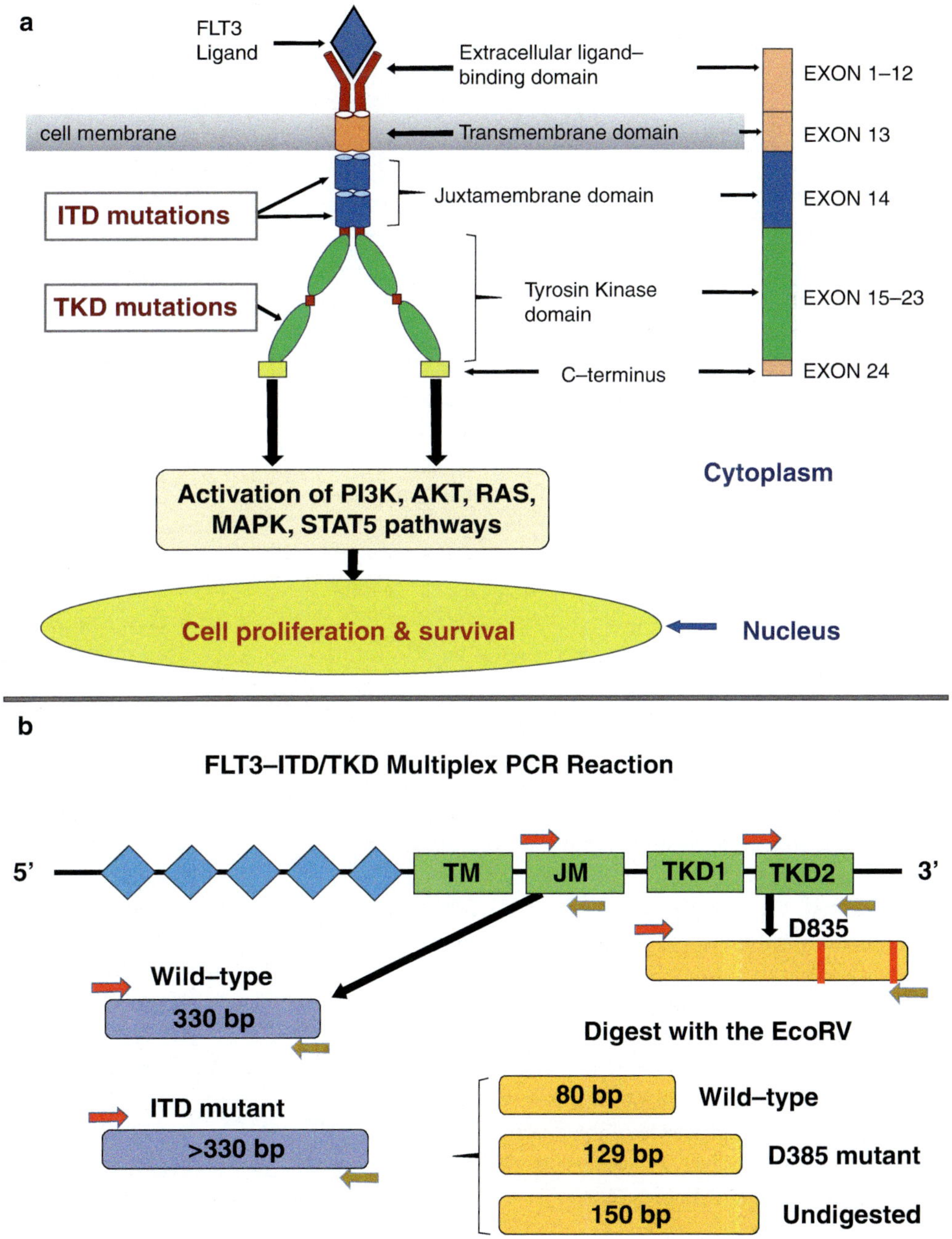

Fig. 13.1 *FLT3* (**a**) from gene/exons to protein domains and functions and (**b**) multiplex PCR detection of *FLT3* mutations. See text for more information

cific for any subtypes of AML and can also be seen in other myeloid neoplasms, as well as an early T-cell precursor (ETP) lymphoblastic leukemia/lymphoma. Three major groups of FLT3 activation mutations have been described: (1) internal tandem duplications (*FLT3*-ITDs) in JM domain (~20–25% of AML cases), (2) tyrosine-kinase domain mutations (*FLT3*-TKD) (~7–10%), and (3) point mutations in the JM domain (JMD) and in the extracellular domain (< 2% of AML patients) [57].

- *FLT3*-ITD usually results from an in-frame insertion in exons 14 and 15, and its size can vary greatly (3~400 bp, most commonly 6–30 bp). *FLT3*-ITD is associated with a high leukemic burden and poor prognosis in AML patients. *FLT3*-TKD mutations are point mutations or deletion most commonly affecting codon D835 in exon 20 of the kinase domain. In contrast to *FLT3*-ITD, the prognostic value of an *FLT3*-TKD mutation is not well established [58, 59].
- Traditionally, *FLT3* mutation assay is performed with a multiplex PCR-based fragment-length analysis. Two sets of fluorescent-labeled primers are designed to simultaneously amplify the regions where ITD and D835 mutations occur [60]; the D835 mutation is recognized by the loss of EcoRV enzyme digestion site (see Fig. 13.1b). The *FLT3*-ITD mutant allelic burden, defined as the mutant to the total *FLT3* ratio, is calculated from the electropherogram data by the areas under the curves (peaks) of mutant and wild-type alleles [61]. The fragment-length analysis is highly specific and has an analytic sensitivity of approximately 5%; the result is available within 3 days. The major limitation is that only a few *FLT3*-TKD point mutations can be detected based on the loss of the EcoRV enzyme site [62].
- The 2017 ELN recommendations and updated NCCN guidelines have incorporated *FLT3*-ITD mutation in risk stratifying patients based on the allelic burden, as well as co-occurring *NPM1* mutation. A high mutant level, defined as an allelic ratio of more than 50%, is associated with significantly worse clinical outcomes [8, 63]. However, in patients treated with FLT3 TKI, the clinical relevance of the allele burden needs further investigation [64].
- More than one mutation in *FLT3* can be seen in a patient with AML. In AML patients treated with TKI, a single, two, and three *FLT3* mutations were present in 47%, 18%, and 35% of cases, respectively. The prognostic significance of the number (single vs multiple) of *FLT3*-ITD variants is still controversial among different studies [65–67].
- To date, several FLT3 TKIs have been clinically approved as monotherapy or combination with conventional chemotherapy [55]. However, resistance to FLT3 inhibitors develops because of the expansion of *FLT3* wild-type clones, emerging clones with secondary mutations, especially those occurring at and around D835 as well as those with "gatekeeper" mutations affecting codon F691, and enhanced proliferation signal from other growth factors [55, 68].
- In view of the therapeutic and prognostic values of *FLT3* mutations, it is recommended that *FLT3* mutation testing should be expedited at the initial diagnosis of AML so that targeted therapy can be initiated in a timely manner [8]. *FLT3* mutation tests have limited value in evaluating MRD because (1) they probably always occur relatively late in leukemogenesis and (2) the mutations are unstable and the mutant allele level fluctuates in the clinical course [69].
- Different protocols of NGS-based tests have been developed to include *FLT3* mutation testing. One advantage of using NGS is that it can detect rare variants, such as TKI resistance-related mutations. The disadvantages include longer turnaround time and high complexity of workflow [62, 70]. Another significant pitfall of using NGS to detect *FLT3* mutations is that most bioinformatics pipelines are designed to detect single or multiple sequence variants (SNVs or MNVs) and short insertions or deletions (indels) and would not routinely identify long indels due to the difficulty in the sequence alignment. Therefore, validation of a pipeline with high sensitivity for long indels is required for *FLT3*-ITD detection [71, 72].

11. **What is the clinical significance of *NPM1* mutation in AML, and how do we test *NPM1* mutations?**
    - Nucleophosmin (NPM1) is a member of the nucleophosmin/nucleoplasmin (NPM) family of nuclear chaperones and in its wild-type state is localized to the nucleolus. NPM1 contains two nuclear export signal (NES) motifs in the N-terminal side, two nuclear localization signals (NLS) in the middle and one nucleolar localization signal (NoLS) at the C-terminus of the protein. These signals aid in shuttling the protein from the cytoplasm to the nucleus and then to the nucleolus, where it serves as a scaffolding protein for rRNA [73].
    - *NPM1* is one of the most commonly mutated genes in AML, present in 20–30% of all AMLs and 50–60% of adult AML with a normal karyotype. AML with mutated *NPM1*, showing characteristic genetic, morphologic, immunophenotypic, and clinical features, has been recognized as a distinct category in the 2016

WHO classification [6]. *NPM1* mutation is mutually exclusive with recurrent genetic abnormalities defining other AML entities; only approximately 15% of the AML with mutated *NPM1* cases carry chromosome aberrations such as trisomy 8 and del(9q) [74]. Of note, multilineage dysplasia is seen in approximately 20% of cases; the presence of multilineage dysplasia does not exclude a diagnosis of AML with mutated *NPM1* (see more discussion in question 16 and Case 1).

- *NPM1* mutations are typically small frameshift insertions (usually of 4 bp, up to 11 bp) in exon 12 (the last exon of *NPM1* coding sequence). These mutations result in the loss of W288 and W290 (or W290 alone), disrupting the NoLS and generating a novel NES at the C-terminus of the protein, leading to an aberrant accumulation of the protein within the cytoplasm [75]. The exact leukemogenesis mechanism of mutated NPM1 is still not well understood. Although more than 50 *NPM1* mutations have been reported so far, the three most common *NPM1* mutations (types A, B, and D) account for approximately 90% of AML cases with mutated *NPM1*. Types A, B, C, and D are all 4-bp insertion at the same location but with different sequences and prevalence, i.e., TCTG (type A, 80%), CATG (type B, ~6%), CGTG (type C, <1%), and CCTG (type D, ~6%), respectively [76, 77].
- About 40% of *NPM1*-mutated AMLs also harbor *FLT3*-ITD. In the context of cytogenetically normal AML, the presence of *NPM1* mutation without a *FLT3*-ITD correlates with a favorable prognosis, although this may not hold true in patients ≥60 years old [23]. In contrast, the coexistence of the *NPM1* mutation with *FLT3*-ITD, especially at an allelic ratio > 0.5, is associated with an intermediate prognosis [8]. The prognostic value of *FLT3*-ITD at a low allelic ratio (< 0.5) is controversial. Recent studies found that the co-existence of other mutations also affects the prognosis, for example, *NPM1/NRAS* of *NPM1/RAD21* combination is associated with good prognosis; *NPM1/WT1*, *NPM1/DNMT3A* double mutations or *NPM1/FLT3-ITD/DNMT3A* triple mutations show a particularly adverse clinical outcome [22, 73, 78]. With the increasing adoption of NGS-based mutation profiling in clinical laboratories and expanding use of targeted therapy, AML with mutated *NPM1* may be fragmented into many small molecular subsets of diverse prognoses [23, 37, 73].
- *NPM1* mutations are considered the driver and "gatekeepers" in the pathogenesis of AML and generally harbored in the whole leukemic population [79], persisted in the post-treatment residual clone, but not detected in the pre-leukemic clonal hematopoiesis of indeterminate potential (CHIP). As such, *NPM1* mutations are considered the ideal leukemia-specific target to monitor disease evolution. According to ELN recommendations, the patients of AML with mutated *NPM1* undergoing standard treatment should be tested with a highly sensitive method at least at diagnosis, after two cycles of therapy, and at the end of treatment. MRD should be measured every 3 months for the first 2 years of follow-up [80] and appropriate intervals determined by clinical presentations for the long-term follow-up.
- Several methods can be used to identify *NPM1* mutations in AML. Because almost all *NPM1* mutations are indels in exon 12, the PCR amplification of the exon followed by fragment-length analysis with capillary electrophoresis or melting curve analysis can be used to screen *NPM1* mutations at initial diagnosis. However, the analytic sensitivity of these methods is not enough for the purpose of monitoring low level mutations. RT-qPCR has been widely used as a sensitive and specific method for the diagnosis and monitoring of AML with mutated *NPM1* [81]. Depending on the multiplex PCR primer design, RT-qPCR testing can cover different percentages of *NPM1* mutations [82, 83]. *NPM1* is invariably included in the NGS panel for mutation profiling of myeloid neoplasms, generally reaching an analytic sensitivity below 5%. With special designs and unique molecular identifiers (UMI or molecular barcode), NGS can also be an excellent method for MRD detection and disease monitoring (see more discussion in question 18).

12. **What are the characteristics of *CEBPA* mutations in AML and how are *CEBPA* mutations detected in the clinical laboratories?**
    - *CEBPA* (CCAAT-enhancer binding protein alpha) is a single-exon gene that maps to chromosome band 19q13.11. It encodes a transcription factor that contains three transactivation elements (most publications described only two transactivation domains) and a basic region leucine zipper (BR-LZ) domain recognizing the CCAAT motif in the promoters of target genes, regulating myeloid cell differentiation and proliferation [84].
    - *CEBPA* gene mutations are detected in approximately 8–15% of all AML and 10% of cytogenetically normal AML [85]. AML patients with *CEBPA* mutations may carry one or two mutations; double *CEBPA* mutations are detected in approximately 60% of all *CEBPA*-mutated cases [86–88]. Most double mutations in *CEBPA* are confirmed to be biallelic [89, 90],

frequently one N-terminal truncating mutation and another C-terminal in-frame insertion/deletion [86, 87, 89]. The majority of AML with double *CEBPA* mutation cases have a normal karyotype; concurrent *FLT3*-ITD [87, 90–92] and *GATA2* [93] mutations are found in 5–9% and ~39% of cases, respectively.

- The N-terminal *CEBPA* mutations usually occur between the major translational start codon and a downstream start codon, leading to the production of only a smaller 30 kD (p30) isoform, in contrast to the full-length 42 kD (p42) CEBPA protein. The p30 protein cannot repress E2F family transcription factor activity, but retains the BR-LZ-binding domain, thus can promote granulocytic lineage commitment and cell proliferation, but not terminal differentiation. The C-terminal mutations usually cause proteins with impaired DNA binding and dimerization; it is thought to have a dominant-negative effect by preventing the heterodimers from binding to DNA [84].
- The possibility of a germline mutation with a predisposition to develop AML should be considered when double *CEBPA* mutations are detected, especially in younger patients [91, 94, 95]. *CEBPA* germline mutations clustered within the N-terminus are highly penetrant, with AML presenting at a median age of 24.5 years. In patients with germline *CEBPA* mutations, somatic C-terminal mutations occur as the "second hit" leading to leukemogenesis. Although familial *CEBPA*-mutated AML has a high recurrent rate, its long-term outcomes are usually favorable [95].
- In the 2016 WHO classification, a new entity is named "acute myeloid leukemia with biallelic mutation of *CEBPA*" and defines a group of AML with favorable prognosis. It is stated that "the favorable prognosis associated with *CEBPA* mutation in AML is now known to be related to biallelic mutations only; therefore, biallelic mutation is now required for assignment to this category" [6]. However, there is currently no clinically available molecular testing to recognize "biallelic" mutations (see below). In the published literature, there are only 2 studies using molecular cloning technique to confirm that 34 of the total 36 patients with double *CEBPA* mutations were in fact biallelic [89, 90]. All other studies with clinical and prognostic correlations reported "double *CEBPA* mutations" without confirming whether they were biallelic or not [87, 88, 91, 96–98]. So far there is no study to characterize the prognosis of rare AML with double but monoallelic *CEBPA* mutations. Therefore, in clinical practice, some hematopathologists prefer to use the diagnosing name "AML with double *CEBPA* mutations."
- Identification of *CEBPA* mutants is challenging for the following reasons: (1) the high GC content of the gene (75% in the coding region), (2) the presence of a trinucleotide repeat region, (3) the complexity of the mutations, and (4) the frequent occurrence of mutations in mononucleotide repeats [86]. So far multiple techniques have been used for *CEBPA* mutational analysis, including PCR-based fragment-length or melting curve analysis, Sanger sequencing, and NGS. Although efficient and sensitive, PCR-based fragment-length analysis can only detect mutations resulting in a net insertion or deletion and not substitution mutations; in addition, these tests also cannot distinguish a common 6-bp duplication polymorphism (p.H195_P196dup) from a pathologic insertion or duplication [99].
- Sequencing the entire coding region of the *CEBPA* gene enables detection of all mutations but is labor-intensive and requires expertise with unusual variants. NGS-based *CEBPA* mutation test can overcome the challenges associated with amplification efficiency and low coverage of *CEBPA* [86, 100]. It is important to note that Sanger sequencing cannot recognize the allelic origin of the mutations. Given the size of the coding region (1077-bp coding for 359 amino acids) and the double mutations usually occur distant from each other, in most cases, NGS reads cannot distinguish *cis* (monoallelic) and *trans* (biallelic) mutations in the *CEBPA* gene. However, double *CEBPA* mutations are usually assumed to be biallelic [89, 90].

13. **What is the clinical significance of *TP53* mutations in AML and how do we test *TP53* mutations?**
    - *TP53* mutations occur in ~8% of de novo AML cases, ~30% of t-AML, and ~ 70% of AML with complex karyotype [101]. In de novo AML, *TP53* mutations are commonly associated with older age, lower blast counts, and adverse risk karyotypes [102, 103]. In myeloid neoplasms, *TP53* mutations are considered as early initiating driver [101]. Studies have confirmed that *TP53* mutations are present in the "preleukemic" states such as CHIP [104, 105]. In therapy-related AML, *TP53* mutations are not acquired during cytotoxic therapy, but preexisted in hematopoietic cells; the mutant clones expand preferentially after treatment [106].
    - While commonly associated with complex cytogenetic abnormalities, frequently involving chromosomes 5, 7, and 17, *TP53*-mutated AMLs have significantly lower incidences of co-mutations in other genes, especially *FLT3*, *RAS*, and *NPM1* [107]. This is especially obvious in pure erythroid leukemia that invariably displays complex karyotypic abnor-

mality yet usually harbors mutation only in *TP53* gene (see example Case 5) [108].

- Despite recent advances and approvals for multiple therapeutic agents for AML, the outcome for *TP53*-mutated AML remains dismal [109]. It is essential to assess *TP53* mutation status at the initial diagnosis of AML for the best treatment decision. Recent studies found AML and MDS patients with *TP53* mutations showed a consistent response to decitabine [110, 111]. Clinical trials combining hypomethylating agents with the BCL2 inhibitor venetoclax for AML reported encouraging results in patients with *TP53* mutations, although the duration of response can be relatively short [112, 113].
- *TP53* mutations are stable during AML evolution [103] and may persist after AML patients achieving hematologic remission [114]. Monitoring *TP53* mutation status, therefore, provides significant prognostic information [103, 114].
- Like in other malignancies, the *TP53* mutations are distributed throughout the coding sequence in AML [115]. Therefore, sequencing the whole gene is the preferred molecular method for *TP53* analysis.
- It has been shown that somatic *TP53* missense mutations cause the nuclear accumulation of the mutant p53 protein in the tumor cells. Immunohistochemistry using various p53 monoclonal antibodies have been studied as a surrogate for *TP53* variant analysis [116–118]. However, some studies revealed that the relation between p53 accumulation and *TP53* variants is not straightforward; thus, some pathologists believe that p53 immunohistochemical staining should not be used as a screening methodology for *TP53* mutation [119].

14. **What are the *RUNX1* mutations frequently seen in AML and their clinical significance?**
    - *RUNX1* gene located on chromosome 21q22.12 was first identified as a part of the fusion gene, *AML1-ETO* (now named as *RUNX1-RUNX1T1*) generated by t(8;21) chromosome translocation associated with AML [120]. It encodes a runt-related transcription factor, RUNX1, a member of the core-binding factor family. The major functional domains of RUNX1 protein include a highly conserved, DNA-binding "runt" homology domain, and a C-terminal transcription activation domain [120].
    - The majority of mutations in *RUNX1* are missense mutations, large deletions, or truncation mutations in the "runt" homology domain, spanning exons 3–5, or transcription activation domain, spanning exons 6–8 [121, 122]. The mutant RUNX1 protein is either nonfunctional or acting with a dominant negative effect. At least one additional mutation is observed in other genes, such as *FLT3-ITD/TKD*, *NRAS*, *MLL-PTD*, *ASXL1*, *IDH1/IDH2*, *TET2*, *BCOR*, *DNMT3A*, *SRSF2*, *SF3B1*, and *WT1*, in 40.8–95% of AML patients with *RUNX1* mutations [122]. However, recurrent cytogenetic abnormalities, *NPM1* and *CEBPA* mutations, are not commonly associated with *RUNX1* mutation [6].
    - *RUNX1* mutations occur in 5.6–17.9% of AML cases [121, 122] more frequently show minimal differentiation (previous FAB M0 [1]). *RUNX1* mutations present in a variety of hematological malignancies, including de novo and secondary AML [123] and other myeloid neoplasms, confer a worse prognosis [124, 125]. Given the prognostic significance, *RUNX1* mutation is defining a new provisional entity of AML in the current WHO classification, when the AML cannot be otherwise classified. However, when occurring in favorable-risk AML subtypes (see discussion in question 4), *RUNX1* mutation is not a significant adverse prognostic marker [8].
    - A subset of *RUNX1* mutations are germline and associated with familial platelet disorder with myeloid malignancy (FPDMM), an autosomal-dominant disorder presenting with quantitative/qualitative platelet defect and a tendency to develop primarily myeloid malignancies, such as myelodysplastic syndrome (MDS) and AML [126] at a median onset age of 33 years old. Additional mutation is required for *RUNX1* germline mutation patients transforming to AML.
15. **What is the role of *GATA1* mutation in transient abnormal myelopoiesis (TAM) and myeloid leukemia associated with Down syndrome (MLADS)?**
    - A pre-leukemic condition known as transient abnormal myelopoiesis (TAM) is diagnosed in approximately 10% of newborns with Down syndrome with a median age at 3–7 days. 20–30% of these children develop nontransient acute myeloid leukemia 1–3 years later [6], commonly following a prolonged myelodysplasia-like phase. *GATA1* mutations are common in TAM and MLADS, as well as some Down syndrome neonates without distinguishing hematologic features [127].
    - GATA1 protein is one of the six zinc-finger transcription factors within the GATA family, which is named after the consensus-binding DNA sequence (A/T) GATA(A/G) [128]. There are at least two GATA1 protein isoforms that exist in normal human hematopoiesis: the well-characterized GATA1 full-length isoform and a truncated GATA1 short isoform (GATA1s). GATA1s lacks the 83 amino acids comprising the N-terminal transcription activation domain [129].

- The majority of *GATA1* somatic mutations observed in TAM and MLADS are deletions, insertions, and point mutations clustered in exon 2 or the beginning of exon 3. These mutations exclusively result in truncated GATA1s in TAM and MLADS blasts, perturbing the transcription of genes involved in erythroid and megakaryocytic differentiation [130].
- When TAM evolves to MLADS, the neoplastic clone usually acquires additional genetic abnormalities. In addition to trisomy 21, trisomy 8 is commonly seen in MLADS, occurring in 13–44% of patients [6]. Acquired mutations in MLADS are found in cohesion components; epigenetic regulators such as *CTCF*, *EZH2*, and *KANSL1*; JAK family kinases *JAK2*, *JAK3*, *MPL*, *SH2B3*; RAS pathway genes [131]; and gain-of-function mutation in myeloid cytokine receptor *CSF2RB* [132]. Further studies are required to determine whether additional mutations can predict disease progression, treatment response, and overall survival.

16. **What ancillary tests should be considered toward a diagnosis of AML with myelodysplasia-related changes?**
    - AML with myelodysplasia-related changes (AML-MRC) is a group of AMLs associated with relatively inferior outcomes compared to other subtypes of AML. By definition, the diagnosis of AML-MRC requires (1) the presence of 20% or more peripheral blood or bone marrow blasts, (2) morphological features of myelodysplasia or a prior history of an MDS or myelodysplastic/myeloproliferative neoplasm (MDS/MPN) or MDS-related cytogenetic abnormalities, and (3) the absence of the specific genetic abnormalities characteristic of AML with recurrent genetic abnormalities [6].
    - Based on the criteria, the diagnosis of AML-MRC first requires to rule out the subtypes of AML with recurrent genetic abnormalities; and a subgroup of AML-MRC is diagnosed based on the presence of the MDS-associated cytogenetic abnormality, even in the absence of morphologic evidence of dysplasia (the complete list of specific abnormalities can be found in the WHO classification book and will not be detailed here). Therefore, conventional and/or molecular karyotyping (FISH or copy number array) is required before making a diagnosis of AML-MRC.
    - Studies showed that multilineage dysplasia in the absence of myelodysplasia-related cytogenetic changes did not appear to be associated with poor prognosis in the presence of an *NPM1* mutation or double *CEBPA* mutations [133, 134]. In light of these findings, the 2016 WHO classification clarifies that the presence of multilineage dysplasia alone is not sufficient to classify a case as AML-MRC; when a mutation in *NPM1* or double mutation of *CEBPA* is present, the case should be classified based on the mutations [4]. In cases lacking these mutations, the morphologic finding of multilineage dysplasia (defined as the presence of 50% or more dysplastic cells in at least two lineages) is still a poor prognostic indicator and is sufficient to render a diagnosis of AML-MRC [135].
    - *NPM1* mutation and biallelic mutation of *CEBPA* are uncommonly seen in AML-MRC; in contrast, *U2AF1*, *ASXL1*, and *TP53* are more frequently mutated. *TP53* mutations are almost always associated with a complex karyotype abnormalities, which indicate an even worse prognosis in this generally poor prognostic group of AML [135]. With the recent advancement in NGS and the discovery of the emerging role that mutations play in AML-MRC and their impact on prognosis, our understanding of AML-MRC is evolving [136]. An MRC-like molecular profile may need to be taken into consideration in the definition of AML-MRC in the future [3].
17. **How frequently should molecular testing or mutation profiling be repeated in the clinical follow up of the AML patients after treatment?**
    - Repeat molecular testing for the signature of leukemic clone(s) is an approach to evaluate the disease status, providing valuable prognostic and predictive information to help further management decisions. Serial tests to monitor the level of AML-specific mutations/fusions transcripts helped inform the treatment response in some studies [83, 137, 138]. See more discussion on MRD testing in question 18.
    - The current NCCN guideline for AML recommends multiplex gene panels or comprehensive NGS analysis for the ongoing management of AML at various phases of treatment [7]. Molecular testing of clinically significant mutations to assess early treatment response in AML can predict relapse hazard and help risk-directed therapy [139]. However, except for RT-qPCR for *PML-RARA* [140], there are no standardized guidelines regarding when and how to repeat molecular testing for most AML patients.
    - NCCN guideline also recommended that comprehensive genomic profiling to determine the mutation status of actionable genes be repeated at relapse or progression as it may facilitate better selection of therapy and appropriate clinical trials [7].
    - For patients in complete remission preparing for allogeneic hematopoietic stem cell transplantation, the presence of leukemic clone(s) in peripheral blood detected by molecular testing was associated with poor survival similar to patients with active bone

marrow disease identified by traditional evaluation [141]. Molecular testing prior to transplantation could be helpful to triage patients for transplantation based on improved risk stratification.

18. **What is the role of molecular methods in the minimal/measurable residual disease (MRD) detection of AML and how are they performed in the clinical laboratories?**
    - Measurable residual disease (AKA minimal residual disease, MRD) refers to the posttreatment persistence of leukemic cells below the level recognizable by routine morphologic examination. The presence of MRD has been recognized as a strong and independent prognostic indicator of increased risk of relapse and shorter survival in most AML patients reported by many studies. MRD detection is used to assess treatment response and refine risk-stratification [142].
    - MRD monitoring has been part of routine clinical practice in the management of patients with APL [140]. Recent studies suggest that MRD monitoring should be considered a part of the standard of care for AML patients for the following purposes [80, 143]:
        1. To establish a deeper remission status, providing a refined outcome prediction and guidance for post-remission treatment
        2. Identifying impending relapse and enabling early intervention
        3. Allowing more robust post-transplant surveillance
        4. Providing a surrogate endpoint to accelerate clinical trial drug testing and approval
    - Many methods have been used for evaluating MRD in AML patients, including multiparameter flow cytometry (MFC), FISH and quantitative PCR (qPCR). Recently, newer technologies, including droplet digital PCR (ddPCR) and NGS, have been developed to detect MRD. Each methodology differs in the proportion of patients to whom it can be applied and in its analytic sensitivity [142].
    - The two most widely applied MRD detection methods in AML are MFC and qPCR. The analytic sensitivity of MFC can reach 10^{-4} to 10^{-5}, with the advantages of wide applicability (>90%), quick turnaround time (within 1 day), and high specificity when leukemia-associated immunophenotype is present [142]. qPCR (or RT-qPCR) can be used to detect gene fusions, insertions/duplications, point mutations, and gene overexpression. PCR-based MRD assessment is easier to standardize in the clinical laboratories than MFC analysis. Optimized qPCR can be more sensitive than MFC for MRD assessment.
    - Gene fusions commonly used as a target for MRD monitoring include *PML-RARA*, *CBFB-MYH11*, and *RUNX1-RUNX1T1*. RT-qPCR is performed to amplify fusion targets. Other fusion genes less commonly seen in AML can also be targeted; however, it would be more challenging to validate and maintain as a clinical test. Of note, the transcript level may not always correlate well with the number of leukemic cells [144, 145].
    - The best example of insertions/duplications for MRD detection is *NPM1* mutations. Multiplex PCR designed for the most common variants of *NPM1* mutations (types A, B, and D) covers 90% of AML-harboring *NPM1* mutations.
    - The main target of gene overexpression in AML is *WT1*; however, it is difficult to obtain an analytic sensitivity to test *WT1* amplification for low-level disease. Given the limited sensitivity and specificity, *WT1* expression should not be used as an MRD marker unless no other markers are available in the patient [80].
    - A major disadvantage of qPCR is that it can only be applied in approximately 50% of AML cases [146]. Currently, qPCR-based MRD detection can be routinely performed only for APL, core-binding factor AML, and AML with *NPM1* mutation. While ddPCR promises much better analytic sensitivity, other limitations are the same as traditional qPCR.
    - NGS, especially targeted-panel deep sequencing combining DNA and RNA with UMI, is becoming a powerful tool for MRD evaluation. Compared to PCR-based methods, targeted panel NGS have the advantage to cover a broader range of genes and as such are applicable for MRD detection in more AML patients. The mutation profile detected by NGS helps trace clonal evolution of the leukemic cells [147] and monitor changes of the mutations with targeted therapies [142, 148].
    - One caveat of NGS-based MRD assessment is that it can be hampered by the presence of mutations not specific for AML clone(s). *DNMT3A*, *TET2*, *ASXL1* (DTA), *IDH1/2*, *TP53*, and *SRSF2* mutations are frequently detected, many times at relatively high allele frequencies, during complete remission [114, 149]. These mutations are considered from "pre-leukemic" CHIP or other myeloid neoplasms [114, 147, 149]. The presence of pre-leukemic DTA mutations may not have independent prognostic value with respect to the risk of relapse and survival rates [114, 149].
    - In addition to DTA mutations, many other mutations are also detected in AML patients at complete remission. Currently, there are not sufficient studies to elucidate the significance of each mutation in asso-

ciation with the risk of relapse or worse prognosis [150]. In the study reported by Morita et al., residual *TP53* mutations at complete remission have a strong prognostic impact [114]. Debarri et al. reported that monitoring of *IDH1/2* mutations allowed the prediction of relapse in the majority of patients [151].

- MRD levels measured after induction and consolidation chemotherapies may not always be predictive of clinical outcome [139, 152]. Studies have found that some AML patients without detectable MRD after induction therapy eventually relapsed; in contrast, a subset of patients with detectable MRD had a long relapse-free survival. Furthermore, with the continuous improvement of the sensitivity of MRD detection methods, MRD levels below a certain threshold may not correlate with relapse [153–155]. More studies on the molecular markers, timing, methods, and optimal sensitivity level or cutoff value of MRD detection are required to correlate with the clinical outcomes; and the MRD detection protocols need to be standardized before implementing as routine clinical tests.

Case Presentations

The clinical histories of these cases are slightly modified to simplify the presentation and avoid the potential association of any protected patient information.

Case 1

Learning Objectives

- Recognize the typical clinical workup for an APL diagnosis usually requires a STAT test for *PML-RARA* fusion.
- Learn the molecular method of RT-qPCR for the fusion transcript detection in APL.

Case History and Laboratory Findings

A 53-year-old male is found to have high blood glucose on a visit to his primary care physician. He is referred to the emergency department. Routine blood tests show pancytopenia with "unidentified cells" on a blood smear.

Laboratory Findings

Blood cell counts:

WBC 20 K/μL with "unidentified cells" on peripheral smear
Hb 9.8 g/dL, RBC 3.26 M/μL, MCV 90.5 fL
Platelets 68 K/μL

Blood coagulation related tests:

PT 14.7 sec (reference <12.5)
D-dimer 19,290 ng/mL (reference <574)
Fibrinogen 141 (200–393)

Pathology

Representative blood smear findings are displayed in Fig. 13.2a and b; the dot plots of flow cytometric analysis are shown in Fig. 13.3. The morphologic and immunophenotypic features are highly suspicious for acute promyelocytic leukemia.

Molecular Genetic Tests

A stat FISH for t(15;17);*PML-RARA* is requested. Abnormal fusion signals were detected (Fig. 13.2c). A molecular test for the quantitation of *PML-RARA* transcript level is also performed (Fig. 13.4).

Final Diagnosis

Acute promyelocytic leukemia with *PML-RARA*

Follow-Up

The patient starts to take all-trans retinoic acid (ATRA) and arsenic trioxide (ATO) and achieves remission 2 months later. A bone marrow biopsy shows 60% cellularity with no blasts by morphologic examination and flow cytometry. The FISH and RT-qPCR for *PML-RARA* both report negative results.

Discussion

This case illustrates the typical laboratory diagnosis of APL. When morphologic and immunophenotypic features suggest the possibility of APL, a STAT FISH or other forms of rapid tests for *PML-RARA* fusion gene or protein is usually performed to confirm the diagnosis. Although RT-qPCR is not necessary for the diagnosis of APL, it is frequently performed to determine the baseline level of the fusion transcript. In recent years, more and more APL cases are diagnosed with blood samples only, without requiring a bone marrow sampling. To follow up on the treatment response, either blood or bone marrow samples, or both, are acceptable. The fusion transcript usually becomes negative after successful induction with ARTA with or without ATO.

Case 2

Learning Objectives

- AML with mutated *NPM1* is a distinct category of AML in the 2016 revised WHO classification and shows dis-

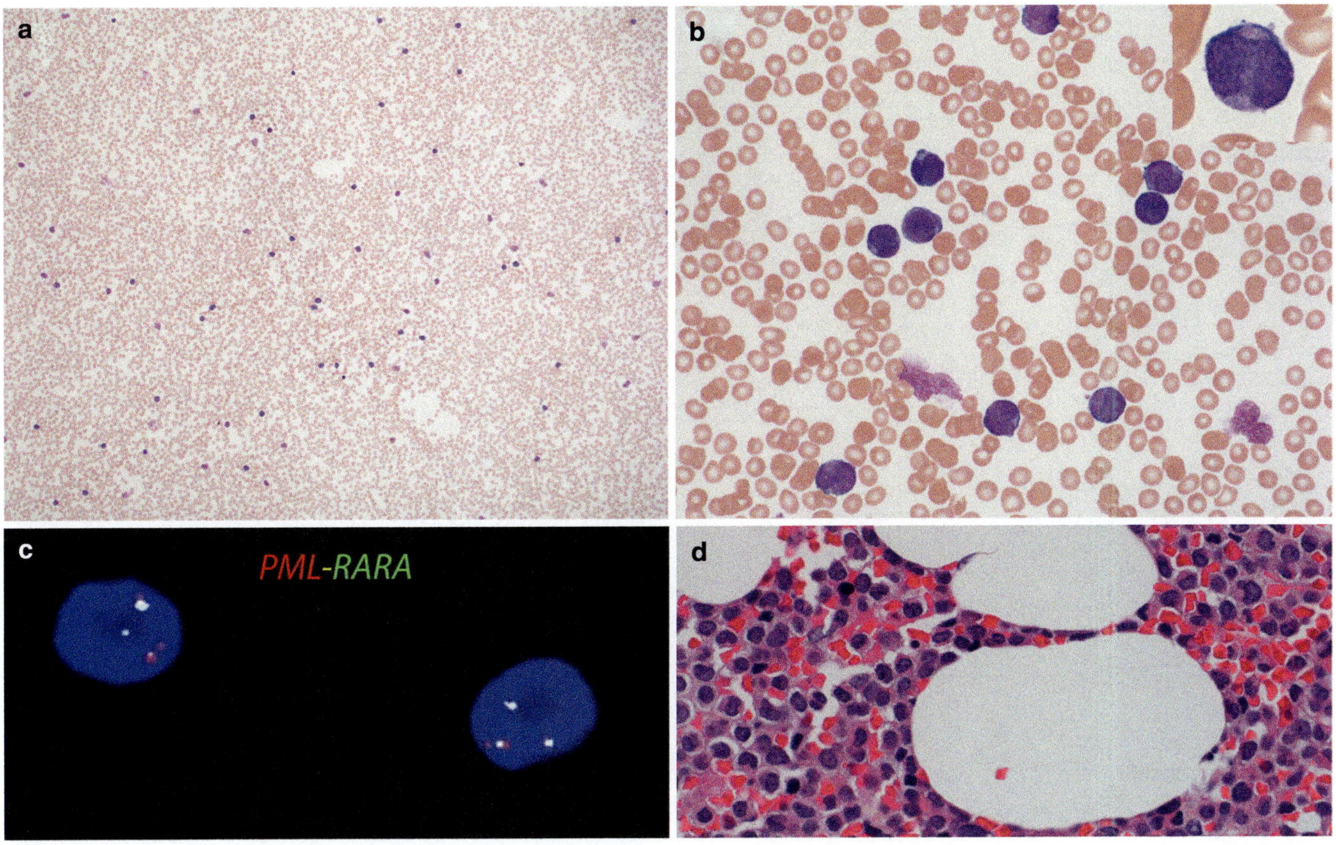

Fig. 13.2 Morphologic features and *PML-RARA* FISH result of APL. (**a**) Blood smear (Wright-Giemsa stain, 100×) shows leukocytosis with mostly blasts and (**b**) (600×) shows most blasts have cleaved nuclei; cytoplasmic granules are seen in some blasts; however, they are not hypergranular (see insert on the right upper corner). The morphologic features are characteristic of a hypogranular (microgranular) acute promyelocytic leukemia (APL). (**c**) Fluorescence in situ hybridization (FISH) shows an abnormal signal pattern (one green, one red, two fusion: FFGR) indicating the presence of *PML-RARA* fusion gene. Of note, the fusion gene may not always be detectable by chromosome analysis (conventional karyotyping); therefore, the current WHO classification have removed t(15;17) from the diagnosing name of APL. A bone marrow biopsy (**d**, H&E stain, 600×) reveals numerous blasts with slightly irregular nuclei, the cleaved nuclei can be seen in some blasts

tinctive genetic, pathologic, immunophenotypic, and clinical features.

- Multilineage dysplasia is seen in approximately 20% of de novo AML with mutated *NPM1*, but it does not result in a worse prognosis as seen in AML-MRC.

Case History

A 78-year-old female presents to the hospital with rapid atrial fibrillation. She is found to have abnormal blood cell counts and thrush.

Laboratory Findings

Blood cell counts:

WBC 24.5 K/μL with absolute monocyte count 13 K/μL
Hemoglobin 10.4 g/dL; platelets 73 K/μL

Flow Cytometry

Flow cytometric analysis performed on the bone marrow aspirate shows a discrete population of blasts with no CD34 and CD117 expression (Fig. 13.5).

Histologic Features

Bone marrow aspirate smears (Fig. 13.6) show a heterogeneous population of large-sized blasts without Auer rods and trilineage dysplasia. Core biopsy (not shown) reveals hypercellular marrow (90%) with sheets of immature mononuclear cells accounting for approximately 80% of cellularity.

Preliminary Diagnosis

Acute myeloid leukemia with myelodysplasia-related changes (AML-MRC)

Cytogenetic and Molecular Tests

- Karyotype: 46,XX [20]
- FISH: negative for core-binding factor gene rearrangements
- Negative for *PML-RARA*, *BCR-ABL1* fusion transcripts, *FLT3*, and *IDH* mutations
- Next-generation sequencing (hematological malignancies panel, 116 genes):

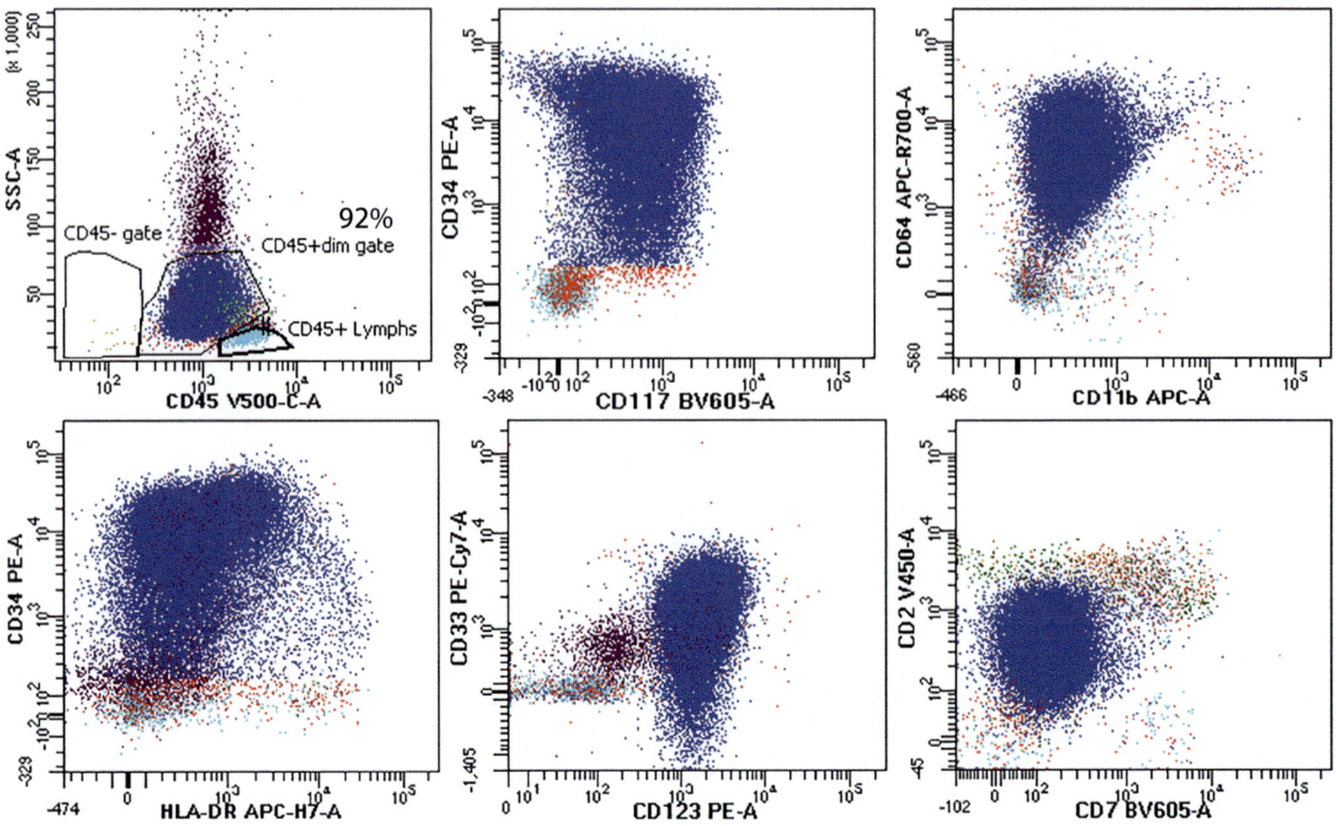

Fig. 13.3 Flow cytometry of the blood sample. The dot plots show a large percentage of cells in the CD45 dim blast gate merged with the granulocytes (high SSC). The blasts are positive for CD2 (dim), CD33, variable CD34, CD64, CD117 (dim), and CD123 and only a small subset positive for HLA-DR; they are negative for CD11b and CD7. Additionally (not shown in the figure), blasts are positive for CD4 (partial), CD13, CD36 (partial), CD38 (dim), CD56, and CD200 and negative for CD3, CD5, CD8, CD10, CD11c, CD14, CD15, CD16, CD19, CD20, CD22, and CD26. The immunophenotype of variable CD34, subset HLA-DR, and partial CD2 expression is frequently seen in microgranular APL

1. *NPM1* [NM_002520.6] c.860_863dupTCTG (p.W288fs*12) (*NPM1* Type A) at 43%
2. *PTPN11* [NM_002834.5] c.182A > G; p.D61G at 44%
3. *TET2* [NM_001127208.3] c.2905C > T; p.Q969* at 46%

Final Diagnosis

AML with mutated *NPM1*

Discussion

This case is initially classified as AML-MRC based on the multilineage dysplasia and normal cytogenetic results. However, a well-defined *NPM1* mutation is detected. Recurrent genetic abnormalities generally have priority over morphologic and immunophenotypic features in classifying AML. AML with mutated *NPM1* accounts for approximately half of adult AML with a normal karyotype and one-fifth of pediatric AML with a normal karyotype [6]. Multilineage dysplasia is seen in approximately one-quarter of cases of de novo AML with mutated *NPM1*. In the 2008 WHO classification, such cases were considered AML-MRC [24]. However, studies showed that the presence of dyspoiesis in this setting does not appear to affect prognosis [121]. WHO reclassified such cases as AML with mutated *NPM1* in the 2016 revised classification.

Therefore, the final diagnosis is modified to AML with mutated *NPM1*. Of note, cases of AML with multilineage dysplasia may also carry *FLT3* of *CEBPA* mutations, in addition to *NPM1* mutation. Cases with both *NPM1* and *FLT3* mutations are still classified as AML with mutated *NPM1*. If double *CEBPA* mutations are present, it should be classified as AML with double/biallelic mutation of *CEBPA*.

Case 3

Learning Objective

Discuss AML with mutated *RUNX1*, a provisional AML category that can only be recognized by sequencing the *RUNX1* gene.

a Sample	Ct APL	Ct APL	Ct Abl	Ct Abl	Avg APL	Avg Abl	Ratio
NTC	UNDET		UNDET				
INV PML RNA POS Control	31.9536	32.1103	29.4295	29.434	32.03195	29.43175	1.00E+00
bcr1	34.7969				34.7969		
NB4 1E-3	33.1631		23.616		33.1631	23.616	8.11E-03
Patient #1	39.614	38.2155	24.4232	24.9725	38.91475	24.69785	3.18E-04
Patient #2	24.1504	24.0267	23.0718	23.2759	24.08855	23.17385	3.22E+00
Patient #3	UNDET	UNDET	24.9154	24.6929	UNDET	24.80415	NEGATIVE
Patient #4	UNDET	UNDET	24.3894	25.2228	UNDET	24.8061	NEGATIVE
Patient #5	UNDET	UNDET	25.084	25.4041	UNDET	25.24405	NEGATIVE
Patient #6	27.4569	27.2769	25.4041	25.4565	27.3669	25.4303	1.58E+00
Patient #7	UNDET	UNDET	25.8531	25.8085	UNDET	25.8308	NEGATIVE

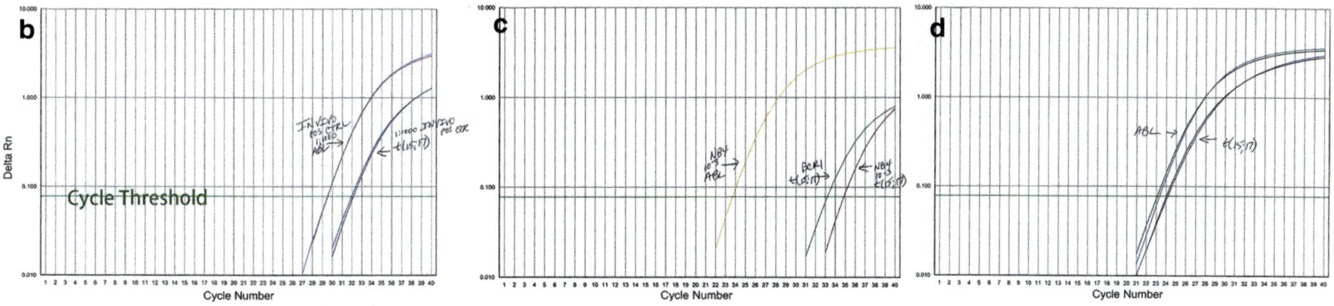

Fig. 13.4 *PML-RARA* RT-qPCR test. This figure displays a complete laboratory run of *PML-RARA* quantitative (real-time) reverse transcription polymerase chain reaction (RT-qPCR) test. (**a**) The table records the cycle threshold of controls and seven patients, as well as the final *PML-RARA* to *ABL* ratio calculation. The test has a negative control (no template control, NTC), a positive (POS) control provided in the test kit, a positive breakpoint control (bcr1), and an NB4 cell line control. **b**, **c**, and **d** show the qPCR amplification curves. The cycle threshold is determined by a horizontal green line. When this line crosses the *PML-RARA* or *ABL* amplification curve, the corresponding cycle number is the Ct value. (**b**) The manufacturer provided positive control, (**c**) bcr1 and NB4 control. (**d**) Patient 2 (the case described above) with relatively high fusion transcript level. The test is designed to detect three breakpoint clusters (*bcr1*, *bcr2*, *bcr3* [160]). However, for each test run, only one breakpoint control is required as long as all three controls are tested periodically. NB4 control is used to verify that the whole experimental process starting from RNA extraction to the calculation of *PML-RARA* to *ABL* ratio is successful

Case History

A 58-year-old woman has a new onset of dizziness then a pre-syncopal episode. She is brought to the emergency department and a blood cell count shows marked pancytopenia (WBC 400/μL, hemoglobin 4.8 g/dL, platelet 2400/μL), and blast type cells are identified by blood smear review, representing 2% of white blood cells.

A bone marrow biopsy is performed. The bone marrow aspirate smear and biopsy section are shown in Fig. 13.7, and flow cytometric analysis of the bone marrow aspirate is displayed in Fig. 13.8.

Cytogenetic Studies

Conventional chromosome analysis and copy number-single nucleotide polymorphism (CN-SNP) array reveal normal female karyotype. FISH for *PML-RARA*, *RUNX1-RUNX1T1*, *CBFB-MYH11*, and *BCR-ABL1* fusion or translocation involving *KMT2A* are all negative.

Based on the morphologic and immunophenotypic features, with no abnormal cytogenetic findings, a preliminary diagnosis of acute myeloid leukemia with minimal differentiation was rendered.

Molecular Genetic Studies

NGS of 75 genes (myeloid neoplasm-panel) identifies the following 4 mutations:

- *FLT3* [NM_004119.2] c.2505 T > G; p.D835E at 4.5%
- *NRAS* [NM_002524.4] c.38G > A; p.G13D at 23.2%
- *RUNX1* [NM_001754.4] c.293_295delTCTinsGACTTCC; p.L98fs at 29.2%
- *WT1* [NM_024426.4] c.1104dupG; p.R369fs at 3.2% and c.1138delCinsGG (p.R380fs) at 1.5%

Final Diagnosis

Acute myeloid leukemia with mutated *RUNX1*

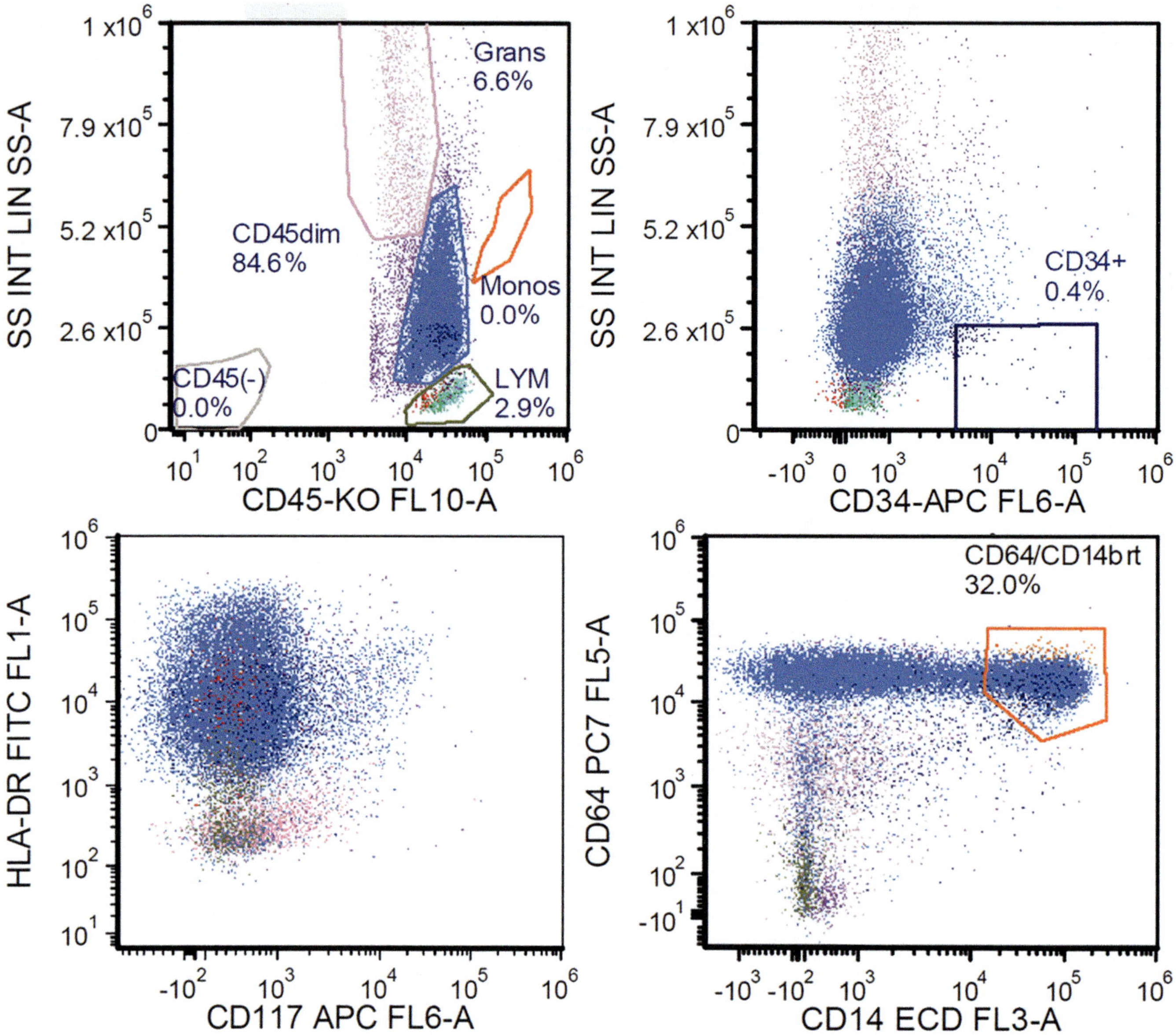

Fig. 13.5 Flow cytometry dot plots. The blasts (84.6%) are positive for partial CD14, CD64, and HLA-DR and negative for CD34 and CD117. Other positive markers (not shown) are CD7, CD11b, CD13 (dim), CD15, CD33, CD56 (dim), CD71 (dim), CD123 (subset), and cMPO

Discussion

- 15–65% of cases of minimally differentiated AML demonstrate *RUNX1* mutation [156]. Without NGS-based mutation profiling, correct classification of this case would not be feasible because *RUNX1* is not routinely tested as a single gene in AML.
- The *RUNX1* c.293_295delTCTinsGACTTCC is a frameshift mutation affecting the runt-homology domain (RHD). This kind of mutation is characteristic in AML with mutated *RUNX1*.
- *RUNX1* mutations in AML have been associated with worse overall survival. Cooperating mutations are common with *RUNX1* mutation. Additional mutations in *FLT3*, *NRAS*, and *WT1* in this case are likely significant for the prognosis but not used for the classification of AML.
- The recurrent cytogenetic abnormalities and mutations of *NPM1*, *CEBPA*, and *JAK2* described in AML are uncommon in *RUNX1*-mutated cases [123, 157–159]. If an AML can be classified based on the other molecular genetic abnormalities, it should not be classified as AML with mutated *RUNX1*.

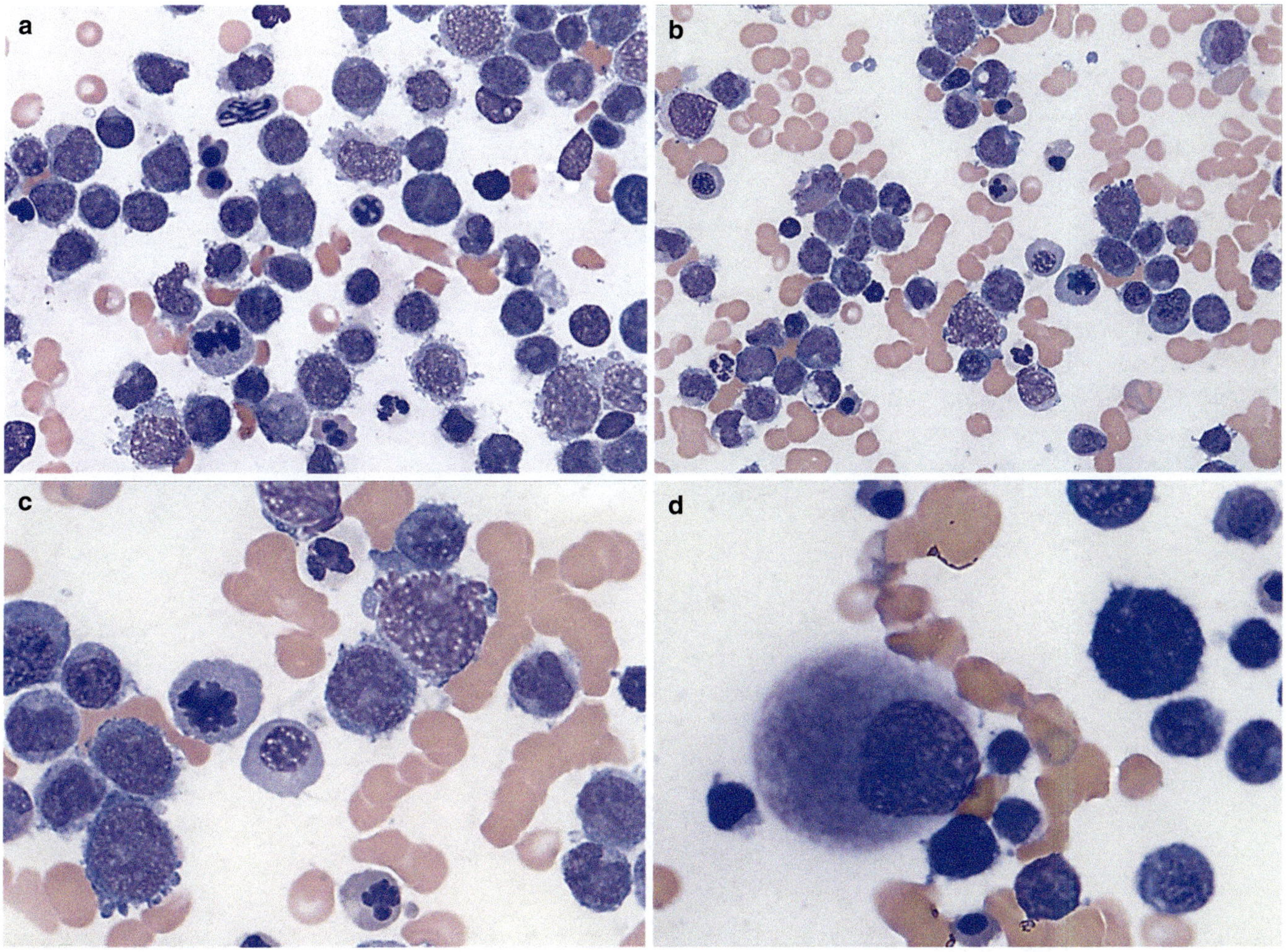

Fig. 13.6 Bone marrow aspirate smear (Wright-Giemsa stain; (**a** and **b**) 400×, (**c** and **d**) 1000×) shows a heterogeneous population of large-sized blasts without Auer rods; the majority contains fine chromatin, small nucleoli, and scant blue cytoplasm. Erythroid precursors are decreased and show significant dyserythropoiesis (megaloblastoid maturation, nuclear blebbing/budding) in greater than 50% of nucleated precursors. Maturing myeloid elements are markedly decreased and show significant dysgranulopoiesis (cytoplasmic hypogranularity and nuclear hyposegmentation) in greater than 50% of precursors (**a**, **b**, and **c**). Megakaryocytes are decreased with occasional small forms (**d**)

Case 4

Learning Objective

The neoplastic clone of AML is evolving after treatment. Following the changes of mutations and their allele frequencies can provide information regarding clonal evolution, residual disease, and potential coexisting clones of other origins.

Case History

A 78-year-old male is found to have a high white cell count (149 K/μL) and 86% "blasts" in the blood smear at a routine clinic visit for his high blood pressure. He denies any symptoms including fever, chills, and shortness of breath or bruising tendency.

Blood and bone marrow sampling confirm marked leukocytosis with numerous blasts (Fig. 13.9).

Flow cytometric immunophenotyping reveals a distinct myeloblast population (Fig. 13.10).

Molecular Genetic Studies

- Chromosome analysis reveals normal male karyotype: 46,XY [20].
- FISH for *PML-RARA* fusion is negative.
- NGS of myeloid neoplasm-related 75 gene panel detects the following 4 mutations:
  - *NPM1* [NM_002520.6] c.860_863dupTCTG (p. W288fs) (*NPM1* Type A) at 37.3%
  - *FLT3-ITD* 27 bp: [NM_0049119.2] c.1758_1784dup (p.F594_R595ins9) at 22.9%
  - *DNMT3A* [NM_022552.4] c.1743G > T (p.W581C) at 44.7%
  - *SMC1A* [NM_006306.3] c.1193G > A (p.R398Q) at 95.9%

Final Diagnosis

Acute myeloid leukemia with mutated *NPM1*

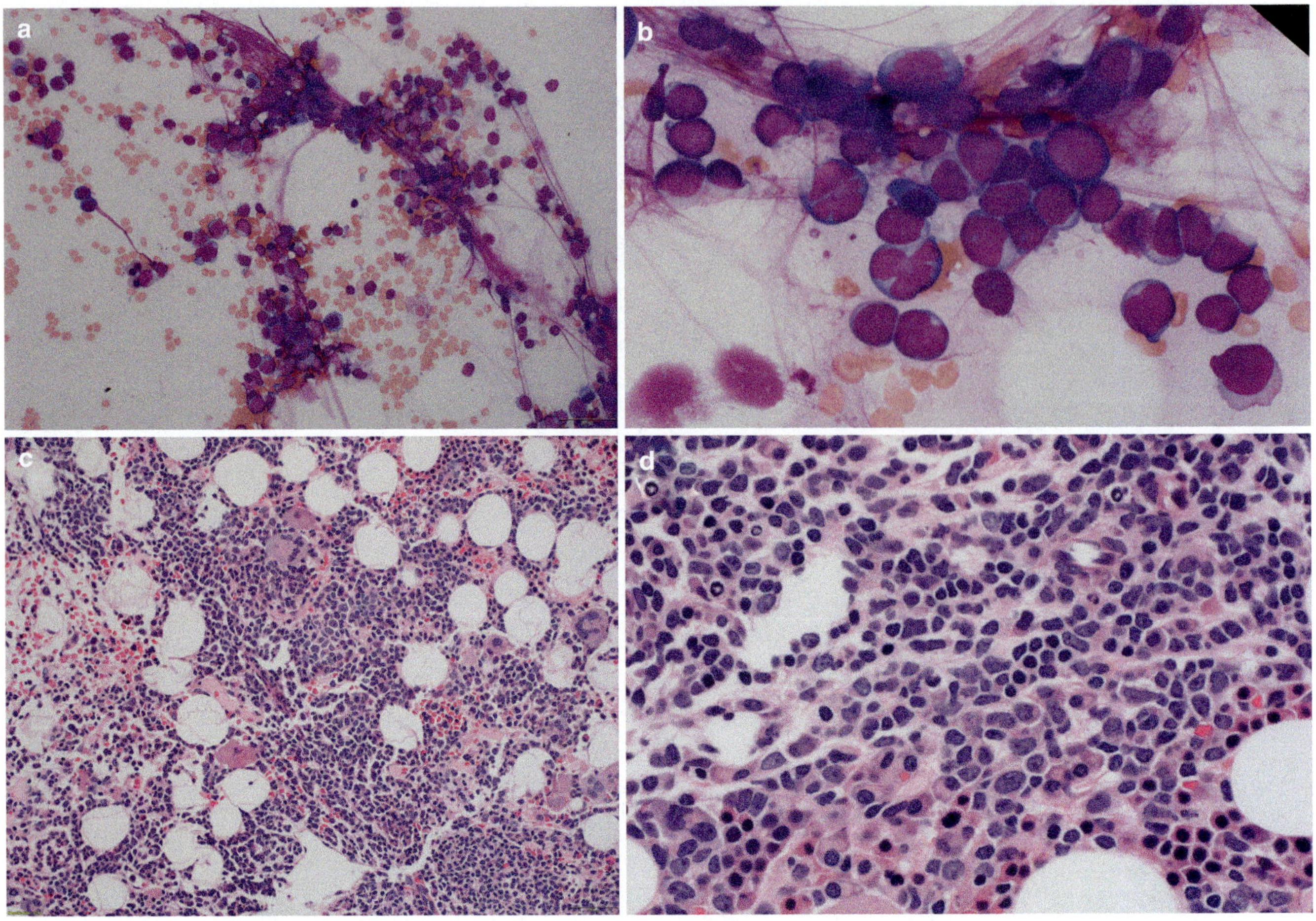

Fig. 13.7 Bone marrow aspirate smear and biopsy section. Wright-Giemsa-stained smears (**a**) (200×) and (**b**) (600×) show blasts with no obvious differentiation features; the sheets of blasts are present in the hypercellular bone marrow ((**c** and **d**) H&E stained biopsy core; (**c**) 200× and (**d**) 600×)

Treatment and Clinical Follow-Up

Considering the advanced age of the patient and the presence of *FLT3-ITD*, the patient is treated with gilteritinib and decitabine. Five months later, a repeated bone marrow sampling reveals no morphologic and immunophenotypic evidence of residual blasts in the hypocellular bone marrow. However, a population of immunoglobulin kappa light chain-restricted B-cells expressing CD19, CD20, CD22 (slightly dimmer than background polytypic B cells), CD200 (dim), HLA-DR, and CD45 is detected by flow cytometry. The monotypic B-cell population is negative for CD5, CD10, and CD11c.

Repeat NGS (75 gene panel) detects the following four mutations:

- *NPM1* [NM_002520.6] c.860_863dupTCTG (p.W288fs) (*NPM1* Type A) at 5.7%
- *DNMT3A* [NM_022552.4] c.1743G > T (p.W581C) at 3.9%
- *SMC1A* [NM_006306.3] c.1193G > A (p.R398Q) at 10.2%
- *MYD88* [NM_002468.4] c.794 T > C (p.L265P) at 4.8%

The *FLT3-ITD* mutation is not identified in this posttreatment bone marrow sample. Therefore, gilteritinib is stopped and only decitabine is continued.

Five more months later, another bone marrow sampling shows hypocellular bone marrow with no evidence of residual leukemia. Several lymphoid aggregates are present with mixed CD3-positive and CD20-positive cells (Fig. 13.11). The NGS of the same 75 gene panel only detected *MYD88* c.794 T > C (p.L265P) at 1% of alleles.

Discussion

- The mutation profile of this AML with mutated *NPM1* case exemplifies that the *NPM1* mutation is an early event in the leukemogenesis and *FLT3*-ITD mutation coexists in a subpopulation of AML cells (clonal evolution result-

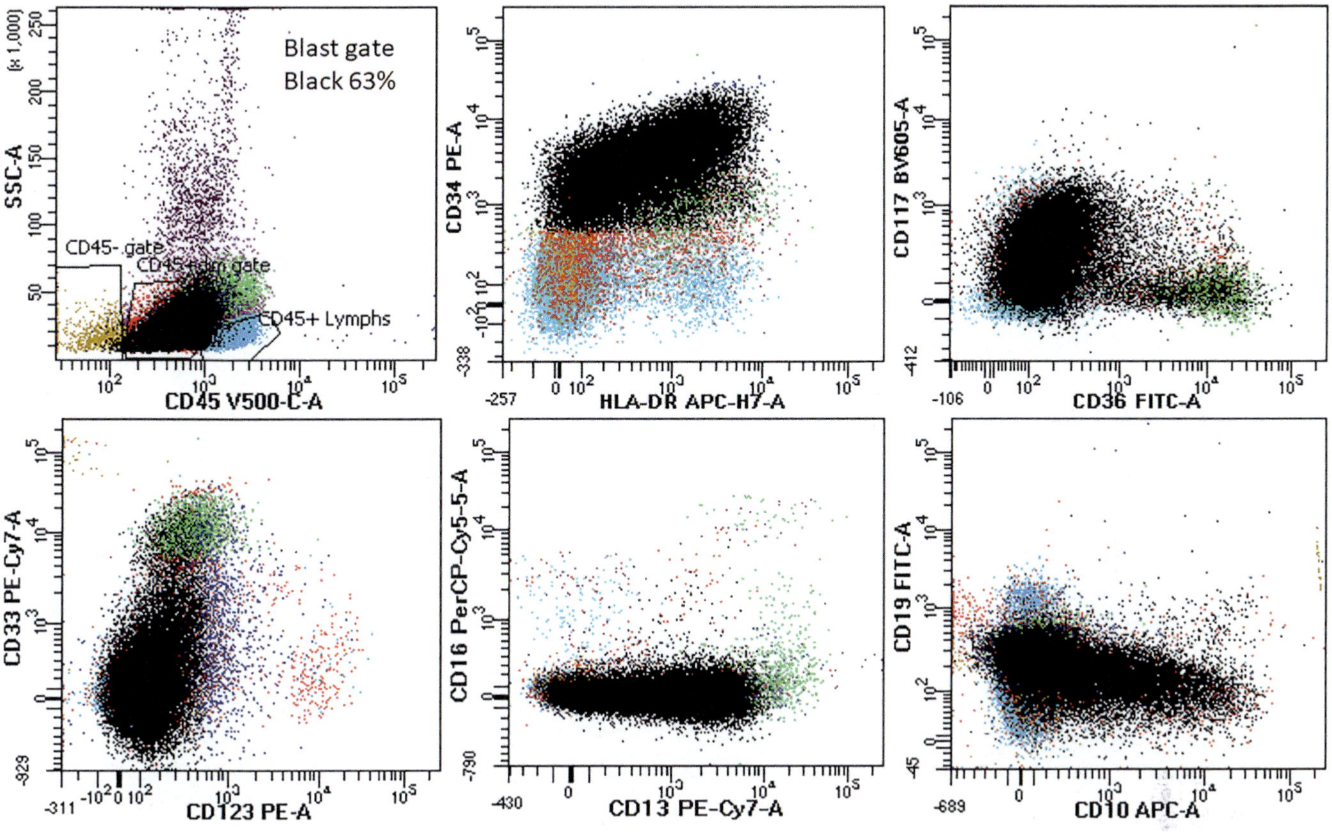

Fig. 13.8 Flow cytometry. The blasts in the CD45 dim gate are positive for partial CD10, variable CD13, partial CD33 (small subset, dim), CD34, CD117, and HLA-DR. Additionally (not shown in the figure), the blasts are positive for CD38; variably positive for CD7 (small subset), CD22, and CD200; and negative for CD2, CD3 (surface and cytoplasmic), CD4, CD5, CD8, CD11b, CD11c, CD14, CD15, CD16, CD20, CD64, myeloperoxidase, and TdT. The phenotype is consistent with acute myeloid leukemia with minimal differentiation

ing in clonal diversity). The additional *DNMT3A* and *SMC1A* mutations probably occur even earlier than *NPM1*, but they are not specific for AML.

- In recent years, hypomethylation therapy and novel therapies targeting AML-related mutations have been considered a potential alternative protocol to replace the standard cytosine arabinoside (7 days) and anthracycline (3 days) chemotherapy (7 + 3 regimen) in old-age patients with AML. It is proven effective in eradicating the AML clone in this case.
- NGS-based mutation profiling detects the persistence of mutation in the bone marrow sample 5 months after treatment. It is more sensitive and specific than the morphologic examination and flow cytometric analysis.
- Interestingly, the reduction of AML cells in this case resurfaces a neoplastic B-cell clone with *MYD88* c.794 T > C (p.L265P) mutation. The *MYD88* mutation is clearly not associated with the AML clone(s); although this mutation is frequently associated with lymphoplasmacytic lymphoma, the low-level involvement in this case likely indicates an evolving B-cell neoplasm at the stage of monoclonal B-cell lymphocytosis.
- Sequential NGS mutation profiling results provide meaningful information to evaluate the clonal evolution, clonal diversity, and residual leukemia. The disappearance of *FLT3*-ITD is a critical information for the decision to stop the targeted therapy drug gilteritinib.

Case 5

Learning Objective

Although mutation profiling is essential for the diagnosis and classification of AML, conventional karyotyping still has critical value in demonstrating complex genetic abnormalities on a large scale.

Case History

A 69-year-old male has fatigue for a few weeks. He is found to have pancytopenia during a clinic visit. A routine blood cell count shows WBC of 1.4 K/μL, RBC of 2.54 M/μL, hemoglobin of 7.5 g/dL, and platelet of 33 K/μL. The bone marrow aspirate smear and biopsy core show numerous blasts with features suggesting either monoblasts or imma-

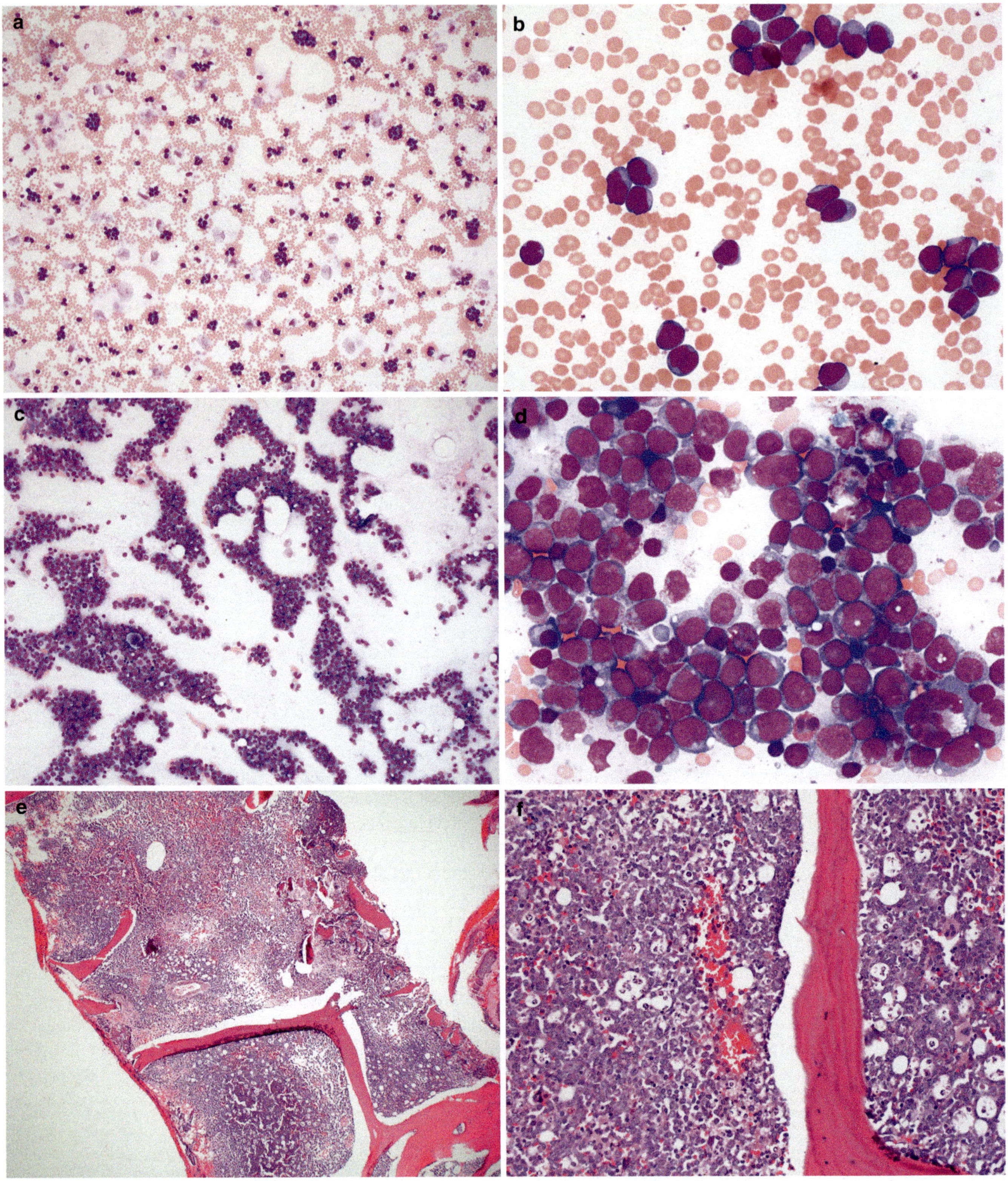

Fig. 13.9 Blood and bone marrow morphologic findings. Wright-Giemsa-stained blood smear (**a**) (100×) and (**b**) (600×) show marked leukocytosis with numerous blasts. The same blast population is present in the bone marrow aspirate ((**c**) 100× and (**d**) 600×). The blasts have a minimal to moderate amount of cytoplasm, and a small subset contains cytoplasmic granules. No nuclear cleft characteristic of APL (see case 1) is seen. The H&E-stained biopsy core shows markedly hypercellular bone marrow (**e**, 40×) with sheets of blasts (**f**, 200×)

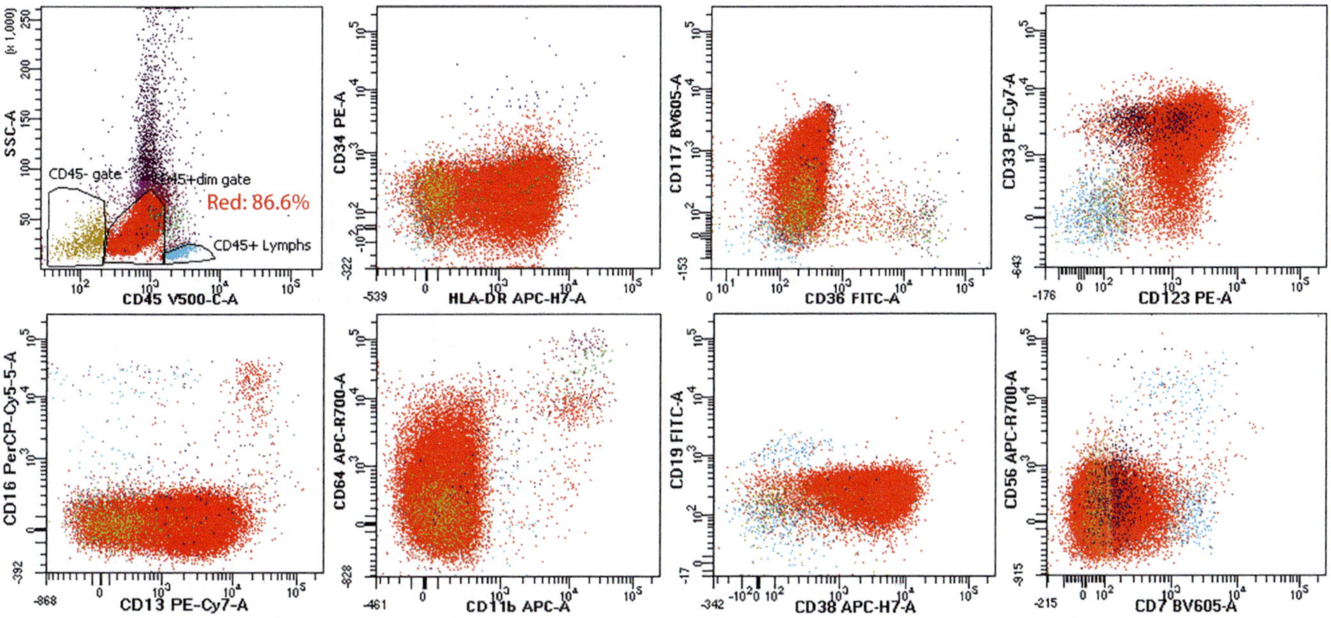

Fig. 13.10 Flow cytometry. The CD45 dim gate blasts comprise 86.6% of the total events and express CD13, CD33, CD38, variable CD117, CD123, variable CD64, and HLA-DR. There is no expression of CD7, CD11b, CD16, CD19, CD34, CD36, and CD56. Additionally (not shown in the figure), blasts are partially positive for CD11c and CD15 and negative for CD2, CD3, CD4, CD5, CD8, CD10, CD11c, CD14, CD15, CD20, CD22, and CD26. Although lacking CD34 expression raises concern for an APL (see Case 1), the morphologic features (see Fig. 13.9 above) and expression of HLA-DR indicate APL is unlikely

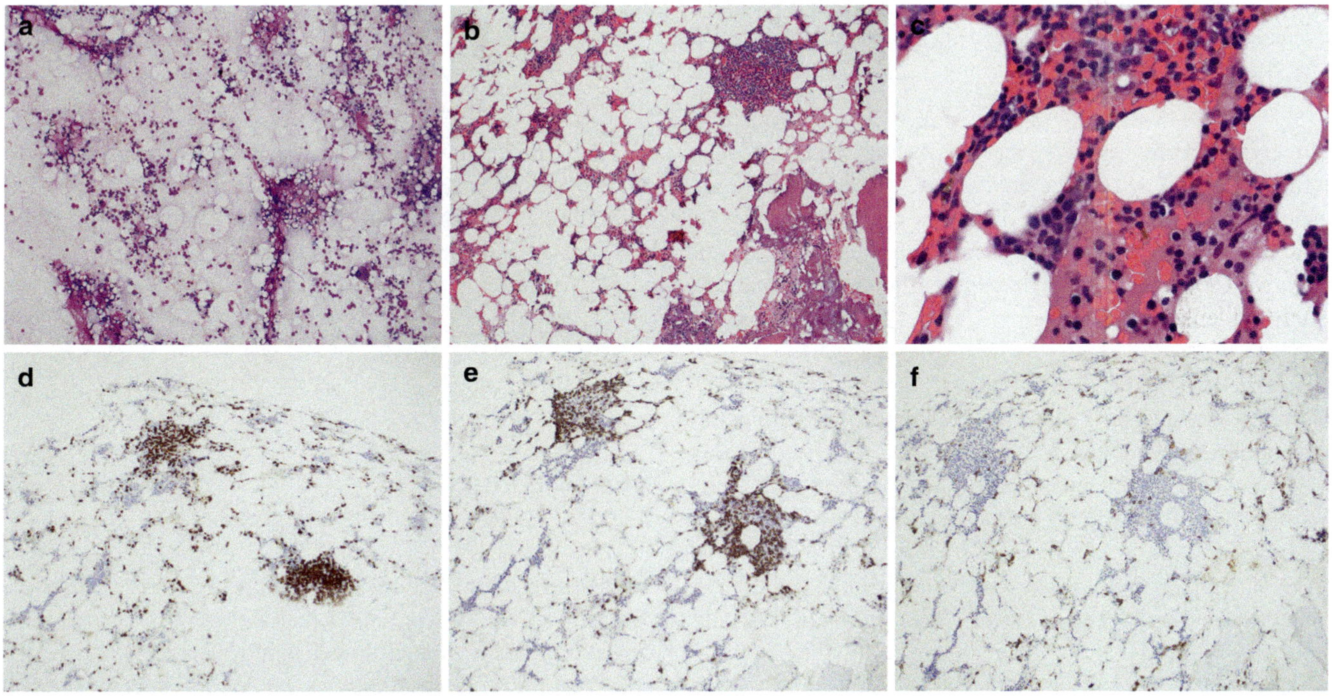

Fig. 13.11 Morphologic and immunohistochemical stains of the follow-up bone marrow. (**a**) Bone marrow aspirate smear (Wright-Giemsa stain, 200×) is hypocellular with predominance of lymphoid cells. Bone marrow biopsy (H&E stain) (**b**) (100×) and (**c**) (600×) confirm the hypocellular bone marrow; interstitial small lymphoid aggregates are present. The lymphoid population shows a mixture of CD3-positive T cells (**d**) and CD20-positive B cells (**e**). Scattered plasma cells are highlighted by CD138 (**f**); they are not increased and show no clustering either ((**d**, **e**, and **f**) 100×)

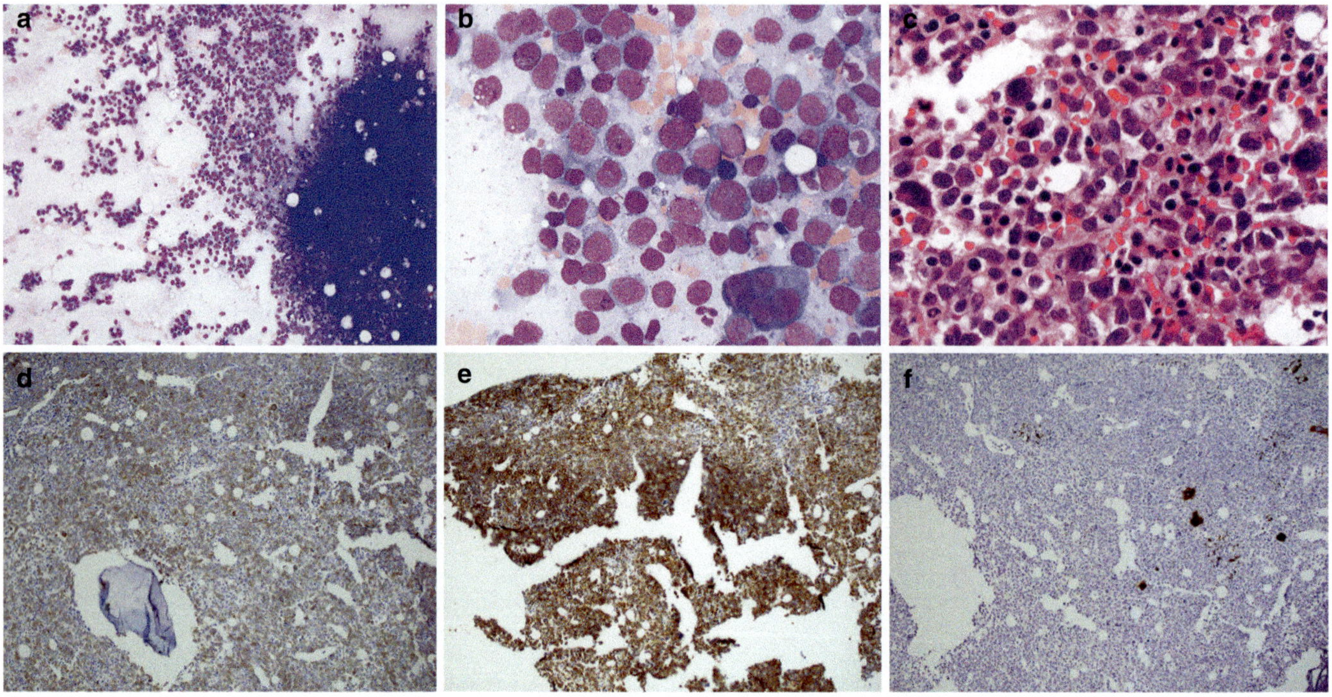

Fig. 13.12 Bone marrow smear, biopsy core, and immunohistochemical stains. The bone marrow aspirate smear ((**a**) 100×, (**b**) 600×, Wright-Giemsa stain) shows numerous blasts (~80%) with blue cytoplasm, frequent cytoplasmic vacuoles, and some multinucleation. The biopsy core (**c**, H&E stain, 600×) is hypercellular with blasts of slight pleomorphism; large nuclei and multinucleation are also present. Background late erythroid precursors are recognizable. Immunohistochemical stains show the blasts are positive for CD117 (**d**) and e-cadherin (**e**) and negative for CD61 (**f**) and factor VIII (not shown). The morphologic features, positive e-cadherin, combining with the flow cytometric immunophenotypic results, are consistent with pure erythroid leukemia

ture erythroid precursors (proerythroblasts) (see Fig. 13.12a, b, and c). Flow cytometric analysis reveals no specific lineage markers, ruling out the diagnosis of monocytic leukemia (Fig. 13.13). A positive e-cadherin (Fig. 13.12e) and negative CD61 (Fig. 13.12f) supports the diagnosis of pure erythroid leukemia.

Genetic and Molecular Studies

Complex chromosome abnormalities with three clones are detected by conventional karyotyping:

44 ~ 45,XY,inv.(1)(p36.3q12),-4,+6,r(6)(p25q27),-9,der(9)ins(9;?)(q13;?),+10,del(10)(p12),-13,add(14)(p11.2),-15,del(17)(p11.2),add(19)(q13.4),+r[cp4]/43 ~ 48,sl,-inv(1), dup(1)(q32q44), −2, del(6)(q26),-18, del(18)(q21),+1 ~ 3mar[cp11]/78 ~ 88,sdl1 x2[cp2]/46,XY [5]

One karyotype image is displayed in Fig. 13.14.

FISH AML panel reveals no abnormality in chromosome 5 (−5 or del(5q)); chromosome 7 (−7 or del(7q)); no *RUNX1-RUNX1T1*, *CBFB-MYH11*, or translocation involving *KMT2A*.

NGS myeloid panel (75 genes) detected two mutations in *TP53* [NM_000546.5]:

- c.524G > A (p.R175H) at 31.4%
- c.578A > G (p.H193R) at 2.0%

Final Diagnosis

AML, NOS, and pure erythroid leukemia

Treatment and Clinical Follow-Up

The patient is treated with azacitidine and venetoclax. A repeat bone marrow sampling 1 month later shows there are still sheets of proerythroblasts in the aspirate and biopsy core.

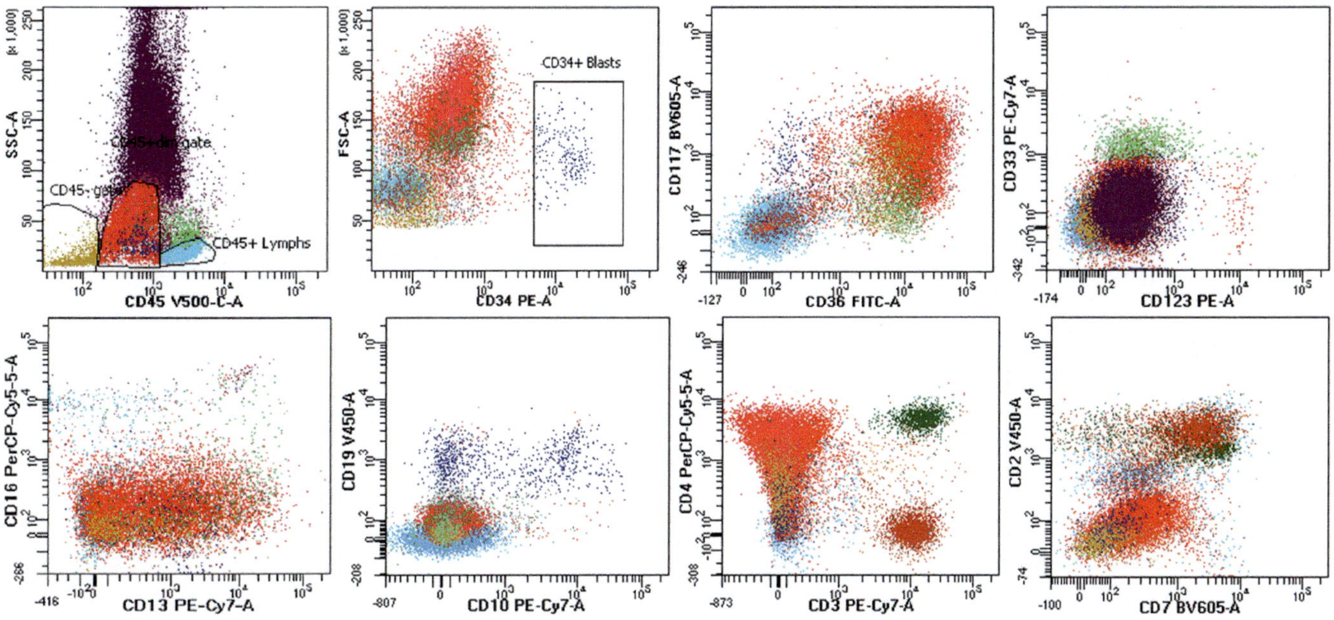

Fig. 13.13 Flow cytometry. The blast population comprises approximately 30% of the total analyzed events (given the high percentage of granulocytes, we can assume that this sample is significantly diluted by blood). The blast population displays a high forward scatter, expresses CD4, variable CD13, CD36, and CD117. They are negative for CD2, CD3, CD7, CD10, CD16, CD19, CD33, CD34, and CD123. Additionally, the blasts are also negative for CD1a, CD5, CD11b, CD11c, CD15, CD20, CD22, CD38, CD56, CD64, CD79a, CD200, HLA-DR, and TdT. The phenotype is not lineage specific; however, the expressions of CD36 and CD117 suggest either erythroid or megakaryocytic lineage

Discussion

- Complex cytogenetic abnormality and simple *TP53* mutation, both associated with poor clinical outcome, are the most frequent genetic findings in pure erythroid leukemia (PEL) [108].
- Similar patterns of genetic abnormalities can be seen in some patients of myelodysplastic syndrome (MDS) with marked erythroid hyperplasia but do not meet the criteria for PEL and AML-MRC. These patients are particularly resistant to chemotherapy. Alternative treatment options like hypomethylation agents may be more effective in these patients [111].
- As we can see in this case, the complex cytogenetic abnormalities do not involve the recurrent changes frequently seen in AML (FISH panel for AML reveals normal result). Therefore, conventional karyotyping still has great clinical value in the prognostic evaluation and guiding treatment decisions of AML.

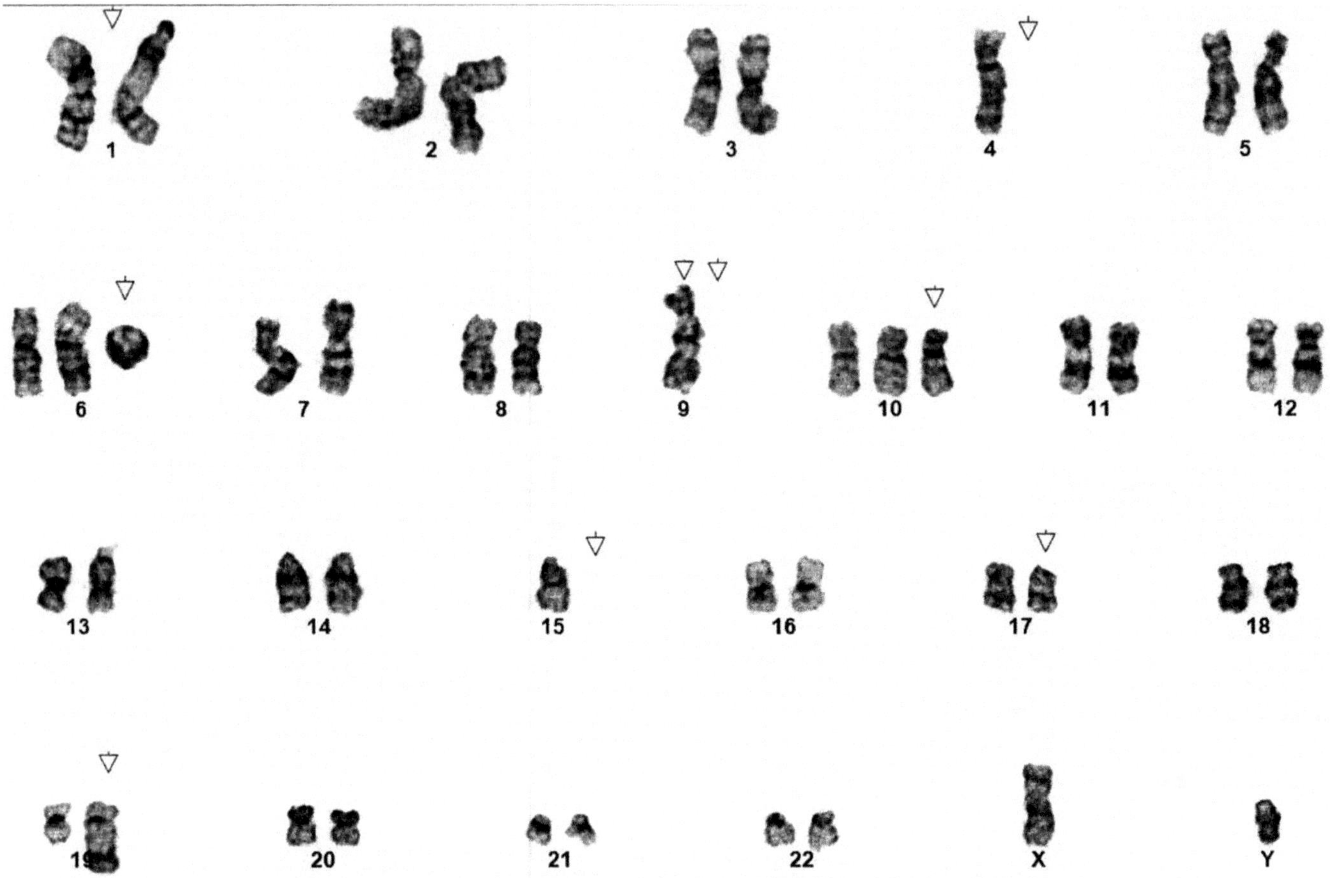

45,XY,inv(1)(p36.3q12),-4,+6,r(6)(p25q27),-9,der(9)ins(9;?)(q13;?),+10,del(10)(p12),-15,del(17)(p11.2),add(19)(q13.4)

Fig. 13.14 Karyotype. The picture is an example of the complex karyotypic abnormalities detected in clone 1 of the blasts

References

1. Bennett JM, et al. Proposals for the classification of the acute leukaemias. French-American-British (FAB) co-operative group. Br J Haematol. 1976;33(4):451–8.
2. Ley TJ, et al. DNA sequencing of a cytogenetically normal acute myeloid leukaemia genome. Nature. 2008;456(7218):66–72.
3. Papaemmanuil E, et al. Genomic classification and prognosis in acute myeloid leukemia. N Engl J Med. 2016;374(23):2209–21.
4. Arber DA, et al. The 2016 revision to the World Health Organization classification of myeloid neoplasms and acute leukemia. Blood. 2016;127(20):2391–405.
5. Grimwade D, et al. Refinement of cytogenetic classification in acute myeloid leukemia: determination of prognostic significance of rare recurring chromosomal abnormalities among 5876 younger adult patients treated in the United Kingdom Medical Research Council trials. Blood. 2010;116(3):354–65.
6. Arber DA, et al. Acute myeloid leukaemia with recurrent genetic abnormalities. In: Swerdlow S, et al., editors. WHO classification of tumours of haematopoietic and lymphoid tissues. Lyon: International Agency for Research on Cancer; 2017. p. 130–45.
7. National Comprehensive Cancer Network (NCCN). Acute Myeloid Leukemia (Version 1.2021). October 14, 2020. Available from: https://www.nccn.org/professionals/physician_gls/pdf/aml.pdf. Accessed 3 Nov 2020.
8. Dohner H, et al. Diagnosis and management of AML in adults: 2017 ELN recommendations from an international expert panel. Blood. 2017;129(4):424–47.
9. Arber DA, et al. Initial diagnostic workup of acute Leukemia: guideline from the college of American pathologists and the American society of hematology. Arch Pathol Lab Med. 2017;141(10):1342–93.
10. Sridhar K, et al. Molecular genetic testing methodologies in hematopoietic diseases: current and future methods. Int J Lab Hematol. 2019;41(Suppl 1):102–16.
11. Li S, et al. Multimodality technologies in the assessment of hematolymphoid neoplasms. Arch Pathol Lab Med. 2017;141(3):341–54.
12. He R, et al. Conventional karyotyping and fluorescence in situ hybridization: an effective utilization strategy in diagnostic adult acute myeloid leukemia. Am J Clin Pathol. 2015;143(6):873–8.
13. Wheeler FC, et al. Limited utility of fluorescence in situ hybridization for recurrent abnormalities in acute myeloid Leukemia at diagnosis and follow-up. Am J Clin Pathol. 2018;149(5):418–24.
14. Mrózek K, et al. Comparison of cytogenetic and molecular genetic detection of t(8;21) and inv(16) in a prospective series of adults with de novo acute myeloid leukemia: a Cancer and Leukemia group B study. J Clin Oncol. 2001;19(9):2482–92.

15. Hammer RD, et al. Is it time for a new gold standard? FISH vs cytogenetics in AML diagnosis. Am J Clin Pathol. 2016;145(3):430–2.
16. Taylor AC. Titration of heparinase for removal of the PCR-inhibitory effect of heparin in DNA samples. Mol Ecol. 1997;6(4):383–5.
17. Do H, Dobrovic A. Sequence artifacts in DNA from formalin-fixed tissues: causes and strategies for minimization. Clin Chem. 2015;61(1):64–71.
18. Lee SH, et al. ICSH guidelines for the standardization of bone marrow specimens and reports. Int J Lab Hematol. 2008;30(5):349–64.
19. Schrijver WA, et al. Influence of decalcification procedures on immunohistochemistry and molecular pathology in breast cancer. Mod Pathol. 2016;29(12):1460–70.
20. Singh VM, et al. Analysis of the effect of various decalcification agents on the quantity and quality of nucleic acid (DNA and RNA) recovered from bone biopsies. Ann Diagn Pathol. 2013;17(4):322–6.
21. Poire X, et al. Allogeneic stem cell transplantation in adult patients with acute myeloid leukaemia and 17p abnormalities in first complete remission: a study from the acute Leukemia working party (ALWP) of the European Society for Blood and Marrow Transplantation (EBMT). J Hematol Oncol. 2017;10(1):20.
22. Bezerra MF, et al. Co-occurrence of DNMT3A, NPM1, FLT3 mutations identifies a subset of acute myeloid leukemia with adverse prognosis. Blood. 2020;135(11):870–5.
23. Straube J, et al. The impact of age, NPM1mut, and FLT3ITD allelic ratio in patients with acute myeloid leukemia. Blood. 2018;131(10):1148–53.
24. Vardiman JW, et al. The 2008 revision of the World Health Organization (WHO) classification of myeloid neoplasms and acute leukemia: rationale and important changes. Blood. 2009;114(5):937–51.
25. Gerstung M, et al. Precision oncology for acute myeloid leukemia using a knowledge bank approach. Nat Genet. 2017;49(3):332–40.
26. Sorror ML, et al. Development and validation of a novel acute myeloid Leukemia-composite model to estimate risks of mortality. JAMA Oncol. 2017;3(12):1675–82.
27. Lagunas-Rangel FA, et al. Acute myeloid leukemia-genetic alterations and their clinical prognosis. Int J Hematol Oncol Stem Cell Res. 2017;11(4):328–39.
28. Tallman MS, Altman JK. How I treat acute promyelocytic leukemia. Blood. 2009;114(25):5126–35.
29. Wu N C-h, et al. A fast and accurate cartridge-based RT-qPCR assay to quantify PML-Rara mRNA fusion transcripts near the point of care. Blood. 2018;132(Supplement 1):1481–1.
30. Kim MJ, et al. FISH-negative cryptic PML-RARA rearrangement detected by long-distance polymerase chain reaction and sequencing analyses: a case study and review of the literature. Cancer Genet Cytogenet. 2010;203(2):278–83.
31. Dimov ND, et al. Rapid and reliable confirmation of acute promyelocytic leukemia by immunofluorescence staining with an antipromyelocytic leukemia antibody: the M. D. Anderson Cancer Center experience of 349 patients. Cancer. 2010;116(2):369–76.
32. Geoffroy MC, de Thé H. Classic and variants APLs, as viewed from a therapy response. Cancers (Basel). 2020;12(4):967.
33. Yin CC, et al. Identification of a novel fusion gene, IRF2BP2-RARA, in acute promyelocytic leukemia. J Natl Compr Cancer Netw. 2015;13(1):19–22.
34. Singh MK, et al. Diagnosis of variant RARA translocation using standard dual-color dual-fusion PML/RARA FISH probes: an illustrative report. Hematol Oncol Stem Cell Ther. 2019;12(1):50–3.
35. Khanal N, Upadhyay Banskota S, Bhatt VR. Novel treatment paradigms in acute myeloid leukemia. Clin Pharmacol Ther. 2020;108(3):506–14.
36. DiNardo CD, Wei AH. How I treat acute myeloid leukemia in the era of new drugs. Blood. 2020;135(2):85–96.
37. Lachowiez CA, et al. Outcomes of older patients with NPM1-mutated AML: current treatments and the promise of venetoclax-based regimens. Blood Adv. 2020;4(7):1311–20.
38. Tiong IS, et al. Venetoclax induces rapid elimination of NPM1 mutant measurable residual disease in combination with low-intensity chemotherapy in acute myeloid leukaemia. Br J Haematol. 2020; Online ahead of print
39. Keung YK, et al. Philadelphia chromosome positive myelodysplastic syndrome and acute myeloid leukemia-retrospective study and review of literature. Leuk Res. 2004;28(6):579–86.
40. Konoplev S, et al. Molecular characterization of de novo Philadelphia chromosome-positive acute myeloid leukemia. Leuk Lymphoma. 2013;54(1):138–44.
41. Paietta E, et al. Biologic heterogeneity in Philadelphia chromosome-positive acute leukemia with myeloid morphology: the eastern cooperative oncology group experience. Leukemia. 1998;12(12):1881–5.
42. Soupir CP, et al. Philadelphia chromosome-positive acute myeloid leukemia: a rare aggressive leukemia with clinicopathologic features distinct from chronic myeloid leukemia in myeloid blast crisis. Am J Clin Pathol. 2007;127(4):642–50.
43. Nacheva EP, et al. Does BCR/ABL1 positive acute myeloid leukaemia exist? Br J Haematol. 2013;161(4):541–50.
44. Neuendorff NR, et al. BCR-ABL(+) acute myeloid leukemia: are we always dealing with a high-risk disease? Blood Adv. 2018;2(12):1409–11.
45. Chantepie SP, et al. Allogeneic stem cell transplantation (Allo-SCT) for de novo Ph+ AML: a study from the French society of bone marrow transplantation and cell therapy. Bone Marrow Transplant. 2015;50(12):1586–8.
46. Lazarevic VL, et al. Relatively favorable outcome after allogeneic stem cell transplantation for BCR-ABL1-positive AML: a survey from the acute leukemia working party of the European society for blood and marrow transplantation (EBMT). Am J Hematol. 2018;93(1):31–9.
47. Han JY, Theil KS. The Philadelphia chromosome as a secondary abnormality in inv(3)(q21q26) acute myeloid leukemia at diagnosis: confirmation of p190 BCR-ABL mRNA by real-time quantitative polymerase chain reaction. Cancer Genet Cytogenet. 2006;165(1):70–4.
48. Kakihana K, et al. Late appearance of Philadelphia chromosome with the p190 BCR/ABL chimeric transcript in acute myelogenous leukemia progressing from myelodysplastic syndrome. Rinsho Ketsueki. 2003;44(4):242–8.
49. Quintás-Cardama A, et al. Association of 3q21q26 syndrome and late-appearing Philadelphia chromosome in acute myeloid leukemia. Leukemia. 2008;22(4):877–8.
50. Shah N, et al. Late-appearing Philadelphia chromosome in childhood acute myeloid leukemia. Pediatr Blood Cancer. 2008;50(5):1052–3.
51. Yagyu S, et al. Late appearance of a Philadelphia chromosome in a patient with therapy-related acute myeloid leukemia and high expression of EVI1. Cancer Genet Cytogenet. 2008;180(2):115–20.
52. Najfeld V, et al. Acquisition of the Ph chromosome and BCR-ABL fusion product in AML-M2 and t(8;21) leukemia: cytogenetic and FISH evidence for a late event. Leukemia. 1998;12(4):517–9.
53. Kurt H, et al. Secondary Philadelphia chromosome acquired during therapy of acute leukemia and myelodysplastic syndrome. Modern Pathology. 2018;31(7):1141–54.
54. Alotaibi AS, et al. Emergence of BCR–ABL1 fusion in AML Post–FLT3 inhibitor-based therapy: a potentially targetable mechanism of resistance – a case series. Front Oncol. 2020;10(588876):1–4.

55. Kiyoi H, Kawashima N, Ishikawa Y. FLT3 mutations in acute myeloid leukemia: therapeutic paradigm beyond inhibitor development. Cancer Sci. 2020;111(2):312–22.
56. Schnittger S. FLT3 (FMS-like tyrosine kinase 3). Atlas Genet Cytogenet Oncol Haematol. 2005;9(4):275–7.
57. Hu X, Chen F. Targeting on glycosylation of mutant FLT3 in acute myeloid leukemia. Hematology. 2019;24(1):651–60.
58. Daver N, et al. Targeting FLT3 mutations in AML: review of current knowledge and evidence. Leukemia. 2019;33(2):299–312.
59. Perry M, et al. FLT3-TKD mutations associated with NPM1 mutations define a favorable-risk group in patients with acute myeloid leukemia. Clin Lymphoma Myeloma Leuk. 2018;18(12):e545–50.
60. Murphy KM, et al. Detection of FLT3 internal tandem duplication and D835 mutations by a multiplex polymerase chain reaction and capillary electrophoresis assay. J Mol Diagn. 2003;5(2):96–102.
61. Kim Y, et al. Quantitative fragment analysis of FLT3-ITD efficiently identifying poor prognostic group with high mutant allele burden or long ITD length. Blood Cancer J. 2015;5:e336.
62. Patnaik MM. The importance of FLT3 mutational analysis in acute myeloid leukemia. Leuk Lymphoma. 2018;59(10):2273–86.
63. Tallman MS, et al. Acute myeloid Leukemia, version 3.2019, NCCN clinical practice guidelines in oncology. J Natl Compr Cancer Netw. 2019;17(6):721–49.
64. Yalniz F, et al. Prognostic significance of baseline FLT3-ITD mutant allele level in acute myeloid leukemia treated with intensive chemotherapy with/without sorafenib. Am J Hematol. 2019;94(9):984–91.
65. Abou Dalle I, et al. Impact of numerical variation, allele burden, mutation length and co-occurring mutations on the efficacy of tyrosine kinase inhibitors in newly diagnosed FLT3- mutant acute myeloid leukemia. Blood Cancer J. 2020;10(5):48.
66. Borthakur G, et al. Impact of numerical variation in FMS-like tyrosine kinase receptor 3 internal tandem duplications on clinical outcome in normal karyotype acute myelogenous leukemia. Cancer. 2012;118(23):5819–22.
67. Meshinchi S, et al. Structural and numerical variation of FLT3/ITD in pediatric AML. Blood. 2008;111(10):4930–3.
68. Eguchi M, et al. Mechanisms underlying resistance to FLT3 inhibitors in acute myeloid Leukemia. Biomedicine. 2020;8(8):245.
69. Kottaridis PD, et al. Studies of FLT3 mutations in paired presentation and relapse samples from patients with acute myeloid leukemia: implications for the role of FLT3 mutations in leukemogenesis, minimal residual disease detection, and possible therapy with FLT3 inhibitors. Blood. 2002;100(7):2393–8.
70. Levis MJ, et al. A next-generation sequencing-based assay for minimal residual disease assessment in AML patients with FLT3-ITD mutations. Blood Adv. 2018;2(8):825–31.
71. Au CH, et al. Clinical evaluation of panel testing by next-generation sequencing (NGS) for gene mutations in myeloid neoplasms. Diagn Pathol. 2016;11:11.
72. Spencer DH, et al. Detection of FLT3 internal tandem duplication in targeted, short-read-length, next-generation sequencing data. J Mol Diagn. 2013;15(1):81–93.
73. Falini B, et al. NPM1-mutated acute myeloid leukemia: from bench to bedside. Blood. 2020;136(15):1707–21.
74. Thiede C, et al. Prevalence and prognostic impact of NPM1 mutations in 1485 adult patients with acute myeloid leukemia (AML). Blood. 2006;107(10):4011–20.
75. Falini B, et al. Altered nucleophosmin transport in acute myeloid leukaemia with mutated NPM1: molecular basis and clinical implications. Leukemia. 2009;23(10):1731–43.
76. Falini B, et al. Cytoplasmic nucleophosmin in acute myelogenous leukemia with a normal karyotype. N Engl J Med. 2005;352(3):254–66.
77. Federici L, Falini B. Nucleophosmin mutations in acute myeloid leukemia: a tale of protein unfolding and mislocalization. Protein Sci. 2013;22(5):545–56.
78. Loghavi S, et al. Clinical features of de novo acute myeloid leukemia with concurrent DNMT3A, FLT3 and NPM1 mutations. J Hematol Oncol. 2014;7:74.
79. Cocciardi S, et al. Clonal evolution patterns in acute myeloid leukemia with NPM1 mutation. Nat Commun. 2019;10(1):2031.
80. Schuurhuis GJ, et al. Minimal/measurable residual disease in AML: a consensus document from the European LeukemiaNet MRD working party. Blood. 2018;131(12):1275–91.
81. Hafez M, et al. Performance and clinical evaluation of a sensitive multiplex assay for the rapid detection of common NPM1 mutations. J Mol Diagn. 2010;12(5):629–35.
82. Forghieri F, et al. Minimal/measurable residual disease monitoring in NPM1-mutated acute myeloid Leukemia: a clinical viewpoint and perspectives. Int J Mol Sci. 2018;19(11):3942.
83. Ivey A, et al. Assessment of minimal residual disease in standard-risk AML. N Engl J Med. 2016;374(5):422–33.
84. Nerlov C. C/EBPalpha mutations in acute myeloid leukaemias. Nat Rev Cancer. 2004;4(5):394–400.
85. Konstandin NP, et al. Genetic heterogeneity of cytogenetically normal AML with mutations of CEBPA. Blood Adv. 2018;2(20):2724–31.
86. Behdad A, et al. A clinical grade sequencing-based assay for CEBPA mutation testing: report of a large series of myeloid neoplasms. J Mol Diagn. 2015;17(1):76–84.
87. Green CL, et al. Prognostic significance of CEBPA mutations in a large cohort of younger adult patients with acute myeloid leukemia: impact of double CEBPA mutations and the interaction with FLT3 and NPM1 mutations. J Clin Oncol. 2010;28(16):2739–47.
88. Wouters BJ, et al. Double CEBPA mutations, but not single CEBPA mutations, define a subgroup of acute myeloid leukemia with a distinctive gene expression profile that is uniquely associated with a favorable outcome. Blood. 2009;113(13):3088–91.
89. Lin LI, et al. Characterization of CEBPA mutations in acute myeloid leukemia: most patients with CEBPA mutations have biallelic mutations and show a distinct immunophenotype of the leukemic cells. Clin Cancer Res. 2005;11(4):1372–9.
90. Dufour A, et al. Acute myeloid leukemia with biallelic CEBPA gene mutations and normal karyotype represents a distinct genetic entity associated with a favorable clinical outcome. J Clin Oncol. 2010;28(4):570–7.
91. Taskesen E, et al. Prognostic impact, concurrent genetic mutations, and gene expression features of AML with CEBPA mutations in a cohort of 1182 cytogenetically normal AML patients: further evidence for CEBPA double mutant AML as a distinctive disease entity. Blood. 2011;117(8):2469–75.
92. Schlenk RF, et al. The value of allogeneic and autologous hematopoietic stem cell transplantation in prognostically favorable acute myeloid leukemia with double mutant CEBPA. Blood. 2013;122(9):1576–82.
93. Greif PA, et al. GATA2 zinc finger 1 mutations associated with biallelic CEBPA mutations define a unique genetic entity of acute myeloid leukemia. Blood. 2012;120(2):395–403.
94. Tawana K, et al. Familial CEBPA-mutated acute myeloid leukemia. Semin Hematol. 2017;54(2):87–93.
95. Tawana K, et al. Disease evolution and outcomes in familial AML with germline CEBPA mutations. Blood. 2015;126(10):1214–23.
96. Hollink IH, et al. Characterization of CEBPA mutations and promoter hypermethylation in pediatric acute myeloid leukemia. Haematologica. 2011;96(3):384–92.
97. Hou HA, et al. Reply to 'Heterogeneity within AML with CEBPA mutations; only CEBPA double mutations, but not single CEBPA mutations are associated with favorable prognosis'. Br J Cancer. 2009;101(4):738–40.
98. Pabst T, et al. Heterogeneity within AML with CEBPA mutations; only CEBPA double mutations, but not single CEBPA mutations are associated with favourable prognosis. Br J Cancer. 2009;100(8):1343–6.

99. Wouters BJ, et al. A recurrent in-frame insertion in a CEBPA transactivation domain is a polymorphism rather than a mutation that does not affect gene expression profiling-based clustering of AML. Blood. 2007;109(1):389–90.
100. Ng CWS, et al. CEBPA mutational analysis in acute myeloid leukaemia by a laboratory-developed next-generation sequencing assay. J Clin Pathol. 2018;71(6):522–31.
101. Prokocimer M, Molchadsky A, Rotter V. Dysfunctional diversity of p53 proteins in adult acute myeloid leukemia: projections on diagnostic workup and therapy. Blood. 2017;130(6): 699–712.
102. Welch JS. Patterns of mutations in TP53 mutated AML. Best Pract Res Clin Haematol. 2018;31(4):379–83.
103. Hou HA, et al. TP53 mutations in de novo acute myeloid leukemia patients: longitudinal follow-ups show the mutation is stable during disease evolution. Blood Cancer J. 2015;5(7):e331.
104. Jaiswal S, et al. Age-related clonal hematopoiesis associated with adverse outcomes. N Engl J Med. 2014;371(26):2488–98.
105. Xie M, et al. Age-related mutations associated with clonal hematopoietic expansion and malignancies. Nat Med. 2014;20(12):1472–8.
106. Wong TN, et al. Role of TP53 mutations in the origin and evolution of therapy-related acute myeloid leukaemia. Nature. 2015;518(7540):552–5.
107. Kadia TM, et al. TP53 mutations in newly diagnosed acute myeloid leukemia: clinicomolecular characteristics, response to therapy, and outcomes. Cancer. 2016;122(22):3484–91.
108. Wang W, et al. Pure erythroid leukemia. Am J Hematol. 2017;92(3):292–6.
109. Asghari H, Talati C. Tumor protein 53 mutations in acute myeloid leukemia: conventional induction chemotherapy or novel therapeutics. Curr Opin Hematol. 2020;27(2):66–75.
110. Chang CK, et al. TP53 mutations predict decitabine-induced complete responses in patients with myelodysplastic syndromes. Br J Haematol. 2017;176(4):600–8.
111. Welch JS, et al. TP53 and decitabine in acute myeloid leukemia and myelodysplastic syndromes. N Engl J Med. 2016;375(21):2023–36.
112. Aldoss I, et al. Venetoclax and hypomethylating agents in TP53-mutated acute myeloid leukaemia. Br J Haematol. 2019;187(2):e45–8.
113. DiNardo CD, et al. Venetoclax combined with decitabine or azacitidine in treatment-naive, elderly patients with acute myeloid leukemia. Blood. 2019;133(1):7–17.
114. Morita K, et al. Clearance of somatic mutations at remission and the risk of relapse in acute myeloid Leukemia. J Clin Oncol. 2018;36(18):1788–97.
115. Kotler E, et al. A systematic p53 mutation library links differential functional impact to cancer mutation pattern and evolutionary conservation. Molecular Cell. 2018;71(1) 178–190.e8
116. Fernandez-Pol S, et al. Immunohistochemistry for p53 is a useful tool to identify cases of acute myeloid leukemia with myelodysplasia-related changes that are TP53 mutated, have complex karyotype, and have poor prognosis. Mod Pathol. 2017;30(3):382–92.
117. McGraw KL, et al. Immunohistochemical pattern of p53 is a measure of TP53 mutation burden and adverse clinical outcome in myelodysplastic syndromes and secondary acute myeloid leukemia. Haematologica. 2016;101(8):e320–3.
118. Ruzinova MB, et al. TP53 immunohistochemistry correlates with TP53 mutation status and clearance in decitabine-treated patients with myeloid malignancies. Haematologica. 2019;104(8): e345–8.
119. Soussi T, Leroy B, Taschner PE. Recommendations for analyzing and reporting TP53 gene variants in the high-throughput sequencing era. Hum Mutat. 2014;35(6):766–78.
120. Ito Y, Bae SC, Chuang LS. The RUNX family: developmental regulators in cancer. Nat Rev Cancer. 2015;15(2):81–95.
121. Schnittger S, et al. RUNX1 mutations are frequent in de novo AML with noncomplex karyotype and confer an unfavorable prognosis. Blood. 2011;117(8):2348–57.
122. Yokota A, et al. The clinical, molecular, and mechanistic basis of RUNX1 mutations identified in Hematological malignancies. Mol Cells. 2020;43(2):145–52.
123. Sood R, Kamikubo Y, Liu P. Role of RUNX1 in hematological malignancies. Blood. 2017;129(15):2070–82.
124. Bellissimo DC, Speck NA. RUNX1 mutations in inherited and sporadic Leukemia. Front Cell Dev Biol. 2017;5:111.
125. Khan M, et al. Clinical outcomes and co-occurring mutations in patients with RUNX1-mutated acute myeloid leukemia. Int J Mol Sci. 2017;18(8):1–15.
126. Hayashi Y, et al. Myeloid neoplasms with germ line RUNX1 mutation. Int J Hematol. 2017;106(2):183–8.
127. Roberts I, et al. GATA1-mutant clones are frequent and often unsuspected in babies with down syndrome: identification of a population at risk of leukemia. Blood. 2013;122(24):3908–17.
128. Ling T, Crispino JD. GATA1 mutations in red cell disorders. IUBMB Life. 2020;72(1):106–18.
129. Halsey C, et al. The GATA1s isoform is normally down-regulated during terminal haematopoietic differentiation and over-expression leads to failure to repress MYB, CCND2 and SKI during erythroid differentiation of K562 cells. J Hematol Oncol. 2012;5:45.
130. Garnett C, Cruz Hernandez D, Vyas P. GATA1 and cooperating mutations in myeloid leukaemia of down syndrome. IUBMB Life. 2020;72(1):119–30.
131. Yoshida K, et al. The landscape of somatic mutations in down syndrome-related myeloid disorders. Nat Genet. 2013;45(11):1293–9.
132. Labuhn M, et al. Mechanisms of progression of myeloid preleukemia to transformed myeloid leukemia in children with down syndrome. Cancer Cell, 2019. 36(2) 123–138.e10
133. Bacher U, et al. Multilineage dysplasia does not influence prognosis in CEBPA-mutated AML, supporting the WHO proposal to classify these patients as a unique entity. Blood. 2012;119(20):4719–22.
134. Falini B, et al. Multilineage dysplasia has no impact on biologic, clinicopathologic, and prognostic features of AML with mutated nucleophosmin (NPM1). Blood. 2010;115(18):3776–86.
135. Arber DA, et al. Acute myeloid leukaemia with myelodysplasia-related change. In: Swerdlow S, et al., editors. WHO classification of tumours of haematopoietic and lymphoid tissues. Lyon: International Agency for Research on Cancer; 2017. p. 150–2.
136. Koenig KL, et al. AML with myelodysplasia-related changes: development, challenges, and treatment advances. Genes (Basel). 2020;11(8):845.
137. Viehmann S, et al. Monitoring of minimal residual disease (MRD) by real-time quantitative reverse transcription PCR (RQ-RT-PCR) in childhood acute myeloid leukemia with AML1/ETO rearrangement. Leukemia. 2003;17(6):1130–6.
138. Schnittger S, et al. Minimal residual disease levels assessed by NPM1 mutation-specific RQ-PCR provide important prognostic information in AML. Blood. 2009;114(11):2220–31.
139. Inaba H, et al. Comparative analysis of different approaches to measure treatment response in acute myeloid leukemia. J Clin Oncol. 2012;30(29):3625–32.
140. Sanz MA, et al. Management of acute promyelocytic leukemia: updated recommendations from an expert panel of the European LeukemiaNet. Blood. 2019;133(15):1630–43.
141. Goswami M, et al. A multigene array for measurable residual disease detection in AML patients undergoing SCT. Bone Marrow Transplant. 2015;50(5):642–51.

142. Ravandi F, Walter RB, Freeman SD. Evaluating measurable residual disease in acute myeloid leukemia. Blood Adv. 2018;2(11):1356–66.
143. Tomlinson B, Lazarus HM. Enhancing acute myeloid leukemia therapy - monitoring response using residual disease testing as a guide to therapeutic decision-making. Expert Rev Hematol. 2017;10(6):563–74.
144. Varella-Garcia M, et al. Minimal residual disease (MRD) in remission t(8;21) AML and in vivo differentiation detected by FISH and CD34+ cell sorting. Leukemia. 2001;15(9):1408–14.
145. Sexauer A, et al. Terminal myeloid differentiation in vivo is induced by FLT3 inhibition in FLT3/ITD AML. Blood. 2012;120(20):4205–14.
146. Ossenkoppele G, Schuurhuis GJ. MRD in AML: does it already guide therapy decision-making? Hematology Am Soc Hematol Educ Program. 2016;2016(1):356–65.
147. Voso MT, et al. MRD in AML: the role of new techniques. Front Oncol. 2019;9:655.
148. Crowgey EL, et al. Error-corrected sequencing strategies enable comprehensive detection of leukemic mutations relevant for diagnosis and minimal residual disease monitoring. BMC Med Genet. 2020;13(1):32.
149. Jongen-Lavrencic M, et al. Molecular minimal residual disease in acute myeloid leukemia. N Engl J Med. 2018;378(13):1189–99.
150. Hartmann L, Metzeler KH. Clonal hematopoiesis and preleukemia – genetics, biology, and clinical implications. Genes Chromosomes Cancer. 2019;58(12):828–38.
151. Debarri H, et al. IDH1/2 but not DNMT3A mutations are suitable targets for minimal residual disease monitoring in acute myeloid leukemia patients: a study by the acute Leukemia French association. Oncotarget. 2015;6(39):42345–53.
152. Lane S, et al. A >or=1 log rise in RQ-PCR transcript levels defines molecular relapse in core binding factor acute myeloid leukemia and predicts subsequent morphologic relapse. Leuk Lymphoma. 2008;49(3):517–23.
153. Yin JA, et al. Minimal residual disease monitoring by quantitative RT-PCR in core binding factor AML allows risk stratification and predicts relapse: results of the United Kingdom MRC AML-15 trial. Blood. 2012;120(14):2826–35.
154. Ommen HB, et al. Strikingly different molecular relapse kinetics in NPM1c, PML-RARA, RUNX1-RUNX1T1, and CBFB-MYH11 acute myeloid leukemias. Blood. 2010;115(2):198–205.
155. Ommen HB, et al. Relapse kinetics in acute myeloid leukaemias with MLL translocations or partial tandem duplications within the MLL gene. Br J Haematol. 2014;165(5):618–28.
156. Swerdlow SH. World health organization, and international agency for research on cancer. In: World Health Organization classification of tumours, editors, editor. WHO classification of tumours of haematopoietic and lymphoid tissues. Revised 4th ed. Lyon: International Agency for Research on Cancer; 2017. 585 pages.
157. Gaidzik VI, et al. RUNX1 mutations in acute myeloid leukemia: results from a comprehensive genetic and clinical analysis from the AML study group. J Clin Oncol. 2011;29(10):1364–72.
158. Mendler JH, et al. RUNX1 mutations are associated with poor outcome in younger and older patients with cytogenetically normal acute myeloid leukemia and with distinct gene and MicroRNA expression signatures. J Clin Oncol. 2012;30(25):3109–18.
159. Tang JL, et al. AML1/RUNX1 mutations in 470 adult patients with de novo acute myeloid leukemia: prognostic implication and interaction with other gene alterations. Blood. 2009;114(26):5352–61.
160. Gabert J, et al. Standardization and quality control studies of 'real-time' quantitative reverse transcriptase polymerase chain reaction of fusion gene transcripts for residual disease detection in leukemia - a Europe against Cancer program. Leukemia. 2003;17(12):2318–57.

Myeloproliferative Neoplasms, Myelodysplastic/Myeloproliferative Neoplasms, and Myelodysplastic Syndromes

14

Julie Li and Gang Zheng

List of Frequently Asked Questions

1. How many *BCR-ABL1* fusion variants are there in chronic myeloid leukemia (CML)?
2. Which molecular genetic techniques are commonly used for the diagnosis of chronic myeloid leukemia (CML)?
3. What cytogenetic abnormalities are commonly seen in accelerated/blast-phase chronic myeloid leukemia (CML)?
4. How is "complete response" to tyrosine kinase inhibitor (TKI) therapy defined in chronic myeloid leukemia (CML)?
5. What tests are useful to monitor tyrosine kinase inhibitor (TKI) therapy in patients with chronic myeloid leukemia (CML)?
6. What is the major cause of resistance to tyrosine kinase inhibitors (TKIs) in chronic myeloid leukemia (CML)? What are the therapeutic options for CML?
7. What are the common molecular alterations in the *BCR-ABL1*-negative myeloproliferative neoplasms?
8. Which molecular genetic abnormality is frequently associated with chronic neutrophilic leukemia (CNL)?
9. How to distinguish chronic neutrophilic leukemia (CNL) from chronic myeloid leukemia (CML)?
10. What molecular changes are associated with systemic mastocytosis?
11. What is the underlying molecular abnormality of *PDGFRA* rearrangement?
12. What are the common underlying genetic abnormalities involved in chronic myelomonocytic leukemia (CMML)?
13. What are the prognostic significance of the genetic changes in chronic myelomonocytic leukemia (CMML)?
14. In the 2017 WHO classification, chronic myelomonocytic leukemia (CMML) is further categorized into "proliferative CMML" and "dysplastic CMML." What are the molecular genetic differences between these two types?
15. Which genetic abnormalities are relatively common in atypical chronic myeloid leukemia (aCML), *BCR-ABL1*-negative?
16. What are the major features to differentiate atypical chronic myeloid leukemia (aCML), *BCR-ABL1*-negative, from chronic neutrophilic leukemia (CNL)?
17. Which genes are most commonly mutated in juvenile myelomonocytic leukemia (JMML)?
18. What are the common molecular genetic abnormalities that are associated with myelodysplastic/myeloproliferative neoplasm with ring sideroblasts and thrombocytosis (MDS/MPN-RS-T)?
19. What are the disease-defining chromosomal abnormalities in myelodysplastic syndrome (MDS)?
20. What are the typical clinicopathological findings in patients with myelodysplastic syndrome (MDS) with isolated del(5q)?
21. What are the common molecular abnormalities associated with MDS?
22. How to differentiate idiopathic cytopenia of undetermined significance (ICUS), clonal hematopoiesis of indeterminate potential (CHIP), clonal cytopenia of undetermined significance (CCUS), and myelodysplastic syndrome (MDS) from each other?

J. Li (✉)
Pathology and Laboratory Medicine Department, Boston University/Boston Medical Center, Boston, MA, USA
e-mail: Julie.li@bmc.org

G. Zheng
Department of Laboratory Medicine and Pathology, Mayo Clinic, Rochester, MN, USA
e-mail: zheng.gang@mayo.edu

Y. Ding, L. Zhang (eds.), *Practical Oncologic Molecular Pathology*, Practical Anatomic Pathology,
https://doi.org/10.1007/978-3-030-73227-1_14

Frequently Asked Questions

1. **How Many *BCR-ABL1* Fusion Variants Are There in Chronic Myeloid Leukemia (CML)?**
   - Chronic myeloid leukemia (CML) is a myeloproliferative disorder and characterized by a reciprocal chromosomal translocation between the Abelson oncogene (*ABL*) on chromosome 9q34.1 and the breakpoint cluster region (*BCR*) gene on chromosome 22q11.2, also known as Philadelphia chromosome (Ph). BCR-ABL is a constitutively active tyrosine kinase that promotes proliferation through several downstream signaling pathways involving RAS, RAF, JUN kinase, MYC, and STAT [1]. The most common conserved breakpoint in *ABL1* gene occurs in the intron before exon 2 (a2) and rarely downstream of exon 2 (a3) [2, 3]. Breakpoints in *ABL1* are mostly located in the 5′ of the second exon. The different breakpoints in the *BCR* gene result in different sizes of *BCR-ABL1* fusion genes. Three breakpoint cluster regions in the *BCR* gene have been identified: major breakpoint cluster region (*M-bcr*), minor breakpoint cluster region (*m-bcr*), and micro-breakpoint cluster region (*μ-bcr*) [4, 5].
   - *M*-bcr breakpoints occur downstream of exon 13 (e13) or exon 14 (e14) and result in a p210 fusion protein. The p210 (*M-bcr*) is detected in majority (97–99%) of CML cases and also presents in B-lymphoblastic leukemia/lymphoma (40% of adults and 10% of pediatric B-ALL patients) [6].
   - *m-bcr* breakpoints occur after the exon 1 (e1) of the *BCR* gene and produce a smaller fusion protein p190. CML with p190 (*m-bcr*) is rare (<1%) and mimics chronic myelomonocytic leukemia with increased numbers of monocytes [7]. p190 is mostly associated with Ph-positive B-ALL (60% of adult and 90% of pediatric patients) [6, 8].
   - *μ-bcr* breakpoints occur beyond the exon 19 (e19) of *BCR* in the micro-region and encode a larger oncoprotein p230. The p230 (*μ-bcr*) is rare and associated with cases of neutrophilic CML that display predominant neutrophilic maturation and/or thrombocytosis [9].
2. **Which Molecular Genetic Techniques Are Commonly Used for the Diagnosis of Chronic Myeloid Leukemia (CML)?**
   - The diagnosis of CML is based on the detection of *BCR-ABL1* or Ph chromosome t(9,22) (q34.1;q11.2) [10]. Screening test is often performed using blood specimen with abnormal high granulocyte count in a proper clinical setting. The commonly used diagnostic methods for CML are summarized in Table 14.1.
   - Conventional cytogenetics is still an important tool for the detection of the Ph chromosome, and the bone marrow aspirate is the commonly used specimen. It's routinely performed at the diagnosis which offers baseline information for monitoring clonal evolution. However, conventional cytogenetics has longer turnaround time due to the cell culture, low sensitivity (5–10%), and failure to detect cryptic translocations [11–13].
   - Fluorescence in situ hybridization (FISH) uses specific probes for *BCR-ABL1* gene and can rapidly identify the abnormality with higher sensitivity and detection cryptic translocations. A wide range of specimens can be used, such as peripheral blood, bone marrow, and paraffin-embedded tissue. To be noted, additional chromosomal changes will be missed by FISH [5]. If the Ph chromosome is detected by conventional cytogenetics, FISH is not mandatory and should not replace conventional cytogenetics.
   - Qualitative reverse transcriptase PCR (RT-PCR) measures *BCR-ABL1* transcripts on the mRNA level. Multiplex RT-PCR and nested RT-PCR are useful for detecting atypical *BCR-ABL1* variants [11, 14–16]. Importantly, qualitative RT-PCR (low sensitivity) should not be used for monitoring molecular response during therapy, which requires quantitative RT-PCR.
   - Quantitative RT-PCR (qPCR) is a highly sensitive assay and required for the initial workup to establish the bassline level for *BCR-ABL1* mRNA transcripts. Peripheral blood is more commonly used than bone marrow and makes monitoring less invasive [17, 18]. An international scale (IS) is recommended to standardize *BCR-ABL1* mRNA level across different laboratories and is defined as the ratio of *BCR-ABL1* transcripts to the internal control (such as *ABL1* and *GUSB*) and reported as *BCR-ABL1* percentage on a log scale (10%, 1%, 0.1%, 0.01%, and 0.032% correspond to 1, 2,3, 4, and 4.5 logs, respectively) [19]. To be noted, the low levels of *BCR-ABL1* can be detected in normal individuals, and interpretation should be used with caution as the results do not indicate the disease of CML [20].
3. **What Cytogenetic Abnormalities Are Commonly Seen in Accelerated/Blast-Phase Chronic Myeloid Leukemia (CML)?**
   - The evolution of CML from chronic to accelerated phase (AP-CML) or blast phase (BP-CML) is caused by the development of subclones with new cytogenetic and molecular changes. Conventional cytogenetics is useful to detect the additional abnormalities when suspicious of accelerated or blast phase [23, 24]. The most common secondary karyotypic abnormalities in CML in the advanced stages include:
     - Trisomy 8
     - Isochromosome 17q

Table 14.1 The molecular techniques for CML diagnosis [12, 13, 16, 18, 21, 22]

	Conventional cytogenetics	FISH	Qualitative RT-PCR	Quantitative RT-PCR (qPCR)
Target	Metaphase chromosome Ph chromosome t(9;22)	DNA *BCR-ABL1*	mRNA *BCR-ABL1*	mRNA
Sensitivity	5–10%	0.1–5%	0.1%	0.001–0.01%
Advantages	Provides the baseline karyotype	Rapid, specific probes; detect complex or cryptic translocation	Rapid; sensitive; cryptic variant; determines breakpoints	Very sensitive
Disadvantages	Time and labor intensive; miss complex and cryptic translocations	Does not detect additional chromosomal abnormalities	Inability to detect rare variants; false positivity; lower specificity with RNA cross contamination	Need to standardize across different laboratories; false positivity

FISH, fluorescence in situ hybridization; Qualitative RT-PCR, qualitative reverse transcription polymerase chain reaction; Quantitative RT-PC, quantitative reverse transcription polymerase chain reaction

  - Trisomy 19
  - Secondary Ph
  - Abnormalities of 3q26.2
  - Complex karyotype
- The additional chromosomal abnormalities (ACAs) are further subgrouped by occurring frequency into "major route" (trisomy 8, iso17q, a second Ph or trisomy 19) and "minor route" (−7, −17, +17. +21, -Y and abnormalities of 3q26) [25]. The presence of major route ACA at diagnosis has been associated with poor prognosis [26, 27]. Wang et al. proposed prognostic risk stratification based on the survival and prognosis with TKI therapy and divided ACAs into two groups. Group 1 includes trisomy 8, -Y, and a second Ph and is associated with good prognosis, whereas Group 2 includes i(17)(q10), −7/del7q, and 3q26.2 rearrangements with poor prognosis [28]. The patients with ACAs need to be monitored carefully for the evidence of therapy failure.

4. **How Is "Complete Response" to Tyrosine Kinase Inhibitor (TKI) Therapy Defined in Chronic Myeloid Leukemia (CML)?**
   - TKIs can competitively bind to the ATP-binding pocket of the ABL1 tyrosine kinase domain (TKD) so that the downstream cascade signaling pathway is halted. TKI therapy is considered the standard first-line treatment for the patients with newly diagnosed chronic-phase CML (CP-CML). Complete response to TKI therapy is determined by three different measurements.
   - Complete hematologic response (CHR) includes WBC < 10×10^9/L, platelets <450×10^9/L, the absence of immature granulocytes in peripheral blood, and impalpable spleen.
   - Complete cytogenetic response (CCyR) is defined as the absence of Ph chromosomes, which correlates with *BCR-ABL1* ≤1%. The goal of TKI therapy is to achieve a CCyR (≤1% *BCR-ABL1* IS) within 12 months after first-line TKI therapy and to prevent disease progression to AP-CML or BP-CML.
   - The major molecular response (MMR) is defined as *BCR-ABL1* (IS) ≤0.1% or 3-log reduction in *BCR-ABL1* mRNA from the standardized baselines, if qPCR (IS) is not available. The deep molecular response (DMR) is defined as MR 4.0 (*BCR-ABL1* IS ≤0.01%) or MR 4.5 (*BCR-ABL1* IS ≤0.0032%) [29, 30].
5. **What Tests Are Useful to Monitor Tyrosine Kinase Inhibitor (TKI) Therapy in the Patients with Chronic Myeloid Leukemia (CML)?**
   - Cytogenetic analysis is valuable to assess the degree of cytogenetic response and possible clonal evolution if there is disease progression or relapse.
   - Quantitative RT-PCR (qPCR) is recommended for all patients after initiating TKI therapy. The majority of CML patients achieve major or even deep molecular remissions with TKI therapy. To be noted, qPCR is the only method to monitor response after the patient has achieved in complete cytogenetic response (CCyR).
   - *BCR-ABL* kinase domain mutational analysis provides additional guidance in the selection of subsequent TKI therapy for patients who do not respond well with TKIs. 1-log increase in *BCR-ABL1* transcript levels without loss of MMR should prompt bone marrow evaluation for loss of complete cytogenetic response (CCyR). The recommended tests to monitor the response to TKI are listed in Table 14.2.
6. **What Is the Major Cause of Resistance to Tyrosine Kinase Inhibitors (TKIs) in CML? What Are the Therapeutic Options for CML?**
   - The introduction of tyrosine kinase inhibitors (TKIs) decreased mortality rates in CML. Point mutations in the BCR-ABL1 kinase domain are the major causes for the resistance of TKIs and associated with poor prognosis and higher risk of disease progression.

Currently, there are five TKIs available: imatinib (first generation); dasatinib, nilotinib, and bosutinib (second generation); and ponatinib (third generation). The T315I mutation confers complete resistance to imatinib, dasatinib, nilotinib, and bosutinib [28–30]. See Table 14.3.

Table 14.2 Tests recommended for monitoring response to TKI therapy

Test	Recommendations
Bone marrow cytogenetics	Failure to reach response milestones Any sign of loss of response (defined as hematologic or cytogenetic relapse)
qPCR using IS	Every 3 months after initiating treatment. After *BCR-ABL1* (IS) ≤ 1% (>0.1%–1%) has been achieved, every 3 months for 2 years and every 3–6 months thereafter If there is 1-log increases in *BCR-ABL1* transcript levels with MMR, qPCR should be repeated in 1–3 months
BCR-ABL kinase domain mutation analysis	Chronic phase Failure to reach response milestones Any sign of loss of response (defined as hematologic or cytogenetic relapse) 1-log increased in *BCR-ABL1* transcript levels and loss of MMR Disease progression to accelerated or blast phase

Modified from NCCN guidelines, CML, version 1.2019 [18]
MMR = major molecular response (≤ 0.1% *BCR-ABL1* IS)

Table 14.3 Therapeutic options based on the *BCR-ABL1* gene mutations

Mutation in *BCR-ABL1* gene	Treatment recommendation
Y253H, E255K/V, or F359V/C/I	Dasatinib
F317L/V/I/C, T315A, or V299L	Nilotinib
E255K/V, F317L/V/I/C, F359V/C/I, T315A, or Y253H	Bosutinib
T315I	Ponatinib, omacetaxine, or allogeneic HCT, or clinical trial

Adapted from NCCN guidelines, CML, version 1.2019 [18]
HCT, hemopoietic cell transplant

7. **What Are the Common Molecular Alterations in the *BCR-ABL1*-Negative Myeloproliferative Neoplasms?**
   - Polycythemia vera (PV), essential thrombocythemia (ET), and primary myelofibrosis (PMF) are collectively known as Philadelphia chromosome-negative myeloproliferative neoplasms. The identification of driver mutations in *JAK2*, *CALR*, and *MPL* provides a better understanding of the pathogenesis as well as therapeutic options.
   - PV is more homogenous in the molecular level, and most of the patients with PV (95–98%) harbor *JAK2* V617F mutation (exon 14), and the remainder of PV cases have small insertion or deletions in *JAK2* exon 12 [31–33].
   - ET and PMF have more heterogeneous molecular abnormalities with the most common mutation being *JAK2* V617F, followed by mutations in *CALR* (exon 9) and *MPL* (exon 10). These mutations are mutually exclusive to each other.
   - "Triple negative" refers to negative mutations in *JAK2*, *CALR*, and *MPL* genes. *CALR* mutations have been shown with favorable clinical courses, while "triple negative" is associated with a worse prognosis in PMF [34–36]. In the triple-negative MPNs, the mutations in *ASXL1*, *EZH2*, *TET2*, *IDH1*, *IDH2*, *SF3B1*, and *SRSF2* are also helpful in determining the clonal nature of the disease [37–40]. The comparison of these three Ph-negative MPNs is summarized in Table 14.4.
8. **Which Molecular Genetic Abnormality Is Frequently Associated with Chronic Neutrophilic Leukemia (CNL)?**
   - Chronic neutrophilic leukemia (CNL) is a rare, aggressive myeloproliferative neoplasm that is characterized with sustained neutrophilic leukocytosis (WBC ≥25 × 10^9/L with mature neutrophils ≥80% of WBC and immature neutrophilic precursors<10% of WBC; ≥ 3 months), bone marrow granulocytic hyperplasia, and frequent splenomegaly. The differential diagnosis between CNL and aCML is listed in Table 14.6 (question 16).

Table 14.4 Ph-negative myeloproliferative neoplasms

		PV	ET	PMF
Laboratory findings		↑Hb (>16.5 g/dL in men; >16 g/dL in women) ↑ Hct (>49% in men; >48% in women) ↑RBC mass (>25% of normal)	↑platelet (≥450 × 10^9/L)	Leukocytosis ≥11 × 10^9/L; anemia; leukoerythroblastosis
Morphological features		Panmyelosis, pleomorphic megakaryocytes	↑enlarged mature megakaryocytes with hyperlobated nuclei	Atypical myeloproliferation, atypical megakaryocytic hyperplasia, fibrosis of bone marrow
Molecular features	*JAK2* V617F	95–98%; *JAK2* exon 12 (2–5%)	50–60%	50–60%
	CALR		20–30%	20–30%
	MPL		3–5%	5–10%
	Triple neg.		10–16%	9–12%

PV, polycythemia vera; *ET*, essential thrombocythemia; *PMF*, primary myelofibrosis

- The colony-stimulating factor 3 receptor (*CSF3R*) mutations were identified in most of the patients with CNL [41–43]. The 2017 WHO diagnostic criteria endorsed the presence of *CSF3R* T618I or another activating *CSF3R* mutation as an important clonal marker for the diagnosis of CNL [44].
- There are two types of mutations in *CSF3R*: point mutations in the extracellular domain (exon 14)-activating JAK-STAT signaling pathway and less frequently, nonsense or frameshift mutations in the cytoplasmic tail (exon 17)-activating SRC tyrosine kinase [45]. In CNL, the most common mutation is the membrane proximal p.Thr618Ile (T618I) point mutation. Mutations in the cytoplasmic truncation mutations are often concurrent with T618I. The two distinct mutation regions and downstream kinases signaling pathways result in the different sensitivity to JAK2 inhibitors (e.g., ruxolitinib) and SRC inhibitors (dasatinib) [45, 46].

9. **How to Distinguish Chronic Neutrophilic Leukemia (CNL) from Chronic Myeloid Leukemia (CML)?**
   - A rare form of CML with p230 BCR-ABL protein may demonstrate prominent neutrophilic maturation and is called neutrophilic-CML (N-CML).
   - Both N-CML and CNL share morphological features such as prominent neutrophilic leukocytosis, minimal granulocytic precursors in the peripheral blood, and hypercellular bone marrow consisting of hyperplastic granulocytic cells.
   - The clinical course of the patients with N-CML is milder with a lower total WBC count, absent or minimal precursors in the peripheral smear, less severe anemia, less prominent splenomegaly, and blastic transformation which occurs much later [9, 43].
   - N-CML is invariably associated with a *BCR-ABL1* fusion and should be easily differentiated from CNL with proper molecular testing.
10. **What Molecular Changes Are Associated with Mastocytosis?**
    - Detection of the *KIT* D816V (exon 17)-activating mutation in the bone marrow, blood, or other extracutaneous organs is counted as a minor criterion for the diagnosis of cutaneous and systemic mastocytosis. *KIT* D816V can be detected in more than 80% of the patients. KIT D816V is considered as a major therapeutic target in advanced systemic mastocytosis (SM). Though D816V mutation is resistant to imatinib and masitinib, several drugs have been developed (e.g., nilotinib, dasatinib, and midostaurin) to target this mutation. Wild-type KIT and other mutations such as K509I or F522C are sensitive to imatinib [47, 48].
    - Besides D816V, other oncogenic variants of *KIT* in exons 8, 9, 10, and 11 have been detected. In advanced systemic mastocytosis (SM) and especially in patients with systemic mastocytosis with associated hematological neoplasm (SM-AHN), somatic mutations have been detected in *KIT* and its signaling pathways [49–51].
11. **What Is the Underlying Molecular Abnormality of *PDGFRA* Rearrangement?**
    - Myeloid/lymphoid neoplasms with eosinophilia involving recurrent genetic abnormalities of *PDGFRA*, *PDGFRB*, *FGFR1*, or *PCM1-JAK2* are a specific disease entity defined by the 2017 WHO [44]. Tyrosine kinase inhibitors have been proven successful for the treatment of *PDGFRA*-, *PDGFRB*-, and *PCM1-JAK2*-related diseases. However, *FGFR1*-associated neoplasms are resistant to imatinib therapy and associated with a poor prognosis [52, 53].
    - *FIP1L1-PDGFRA* fusion gene results from an 800-kb cryptic interstitial deletion that includes the cysteine-rich hydrophobic domain 2 (*CHIC2*) loci at 4q12. The deletion disrupts the *FIP1L1* and *PDGFRA* genes and fuses the 5′ part of *FIP1L1* to the 3′ part of *PDGFRA* [53, 54].
    - *FIP1L1-PDGFRA* fusion gene can only be detected by break-apart FISH or RT-PCR due to cryptic deletion [Fig. 14.1]. Since the *CHIC2* gene is in this deleted region, the test is also referred as "FISH for *CHIC2* deletion" [55, 56]. The *FIP1L1-PDGFRA* fusion has been identified in patients with increased eosinophilia associated with acute myeloid leukemia, mast cell neoplasms, and T-cell lymphoblastic lymphoma [57, 58].
12. **What Are the Common Underlying Genetic Abnormalities Involved in Chronic Myelomonocytic Leukemia (CMML)?**
    - Chronic myelomonocytic leukemia (CMML) is a clonal hematopoietic stem cell disorder with overlapping features of MDS and MPN and potential evolution to acute myeloid leukemia. It is characterized by the presence of sustained (>3 months) peripheral blood monocytosis ($\geq 1 \times 10^9$/L; monocytes $\geq$10% of white blood cells count) with or without dysplastic changes in the bone marrow [44]. The *BCR-ABL1* fusion and rearrangements of *PDGFRA*, *PDGFRB*, or *FGFR1* are absent.
    - Clonal cytogenetic abnormalities are seen in about 20–40% of patients. Most common abnormalities include trisomy 8, monosomy 7, del (7q), trisomy 21, and complex karyotypes [59, 60].
    - Recurrent somatic gene mutations have been identified in up to 90% of CMML cases. These gene muta-

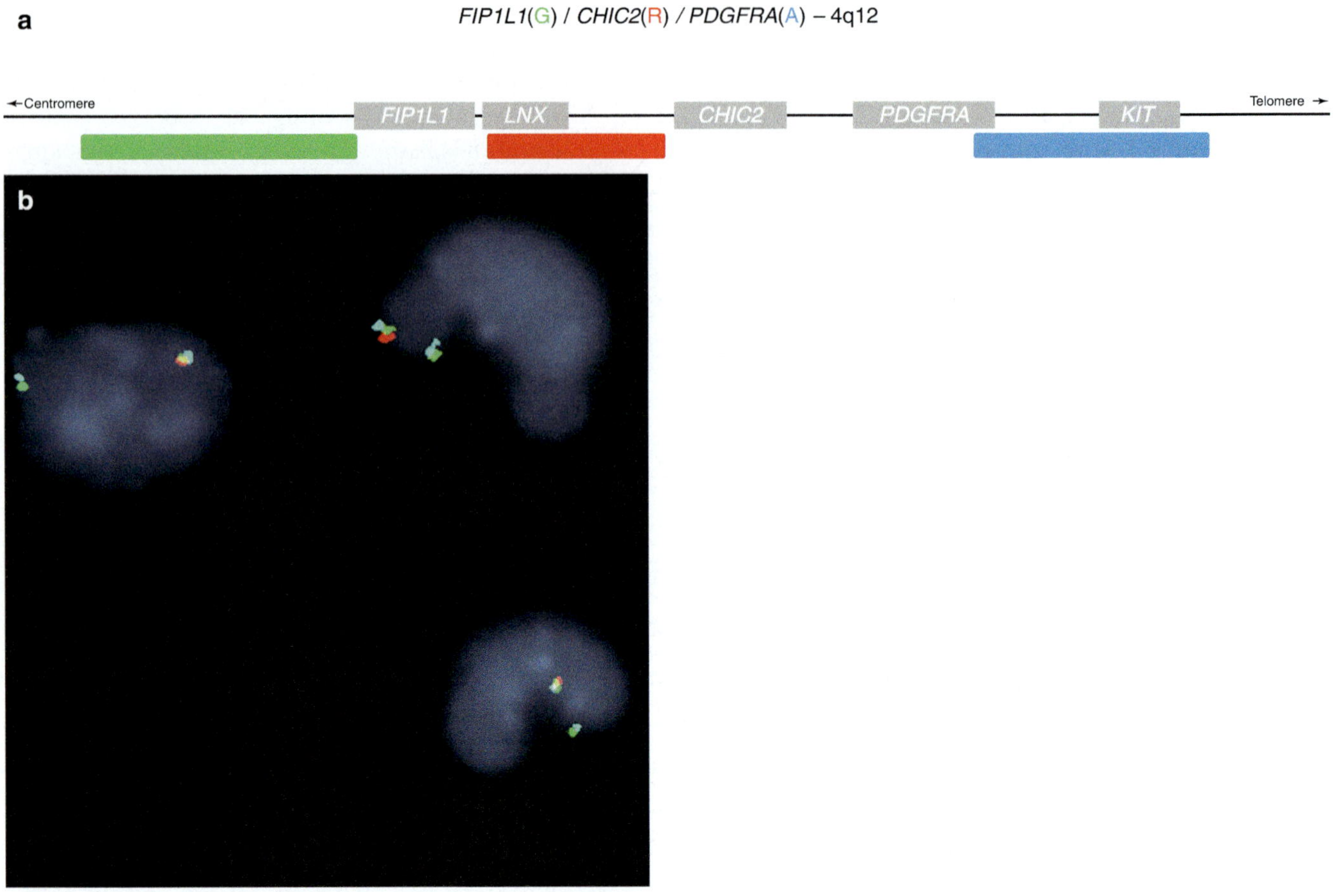

Fig. 14.1 (**a**) Schematic representation of the three probes for FIP1L1 (green), CHIC2 (red), and PDGFRA genes(aqua) that flank the 4q12 region. (**b**) The deletion of CHIC2 resulted in the fusion of 5′ of FIP1L1 to the 3′ part of PDGFRA. The absence of CHIC (red) signaling and the presence of the two flaking probes is indicative of the deletion of CHIC gene. (Credit for Jason Yuhas, Genomics Laboratory, Mayo Clinic, MN)

tions in CMML are divided into three groups: regulate cell signaling molecules (*KRAS*, *NRAS*, *CBL*, *PTPN11*, *FLT3*, *JAK2*), splicing factors (*SRSF2*, *SF3B1*, *ZRSF2*, *U2AF1*), and epigenetic control of transcription such as DNA methylation (*DNMT3A*, *IDH1*, *IDH2*, and *TET2*) and histone modification (*ASXL1*, *EZH2*, and *BCOR*) [61–71]. Of these, the most frequent mutations involve *TET2* (~60%), *SRSF2* (~50%), *ASXl1* (~40%), and the RAS signaling pathway (~30%). The triad of *TET2*, *SRSF2*, and *ASXL1* mutations is very specific for CMML [72, 73].

13. **What Is the Prognostic Significance of the Genetic Changes in Chronic Myelomonocytic Leukemia (CMML)?**
    - Karyotypic abnormalities occur in 20–30% of patients with CMML. The Spanish CMML-specific cytogenetic risk stratification (CPSS) system separates the patients into three prognostic groups: low risk (normal karyotype and isolated loss of Y chromosome), high risk (trisomy 8, chromosome 7 abnormalities and complex karyotype), and intermediate (all other karyotypic abnormalities). The 5-year overall survival (OS) was 35% for low-risk, 26% for intermediate, and 4% for high-risk groups [60, 74].
    - Mayo molecular model (MMM) that focused on the combination of hemoglobin, absolute monocyte, circulating immature myeloid cells and platelet values, and *ASXL1*. The univariate analysis showed a poor prognostic value of nonsense/frameshift *ASXL1* mutations [75, 76].
    - CMML-specific prognostic scoring system (CPSS) was updated to include molecular mutations in *RUNX1*, *NRAS*, *SETBP1*, and *ASXL1* in addition to the prior CPSS cytogenetic scores. The CPSS-Mol stratified CMML into four risk groups: low (0 risk factors), intermediate-1 (1 risk factor), intermediate-2 (2–3 risk factors), and high (≥4 risk factors) [77, 78]. *NPM1* mutation in CMML is rare and tends to be associated with normal cytogenetics, dysplastic CMML, *DNTM3A* mutations, and high risk of AML transformation [79, 80].

14. **In the 2017 WHO Classification, Chronic Myelomonocytic Leukemia (CMML) Is Further Categorized into "Proliferative CMML" and "Dysplastic CMML." What Are the Clinical and Molecular Genetic Differences Between These Two Types?**
    - CMML is heterogeneous with different clinical manifestations and underlying molecular changes. CMML is further divided into "dysplastic CMML (WBC < 13 × 10^9/L)" and "proliferative CMML" (WBC ≥ 13 × 10^9/L) [Table 14.5]. If myelodysplasia is absent or minimal, a diagnosis of CMML can still be made if clonal cytogenetic or molecular abnormalities are present [44, 61, 81, 82].
15. **Which Genetic Abnormalities Are Relatively Common in Atypical Chronic Myeloid Leukemia (aCML), *BCR-ABL1*-Negative?**
    - Atypical chronic myeloid leukemia (aCML) is a rare subtype of MDS/MPN. Patients tend to have severe anemia, thrombocytopenia, neutrophilic leukocytosis, granulocytic dysplasia, and splenomegaly. *BCR-ABL1* fusions as well as the rearrangements of *PDGFRA*, *PDGFRB*, or *FGFR1* are absent in aCML.
    - The most common cytogenetic abnormalities are gain of chromosome 8 and del(20q) [84, 85]. The other reported changes included −7/−7q and i17 (q); deletions of 5q, 13q, 17p, 12q, and 11q; t(6,8)(p23;q22); trisomy 14, 21, and 19; and complex karyotype [86]. However, none of these abnormalities is specific for aCML.
    - Currently, no specific molecular changes have been identified for aCML. Recurrent *SETBP1* mutations, which are encountered in 12–33% of aCML patients, are associated with worse prognosis than aCMLs with wild-type *SETBP1* [87–89]. However, *SETBP1* mutations have also been described in patients with CMML (15%) and JMML (<3%) [89–92].

Table 14.5 Dysplastic CMML and proliferative CMML [44, 61, 72, 83]

	Dysplastic CMML	Proliferative CMML
Clinical features and prognosis	Easy bruising, recurrent infection, transfusion dependent	Fatigue, night sweats, organomegaly, worse prognosis than dysplastic CMML
Peripheral blood	WBC < 13 × 10^9/L Cytopenia	WBC ≥ 13 × 10^9/L Leukocytosis, monocytosis
Molecular	More mutations in splicing pathway (*SF3B1*, *SRSF2*, *ZRSR2*, and *U2AF35*)	More mutations in RAS-signaling pathway (*JAK2*, *NRAS*, *KRAS*, *CBL*, and *PTPN11*)

CMML, chronic myelomonocytic leukemia

    - Somatic missense mutations involving ETNK1 have been found in 8.8% of aCML cases [93]. Other somatic mutations involving *NRAS*, *KRAS*, *TET2*, *EZH2*, *JAK2*, *IDH2*, *CSF3R*, *SRSF2*, *RUNX1*, *CEBPA*, *ASXL1*, and *CBL* have also been detected in aCML, although at a much lower frequency [72, 86, 88, 94].
16. **What Are the Major Features to Differentiate Atypical Chronic Myeloid Leukemia (aCML), *BCR-ABL1*-Negative, from Chronic Neutrophilic Leukemia (CNL)?**

    There are strong morphological and clinical resemblances between aCML and CNL. Lack of specific molecular markers makes the diagnosis challenging in some cases. It is important to incorporate clinical presentations, morphology, and molecular markers for an accurate diagnosis [Table 14.6].

17. **Which Genes Are Most Commonly Mutated in Juvenile Myelomonocytic Leukemia (JMML)?**
    - Juvenile myelomonocytic leukemia (JMML) is a rare MDS/MPN disorder that occurs during infancy and early childhood, clinically characterized by the overproduction of myelomonocytic cells. It is associated

Table 14.6 The WHO 2017 revised diagnostic criteria for CNL and aCML [44]

	aCML	CNL
Peripheral blood	WBC ≥ 13 × 10^9/L	WBC ≥ 25 × 10^9/L;
	↑ numbers of neutrophils	Segmented neutrophils plus bands ≥80% of WBC
	Neutrophil precursors ≥10% of WBC No/minimal absolute basophilia	Neutrophil precursors <10% of WBC Myeloblasts rare or absent
	No/minimal monocytosis[b]	
Bone marrow	Hypercellular BM, ↑neutrophils	Hypercellular BM, ↑neutrophils
	Dysgranulopoiesis; ± erythroid and megakaryocytic dysplasia	No dysgranulopoiesis
	Myeloblasts <20%	Myeloblasts<5%
Molecular Genetics	No specific alteration. See question 15	Presence of *CSF3R*T618I or other activating *CSF3R* mutation[a]
	Not meeting WHO criteria for *BCR-ABL1*+ CML, PMF, PV or ET[b] No rearrangement of *PDGFRA*, *PDGFRB*, or *FGFR1* or *PCM1-JAK2*[b]	

CML, atypical chronic myeloid leukemia, *BCR-ABL1*-negative; *CNL*, chronic neutrophilic leukemia

[a]For CNL, in the absence of a *CSF3R* mutation, alternative diagnostic criteria requires persistent neutrophilia (≥3 months) and no identifiable cause of reactive neutrophilia, including absence of a plasma cell neoplasm or if present, demonstration of clonality of myeloid cells by cytogenetic of molecular studies

[b]Common features present in both aCML and CNL

with a poor prognosis and shares some clinical and molecular features with CMML.

- The recurrent mutations in the RAS signaling pathway are the main driving events in JMML. About 90% of the patients harbor either a somatic or germline mutation in the genes of *PTPN11*, *NF1*, *NRAS*, *KRAS*, and *CBL*; these genetic mutations are largely mutually exclusive. Among these, the gain-of-function mutations in *PTPN11* are the most common molecular genetic changes (35%) in JMML [95–97]. A recent study with RNA-sequencing detected ALK/ROS1 tyrosine kinase fusion (18%) in JMML patients without RAS pathway mutations [98]. Germline mutations in *NF1* are present in 10% of children with JMML. In some cases, JMML may be the first sign of neurofibromatosis 1. The patients are mostly diagnosed after 5 years and have a higher blast count in BM and higher platelet count than the patients without NF1 [98, 99].
- Noonan syndrome is the most common RASopathy, involving germline mutations in *PTPN11* (~50%), *SOS1*, *RAF1*, *RIT1*, *KRAS*, or other genes of the RAS signaling pathway. Approximately 3% of neonates and infants with Noonan syndrome develop JMML [100].

18. **What Are the Common Molecular Genetic Abnormalities That Are Associated with Myelodysplastic/Myeloproliferative Neoplasm with Ring Sideroblasts and Thrombocytosis (MDS/MPN-RS-T)?**
    - MDS/MPN-RS-T is characterized by thrombocytosis ($\geq 450 \times 10^9$/L), refractory anemia and dyserythropoiesis with ring sideroblasts (≥15% of erythroid precursors) in the bone marrow. Somatic mutations in the spliceosome gene SF3B1 are associated with ring sideroblasts and are highly associated (65–90%) with MDS/MPN-RS-T [101–103].
    - *SF3B1* mutations often coexist with *JAK2* V617F (~50%) and less commonly *CALR* (0–3%) or *MPL* (1–3%) in MDS/MPN-RS-T [104–106]. *SF3B1* mutations confer increased risk of thrombosis in patients with MDS/MPN-RS-T [107]. Mutations of *TET2*, *ASXL1*, *SETBP1*, and *DNMT3A* were also detected in several cohort studies [105].
    - The prognosis of MDS/PMN-RS-T is better than that of MDS-RS but inferior to that of ET. The patients with *SF3B1* mutations had fewer cytopenias and longer event-free survival than those with wild-type [102]. The presence of a *SF3B1* mutation is an independent predictor for a favorable clinical outcome, while *ASXL1* or *SETBP1* mutations are associated with poor prognosis [101, 105].

19. **What Are the Disease-Defining Chromosomal Abnormalities in Myelodysplastic Syndrome (MDS)?**
    - Chromosomal abnormalities can be detected by cytogenetics in 50% of de novo MDS cases [110]. Of these, the most common abnormalities are monosomy 5/del(5q), trisomy 8, and monosomy 7/del(7q) [111]. Balanced chromosomal translocations are relatively rare (<2–3%) in MDS and are also important to help the diagnosis of MDS with equivocal morphological dysplastic features [112, 113]. The recurrent chromosomal abnormalities are summarized in Table 14.7. Presence of one of these chromosomal abnormalities is presumptive evidence of MDS in patients with otherwise unexplained refractory cytopenia and no morphologic evidence of dysplasia [45]. Complex chromosomal abnormalities are defined as multiple (≥3) chromosomal abnormalities and often associated with TP53 mutation and a poor clinical course [114].
    - It should be noted that certain cytogenetic alterations have been found in the normal elderly population, such as -Y. Without definitive morphological evidence, these cytogenetic changes are insufficient to establish a diagnosis of MDS.

20. **What Are the Typical Clinicopathological Findings in Patients with Myelodysplastic Syndrome (MDS) with Isolated del(5q)?**
    - MDS with isolated del(5q) is defined by the presence of cytogenetic abnormality involving an interstitial deletion of the long arm of chromosome 5 (5q) with or without one additional cytogenetic abnormality (except del(7q) or monosomy 7) and in the absence of increased blasts [110, 111]. There are two common deleted regions (CDR): one is the region flanking 5q32–33.1 which is with 5q-syndrome that confers a good clinical course; the other one is 5q31.2 which is more common in patients with high-risk MDS and therapy-related myeloid neoplasms [112–114]. In the 2017 WHO classification, isolated del(5q) is the only cytogenetic abnormality to define a specific MDS subtype.
    - MDS with isolated del(5q) is one of the most common cytogenetic changes in patients with MDS (10–15%), and mostly affect elderly women and typically present macrocytic anemia, thrombocytosis, neutropenia, and hypolobated small megakaryocytes in the bone marrow [115].
    - Patients with MDS with isolated del(5q) generally have a favorable prognosis with a median survival and a low risk of transformation to AML [116, 117]. Gain of an additional clonal aberration with monosomy 7 or del(7q) was shown to confer a poor prog-

Table 14.7 The cytogenetic scoring system in MDS, revised [44, 108, 109]

Chromosomal abnormalities		Prognosis	Frequency (%)
Unbalanced	del(11q)	Very good	3
	Loss Y[b]	Very good	5
	del(5q)[a]	Good	10
	del(12p)	Good	3
	del(20q)[b]	Good	5–8
	Double, including del(5q)	Good	
	Trisomy 8[b]	Intermediate	10
	Isochromosome 17 or t(17p)	Intermediate	3–5
	Trisomy 19	Intermediate	
	Any other single- or double-independent abnormalities	Intermediate	
	inv(3), t(3q), or del(3q)	Poor	
	Monosomy 7[c]	Poor	[c]
	Double including loss of 7 or del(7)	Poor	
	Complex karyotype (>3)	Very poor	
	Loss of chromosome 13 or del(13q)	Favorable	3
	del(9q)		1–2
	Idic(X)(q13)		1–2
Balanced	t(3;21)(q26.2;q22.1)		
	t(1;3)(p36.3;q21.3)		1
	t(2;11)(p21;q23.3)		1
	Inv(3)(q21.3q26.2)		1
	t(6;9)(p23.3;q34.1)		1
	t(11;16)(q23.3;p13.3)		

[a]Isolated del(5q)/del(5q) plus one other abnormality (with the exception of monosomy7/del(7q))
[b]Without definitive morphological evidence, trisomy8, -Y, and del(20q) cannot be used for establishing diagnosis of MDS
[c]The combined frequency for monosomy7 and del(7q) is 10%

nosis [118]. TP53 mutation has been found to correlate with a significantly worse outcome, which is helpful to further refine the prognostic risk [119, 120]. *ASXL1* mutation is associated with a higher risk of AML transformation [111].

- Lenalidomide, an immunomodulatory drug with efficacy in multiple myeloma (MM), is the standard therapy for the patients with MDS with isolated del(5q). However *TP53* mutation has been shown to confer lenalidomide resistance [115].

21. **What Are the Common Molecular Abnormalities Associated with MDS?**
    - Gene mutations in MDS can occur with or without chromosomal abnormalities and have been shown to have prognostic and therapeutic significance. The common driver genes mutated in MDS with mutational frequency and respective common associations are summarized in Table 14.8.
    - The driver genes are classified into several functional pathways including DNA methylation, RNA spliceosome machinery, histone modification, transcription, signal transduction, DNA repair, and cohesion complexes [121].
    - The most frequently mutated genes are *SF3B1*, *TET2*, *SRSF2*, and *ASXL1* (>10%), followed by *DNMT3A* and *RUNX1* (5–10%) [122]. Most of these mutations are associated with functional loss, instead of activating mutations. The wide spectrum of the mutations contributes to the different clinical courses in the patients with MDS.
    - Keep in mind that germline mutations in *DDX41*, *RUNX1*, *GATA2*, and *TP53* may also occur, and it is crucial to screen the family members when bone marrow transplant is the treatment of choice.

22. **How to Differentiate Idiopathic Cytopenia of Undetermined Significance (ICUS), Clonal Hematopoiesis of Indeterminate Potential (CHIP), Clonal Cytopenia of Undetermined Significance (CCUS), and Myelodysplastic Syndrome from Each Other?**
    - ICUS, CHIP, and CCUS are considered precursor conditions that can progress to MDS, AML, or other hematologic malignancies [Table 14.9]. It is important to make accurate diagnosis for monitoring cytopenia and clinical follow-up.
    - ICUS is defined as persistent cytopenia (≥6 months) in one or more lineages and absence of fulfillment of the diagnostic criteria for MDS. CCUS is defined as persistent cytopenia (≥4 months) in one or more lineages as well as at least one somatic mutation in

Table 14.8 Common recurrent mutations in MDS

Mutated genes		Prognostic impact	Frequency (%)	Associations with
RNA splicing	*SF3B1*	Favorable	20–30	Ring sideroblasts; *DNMT3A* mutation
	SRSF2	Adverse	10–20	*RUNX1*, *TET2*, *IDH1* mutations *RUNX1* overexpression
	U2AF1	Unknown	5–10	*ASXL1*, *IDH2* mutations
	ZRSR2	Unknown	<5	*TET2* mutations
DNA methylation	*TET2*	Unknown	20–30	60% CMML
	DNMT3A	Unfavorable	5–10	*IDH2* mutations
	IDH1/2	Unfavorable	5	*DNMT3A*, *ASXL1*, and *SRSF* mutations
Histone modification	*EZH2*	Unfavorable	5	*U2AF1* mutations
	ASXL1	Unfavorable	15–20	
Transcription	*RUNX1*	Unfavorable	5–10	t-MN, *SRSF2* mutations, −7/del(7)
	NRAS	Unfavorable	5	−7/del(7)
	ETV6	Unfavorable	<5	
	SETBP1	Unfavorable	2–5	del(7q) and *ASXL1* mutations
	BCOR	Unfavorable	5	
	GATA2	Unfavorable	Rare	
Signaling	*CBL*	Unfavorable	5	
	JAK2		5%	In 50% of cases of MDS/MPN-RS-T
	FLT3	Unfavorable	<5	
	KIT		Rare	
DNA repair	*TP53*	Unfavorable	5–10	Poor prognosis; rarely a/w spliceosome mutations
Cohesion complex	*STAG2*	Unfavorable	5–7	Rarely identified as a founding clone
	SMC3		<3	
	RAD21		<3	

Modified [109, 121, 123]

Table 14.9 Comparison of ICUS, CHIP, CCUS, and MDS

	ICUS	CHIP	CCUS	MDS
Dysplasia	–	–	–	+
Cytopenia	+	–	+	+
Clonality	–	+	+	+

ICUS, idiopathic cytopenia of undetermined significance; *CHIP*, clonal hematopoiesis of indeterminate potential (CHIP); *CCUS*, clonal cytopenia of undetermined significance; *MDS*, myelodysplastic syndrome

MDS-associated genes (allele burden ≥2% in bone marrow or peripheral blood).

- CHIP is defined as the absence of persistent cytopenia but presents ≥1 somatic mutation in MDS-associated genes (≥2% variant allele frequency) [124, 125].

Case Presentation

Case 1

Learning Objectives

To become familiar with the underlying cytogenetic abnormalities for CML accelerated and blast phase.

Case History

A 30-year-old male with a history of CML (Philadelphia chromosome-positive, p210) presented with fever and diarrhea with CBC: Hb 10.9 g/dL; RBC 3.79 × 10^{12}/L; MCV 89.7 fL; RDW 20.8%; WBC 11.0 × 10^9/L; and platelet 341 × 10^9/L. Peripheral blood smear was reviewed as no cytological abnormalities with no blasts identified.

Bone Marrow, Biopsy, and Aspirate

- Bone marrow core biopsy with hypercellular bone marrow with abnormal interstitial infiltration of immature cells [Fig. 14.2a].
- Bone marrow aspirate smear showed the immature cells have high N/C ratio, scant basophilic cytoplasm, fine chromatin, and conspicuous nucleoli, consistent with blast cells [Fig. 14.2b].

Differential Diagnosis

- CML chronic phase
- CML blast phase
- CML accelerated phase

Ancillary Studies

- IHC demonstrated that the blasts are mostly negative for CD34 and positive for TdT. On the flow cytometry analysis, the blasts are positive for CD19 and CD10 but are negative for CD20 and MPO.

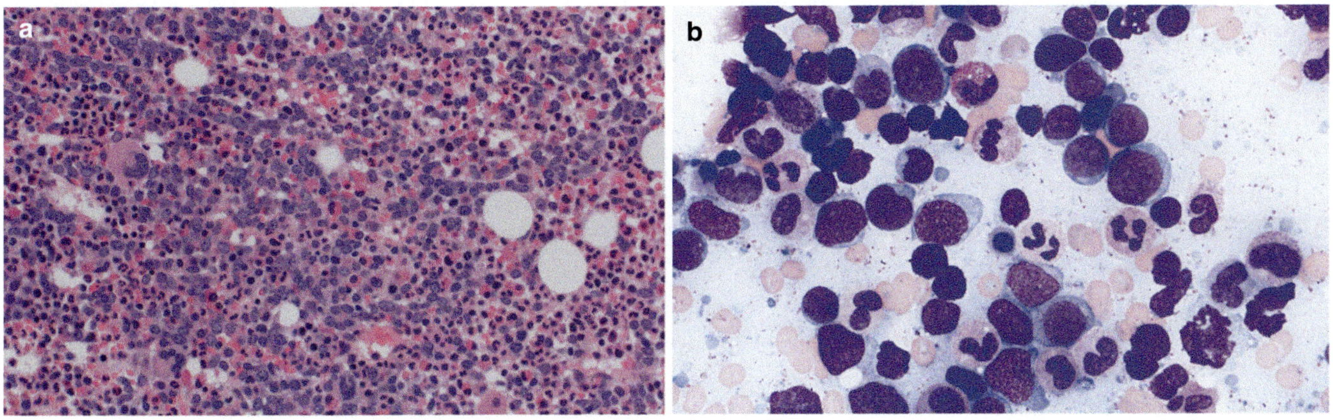

Fig. 14.2 (**a**) Bone marrow biopsy (40×). (**b**) Bone marrow aspirate smear (100×)

- Flow cytometry on the bone marrow showed 22% blasts with B-ALL phenotype that are positive for CD34 (partial), CD19, CD10 (partial), CD45 (dim), CD13 (partial), CD33 (dim), HLA-DR, CD38, and CD9 (partial) and negative for CD3, CD15, CD16, CD117, CD2, CD7, CD56, CD36, CD64, CD20, and MPO.
- Cytogenetic: 46,XY,add(5)(q13),t(9;22)(q34;q11.2) [4]/46,Y,t(X;5)(p10;p10),add(5)(q13),t(9;22)(q34;q11.2),der(17)t(5;17)(q13;q21) [4]/46,XY,t(2;21)(p13;q22),add(5)(q13),t(9;22)(q34;q11.2) [1]/46,XY [10]. Of the 20 metaphases, 10 were normal, and 10 had a t(9,22)(q34;q11.2) and additional abnormalities.
- FISH analysis: 1.8% of nuclei had *BCR-ABL1* fusion.
- Molecular studies: *BCR-ABL1* RT-qPCR result of 1.47 (IS).

Final Diagnosis

Chronic myeloid leukemia, *BCR-ABL1*-positive, blast phase (22% B-lymphoblasts)

Take Home Messages

1. CML can progress into blast phase with increased blast, ≥ 20% in the blood or bone marrow, or the presence of extramedullary blast proliferation.
2. Progression is often associated with additional cytogenetic changes including a second Ph chromosome, trisomy 8, trisomy 19, and isochromosome 17q.
3. The blast lineage can be myeloid (70–80%) or lymphoid (20–30%). The prognosis of the blast phase is poor.

Case 2

Learning Objectives

To become familiar with the molecular basis of essential thrombocythemia.

Case History

A 46-year-old male presented with thrombocytosis for a few years. He denies headaches, dizziness, blurred vision, fevers, chills, weight loss, or night sweat. *JAK2* mutation analysis from outside the hospital showed negative for V617F. Current CBC: Hb 15.4 g/dL; RBC 4.70 × 10^{12}/L; MCV 94.5 fL; RDW 12.9%; WBC 6.6 × 10^9/L; platelet 1151 × 10^9/L.

Bone Marrow, Biopsy and Aspirate

- Normocellular bone marrow with trilineage hematopoietic maturation and increased number of large megakaryocytes dispersed throughout. No significant increase in erythropoiesis or granulopoiesis [Fig. 14.3a].
- The megakaryocytes are presented with abundant mature cytoplasm and hypersegmented (staghorn-like) nuclei. Some form loose clusters [Fig. 14.3b].

Differential Diagnosis

- Reactive thrombocytosis
- Essential thrombocythemia
- Primary myelofibrosis
- Polycythemia vera

Ancillary Studies

- Iron stain, bone marrow aspirate: increased storage iron. Sideroblasts present. No ring sideroblasts seen
- Reticulin stain, bone marrow biopsy: no increase in reticulin fibrosis, grade 0 of 3
- Cytogenetics (bone marrow): 46, XY [20]
- Molecular analysis (*JAK2*, *CALR*, and *MPL* mutation): positive for *CALR* mutation [Fig. 14.3c]. Negative for *JAK2* V617F and *MPL* mutation

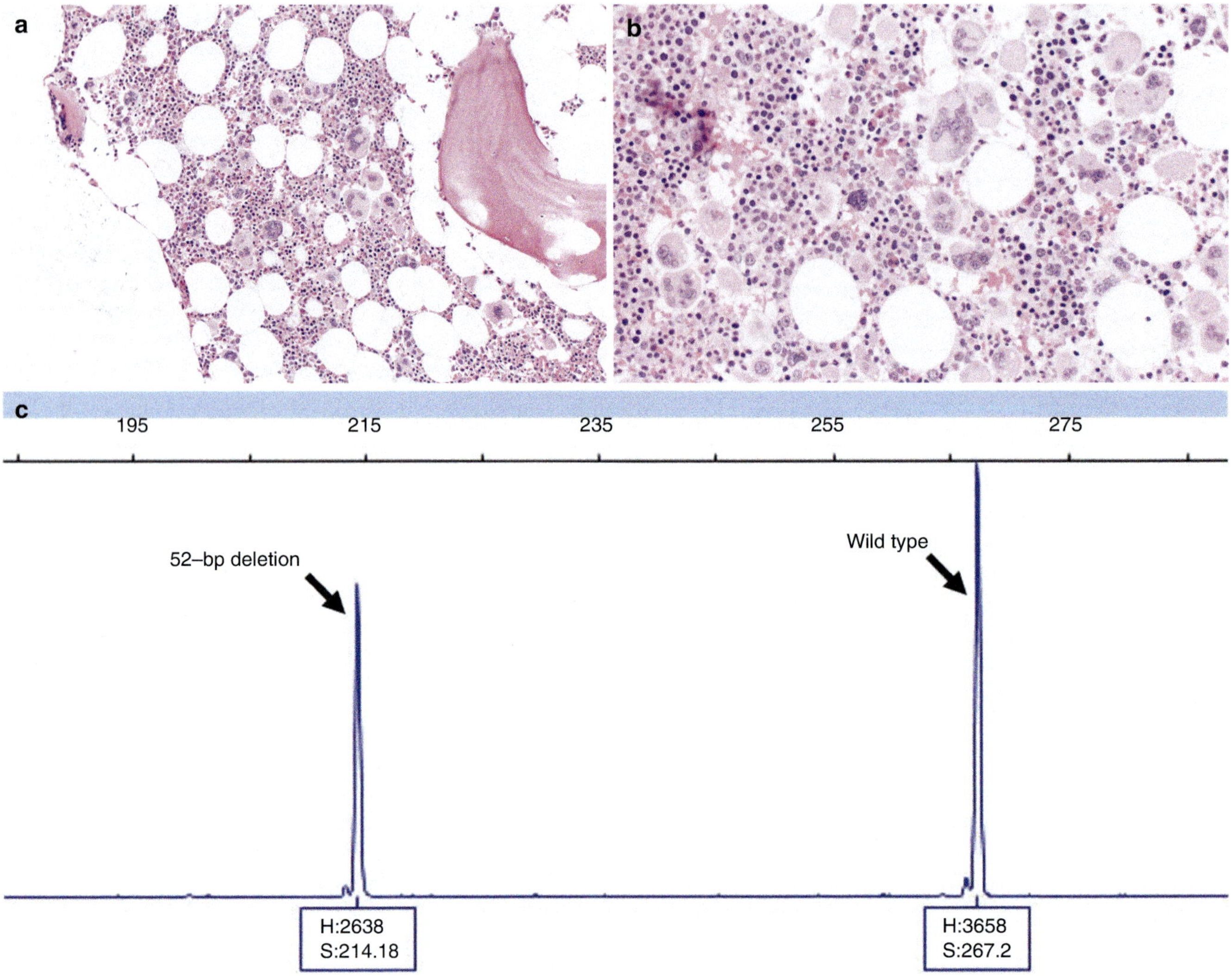

Fig. 14.3 (**a**) Bone marrow biopsy (20×). (**b**) Bone marrow biopsy (40×). (**c**) CALR mutation result

Final Diagnosis

Essential Thrombocythemia

Take Home Messages

1. ET is characterized with an elevated platelet count ($\geq$ 450 × 10^9/L) on routine CBC and presence of a clonal marker. In most cases (>95%), mutations of one of the three genes (*JAK2*, *CALR*, and *MPL*) can be detected, and they are mutually exclusive.
2. The majority of *CALR* mutational changes are insertion or deletion in exon 9 resulting in truncated protein. The 52-bp deletion (type 1) and the 5-bp insertion (type 2) are the most frequent *CALR* mutations.
3. Triple-negative ETs have a better prognosis, whereas triple-negative PMFs are associated with a worse survival rate.
4. Morphology is important to distinguish ET from prefibrotic/early primary myelofibrosis (PMF), which may also present as thrombocytosis [Table 14.4]. The patients with ET have a low risk of progression to acute leukemia and superior overall survival than those with pre-PMF.

Case 3

Learning Objectives

To become familiar with the diagnostic criteria for systemic mastocytosis.

Case History

A 56-year-old female with a history of urticaria pigmentosa presented with persistent diarrhea. Image studies showed mild hepatomegaly, significant splenomegaly, and mild thickening of the stomach walls. The biopsy of the colon demonstrated mast cell infiltration. The tryptase level was

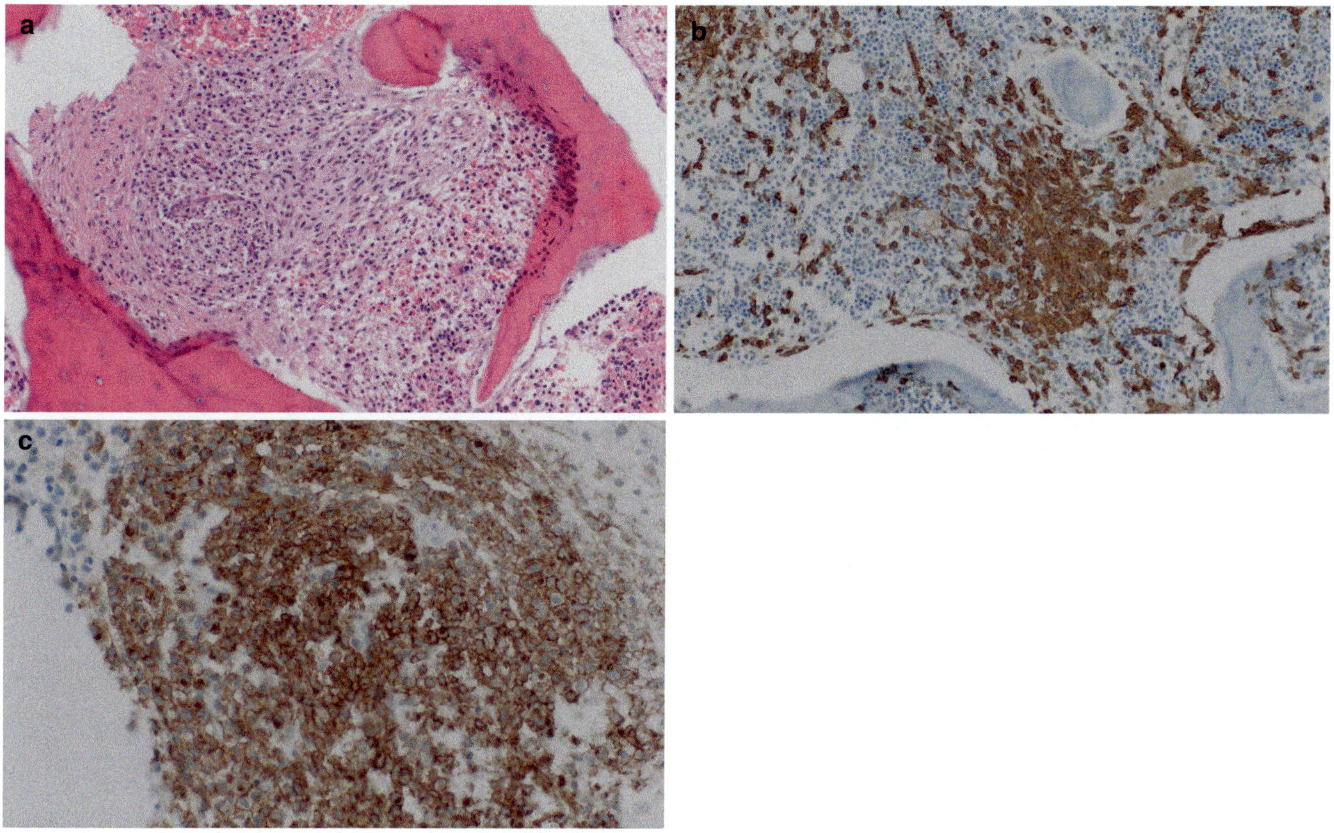

Fig. 14.4 (**a**) Bone marrow biopsy (20×). (**b** and **c**) Immunohistochemical stains for CD117 and CD25, respectively

498 ng/ml. Current CBC: Hb 8.2 g/dL; RBC 2.6 × 10^{12}/L; MCV 91.7 fL; RDW 16.2%; WBC 2.7 × 10^9/L (lymphocytes 1%, monocytes 9%, eosinophil 17%); platelet 23 × 10^9/L.

Bone Marrow, Biopsy, and Aspirate (BM-184793)

- Abnormal paratrabecular infiltration of dense spindle-shaped cells with increased eosinophils [Fig. 14.4a]

Differential Diagnosis

1. Reactive mastocytosis
2. Systemic mastocytosis

Ancillary Studies

- On immunohistochemistry stain, the neoplastic cells are strongly positive for CD117 [Fig. 14.4b] and CD25 [Fig. 14.4c].
- Cytogenetics (bone marrow): 46,XX [20].
- Molecular analysis (bone marrow): positive for KIT p. Asp816Val.

Final Diagnosis

Systemic mastocytosis

Take Home Messages

1. The diagnosis for systemic mastocytosis requires one major criterion and at least one minor criterion; or ≥ 3 minor criteria are met.
2. The major criterion is the presence of multifocal clusters of mast cells (≥15 mast cells in aggregates) in the bone marrow and/or extramedullary site(s).
3. The minor criteria include atypical morphology of mast cells (≥25% of mast cells), activating mutation at codon 816 of *KIT*, abnormal expression CD25, with or without CD2, and serum total tryptase >20 ng/ml.

Case 4

Learning Objectives

To become familiar with the diagnostic criteria for chronic myelomonocytic leukemia.

Case History

A 64-year-old male was referred with progressive drop in hemoglobin, white blood cell count, and platelet count over several years. He also complained of intermittent left-sided abdominal pain and low back pain. He denied any recurrent

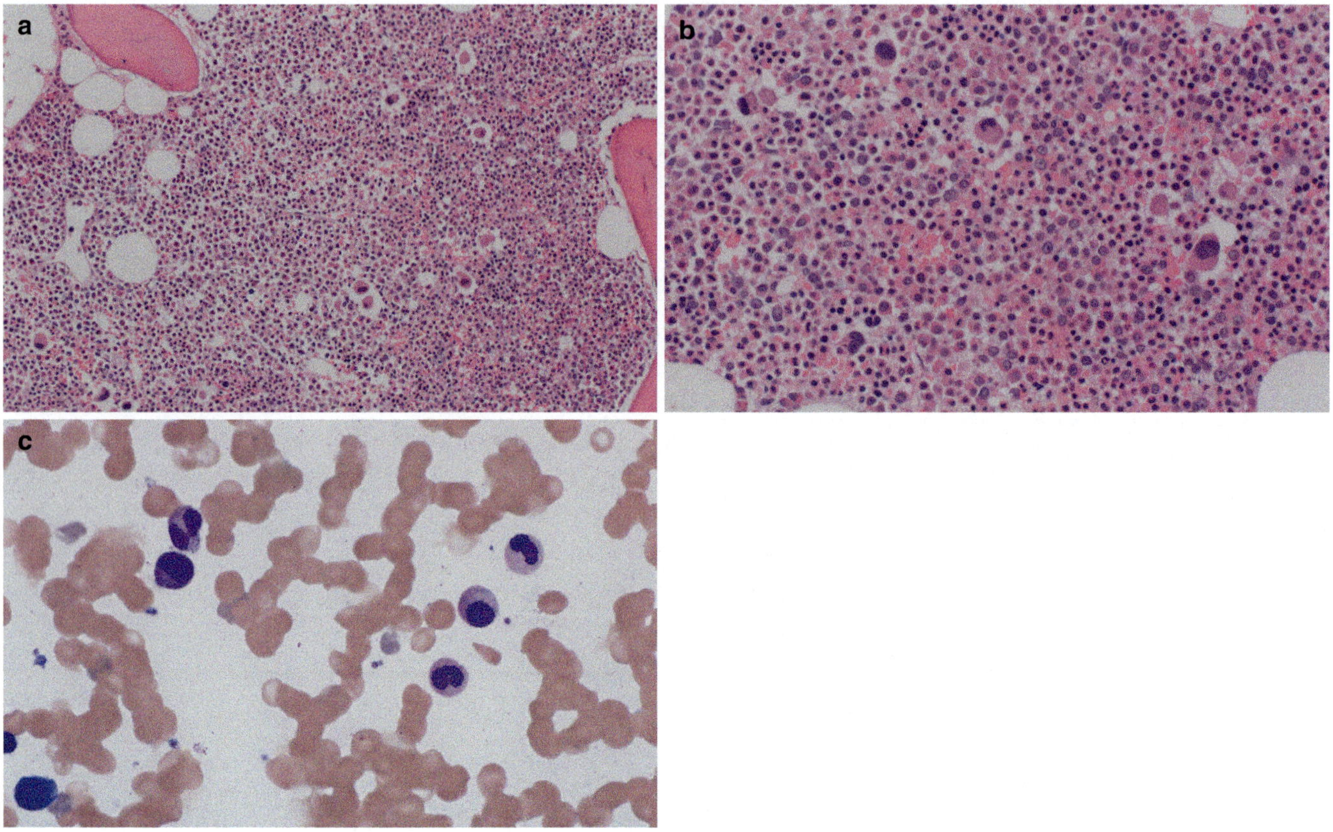

Fig. 14.5 (**a**) Bone marrow biopsy (20×). (**b**) Bone marrow biopsy (40×). (**c**) Bone marrow aspirate smear (100×)

infection or bleeding tendencies. Imaging showed mild splenomegaly. Current CBC: Hb 8.1 g/dL; RBC 2 × 10^{12}/L; MCV 90 fL; RDW 14%; WBC 3.2 × 10^9/L; platelet 106 × 10^9/L. White blood cell differential showed absolute monocytosis with monocytes 36%.

Bone Marrow, Biopsy, and Aspirate

- Hypercellular marrow with granulocytic and megakaryocytic proliferation. Frequent small forms dysplastic megakaryocytes with monolobated and/or hyperchromatic nuclei are noted [Fig. 14.5a and b].
- Marrow aspirate smear demonstrated the dysgranulopoiesis with hypolobated/pseudo-Pelger-Huet and hypogranular forms. Blasts are minimally increased (4%) [Fig. 14.5c].

Differential Diagnosis

1. Atypical chronic myeloid leukemia, *BCR-ABL1*-negative
2. Chronic myelomonocytic leukemia
3. Myelodysplastic syndrome with multilineage dysplasia
4. Reactive monocytosis

Ancillary Studies

Iron stains (bone marrow aspirate): normal stainable storage iron. Sideroblasts present. Rare ring sideroblasts are not seen.

Cytogenetics (bone marrow): 46, XY [20].

Molecular analysis: pathogenic mutations detected as follows:

1. *TET2*: c.538C > T; p.Gln180* (6%)
   c.774dup; p.Glu259* (14%)
   c.2524dup; p.Ser842Phefs*4 (6%)
   c.4546C > T; p.Arg1516* (7%)
2. *ZRSR2*: c.122-1G > A; p.? (89%)

Final Diagnosis

Chronic myelomonocytic leukemia-0 (CMML-0)

Take Home Messages

1. CMML is characterized by persistent monocytosis (≥1 × 10^9/L and ≥ 10% of WBC) in the peripheral blood as well as dysplastic changes in the bone marrow. Cytopenias and splenomegaly are common. It is divided

into proliferative type (WBC $\geq 13 \times 10^9$/L) and dysplastic type ($<13 \times 10^9$/L).
2. The most common molecular mutations in CMML are *TET2*, *SRSF2*, *ASXL1*, and *SETBP1*.
3. The mutation profile of this case provides clonal evidence; although not entirely specific, is extremely helpful for the definitive diagnosis.

Case 5

Learning Objectives

To become familiar with the clinical presentation and diagnostic criteria for MDS with isolated del(5q) (correlation and comparison with Case 6).

Case History

A 80-year-old female presented with fatigue, and she denies any recent weight loss, night sweats, or fever. No history of pulmonary or cardiovascular diseases. No exposure to chemotherapy, radiation, or mutagens and normal levels of folate, vitB12, copper, iron/ferritin, TSH, and LDH. Current CBC: Hb 7.2 g/dL; RBC 1.8×10^{12}/L; MCV 122.7 fL; RDW17%; WBC 2.5×10^9/L; PLT 159×10^9/L.

Bone Marrow, Biopsy, and Aspirate

- Many small and monolobated forms distributed in loose clusters [Fig. 14.6a]
- Bone marrow smears of the same case [Fig. 14.6b]

Differential Diagnosis

1. Myelodysplastic syndrome with isolated del(5q)
2. Myelodysplastic syndrome with single lineage dysplasia

Ancillary Studies

Iron stain (bone marrow aspirate): normal storage iron, sideroblasts are present, no ring sideroblasts.

On immunohistochemical stain, CD61 highlights many small hypolobated/monolobated megakaryocytes [Fig. 14.6c]

Cytogenetic (bone marrow): 46,XX,del(5)(q15q33)[18]/46,XX [1]

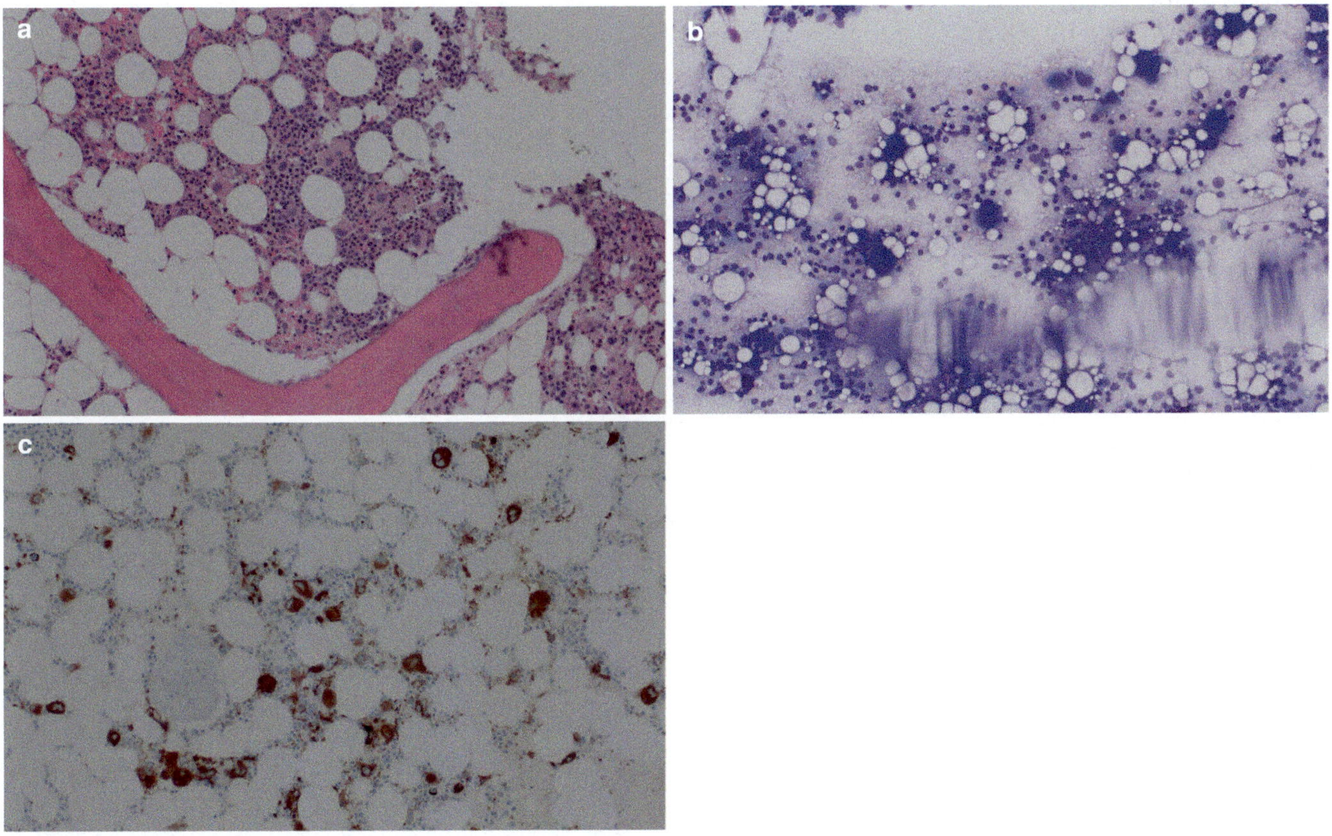

Fig. 14.6 (**a**) Bone marrow biopsy (20×). (**b**) Bone marrow smear (100×). (**c**) Immunohistochemical stain for CD61

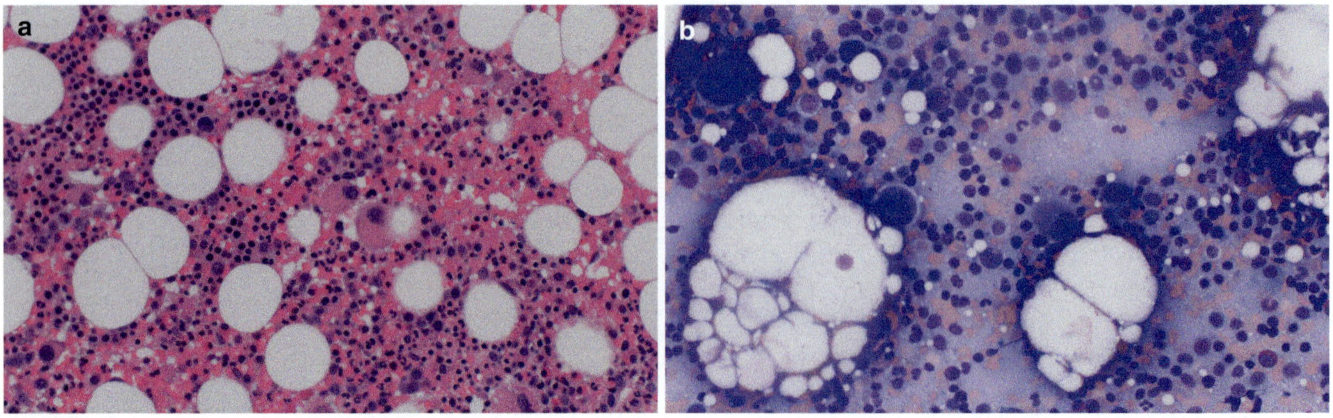

Fig. 14.7 (**a**) Bone marrow biopsy (40×). (**b**) Bone marrow smear (100×)

Molecular analysis (bone marrow): negative for *TP53* gene mutation

Final Diagnosis

Myelodysplastic syndrome with isolated del(5q).

Take Home Messages

1. MDS syndrome with isolated del(5q) is characterized by macrocytic anemia with or without other cytopenia and/or thrombocytosis with female predominance.
2. Bone marrow shows increased megakaryocytes with non-lobated and hypolobated nuclei. Blast count<5%. Of note, similar findings can be seen in MDS with inv(3).
3. Can present with one additional cytogenetic abnormality, other than monosomy 7 or del(7q).
4. *TP53* mutation is associated with increased risk of leukemia and poor survival.

Case 6

Learning Objectives

To become familiar with the classification for MDS.

Case History

An 80-year-old male presented with fatigue for several months. He has been followed up for several years for a history of mild asymptomatic splenomegaly without any demonstrable underlying hematological disorder. He denies having recurrent infections, fevers, chills, nausea, vomiting, diarrhea, overt bleeding, skin changes, lymphadenopathy, unintentional weight loss, and drenching night sweats. Current CBC: Hb 8.4 g/dL; RBC 2.2×10^{12}/L; MCV 110.4 fL; RDW 18.8%; WBC 5×10^9/L; platelet 166×10^9/L.

Bone Marrow, Biopsy, and Aspirate

- Both erythroid and myeloid lineages show full range of maturation with normal morphology. Blasts are not increased.
- Abnormal megakaryocytes with many monolobated forms [Fig. 14.7a and b].
- Iron stain shows storage iron present without ring sideroblasts.

Differential Diagnosis

1. Myelodysplastic syndrome with single lineage dysplasia
2. Myelodysplastic syndrome with isolated del(5q)

Ancillary Studies

Iron stains (bone marrow aspirate): normal stainable storage iron. Sideroblasts present. Rare ring sideroblasts seen (1% of erythroid precursors)

Cytogenetics (bone marrow): 46,XY,del(5)(q13q33)[1]/46,idem,del(7)(q22q34) [7]/46, XY [11]

Molecular analysis: *TP53* Arg175Cys, a variant of uncertain clinical significance

Final Diagnosis

Myelodysplastic syndrome with single lineage dysplasia (MDS-SLD).

Take Home Messages

1. The diagnostic criteria for MDS-SLD include single cytopenia or bicytopenia and ≥ 10% dysplastic cells in one cell line and blasts <5%. The diagnosis requires correlation with clinical and other laboratory tests to exclude nutrition, toxic metals, medications, and other factors that can also cause dysplastic changes.

2. Patients with MDS with isolated del(5q) have a relatively better prognosis and reduced risk of progression to AML. Chromosomal 7 abnormalities are associated with worse prognosis and reduced overall survival. MDS with isolated del(5q) as well as del7q/monosomy 7 should be best diagnosed as MDS-SLD.

References

1. Jabbour E, Kantarjian H. Chronic myeloid leukemia: 2014 update on diagnosis, monitoring, and management. Am J Hematol. 2014;89(5):547–56.
2. Melo JV. The diversity of BCR-ABL fusion proteins and their relationship to leukemia phenotype. Blood. 1996;88(7):2375–84.
3. Foroni L, et al. Guidelines for the measurement of BCR-ABL1 transcripts in chronic myeloid leukaemia. Br J Haematol. 2011;153(2):179–90.
4. Bennour A, et al. Comprehensive analysis of BCR/ABL variants in chronic myeloid leukemia patients using multiplex RT-PCR. Clin Lab. 2012;58(5–6):433–9.
5. Bennour A, Saad A, Sennana H. Chronic myeloid leukemia: relevance of cytogenetic and molecular assays. Crit Rev Oncol Hematol. 2016;97:263–74.
6. Faderl S, Jeha S, Kantarjian HM. The biology and therapy of adult acute lymphoblastic leukemia. Cancer. 2003;98(7):1337–54.
7. Melo JV, et al. P190BCR-ABL chronic myeloid leukaemia: the missing link with chronic myelomonocytic leukaemia? Leukemia. 1994;8(1):208–11.
8. Hochhaus A, et al. A novel BCR-ABL fusion gene (e6a2) in a patient with Philadelphia chromosome-negative chronic myelogenous leukemia. Blood. 1996;88(6):2236–40.
9. Pane F, et al. Neutrophilic-chronic myeloid leukemia: a distinct disease with a specific molecular marker (BCR/ABL with C3/A2 junction). Blood. 1996;88(7):2410–4.
10. Rowley JD. Letter: a new consistent chromosomal abnormality in chronic myelogenous leukaemia identified by quinacrine fluorescence and Giemsa staining. Nature. 1973;243(5405):290–3.
11. Jabbour E, Kantarjian H. Chronic myeloid leukemia: 2020 update on diagnosis, therapy and monitoring. Am J Hematol. 2020; 96(6):691–709.
12. Yeung CC, Egan D, Radich JP. Molecular monitoring of chronic myeloid leukemia: present and future. Expert Rev Mol Diagn. 2016;16(10):1083–91.
13. Chereda B, Melo JV. Natural course and biology of CML. Ann Hematol. 2015;94(Suppl 2):S107–21.
14. Mondal BC, et al. e19a2 BCR-ABL fusion transcript in typical chronic myeloid leukaemia: a report of two cases. J Clin Pathol. 2006;59(10):1102–3.
15. Schoch C, et al. Comparison of chromosome banding analysis, interphase- and hypermetaphase-FISH, qualitative and quantitative PCR for diagnosis and for follow-up in chronic myeloid leukemia: a study on 350 cases. Leukemia. 2002;16(1):53–9.
16. Tohami T, Nagler A, Amariglio N. Laboratory tools for diagnosis and monitoring response in patients with chronic myeloid leukemia. Isr Med Assoc J. 2012;14(8):501–7.
17. Akard LP, et al. Correlations between cytogenetic and molecular monitoring among patients with newly diagnosed chronic myeloid leukemia in chronic phase: post hoc analyses of the rationale and insight for Gleevec high-dose therapy study. Arch Pathol Lab Med. 2014;138(9):1186–92.
18. Radich JP, et al. Chronic myeloid Leukemia, version 1.2019, NCCN clinical practice guidelines in oncology. J Natl Compr Cancer Netw. 2018;16(9):1108–35.
19. Hughes T, et al. Monitoring CML patients responding to treatment with tyrosine kinase inhibitors: review and recommendations for harmonizing current methodology for detecting BCR-ABL transcripts and kinase domain mutations and for expressing results. Blood. 2006;108(1):28–37.
20. Bose S, et al. The presence of typical and atypical BCR-ABL fusion genes in leukocytes of normal individuals: biologic significance and implications for the assessment of minimal residual disease. Blood. 1998;92(9):3362–7.
21. Deininger MW. Milestones and monitoring in patients with CML treated with imatinib. Hematology Am Soc Hematol Educ Program. 2008;(1):419–26.
22. Apperley JF. Chronic myeloid leukaemia. Lancet. 2015;385(9976):1447–59.
23. Feldman E, et al. The emergence of Ph-, trisomy −8+ cells in patients with chronic myeloid leukemia treated with imatinib mesylate. Exp Hematol. 2003;31(8):702–7.
24. Griesshammer M, et al. Karyotype abnormalities and their clinical significance in blast crisis of chronic myeloid leukemia. J Mol Med (Berl). 1997;75(11–12):836–8.
25. Mitelman F. The cytogenetic scenario of chronic myeloid leukemia. Leuk Lymphoma. 1993;11(Suppl 1):11–5.
26. Fabarius A, et al. Impact of unbalanced minor route versus major route karyotypes at diagnosis on prognosis of CML. Ann Hematol. 2015;94(12):2015–24.
27. Verma D, et al. Survival outcomes for clonal evolution in chronic myeloid leukemia patients on second generation tyrosine kinase inhibitor therapy. Cancer. 2010;116(11):2673–81.
28. Wang W, et al. Risk stratification of chromosomal abnormalities in chronic myelogenous leukemia in the era of tyrosine kinase inhibitor therapy. Blood. 2016;127(22):2742–50.
29. Thompson PA, Kantarjian HM, Cortes JE. Diagnosis and treatment of chronic myeloid leukemia in 2015. Mayo Clin Proc. 2015;90(10):1440–54.
30. Vinhas R, et al. Current trends in molecular diagnostics of chronic myeloid leukemia. Leuk Lymphoma. 2017;58(8):1791–804.
31. Baxter EJ, et al. Acquired mutation of the tyrosine kinase JAK2 in human myeloproliferative disorders. Lancet. 2005;365(9464):1054–61.
32. Kralovics R, et al. A gain-of-function mutation of JAK2 in myeloproliferative disorders. N Engl J Med. 2005;352(17):1779–90.
33. Pietra D, et al. Somatic mutations of JAK2 exon 12 in patients with JAK2 (V617F)-negative myeloproliferative disorders. Blood. 2008;111(3):1686–9.
34. Michiels JJ, et al. 2016 WHO clinical molecular and pathological criteria for classification and staging of Myeloproliferative neoplasms (MPN) caused by MPN driver mutations in the JAK2, MPL and CALR genes in the context of new 2016 WHO classification: prognostic and therapeutic implications. Maedica. 2016;11(1):5–25.
35. Tefferi A, et al. CALR vs JAK2 vs MPL-mutated or triple-negative myelofibrosis: clinical, cytogenetic and molecular comparisons. Leukemia. 2014;28(7):1472–7.
36. Barbui T, et al. The 2016 revision of WHO classification of myeloproliferative neoplasms: clinical and molecular advances. Blood Rev. 2016;30(6):453–9.
37. Lundberg P, et al. Clonal evolution and clinical correlates of somatic mutations in myeloproliferative neoplasms. Blood. 2014;123(14):2220–8.
38. Vannucchi AM, et al. Mutations and prognosis in primary myelofibrosis. Leukemia. 2013;27(9):1861–9.

39. Guglielmelli P, et al. The number of prognostically detrimental mutations and prognosis in primary myelofibrosis: an international study of 797 patients. Leukemia. 2014;28(9):1804–10.
40. Swerdlow SH, Campo E, Harris N, Jaffe E, Pileri S, Stein H. WHO classification of tumours of haematopoietic and lymphoid tissues, vol. 2. 4th ed; IRAC: Lyon 2017.
41. Pardanani A, et al. CSF3R T618I is a highly prevalent and specific mutation in chronic neutrophilic leukemia. Leukemia. 2013;27(9):1870–3.
42. Szuber N, Tefferi A. Chronic neutrophilic leukemia: new science and new diagnostic criteria. Blood Cancer J. 2018;8(2):19.
43. Maxson JE, et al. Oncogenic CSF3R mutations in chronic neutrophilic leukemia and atypical CML. N Engl J Med. 2013;368(19):1781–90.
44. Arber DA, et al. The 2016 revision to the World Health Organization classification of myeloid neoplasms and acute leukemia. Blood. 2016;127(20):2391–405.
45. Elliott MA, Tefferi A. Chronic neutrophilic leukemia: 2018 update on diagnosis, molecular genetics and management. Am J Hematol. 2018;93(4):578–87.
46. Fleischman AG, et al. The CSF3R T618I mutation causes a lethal neutrophilic neoplasia in mice that is responsive to therapeutic JAK inhibition. Blood. 2013;122(22):3628–31.
47. Valent P, Akin C, Metcalfe DD. Mastocytosis: 2016 updated WHO classification and novel emerging treatment concepts. Blood. 2017;129(11):1420–7.
48. Pardanani A. Systemic mastocytosis in adults: 2019 update on diagnosis, risk stratification and management. Am J Hematol. 2019;94(3):363–77.
49. Wilson TM, et al. Clonal analysis of NRAS activating mutations in KIT-D816V systemic mastocytosis. Haematologica. 2011;96(3):459–63.
50. Traina F, et al. Single nucleotide polymorphism array lesions, TET2, DNMT3A, ASXL1 and CBL mutations are present in systemic mastocytosis. PLoS One. 2012;7(8):e43090.
51. Schwaab J, et al. Comprehensive mutational profiling in advanced systemic mastocytosis. Blood. 2013;122(14):2460–6.
52. Reiter A, Gotlib J. Myeloid neoplasms with eosinophilia. Blood. 2017;129(6):704–14.
53. Gotlib J. World Health Organization-defined eosinophilic disorders: 2017 update on diagnosis, risk stratification, and management. Am J Hematol. 2017;92(11):1243–59.
54. Vardiman JW. The World Health Organization (WHO) classification of tumors of the hematopoietic and lymphoid tissues: an overview with emphasis on the myeloid neoplasms. Chem Biol Interact. 2010;184(1–2):16–20.
55. Gotlib J, et al. The FIP1L1-PDGFRalpha fusion tyrosine kinase in hypereosinophilic syndrome and chronic eosinophilic leukemia: implications for diagnosis, classification, and management. Blood. 2004;103(8):2879–91.
56. Cools J, et al. A tyrosine kinase created by fusion of the PDGFRA and FIP1L1 genes as a therapeutic target of imatinib in idiopathic hypereosinophilic syndrome. N Engl J Med. 2003;348(13):1201–14.
57. Schwaab J, et al. Diagnostic challenges in the work up of hypereosinophilia: pitfalls in bone marrow core biopsy interpretation. Ann Hematol. 2016;95(4):557–62.
58. Metzgeroth G, et al. Recurrent finding of the FIP1L1-PDGFRA fusion gene in eosinophilia-associated acute myeloid leukemia and lymphoblastic T-cell lymphoma. Leukemia. 2007;21(6):1183–8.
59. Patnaik MM, et al. Chronic myelomonocytic leukaemia: a concise clinical and pathophysiological review. Br J Haematol. 2014;165(3):273–86.
60. Such E, et al. Cytogenetic risk stratification in chronic myelomonocytic leukemia. Haematologica. 2011;96(3):375–83.
61. Cervera N, et al. Gene mutations differently impact the prognosis of the myelodysplastic and myeloproliferative classes of chronic myelomonocytic leukemia. Am J Hematol. 2014;89(6):604–9.
62. Damm F, et al. BCOR and BCORL1 mutations in myelodysplastic syndromes and related disorders. Blood. 2013;122(18):3169–77.
63. Daver N, et al. FLT3 mutations in myelodysplastic syndrome and chronic myelomonocytic leukemia. Am J Hematol. 2013;88(1):56–9.
64. Ernst T, et al. Transcription factor mutations in myelodysplastic/myeloproliferative neoplasms. Haematologica. 2010;95(9):1473–80.
65. Gelsi-Boyer V, et al. Genome profiling of chronic myelomonocytic leukemia: frequent alterations of RAS and RUNX1 genes. BMC Cancer. 2008;8:299.
66. Grossmann V, et al. Molecular profiling of chronic myelomonocytic leukemia reveals diverse mutations in >80% of patients with TET2 and EZH2 being of high prognostic relevance. Leukemia. 2011;25(5):877–9.
67. Itzykson R, et al. Prognostic score including gene mutations in chronic myelomonocytic leukemia. J Clin Oncol. 2013;31(19):2428–36.
68. Kohlmann A, et al. Next-generation sequencing technology reveals a characteristic pattern of molecular mutations in 72.8% of chronic myelomonocytic leukemia by detecting frequent alterations in TET2, CBL, RAS, and RUNX1. J Clin Oncol. 2010;28(24):3858–65.
69. Makishima H, et al. Mutations of e3 ubiquitin ligase cbl family members constitute a novel common pathogenic lesion in myeloid malignancies. J Clin Oncol. 2009;27(36):6109–16.
70. Onida F, et al. Prognostic factors and scoring systems in chronic myelomonocytic leukemia: a retrospective analysis of 213 patients. Blood. 2002;99(3):840–9.
71. Patnaik MM, et al. Spliceosome mutations involving SRSF2, SF3B1, and U2AF35 in chronic myelomonocytic leukemia: prevalence, clinical correlates, and prognostic relevance. Am J Hematol. 2013;88(3):201–6.
72. Mughal TI, et al. An international MDS/MPN working Group's perspective and recommendations on molecular pathogenesis, diagnosis and clinical characterization of myelodysplastic/myeloproliferative neoplasms. Haematologica. 2015;100(9):1117–30.
73. Padron E, et al. An international data set for CMML validates prognostic scoring systems and demonstrates a need for novel prognostication strategies. Blood Cancer J. 2015;5:e333.
74. Tang G, et al. Cytogenetic risk stratification of 417 patients with chronic myelomonocytic leukemia from a single institution. Am J Hematol. 2014;89(8):813–8.
75. Patnaik MM, et al. ASXL1 and SETBP1 mutations and their prognostic contribution in chronic myelomonocytic leukemia: a two-center study of 466 patients. Leukemia. 2014;28(11):2206–12.
76. Wassie EA, et al. Molecular and prognostic correlates of cytogenetic abnormalities in chronic myelomonocytic leukemia: a Mayo Clinic-French consortium study. Am J Hematol. 2014;89(12):1111–5.
77. Elena C, et al. Integrating clinical features and genetic lesions in the risk assessment of patients with chronic myelomonocytic leukemia. Blood. 2016;128(10):1408–17.
78. Laborde RR, et al. SETBP1 mutations in 415 patients with primary myelofibrosis or chronic myelomonocytic leukemia: independent prognostic impact in CMML. Leukemia. 2013;27(10):2100–2.
79. Peng J, et al. Chronic myelomonocytic leukemia with nucleophosmin (NPM1) mutation. Eur J Haematol. 2016;96(1):65–71.
80. Vallapureddy R, et al. Nucleophosmin 1 (NPM1) mutations in chronic myelomonocytic leukemia and their prognostic relevance. Am J Hematol. 2017;92(10):E614–e618.
81. Ricci C, et al. RAS mutations contribute to evolution of chronic myelomonocytic leukemia to the proliferative variant. Clin Cancer Res. 2010;16(8):2246–56.
82. Tanaka TN, Bejar R. MDS overlap disorders and diagnostic boundaries. Blood. 2019;133(10):1086–95.

83. Abdel-Wahab O, et al. Concomitant analysis of EZH2 and ASXL1 mutations in myelofibrosis, chronic myelomonocytic leukemia and blast-phase myeloproliferative neoplasms. Leukemia. 2011;25(7):1200–2.
84. Hernandez JM, et al. Clinical, hematological and cytogenetic characteristics of atypical chronic myeloid leukemia. Ann Oncol. 2000;11(4):441–4.
85. Talati C, Padron E. An exercise in extrapolation: clinical Management of Atypical CML, MDS/MPN-unclassifiable, and MDS/MPN-RS-T. Curr Hematol Malig Rep. 2016;11(6):425–33.
86. Wang SA, et al. Atypical chronic myeloid leukemia is clinically distinct from unclassifiable myelodysplastic/myeloproliferative neoplasms. Blood. 2014;123(17):2645–51.
87. Meggendorfer M, et al. Specific molecular mutation patterns delineate chronic neutrophilic leukemia, atypical chronic myeloid leukemia, and chronic myelomonocytic leukemia. Haematologica. 2014;99(12):e244–6.
88. Patnaik MM, et al. Targeted next generation sequencing and identification of risk factors in World Health Organization defined atypical chronic myeloid leukemia. Am J Hematol. 2017;92(6): 542–8.
89. Piazza R, et al. Recurrent SETBP1 mutations in atypical chronic myeloid leukemia. Nat Genet. 2013;45(1):18–24.
90. Kosmider O, et al. Mutation of the colony-stimulating factor-3 receptor gene is a rare event with poor prognosis in chronic myelomonocytic leukemia. Leukemia. 2013;27(9):1946–9.
91. Trimarchi T, Ntziachristos P, Aifantis I. A new player SETs in myeloid malignancy. Nat Genet. 2013;45(8):846–7.
92. Makishima H, et al. Somatic SETBP1 mutations in myeloid malignancies. Nat Genet. 2013;45(8):942–6.
93. Gambacorti-Passerini CB, et al. Recurrent ETNK1 mutations in atypical chronic myeloid leukemia. Blood. 2015;125(3):499–503.
94. Reiter A, et al. Molecular basis of myelodysplastic/myeloproliferative neoplasms. Haematologica. 2009;94(12):1634–8.
95. Caye A, et al. Juvenile myelomonocytic leukemia displays mutations in components of the RAS pathway and the PRC2 network. Nat Genet. 2015;47(11):1334–40.
96. Niemeyer CM. JMML genomics and decisions. Hematology Am Soc Hematol Educ Program. 2018;2018(1):307–12.
97. Stieglitz E, et al. The genomic landscape of juvenile myelomonocytic leukemia. Nat Genet. 2015;47(11):1326–33.
98. Murakami N, et al. Integrated molecular profiling of juvenile myelomonocytic leukemia. Blood. 2018;131(14):1576–86.
99. Niemeyer CM, et al. Chronic myelomonocytic leukemia in childhood: a retrospective analysis of 110 cases. European working group on Myelodysplastic syndromes in childhood (EWOG-MDS). Blood. 1997;89(10):3534–43.
100. Strullu M, et al. Juvenile myelomonocytic leukaemia and Noonan syndrome. J Med Genet. 2014;51(10):689–97.
101. Malcovati L, Cazzola M. Refractory anemia with ring sideroblasts. Best Pract Res Clin Haematol. 2013;26(4):377–85.
102. Papaemmanuil E, et al. Somatic SF3B1 mutation in myelodysplasia with ring sideroblasts. N Engl J Med. 2011;365(15):1384–95.
103. Malcovati L, et al. SF3B1 mutation identifies a distinct subset of myelodysplastic syndrome with ring sideroblasts. Blood. 2015;126(2):233–41.
104. Ceesay MM, et al. The JAK2 V617F mutation is rare in RARS but common in RARS-T. Leukemia. 2006;20(11):2060–1.
105. Patnaik MM, Tefferi A. Refractory anemia with ring sideroblasts (RARS) and RARS with thrombocytosis: "2019 update on diagnosis, risk-stratification, and management". Am J Hematol. 2019;94(4):475–88.
106. Jeromin S, et al. Refractory anemia with ring sideroblasts and marked thrombocytosis cases harbor mutations in SF3B1 or other spliceosome genes accompanied by JAK2V617F and ASXL1 mutations. Haematologica. 2015;100(4):e125–7.
107. Visconte V, et al. SF3B1, a splicing factor is frequently mutated in refractory anemia with ring sideroblasts. Leukemia. 2012;26(3):542–5.
108. Haase D. Cytogenetic features in myelodysplastic syndromes. Ann Hematol. 2008;87(7):515–26.
109. Shallis RM, Ahmad R, Zeidan AM. The genetic and molecular pathogenesis of myelodysplastic syndromes. Eur J Haematol. 2018;101(3):260–71.
110. Nagata Y, Maciejewski JP. The functional mechanisms of mutations in myelodysplastic syndrome. Leukemia. 2019;33(12):2779–94.
111. List A, Ebert BL, Fenaux P. A decade of progress in myelodysplastic syndrome with chromosome 5q deletion. Leukemia. 2018;32(7):1493–9.
112. Ogawa S. Genetics of MDS. Blood. 2019;133(10):1049–59.
113. Ribezzo F, et al. Rps14, Csnk1a1 and miRNA145/miRNA146a deficiency cooperate in the clinical phenotype and activation of the innate immune system in the 5q-syndrome. Leukemia. 2019;33(7):1759–72.
114. McNerney ME, Godley LA, Le Beau MM. Therapy-related myeloid neoplasms: when genetics and environment collide. Nat Rev Cancer. 2017;17(9):513–27.
115. Lee JH, List A, Sallman DA. Molecular pathogenesis of myelodysplastic syndromes with deletion 5q. Eur J Haematol. 2019;102(3):203–9.
116. Germing U, et al. Survival, prognostic factors and rates of leukemic transformation in 381 untreated patients with MDS and del(5q): a multicenter study. Leukemia. 2012;26(6):1286–92.
117. Mallo M, et al. Impact of adjunct cytogenetic abnormalities for prognostic stratification in patients with myelodysplastic syndrome and deletion 5q. Leukemia. 2011;25(1):110–20.
118. Schanz J, et al. New comprehensive cytogenetic scoring system for primary myelodysplastic syndromes (MDS) and oligoblastic acute myeloid leukemia after MDS derived from an international database merge. J Clin Oncol. 2012;30(8):820–9.
119. Pellagatti A, et al. Whole-exome sequencing in del(5q) myelodysplastic syndromes in transformation to acute myeloid leukemia. Leukemia. 2014;28(5):1148–51.
120. Jädersten M, et al. TP53 mutations in low-risk myelodysplastic syndromes with del(5q) predict disease progression. J Clin Oncol. 2011;29(15):1971–9.
121. Gill H, Leung AY, Kwong YL. Molecular and cellular mechanisms of myelodysplastic syndrome: implications on targeted therapy. Int J Mol Sci. 2016;17(4):440.
122. Papaemmanuil E, et al. Clinical and biological implications of driver mutations in myelodysplastic syndromes. Blood. 2013;122(22):3616–27. quiz 3699
123. Greenberg PL. Molecular and genetic features of myelodysplastic syndromes. Int J Lab Hematol. 2012;34(3):215–22.
124. DeZern AE, Malcovati L, Ebert BL. CHIP, CCUS, and other acronyms: definition, implications, and impact on practice. Am Soc Clin Oncol Educ Book. 2019;39:400–10.
125. Steensma DP, et al. Clonal hematopoiesis of indeterminate potential and its distinction from myelodysplastic syndromes. Blood. 2015;126(1):9–16.

Precursor Lymphoid Neoplasms

15

Xiaohui Zhang

List of Frequently Asked Questions

1. What are the recommendations for initial molecular genetic workup of B lymphoblastic leukemia/lymphoma (B-ALL)?
2. What are the recommendations for initial molecular genetic workup of T lymphoblastic leukemia/lymphoma (T-ALL)?
3. What are the most common cytogenetic abnormalities in B-ALL? How are these changes integrated into the subclassification of B-ALL?
4. Why *BCR-ABL1* fusion and *KMT2A* (*MLL*) translocations are important in B-ALL subtyping?
5. What genetic alterations are associated with TKI resistance and relapse of B-ALL with *BCR-ABL1*?
6. What are the cytogenetic features of *KMT2A/MLL* translocation?
7. What are the prognostic implications of the chromosomal numerical abnormalities in B-ALL?
8. What is the significance of *TP53* mutations in hypodiploid B-ALL?
9. What are some other rare cytogenetic changes associated with poor prognosis in B-ALL?
10. What are the clinicopathological features of B-ALL with t(12;21)/*ETV6-RUNX1*?
11. How is B-ALL with intrachromosomal amplification of chromosome 21 (iAMP21) diagnosed and what are its clinical features?
12. What is *BCR-ABL1*-like B-ALL, and how can the diagnosis be made?
13. What are the specific molecular genetic changes in *BCR-ABL1*-like B-ALL?
14. What is the mutational landscape of B-ALL?
15. What is the significance of *IKZF1* mutations in B-ALL?
16. What is the significance of *CRLF2* alterations in B-ALL?
17. What is the significance of *PAX5* alterations in B-ALL?
18. What is the significance of *CREBBP* mutations in B-ALL?
19. What is the significance of *ERG* mutations in B-ALL?
20. What are the molecular methods to assess ALL minimal residual disease (MRD)?
21. What are the molecular genetic changes in T lymphoblastic leukemia (T-ALL)?
22. What are the molecular genetic changes in early T-cell precursor lymphoblastic leukemia (ETP-ALL)?

Frequently Asked Questions

1. **What are the recommendations for initial molecular genetic workup of B lymphoblastic leukemia/lymphoma (B-ALL)?**
   - The most recently published guidelines by College of American Pathologists and American Society of Hematology (CAP/ASH) recommend the below initial molecular genetic workup for B-ALL [1]:
     – Conventional cytogenetic analysis (i.e., karyotype), appropriate molecular genetic testing, and/or fluorescence in situ hybridization (FISH) testing should be performed.
     – Testing for t(12;21)(p13.2;q22.1); *ETV6-RUNX1*, t(9;22)(q34.1;q11.2); *BCR-ABL1, KMT2A (MLL)* translocation, iAMP21, and trisomy 4 and 10 is recommended for pediatric cases with suspected or confirmed B-ALL.
     – Testing for t(9;22)(q34.1;q11.2); *BCR-ABL1* is recommended for adult cases with suspected or confirmed B-ALL. Testing for *KMT2A* (*MLL*) translocations may be performed.
     – Mutational analysis for selected genes that influence diagnosis, prognosis, and/or therapeutic man-

X. Zhang (✉)
Department of Pathology, H. Lee Moffitt Cancer Center and Research Institute, Tampa, FL, USA
e-mail: xiaohui.zhang@moffitt.org

Y. Ding, L. Zhang (eds.), *Practical Oncologic Molecular Pathology*, Practical Anatomic Pathology,
https://doi.org/10.1007/978-3-030-73227-1_15

agement, which include, but are not limited to, *PAX5, JAK1, JAK2,* and/or *IKZF1*, is recommended for B-ALL. Testing for overexpression of *CRLF2* may also be performed.

- National Comprehensive Cancer Network (NCCN) guidelines have similar recommendations of karyotype and appropriate FISH, as well as reverse transcription polymerase chain reaction (RT-PCR) for *BCR-ABL1* product (i.e., p190 vs. p210) in *BCR-ABL1*-positive B-ALL. When *BCR-ABL1* is negative, NCCN guidelines encourage testing for gene mutations associated with *BCR-ABL1*-like B-ALL including gene fusions of *ABL1, ABL2, CRLF2, CSF1R, EPOR, JAK2,* or *PDGFRB* and mutations of *FLT3, IL7R, SH2B3, JAK1, JAK3,* and *JAK2* (in combination with *CRLF2* gene fusions). Additional optional tests include genomic assessment (comparative genomic hybridization array, CGH array) in cases of aneuploidy or failed karyotype [2].

2. **What are the recommendations for initial molecular genetic workup of T lymphoblastic leukemia/lymphoma (T-ALL)?**
   CAP/ASH and NCCN guidelines recommend the below testing [3]:
   - Conventional cytogenetic analysis.
   - Mutational analysis for selected genes that influence diagnosis, prognosis, and/or therapeutic management, such as *NOTCH1* and/or *FBXW7.*
3. **What are the most common cytogenetic abnormalities in B-ALL? How are these changes integrated into the subclassification of B-ALL?**
   - B-ALL is a heterogeneous disease that is associated with a plethora of chromosomal abnormalities, involving both numerical and structural alterations, such as hyperdiploidy, hypodiploidy, translocation, and intrachromosomal amplification. Approximately 75% of B-ALL cases have recurrent chromosomal changes detectable by conventional cytogenetic analysis [4], many of which have impacts on prognosis and are used for risk stratification on some treatment protocols [4–6] (Table 15.1, Fig. 15.1).
   - The cytogenetic changes have also been integrated into the 2017 revision of WHO classification of tumors of hematopoietic and lymphoid tissues [7]. They have been categorized as such because the recurrent cytogenetic changes are associated with distinctive clinical or phenotypic properties, have important prognostic implications, demonstrate other biologically distinct features, and are generally mutually exclusive with other entities. The subclassification of acute lymphoblastic leukemia/lymphoma includes the below entities:
     - B-lymphoblastic leukemia/lymphoma, not otherwise specified (NOS)
     - B-lymphoblastic leukemia/lymphoma with recurrent genetic abnormalities

Table 15.1 Common recurrent cytogenetic abnormalities in pediatric and adult B-ALL [5, 7, 8]

Risk groups	Cytogenetic abnormalities	Clinical significance	Frequency
Good risk	Hyperdiploidy (>50 chromosomes)	Favorable prognosis	25–30% in children; 7–8% in adults
	t(12;21)/*ETV-RUNX1*	Favorable prognosis in children, undetermined in adults	25% in children; 0–4% in adults
Intermediate risk	t(1;19)/*E2A-PBX1*	Intermediate to favorable prognosis	1–6% in children; 1–3% in adults
	t(5;14)/*IL3-IGH*	Intermediate	Rare
Poor risk	t (9; 22)/*BCR-ABL1*	Poor prognosis	1–3% in children; 25–30% in adults
	t(v;11q23)/*KMT2A (MLL)* Rearrangements	Poor prognosis	2/3 in infants; 1–2% in older children; 4–9% in adults
	Hypodiploidy (<44 chromosomes)	Poor prognosis	6% in children, 7–8% in adults

     - B-lymphoblastic leukemia/lymphoma with t(9;22)(q34.1;q11.2); *BCR-ABL1*
     - B-lymphoblastic leukemia/lymphoma with t(v;11q23.3); *KMT2A* rearranged
     - B-lymphoblastic leukemia/lymphoma with t(12;21)(p13.2;q22.1); *ETV6-RUNX1*
     - B-lymphoblastic leukemia/lymphoma with hyperdiploidy
     - B-lymphoblastic leukemia/lymphoma with hypodiploidy
     - B-lymphoblastic leukemia/lymphoma with t(5;14)(q31.1;q32.3); *IL3-IGH*
     - B-lymphoblastic leukemia/lymphoma with t(1;19)(q23;p13.3); *TCF3-PBX1*
     - Provisional: B-lymphoblastic leukemia/lymphoma, *BCR-ABL1*-like
     - Provisional: B-lymphoblastic leukemia/lymphoma with iAMP21
4. **Why *BCR-ABL1* fusion and *KMT2A* (*MLL*) translocations are important in B-ALL subtyping?**
   - *BCR-ABL1* fusion (also known as t(9;22) translocation, Philadelphia chromosome, and Ph chromosome) and *KMT2A/MLL* translocations are associated with an increased risk of disease relapse or worse prognosis.

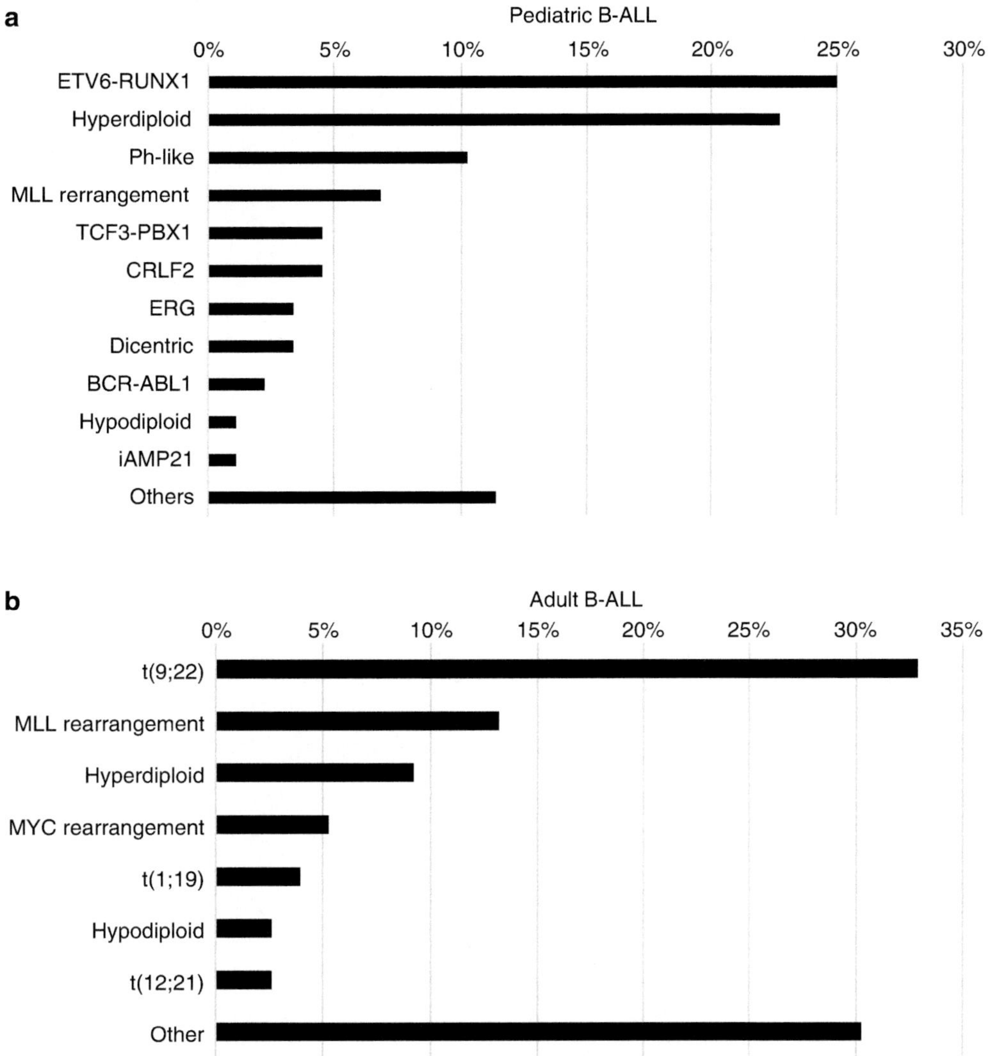

Fig. 15.1 Frequency of cytogenetic and molecular genetic abnormalities in pediatric B-ALL (**a**) and adult B-ALL (**b**)

- The clinical outcome with conventional chemotherapy in the patient group with *BCR-ABL1* is extremely poor. However, tyrosine kinase inhibitors (TKIs) such as imatinib mesylate, in combination with intensive chemotherapy, have been used successfully, although primary or secondary drug resistance and high rates of relapse are problematic [9].
- Rearrangements involving the *KMT2A/MLL* gene and partner genes are associated with poor prognosis. There is also a high frequency of central nervous system involvement at diagnosis.

5. **What genetic alterations are associated with TKI resistance and relapse of B-ALL with *BCR-ABL1*?**
   - Point mutations within the *ABL*1 kinase domain and alternative signaling pathways mediated by the Src family kinase are implicated in the mechanism of resistance to TKI therapy [10, 11].
   - *ABL1* mutations (frequently T315I, Y253F/H, E255K/V, M351T, G250E, F359C/V, H396R/P, M244V, E355G, F317L, M237I, Q252H/R, D276G, L248V, F486S, etc.) are the major contributors to the TKI resistance [12], for which new TKIs have been developed to bypass the signaling pathways or to bind to alternative sites, including bosutinib, dasatinib, nilotinib, and ponatinib. They have shown great improvement on the clinical response in certain patients [13].
   - Clonal evolution and secondary gene aberrations such as deletions or mutations of *IKZF1* or other genes are found to be significantly associated with the resistance and relapse [14, 15].
6. **What are the cytogenetic features of *KMT2A/MLL* translocation?**
   - The *mixed-lineage leukemia 1* (*MLL1*) gene (now renamed *lysine [K]-specific MethylTransferase 2A* or *KMT2A*) has more than 100 different partner genes described.
   - Most cases show *MLL1* fusions with one of the six common partner genes: *AFF1/AF4* [t(4,11)], *MLLT3/*

AF9 [t(9,11)], *MLLT1/ENL* [t(11,19)(q23,p13.3)], *AF10* [t(10,11)], *ELL* [t(11,19)(q23,p13.1)], and *AF6* [t(6,11)] [16, 17].
- The translocation may be missed by conventional karyotyping, and FISH with a *KMT2A/MLL* break-apart probe can be performed. PCR may be used to identify major translocation partners.

7. **What are the prognostic implications of the chromosomal numerical abnormalities in B-ALL?**
   - Conventional cytogenetic analysis can identify changes in chromosome number. Numerical abnormalities may involve the whole chromosome set, resulting in ploidy changes or the gain or loss of individual chromosomes (aneuploidy).
   - Chromosomal numerical changes have prognostic significance.
   - High hyperdiploidy (51–65 chromosomes) is an independent indicator in childhood ALL with favorable prognosis [18].
   - Hypodiploidy (<46 chromosomes, with some people suggesting a stricter criteria with <44 chromosomes [19]) is a poor prognostic indicator.
   - Hypodiploidy can be further classified into different categories: high hypodiploidy (40–43 chromosomes), low hypodiploidy (33–39 chromosomes), and near haploidy (23–29 chromosomes) [20]. The patient has progressively poor prognosis with decreasing chromosome numbers. Near-haploidy and low-hypoploidy B-ALL patients have extremely poor prognosis [21]. Near-diploid (44–45 chromosomes) B-ALL is usually not included in hypodiploid B-ALL.
   - B-ALL cases with hypodiploid karyotype may appear to be hyperdiploid by conventional karyotyping, when the hypodiploid cells undergo endoreduplication. The set of chromosomes is often doubled, which allows a distinction between hypodiploid ALL with doubled chromosome set and hyperdiploid B-ALL [7, 22]. SNP microarray, FISH, and DNA content flow cytometry may be helpful in differentiating the ploidy level (see case study #2).
8. **What is the significance of *TP53* mutations in B-ALL, particularly hypodiploid B-ALL?**
   - *TP53* deletions and mutations are initially found in 2–4% of pediatric patients [23] and 8% of adult patients [24] at initial diagnosis of B-ALL. Next-generation sequencing (NGS) data revealed that overall *TP53* mutations were present in up to 16% of B-ALL cases [25–27].
   - *TP53* alterations, often germline as seen in Li-Fraumeni syndrome [27], are present in almost all cases of B-ALL with low hypodiploidy [28].
   - *TP53* germline mutations are associated with early relapse and poor overall survival in pediatric and adult B-ALL [24, 29–31].
   - *TP53* alterations are associated with alterations of the lymphoid transcription factor *IKZF2* and the tumor suppressor gene loci *CDKN2A* and *CDKN2B* [28].
9. **What are some other rare cytogenetic changes associated with poor prognosis in B-ALL?**
   - B-ALL with rearrangement of *IGH* locus occurs in less than 5% of the cases and confers poor prognosis [32]. The most common partner gene is cytokine receptor-like factor 2 (*CRLF2*) located at chromosome X, and other partner genes can be inhibitor of DNA binding 4 (*ID4*), *EPOR*, CCAAT/enhancer-binding protein (CEBP) family members, *BCL2*, and the LIM domain homeobox 4 (*LHX4*) [33].
   - Some other genetic changes that are associated with poor prognosis include the very rare t(17;19)/*E2A-HLF* translocation [34], abnormal 17p, and loss of 13q [5], as well as complex karyotype with five or more abnormalities in adult B-ALL patients [35].
10. **What should be considered when testing for t(12;21)/*ETV6-RUNX1* in B-ALL?**
    - Cytogenetic testing for t(12;21)/*ETV6-RUNX1* is important since B-ALL with the t(12;21)/*ETV6-RUNX1* (>90% are pediatric cases) has a very favorable prognosis.
    - Abnormality of t(12;21)/*ETV6-RUNX1* is usually cryptic by conventional karyotyping but detectable by FISH or PCR.
    - FISH for t(12;21) can actually detect copy number changes of chromosome 21 in B-ALL with iAMP21.
11. **How is B-ALL with intrachromosomal amplification of chromosome 21 (iAMP21) diagnosed and what are its clinical features?**
    - iAMP21 is amplification of a large but variable region of chromosome 21.
    - iAMP21 can be detected by FISH with a RUNX1 probe that reveals extra signals (five or more copies per interphase nucleus or three or more copies on a single abnormal chromosome 21 in metaphase FISH).
    - The abnormality can be detected by conventional karyotyping analysis with finding of the absence of a second normal copy of chromosome 21, which may not always be present [36].
    - B-ALL with iAMP21 is present in about 2% of pediatric B-ALL, mostly in older children and adolescents (median age 9 years), but is uncommon in adults. The patients are characterized by lower white blood cell and blast cell counts, older age, the French-American-British classification (FAB) L1 morphology, and common B-lymphoblast immunophenotype with a subset showing aberrant myeloid-associated antigen expression [36].
    - B-ALL with iAMP21 patients demonstrated a consistently poor prognosis with worse event-free survival

and overall survival when treated with standard-risk chemotherapy regimens [37]. It is justified to assign such patients in the very-high-risk group and treat them with more intensive chemotherapy. The clinical outcome has been significantly improved with more aggressive therapy [21, 38].
- B-ALL with iAMP21 is extremely rare in adults, and its prognostic effect in adult group is undetermined.

12. **What is *BCR-ABL1*-like B-ALL, and how can the diagnosis be made?**
    - *BCR-ABL1*-like ALL is a subgroup of *BCR-ABL1*-negative B-ALL exhibiting similar gene expression profile to that of B-ALL with *BCR-ABL1* rearrangement [39, 40]. The patients have similar poor prognosis and high risk for relapse to *BCR-ABL1*-positive B-ALL [41, 42]. Patients in this group, particularly those with translocations involving tyrosine kinases, show improved clinical outcome with remarkable responses to TKI therapy [43, 44] or JAK inhibitors such as ruxolitinib [45].
    - *BCR-ABL1*-like ALL demonstrates a number of different genetic alterations: translocation involving cytokine receptor genes such as *CRLF2* (leading to CRLF2 overexpression), translocations involving tyrosine kinases (other than *BCR-ABL1*), and activating mutations or deletions of critical genes (*ABL1, JAK2*, etc.) leading to activation of the *Ras* or *JAK-STAT* pathway [43]. The gene fusions and mutations include *ABL1, ABL2, CRLF2, CSF1R, EPOR, JAK1, JAK2, JAK3, PDGFRB, EBF1, FLT3, IL7R, NIRK3,* and *SH2B3* genes [39].
    - There is no consensus regarding the approach to screen and diagnose *BCR-ABL1*-like B-ALL. It is difficult to screen for every case for all possible fusions and mutations and not practically feasible due to inaccessible genetic testing (such as gene expression profiling assays) to most labs and excessive cost.
    - It has been reported that 50% of *BCR-ABL1*-like B-ALL cases harbor *CRLF2* rearrangements. Flow cytometry may be used to detect CRLF2 overexpression, and a subsequent FISH study can be performed to confirm *CRLF2* rearrangement.
    - NGS-based targeted RNA sequencing is widely available and can be used to identify a broad variety of gene fusions including those related to *BCR-ABL1*-like B-ALL.
    - Other less readily available methodologies to identify *BCR-ABL1*-like B-ALL include gene expression profiling assay, low-density gene expression arrays, RT-PCR, and FISH for known translocations.
    - Different centers around the world use different approaches to screen and confirm *BCR-ABL1*-like B-ALL. Some groups in Europe use multiplex PCR or commercially available targeted RNA sequencing kits, while others use a FISH for primary screening. Some group in the USA uses low-density microarray (LDA) as the screening approach. Some others use comprehensive RNA sequencing [46].
    - Although there has been no standard guideline established for *BCR-ABL1*-like ALL diagnosis at initial workup of B-ALL, different algorithms have been proposed by different authors. Below is an algorithm modified from several literatures [46, 47] (Fig. 15.2).

13. **What are the specific molecular genetic changes in *BCR-ABL1*-like B-ALL?**
    - *ABL1*-like rearrangements involving *ABL1, ABL2, CSF1R*, and *PDGFRB.*
    - *JAK2* or *EPOR* rearrangements.
    - *CRLF2* rearrangements (often with *JAK* gene mutations and activation of *JAK-STAT* signaling).
    - *Ras* signaling pathway gene mutations.
    - Uncommon kinase alterations including *NTRK3, PTK2B TYK2*, etc. [43].
    - They usually have a high frequency of *IKZF1* deletion (~70%), *CRLF2* overexpression (~50%), and *JAK* mutations (~30%) [43, 48].
    - See Fig. 15.3 for the breakdown of the molecular genetic alterations [43, 49].

14. **What is the mutational landscape of B-ALL?**
    - Genome-wide genetic profiling studies on B-ALL have extended our understanding of the genetic landscape of B-ALL in children and young adults over the past decade. Mutations involved in various key pathways are found in different subtypes of B-ALL.
    - The mutated genes include transcriptional factors promoting early lymphoid cell development, e.g., *PAX5, IKZF1, EBF1, ETV6*, and *LMO2,* which were detected in ~40% of B-ALL cases [50], and other genes including tumor suppressor genes and cell cycle regulators (e.g., *TP53, RB1, CDKN2A/CDKN2B*), cytokine receptor (e.g., *CRLF2, RPOR*), kinase (e.g., *ABL1, ABL2, CSF1R, JAK2, PDGFRB*), *Ras* signaling pathway (e.g., *KRAS, NF1, NRAS, PTPN11*), lymphoid signaling (e.g., *BTLA, CD200*), and epigenetic modification (e.g., *EZH2, CREBBP, SETD2, MLL2, NSD2*) [43, 50].
    - Among them, some genetic alterations are found to be associated with adverse or favorable clinical outcome [51] such as *IKZF1, CREBBP*, and *ERG* mutations or alterations (see Questions 15–19).

15. **What is the significance of *IKZF1* mutations in B-ALL?**
    - Mutations of transcription factors involved in early lymphoid development are considered a hallmark of

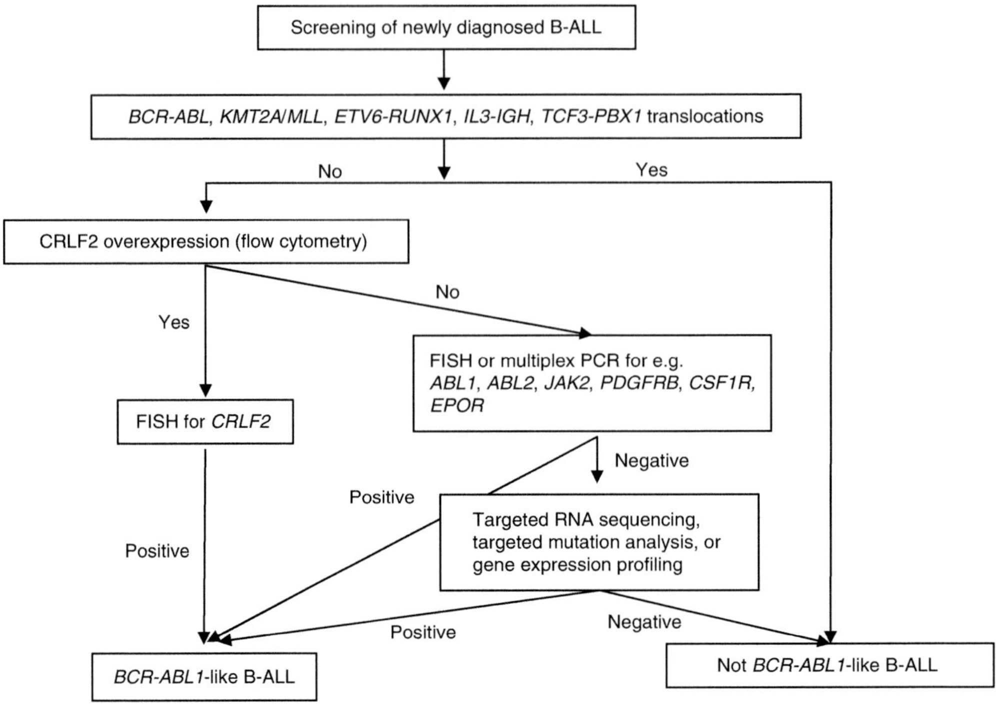

Fig. 15.2 Proposed flowchart for the initial *BCR-ABL1*-like ALL workup

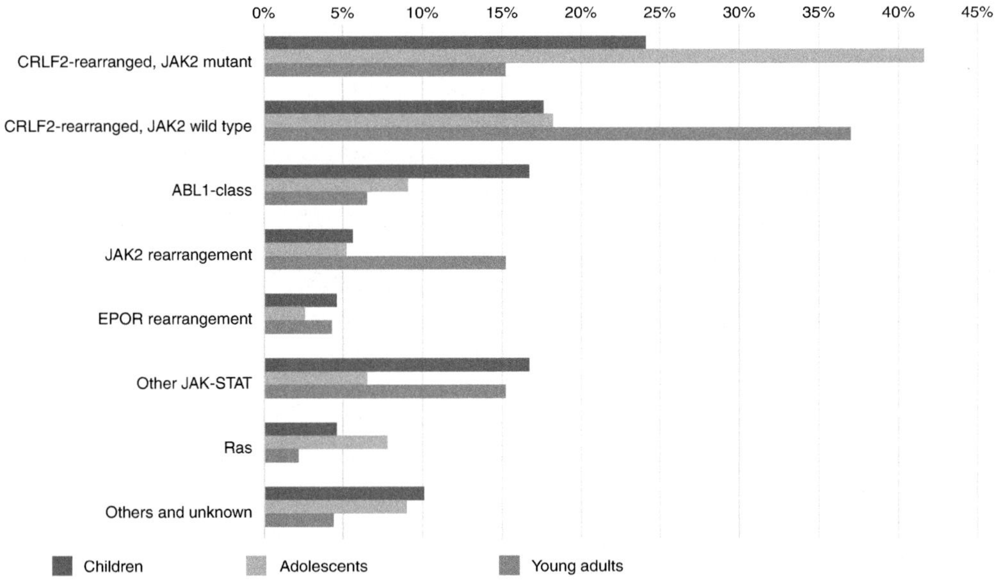

Fig. 15.3 Breakdown of kinase alterations in children, adolescents, and young adults *BCR-ABL1*-like ALL

B-ALL genetic changes. The transcription factors include *IKZF1*, *PAX5*, *EBF1*, *ETV6*, *LMO2*, etc.

- *IKZF1* mutation is one of the most frequent genetic aberrations in B-ALL. *IKZF1* gene encodes the Ikaros transcription factor that is an important regulator of normal lymphoid development and differentiation [52, 53].
- *IKZF1* gene mutation is observed in high-risk B-ALL, including approximately 80% of *BCR-ABL1*-positive B-ALL cases and 70% of *BCR-ABL1*-like B-ALL cases [54, 55].
- *IKZF1* mutations are often deletions and rarely point mutations [56, 57]. Most deletions are monoallelic and involve exons 3–6, which encode the N-terminal zinc finger DNA-binding domain [56]. The deletions result in dominant negative form of the Ikaros protein that inhibits the function of wild-type Ikaros. It has been shown that induction of mutant, dominant negative Ikaros in early pre-B cells arrests the cell differentiation, suggesting that loss of Ikaros activity contributes to B-ALL leukemogenesis and *IKZF1* mutations are likely driver mutations [58].

- Multiple studies support that *IKZF1* mutation/deletion is an independent indicator of B-ALL unfavorable clinical outcome including chemotherapy resistance and higher risk for relapse [15, 43, 59–61].
- Different methodologies including single-nucleotide polymorphism (SNP) microarray, transcriptional profiling, sequencing, and CGH can be used to detect *IKZF1* mutation/deletion [40, 62].

16. **What is the significance of *CRLF2* alterations in B-ALL?**
    - *CRLF2* alterations are found in approximately 8% of pediatric B-ALL patients, and more than 50% of patients with Down syndrome-associated B-ALL [63].
    - *CRLF2* alterations are commonly gene rearrangement with immunoglobulin heavy chain locus resulting in *IGH-CRLF2* fusion gene, less often interstitial deletions resulting in *P2RY8-CRLF2* fusion gene, and rarely can be point mutations [48, 64].
    - These changes usually result in overexpression of CRLF2 (therefore can be analyzed by flow cytometry). *CRLF2* alterations are associated with constitutive activation in the *JAK-2* pathway such as *JAK-STAT*, *PI3K*/mTOR, and *BCL-2* transduction [65].
    - The alterations are often found in high-risk B-ALL [48], although the prognostic significance of *CRLF2* deregulation in B-ALL remains controversial [64].
17. **What is the significance of *PAX5* alterations in B-ALL?**
    - Alterations of *PAX5* have been found in ~30% of B-ALL cases [50].
    - The alterations include acquired mutations, rearrangements involving various partner genes such as *ETV6* and *JAK2*, and germline mutations [50, 66, 67].
    - Unlike *IKZF1*, *PAX5* alterations do not appear to impact clinical outcomes; however, the *PAX5* mutations may be driver mutations in B-ALL leukemogenesis and play a role in susceptibility to B-ALL [67, 68].
    - Sequencing is usually the methodology to detect *PAX5* mutations [50].
18. **What is the significance of *CREBBP* mutations in B-ALL?**
    - Deletions and mutations of *CREBBP*, which encodes the transcriptional coactivators and acetyltransferase CREB binding protein, are found in 18% of relapsed pediatric B-ALL patients, but less than 1% at diagnosis in those who did not relapse [69], suggesting *CREBBP* gene mutations are associated with relapse of the disease.
    - The mutations result in loss of function of CREBBP. In one study, *CREBBP* mutations were associated with hyperdiploid B-ALL relapse. Up to 60% of high-hyperdiploid relapse cases show *CREBBP* mutation, altering the clinical outcome in the favorable B-ALL group [70]. It might be a marker that can be integrated into risk stratification system after large cohort study.
19. **What is the significance of *ERG* mutations in B-ALL?**
    - Several studies have identified a subgroup of pediatric B-ALL patients, comprising 3–5% of B-ALL cases, with monoallelic deletion of *ERG* gene, which encodes an ETS-domain-containing transcription factor [71, 72].
    - The deletions result in an aberrant ERG protein that functions as a competitive inhibitor of wild-type *ERG* [73].
    - The *ERG* deletion and other known classifying genetic lesions are mutually exclusive, suggesting that B-ALL with *ERG* deletion may be a distinct subtype.
    - These patients generally have excellent prognosis, despite an association with frequent *IKZF1* deletions, which is different from *BCR-ABL1*-positive and *BCR-ABL1*-like B-ALL cases [72]. Whether or not the *ERG* mutations function as a negative regulator under *IKZF1* mutated status needs to be explored.
20. **What are the molecular methods to assess ALL minimal residual disease (MRD)?**
    - The most frequently used molecular methods to assess ALL MRD are 1) antigen-receptor (immunoglobulin/IG and T-cell receptor/TCR) gene rearrangement analysis, 2) real-time quantitative polymerase chain reaction (RQ-PCR) to detect known fusion genes such as *BCR-ABL1*, and 3) NGS-based assay to detect clonal immunoglobulin heavy-chain gene or T-cell receptor gene rearrangements [2].
    - RQ-PCR-based IG and TCR gene rearrangement analyses and RQ-PCR-based fusion gene assay can detect MRD at a level of 1×10^{-5} sensitivity [74], and NGS-based MRD assay to detect clone-specific IG or TCR index sequence can reach a sensitivity level of 1×10^{-6}, comparing to a sensitivity of 1×10^{-4} cells by using six-color flow cytometry [2, 74].
    - About 5–10% ALL cases do not carry clonal IG or TR gene rearrangements.
    - Examples of fusion genes that can be used in RQ-PCR to detect MRD include *BCR-ABL1, ETV6-RUNX1, KMT2A/MLL* rearrangement, and *TCF3-PBX1* in B-ALL and *TAL1* deletions (*SIL/TAL1*) in T-ALL. The detection of these potential MRD markers should be performed at diagnosis and monitored throughout the course of disease.
    - Novel technologies and applications are under further investigation and validation. Examples are

droplet digital PCR [75, 76] and deep sequencing NGS [77].

- Table 15.2 is the comparison of different methods commonly used to detect ALL MRD [74, 78–81].

21. **What are the molecular genetic changes in T lymphoblastic leukemia (T-ALL)?**
    - Rearrangements between the regulatory region of a T-cell receptor locus (alpha and delta *TR* loci at 14q11.2, beta locus at 7q35, and gamma locus at 7p14-15) and an oncogenic transcription factor (such as *TAL1* at 1p32, *TLX1* at 10q24, *MYC* at 8q24.1, *LMO1* at 11p15, *LMO2* at 11p13, and *LYL1* at 19p13) are also common [7].
    - Rearrangements of *MLLT10*, *KMT2A*, *ABL1*, or *NIP98* with a variety of different partner genes result in deregulated expression of the transcription factor [82].
    - Most of the translocations can only be detected by molecular genetic studies, but not by conventional karyotyping. For example, *TAL1* is fused to *SIL/STIL* as a result of a cryptic interstitial deletion at chromosome 1p32 [7].
    - *NOTCH1* activating mutations and loss of *CDKN2A* locus occur in over 70% of the T-ALL cases. *NOTCH1* pathway activation (*NOTCH1* mutations, *FBXW7* mutations (resulting in increased half-life of *NOTCH1*) or, rarely, *NOTCH1* rearrangement) is present in >50% of T-ALL cases [3]. *CDKN2A/2B* mutations and deletion of chromosome 9p that result in inactivation of *CDKN2A/2B* occur in >50% of the T-ALL cases [83].
    - Genome-wide sequencing has revealed a broad spectrum of mutations and copy number alterations of genes involving *JAK-STAT* (*IL7R, JAK1, JAK3, DNM2*), *RAS* (*NRAS, KRAS,* and *NF1*), *PI3K-AKT* (*PTEN, AKT1, PIK3CA, PIK3CD*), epigenetic regulators (*PHF6, SUZ12, EZH2, KDM6A*), transcription factors and regulators (*ETV6, GATA3, RUNX1, LEF1, WT1, BCL11B*), and translation regulators (*CNOT3, RPL5, RPL10*) [83, 84].
22. **What are the molecular genetic changes in early T-cell precursor lymphoblastic leukemia (ETP-ALL)?**
    - The mutational landscape of ETP-ALL includes alterations in genes involved in cytokine and *RAS* signaling (e.g., *NRAS*, *KRAS*, FLT3, and *JAK1*), epigenetic regulation (e.g., *EZH2*, *DNMT3A*, and *SUZ12*), and hematopoietic development (e.g., *ETV6*, *RUNX1*, and *IKZF1*) [85].
    - The mutation profile of ETP-ALL is more similar to that of myeloid leukemias, with high frequency mutations of *FLT3*, the *RAS* family of genes, *DNMT3A*, *IDH1*, and *IDH2* [7].
    - The incidence of activating *NOTCH1* mutations is lower in ETP-ALL (15%) than that of T-ALL (higher than 50%) [85].
    - ETP-ALL shares some genomic and epigenomic features with T/myeloid mixed phenotype acute leukemia, with frequent biallelic *WT1* alterations, and alterations in other several transcription factors (*ETV6, RUNX1, CEBPA*) and signaling pathways (*JAK-STAT, FLT3, RAS*) [84].

Case Presentations

Case 1

Learning Objective

- Review CAP/ASH and NCCN guidelines for initial ALL workup recommendations.
- *KMT2A/MLL* translocation may be missed by conventional karyotyping.
- B-ALL with *KMT2A/MLL* translocation cases can show peculiar immunophenotype.

Table 15.2 Comparison of characteristics of the commonly used MRD detection methods

MRD detection technique	Conventional flow cytometry	RQ-PCR for IG/TCR genes	RQ-PCR for fusion genes (e.g., *BCR-ABL1*)	NGS for IG/TCR genes
Estimated sensitivity	3–4 colors: 10^{-3}–10^{-4} 6–8 colors: 10^{-4}	10^{-4}–10^{-5}	10^{-4}–10^{-6}	10^{-6}
Applicability	>90%	90–95%	B-ALL: 25–40% T-ALL: 10–15%	95%
Advantages	Fast Widely used	Relatively sensitive Standardized	Relatively sensitive Rapid Relatively easy Stable throughout treatment Standardized	High sensitivity High specificity Able to detect subclones
Disadvantages	Variable sensitivity due to operator variation Limited standardization Viable cells required	Time-consuming Affected by clonal evolution	Limited applicability RNA instability Patient specific	Expensive Not widely used Standardization and validation ongoing [79]

Case History

A 34-year-old female complained of vague symptoms including dyspnea, headache, and fatigue. She was diagnosed with COVID-19 in 2020 and started developing new symptoms after that. She was found to have an elevated white blood cell count of 15.9 K/μL and circulating immature mononuclear cells in the peripheral blood.

Laboratory Findings

Blood cell counts: WBC 9.39 K/μL; hemoglobin 7.9 g/dL; platelets 332 K/μL

Peripheral blood smear showed 3% circulating blasts. The bone marrow was hypercellular with sheets of blasts (Fig. 15.4a, b). By immunohistochemical staining, the blasts were positive for CD34, CD19, and PAX5 and negative for TdT, CD117, CD3, CD20, and myeloperoxidase (Fig. 15.4c–f).

Flow cytometric analysis demonstrated a population of blasts expressing dim CD45, CD19, CD34, CD38, and cytoplasmic CD79a and lacking cytoplasmic CD3, CD10, CD20, CD22, CD117, myeloperoxidase, and terminal deoxynucleotidyl transferase (TdT).

Genetic Study

Chromosome analysis revealed a normal karyotype: 46,XX [10]. FISH study for *BCR-ABL1* was negative. NGS analysis (targeted gene DNA sequencing and RNA sequencing) detected *KMT2A (MLL)/MLLT1 (ENL)* fusion. Multiple variants of unknown significance (VUS) were also detected,.

Final Diagnosis

B lymphoblastic leukemia/lymphoma, with *KMT2A-MLLT1* rearrangement

Discussion

CAP/ASH and NCCN guidelines recommend initial molecular genetic workup for B-ALL to include conventional cytogenetic analysis (i.e., karyotype), appropriate molecular genetic testing, and/or FISH testing. FISH for *KMT2A/MLL* translocation is optional. However, conventional cytogenetic analysis may miss the *KMT2A/MLL* aberrancy. Some commercially available NGS-based mutational assays include both DNA sequencing and RNA sequencing and can detect certain gene rearrangements. In this case, the *KMT2A -MLLT1* translocation was detected by NGS-based mutational analysis.

Additionally, B-ALL with *KMT2A* rearrangements may show immunophenotypic variation different from the other B-ALL cases, usually with more mature phenotype, positive for CD19, negative for CD10 and CD24, and variable expression of CD34 and TdT [86]. In this case, the immunophenotype was unusual, with negative CD10 and TdT.

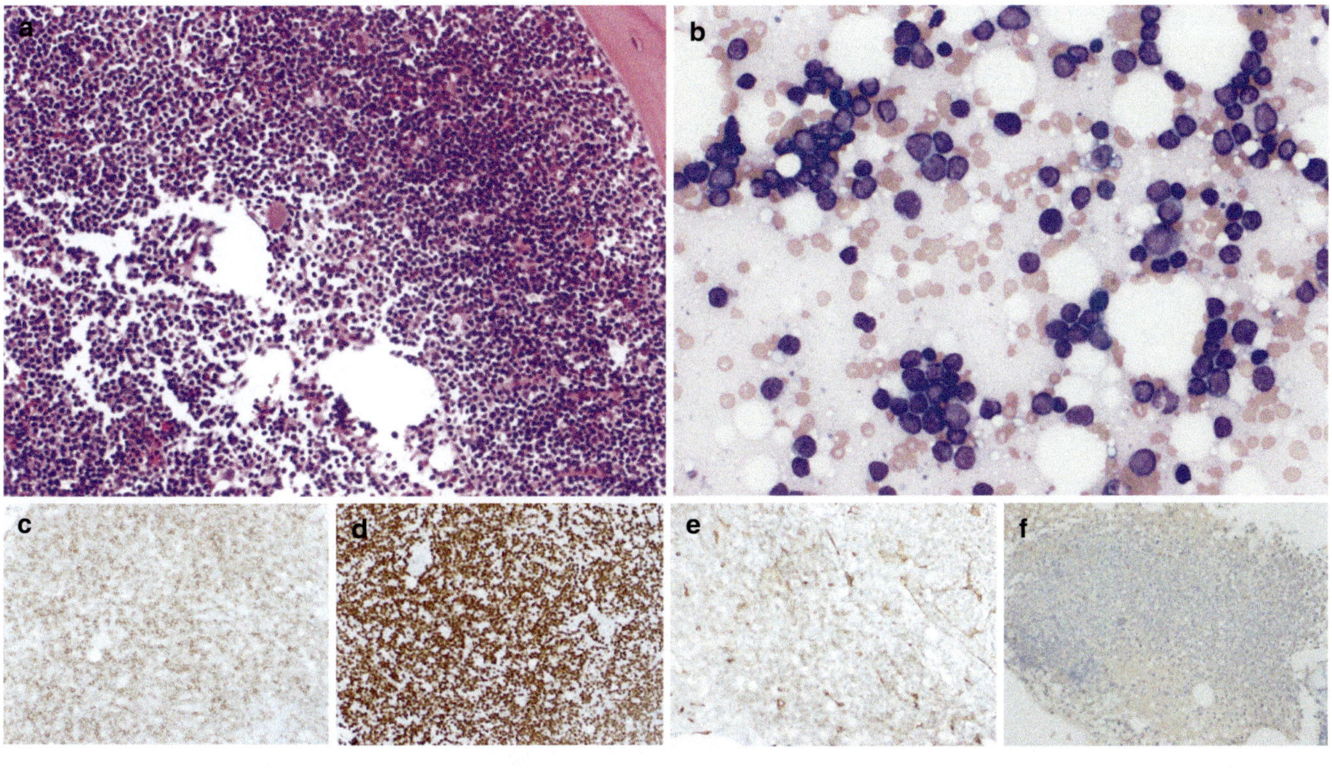

Fig. 15.4 The bone marrow biopsy and aspirate smear showed sheets of blasts (**a, b**). By immunohistochemical staining, the blasts were positive for CD19 (**c**), PAX5 (**d**), and CD34 (**e**) and negative for TdT (F)

Case 2 (Courtesy of Dr. Peter Papenhausen at LabCorp)

Learning Objective

- Hypodiploidy in B-ALL can present as pseudo-hyperdiploidy.
- SNP microarray may be helpful in differentiating the ploidy level.

Case History

A 10-year-old boy complained of fatigue and bone pain. He was found to have an elevated WBC count, anemia, and thrombocytopenia. A bone marrow aspiration was performed.

Laboratory Findings

Blood cell counts: WBC 17.5 K/μL, 60% blasts

The bone marrow aspirate smears show hypercellular marrow with greater than 90% blasts.

Flow cytometric analysis demonstrated a population of blasts (97% of total events) positive for CD45 (dim), CD19, CD10, CD22, CD34, CD38, HLA-DR, TdT, CD52, CD58, and CD123 and negative for CD2, CD3, CD4, CD5, CD7, CD8, CD11c, CD13, CD15, CD20, CD23, CD25, CD35, CD41, CD61, CD64, CD79b, CD235a, sIgM, cIgM, MPO, kappa light chain, and lambda light chain.

Genetic Study

Chromosome analysis revealed an abnormal karyotype: 52,XY,+X,+Y,+14,+14,+21,+21[cp20] (Fig. 15.5).

FISH studies demonstrated no *ETV6(TEL)/RUNX1*, *MLL*, *BCR/ABL1*, or *TCF3* gene rearrangements, but 95% of nuclei showed four copies of the *RUNX1* (*AML1*) gene locus on chromosome 21q22.

SNP microarray analysis was performed and demonstrated near-haploid clone (26 chromosomes with two copies of chromosomes 14 and 21 and single copies of all other chromosomes).

Final Diagnosis

B lymphoblastic leukemia/lymphoma, with hypodiploidy

Discussion

The conventional cytogenetics in this case showed a karyotype appearing to be hyperdiploid. However, tetrasomy 14 and 21 suggested that the karyotype might actually have evolved from hypodiploid karyotype, with chromosomes doubled from a near-haploid karyotype. SNP microarray, FISH, and DNA content flow cytometry may be helpful in differentiating the ploidy level.

B-ALL cases with hypodiploid karyotype may appear to be hyperdiploid by conventional karyotyping, when the hypodiploid cells undergo endoreduplication. The set of chromosomes is often doubled (so-called hypotriploidy, or very low tetraploid chromosome set). This results in a typical pattern of two or four chromosomes, which allows a distinction between hypodiploid ALL with doubled chromosome set and hyperdiploid B-ALL [7, 22]. Hypodiploidy is a poor prognostic indicator, while hyperdiploidy is a favorable prognostic indicator in pediatric B-ALL patients. Importantly, the subsequent therapy selection for these two subtypes is

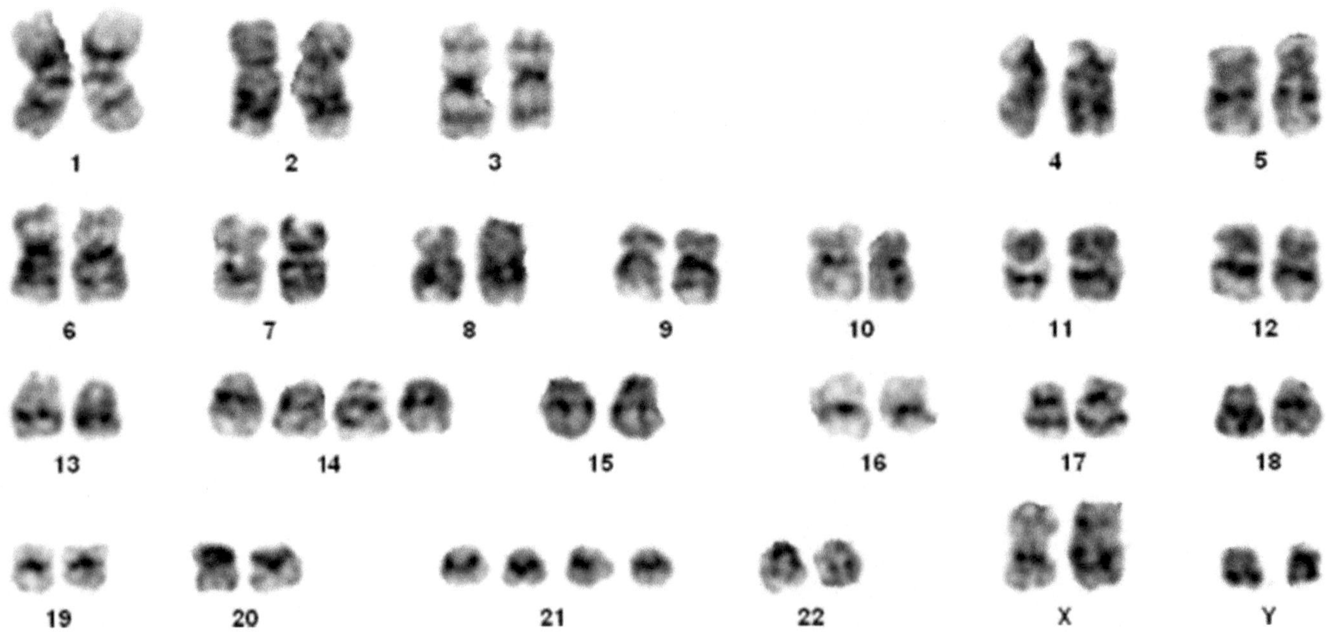

Fig. 15.5 Chromosome analysis showed a karyotype with tetrasomies, which actually evolved from a hypodiploid karyotype

different. Current recommendations for pediatric B-ALL patients with near haploid are to proceed to allogeneic stem cell transplant at the first complete remission.

Case 3

Learning Objective

- Diagnosis of *BCR-ABL1*-like B-ALL requires molecular genetic workup.

Case History

A 46-year-old female presented with progressing weakness and fatigue. Initial CBC showed leukocytosis. Peripheral blood smear showed 90% circulating blasts. CT scan showed axillary adenopathy.

Laboratory Findings

Blood cell counts: WBC 112 K/μL; hemoglobin 9.2 g/dL; platelets 103 K/μL.

The bone marrow was hypercellular with sheets of blasts (85%).

Flow cytometric analysis demonstrated a population of lymphoblasts (88% of total events) expressing dim CD45, CD19, CD10 (bright), CD22 (dim), CD58, CD200, cytoplasmic CD79a, CD33 (dim), CD99 (dim), CD34, and TdT and lacking cytoplasmic CD3, CD117, and myeloperoxidase.

Genetic Study

Chromosome analysis revealed an abnormal karyotype: 46,XX [20]. FISH for *BCR-ABL1* translocation was negative.

NGS analysis (targeted gene DNA sequencing and RNA sequencing) detected *JAK2* R683S mutation and *IGH-CRLF2* rearrangement. Multiple VUS was also detected, including *CHEK2* L236P, *HDAC4* P64A, *IKZF1* F145L, *KMT2A* A53V *TNFRSF14* T160A, and *TSC1* K587R.

Final Diagnosis

B lymphoblastic leukemia/lymphoma, *BCR-ABL1*-like

Follow-Up

The patient received hyper-CVAD chemotherapy (hyperfractionated cyclophosphamide, vincristine, doxorubicin, and dexamethasone), and a repeat bone marrow biopsy showed residual disease. The treatment was switched to augmented hyper-CVAD (plus PEG-asparaginase with higher dose of vincristine). Follow-up bone marrow biopsy showed evidence of minimal residual disease. She was then treated with blinatumomab and POMP (6-mercaptopurine (Purinethol), vincristine (Oncovin), methotrexate, and prednisone) maintenance. Unfortunately, the disease relapsed after 3 years at the last follow-up.

Discussion

This is an example of *BCR-ABL1*-negative B-ALL, with findings of *JAK2* mutation and *IGH-CRLF2* rearrangement by molecular study, consistent with *BCR-ABL1*-like B-ALL. *JAK2* mutation and coexistent *IGH-CRLF2* rearrangement (therefore high level expression of CRLF2) occur in 47% of *BCR-ABL1*-like B-ALL [43].

Currently there is no consensus as to the approach to diagnose *BCR-ABL1*-like B-ALL, and it is somehow challenging in the practice to screen and confirm this subtype of B-ALL. Mutational analysis for selected genes including the genes frequently found in *BCR-ABL1*-like B-ALL is recommended in *BCR-ABL1*-negative B-ALL. In the labs where there are resources, certain diagnostic algorithm may be adopted to be more cost-effective, such as performing FISH and CRLF2 flow cytometry analysis before mutational testing. It is clinically significant to diagnose *BCR-ABL1*-like B-ALL since this subtype of B-ALL shows poor prognosis and high relapse rate and, more importantly, may be treated with TKI.

Case 4

Learning Objective

- The molecular profiling study can assist in the diagnosis of ETP-ALL.

Case History

A 70-year-old male presented with weakness and falls and CT scan of abdomen and pelvic areas showed lymphadenopathy and splenomegaly.

Laboratory Findings

Blood cell counts: WBC 14.58 K/μL; hemoglobin 9.8 g/dL; platelets 33 K/μL.

Peripheral blood shows circulating blasts (73%). The bone marrow was 60% cellular with 80% blasts (Fig. 15.6a).

Flow cytometric analysis demonstrated a population of lymphoblasts (70% of total events) expressing dim CD45, CD34, CD117 (partial), cytoplasmic CD3, CD7, CD13, CD33, CD56, and TdT (dim) and negative for CD1a, CD5, CD4, CD8, CD2, HLA-DR, CD19, CD10, CD20, CD79a, cytoplasmic CD22, cytoplasmic CD79a, and cytoplasmic myeloperoxidase (Fig. 15.6b).

Genetic Study

NGS analysis (targeted gene DNA sequencing) detected the following mutations: *NRAS* G12D, VAF 38.8%; *DNMT3A* R882H, VAF 37.25%; *DNMT3A* E30A, VAF 50.59%; *RAD21*, D276Vfs*15, VAF 20%; *NOTCH1* Q2184*, VAF 8.11%; and *ETV6* G91D, VAF 39.94%.

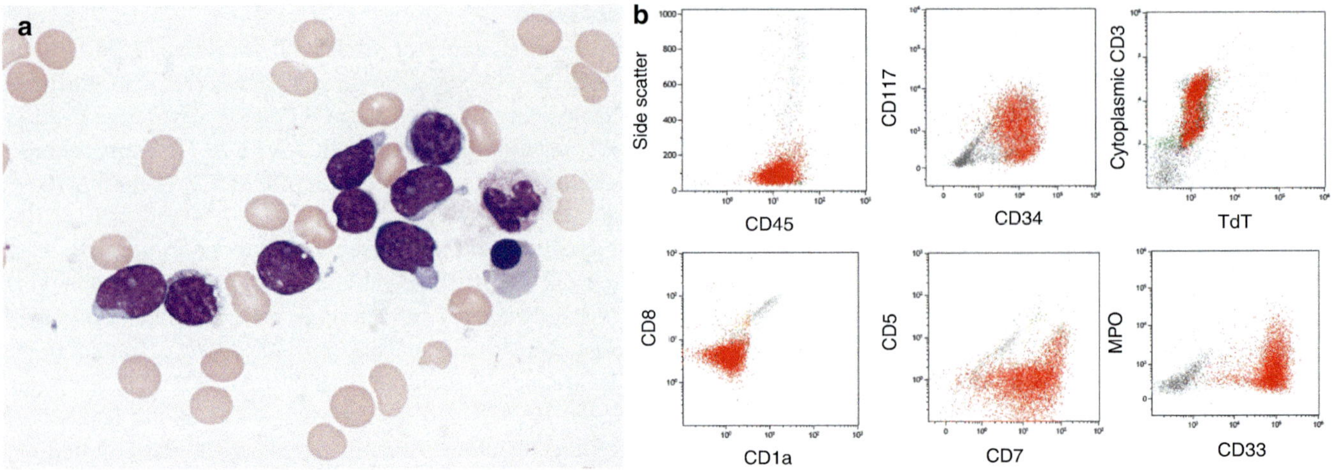

Fig. 15.6 The bone marrow aspirate smear showed increased medium-sized lymphoblasts (**a**, 1000×). Flow cytometry analysis demonstrated characteristic immunophenotype (CD45dim+, CD34+, CD117 partial+, cytoplasmic CD3+, CD7+, CD33+, TdT dim+, CD1a-, CD5-, CD8-, and cytoplasmic myeloperoxidase-) (**b**)

Final Diagnosis

Early T-cell precursor lymphoblastic leukemia

Follow-Up

The patient was treated with hyper-CVAD and intrathecal methotrexate and cytarabine. Two months later, repeat peripheral blood testing showed recurrent/persistent disease. He was given comfort measures and deceased 3 months after the initial diagnosis.

Discussion

By definition, ETP-ALL cases show characteristic immunophenotype. The T lymphoblasts express CD7 but lack CD1a and CD8 and are positive for one or more of the myeloid/stem cell markers (CD34, CD117, HLA-DR, CD13, CD33, CD11b, and CD65). CD5 is either negative or positive in < 75% of the blasts [7]. Different from the classic T lymphoblastic leukemia, the molecular mutation profile is similar to T/myeloid mixed phenotype acute leukemia. Besides the mutation in genes usually associated with T-ALL such as *NOTCH1*, there can be mutations frequently seen in myeloid neoplasms, like *DNMT3A*, *RAS* and *ETV6* mutations, as what we see in this case.

In this case, findings from flow cytometry, together with the molecular study results, are consistent with the final diagnosis of ETP-ALL. ETP-ALL is derived from cells committed to the T-cell lineage but retain the potential for myeloid/dendritic cell differentiation. The clinical outcomes of adult ETP-ALL to standard chemotherapy are suboptimal, and different clinical regimen and management including molecular targeting therapy may be pursued [87].

References

1. de Haas V, et al. Initial diagnostic work-up of acute leukemia: ASCO clinical practice guideline endorsement of the College of American Pathologists and American Society of hematology guideline. J Clin Oncol. 2019;37(3):239–53.
2. National Comprehensive Cancer Network. NCCN clinical practice guidelines in oncology (NCCN guidelines) acute lymphoblastic leukemia (Version 2.2020). 2020 [cited 2020 Nov 19]; Available from: https://www.nccn.org/professionals/physician_gls/pdf/all.pdf.
3. Harris MH, et al. Genetic testing in the diagnosis and biology of acute leukemia. Am J Clin Pathol. 2019;152(3):322–46.
4. Mullighan CG. Molecular genetics of B-precursor acute lymphoblastic leukemia. J Clin Invest. 2012;122(10):3407–15.
5. Moorman AV, et al. Prognostic effect of chromosomal abnormalities in childhood B-cell precursor acute lymphoblastic leukaemia: results from the UK Medical Research Council ALL97/99 randomised trial. Lancet Oncol. 2010;11(5):429–38.
6. Pui CH, Jeha S. New therapeutic strategies for the treatment of acute lymphoblastic leukaemia. Nat Rev Drug Discov. 2007;6(2):149–65.
7. Swerdlow S, et al., editors. World Health Organization classification of tumours of haematopoietic and lymphoid tissues, World Health Organization classification of tumours. Revised 4th ed. Lyon: International Agency for Research on Cancer; 2017.
8. Mrozek K, Harper DP, Aplan PD. Cytogenetics and molecular genetics of acute lymphoblastic leukemia. Hematol Oncol Clin North Am. 2009;23(5):991–1010. v
9. Liu-Dumlao T, et al. Philadelphia-positive acute lymphoblastic leukemia: current treatment options. Curr Oncol Rep. 2012;14(5):387–94.
10. Branford S, et al. High frequency of point mutations clustered within the adenosine triphosphate-binding region of BCR/ABL in patients with chronic myeloid leukemia or Ph-positive acute lymphoblastic leukemia who develop imatinib (STI571) resistance. Blood. 2002;99(9):3472–5.
11. Soverini S, et al. Contribution of ABL kinase domain mutations to imatinib resistance in different subsets of Philadelphia-positive

patients: by the GIMEMA working party on chronic myeloid leukemia. Clin Cancer Res. 2006;12(24):7374–9.
12. Shah NP, et al. Multiple BCR-ABL kinase domain mutations confer polyclonal resistance to the tyrosine kinase inhibitor imatinib (STI571) in chronic phase and blast crisis chronic myeloid leukemia. Cancer Cell. 2002;2(2):117–25.
13. Bitencourt R, Zalcberg I, Louro ID. Imatinib resistance: a review of alternative inhibitors in chronic myeloid leukemia. Rev Bras Hematol Hemoter. 2011;33(6):470–5.
14. Wetzler M, et al. Additional cytogenetic abnormalities in adults with Philadelphia chromosome-positive acute lymphoblastic leukaemia: a study of the Cancer and Leukaemia group B. Br J Haematol. 2004;124(3):275–88.
15. Martinelli G, et al. IKZF1 (Ikaros) deletions in BCR-ABL1-positive acute lymphoblastic leukemia are associated with short disease-free survival and high rate of cumulative incidence of relapse: a GIMEMA AL WP report. J Clin Oncol. 2009;27(31):5202–7.
16. Meyer C, et al. The MLL recombinome of acute leukemias in 2013. Leukemia. 2013;27(11):2165–76.
17. Winters AC, Bernt KM. MLL-rearranged leukemias-an update on science and clinical approaches. Front Pediatr. 2017;5:4.
18. Harrison CJ. Cytogenetics of paediatric and adolescent acute lymphoblastic leukaemia. Br J Haematol. 2009;144(2):147–56.
19. Nachman JB, et al. Outcome of treatment in children with hypodiploid acute lymphoblastic leukemia. Blood. 2007;110(4):1112–5.
20. Harrison CJ, et al. Three distinct subgroups of hypodiploidy in acute lymphoblastic leukaemia. Br J Haematol. 2004;125(5):552–9.
21. Safavi S, et al. Loss of chromosomes is the primary event in near-haploid and low-hypodiploid acute lymphoblastic leukemia. Leukemia. 2013;27(1):248–50.
22. Charrin C, et al. A report from the LALA-94 and LALA-SA groups on hypodiploidy with 30 to 39 chromosomes and near-triploidy: 2 possible expressions of a sole entity conferring poor prognosis in adult acute lymphoblastic leukemia (ALL). Blood. 2004;104(8):2444–51.
23. Zhang J, et al. Key pathways are frequently mutated in high-risk childhood acute lymphoblastic leukemia: a report from the Children's Oncology Group. Blood. 2011;118(11):3080–7.
24. Chiaretti S, et al. TP53 mutations are frequent in adult acute lymphoblastic leukemia cases negative for recurrent fusion genes and correlate with poor response to induction therapy. Haematologica. 2013;98(5):e59–61.
25. Stengel A, et al. TP53 mutations occur in 15.7% of ALL and are associated with MYC-rearrangement, low hypodiploidy, and a poor prognosis. Blood. 2014;124(2):251–8.
26. Muhlbacher V, et al. Acute lymphoblastic leukemia with low hypodiploid/near triploid karyotype is a specific clinical entity and exhibits a very high TP53 mutation frequency of 93%. Genes Chromosomes Cancer. 2014;53(6):524–36.
27. Holmfeldt L, et al. The genomic landscape of hypodiploid acute lymphoblastic leukemia. Nat Genet. 2013;45(3):242–52.
28. Comeaux EQ, Mullighan CG. TP53 mutations in hypodiploid acute lymphoblastic leukemia. Cold Spring Harb Perspect Med. 2017;7(3):a026286.
29. Qian M, et al. TP53 germline variations influence the predisposition and prognosis of B-cell acute lymphoblastic leukemia in children. J Clin Oncol. 2018;36(6):591–9.
30. Salmoiraghi S, et al. Mutations of TP53 gene in adult acute lymphoblastic leukemia at diagnosis do not affect the achievement of hematologic response but correlate with early relapse and very poor survival. Haematologica. 2016;101(6):e245–8.
31. Hof J, et al. Mutations and deletions of the TP53 gene predict nonresponse to treatment and poor outcome in first relapse of childhood acute lymphoblastic leukemia. J Clin Oncol. 2011;29(23):3185–93.
32. Dyer MJ, et al. Immunoglobulin heavy chain locus chromosomal translocations in B-cell precursor acute lymphoblastic leukemia: rare clinical curios or potent genetic drivers? Blood. 2010;115(8):1490–9.
33. Ghazavi F, et al. Molecular basis and clinical significance of genetic aberrations in B-cell precursor acute lymphoblastic leukemia. Exp Hematol. 2015;43(8):640–53.
34. de Boer J, et al. The E2A-HLF oncogenic fusion protein acts through Lmo2 and Bcl-2 to immortalize hematopoietic progenitors. Leukemia. 2011;25(2):321–30.
35. Moorman AV. The clinical relevance of chromosomal and genomic abnormalities in B-cell precursor acute lymphoblastic leukaemia. Blood Rev. 2012;26(3):123–35.
36. Johnson RC, et al. Cytogenetic variation of B-lymphoblastic leukemia with intrachromosomal amplification of chromosome 21 (iAMP21): a multi-institutional series review. Am J Clin Pathol. 2015;144(1):103–12.
37. Moorman AV, et al. Prognosis of children with acute lymphoblastic leukemia (ALL) and intrachromosomal amplification of chromosome 21 (iAMP21). Blood. 2007;109(6):2327–30.
38. Harrison CJ. Blood spotlight on iAMP21 acute lymphoblastic leukemia (ALL), a high-risk pediatric disease. Blood. 2015;125(9):1383–6.
39. Den Boer ML, et al. A subtype of childhood acute lymphoblastic leukaemia with poor treatment outcome: a genome-wide classification study. Lancet Oncol. 2009;10(2):125–34.
40. Mullighan CG, et al. Deletion of IKZF1 and prognosis in acute lymphoblastic leukemia. N Engl J Med. 2009;360(5):470–80.
41. Boer JM, et al. Expression profiling of adult acute lymphoblastic leukemia identifies a BCR-ABL1-like subgroup characterized by high non-response and relapse rates. Haematologica. 2015;100(7):e261–4.
42. Moorman AV. New and emerging prognostic and predictive genetic biomarkers in B-cell precursor acute lymphoblastic leukemia. Haematologica. 2016;101(4):407–16.
43. Roberts KG, et al. Targetable kinase-activating lesions in Ph-like acute lymphoblastic leukemia. N Engl J Med. 2014;371(11):1005–15.
44. Weston BW, et al. Tyrosine kinase inhibitor therapy induces remission in a patient with refractory EBF1-PDGFRB-positive acute lymphoblastic leukemia. J Clin Oncol. 2013;31(25):e413–6.
45. Ding YY, et al. Clinical efficacy of ruxolitinib and chemotherapy in a child with Philadelphia chromosome-like acute lymphoblastic leukemia with GOLGA5-JAK2 fusion and induction failure. Haematologica. 2018;103(9):e427–31.
46. Frisch A, Ofran Y. How I diagnose and manage Philadelphia chromosome-like acute lymphoblastic leukemia. Haematologica. 2019;104(11):2135–43.
47. Herold T, Gokbuget N. Philadelphia-like acute lymphoblastic leukemia in adults. Curr Oncol Rep. 2017;19(5):31.
48. Harvey RC, et al. Identification of novel cluster groups in pediatric high-risk B-precursor acute lymphoblastic leukemia with gene expression profiling: correlation with genome-wide DNA copy number alterations, clinical characteristics, and outcome. Blood. 2010;116(23):4874–84.
49. Roberts KG, Mullighan CG. Genomics in acute lymphoblastic leukaemia: insights and treatment implications. Nat Rev Clin Oncol. 2015;12(6):344–57.
50. Mullighan CG, et al. Genome-wide analysis of genetic alterations in acute lymphoblastic leukaemia. Nature. 2007;446(7137):758–64.

51. Liu YF, et al. Genomic profiling of adult and pediatric B-cell acute lymphoblastic leukemia. EBioMedicine. 2016;8:173–83.
52. Rebollo A, Schmitt C. Ikaros, Aiolos and Helios: transcription regulators and lymphoid malignancies. Immunol Cell Biol. 2003;81(3):171–5.
53. Georgopoulos K, et al. The Ikaros gene is required for the development of all lymphoid lineages. Cell. 1994;79(1):143–56.
54. Ensor HM, et al. Demographic, clinical, and outcome features of children with acute lymphoblastic leukemia and CRLF2 deregulation: results from the MRC ALL97 clinical trial. Blood. 2011;117(7):2129–36.
55. Hertzberg L, et al. Down syndrome acute lymphoblastic leukemia, a highly heterogeneous disease in which aberrant expression of CRLF2 is associated with mutated JAK2: a report from the international BFM study group. Blood. 2010;115(5):1006–17.
56. Mullighan CG, et al. BCR-ABL1 lymphoblastic leukaemia is characterized by the deletion of Ikaros. Nature. 2008;453(7191):110–4.
57. Olsson L, Johansson B. Ikaros and leukaemia. Br J Haematol. 2015;169(4):479–91.
58. Joshi I, et al. Loss of Ikaros DNA-binding function confers integrin-dependent survival on pre-B cells and progression to acute lymphoblastic leukemia. Nat Immunol. 2014;15(3):294–304.
59. Yao QM, et al. Prognostic impact of IKZF1 deletion in adults with common B-cell acute lymphoblastic leukemia. BMC Cancer. 2016;16(1):269.
60. Boer JM, et al. Prognostic value of rare IKZF1 deletion in childhood B-cell precursor acute lymphoblastic leukemia: an international collaborative study. Leukemia. 2016;30(1):32–8.
61. Clappier E, et al. IKZF1 deletion is an independent prognostic marker in childhood B-cell precursor acute lymphoblastic leukemia, and distinguishes patients benefiting from pulses during maintenance therapy: results of the EORTC Children's Leukemia Group study 58951. Leukemia. 2015;29(11):2154–61.
62. Stanulla M, Cave H, Moorman AV. IKZF1 deletions in pediatric acute lymphoblastic leukemia: still a poor prognostic marker? Blood. 2020;135(4):252–60.
63. Buitenkamp TD, et al. Outcome in children with Down's syndrome and acute lymphoblastic leukemia: role of IKZF1 deletions and CRLF2 aberrations. Leukemia. 2012;26(10):2204–11.
64. Zhou Y, et al. Advances in B-lymphoblastic leukemia: cytogenetic and genomic lesions. Ann Diagn Pathol. 2016;23:43–50.
65. Tasian SK, et al. Aberrant STAT5 and PI3K/mTOR pathway signaling occurs in human CRLF2-rearranged B-precursor acute lymphoblastic leukemia. Blood. 2012;120(4):833–42.
66. Nebral K, et al. Incidence and diversity of PAX5 fusion genes in childhood acute lymphoblastic leukemia. Leukemia. 2009;23(1):134–43.
67. Shah S, et al. A recurrent germline PAX5 mutation confers susceptibility to pre-B cell acute lymphoblastic leukemia. Nat Genet. 2013;45(10):1226–31.
68. Auer F, et al. Inherited susceptibility to pre B-ALL caused by germline transmission of PAX5 c.547G>A. Leukemia. 2014;28(5):1136–8.
69. Mullighan CG, et al. CREBBP mutations in relapsed acute lymphoblastic leukaemia. Nature. 2011;471(7337):235–9.
70. Inthal A, et al. CREBBP HAT domain mutations prevail in relapse cases of high hyperdiploid childhood acute lymphoblastic leukemia. Leukemia. 2012;26(8):1797–803.
71. Zaliova M, et al. ERG deletion is associated with CD2 and attenuates the negative impact of IKZF1 deletion in childhood acute lymphoblastic leukemia. Leukemia. 2014;28(1):182–5.
72. Clappier E, et al. An intragenic ERG deletion is a marker of an oncogenic subtype of B-cell precursor acute lymphoblastic leukemia with a favorable outcome despite frequent IKZF1 deletions. Leukemia. 2014;28(1):70–7.
73. Mullighan CG. The molecular genetic makeup of acute lymphoblastic leukemia. Hematology Am Soc Hematol Educ Program. 2012;2012:389–96.
74. Della Starza I, et al. Minimal residual disease in acute lymphoblastic leukemia: technical and clinical advances. Front Oncol. 2019;9:726.
75. Jennings LJ, et al. Detection and quantification of BCR-ABL1 fusion transcripts by droplet digital PCR. J Mol Diagn. 2014;16(2):174–9.
76. Coccaro N, et al. Droplet digital PCR is a robust tool for monitoring minimal residual disease in adult Philadelphia-positive acute lymphoblastic leukemia. J Mol Diagn. 2018;20(4):474–82.
77. Faham M, et al. Deep-sequencing approach for minimal residual disease detection in acute lymphoblastic leukemia. Blood. 2012;120(26):5173–80.
78. van Dongen JJ, et al. Minimal residual disease diagnostics in acute lymphoblastic leukemia: need for sensitive, fast, and standardized technologies. Blood. 2015;125(26):3996–4009.
79. Bruggemann M, et al. Standardized next-generation sequencing of immunoglobulin and T-cell receptor gene recombinations for MRD marker identification in acute lymphoblastic leukaemia; a EuroClonality-NGS validation study. Leukemia. 2019;33(9):2241–53.
80. Kim IS. Minimal residual disease in acute lymphoblastic leukemia: technical aspects and implications for clinical interpretation. Blood Res. 2020;55(S1):S19–26.
81. Reyes-Barron C, et al. Next-generation sequencing for minimal residual disease surveillance in acute lymphoblastic leukemia: an update. Crit Rev Oncog. 2017;22(5–6):559–67.
82. Liu Y, et al. The genomic landscape of pediatric and young adult T-lineage acute lymphoblastic leukemia. Nat Genet. 2017;49(8):1211–8.
83. Girardi T, et al. The genetics and molecular biology of T-ALL. Blood. 2017;129(9):1113–23.
84. Kimura S, Mullighan CG. Molecular markers in ALL: clinical implications. Best Pract Res Clin Haematol. 2020;33(3):101193.
85. Fransecky L, et al. Silencing of GATA3 defines a novel stem cell-like subgroup of ETP-ALL. J Hematol Oncol. 2016;9(1):95.
86. Sajaroff EO, et al. B-cell acute lymphoblastic leukemia with mature phenotype and MLL rearrangement: report of five new cases and review of the literature. Leuk Lymphoma. 2016;57(10):2289–97.
87. Castaneda Puglianini O, Papadantonakis N. Early precursor T-cell acute lymphoblastic leukemia: current paradigms and evolving concepts. Adv Hematol. 2020;11:2040620720929475.

Mature B-Cell Neoplasms

16

Yi Ding

List of Frequently Asked Questions

1. What are commonly used molecular techniques in diagnosis of mature B-cell neoplasms?
2. How to choose the molecular techniques in lymphoid neoplasms?
3. What are the principles of B-cell (immunoglobulin gene) clonality determination?
4. What are the indications of B-cell (immunoglobulin gene) clonality determination?
5. What methods are commonly used for clonality determination?
6. What are the limitations of clonality testing we should keep in mind?
7. Can we use immunoglobulin kappa and lambda light chain stainings by chromogenic in situ hybridization (CISH) to replace clonality test by molecular methods?
8. Are both *IGH* and *IGK* clonal gene rearrangement required to call a positive clonality result?
9. Is the positive immunoglobulin (Ig) gene rearrangement result required or by itself enough to diagnose a B-cell neoplasm?
10. What are the advantages of NGS-based clonality test over length-based analysis, and when should I consider it for clinical samples?
11. What are the prognostic molecular biomarkers in chronic lymphocytic leukemia (CLL)?
12. Besides those established prognostic biomarkers, what are the emerging prognostic biomarkers in CLL?
13. What are the clinical implications for *MYD88* L265P mutation in B-cell neoplasms?
14. What methods are commonly used for *MYD88* mutation detection?
15. What genetic changes are largely seen in extranodal marginal zone lymphoma of mucosa-associated lymphoid tissue (MALT lymphoma) but not in other types of marginal zone lymphomas?
16. What are the clinical implications for *EZH2* mutation in B-cell neoplasms?
17. When should the mutational analysis be considered in lymphoma diagnosis?

Y. Ding (✉)
Department of Laboratory Medicine,
Geisinger Health, Danville, PA, USA
e-mail: yding1@geisinger.edu

Frequently Asked Questions

1. **What are commonly used molecular techniques in diagnosis of mature B-cell neoplasms?**
   - Hematopathology has always been the best representative for pathology evolution and on the forefront of integration of diagnostic application of molecular technology.
   - Mature B-cell neoplasms can usually be diagnosed with routine histologic evaluation, combined with flow cytometry and immunohistochemistry (IHC). Molecular techniques, including fluorescence in situ hybridization (FISH), PCR, Sanger sequencing, and next-generation sequencing (NGS), are getting more widely used to determine subclassification of malignancy and provide prognostic or therapeutic information for clinical management (Table 16.1).
2. **How to choose the molecular techniques in lymphoid neoplasms?**
   - The choice of technique should be decided by multiple factors [1], including:
   - The type and amount of available material
   - The desired sensitivity levels
   - The type of target(s) to be analyzed
   - Turnaround time requirement
   - Cost and volumes of the tests
   - Fresh or frozen samples generally show higher quality of nucleic acids and are less prone to artifacts introduced by DNA and RNA degradation, which are

Y. Ding, L. Zhang (eds.), *Practical Oncologic Molecular Pathology*, Practical Anatomic Pathology,
https://doi.org/10.1007/978-3-030-73227-1_16

Table 16.1 Examples of commonly used molecular assays in mature B-cell neoplasms

Molecular assays	Method	Target	Utility	Tissue
Clonality test	PCR, NGS	*IGH, IGK*	Detection of B-cell clonality	FFPE tissue, fresh tissue
Translocation analysis	FISH, PCR, NGS	t(14;18)	Aid in diagnosis of FL	FFPE tissue
	FISH	*BCL2, BCL6, MYC*	Subclassification of DLBCL	FFPE tissue
Mutational analysis	PCR,	*TP53*	Therapy decisions in CLL	FFPE tissue, fresh tissue
	Sanger sequencing, pyrosequencing NGS	*MYD88* *BRAF*	Differentiate between LPL and MZL	FFPE tissue

FL Follicular lymphoma; *DLBCL* Diffuse large B-cell lymphoma; *CLL* Chronic lymphocytic leukemia; *LPL* Lymphoplasmacytic lymphoma; *MZL* Marginal zone lymphoma; *FFPE* Formalin-fixed paraffin-embedded

generally preferred for RNA-based studies. However, fresh or frozen samples are usually unavailable during the workups of mature B-cell neoplasms due to the traditional workflow setup in the pathology laboratory. Additionally, frozen tissues are not evaluated morphologically. When the lymphoid tissue is only partially involved by a neoplastic process, there might be sampling bias resulting in false-negative results.

- In general, formalin-fixed, paraffin-embedded (FFPE) samples are suitable for most diagnostic purposes. Compared to blood and fresh tissues which are considered biohazards, FFPE tissue is regarded safer for handling.
- Chromosome translocations associated with mature B-cell lymphomas (e.g., *IGH/BCL2*, *IGH/CCND1*) do not usually create fusion transcripts. Therefore, molecular testing to detect these fusion genes will require DNA as a template, which is technically challenging. FISH tests have better diagnostic (not analytic) sensitivity in detecting these chromosome translocations.
- With the development of technologies, there is a move away from single-gene assays toward panel testing in many laboratories because although most diagnostic biopsies are small, the list of requested predictive biomarkers keeps growing. It is more practical to use a panel-based testing approach for economical, time-saving, and material preservation consideration.

3. **What are the principles of B-cell (immunoglobulin gene) clonality tests?**
   - In the development of the lymphoid system, B cells undergo a series of strictly programmed genetic recombination of the surface antigen receptor (immunoglobulin (Ig) in B cells) genes which encode for the various parts of antigen receptor molecules.
   - In bone marrow, the recombination process takes place in committed precursor B cells and follows a sequential order primarily involving different variable (V), diversity (D), and joining (J) gene segments. This process is antigen independent (Fig. 16.1a–b).
   - In periphery, mature B lymphocytes further extend their Ig repertoire upon antigen recognition in germinal centers via somatic hypermutation, a process leading to affinity maturation of the Ig molecules.
   - A normal or reactive immune response typically generates a polyclonal population of lymphocytes with a multitude of different antibodies, whereas a monoclonal proliferation is assumed to be the hallmark of neoplasms.
   - The clonality tests are based on the principle that rearrangement of antigen receptor genes occurs during lymphoid proliferation and each lymphocyte clone has a unique coding sequence for its antigen receptor. The receptor DNA sequences are amplified by multiplex PCR reactions that contain primers binding to the conserved regions. Due to the size difference of the antigen receptor gene in a diversified lymphoid population, the PCR products (amplicons) will have a variety of sizes in Gaussian distribution pattern when running through size differentiating electrophoresis.
   - During a clonal proliferation, such as B-cell neoplasms, the clonal population will be amplified, and its product is also called as "clonal rearrangement positive."
4. **When should I consider a B-cell (immunoglobulin gene) clonality test?**
   - Benign versus malignant lymphoproliferative disorder: Because it can be performed on FFPE tissue, clonality test has been a useful adjunctive method for diagnosis of lymphoproliferative disorder, especially in some cases that morphological and immunophenotypic features can be difficult to interpret between benign versus malignant lesions. It should be particularly considered when biopsy is very small but with predominant B-cell proliferation, without accompanied flow cytometry study due to lack of fresh tissue, appreciable histological architecture, or limited material to complete the immunohistochemistry workup.
   - Lineage verification between T- and B-cell neoplasms, when morphologic and immunophenotypic features are not sufficient to characterize the cell lineage.
   - Clonal relationship determination between two and multiple neoplasms. The test will be valuable in several situations, such as:
     - To determine if a new lymphoproliferative neoplasm in a patient with history of lymphoma is an actual relapse or a de novo malignancy
     - To determine if a higher-grade lymphoma in a patient with a history of low-grade B-cell lymphoma is a disease progression or a separate process

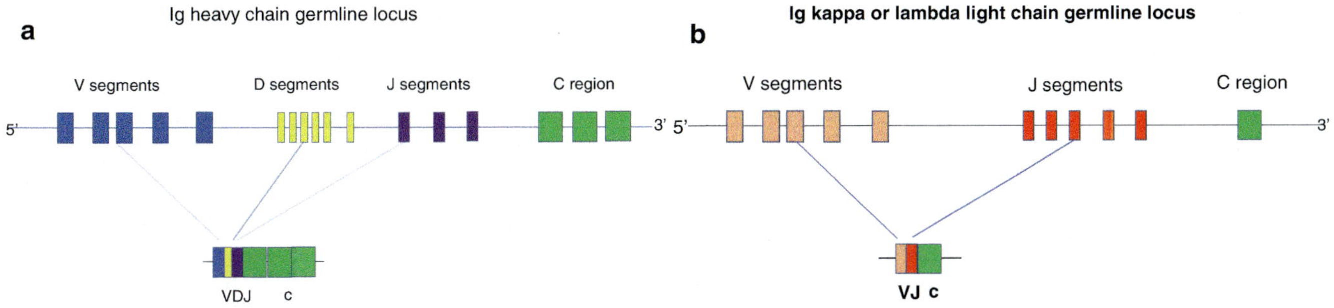

Fig. 16.1 B-cell gene rearrangement (**a**) V-DJ rearrangement in immunoglobulin heavy chain; (**b**) V-J rearrangement in immunoglobulin light chain

Table 16.2 Comparison of different methods of clonality test

	Advantages	Disadvantages
Southern blot	Used to be the gold standard method for clonality testing and now being largely replaced by PCR-based methods Primarily used for TRA tests (too large for PCR or NGS) in research setting	Slow and laborious Large amount of DNA required Relatively insensitive
PCR (Most commonly used)	Fast and inexpensive Much less DNA required Better sensitivity (5–10%) Available and easily instituted into most labs	Separated PCR product by size not by sequence Subjective interpretation Not sensitive enough MRD detection
NGS	Similar DNA input but resulted with sequence data Less subjective More sensitive, suitable for MRD detection	Relative expensive Longer TAT depending on volume

NGS Next-generation sequencing; *MRD* Minimal residual diseases; *TAT* Turnaround time; *TRA* test, T-cell receptor gene rearrangement alpha locus

5. **What methods are commonly used for clonality determination?**
   - Southern blot hybridization-based clonality test for Ig gene rearrangement was introduced to research and later clinical practice in the mid-1990s [2]. It has been replaced by PCR-based assay due to its intrinsic limitations (Table 16.2).
   - Currently multiplex PCR-based clonality assay is commonly used in the clinical practice. The European BIOMED-2 collaborative study has developed and standardized the immunoglobulin gene rearrangement assay, and the BIOMED-2 primer set and kits are commercially available for Ig heavy chain *(IGH)*, kappa light chain (*IGK*), and lambda light chain (*IGL*) genes.
   - B lineage cells can express with kappa or lambda Ig light chain; however, the gene rearrangement is programmed to prefer the kappa locus by the recombinase machinery so that *IGK* gene rearrangement begins before *IGL* gene. In addition, *IGK* gene is rearranged in the lambda light chain expressing B cells or plasma cells. Thus, there are more B lineage cells that express kappa than lambda light chain in a healthy individual.
   - B-cell clonality test usually includes both *IGH* and *IGK* but not *IGL* gene rearrangement to keep the balance of higher detection sensitivity yet not too complicated test itself. Studies have shown that testing in both *IGH* and *IGK* will not only ensure the detection of Ig-gene rearrangements in mantle cell lymphomas (MCL) and chronic lymphocytic leukemia/small lymphocytic lymphomas (CLL/SLL) but also increase the detection rate to close to 100% in the heavily somatically mutated follicular lymphomas (FL), marginal zone lymphomas (MZL), and diffuse large B-cell lymphomas (DLBCL) [3].
   - NGS-based clonality tests have been developed in recent years and slowly gain its popularity because of its advantages over traditional PCR-based assays.
6. **What are the limitations of clonality testing we should keep in mind?**
   - During selection of FFPE block or area of slide for testing, we should circle B cell-rich areas or choose B-cell-rich blocks. If only low numbers of B cells are present in the sample tested, there is a possibility of pseudoclonality or false-negative result due to failed amplification or high reactive background.
   - Pseudoclonality, defined as the erroneous detection of a pseduoclonal lymphoid population, is an important pitfall and a major consideration when performing PCR clonality assays on low numbers of lymphocytes. The possibility of pseudoclonality increases when there is less than 20–40 ng of DNA or 800–2000 lymphocytes being analyzed which is more often seen in the interpretation of small biopsies, especially in lymphocytic cutaneous infiltrates [4–8].
   - Duplicate or triplicate tests should be required as the standard procedure, especially for low template samples, to avoid misinterpretation or false diagnosis of a

clonal population. In addition, background knowledge of the sample, including clinical history and histological differential diagnosis, etc., and ample experience are required for accurate interpretation of the clonality tests [9, 10].

- Many factors could affect the sensitivity of the clonality test, for example, type of lymphoma and length of tissue fixation. It is well known that the sensitivity of clonality test is higher in MCL and CLL/SLL than that of FL [4].
- A positive clonal rearrangement result by itself is supportive but not enough to diagnose a neoplastic lesion, and the clonality test should be used as a valuable tool to clarify morphologic ambiguities. Oligoclonal or monoclonal patterns can be observed in some reactive conditions or B-cell-poor lesions, especially in some small cutaneous biopsy samples [11–13].

7. **Can we use immunoglobulin kappa and lambda light chain stainings by chromogenic in situ hybridization (CISH) to replace clonality tests by molecular methods?**
    - In mature B-cell neoplasms, the majority of immunoglobulin gene rearrangement involves the heavy chain (*IGH*) locus, while a minor part involves the light chain loci, either the kappa light chain (*IGK*) or the lambda light chain (*IGL*).
    - *IGK* and *IGL* by conventional CISH can be used in helping the diagnosis of a mature B-cell neoplasm which expresses abundant kappa or lambda light chains, such as plasma cell neoplasm and marginal B-cell lymphoma with plasma cell differentiation.
    - Majority of B-cell neoplasm, such as follicular lymphoma (FL), diffuse large B-cell lymphoma (DLBCL), chronic lymphocytic leukemia/small lymphocytic lymphoma (CLL/SLL), nodal and splenic marginal zone lymphoma (MZL), and mantle cell lymphoma (MCL), have lower levels of light chain mRNA expression and do not typically demonstrate an *IGK* or *IGL* restriction by CISH in FFPE tissue.
    - To determine clonality, CISH-based assay is generally less sensitive and specific compared to molecular methods and should not be used as a replacement of the latter.
8. **Are both IGH and IGK clonal gene rearrangement required to call a positive clonality result?**
    - If a clonal gene rearrangement of either *IGH* or *IGK* gene is detected, it is called that the clonality result is positive (aka there is a clonal B-cell population). Although sometimes, if not more common, both *IGH* and *IGK* gene rearrangement can be detected in the same sample, it is not necessary or required for both *IGH* and *IGK* clonal gene rearrangement detected to demonstrate a clonal B-cell population present.
    - However, depending on the detection method used, a standardized interpretation algorithm should be established for result interpretation. For example, in PCR-capillary electrophoresis-based clonality test, it should be considered of peak heights and peak ratio to define "truly clonal" rearrangements.
9. **Is the positive immunoglobulin (Ig) gene rearrangement result required or by Itself enough to diagnose a B-cell neoplasm?**
    - As mentioned above, a positive *IGH* and/or *IGK* gene rearrangement result provides supportive evidence to aid the diagnosis of a B-cell neoplasm. However, it should not be used as the sole evidence to make such diagnosis.
    - In some cases, particularly when biopsy tissues are tiny, determination of the difference between reactive and neoplastic lesions can be challenging. In these cases, the value of immunohistochemistry stains can be limited too due to lack of appropriate architecture. If a B-cell neoplasm is suspected but histological criteria for neoplasia are not met, the clonality analysis would be most useful.
    - The positive clonality test result is not required to establish the diagnosis of a B-cell neoplasm. Histomorphology has a long history and has been essential in the diagnosis of diseases. Additional ancillary tests, such as a clonality test, are not indicated if the histological evidence is clear and enough. In addition, not every B-cell neoplasm has an identifiable Ig gene rearrangement by currently available technology. The cause of the observed difference includes differences in somatic hypermutation rates in the *IGH* locus which result in different recognition and binding efficiency of the PCR primers to their target sequences.
    - Neoplastic B-cell neoplasms could contain cross-lineage T-cell receptor (*TCR*) gene rearrangement. It has been reported that clonal *TCR* gene rearrangement could be detected in up to 90% of children and adults with precursor B-cell lymphoblastic leukemia [14]. This lineage infidelity phenomenon is usually more commonly seen in precursor lymphocytic malignancies than in mature B-cell neoplasms or normal B cells.
10. **What are the advantages of NGS-based clonality tests over length-based analysis, and when should I consider it for clinical samples?**
    - Advantages of NGS-based clonality test include:
        - Allowing identification of the full range of clonal populations

- Determination of the unique DNA/RNA sequence of clonal rearrangement, in additional to the size of the rearrangement product
- Detection of clonal events hidden in a polyclonal distribution

- Because of the cost of the test and turnaround time requirement, currently PCR-based clonality test is still the most used method. Detection of clonality using NGS of the immunoglobulin genes has a relatively infrequent but occasionally critical niche in the clinical workup of mature B-cell neoplasms. It should be considered in the following circumstance:
  - By recognizing the unique clonal DNA sequence, it can help determine the clonal relationship between neoplasms of different anatomic sites and time.
  - It can be used for disease monitoring or minimal/measurable residual disease (MRD) detection by comparing to the unique sequence of the original diagnostic sample.

11. **What are the established prognostic biomarkers in chronic lymphocytic leukemia (CLL)?**
    - CLL is a mature B-cell malignancy and the most common lymphocytic leukemia [15].
    - The major diagnostic criteria of CLL include the presence of a circulating clonal B-cell population (>5000/microliter in peripheral blood) with surface co-expression of CD5 and CD23.
    - To assess CLL prognosis, NCCN guideline and iwCLL criteria recommend using several biomarkers, including cytogenetic changes and gene mutation status, which are summarized in Table 16.3 and should be tested in all CLL patients upon diagnosis to facilitate therapy determination [16–20].
    - Because CLL could have different clinical courses and many patients may have an indolent presentation which does not require treatment for many years while others may have more aggressive courses, for patients with newly diagnosed CLL, International Prognostic Index for CLL (CLL-IPI) (Table 16.4) can be used to estimate prognosis and time for start treatment (Table 16.5).
    - In addition, both NCCN and iwCLL also recommend retesting previously treated CLL patients before starting patients on a new treatment.
12. **Besides those established prognostic biomarkers, what are the emerging prognostic biomarkers for CLL?**
    - With advances in DNA sequencing technology and its application in clinical practice, the last decade has seen significant advances in the development of biomarkers in oncology. More predictive biomarkers have been identified and the landscape of CLL therapeutics has changed drastically over the last few years.
    - Among the new markers, *NOTCH1, SF3B1*, and *BIRC3* mutations are present in relatively lower frequency compared to above established biomarkers (*TP53, IGHV*, and cytogenetic abnormalities) in untreated CLL; however, the incidence increases to nearly 25% in patient refractory to chemotherapy, especially fludarabine. Although currently there are limited and conflicting evidence regarding their prognostic significance, it has been demonstrated that *NOTCH1* mutation is independently associated with Richter's transformation of CLL.
    - Recurrent *BTK* and *PLCG2* mutations are usually not detectable at baseline but identified in most patients with CLL progressing on ibrutinib therapy. Activating mutations in *BTK* and *PLCG2* induce increased B-cell receptor signaling and ibrutinib resistance. Because these resistance mutations can usually be detected months prior to clinical disease progression, they could be used for disease/treatment monitoring. Studies have been reported to incorporate these biomarkers into the prognostic and risk stratification model for CLL patients [48].
13. **What are the clinical implications for *MYD88* L265P mutation in B-cell neoplasms?**
    - *MYD88* is a driver gene found in B-cell neoplasms. L265P is a highly recurrent hot spot mutation in *MYD88* which changes leucine at position 265 to proline [49].

Table 16.3 Established CLL prognostic biomarkers and commonly used testing methods [16, 21–47]

Category	Biomarkers	Mean frequency (range) (%)	Prognosis	Methods of detection
Gene	*TP53* mutation	8 (4–12)	Unfavorable	Sequencing
	IGHV mutation[a]	60 (37–78)	Favorable	Sequencing
Cytogenetics	Complex karyotype[b]	–	Unfavorable	Karyotype
	Del(11q)	17 (5–25)	Unfavorable	FISH
	Trisomy 12	14 (12–19)	Intermediate	FISH
	Del(13q)	55 (35–60)	Favorable	FISH
	Del(17p)	6 (3–8)	Unfavorable	FISH

[a]*IGHV* mutated is defined as 98% or less homology with germline gene sequence

[b]Complex karyotype is defined by the presence of at least three unrelated chromosomal abnormalities in more than one cell on karyotype

Table 16.4 International Prognostic Index for Chronic Lymphocytic Leukemia (CLL-IPI)

Variable	Description	Score
Age	≤65 years	0
	>65 years	+1
Clinical stage	Binet A or Rai 0	0
	Binet B-C or Rai I-IV	+1
Serum β2 microglobulin (mg/L)	≤3.5	0
	>3.5	+2
IGHV mutational status	Mutated	0
	Unmutated	+2
TP53 mutational status	Wild type	0
	Del(17p) by FISH and/or *TP53* mutation by sequencing	+4

Table 16.5 Using CLL-IPI to estimate CLL prognosis and time for start treatment

CLL-IPI total score	Risk group	Treatment recommendation[a]	5-yr overall survival (%)
0–1	Low	Do not treat	93.2
2–3	Intermediate	Do not treat unless symptomatic	79.3
4–6	High	Treatment indicated unless asymptomatic	63.3
7–10	Very high	Do not use chemotherapy. Treat on clinical trial or novel targeted inhibitor	23.3

[a]The decision to treat should not be based solely on the risk group. Risk categories should be used to estimate prognosis, and for patients in higher-risk groups, closer monitoring should be considered

- *MYD88* L265P is found in 90–97% of Waldenström macroglobulinemia (WM) or lymphoplasmacytic lymphoma (LPL) and has helped to differentiate these entities from other B-cell neoplasms, particularly marginal zone lymphomas. Besides *MYD88*, other recurrent somatic mutations, including *CXCR4* (30–40%), *ARID1A* (17%), and *CD79B* (8–15%), and deletions in chromosome 6q were also commonly identified in the lymphoplasmacytic cells in WM [50]. In the small number of WM patients who lack *MYD88* L265P mutation, they might have increased risk of disease transformation, poor response to ibrutinib, and shorter overall survival [51, 52].
- *MYD88* L265P also occurs in a small percentage of IgM but not IgG or IgA monoclonal gammopathy of undetermined significance (MGUS), splenic marginal zone lymphoma, 25–30% of DLBCL of activated B cell (ABC) type, and 60–70% of primary large B cell lymphoma of the central nervous system [53, 54]. *MYD88* L265P-positive IgM MGUS patients have shown an increased risk of disease progression to WM [55].
- Because of the above clinical implication and its impact on treatment strategies, it is important to distinguish patients with *MYD88* wild-type WM from those with other IgM-secreting neoplasms, such as plasma cell myeloma.

14. **What methods are commonly used for *MYD88* mutation detection?**
    - Like detection of other gene mutations, *MYD88* L265P can be detected using different molecular methods such as relatively simple, straightforward techniques like allele-specific PCR (AS-PCR), pyrosequencing, and Sanger sequencing or more complicated but comprehensive analysis techniques such as NGS.
    - The selection of the specific method depends on many factors, which usually include the following:
      1. Desired test sensitivity or lower limit of detection.
      2. Volume of the test.
      3. Cost of the test, including instrument, reagent, technologists, quality control, proficiency test, and maintenance of the equipment.
      4. Is it usually ordered as a single biomarker or combined with other biomarkers?
      5. Requirement of turnaround time.
15. **What genetic changes are largely seen in extranodal marginal zone lymphoma of mucosa-associated lymphoid tissue (MALT lymphoma) but not in other types of marginal zone lymphomas?**
    - There are three main groups of marginal zone lymphoma (MZL), including MALT lymphoma, nodal marginal zone lymphoma (NMZL), and splenic marginal zone lymphoma (SMZL).
    - Chromosomal translocations are commonly associated with certain types of MALT lymphomas but not in SMZL or NMZL. For example, t(11;18)(q21;q21) is associated with pulmonary and gastric MALT, whereas t(3;14)(p14.1;q32) is more commonly associated with MALT lymphoma arising in the thyroid, ocular adnexa, orbit, and skin. A summary of commonly seen chromosomal translocation in MALT is listed in Table 16.6.
16. **What are the clinical implications for *EZH2* mutation in B-cell neoplasms?**
    - *EZH2* (enhancer of zeste homolog 2) gene plays an essential role in the development of lymphocytes and is required for germinal center formation. When deregulated, mutant *EZH2* can induce germinal center hyperplasia and B cell neoplasm, which mainly includes FL and germinal center type DLBCL [56, 57].
    - Activating *EZH2* mutation resulting in aberrant methylation of histone H3 lysine 27 (H3K27) can be identified in 20–25% of FL. The *EZH2* mutations can also be detected by sequencing methods. Copy num-

Table 16.6 Recurrent chromosomal translocation in MALT lymphoma

Chromosome translocation	Gene partners	Site of disease	Detection methods
t(11;18)(q22;q21)	*BIRC3-MALT1*	Lung and stomach	FISH, RT-PCR, NGS
t(3;14)(p14.1;q32)	*FOXP1-IGH*	Thyroid, ocular adnexa, orbit, and skin	FISH, RT-PCR, NGS
t(1;14)(p22;q32)	*BCL10-IGH*	GI tract and lung	FISH, RT-PCR, NGS
t(14;18)(q32;q21)	*IGH-MALT1*	Ocular, salivary gland, and skin	FISH, RT-PCR, NGS

GI tract gastrointestinal tract

ber changes of *EZH2*, which is also clinically relevant, can be detected by SNP arrays when indicated. Immunohistochemical stain for EZH2 expression or H3K27 methylation may be a useful surrogate for *EZH2* mutation analysis [58].

- There are emerging interests in recent years to investigate the role of *EZH2* in lymphomagenesis with dozens of therapeutic agents that have been developed to target the EZH2 enzymatic domain. For example, tazemetostat (TAZVERIK™) is a protein known as a methyltransferase, which is an *EZH2* gene inhibitor and works by targeting *EZH2* and can be used to treat *EZH2* mutation bearing follicular lymphoma, after other treatments have been tried. However, further studies and clinical trials are still required to advance our knowledge in the tumorigenesis of *EZH2* mutants.

17. **When should the mutational analysis be considered in mature B-cell neoplasm diagnosis, prognosis, and treatment?**
    - Besides the molecular biomarkers discussed above, high-throughput technology has identified many emerging markers with prognostic potentials in other mature B-cell neoplasms, such as MCL and DLBCL.
      – Besides traditional *CCND1* gene rearrangement in MCL, molecular aberrations such as *ATM*, *TP53*, *CDKN2A*, and *MYC* are also frequently seen in at least 20% of patients [59].
      – In DLBCL, somatic mutations in *MYD88*, *CD79B*, *EZH2*, *NOTCH1*, and *NOTCH2* and gene rearrangement in *BCL2* and *BCL6* genes could further distinguish DLBCL into genetic subtypes with different clinical courses [60, 61].
    - Although the understanding of the genetic landscape of mature B-cell neoplasm has grown rapidly in recent years and had a significant impact on our understanding of lymphoma pathobiology and by extension on the current WHO classification, mutational analysis has not been a standard clinical practice in mature B-cell neoplasm diagnosis and currently being used only in a few entities and specific clinical situations, such as *BRAF* V600E in hairy cell leukemia and *MYD88* L265P in lymphoplasmacytic lymphoma. This is mainly because:
      – Lymphoma diagnosis can usually be achieved with routine histologic evaluation, combined with immunohistochemistry (IHC), flow cytometry (FCM), and sometimes with addition of fluorescence in situ hybridization (FISH) assay.
      – Mutational analysis has limited direct impact on lymphoma prognostic purpose and therapy decisions.
      – As the newer member of ancillary tests, the current cost of mutational analysis is similar or more expensive compared to IHC, FISH, or FCM.
    - It is likely that we will experience a significant increase in molecular testing, especially sequencing-based mutational analysis, in B-cell neoplasm for subclassification of lymphoma, as well as prognostic and treatment stratification. It will bring many benefits in practical applications such as:
      – Mutational analysis, especially panel-based NGS testing, is a more efficient and timely technology for genomic profiling of mature B-cell neoplasm. As we see more cytology and core biopsy samples in lymphoma workup, NGS test minimizes the amount of tissue consumed and avoids the need for iterative reflex testing.
      – Greater use of panel-based mutational analysis will allow the discovery of more driver mutations.
      – Utilization of molecular tumor boards allows molecular pathologists and oncologists to integrate genomic reports in the context of a broader knowledge base and the patient to support better treatment decisions.

Cases Presentation

Case 1

Learning Objectives

1. Indication of clonality test in mature B-cell neoplasm
2. The utility and limitation of PCR-based clonality assay
3. Use of NGS-based clonality assay in determination of clonal relationship

Case History

A 70-year-old male presented to his primary care physician complaining of several days of black tarry stools, occasional bright red blood per rectum, fatigue, and abdominal pain. Patient's past medical history includes basal cell carcinoma diagnosed 10 years ago which was treated with resection.

Initial Workup

His complete blood count (CBC) was significant for mild anemia with a hemoglobin of 11.7 g/dL (reference 13.7–17.5), hematocrit of 30% (reference 40–51%), and leukocytosis of 14.5 thousand/uL (reference 4.2–9.1). An esophagogastroduodenoscopy revealed a 5–6 cm mass with central ulceration in the lesser curvature of the stomach which was biopsied.

Histologic Findings

The biopsy of the gastric lesion showed intact gastric mucosa with a diffuse atypical infiltrate of small lymphoid cells with scattered larger forms in the submucosa (Fig. 16.2a–b). The atypical infiltrates were positive for B-cell markers CD20 (Fig. 16.2c) and CD79a while negative for CD5 (Fig. 16.2d), cyclin D1, and CD10. Flow cytometry was not performed.

Question 1: After reviewing this preliminary information, which hematologic diseases are in the differential diagnosis?

Question 2: Which molecular studies could be ordered to help the diagnosis?

Based on the described findings, there are two primary considerations: reactive lymphoid proliferation and a mature B-cell neoplasm. Testing for *IGH* and *IGK* gene rearrangement was ordered, and the result was positive for clonal proliferation of both *IGH* and *IGK* genes. Taken together with its immunophenotype, a diagnosis of low-grade extranodal marginal zone B cell lymphoma/mucosa-associated lymphoid tissue (MALT) lymphoma was made. Fluorescence in situ hybridization (FISH) for t(11;18) *BIRC/MALT1* fusion was performed on the gastric biopsy with no translocation detected. However, approximately 90% of the nuclei had trisomy 18 at 18q21 resulting in three copies of the *MALT1* gene.

Next, positron emission tomography (PET) scan and bone marrow biopsy were performed for staging purposes. PET identified increased fluorodeoxyglucose (FDG) uptake and gastric thickening in the region of the gastric cardia with max SUV of 8.6 consistent with known diagnosis of MALT lymphoma. No other abnormal regional FDG uptake is identified.

The bone marrow biopsy was mildly hypocellular for age with progressive trilineage hematopoiesis (Fig. 16.3a). Flow cytometry identified a population of clonal B-cell population which expresses CD19, CD20 (dim), CD5, and CD23 with dim kappa light chain restriction (Fig. 16.3b). The monoclonal B-cell population has an immunophenotype most typical of chronic lymphocytic leukemia (CLL). However, the absolute count of clonal B cells is too low to reach formal criteria for a diagnosis of CLL in the absence of symptoms or adenopathy. Given the disparity between this phenotype and the impression based on the gastric biopsy, additional molecular studies were ordered.

Question 3: Is the monoclonal B-cell proliferation identified in marrow related to the patient's gastric MALT lymphoma? Which molecular studies could be ordered now?

Because the flow cytometry was not performed on the gastric biopsy, the immunophenotype cannot be compared with that of the patient's bone marrow. The gastric B-cell lymphoma was CD5 negative by IHC, whereas the clonal B cells in bone marrow were expressing CD5 and CD23.

Molecular Genetic Study

First, the PCR-based gel detection of *IGH* and *IGK* gene rearrangements was also performed on the bone marrow aspirate, and the result was also positive for clonal proliferation. Although clonal amplification products were detected in both gastric lymphoma and bone marrow B-cell proliferation, the sizes of the products are not identical, and it is inconclusive that the marrow B cell lymphocytosis was originated from the same clone of the gastric lymphoma (Fig. 16.4a–b).

Question 4: What else could we do to clarify this inconclusive result?

NGS-based IGH clonality assay was next performed on the gastric lymphoma and marrow B-cell lymphocytosis samples. In bone marrow, the only clone identified is a 302 bp sequence using *IGHV3* and *IGHJ6* segments with cumulative of 51.7% of total reads. In the gastric MALT lymphoma, the dominant clone identified is a 303 bp sequence using *IGHV4* and *IGHJ5* segments with cumulative of 58.3% of total reads. Interestingly, another small clone (3.1% of total reads) is also identified in this sample which is using the same V and J segments as in the clone identified in the marrow (Fig. 16.5a-b) with 100% match of their sequence (Fig. 16.5c).

Final Diagnosis

1. Gastric MALT lymphoma without bone marrow involvement
2. Monoclonal B-cell lymphocytosis (MBL) with CLL type

Follow-Up

The patient completed radiation therapy for gastric MALT lymphoma and is doing well. A recent PET scan indicated complete remission. His monoclonal B-cell lymphocytosis, CLL type, was monitored clinically on blood-based flow cytometry test every 6 months without any treatment.

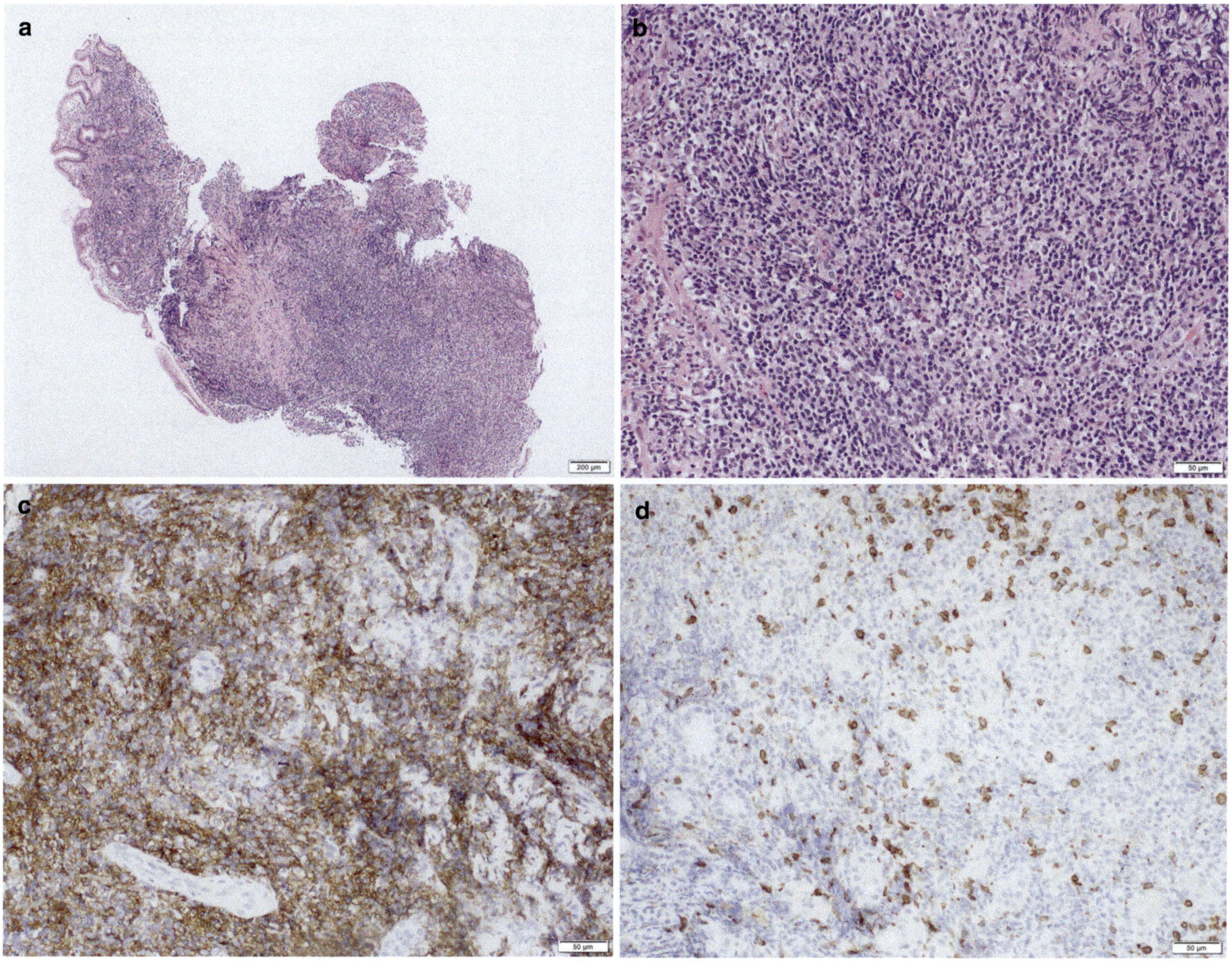

Fig. 16.2 Gastric biopsy showing sheets of atypical lymphoid cells in the gastric submucosa. (**a**) Hematoxylin and eosin, 40×; (**b**) hematoxylin and eosin, 200×; (**c**) CD20 was positive in atypical cells, 200×; (**d**) CD5 highlighted scattered small T lymphocytes and was negative in atypical cells, 200×

Discussion

This interesting but not uncommon case illustrates the utility and limitation of PCR-based clonality assay. It also highlights the advantage of NGS-based tests in determination of clonal relationship of mature B-cell neoplasms. In summary, there were two clonally unrelated neoplastic diseases identified in this patient: a MALT lymphoma which is localized at the stomach only and another MBL of CLL type which involves the patient's blood and bone marrow. The B-cell clone identified in the bone marrow which was also identified in the patient's gastric sample could be explained by blood circulating neoplastic cells in the stomach. Clonality test should not be performed on clear-cut lymphomas; however, because NGS-based clonality assay can identify the unique DNA sequence, clonal prevalence, and V-J family identity for each gene rearrangement, it is a power tool in the determination of clonal relationship. In this case, it has helped the clinical treatment stratification and patients did not need to receive systemic treatment.

a

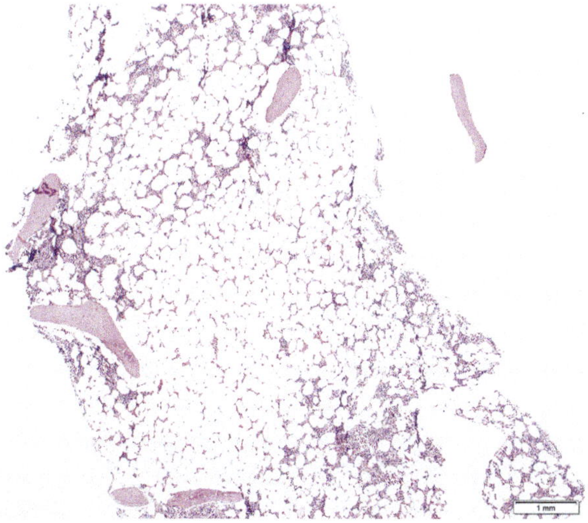

Fig. 16.3 Bone marrow biopsy. (**a**) Mildly hypocellular bone marrow for age with trilineage hematopoiesis; (**b**) flow cytometry results showing a population of lymphocytes expressing CD19, CD20 (dim), CD5, and dim kappa light chain restriction

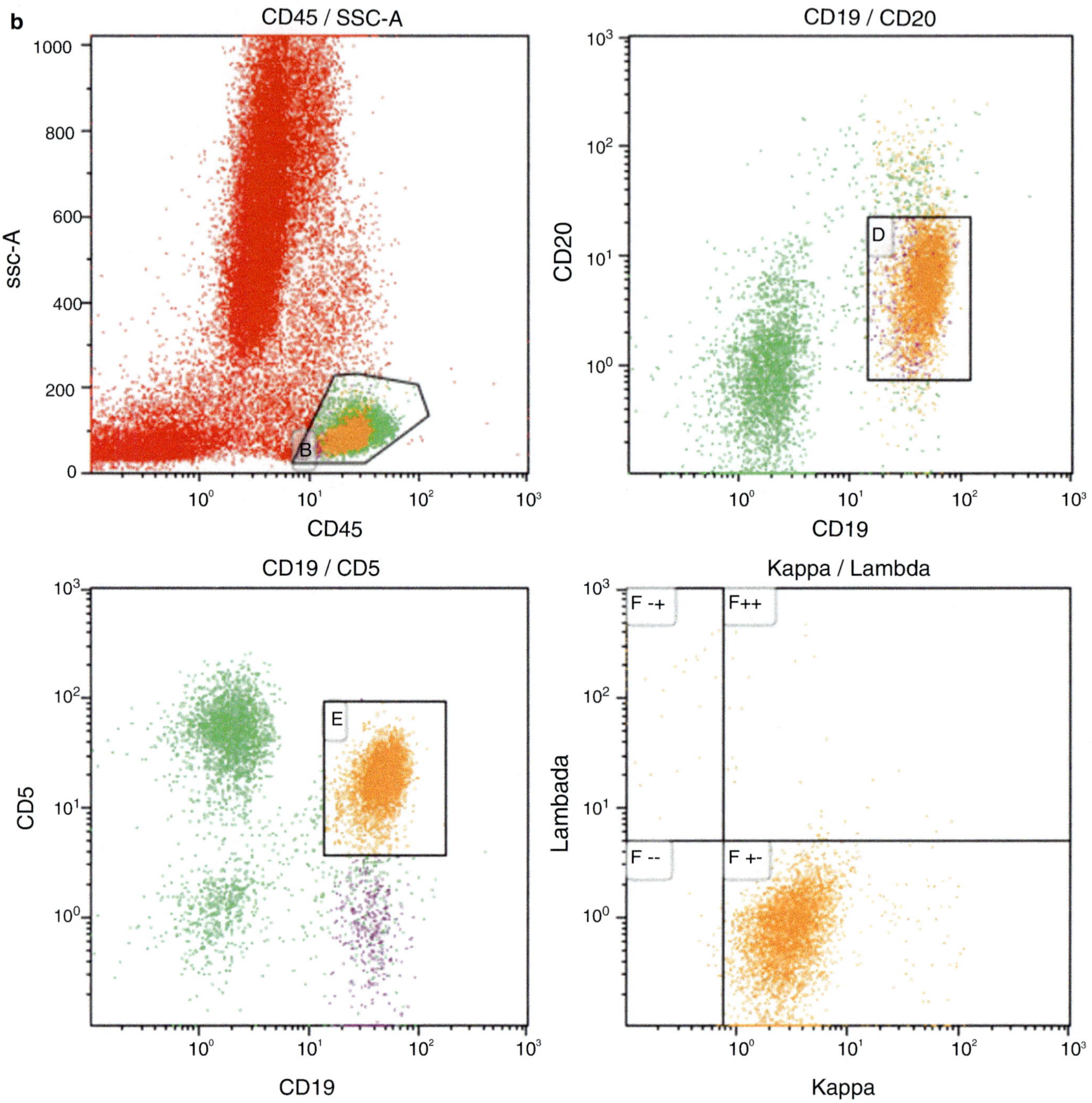

Fig. 16.3 (continued)

Case 2

Learning Objectives

1. Use of NGS-based clonality assay in determination of clonal relationship and help on clinical management
2. The utility of clonality assay in Hodgkin lymphoma

Case History

A 26-year-old female, with no past medical history, presented to the emergency department complaining of acute chest pain radiating to her shoulder accompanied by shortness of breath. Deep inspiration provoked pain radiating to the middle of her back. In addition, she was experiencing general malaise, recent drenching night sweats, and weight loss.

Chest x-ray showed a widened mediastinum, most prevalent on the right. A subsequent CT scan revealed a 7 cm mass in the anterior mediastinum compressing the medial aspect of the lung right upper lobe. A video-assisted thoracoscopic (VATS) biopsy of the mass was performed and sent to pathology for evaluation.

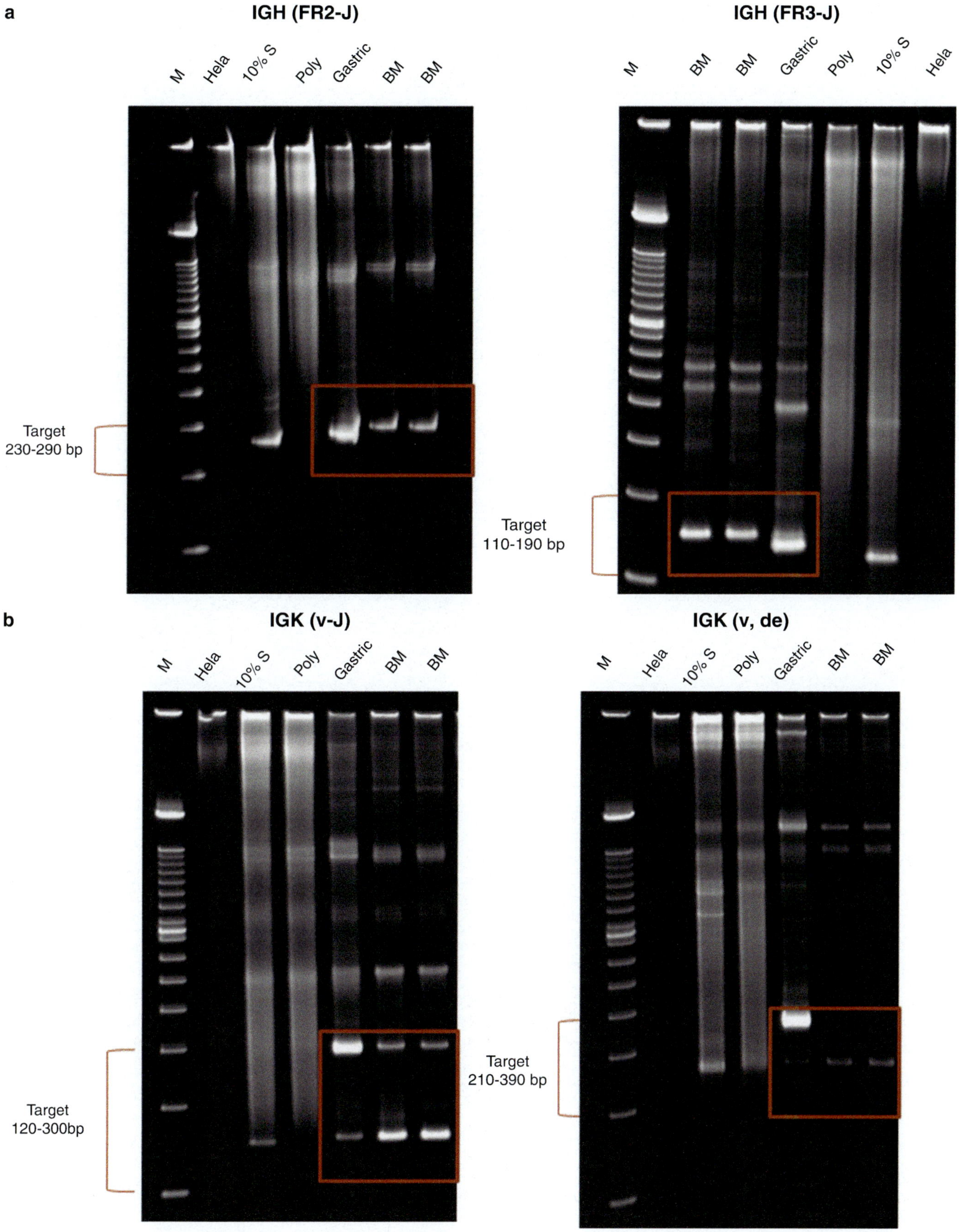

Fig. 16.4 PCR-based clonality assay with gel detection. (**a**) *IGH* gene rearrangement, FR2 primers, and FR3 primers. (**b**) *IGK* gene rearrangement, two sets of primers. (M, DNA size marker; BM, bone marrow aspirate; Gastric, gastric biopsy; Poly, polyclonal control; 10% S, 10% sensitivity and positive control; Hela, negative control)

a

Rank	Sequence	Length	Raw count	V-gene	J-gene	% total reads	Cumulative %	V-coverage
1	CGCTGTCTATGGT	303	1161654	IGHV4-34_02	IGHJ5_02	58.3908871	58.3908871	97.3700000
2	GCCTCTGGATTCA	302	61085	IGHV3-21_02	IGHJ6_03	3.0704559	61.4613430	98.6800000
3	CGCTGTCTATGGT	303	52868	IGHV4-34_02	IGHJ5_02	2.6574259	64.1187689	97.3700000
4	CGCTGTCTATGGT	303	22331	IGHV4-34_02	IGHJ5_02	1.1224744	65.2412433	97.3700000
5	CGCTGTCTATGGT	303	20798	IGHV4-34_02	IGHJ5_02	1.0454177	66.2866610	97.3700000
6	CGCTGTCTATGGT	303	20636	IGHV4-34_02	IGHJ5_02	1.0372747	67.3239357	97.3700000
7	CGCTGTCTATGGT	303	8019	IGHV4-34_02	IGHJ5_02	0.4030774	67.7270132	97.3700000
8	CGCTGTCTATGGT	303	7441	IGHV4-34_02	IGHJ5_02	0.3740241	68.1010373	97.3700000
9	CGCTGTCTATGGT	303	7345	IGHV4-34_02	IGHJ5_02	0.3691986	68.4702359	97.3700000
10	CGCTGTCTATGGT	303	6598	IGHV4-34_02	IGHJ5_02	0.3316505	68.8018864	97.3700000

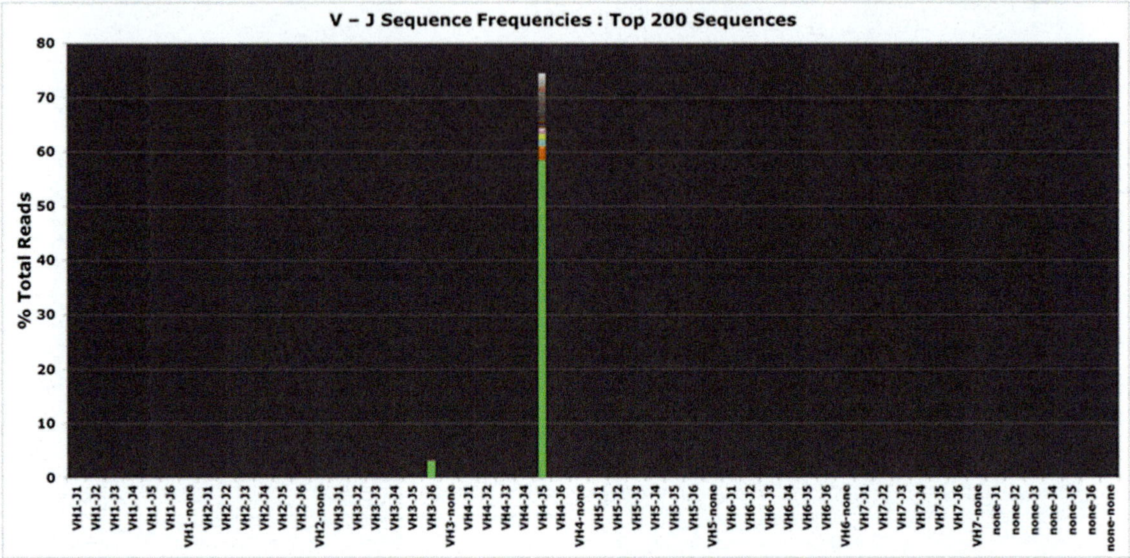

b

Rank	Sequence	Length	Raw count	V-gene	J-gene	% total reads	Cumulative %	V-coverage
1	GCCTCTGGATTCA	302	981752	IGHV3-21_02	IGHJ6_03	51.6529706	51.6529706	98.6800000
2	GCCTCTGGATTCA	302	25127	IGHV3-21_02	IGHJ6_03	1.3220082	52.9749788	98.6800000
3	GCCTCTGGATTCA	302	16418	IGHV3-21_02	IGHJ6_03	0.8638011	53.8387799	98.6800000
4	GCCTCTGGATTCA	302	13290	IGHV3-21_02	IGHJ6_03	0.6992275	54.5380074	98.6800000
5	GCCTCTGGATTCA	269	9991	IGHV3-7_01	IGHJ4_02	0.5256570	55.0636644	99.5600000
6	GCCTCTGGATTCA	256	9137	IGHV3-20_01	IGHJ4_02	0.4807255	55.5443899	95.5900000
7	GCCTCTGGATTCA	299	8735	IGHV3-21_02	IGHJ6_03	0.4595750	56.0039649	97.3600000
8	GCCTCTGGATTCA	281	8407	IGHV3-74_02	IGHJ4_02	0.4423179	56.4462829	99.5600000
9	GCCTCTGGATTCA	302	8028	IGHV3-21_02	IGHJ6_03	0.4223776	56.8686605	98.6800000
10	GCCTCTGGATTCA	269	7351	IGHV3-74_02	IGHJ4_02	0.3867586	57.2554190	99.5600000

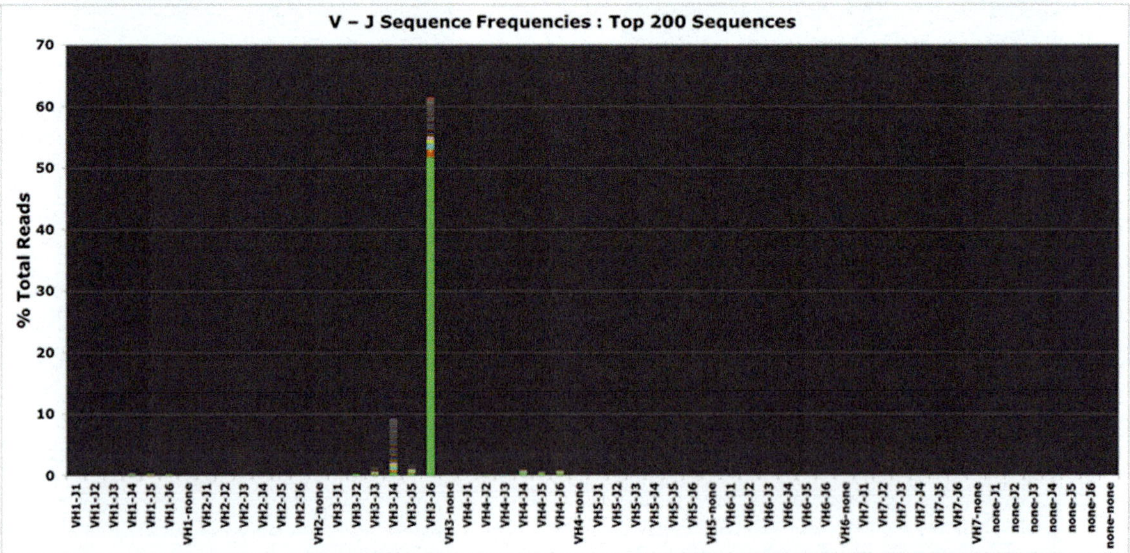

Fig. 16.5 NGS-based clonality assay. (**a**) Gastric MALT lymphoma. (**b**) Bone marrow. (**c**) 100% identical sequence match between rank 2 clone from gastric lymphoma to that of rank 1 clone from bone marrow

c

```
gastric    1 GCCTCTGGATTCACCTTCAGTAGTTATAACATGAACTGGGTCCGTCAGGC   50
             ||||||||||||||||||||||||||||||||||||||||||||||||||
BM         1 GCCTCTGGATTCACCTTCAGTAGTTATAACATGAACTGGGTCCGTCAGGC   50

gastric   51 TCCAGGGAAGGGGCTGGAGTGGGTCTCATCCATTAGTAGTAGTAGTACTT  100
             ||||||||||||||||||||||||||||||||||||||||||||||||||
BM        51 TCCAGGGAAGGGGCTGGAGTGGGTCTCATCCATTAGTAGTAGTAGTACTT  100

gastric  101 ACATATACTACGCAGACTCACTGAAGGGCCGATTCACCATCTCCAGAGAC  150
             ||||||||||||||||||||||||||||||||||||||||||||||||||
BM       101 ACATATACTACGCAGACTCACTGAAGGGCCGATTCACCATCTCCAGAGAC  150

gastric  151 AACGCCAACAACTCACTGTATCTGCAAATGAACAGCCTGAGAGCCGAGGA  200
             ||||||||||||||||||||||||||||||||||||||||||||||||||
BM       151 AACGCCAACAACTCACTGTATCTGCAAATGAACAGCCTGAGAGCCGAGGA  200

gastric  201 CACGGCTGTGTATTACTGTGCGAGGTCCCCGTCTGACTATTTTTGGACTG  250
             ||||||||||||||||||||||||||||||||||||||||||||||||||
BM       201 CACGGCTGTGTATTACTGTGCGAGGTCCCCGTCTGACTATTTTTGGACTG  250

gastric  251 GTTATTCTTCGACTTACTATTACTACATGGACGTCTGGGGCAAAGGGACC  300
             ||||||||||||||||||||||||||||||||||||||||||||||||||
BM       251 GTTATTCTTCGACTTACTATTACTACATGGACGTCTGGGGCAAAGGGACC  300

gastric  301 AC   302
             ||
BM       301 AC   302
```

Fig. 16.5 (continued)

Histologic Findings

Biopsy sections showed sheets of large atypical cells, with abundant pale cytoplasm and relative round or ovoid nuclei. The mass had a vaguely nodular growth pattern with coarse fibrotic band (Fig. 16.6a-b). The neoplastic cells were positive for CD45, CD20, and CD79a while negative for pancytokeratin, CD3, CD30, and TdT (Fig. 16.6c–d). The Ki67 proliferation index was approximately 60% (Fig. 16.6e).

Question 1: After reviewing this histology and its immunophenotype, what is the diagnosis?

A diagnosis of primary mediastinal (thymic) large B-cell lymphoma was rendered. The patient received six cycles of R-CHOP treatment and achieved complete remission. Five years after the completion of her treatment, routine surveillance imaging revealed a new development of anterior mediastinal soft tissue adjacent to the left brachiocephalic vein, suspicious for a recurrence of lymphoma. PET scan showed increased uptake in the mediastinum and multiple lymph nodes. Excisional biopsy of a supraclavicular lymph node was performed. Biopsy sections consisted of enlarged lymph node with effaced architecture. Numerous large cells with amphophilic cytoplasm, two to multiple nuclei or one large lobated nucleus with clear karyoplasm, and huge viral inclusion-like nucleoli were present in a background of mixed inflammatory cells which consist mainly of small lymphocytes, histiocytes, eosinophils, and plasma cells (Fig. 16.7a). These large neoplastic cells were positive for CD30, CD15, MUM-1, and weakly positive for PAX5 while negative for CD20 and CD3 (Fig. 16.7b–f).

Question 2: In a patient with a known history of primary mediastinal large B-cell lymphoma, chemotherapy, and current findings in the enlarged lymph node, which hematologic diseases are in the differential diagnosis?

Although the relapse of a patient's previously diagnosed primary mediastinal large B-cell lymphoma was suspected at

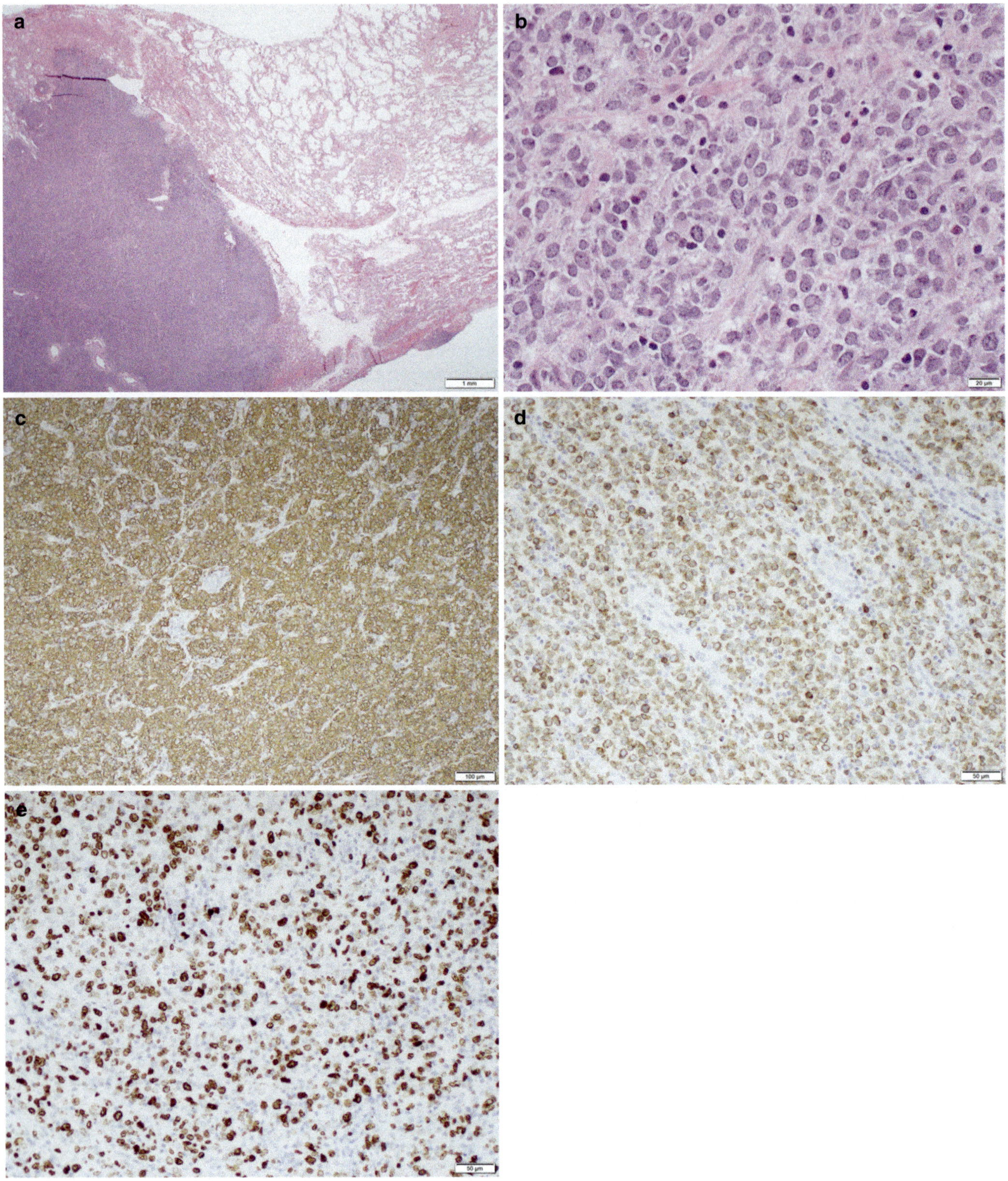

Fig. 16.6 Biopsy of mediastinal mass showed sheets of large atypical cells, (**a**) Hematoxylin and eosin, 20×; (**b**) hematoxylin and eosin, 400×; (**c**) CD20, strongly positive, 100×; (**d**) CD79a, positive, 200×; (**e**) proliferation index Ki67, approximately 60%, 200×

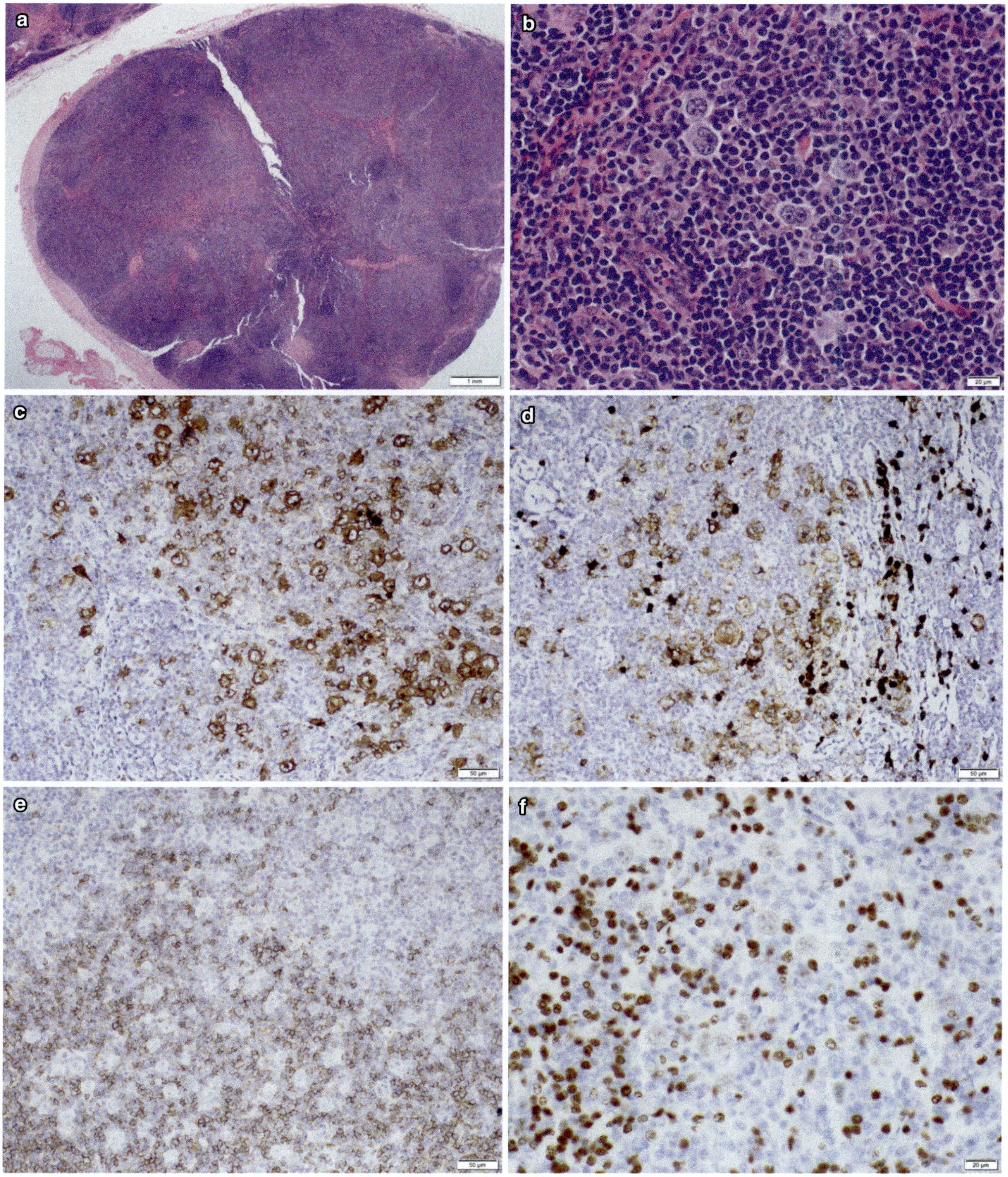

Fig. 16.7 Biopsy of supraclavicular lymph node with Reed-Sternberg cells in a background of mixed inflammation, (**a**) enlarged lymph node with effaced architecture, hematoxylin and eosin, 20×; (**b**) Reed-Sternberg cells, hematoxylin and eosin, 400×; (**c**) CD30 positive in neoplastic cells, 200×; (**d**) CD15, positive in neoplastic cells, 200×; (**e**) CD20 negative in neoplastic cells, 200×; (**f**) PAX5, weakly positive in neoplastic cells, 200×

first, the histologic finding and immunophenotype of this subsequent lesion did not support that diagnosis. Instead, a diagnosis of nodular sclerosis classical Hodgkin lymphoma (cHL) was rendered for this subsequent mass after careful review of the previous lymphoma and comparison of the overall presentation of two tumors.

Question 3: For treatment purposes, the patient's oncologist would like to know if these two lymphomata were clonally related. Which molecular studies could be ordered to help answer this question?

Molecular Genetic Study

NGS-based clonality assay was used to determine the clonal relationship of these two tumors in this patient. A clone was identified in each sample; however, the clones were clearly distinct (Fig. 16.8a–b) with 84.2% of nucleotide difference. Thus, the molecular study supported the presence of two separate metachronous lymphomas in this patient.

Final Diagnosis

1. Primary mediastinal large B- cell lymphoma and several years later
2. Classical Hodgkin Lymphoma, Nodular Sclerosis Type

Follow-Up

The patient completed ABVD chemotherapy and radiation therapy for Hodgkin lymphoma and is currently in complete remission for both lymphomas.

Discussion

The patient was diagnosed with primary mediastinal large B-cell lymphoma first, received chemotherapy, and was in remission for several years before another new mass, classical Hodgkin lymphoma, was diagnosed. Although histologically these two lymphomata could share some overlapping features, their immunophenotypes are distinctly different. Because of the young age of the patient, the oncologist was considering using more aggressive treatment if it is proved that these two tumors were clonally related.

Due to the scarcity of tumor cells (Reed-Sternberg (RS) cells and Hodgkin cells) in cHL and lack of immunoglobulin expression [62], although being classified as a B-cell lymphoma, it has been challenging to detect the clonal rearrangement in cHL by standard CISH, flow cytometry, or molecular techniques. Therefore, clonality assay has generally been considered as a supportive ancillary test for only B-cell non-Hodgkin lymphomas (NHL). With the advancement of research in defining the immunophenotype of the HRS cells as well as the background cells found in Hodgkin lymphoma (HL), Fromm et al. have demonstrated a six-color flow panel to diagnose HL in clinical practice [63, 64]. However, standard PCR-based clonality assay has not been useful in the past in HL diagnosis. The NGS-based clonality assay successfully detected clonal proliferation in this case could be resulted from its relatively high tumor cell load. Based on the completely different clonal origins, standard chemotherapy for Hodgkin lymphoma was selected for treatment.

Case 3

Learning Objectives

1. Established prognostic biomarkers in chronic lymphocytic leukemia (CLL)
2. Role of genetics and risk-stratified approach in CLL treatment

Case History

A 75-year-old female presented to her primary care physician for routine annual checkup. Her past medical history included hypertension, hypothyroidism, remote history of colon cancer, and uterine cancer treated with surgery and chemotherapy. Patient had no current complaint. No swollen lymph nodes or spleen was detected during physical examination.

Initial Workup

Her CBC was significant for mild anemia with a hemoglobin of 8.9 g/dL (reference 13.7–17.5), hematocrit of 29% (reference 40–51%), and leukocytosis of 118.6K/μL (reference 4.2–9.1) with lymphocytosis of 100.81K/μL (reference 1.0–4.8). Peripheral blood smear review is referred. Her serum β2 microglobulin was 9.3 mg/L (reference ≤2.51) and elevated.

Histologic Findings

Peripheral blood smear slides showed significant increase in small lymphocytes with round nuclei, scant cytoplasm, and clumped chromatin. Also noted were numerous "smudge" or "basket" cells where the cellular remnants form a lattice-like pattern. An albumin preparation slide removed these smudge cells which showed the majority of WBCs were small lymphocytes mixed with a few unremarkable neutrophils and monocytes (Fig. 16.9). Multicolor flow cytometry study was performed and on CD45 versus dot plot histogram, the lymphoid population comprises approximately 87% of the total events, which contained a predominant population of monoclonal B-lymphoid cells of small to medium cells. The clonal B-lymphoid population was positive for CD45, CD19, CD20 (low), CD5, CD23, CD38, and CD43, and reveals surface kappa immunoglobulin light chain restriction, and the population of B cells is negative for FMC7, CD10, Zap70, and

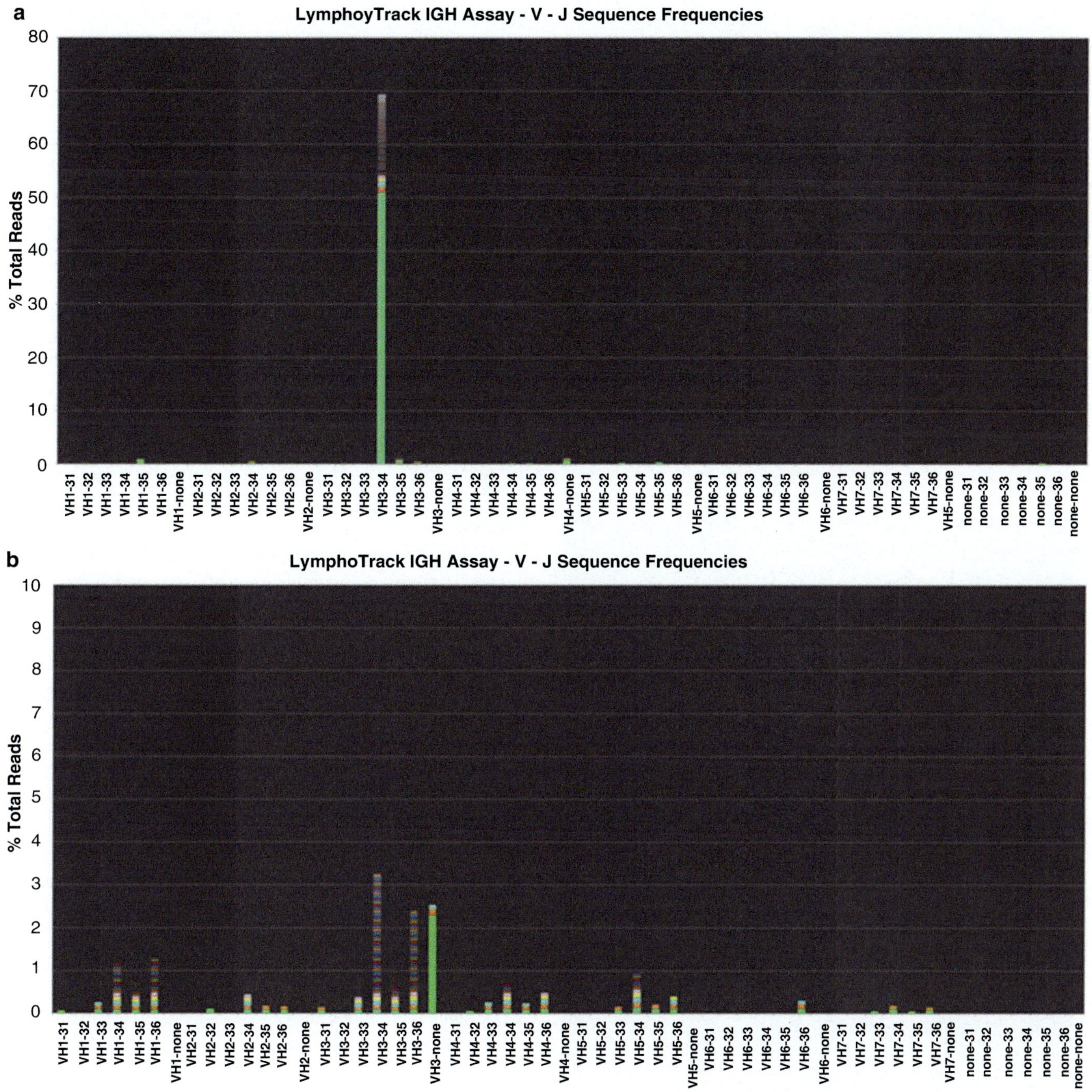

Fig. 16.8 NGS-based clonality assay showing two distinct clonal populations in the (**a**) mediastinal mass and (**b**) supraclavicular lymph node

other T-cell markers tested from this study. There was no increase in the blast population.

Question 1: After reviewing this preliminary information, what neoplastic hematologic disease is most likely?

Question 2: What additional laboratory studies might be helpful?

Data from CBC, peripheral blood smear, and flow cytometry demonstrated a phenotypically distinct population of chronic lymphocytic leukemia (CLL). A typical workup for a patient with CLL includes cytogenetic analysis on the peripheral blood and molecular testing.

Molecular Genetic Study

Cytogenetic analysis on the patient's blood showed a complex karyotype, and FISH studies, performed using a panel of DNA probes for chromosomes 6q, 11,12,13, and 17 to detect abnormalities frequently involved in CLL, were positive for deletion of chromosome 13q (Fig. 16.10). Next-generation

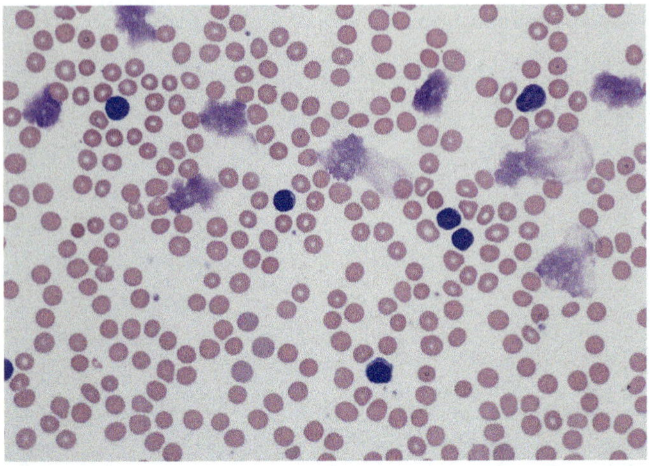

Fig. 16.9 Peripheral blood showed predominant small lymphocytes with round nuclei and clumped chromatin. Numerous "smudge" cells are present. Wright-Giemsa stain, 400×

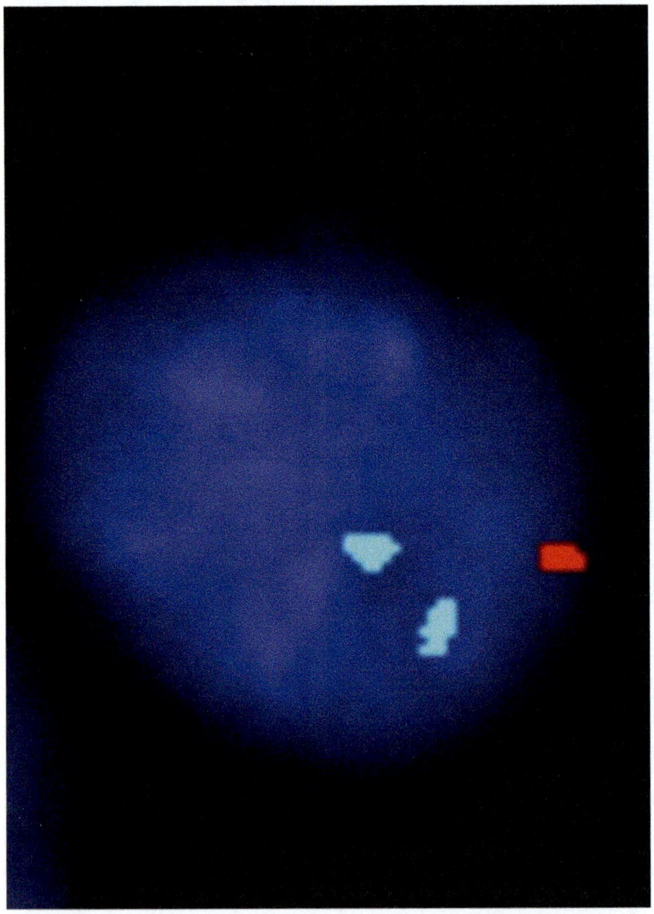

Fig. 16.10 FISH for CLL prognostic panel detected deletion of chromosome 13q with signal pattern of 1 red and 2 aqua. Probe color red for *DLEU1&2* gene at 13q14.3 and probe color aqua for *LAMP1* gene at 13q34

sequencing for *TP53* was positive for p.R342* (c.1024C > T) mutation with allele frequency of 81.2% and unmutated IgVH with expressed VH5–10 family (Fig. 16.11).

Final Diagnosis

Chronic lymphocytic leukemia with complex karyotype, *TP53* mutation, and unmutated IgVH

Follow-Up

According to CLL-IPI (Table 16.7), this patient got a total score of 9, which was in the very-high-risk group. The current treatment recommendation for the very-high-risk group is to treat on clinical trial or novel targeted inhibitor instead of regular chemotherapy. Patient was enrolled in the clinical trial A041702 (a randomized phase III study of ibrutinib plus obinutuzumab versus ibrutinib plus venetoclax and obinutuzumab in untreated older patients (>70 years of age) with CLL).

Discussion

As one of the most common leukemias in adults, chronic lymphocytic leukemia is incurable in most cases, and the standard approach used to be a "watch and wait" strategy based on the majority of cases being diagnosed in early stage and irrespective of risk factors [65]. Although the pathogenesis of CLL is not fully understood, it is known associated with constitutive activation of the B-cell receptor (BCR) signaling pathway but also with substantial heterogeneity in the disease course. For active disease, combined chemoimmunotherapy of CD20 antibody (rituximab, ofatumumab or obinutuzumab) and chemotherapy (fludarabine, cyclophosphamide and rituximab (FCR)) have been the main choice and widely used [66]. However, this approach does not have satisfactory efficacy in CLL patients with older age, comorbidity, or del [17] or *TP53* mutations [67]. The CLL-IPI was developed using patient data from before and categorizes CLL patients into different risk groups. This scoring system has not been incorporated into CLL management guidelines and should be used with caution to provide prognosis information and at least may warrant closer initial monitoring for patients with higher risk.

Bruton's tyrosine kinase (BTK), a kinase in the downstream of BCR signaling, plays a crucial role in the survival of neoplastic cells, and more recently, small-molecular inhibitors of BTK, such as ibrutinib, have shown excellent antitumor activity and induce prolongation of progression free with CLL and MCL, including patients with high-risk genetic changes [68, 69].

In summary, a standard CLL workup is strongly recommended for every CLL patient at the time of diagnosis to facilitate risk evaluation and treatment stratification [70].

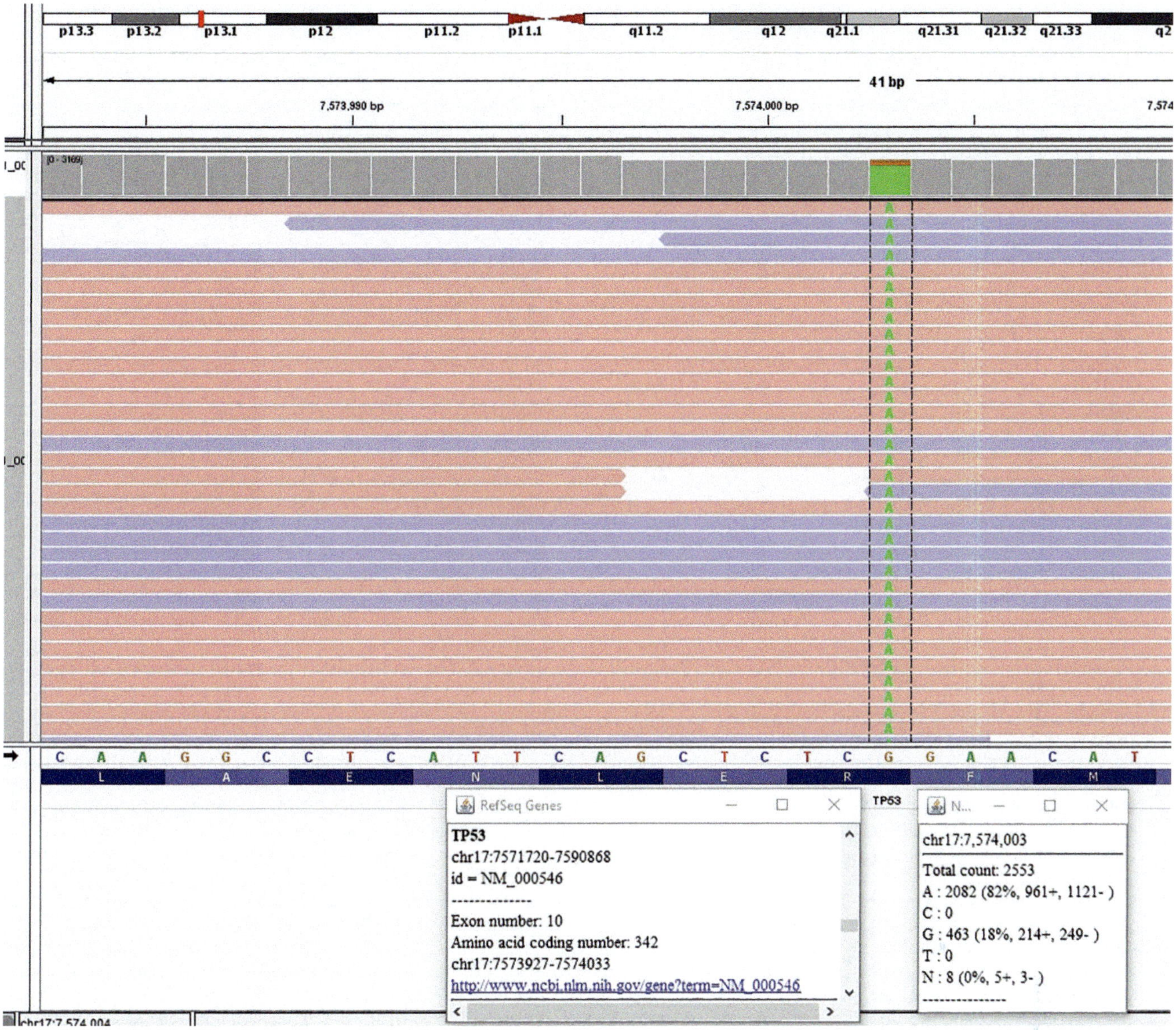

Fig. 16.11 Aligned next-generation sequencing data revealed *TP53* p.R342* mutation with allele frequency of 81.2%

Table 16.7 CLL-IPI risk score calculation for Case 3

Variable	Description	Patient	Score
Age	≤65 years	75 years	+1
	>65 years		
Clinical stage	Binet A or Rai 0	Rai 0	0
	Binet B-C or Rai I-IV		
Serum β2 microglobulin (mg/L)	≤3.5	9.3	+2
	>3.5		
IGHV mutational status	Mutated	Unmutated	+2
	Unmutated		
TP53 mutational status	Wild type	*TP53* R342* detected	+4
	Del(17p) by FISH and/or *TP53* mutation by sequencing		
International Prognostic Index for Chronic Lymphocytic Leukemia (CLL-IPI) Total score			9

References

1. Cree IA, Deans Z, Ligtenberg MJ, Normanno N, Edsjo A, Rouleau E, et al. Guidance for laboratories performing molecular pathology for cancer patients. J Clin Pathol. 2014;67(11):923–31.
2. Sioutos N, Bagg A, Michaud GY, Irving SG, Hartmann DP, Siragy H, et al. Polymerase chain reaction versus southern blot hybridization. Detection of immunoglobulin heavy-chain gene rearrangements. Diagn Mol Pathol. 1995;4(1):8–13.
3. van Krieken JH, Langerak AW, Macintyre EA, Kneba M, Hodges E, Sanz RG, et al. Improved reliability of lymphoma diagnostics via PCR-based clonality testing: report of the BIOMED-2 concerted action BHM4-CT98-3936. Leukemia. 2007;21(2):201–6.
4. van Dongen JJ, Langerak AW, Bruggemann M, Evans PA, Hummel M, Lavender FL, et al. Design and standardization of PCR primers and protocols for detection of clonal immunoglobulin and T-cell receptor gene recombinations in suspect lymphoproliferations: report of the BIOMED-2 concerted action BMH4-CT98-3936. Leukemia. 2003;17(12):2257–317.

5. Hoeve MA, Krol AD, Philippo K, Derksen PW, Veenendaal RA, Schuuring E, et al. Limitations of clonality analysis of B cell proliferations using CDR3 polymerase chain reaction. Mol Pathol. 2000;53(4):194–200.
6. Taylor JM, Spagnolo DV, Kay PH. B-cell target DNA quantity is a critical factor in the interpretation of B-cell clonality by PCR. Pathology. 1997;29(3):309–12.
7. Zhou XG, Sandvej K, Gregersen N, Hamilton-Dutoit SJ. Detection of clonal B cells in microdissected reactive lymphoproliferations: possible diagnostic pitfalls in PCR analysis of immunoglobulin heavy chain gene rearrangement. Mol Pathol. 1999;52(2):104–10.
8. Elenitoba-Johnson KS, Bohling SD, Mitchell RS, Brown MS, Robetorye RS. PCR analysis of the immunoglobulin heavy chain gene in polyclonal processes can yield pseudoclonal bands as an artifact of low B cell number. J Mol Diagn. 2000;2(2):92–6.
9. Groenen PJ, Langerak AW, van Dongen JJ, van Krieken JH. Pitfalls in TCR gene clonality testing: teaching cases. J Hematop. 2008;1(2):97–109.
10. Langerak AW, Groenen PJ, Bruggemann M, Beldjord K, Bellan C, Bonello L, et al. EuroClonality/BIOMED-2 guidelines for interpretation and reporting of Ig/TCR clonality testing in suspected lymphoproliferations. Leukemia. 2012;26(10):2159–71.
11. Boer A, Tirumalae R, Bresch M, Falk TM. Pseudoclonality in cutaneous pseudolymphomas: a pitfall in interpretation of rearrangement studies. Br J Dermatol. 2008;159(2):394–402.
12. Evans PA, Pott C, Groenen PJ, Salles G, Davi F, Berger F, et al. Significantly improved PCR-based clonality testing in B-cell malignancies by use of multiple immunoglobulin gene targets. Report of the BIOMED-2 concerted action BHM4-CT98-3936. Leukemia. 2007;21(2):207–14.
13. Langerak AW, Molina TJ, Lavender FL, Pearson D, Flohr T, Sambade C, et al. Polymerase chain reaction-based clonality testing in tissue samples with reactive lymphoproliferations: usefulness and pitfalls. A report of the BIOMED-2 concerted action BMH4-CT98-3936. Leukemia. 2007;21(2):222–9.
14. Krejci O, Prouzova Z, Horvath O, Trka J, Hrusak O. Cutting edge: TCR delta gene is frequently rearranged in adult B lymphocytes. J Immunol. 2003;171(2):524–7.
15. Jemal A, Siegel R, Ward E, Murray T, Xu J, Thun MJ. Cancer statistics, 2007. CA Cancer J Clin. 2007;57(1):43–66.
16. Hallek M, Cheson BD, Catovsky D, Caligaris-Cappio F, Dighiero G, Dohner H, et al. iwCLL guidelines for diagnosis, indications for treatment, response assessment, and supportive management of CLL. Blood. 2018;131(25):2745–60.
17. Nabhan C, Rosen ST. Chronic lymphocytic leukemia: a clinical review. JAMA. 2014;312(21):2265–76.
18. Rai KR, Jain P. Chronic lymphocytic leukemia (CLL)-then and now. Am J Hematol. 2016;91(3):330–40.
19. Bosch F, Dalla-Favera R. Chronic lymphocytic leukaemia: from genetics to treatment. Nat Rev Clin Oncol. 2019;16(11):684–701.
20. Crassini K, Stevenson WS, Mulligan SP, Best OG. Molecular pathogenesis of chronic lymphocytic leukaemia. Br J Haematol. 2019;186(5):668–84.
21. Abruzzo LV, Herling CD, Calin GA, Oakes C, Barron LL, Banks HE, et al. Trisomy 12 chronic lymphocytic leukemia expresses a unique set of activated and targetable pathways. Haematologica. 2018;103(12):2069–78.
22. Dohner H, Stilgenbauer S, Benner A, Leupolt E, Krober A, Bullinger L, et al. Genomic aberrations and survival in chronic lymphocytic leukemia. N Engl J Med. 2000;343(26):1910–6.
23. Migliazza A, Bosch F, Komatsu H, Cayanis E, Martinotti S, Toniato E, et al. Nucleotide sequence, transcription map, and mutation analysis of the 13q14 chromosomal region deleted in B-cell chronic lymphocytic leukemia. Blood. 2001;97(7):2098–104.
24. Calin GA, Dumitru CD, Shimizu M, Bichi R, Zupo S, Noch E, et al. Frequent deletions and down-regulation of micro-RNA genes miR15 and miR16 at 13q14 in chronic lymphocytic leukemia. Proc Natl Acad Sci U S A. 2002;99(24):15524–9.
25. Chigrinova E, Rinaldi A, Kwee I, Rossi D, Rancoita PM, Strefford JC, et al. Two main genetic pathways lead to the transformation of chronic lymphocytic leukemia to Richter syndrome. Blood. 2013;122(15):2673–82.
26. Parker H, Rose-Zerilli MJ, Parker A, Chaplin T, Wade R, Gardiner A, et al. 13q deletion anatomy and disease progression in patients with chronic lymphocytic leukemia. Leukemia. 2011;25(3):489–97.
27. Klein U, Lia M, Crespo M, Siegel R, Shen Q, Mo T, et al. The DLEU2/miR-15a/16-1 cluster controls B cell proliferation and its deletion leads to chronic lymphocytic leukemia. Cancer Cell. 2010;17(1):28–40.
28. Guieze R, Robbe P, Clifford R, de Guibert S, Pereira B, Timbs A, et al. Presence of multiple recurrent mutations confers poor trial outcome of relapsed/refractory CLL. Blood. 2015;126(18): 2110–7.
29. Rossi D, Cerri M, Deambrogi C, Sozzi E, Cresta S, Rasi S, et al. The prognostic value of TP53 mutations in chronic lymphocytic leukemia is independent of Del17p13: implications for overall survival and chemorefractoriness. Clin Cancer Res. 2009;15(3):995–1004.
30. Rozovski U, Keating MJ, Estrov Z. Why is the immunoglobulin heavy chain gene mutation status a prognostic Indicator in chronic lymphocytic Leukemia? Acta Haematol. 2018;140(1):51–4.
31. Rosenquist R, Ghia P, Hadzidimitriou A, Sutton LA, Agathangelidis A, Baliakas P, et al. Immunoglobulin gene sequence analysis in chronic lymphocytic leukemia: updated ERIC recommendations. Leukemia. 2017;31(7):1477–81.
32. Cerami E, Gao J, Dogrusoz U, Gross BE, Sumer SO, Aksoy BA, et al. The cBio cancer genomics portal: an open platform for exploring multidimensional cancer genomics data. Cancer Discov. 2012;2(5):401–4.
33. Quesada V, Conde L, Villamor N, Ordonez GR, Jares P, Bassaganyas L, et al. Exome sequencing identifies recurrent mutations of the splicing factor SF3B1 gene in chronic lymphocytic leukemia. Nat Genet. 2011;44(1):47–52.
34. Malcikova J, Smardova J, Rocnova L, Tichy B, Kuglik P, Vranova V, et al. Monoallelic and biallelic inactivation of TP53 gene in chronic lymphocytic leukemia: selection, impact on survival, and response to DNA damage. Blood. 2009;114(26):5307–14.
35. Yu L, Kim HT, Kasar S, Benien P, Du W, Hoang K, et al. Survival of Del17p CLL depends on genomic complexity and somatic mutation. Clin Cancer Res. 2017;23(3):735–45.
36. Damle RN, Wasil T, Fais F, Ghiotto F, Valetto A, Allen SL, et al. Ig V gene mutation status and CD38 expression as novel prognostic indicators in chronic lymphocytic leukemia. Blood. 1999;94(6):1840–7.
37. Hamblin TJ, Davis Z, Gardiner A, Oscier DG, Stevenson FK. Unmutated Ig V(H) genes are associated with a more aggressive form of chronic lymphocytic leukemia. Blood. 1999;94(6):1848–54.
38. Guo A, Lu P, Galanina N, Nabhan C, Smith SM, Coleman M, et al. Heightened BTK-dependent cell proliferation in unmutated chronic lymphocytic leukemia confers increased sensitivity to ibrutinib. Oncotarget. 2016;7(4):4598–610.
39. Rossi D, Terzi-di-Bergamo L, De Paoli L, Cerri M, Ghilardi G, Chiarenza A, et al. Molecular prediction of durable remission after first-line fludarabine-cyclophosphamide-rituximab in chronic lymphocytic leukemia. Blood. 2015;126(16):1921–4.
40. Landau DA, Tausch E, Taylor-Weiner AN, Stewart C, Reiter JG, Bahlo J, et al. Mutations driving CLL and their evolution in progression and relapse. Nature. 2015;526(7574):525–30.
41. Puente XS, Bea SR, Villamor N, Gutierrez-Abril J, Martin-Subero JI, et al. Non-coding recurrent mutations in chronic lymphocytic leukaemia. Nature. 2015;526(7574):519–24.
42. Stilgenbauer S, Schnaiter A, Paschka P, Zenz T, Rossi M, Dohner K, et al. Gene mutations and treatment outcome in chronic

lymphocytic leukemia: results from the CLL8 trial. Blood. 2014;123(21):3247–54.
43. Chiaretti S, Marinelli M, Del Giudice I, Bonina S, Piciocchi A, Messina M, et al. NOTCH1, SF3B1, BIRC3 and TP53 mutations in patients with chronic lymphocytic leukemia undergoing first-line treatment: correlation with biological parameters and response to treatment. Leuk Lymphoma. 2014;55(12):2785–92.
44. Winkelmann N, Rose-Zerilli M, Forster J, Parry M, Parker A, Gardiner A, et al. Low frequency mutations independently predict poor treatment-free survival in early stage chronic lymphocytic leukemia and monoclonal B-cell lymphocytosis. Haematologica. 2015;100(6):e237–9.
45. Rossi D, Rasi S, Spina V, Bruscaggin A, Monti S, Ciardullo C, et al. Integrated mutational and cytogenetic analysis identifies new prognostic subgroups in chronic lymphocytic leukemia. Blood. 2013;121(8):1403–12.
46. Jeromin S, Weissmann S, Haferlach C, Dicker F, Bayer K, Grossmann V, et al. SF3B1 mutations correlated to cytogenetics and mutations in NOTCH1, FBXW7, MYD88, XPO1 and TP53 in 1160 untreated CLL patients. Leukemia. 2014;28(1):108–17.
47. Houldsworth J, Guttapalli A, Thodima V, Yan XJ, Mendiratta G, Zielonka T, et al. Genomic imbalance defines three prognostic groups for risk stratification of patients with chronic lymphocytic leukemia. Leuk Lymphoma. 2014;55(4):920–8.
48. Ahn IE, Tian X, Ipe D, Cheng M, Albitar M, Tsao LC, et al. Prediction of outcome in patients with chronic lymphocytic leukemia treated with Ibrutinib: development and validation of a four-factor prognostic model. J Clin Oncol. 2020:JCO2000979.
49. Treon SP, Xu L, Yang G, Zhou Y, Liu X, Cao Y, et al. MYD88 L265P somatic mutation in Waldenstrom's macroglobulinemia. N Engl J Med. 2012;367(9):826–33.
50. Treon SP, Xu L, Guerrera ML, Jimenez C, Hunter ZR, Liu X, et al. Genomic landscape of Waldenstrom macroglobulinemia and its impact on treatment strategies. J Clin Oncol. 2020;38(11):1198–208.
51. Hunter ZR, Xu L, Tsakmaklis N, Demos MG, Kofides A, Jimenez C, et al. Insights into the genomic landscape of MYD88 wild-type Waldenstrom macroglobulinemia. Blood Adv. 2018;2(21):2937–46.
52. Abeykoon JP, Paludo J, King RL, Ansell SM, Gertz MA, LaPlant BR, et al. MYD88 mutation status does not impact overall survival in Waldenstrom macroglobulinemia. Am J Hematol. 2018;93(2):187–94.
53. Kraan W, Horlings HM, van Keimpema M, Schilder-Tol EJ, Oud ME, Scheepstra C, et al. High prevalence of oncogenic MYD88 and CD79B mutations in diffuse large B-cell lymphomas presenting at immune-privileged sites. Blood Cancer J. 2013;3:e139.
54. Yu X, Li W, Deng Q, Li L, Hsi ED, Young KH, et al. MYD88 L265P mutation in lymphoid malignancies. Cancer Res. 2018;78(10):2457–62.
55. Varettoni M, Zibellini S, Arcaini L, Boveri E, Rattotti S, Pascutto C, et al. MYD88 (L265P) mutation is an independent risk factor for progression in patients with IgM monoclonal gammopathy of undetermined significance. Blood. 2013;122(13):2284–5.
56. Li B, Chng WJ. EZH2 abnormalities in lymphoid malignancies: underlying mechanisms and therapeutic implications. J Hematol Oncol. 2019;12(1):118.
57. Beguelin W, Popovic R, Teater M, Jiang Y, Bunting KL, Rosen M, et al. EZH2 is required for germinal center formation and somatic EZH2 mutations promote lymphoid transformation. Cancer Cell. 2013;23(5):677–92.
58. Huet S, Xerri L, Tesson B, Mareschal S, Taix S, Mescam-Mancini L, et al. EZH2 alterations in follicular lymphoma: biological and clinical correlations. Blood Cancer J. 2017;7(4):e555.
59. Hill HA, Qi X, Jain P, Nomie K, Wang Y, Zhou S, et al. Genetic mutations and features of mantle cell lymphoma: a systematic review and meta-analysis. Blood Adv. 2020;4(13):2927–38.
60. Schmitz R, Wright GW, Huang DW, Johnson CA, Phelan JD, Wang JQ, et al. Genetics and pathogenesis of diffuse large B-cell lymphoma. N Engl J Med. 2018;378(15):1396–407.
61. Chapuy B, Stewart C, Dunford AJ, Kim J, Kamburov A, Redd RA, et al. Molecular subtypes of diffuse large B cell lymphoma are associated with distinct pathogenic mechanisms and outcomes. Nat Med. 2018;24(5):679–90.
62. Tamaru J, Hummel M, Zemlin M, Kalvelage B, Stein H. Hodgkin's disease with a B-cell phenotype often shows a VDJ rearrangement and somatic mutations in the VH genes. Blood. 1994;84(3):708–15.
63. Fromm JR, Wood BL. A six-color flow cytometry assay for immunophenotyping classical Hodgkin lymphoma in lymph nodes. Am J Clin Pathol. 2014;141(3):388–96.
64. Wu D, Wood BL, Fromm JR. Flow cytometry for non-Hodgkin and classical Hodgkin lymphoma. Methods Mol Biol. 2013;971: 27–47.
65. Stilgenbauer S. Prognostic markers and standard management of chronic lymphocytic leukemia. Hematology Am Soc Hematol Educ Program. 2015;2015:368–77.
66. Cohen JA, Bomben R, Pozzo F, Tissino E, Harzschel A, Hartmann TN, et al. An updated perspective on current prognostic and predictive biomarkers in chronic lymphocytic leukemia in the context of chemoimmunotherapy and novel targeted therapy. "Cancers (Basel). 2020;12(4):894.
67. Woyach JA, Ruppert AS, Heerema NA, Zhao W, Booth AM, Ding W, et al. Ibrutinib regimens versus chemoimmunotherapy in older patients with untreated CLL. N Engl J Med. 2018;379(26):2517–28.
68. Scheffold A, Stilgenbauer S. Revolution of chronic lymphocytic Leukemia therapy: the chemo-free treatment paradigm. Curr Oncol Rep. 2020;22(2):16.
69. Pal Singh S, Dammeijer F, Hendriks RW. Role of Bruton's tyrosine kinase in B cells and malignancies. Mol Cancer. 2018;17(1):57.
70. Zenz T, Mertens D, Dohner H, Stilgenbauer S. Molecular diagnostics in chronic lymphocytic leukemia – pathogenetic and clinical implications. Leuk Lymphoma. 2008;49(5):864–73.

Plasma Cell Neoplasms

17

Vikas A. Gupta, Nisha S. Joseph, and David L. Jaye

List of Frequently Asked Questions

1. What diagnostics tests are used to establish the diagnosis of multiple myeloma?
2. What are common primary and secondary genetic events observed in myelomagenesis?
3. What genetic tests should be ordered at diagnosis?
4. How are the results of genetic testing incorporated into risk stratification of multiple myeloma?
5. What is the role of genetic testing in the risk stratification and approach to management of precursor states, monoclonal gammopathy of uncertain significance, and smoldering myeloma?
6. How do genetic findings impact the treatment of multiple myeloma?
7. How often are genetic studies repeated for multiple myeloma?
8. When and how is minimal residual disease testing performed?
9. What is the role for copy number-single nucleotide polymorphism microarrays in analysis of multiple myeloma?
10. When should there be concern for therapy-related myeloid neoplasms and what tests should be ordered for their evaluation?
11. What molecular and genetic testing is useful for light chain amyloidosis?
12. How does plasma cell leukemia differ from typical multiple myeloma? Are there different genetic features?
13. How do extramedullary plasma cell neoplasms differ from typical multiple myeloma? Are there different genetic features?
14. Do results of mutation analysis guide therapy?
15. What are some potential new genomic markers for high-risk multiple myeloma that are not yet employed clinically?

Frequently Asked Questions

1. **What diagnostics tests are used to establish the diagnosis of multiple myeloma?**
   - Multiple myeloma (MM) is a plasma cell neoplasm and the second most common hematologic malignancy, accounting for an estimated 32,270 new diagnoses in 2020 and 12,830 deaths worldwide [1]. MM is defined as a clonal, malignant proliferation of plasma cells that can lead to the development of hypercalcemia, anemia, renal dysfunction, and lytic bone disease attributable to the underlying plasma cell clone.
   - The diagnosis of MM, as defined by the International Myeloma Working Group in 2014 [2] and largely echoed by the National Comprehensive Cancer Network (NCCN) guidelines [3] and the 2016 WHO definitions, [4] requires the confirmation of clonal plasma cells either in the bone marrow biopsy (≥10%) or in a bony or extramedullary plasmacytoma and the presence of at least one of the SLiM-CRAB criteria. These criteria consist of the traditional CRAB criteria (serum **C**alcium > 11 mg/dL, **R**enal insufficiency defined as creatinine clearance of <40 mL/min, **A**nemia defined as Hgb <10 g/dL or drop in <2 g/dL from baseline, and **B**one lesions detected on plain film, PET-CT or MRI), plus three additional criteria that individually predict an approximately 80% risk of progression to

V. Gupta and N. Joseph contributed equally to this chapter and are treated as co-first authors.

V. A. Gupta · N. S. Joseph
Department of Hematology and Medical Oncology, Emory University School of Medicine, Atlanta, GA, USA
e-mail: vikas.gupta@emory.edu; nisha.sara.joseph@emory.edu

D. L. Jaye (✉)
Department of Pathology and Laboratory Medicine, Emory University School of Medicine, Atlanta, GA, USA
e-mail: dljaye@emory.edu

Y. Ding, L. Zhang (eds.), *Practical Oncologic Molecular Pathology*, Practical Anatomic Pathology,
https://doi.org/10.1007/978-3-030-73227-1_17

symptomatic myeloma at 2 years. These risk factors include ≥ **S**ixty percent bone marrow plasmacytosis, a serum involved-to-uninvolved free **Li**ght chain ratio of ≥100 with the involved free light chain concentration of ≥10 mg/dL, and more than one focal lesion on **M**RI ≥ 5 mm in size. These revised criteria shift a subset of asymptomatic patients previously classified as smoldering multiple myeloma (SMM) as now meeting the diagnostic criteria for MM given the ultra-high risk of disease progression and the benefit of receiving therapy in terms of preventing end-organ damage.

- To evaluate the diagnostic criteria, testing modalities employed to establish the diagnosis of MM include (1) bone marrow aspirate and biopsy core for morphology and immunophenotyping; (2) bone imaging with a PET-CT or whole body MRI; (3) serum chemistry panel and complete blood count to evaluate creatinine, calcium, and hemoglobin levels as well as a serum beta-2 microglobulin and serum lactate dehydrogenase (LDH) for staging; and (4) immunologic studies including serum protein electrophoresis with immunofixation, urine protein electrophoresis with immunofixation, serum free light chain assay, and quantitative immunoglobulin levels (IgA, IgG, and IgM).
- Of note, current diagnostic criteria for MM, as well as other plasma cell neoplasms, do not specify results of molecular and cytogenetic testing. Nonetheless, these laboratory approaches, particularly cytogenetic studies, including traditional karyotyping and interphase fluorescence in situ hybridization (FISH) analyses, yield key staging and prognostic data which help guide therapy and can serve as an additional method to detect clonality [5, 6].

2. **What are common primary and secondary genetic events observed in myelomagenesis?**
   - Primary genetic events represent initial driver abnormalities in the development of the malignant plasma cell clone and are thus generally present in all neoplastic cells. Approximately half of newly diagnosed MM have aneuploidy of several odd numbered chromosomes, including chromosomes 3, 5, 7, 9, 11, 15, 19, and 21, referred to as hyperdiploidy. The other common primary genetic event involves translocations of the immunoglobulin heavy chain locus (*IGH*) with cyclin D genes (*CCND1, CCND2, CCCND3*), *MMSET, MAF,* or *MAFB* loci. These recurrent cytogenetic abnormalities are displayed in Table 17.1 with their relative frequency in newly diagnosed MM, methods of detection, and their prognostic impact.
   - These alterations are clonal and are often found as well in MM precursor states which include monoclonal gammopathy of undetermined significance (MGUS), and SMM [7].
   - Common secondary genetic events in MM include 13q deletion, 1q21 gain, 1p deletion, and 17p deletion [Table 17.1], all of which may be clonal (involve all neoplastic cells) or sub-clonal (involve a subset of neoplastic cells). Several putative tumor suppressors and oncogenes that may contribute to disease pathogenesis are in these regions of the genome.
   - Several recurrent genetic alterations are associated with myeloma progression. *MYC* translocations, *TP53*

Table 17.1 Recurrent genetic abnormalities in multiple myeloma

Abnormality	Genes	Standard detection method(s)	Frequency in newly diagnosed (%)	Prognosis	Primary vs. secondary event
Translocations	–				
t(11;14)(q13;q32)	*CCND1/IGH*	FISH	15–20	Neutral	Primary
t(6;14)(p21;q32)	*CCND3/IGH*	FISH	1–2	Neutral	Primary
t(4;14)(p16;q32)	*FGFR3/IGH*	FISH	10–15	Unfavorable	Primary
t(14;16)(q32;q23)	*MAF/IGH*	FISH	2–5	Unfavorable	Primary
t(14;20)(q32;q12)	*MAFB/IGH*	FISH	<1	Unfavorable	Primary
MYC (multiple partners)	*MYC*	FISH	15–20	Unfavorable	Secondary
Copy number changes	–				
Hyperdiploidy[a]	–	FISH, CN-SNP	50	Good	Primary
13q deletion	–	FISH, CN-SNP	45–50	Variable	Primary
1q21 gain	–	FISH, CN-SNP	35–40	Unfavorable	Secondary
1p deletion	–	FISH, CN-SNP	30	Unfavorable	Secondary
17p deletion	*TP53*	FISH, CN-SNP	10	Unfavorable	Secondary
Non-hyperdiploidy[b]	–	CN-SNP	–	Unfavorable	–
Complex karyotype (> = 3 abnormalities)	–	Karyotyping	–	Unfavorable	–

[a]Involves chromosomes 3, 5, 7, 9, 11, 15, 19, and/or 21, with 47–74 total chromosomes. Rare patients (5%) show hyperdiploidy and an IgH translocation at diagnosis

[b]Includes hypodiploidy (≤ 44 chromosomes), pseudodiploidy (45–46 chromosomes), and near-tetraploidy (>75 chromosomes)

References: [6, 7, 12–14]

loss via 17p deletion or mutation, and activation of the NFkB and RAS pathways are observed with increasing frequency in relapsed MM, in contrast with MGUS and newly diagnosed MM.

- Exploratory next-generation sequencing has revealed the highly heterogeneous landscape of mutations in MM. However, precision medicine-based approaches targeting these mutations are still under investigation [8–11].

3. **What genetic tests should be ordered at diagnosis for multiple myeloma?**
   - At diagnosis, current guidelines recommend testing to assess for specific recurrent genetic abnormalities that are typically identified using traditional karyotyping and FISH analysis on bone marrow biopsy samples [2, 3].
   - Traditional karyotyping affords analysis of the whole genome but requires dividing cells. Yet, plasma cell neoplasms typically proliferate slowly which reduces the odds of identifying cytogenetic anomalies by this method, and it can be unclear if an identified metaphase is from a plasma cell or not. Moreover, some MM-associated abnormalities are below the resolution of conventional karyotyping. FISH analysis, by contrast, does not require dividing cells and can detect much smaller genomic aberrations, but it is limited to interrogation of the portion of the genome to which the FISH probes are directed [12]. Thus, these methods can provide non-overlapping as well as corroborative genomic information in the analysis of plasma cell neoplasms.
   - In the absence of mandated standards for which genomic loci are tested, laboratories vary in which recurrent MM-associated genetic abnormalities they assess by FISH and the specific probe sets employed for a given abnormality [12]. Nonetheless, a comprehensive panel at diagnosis would include assessment for two major classes of abnormalities including *IGH* locus translocations (t(11;14), t(4;14), t(14;16), t(6;14), t(14,20)) and copy number aberrations (hyperdiploidy of chromosome 3, 7, and 9, 13q deletion, 1q21 gain, 1p deletion, and 17p deletion) [6]. Some laboratories employ an *IGH* break-apart probe, or test initially for t(11;14), to screen for any *IGH* rearrangement before using other translocation-specific probes.
   - To increase the sensitivity of FISH analysis and other DNA-based molecular genetic analyses, enrichment of bone marrow plasma cells is recommended using cell separation technologies with antibodies to the plasma cell-selective surface marker, CD138 [3]. CD138 enrichment has been demonstrated to significantly increase detection rates, up to 50%, compared to cultured, unenriched whole bone marrow specimens [15, 16].

4. **How are the results of genetic testing incorporated into risk stratification of multiple myeloma?**
   - The Durie-Salmon staging system was the first risk stratification model for newly diagnosed MM. It relied heavily on the degree of tumor burden as reflected in hemoglobin, serum calcium level, bone involvement, and serum and urine paraprotein levels [17].
   - In 2005, a new model termed the International Staging System (ISS) was developed by the International Myeloma Working Group based on retrospective data from over 10,000 patients. The most significant prognostic factors from this analysis were serum β2-microglobulin level, serum albumin, platelet count, and serum creatinine. β2-microglobulin and albumin emerged as the strongest outcome predictors [18].
   - Importantly, in 2015, the revised ISS (R-ISS) recognized the importance of genetic abnormalities in the risk stratification of newly diagnosed myeloma. The R-ISS builds upon the ISS and adds the specific genetic abnormalities t(4;14), t(14;16), and 17p deletion and/or the presence of an elevated serum LDH as additional markers of more aggressive (high-risk) disease [5].

5. **What is the role of genetic testing in the risk stratification and approach to the management of precursor states, monoclonal gammopathy of uncertain significance, and smoldering multiple myeloma?**
   - Almost all cases of MM are thought to be preceded by a continuum of asymptomatic precursor states, the premalignant monoclonal gammopathy of uncertain significance (MGUS), and smoldering multiple myeloma (SMM) [19, 20]. The rate of progression of MGUS to symptomatic myeloma is roughly 1% per year; the rate of progression of SMM to MM is roughly 10% per year for the first 3 years, 3% per year for the next 5 years, followed by 1% per year for the subsequent 10 years [21].
   - Genetic testing is not currently used in the risk stratification MGUS. Currently, MGUS is delineated into risk groups by the presence of the following factors: (1) non-IgG paraprotein (IgM or IgA), (2) M-protein >1.5 g/dL, and (3) an abnormal free light chain ratio < 0.26 or > 1.65. The presence of either 0, 1, 2, or 3 of these factors divides patients into low, low-intermediate, high-intermediate, and high-risk MGUS corresponding to a 20-year risk of progression to MM of 58%, 37%, 21%, and 5%, respectively [22]. Of note, while many of the same MM-associated driver genetic abnormalities [Table 17.1] can be identified in MGUS, these abnormalities do not serve as accurate predictors of progression to MM [23, 24].

- Results of genetic testing have a clearer impact on the risk of progression of SMM. The Mayo 2018 criteria, known also as the 20-2-20 criteria, revised the current classification of SMM based on three independent risk factors for progression: (1) bone marrow plasmacytosis (BMPC) >20%, (2) serum free light chain ratio (FLCr) > 20, and (3) M-protein >2 g/dL [25]. The International Myeloma Working Group validated these criteria with the additional presence of high-risk cytogenetic features 1q21 gain, t(4;14), t(14;16), and 13q deletion. Using these four criteria, SMM patients can be grouped into low-risk, low-intermediate, high-intermediate, and high-risk corresponding with a 2-year risk of progression to MM of 8%, 21%, 37%, and 59%, respectively [26].
- For clinical management, the ECOG E3A06 trial randomized intermediate- and high-risk SMM patients to observation or lenalidomide treatment groups until disease progression and found a 72% risk reduction in the treatment arm. This effect was most pronounced in the high-risk subgroup categorized using the 20-2-20 criteria [27].

6. **How do genetic findings impact the treatment of multiple myeloma?**
   - Genetic testing at diagnosis is critical as it allows for accurate risk stratification by the R-ISS and, importantly, appropriate selection of induction therapy and an overall treatment plan based on the patient's risk category.
   - Patients classified as high risk by either the R-ISS or presence of other high-risk cytogenetic findings, including t(14;20) or a complex karyotype (≥3 abnormalities by traditional karyotyping), are considered for more intensive induction therapies and potential upfront autologous stem cell transplant, if the patient is eligible, as these improve overall survival. The ENDURANCE trial recently compared induction therapy with either RVD (lenalidomide (R), bortezomib (V), dexamethasone(D)) or KRD (carfilzomib (K), lenalidomide (R), dexamethasone (D)) and found no significant difference between the two regimens. However, notably, high-risk myeloma patients were excluded from this trial [6]. Conversely, several other studies have demonstrated benefit with carfilzomib in high-risk myeloma patients, a drug that is often used in induction and maintenance regimens for these patients [28].
   - High-risk cytogenetic findings also impact the selection of maintenance therapy. Patients with high-risk cytogenetic features are recommended for triplet maintenance therapy post-transplant with either RVD or other triplet regimens such as KRD or carfilzomib, pomalidomide, and dexamethasone, per physician preference. This approach was validated in a retrospective analysis of MM patients with high-risk cytogenetic findings who received 3 years of RVD maintenance therapy with a very good partial response or better rate of 96% with a stringent complete response rate of 51% corresponding to a median progression-free survival of 32 months and 3-year overall survival of 93% [29].
7. **How often are genetic studies repeated for multiple myeloma?**
   - MM patients on therapy are monitored for disease response by serial immunologic studies on blood. The testing interval depends on the patient's disease state. For example, serologic testing for M-protein and serum free light chains can be done every 3 months for patients with controlled disease on maintenance therapy, whereas for patients undergoing induction therapy or with active relapsed disease, serum markers are generally checked monthly.
   - Repeat genetic testing, specifically by FISH and traditional karyotyping and/or CN-SNP array, is performed on bone marrow biopsy samples at select time points, such as at the completion of induction therapy and post-transplant or at annual restaging using the International Myeloma Working Group Response Criteria to test for residual clonal plasma cells [2] and clonal evolution [30]. For patients with relapsed and/or refractory disease, repeat FISH and karyotyping is considered at the time of disease progression to identify new potential therapeutic targets and to better predict the biologic behavior of the disease.
8. **When and how is minimal residual disease testing performed?**
   - More ambitious and effective therapeutic protocols, designed to further minimize residual malignant plasma cells after treatment, have driven a need for ever more sensitive laboratory tools to detect residual tumor, referred to as minimal residual disease (MRD).
   - MRD testing utilizes highly sensitive techniques such as multiparameter flow cytometry or next-generation sequencing (NGS) to identify the presence of MM cells at a level of 10^{-4} to 10^{-6} neoplastic cells per nucleated cell [31]. NGS involves targeted sequencing of the *IGH* rearrangement to identify a VDJ rearrangement specific to the myeloma clone [32]. Two validated flow cytometry panels, one utilizing eight markers and a second with ten markers, are currently in use in specialized laboratories [33–35]. The use of mass spectroscopy for detection of ultralow levels of paraprotein in serum is a newer technique that is still in experimental development [31, 36].
   - NGS testing requires an initial sample with a relatively high quantity of neoplastic cells from which to define the signature *IGH* VDJ rearrangement. As a DNA-based method of analysis, testing can be per-

formed on archived formalin-fixed paraffin-embedded tissue and fresh samples.
- Hemodilution of the sample, a preanalytical variable that can be difficult to control, can impact the accuracy of MRD testing whether performed by flow cytometry or NGS.
- Numerous studies have demonstrated improved progression-free survival (PFS) and overall survival (OS) in patients who achieve a complete response in the absence of MRD compared to patients who remain MRD positive. However, the most appropriate timing and frequency of MRD testing has yet to be determined. Sustained MRD negativity, defined by two negative MRD tests separated by 1 year, may have the greatest impact on PFS and OS, but long-term follow-up and validation of these results are ongoing [31, 37].
- Future studies of MRD in clinical decision-making include the timing and frequency of testing as well as de-escalation or cessation of maintenance therapy in patients with sustained MRD negativity [31].

9. **What is the role for copy number-single nucleotide polymorphism microarrays in analysis of multiple myeloma?**
    - Copy number variants in MM encompass a broad range of fragment sizes, involving small deletions and amplifications to whole chromosomes. Copy number-single nucleotide polymorphism (CN-SNP) arrays can replace currently employed FISH analysis of select copy number abnormalities, such as those noted in Table 17.1 and similarly can make use of DNA harvested from even small numbers of CD138-enriched plasma cell preparations.
    - In contrast to FISH and traditional karyotyping, CN-SNP arrays not only afford sensitive, genome-scale coverage of aberrations but also can detect copy neutral loss of heterozygosity and other complex genomic abnormalities, such as chromothripsis and chromoanasynthesis. However, in the absence of validated clinical correlates, this additional information does not currently change the approach to patient care [12, 13].
    - Importantly, SNP-CN arrays cannot detect balanced translocations. Thus, while this technology allows a potentially cost-effective reduction in the use of some FISH probes and provides a broader assessment of the genome, it does not entirely obviate the need for FISH testing in MM to assess for IgH translocations [16].
10. **When should there be concern for therapy-related myeloid neoplasms and what tests should be ordered for their evaluation?**
    - Secondary primary malignancies (SPMs), also known as therapy-related malignancies, in MM are likely the result of numerous interacting factors, including predisposition to malignancy, dysfunctional immune surveillance, and use of therapeutics such as alkylating and immunomodulatory agents. The overall incidence of SPMs is reported to be 1–10% and can include solid tumors and hematologic malignancies [38].
    - A conventional karyotype is essential in the workup for suspected hematologic SPMs which are most commonly therapy-related MDS (t-MDS) and AML (t-AML). FISH analysis for recurrent abnormalities associated with MDS and AML may be most useful in cases associated with a negative conventional karyotype or when there is a lack of cell growth [39]. In a study of 41 secondary myeloid neoplasms in MM patients, chromosome analysis revealed a clonal cytogenetic abnormality in 89.2% of cases, with complex karyotype observed in 59.5% and loss of 5q or 7q in 10.8% [40]. Median overall survival in this group of patients was quite low at 19 months. In another study of 55 patients with t-MDS or t-AML, the median overall survival from diagnosis of the SPM was only 6.7 months [41].
    - Although deletion (20q) as a sole abnormality is usually associated with myeloid neoplasia [4], this association might not be the case for patients with plasma cell neoplasms. Recent studies have shown that in such patients, even though the deletion (20q) is not present in the plasma cell population, its presence is not considered by itself diagnostic of a myeloid neoplasm [42].
    - Lenalidomide, now commonly used for long-term maintenance therapy, has been reported to increase the risk of SPMs. However, a meta-analysis of over 3000 patients on randomized phase 3 trials, in which one group received lenalidomide, reported this increased risk is driven primarily by the combination of lenalidomide with oral melphalan [43]. Patients in these trials received various induction regimens, which likely influence the risk of SPMs.
11. **What molecular and genetic testing is useful for light chain amyloidosis?**
    - Light chain (AL) amyloidosis is caused by a plasma cell neoplasm that results in end-organ damage due to deposition of toxic monoclonal immunoglobulin light chain. It can be a diagnostic challenge given the nonspecific presenting signs and symptoms. In patients with suspected light chain amyloidosis, key screening diagnostic tests include serum immunofixation, urine immunofixation, and free light chain quantification. Reference range results make amyloidosis highly unlikely. The presence of a light chain abnormality, or high clinical suspicion with negative results, should prompt a biopsy, typically of fat pad and bone marrow, to be stained with Congo red to confirm the diagnosis. The combination of fat pad and bone marrow biopsy has been reported to iden-

tify 85% of amyloid cases [44]. Amyloid detection by Congo red stain should be followed by mass spectrometry to distinguish light chain amyloidosis from other amyloid subtypes. Biopsy of involved organs is only necessary if fat pad and bone marrow biopsies are negative, but the clinical suspicion remains high.

- In light chain amyloidosis, bone marrow plasma cell content is usually less than 10% [45]. The same set of genetic tests employed for initial evaluation of non-amyloid MM should be considered. By FISH analysis, t(11;14) is identified in approximately 55% of cases, a frequency much higher relative to non-amyloid-related myeloma, and is associated with worse outcomes [46, 47].
- In about 75% of cases, a lambda immunoglobulin light chain is expressed by the plasma cell clone. Interestingly, certain amino acid sequences within the variable regions of lambda light chains demonstrate a biochemical predisposition toward amyloid formation. However, light chain sequencing is not currently part of routine clinical care [48–50].
- Cardiac biomarker testing with troponin-T and N-terminal pro-B type natriuretic peptide is essential for determining the degree of cardiac involvement, staging, prognosis, and appropriate therapy [51].

12. **How does plasma cell leukemia differ from typical multiple myeloma? Are there different genetic features?**
    - Plasma cell leukemia (PCL) is an aggressive plasma cell neoplasm defined as the presence in the blood of greater than 20% clonal plasma cells or an absolute plasma cell count greater than 2×10^9/L [52]. When present at initial diagnosis, PCL is referred to as primary PCL (pPCL), in contrast to secondary PCL (sPCL) that is identified at relapse of MM. sPCL often represents an end-stage disease progression that is highly refractory to treatment and thus has a very poor prognosis with a median overall survival of less than 6 months [53].
    - Median overall survival for PCL is approximately 3 years with modern treatment regimens, which often include aggressive induction treatments with combination chemotherapy such as bortezomib, thalidomide, dexamethasone, cisplatin, doxorubicin, cyclophosphamide, and etoposide (VTD-PACE) [54]. However, patients with just 2% or more circulating plasma cells on blood smear differential counts or as few as 400 plasma cells/150,000 total nucleated cells by flow cytometry had similar outcomes to patients with >20% plasma cells. This finding suggests that patients with circulating plasma cells who do not meet the current WHO definition of PCL still have high-risk disease [55].
    - In contrast to MM, a higher proportion of PCL presents as light chain only disease (30%), while another 15% are non-secretory [56].
    - Cells from both PCL and MM express comparable levels of CD138 and CD38; however PCL is more likely to express CD20, CD23, CD44, and CD45, while less likely to express CD9, CD56, CD71, CD117, and HLA-DR [54].
    - Hyperdiploidy is less common in pPCL (20%) than in MM (60%), whereas *IGH* translocations are more common (87%), in particular t(11;14) (26%) [52, 56]. In addition, high-risk translocations t(4;14) and t(14;16) are present more frequently in sPCL compared to MM [57]. Consistent with their aggressive phenotype, PCL manifests frequent deletion and/or mutation of the *TP53* locus and upregulation of *MYC* [56, 58, 59]. sPCL likely represents a clonal selection process of accumulated genetic alterations through numerous courses of therapy [60, 61].
13. **How do extramedullary plasma cell neoplasms differ from typical multiple myeloma? Are there different genetic features?**
    - Solitary plasmacytomas are a form of plasma cell neoplasm involving a single bone (solitary bone plasmacytoma (SBP)) or soft tissue site (solitary extramedullary plasmacytoma), occurring in approximately 5% of cases [62]. The diagnosis of a solitary plasmacytoma requires demonstration of clonal plasma cells in a lesional biopsy specimen, the absence of both end-organ damage, and evidence of other sites of involvement by imaging and no or less than 10% clonal plasma cells on separate bone marrow biopsy specimen as demonstrated, for example, by immunohistochemistry.
    - The cytogenetic findings in solitary plasmacytomas are like those of MM. Therefore, a similar panel of genetic testing [Table 17.1] would be reasonable in the analysis of the initial bone marrow biopsy specimen. Genetic testing can alternatively be performed on the plasmacytoma cells.
    - Cases with no clonal plasma cells on bone marrow biopsy show roughly 10% progression to MM over 3 years. Cases with less than 10% clonal plasma cells identified on bone marrow biopsy are classified as solitary plasmacytoma with minimal marrow involvement. These latter cases display a risk of progression to MM of about 60% over the first 3 years [63]. Even if morphologically and immunohistochemically inconspicuous, the presence of minimal bone marrow involvement as detected by flow cytometry has also been correlated with increased risk of progression to MM [63, 64]. NGS or other molecular testing for detecting minimal involvement

of the bone marrow at initial diagnosis has not been recommended.

- Treatment of SBP involves radiation therapy, typically without adjuvant systemic therapy. The persistence of the paraprotein 1 year after completion of radiation is associated with increased risk of relapse [65].
- Multifocal extramedullary multiple myeloma (EMM) is identified at diagnosis in up to 4.5% of patients and in up to 10% at relapse [66]. The presence of EMM confers a poor prognosis, particularly in the setting of relapsed MM, where it generally represents end-stage, aggressive disease with a median overall survival of less than 1.3 years [67–69]. The biology of EMM is not fully understood, but EMM is associated with high-risk cytogenetic findings, including increased incidence of t(4;14) and *TP53* mutation [70, 71]. *RAS* mutations have also been reported to be increased in EMM compared to bone marrow-restricted MM. EMM has been found to display decreased expression of CD56 and increased expression of CD44, molecules which are associated with cell adhesion and migration [72, 73].

14. **Do Results of Mutation Analysis Guide Therapy?**
    - All currently approved MM-directed therapies, including proteasome inhibitors, immunomodulatory agents, and monoclonal antibodies, target aspects of plasma cell biology rather than tumor-specific molecular and genetic abnormalities [74].
    - Venetoclax, a Bcl-2-specific inhibitor, is currently being studied in MM and has shown increased efficacy in t(11;14) patients with a single agent response rate of 40%, compared to 6% in non-t(11;14) patients [75]. Expression of Bcl-2 and the ratio of Bcl-2 to the related anti-apoptotic proteins Bcl-xL and Mcl-1 have also been reported to stratify patients more likely to respond to venetoclax [76–79].
    - The genomes of MM patients are highly heterogeneous. Numerous studies have utilized NGS analysis to catalog the mutational spectrum in MM [9, 10, 80]. Clinical trials using mutational profiling are underway to investigate the benefit of therapies targeting common MM mutations present in BRAF (vemurafenib), the RAS/MAPK pathway (cobimetinib), the CDK pathway (abemaciclib), FGFR3 (erdafitinib), and IDH2 (enasidenib) [3]. Thus, mutational profiling does not currently play a role outside of clinical trials for therapy decisions for MM or other plasma cell neoplasms.
15. **What are some potential new genomic markers for high-risk multiple myeloma that are not yet employed clinically?**
    - Despite the utility of current cytogenetics and FISH studies for identifying high-risk patients, and the therapeutic effectiveness of modern induction regimens, 20% of standard-risk patients still relapse within 2 years of diagnosis, highlighting the limitations of relying solely on t(4;14), t(14;16), and deletion 17p FISH for risk stratification.
    - Approximately 25% of patients with deletion 17p also have a *TP53* mutation, resulting in biallelic disruption of *TP53*. Early studies suggest that biallelic disruption yields a significantly higher risk of disease progression within the first 18 months of diagnosis, compared to deletion 17p alone (50% vs. 17.1%) [81, 82]. Monoallelic deletion 17p without *TP53* mutation has outcomes closer to those with wild-type *TP53*, and therefore only those patients with a "double-hit" may be high risk. Thus, combined testing for 17p deletion and TP53 mutation may at some point be recommended for routine clinical evaluation of MM.
    - Gene expression profiling (GEP) by either cDNA microarray or, more recently, RNA sequencing has been used to identify gene sets that correlate with novel biologic and prognostic categories in MM. Three gene sets consisting of 15, 70, and 92 genes have been reported to distinguish low-risk from high-risk patients [83, 84]. However, this GEP analysis has not been adopted clinically due to its technical complexity, including purification of plasma cells, and the heterogeneity in the gene sets reported [85].

Case Presentations

Case 1

Learning Objective(s)

- Review the initial workup and diagnostic criteria for symptomatic myeloma.
- Understand the process of staging and risk stratification.
- Correlate risk stratification with treatment selection and plan.

Case History

A 64-year-old female initially presented to the emergency department with worsening back pain. A plain film of the thoracic spine revealed an acute T10 vertebral compression fracture. A subsequent MRI T-spine confirmed the lesion showing 20% height loss at T10. She underwent palliative vertebroplasty. Based on clinical concern for multiple myeloma, additional evaluation included serum protein electrophoresis and immunofixation, urine protein electrophoresis and immunofixation, serum free light chains, quantitative immunoglobulins, β2-microglobulin, complete blood count, comprehensive metabolic panel, bone imaging with PET-CT, and a bone marrow biopsy with a myeloma FISH panel and traditional karyotyping.

Laboratory and Morphology Findings

Immunologic studies were notable for a paraprotein of 5.3 g/dL of IgG kappa isotype. Serum free kappa light chains were elevated at 443 mg/L with an abnormal free light chain ratio of 211 and an elevated IgG of 6670. Her Hgb was low at 9.9 g/dL, while serum calcium and creatinine levels were within reference range. Serum albumin 3.8, β2-microglobulin 3.2, and serum LDH were within reference ranges. Urine protein electrophoresis and immunofixation showed 184 mg/24 hr. of free kappa light chain paraprotein.

Bone marrow biopsy was notable for a hypercellular marrow with 60% clonal plasma cells.

Imaging Studies

PET-CT again demonstrated the T10 lesion as well as additional compression fractures at T12, L1, L2, and L3.

Genetic Study

Myeloma FISH analysis was notable for monosomy 13 as well as trisomies of chromosomes 9 and 11. FISH analysis was negative for deletion (17p), t(4;14), and t(14;16).

Chromosome analysis showed a normal female 46, XX [20] karyotype.

Final Diagnosis

Multiple myeloma (plasma cell myeloma) with standard-risk genetic features

Discussion

The finding of 60% clonal plasma cells on bone marrow meets criteria for a diagnosis of multiple myeloma. The lack of detected high-risk genetic abnormalities [Table 17.1] as well as serum albumin >3.5, β2M < 3.5, and a normal LDH stages this patient as R-ISS stage 1. Induction therapy was initiated with daratumumab, lenalidomide, bortezomib, and dexamethasone (Dara-RVD). The patient displayed a complete response by the International Myeloma Working Group response criteria [37]. She subsequently underwent successful stem cell mobilization and collection followed by an autologous stem cell transplant. She is currently receiving lenalidomide maintenance therapy and remains in a CR.

Case 2

Learning Objectives

- Review genetic markers of high-risk myeloma.
- Understand stratification of high-risk disease based on cytogenetics.
- Apply genetic information to determine treatment strategy.

Case History

A 46-year-old female with a history of seasonal allergies presented to her primary care physician with complaints of worsening fatigue and was found to be anemic with a hemoglobin of 8.0 g/dL. She was subsequently referred to hematology, and a full workup was initiated including immunologic studies for plasma cell neoplasms.

Laboratory and Morphology Findings

Serum protein electrophoresis and immunofixation revealed an M-spike of 3.5 g/dL of an IgA kappa paraprotein with a free kappa light chain of 56 mg/L and an abnormal free light chain ratio of 31.5. β2M was 2.77, serum albumin was 4.5, and LDH was 113. Calcium and creatinine levels were within reference range. Anemia workup was also unrevealing with a normal iron panel, B12, and folic acid levels.

Bone marrow biopsy and aspirate demonstrated a hypercellular marrow with 70% clonal plasma cells.

Imaging Studies

Skeletal survey was negative for lytic bone disease.

Genetic Studies

Myeloma FISH panel was positive for gain of 1q21, monosomy 13, and t(4;14).

Chromosome analysis showed a normal female karyotype 46,XX [20].

Final Diagnosis

Multiple myeloma (plasma cell myeloma) with high-risk features (R-ISS 2)

Follow-Up

She was initiated on therapy with carfilzomib, lenalidomide and dexamethasone and achieved a stringent complete response after four cycles. Her hemoglobin, which had dropped to 5.9 g/dL by the time of therapy initiation, had improved to 13 g/dL. She underwent stem cell mobilization and collection followed by autologous stem cell transplant and was resumed on a more intensive carfilzomib-based triplet maintenance therapy.

Discussion

This patient has high-risk disease due to the presence of both t(4;14) and + 1q21 by FISH. As demonstrated in an analysis by Schmidt et al., patients with +1q21 with another high-risk feature show significantly shorter progression-free survival when compared to patients with +1q21 alone, when treated with lenalidomide, bortezomib, and dexamethasone (RVD) induction alone [86]. Thus, as previously discussed in terms of efficacy in the high-risk population, a carfilzomib-based induction regimen was employed, followed by autologous stem cell transplant. Furthermore, a triplet maintenance strategy was chosen given her high-risk features, as data have shown improved progression-free survival when compared to high-risk patients treated with lenalidomide maintenance alone. The identification of the genetic abnormalities was critical in directing this patient to the appropriate, more aggressive treatment.

Case 3

Learning Objective(s)

- Review the definition of plasma cell leukemia.
- Recognize the association of t(11;14) with PCL.

Case History

A 70-year-old female with a history of hypertension and hyperlipidemia initially presented to the emergency department with complaints of progressively worsening back pain and lower extremity weakness. With laboratory abnormalities already suspicious for an underlying diagnosis of myeloma, a skeletal survey was obtained and demonstrated numerous lytic lesions throughout the axial and appendicular skeleton.

Laboratory and Morphologic Findings

Laboratory evaluation was notable for a serum creatinine of 2.44 mg/dL, BUN 44 mg/dL, serum calcium of 12.1 mg/dL, LDH 278 U/L, WBC 11.5 × 10^3/μL, hemoglobin 6.7 g/dL, and platelet count of 80 × 10^3/μL. Serum protein electrophoresis was negative for paraprotein, but serum immunofixation identified a free kappa light chain band. Serum free kappa light chains were elevated (603 mg/L) with a free light chain ratio of 215. Urine protein immunofixation detected a free kappa light chain paraprotein.

Blood smear review showed numerous atypical plasmacytoid cells [Fig. 17.1a]. Blood flow cytometry analysis identified a population of cells that comprised approximately 77% of the sample and expressed CD81, CD38 (bright), and CD138 and exhibited cytoplasmic kappa light chain restriction, but lacked CD19, CD20, CD56, and CD45.

Imaging Studies

A CT-guided biopsy of a left femoral lytic lesion was consistent with a plasma cell neoplasm.

Genetic Studies

The MM FISH panel was applied to a blood sample given the high percentage of circulating plasma cells and was positive for deletion of both copies of 1p in 84% of cells, positive for loss of one copy of 1q and loss of both copies of 1p in 3% of cells, positive for t(11;14) in 82% of cells [Fig. 17.1b], and positive for monosomy 13 in 84% of cells.

Final Diagnosis

Plasma cell leukemia

Follow-Up

The patient was admitted to the hospital and given aggressive intravenous chemotherapy with VDT-PACE (bortezomib, dexamethasone, thalidomide, cisplatin, doxorubicin, cyclophosphamide, and etoposide). Her course was complicated by a catheter-associated bacteremia treated with intra-

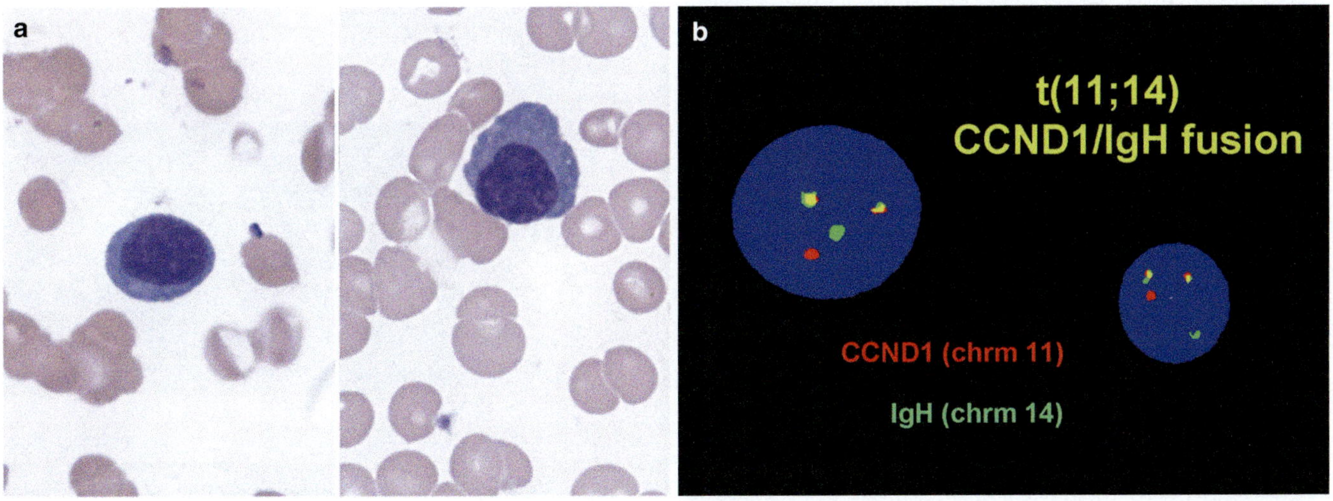

Fig. 17.1 (**a**) Typical of plasma cell leukemia, atypical plasmacytoid cells are numerous on a Wright-stained blood smear. (**b**) FISH analysis, using dual-color, dual-fusion probes against the *CCND1* locus (red) and *IGH* locus (green), demonstrates two fusion signals (yellow) per nucleus, consistent with a t(11;14) balanced translocation, found with increased frequency in plasma cell leukemia

venous antibiotics. She recovered her counts and was discharged to follow up in the clinic, where she began induction therapy followed by autologous stem cell transplant.

Discussion

Plasma cell leukemia is defined by either >20% or > 2×10^9 plasma cells in the blood [4]. This patient presented with diffuse lytic disease, anemia, renal dysfunction, and hypercalcemia with the presence of clonal plasma cells and 80% circulating plasma cells. This is a high-risk presentation, and this is further reflected by the multiple FISH abnormalities and complex karyotype. Of note, t(11;14) was detected, and this translocation is the most common MM-associated translocation identified in primary plasma cell leukemia.

Case 4

Learning Objectives

- Review presentation and diagnosis including molecular testing of therapy-related myeloid neoplasms.
- Discuss the correlation between lenalidomide therapy in myeloma patients and the risk of developing therapy-related myeloid neoplasms.

Case History

A 73-year-old man with a more than 7-year history of multiple myeloma is now status post-autologous stem transplant and currently in a complete response on lenalidomide maintenance therapy. On routine laboratory evaluation, he is noticed to have new-onset pancytopenia. His immunologic studies remain negative with an undetectable serum and urine protein. To further evaluate the etiology of his cytopenias, a bone marrow biopsy is performed.

Laboratory and Morphology Findings

Blood smear and CBC data confirmed pancytopenia. Bone marrow morphology showed dysplastic erythroid precursors and megakaryocytes, about 15% blasts, and rare plasma cells [Fig. 17.2a].

Flow cytometric immunophenotyping demonstrated a population that comprised 20% of the sample and expressed partial CD7 (dim), CD13, CD33, CD34, partial CD36, partial CD38 (dim), partial CD56 (dim), CD117, CD123 (dim), HLA-DR (dim), and CD45 (dim) and polytypic plasma cells.

Genetic Studies

Conventional cytogenetics demonstrated a complex abnormal male karyotype that included deletion 7q [Fig. 17.2b].

An MDS FISH panel was positive for deletion 7q in 85% of cells [Fig. 17.2c], though negative for trisomy 8, deletion 5q, and abnormality of 11q23 *KMT2A* (*MLL*). A FISH panel for MM-associated abnormalities was negative.

Final Diagnosis

Therapy-related myeloid neoplasm (t-MDS)

Follow-Up

Hypomethylating therapy with azacitidine was initiated. After four cycles of azacitidine, repeat bone marrow biopsy was done which unfortunately noted 40% increased blasts with >5% plasma cells in the aspirate smear and core biopsy. Flow cytometry confirmed a large population of myeloblasts supporting progressing to acute myeloid leukemia. A subsequent NGS myeloid mutation gene panel identified a tier 1 *IDH1* mutation that was detected in approximately 44% of alleles. The patient was enrolled on a clinical trial with the IDH1 inhibitor ivosidenib and remains on study to date.

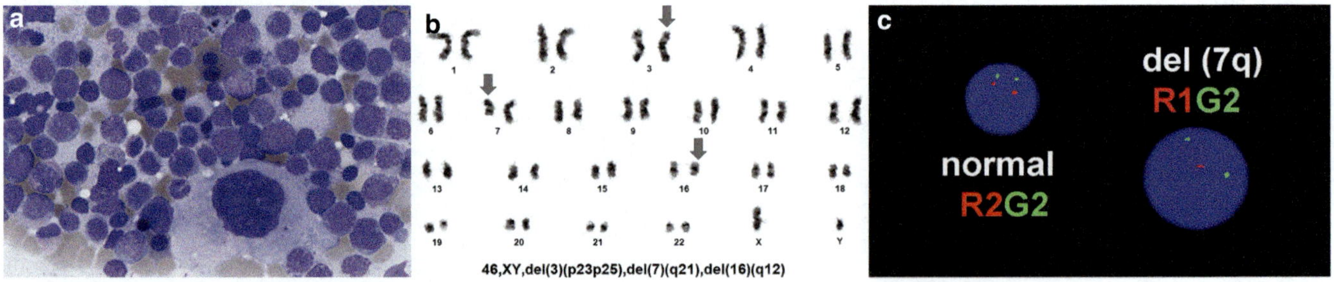

Fig. 17.2 (**a**) Cytomorphologic features of myelodysplasia, including increased blasts, left-shifted myeloid precursors, and a dysplastic megakaryocyte, can be observed in this Wright-stained bone marrow aspirate smear, from a patient treated for many years for multiple myeloma. (**b**) G-banded chromosomes are shown with the karyotype, for this representative cell, that includes several chromosomal deletions (red arrows) that can be observed in therapy-related myeloid neoplasms. (**c**) FISH analysis of chromosome 7 demonstrates deletion of one copy of 7q (red signal) with retention of the centromere of chromosome 7 (green signal) in the cell on the right and a normal pattern (two red and two green signals) in the cell on the left. Loss of 7q is a common adverse prognostic finding in therapy-related myeloid neoplasms

Discussion

Long-term therapy with lenalidomide is associated with an increased risk of second primary malignancies (SPMs). A meta-analysis of over 3000 newly diagnosed myeloma patients treated with lenalidomide demonstrated a cumulative incidence of SPMs at 5 years of 6.9% compared to 4.8% in patients that did not receive lenalidomide. The cumulative incidence specifically of hematologic second primary malignancies was 3.8% versus 3.4%; however [43], another meta-analysis specifically investigated the rate of second primary malignancies in patients on lenalidomide maintenance and found an increased rate of hematologic SPMs of 5.3% versus 0.8% prior to disease progression [87]. Multiple studies have demonstrated the progression-free survival and the overall survival benefit of continuous lenalidomide maintenance, and ongoing research is seeking to understand the optimal length of maintenance and to identify subsets of patients who could discontinue maintenance therapy after certain length of time [87–89]. However, for now, and though uncommon, SPMs are a worrying complication of lenalidomide maintenance therapy, and unexplained cytopenias should prompt an expedient workup including bone marrow evaluation with cytogenetic studies and, if indicated, a myeloid mutation panel. Therapy-related myeloid neoplasms portend a poor prognosis despite improved therapy options.

Case 5

Learning Objectives

- Understand the development and implication of secondary genetic events in relapsed and refractory myeloma.

Case History

A 65-year-old man with a long-standing history of standard risk myeloma, ISS stage 2, presents with progressive disease. After induction therapy following his initial diagnosis, he received an autologous bone marrow transplant and was initiated on lenalidomide maintenance therapy. Four years post-transplant, he experienced disease progression and was started on therapy with daratumumab, pomalidomide, and dexamethasone. FISH analysis on the bone marrow at the time of disease relapse demonstrated trisomy of chromosomes 7, 9, and 11 and was negative for deletion 17p. He now presents to for routine follow-up and is noted to have an increased paraprotein level. A restaging bone marrow biopsy was performed.

Laboratory and Morphology Findings

The blood smear and CBC data showed mild leukopenia. The bone marrow biopsy demonstrated a normocellular marrow with 5% plasma cells on the aspirate rate smear. Flow cytometric immunophenotyping showed a 1% clonal population of plasma cells that expressed CD38 (bright), CD56 (bright), CD117 (dim), and lambda light chain.

Genetic Studies

CD138-enriched plasma cells from bone marrow were prepared. FISH studies were positive for trisomy of chromosomes 7 and 9 [Fig. 17.3a] and for gain of 11q consistent with trisomy 11. In addition, gain of 1q, deletion 17p, and monosomy 13 were detected. A CN-SNP microarray confirmed the copy number abnormalities and additionally showed more complex findings including copy neutral loss of heterozygosity of chromosome 17 in most cells with deletion of 17p in a subset of cells [Fig. 17.3b].

Karyotyping showed a hyperdiploidy with 53,X,-Y, +4, +5, +7, add(8)(p11.2), +9, +9,+11,del(17)(p13),+21, and +mar[cp2]/46,XY [18].

Final Diagnosis

Relapsed, refractory multiple myeloma

Follow-Up

Based on disease relapse with acquisition of aggressive genetic features including deletion 17p and gain of 1q, the patient was offered combination therapy regimens versus clinical trial options. He was enrolled on a CAR-T cell therapy clinical trial for relapsed and refractory myeloma.

Discussion

This case demonstrates the importance of including analysis for secondary events that can predict a more aggressive phase of disease. Initial primary events, such as hyperdiploidy, are often detected initially at diagnosis and continue to be identified on subsequent bone marrow samples, as seen in the case. However, secondary events such as gain of additional copies of chromosome 1q and deletion 17p can appear as the plasma cell clone evolves through multiple relapses. This highlights the relevance of having a broad FISH panel that includes probes for secondary events, and points to the unique information provided by CN-SNP arrays. These acquired genetic abnormalities signal an aggressive transformation of the disease and can help inform treatment decisions.

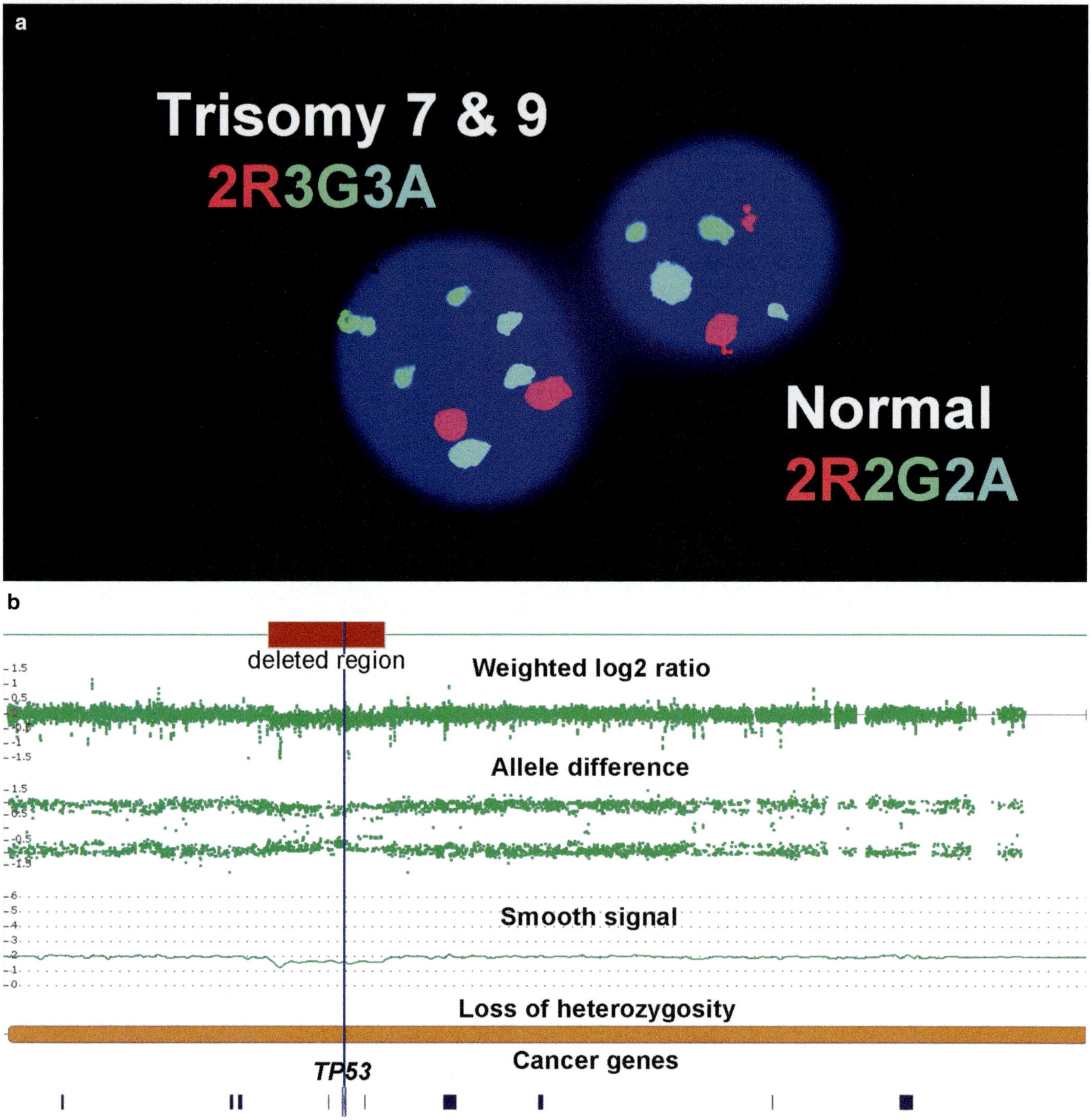

Fig. 17.3 (**a**) Using centromere probes, FISH studies displayed three copies of chromosomes 7 (green) and 9 (aqua) and two copies of chromosome 3 (red), in the cell on the left. The cell on the right demonstrates a normal pattern with two signals for all probes. Hyperdiploidy is considered a primary genetic event in multiple myeloma that often includes trisomy of chromosomes 3, 7, and/or 9. (**b**) Analysis of chromosome 17 from CD138-enriched multiple myeloma cells by CN-SNP microarray is shown. The array result defines a deleted region of 17p (red bar), including the *TP53* gene locus (blue line). Deletion of the *TP53* locus is considered an adverse secondary genetic event in multiple myeloma. The deleted region is identified in different ways by the weighted log2 ratio, the allele difference track, and smooth signal, which together suggest involvement in a subset of cells. The allele difference track, largely lacking AB signal across the chromosome, furthermore, indicates copy neutral loss of heterozygosity (orange bar), an additional adverse prognostic finding that is not apparent in routine FISH and karyotyping

References

1. Mathur P, Sathishkumar K, Chaturvedi M, Das P, Sudarshan KL, Santhappan S, et al. Cancer statistics, 2020: report from national cancer registry programme, India. JCO Glob Oncol. 2020;6:1063–75. https://doi.org/10.1200/GO.20.00122.
2. Rajkumar SV, Dimopoulos MA, Palumbo A, Blade J, Merlini G, Mateos MV, et al. International myeloma working group updated criteria for the diagnosis of multiple myeloma. Lancet Oncol. 2014;15(12):e538–48. https://doi.org/10.1016/S1470-2045(14)70442-5.
3. Kumar SK, Callander NS, Hillengass J, Liedtke M, Baljevic M, Campagnaro E, et al. NCCN guidelines insights: multiple myeloma, version 1.2020. J Natl Compr Cancer Netw. 2019;17(10):1154–65. https://doi.org/10.6004/jnccn.2019.0049.
4. Swerdlow SH, Campo E, Harris NL, Jaffe ES, Pileri SA, Stein H, et al., editors. WHO classification of tumours of haematopoietic and lymphoid tissues. 4th ed. Lyon: IARC publications; 2017.
5. Palumbo A, Avet-Loiseau H, Oliva S, Lokhorst HM, Goldschmidt H, Rosinol L, et al. Revised international staging system for multiple myeloma: a report from international myeloma working group. J Clin Oncol. 2015;33(26):2863–9. https://doi.org/10.1200/JCO.2015.61.2267.
6. Kumar SK, Jacobus SJ, Cohen AD, Weiss M, Callander N, Singh AK, et al. Carfilzomib or bortezomib in combination with lenalidomide and dexamethasone for patients with newly diagnosed multiple myeloma without intention for immediate autologous stem-cell transplantation (ENDURANCE): a multicentre, open-label, phase 3, randomised, controlled trial. Lancet Oncol. 2020; https://doi.org/10.1016/S1470-2045(20)30452-6.
7. Barwick BG, Gupta VA, Vertino PM, Boise LH. Cell of origin and genetic alterations in the pathogenesis of multiple myeloma. Front Immunol. 2019;10:1121. https://doi.org/10.3389/fimmu.2019.01121.
8. Barwick BG, Neri P, Bahlis NJ, Nooka AK, Dhodapkar MV, Jaye DL, et al. Multiple myeloma immunoglobulin lambda translocations portend poor prognosis. Nat Commun. 2019;10(1):1911. https://doi.org/10.1038/s41467-019-09555-6.
9. Chapman MA, Lawrence MS, Keats JJ, Cibulskis K, Sougnez C, Schinzel AC, et al. Initial genome sequencing and analysis of multiple myeloma. Nature. 2011;471(7339):467–72. https://doi.org/10.1038/nature09837.
10. Lohr JG, Stojanov P, Carter SL, Cruz-Gordillo P, Lawrence MS, Auclair D, et al. Widespread genetic heterogeneity in multiple myeloma: implications for targeted therapy. Cancer Cell. 2014;25(1):91–101. https://doi.org/10.1016/j.ccr.2013.12.015.
11. Walker BA, Wardell CP, Melchor L, Brioli A, Johnson DC, Kaiser MF, et al. Intraclonal heterogeneity is a critical early event in the development of myeloma and precedes the development of clinical symptoms. Leukemia. 2014;28(2):384–90. https://doi.org/10.1038/leu.2013.199.
12. Saxe D, Seo EJ, Bergeron MB, Han JY. Recent advances in cytogenetic characterization of multiple myeloma. Int J Lab Hematol. 2019;41(1):5–14. https://doi.org/10.1111/ijlh.12882.
13. Manier S, Salem KZ, Park J, Landau DA, Getz G, Ghobrial IM. Genomic complexity of multiple myeloma and its clinical implications. Nat Rev Clin Oncol. 2017;14(2):100–13. https://doi.org/10.1038/nrclinonc.2016.122.
14. Van Wier S, Braggio E, Baker A, Ahmann G, Levy J, Carpten JD, et al. Hypodiploid multiple myeloma is characterized by more aggressive molecular markers than non-hyperdiploid multiple myeloma. Haematologica. 2013;98(10):1586–92. https://doi.org/10.3324/haematol.2012.081083.
15. Stevens-Kroef M, Weghuis DO, Croockewit S, Derksen L, Hooijer J, Elidrissi-Zaynoun N, et al. High detection rate of clinically relevant genomic abnormalities in plasma cells enriched from patients with multiple myeloma. Genes Chromosomes Cancer. 2012;51(11):997–1006. https://doi.org/10.1002/gcc.21982.
16. Berry NK, Bain NL, Enjeti AK, Rowlings P. Genomic profiling of plasma cell disorders in a clinical setting: integration of microarray and FISH, after CD138 selection of bone marrow. J Clin Pathol. 2014;67(1):66–9. https://doi.org/10.1136/jclinpath-2013-201691.
17. Durie BG, Salmon SE. Cellular kinetics staging, and immunoglobulin synthesis in multiple myeloma. Annu Rev Med. 1975;26:283–8. https://doi.org/10.1146/annurev.me.26.020175.001435.
18. Greipp PR, San Miguel J, Durie BG, Crowley JJ, Barlogie B, Blade J, et al. International staging system for multiple myeloma. J Clin Oncol. 2005;23(15):3412–20. https://doi.org/10.1200/JCO.2005.04.242.
19. Weiss BM, Abadie J, Verma P, Howard RS, Kuehl WM. A monoclonal gammopathy precedes multiple myeloma in most patients. Blood. 2009;113(22):5418–22. https://doi.org/10.1182/blood-2008-12-195008.
20. Landgren O, Kyle RA, Pfeiffer RM, Katzmann JA, Caporaso NE, Hayes RB, et al. Monoclonal gammopathy of undetermined significance (MGUS) consistently precedes multiple myeloma: a prospective study. Blood. 2009;113(22):5412–7. https://doi.org/10.1182/blood-2008-12-194241.
21. Kyle RA, Remstein ED, Therneau TM, Dispenzieri A, Kurtin PJ, Hodnefield JM, et al. Clinical course and prognosis of smoldering (asymptomatic) multiple myeloma. N Engl J Med. 2007;356(25):2582–90. https://doi.org/10.1056/NEJMoa070389.
22. Rajkumar SV, Kyle RA, Therneau TM, Melton LJ 3rd, Bradwell AR, Clark RJ, et al. Serum free light chain ratio is an independent risk factor for progression in monoclonal gammopathy of undetermined significance. Blood. 2005;106(3):812–7. https://doi.org/10.1182/blood-2005-03-1038.
23. Fonseca R, Bailey RJ, Ahmann GJ, Rajkumar SV, Hoyer JD, Lust JA, et al. Genomic abnormalities in monoclonal gammopathy of undetermined significance. Blood. 2002;100(4):1417–24.
24. Mouhieddine TH, Weeks LD, Ghobrial IM. Monoclonal gammopathy of undetermined significance. Blood. 2019;133(23):2484–94. https://doi.org/10.1182/blood.2019846782.
25. Lakshman A, Rajkumar SV, Buadi FK, Binder M, Gertz MA, Lacy MQ, et al. Risk stratification of smoldering multiple myeloma incorporating revised IMWG diagnostic criteria. Blood Cancer J. 2018;8(6):59. https://doi.org/10.1038/s41408-018-0077-4.
26. San Miguel J, Mateos MV, Gonzalez V, Dimopoulos MA, Kastritis E, Hajek R, et al. Updated risk stratification model for smoldering multiple myeloma (SMM) incorporating the revised IMWG diagnostic criteria. J Clin Oncol. 2019;37(15_suppl) 8000.
27. Lonial S, Jacobus S, Fonseca R, Weiss M, Kumar S, Orlowski RZ, et al. Randomized trial of lenalidomide versus observation in smoldering multiple myeloma. J Clin Oncol. 2019:JCO1901740. https://doi.org/10.1200/JCO.19.01740.
28. Avet-Loiseau H, Fonseca R, Siegel D, Dimopoulos MA, Spicka I, Masszi T, et al. Carfilzomib significantly improves the progression-free survival of high-risk patients in multiple myeloma. Blood. 2016;128(9):1174–80. https://doi.org/10.1182/blood-2016-03-707596.
29. Nooka AK, Kaufman JL, Muppidi S, Langston A, Heffner LT, Gleason C, et al. Consolidation and maintenance therapy with lenalidomide, bortezomib and dexamethasone (RVD) in high-risk myeloma patients. Leukemia. 2014;28(3):690–3. https://doi.org/10.1038/leu.2013.335.
30. Fakhri B, Vij R. Clonal evolution in multiple myeloma. Clin Lymphoma Myeloma Leuk. 2016;16(Suppl):S130–4. https://doi.org/10.1016/j.clml.2016.02.025.
31. Diamond BT, Rustad E, Maclachlan K, Thoren K, Ho C, Roshal M, et al. Defining the undetectable: the current landscape of mini-

mal residual disease assessment in multiple myeloma and goals for future clarity. Blood Rev. 2020:100732. https://doi.org/10.1016/j.blre.2020.100732.
32. Faham M, Zheng J, Moorhead M, Carlton VEH, Stow P, Coustan-Smith E, et al. Deep-sequencing approach for minimal residual disease detection in acute lymphoblastic leukemia. Blood. 2012;120(26):5173–80. https://doi.org/10.1182/blood-2012-07-444042.
33. Flores-Montero J, Sanoja-Flores L, Paiva B, Puig N, García-Sánchez O, Böttcher S, et al. Next generation flow for highly sensitive and standardized detection of minimal residual disease in multiple myeloma. Leukemia. 2017;31(10):2094–103. https://doi.org/10.1038/leu.2017.29.
34. Sanoja-Flores L, Flores-Montero J, Puig N, Contreras-Sanfeliciano T, Pontes R, Corral-Mateos A, et al. Blood monitoring of circulating tumor plasma cells by next generation flow in multiple myeloma after therapy. Blood. 2019;134(24):2218–22. https://doi.org/10.1182/blood.2019002610.
35. Roshal M, Flores-Montero JA, Gao Q, Koeber M, Wardrope J, Durie BGM, et al. MRD detection in multiple myeloma: comparison between MSKCC 10-color single-tube and EuroFlow 8-color 2-tube methods. Blood Adv. 2017;1(12):728–32. https://doi.org/10.1182/bloodadvances.2016003715.
36. Bergen HR III, Dasari S, Dispenzieri A, Mills JR, Ramirez-Alvarado M, Tschumper RC, et al. Clonotypic light chain peptides identified for monitoring minimal residual disease in multiple myeloma without bone marrow aspiration. Clin Chem. 2016;62(1):243–51. https://doi.org/10.1373/clinchem.2015.242651.
37. Kumar S, Paiva B, Anderson KC, Durie B, Landgren O, Moreau P, et al. International myeloma working group consensus criteria for response and minimal residual disease assessment in multiple myeloma. Lancet Oncol. 2016;17(8):e328–e46. https://doi.org/10.1016/S1470-2045(16)30206-6.
38. Musto P, Anderson KC, Attal M, Richardson PG, Badros A, Hou J, et al. Second primary malignancies in multiple myeloma: an overview and IMWG consensus. Ann Oncol. 2017;28(2):228–45. https://doi.org/10.1093/annonc/mdw606.
39. Yang W, Stotler B, Sevilla DW, Emmons FN, Murty VV, Alobeid B, et al. FISH analysis in addition to G-band karyotyping: utility in evaluation of myelodysplastic syndromes? Leuk Res. 2010;34(4):420–5. https://doi.org/10.1016/j.leukres.2009.09.013.
40. Reddi DM, Lu CM, Fedoriw G, Liu Y-C, Wang FF, Ely S, et al. Myeloid neoplasms secondary to plasma cell myeloma: an intrinsic predisposition or therapy-related phenomenon?: a Clinicopathologic study of 41 cases and correlation of cytogenetic features with treatment regimens. Am J Clin Pathol. 2012;138(6):855–66. https://doi.org/10.1309/AJCPOP7APGDT9JIU.
41. Gertz MA, Terpos E, Dispenzieri A, Kumar S, Shah RA, Orlowski R, et al. Therapy-related myelodysplastic syndrome/acute leukemia after multiple myeloma in the era of novel agents. Leuk Lymphoma. 2015;56(6):1723–6. https://doi.org/10.3109/10428194.2014.970543.
42. White JS, Zordan A, Batzios C, Campbell LJ. Deletion(20q) as the sole abnormality in plasma cell myeloma is not associated with plasma cells as identified by cIg FISH. Cancer Genet. 2012;205(12):644–52. https://doi.org/10.1016/j.cancergen.2012.10.007.
43. Palumbo A, Bringhen S, Kumar SK, Lupparelli G, Usmani S, Waage A, et al. Second primary malignancies with lenalidomide therapy for newly diagnosed myeloma: a meta-analysis of individual patient data. Lancet Oncol. 2014;15(3):333–42. https://doi.org/10.1016/S1470-2045(13)70609-0.
44. Gertz MA. Immunoglobulin light chain amyloidosis: 2018 update on diagnosis, prognosis, and treatment. Am J Hematol. 2018;93(9):1169–80. https://doi.org/10.1002/ajh.25149.
45. Dispenzieri A, Merlini G. Immunoglobulin light chain systemic amyloidosis. Cancer Treat Res. 2016;169:273–318. https://doi.org/10.1007/978-3-319-40320-5_15.
46. Hayman SR, Bailey RJ, Jalal SM, Ahmann GJ, Dispenzieri A, Gertz MA, et al. Translocations involving the immunoglobulin heavy-chain locus are possible early genetic events in patients with primary systemic amyloidosis. Blood. 2001;98(7):2266–8. https://doi.org/10.1182/blood.v98.7.2266.
47. Bochtler T, Hegenbart U, Kunz C, Granzow M, Benner A, Seckinger A, et al. Translocation t(11;14) is associated with adverse outcome in patients with newly diagnosed AL amyloidosis when treated with bortezomib-based regimens. J Clin Oncol. 2015;33(12):1371–8. https://doi.org/10.1200/jco.2014.57.4947.
48. Abraham RS, Geyer SM, Price-Troska TL, Allmer C, Kyle RA, Gertz MA, et al. Immunoglobulin light chain variable (V) region genes influence clinical presentation and outcome in light chain-associated amyloidosis (AL). Blood. 2003;101(10):3801–8. https://doi.org/10.1182/blood-2002-09-2707.
49. Kumar S, Dispenzieri A, Katzmann JA, Larson DR, Colby CL, Lacy MQ, et al. Serum immunoglobulin free light-chain measurement in primary amyloidosis: prognostic value and correlations with clinical features. Blood. 2010;116(24):5126–9. https://doi.org/10.1182/blood-2010-06-290668.
50. Perfetti V, Palladini G, Casarini S, Navazza V, Rognoni P, Obici L, et al. The repertoire of λ light chains causing predominant amyloid heart involvement and identification of a preferentially involved germline gene, IGLV1-44. Blood. 2012;119(1):144–50. https://doi.org/10.1182/blood-2011-05-355784.
51. Kumar S, Dispenzieri A, Lacy MQ, Hayman SR, Buadi FK, Colby C, et al. Revised prognostic staging system for light chain amyloidosis incorporating cardiac biomarkers and serum free light chain measurements. J Clin Oncol. 2012;30(9):989–95. https://doi.org/10.1200/jco.2011.38.5724.
52. Fernández de Larrea C, Kyle RA, Durie BG, Ludwig H, Usmani S, Vesole DH, et al. Plasma cell leukemia: consensus statement on diagnostic requirements, response criteria and treatment recommendations by the International Myeloma Working Group. Leukemia. 2013;27(4):780–91. https://doi.org/10.1038/leu.2012.336.
53. Jurczyszyn A, Castillo JJ, Avivi I, Czepiel J, Davila J, Vij R, et al. Secondary plasma cell leukemia: a multicenter retrospective study of 101 patients. Leuk Lymphoma. 2019;60(1):118–23. https://doi.org/10.1080/10428194.2018.1473574.
54. Mina R, D'Agostino M, Cerrato C, Gay F, Palumbo A. Plasma cell leukemia: update on biology and therapy. Leuk Lymphoma. 2017;58(7):1538–47. https://doi.org/10.1080/10428194.2016.1250263.
55. Gonsalves WI, Rajkumar SV, Go RS, Dispenzieri A, Gupta V, Singh PP, et al. Trends in survival of patients with primary plasma cell leukemia: a population-based analysis. Blood. 2014;124(6):907–12. https://doi.org/10.1182/blood-2014-03-565051.
56. Gundesen MT, Lund T, Moeller HEH, Abildgaard N. Plasma cell leukemia: definition, presentation, and treatment. Curr Oncol Rep. 2019;21(1):8. https://doi.org/10.1007/s11912-019-0754-x.
57. Tiedemann RE, Gonzalez-Paz N, Kyle RA, Santana-Davila R, Price-Troska T, Van Wier SA, et al. Genetic aberrations and survival in plasma cell leukemia. Leukemia. 2008;22(5):1044–52. https://doi.org/10.1038/leu.2008.4.
58. Chiecchio L, Dagrada GP, White HE, Towsend MR, Protheroe RK, Cheung KL, et al. Frequent upregulation of MYC in plasma cell leukemia. Genes Chromosomes Cancer. 2009;48(7):624–36. https://doi.org/10.1002/gcc.20670.
59. Cifola I, Lionetti M, Pinatel E, Todoerti K, Mangano E, Pietrelli A, et al. Whole-exome sequencing of primary plasma cell leukemia discloses heterogeneous mutational patterns. Oncotarget. 2015;6(19):17543–58. https://doi.org/10.18632/oncotarget.4028.
60. Egan JB, Shi CX, Tembe W, Christoforides A, Kurdoglu A, Sinari S, et al. Whole-genome sequencing of multiple myeloma from diagnosis to plasma cell leukemia reveals genomic initiating events, evolution, and clonal tides. Blood. 2012;120(5):1060–6. https://doi.org/10.1182/blood-2012-01-405977.

61. Keats JJ, Chesi M, Egan JB, Garbitt VM, Palmer SE, Braggio E, et al. Clonal competition with alternating dominance in multiple myeloma. Blood. 2012;120(5):1067–76. https://doi.org/10.1182/blood-2012-01-405985.
62. Pham A, Mahindra A. Solitary plasmacytoma: a review of diagnosis and management. Curr Hematol Malig Rep. 2019;14(2):63–9. https://doi.org/10.1007/s11899-019-00499-8.
63. Hill QA, Rawstron AC, de Tute RM, Owen RG. Outcome prediction in plasmacytoma of bone: a risk model utilizing bone marrow flow cytometry and light-chain analysis. Blood. 2014;124(8):1296–9. https://doi.org/10.1182/blood-2014-04-566521.
64. Paiva B, Chandia M, Vidriales MB, Colado E, Caballero-Velázquez T, Escalante F, et al. Multiparameter flow cytometry for staging of solitary bone plasmacytoma: new criteria for risk of progression to myeloma. Blood. 2014;124(8):1300–3. https://doi.org/10.1182/blood-2014-04-567909.
65. Wilder RB, Ha CS, Cox JD, Weber D, Delasalle K, Alexanian R. Persistence of myeloma protein for more than one year after radiotherapy is an adverse prognostic factor in solitary plasmacytoma of bone. Cancer. 2002;94(5):1532–7. https://doi.org/10.1002/cncr.10366.
66. Bhutani M, Foureau DM, Atrash S, Voorhees PM, Usmani SZ. Extramedullary multiple myeloma. Leukemia. 2020;34(1):1–20. https://doi.org/10.1038/s41375-019-0660-0.
67. Pour L, Sevcikova S, Greslikova H, Kupska R, Majkova P, Zahradova L, et al. Soft-tissue extramedullary multiple myeloma prognosis is significantly worse in comparison to bone-related extramedullary relapse. Haematologica. 2014;99(2):360–4. https://doi.org/10.3324/haematol.2013.094409.
68. Weinstock M, Aljawai Y, Morgan EA, Laubach J, Gannon M, Roccaro AM, et al. Incidence and clinical features of extramedullary multiple myeloma in patients who underwent stem cell transplantation. Br J Haematol. 2015;169(6):851–8. https://doi.org/10.1111/bjh.13383.
69. Beksac M, Seval GC, Kanellias N, Coriu D, Rosiñol L, Ozet G, et al. A real world multicenter retrospective study on extramedullary disease from Balkan myeloma study group and Barcelona university: analysis of parameters that improve outcome. Haematologica. 2020;105(1):201–8. https://doi.org/10.3324/haematol.2019.219295.
70. Rasche L, Bernard C, Topp MS, Kapp M, Duell J, Wesemeier C, et al. Features of extramedullary myeloma relapse: high proliferation, minimal marrow involvement, adverse cytogenetics: a retrospective single-center study of 24 cases. Ann Hematol. 2012;91(7):1031–7. https://doi.org/10.1007/s00277-012-1414-5.
71. Deng S, Xu Y, An G, Sui W, Zou D, Zhao Y, et al. Features of extramedullary disease of multiple myeloma: high frequency of p53 deletion and poor survival: a retrospective single-center study of 834 cases. Clin Lymphoma Myeloma Leuk. 2015;15(5):286–91. https://doi.org/10.1016/j.clml.2014.12.013.
72. Pellat-Deceunynck C, Barillé S, Puthier D, Rapp MJ, Harousseau JL, Bataille R, et al. Adhesion molecules on human myeloma cells: significant changes in expression related to malignancy, tumor spreading, and immortalization. Cancer Res. 1995;55(16):3647–53.
73. Dahl IM, Rasmussen T, Kauric G, Husebekk A. Differential expression of CD56 and CD44 in the evolution of extramedullary myeloma. Br J Haematol. 2002;116(2):273–7. https://doi.org/10.1046/j.1365-2141.2002.03258.x.
74. Boise LH, Kaufman JL, Bahlis NJ, Lonial S, Lee KP. The Tao of myeloma. Blood. 2014;124(12):1873–9. https://doi.org/10.1182/blood-2014-05-578732.
75. Kumar S, Kaufman JL, Gasparetto C, Mikhael J, Vij R, Pegourie B, et al. Efficacy of venetoclax as targeted therapy for relapsed/refractory t(11;14) multiple myeloma. Blood. 2017;130(22):2401–9. https://doi.org/10.1182/blood-2017-06-788786.
76. Gong J-N, Khong T, Segal D, Yao Y, Riffkin CD, Garnier J-M, et al. Hierarchy for targeting prosurvival BCL2 family proteins in multiple myeloma: pivotal role of MCL1. Blood. 2016;128(14):1834.
77. Punnoose EA, Leverson JD, Peale F, Boghaert ER, Belmont LD, Tan N, et al. Expression profile of BCL-2, BCL-XL, and MCL-1 predicts pharmacological response to the BCL-2 selective antagonist Venetoclax in multiple myeloma models. Mol Cancer Ther. 2016;15(5):1132–44. https://doi.org/10.1158/1535-7163.MCT-15-0730.
78. Touzeau C, Moreau P. How I treat extramedullary myeloma. Blood. 2016;127(8):971–6. https://doi.org/10.1182/blood-2015-07-635383.
79. Gomez-Bougie P, Maiga S, Tessoulin B, Bourcier J, Bonnet A, Rodriguez MS, et al. BH3-mimetic toolkit guides the respective use of BCL2 and MCL1 BH3-mimetics in myeloma treatment. Blood. 2018;132(25):2656–69. https://doi.org/10.1182/blood-2018-03-836718.
80. Walker BA, Mavrommatis K, Wardell CP, Ashby TC, Bauer M, Davies FE, et al. Identification of novel mutational drivers reveals oncogene dependencies in multiple myeloma. Blood. 2018;132(6):587–97. https://doi.org/10.1182/blood-2018-03-840132.
81. Walker BA, Mavrommatis K, Wardell CP, Ashby TC, Bauer M, Davies F, et al. A high-risk, double-hit, group of newly diagnosed myeloma identified by genomic analysis. Leukemia. 2019;33(1):159–70. https://doi.org/10.1038/s41375-018-0196-8.
82. D'Agostino M, Zaccaria GM, Ziccheddu B, Rustad EH, Genuardi E, Capra A, et al. Early relapse risk in newly diagnosed multiple myeloma patients characterized by next-generation sequencing. Clin Cancer Res. 2020; https://doi.org/10.1158/1078-0432.Ccr-20-0951.
83. Decaux O, Lodé L, Magrangeas F, Charbonnel C, Gouraud W, Jézéquel P, et al. Prediction of survival in multiple myeloma based on gene expression profiles reveals cell cycle and chromosomal instability signatures in high-risk patients and hyperdiploid signatures in low-risk patients: a study of the Intergroupe Francophone du Myélome. J Clin Oncol. 2008;26(29):4798–805. https://doi.org/10.1200/jco.2007.13.8545.
84. Kuiper R, Broyl A, de Knegt Y, van Vliet MH, van Beers EH, van der Holt B, et al. A gene expression signature for high-risk multiple myeloma. Leukemia. 2012;26(11):2406–13. https://doi.org/10.1038/leu.2012.127.
85. Szalat R, Avet-Loiseau H, Munshi NC. Gene expression profiles in myeloma: ready for the real world? Clin Cancer Res. 2016;22(22):5434–42. https://doi.org/10.1158/1078-0432.ccr-16-0867.
86. Schmidt TM, Barwick BG, Joseph N, Heffner LT, Hofmeister CC, Bernal L, et al. Gain of chromosome 1q is associated with early progression in multiple myeloma patients treated with lenalidomide, bortezomib, and dexamethasone. Blood Cancer J. 2019;9(12):94. https://doi.org/10.1038/s41408-019-0254-0.
87. McCarthy PL, Holstein SA, Petrucci MT, Richardson PG, Hulin C, Tosi P, et al. Lenalidomide maintenance after autologous stem-cell transplantation in newly diagnosed multiple myeloma: a meta-analysis. J Clin Oncol. 2017;35(29):3279–89. https://doi.org/10.1200/JCO.2017.72.6679.
88. Joseph N, Kaufman J, Dhodapkar M, Hofmeister C, Almaula D, Heffner L, et al. Long-term follow-up results of lenalidomide, bortezomib, and dexamethasone induction therapy and risk-adapted maintenance approach in newly diagnosed multiple myeloma. J Clin Oncol. 2020;38:JCO.19.02515. https://doi.org/10.1200/JCO.19.02515.
89. Jackson GH, Davies FE, Pawlyn C, Cairns DA, Striha A, Collett C, et al. Lenalidomide maintenance versus observation for patients with newly diagnosed multiple myeloma (myeloma XI): a multicentre, open-label, randomised, phase 3 trial. Lancet Oncol. 2019;20(1):57–73. https://doi.org/10.1016/S1470-2045(18)30687-9.

Mature T- and NK-Cell Neoplasms

18

Patricia C. Tsang

List of Frequently Asked Questions

1. What are the key takeaways for using T-cell receptor (TCR) gene rearrangement in the diagnostic evaluation of T-cell lymphomas/leukemias?
2. What are the characteristic genetic alterations seen in T-cell prolymphocytic leukemia (T-PLL)?
3. What makes adult T-cell leukemia/lymphoma pathogenically unique among mature T-cell neoplasms?
4. Given the following scenario, what are the genetic abnormalities commonly associated with this disorder? A young adult male presenting with B symptoms and abdominal pain is found to have hepatosplenomegaly and pancytopenia. Bone marrow biopsy reveals sinusoidal infiltration by atypical medium-sized lymphoid cells with the following flow cytometric phenotype: CD2+, surface and cytoplasmic CD3+, CD4-, CD5-, CD7+, CD8-, CD34-, CD56+, TdT-, TCR αβ-, and TCR γδ +.
5. What is the role of molecular testing in the diagnosis and prognosis of mycosis fungoides?
6. How can T-cell large granular lymphocytic leukemia (T-LGLL) be distinguished from chronic lymphoproliferative disorder of NK cells (CLPD-NK) and reactive large granular lymphocytosis?
7. What are the characteristic genetic alterations of extranodal NK/T-cell lymphoma, nasal type (ENKTL-nasal)?
8. What are the molecular genetic links among the following three NK-cell neoplasms – aggressive NK-cell leukemia (ANKL), extranodal NK/T-cell lymphoma-nasal type (ENKTL-nasal), and chronic NK-cell lymphoproliferative disorder (CLPD-NK)?
9. What role does the *ALK* gene play in lymphomagenesis?
10. What are the key molecular features that can be used to distinguish primary cutaneous anaplastic large cell lymphoma (PC-ALCL) from systemic anaplastic large cell lymphoma (ALCL) with cutaneous involvement?
11. How does molecular genetic testing play a role in the diagnosis and prognosis of ALK-negative anaplastic large cell lymphoma (ALK-negative ALCL)?
12. What are the characteristic molecular genetic findings associated with breast implant-associated anaplastic large cell lymphoma (i-ALCL)?
13. What genetic markers are important in the pathologic evaluation of peripheral T-cell lymphomas, not other specified (PTCLs-NOS)?
14. What are the molecular genetic characteristics of angioimmunoblastic T-cell lymphoma (AITL) in comparison and contrast to PTCL-NOS?
15. What are the key molecular genetic aberrations that are characteristic of the two main subtypes of intestinal T-cell lymphoma – enteropathy-associated T-cell lymphoma (EATL) and monomorphic epitheliotropic intestinal T-cell lymphoma (MEITL)?
16. How can subcutaneous panniculitis-like T-cell lymphoma (SPTCL) be distinguished from primary cutaneous gamma delta T-cell lymphoma (PCGD-TCL) at the molecular level?

Frequently Asked Questions

1. **What are the key takeaways for using T-cell receptor (TCR) gene rearrangement in the diagnostic evaluation of T-cell lymphomas/leukemias?**
   - TCR gene rearrangement to assess the clonality of the T cells can be used as an adjunctive tool for cases with equivocal morphology and for minimal residual disease monitoring. While there is a tendency for mature and precursor T-cell lymphomas/leukemias to exhibit TCR gene rearrangements, the assay is far

P. C. Tsang (✉)
Department of Pathology and Laboratory Medicine, Geisinger Commonwealth School of Medicine, Danville, PA, USA
e-mail: ptsang@geisinger.edu

Y. Ding, L. Zhang (eds.), *Practical Oncologic Molecular Pathology*, Practical Anatomic Pathology,
https://doi.org/10.1007/978-3-030-73227-1_18

from being a perfect indicator for confirming or excluding T-cell malignancies. The results should always be interpreted in conjunction with clinical, morphologic, and immunophenotypic features.

- The performance characteristics of the TCR gene rearrangement assay should be validated in-house for each specimen type (e.g., whole blood or formalin-fixed paraffin-embedded (FFPE) tissue). To overcome the effect of potential inhibitors associated with tissue processing, it is advisable to test FFPE DNA at different concentrations (at least two) in the PCR reactions [1]. The overall sensitivity for identifying T-cell malignancies has been reported to range from 76% to 88% using the BIOMED-2 consensus multiplex PCR protocol for TCRγ gene (*TRG*) [2–4].
- Clonality does not equate malignancy. Certain reactive conditions, such as autoimmune diseases, chronic infections, and bone marrow transplantation, are prone to exhibiting clonal TCR patterns due to antigen-driven T-cell expansion [5].
- TCR clonal gene rearrangements are not specific for T-cell lineage neoplasms. For example, B-lymphoblastic leukemias/lymphomas can harbor positive TCR gene rearrangements concurrently with *IGH* gene rearrangements in about 60% to 80% of cases [6, 7]. Likewise, certain T-cell lymphomas, such as angioimmunoblastic T-cell lymphoma, are known to show concurrent TCR and *IGH* gene rearrangements.
- TCR is composed of two different protein chains – αβ and γδ. While each β or δ chain contains V (variable), D (diversity), and J (joining) segments, each α and γ chain contains only V and J segments [5]. Somatic recombination events join gene segments that are spatially separated in the germline configuration. Gene rearrangement begins with *TRD*, followed by *TRG*, *TRB*, and *TRA* [8]. Rearrangement of *TRA* results in deletion of *TRD* [9]. Thus, expression of TCR αβ or γδ is mutually exclusive.
- The gold standard methodology is PCR which is based on the principle that somatic TCR gene rearrangements bring the V, (D), and J segments together, enabling their amplification, while the germline configuration does not yield any PCR product. Standardized PCR primer protocol has been published by a European consortium of over 45 laboratories (EuroClonality/BIOMED-2 Concerted Action) [1, 5]. The protocol involved two multiplex PCR tubes. Alternative primer strategies involving a single multiplex tube have also been devised [10]. PCR reagents for TCR gene rearrangement assays are available as analytic-specific reagents from vendors such as Invivoscribe. After the PCR reactions are complete, fractionation can be done by capillary electrophoresis based on amplicon size and detection achieved by fluorescence.
- The TCRγ (*TRG*) gene is a preferential amplification target for T-lineage clonality as it is rearranged in all but the most immature T lymphocytes of both the TCR γδ and αβ lineages [5]. The limited number of Vγ and Jγ segments and the absence of a Dγ segment help to simplify the PCR design. The Jγ1.2 segment is rarely involved in clonal rearrangements and is excluded from the primer design in order to minimize false-positive results due to amplification of canonical Vγ9-Jγ1.2 rearrangements [1]. See example of a *TRG* test result in case #5 at the end of this chapter.
- Compared to *TRG*, TCRβ (*TRB*) shows significantly more combinatorial and junctional diversity which renders the PCR design more challenging. When added to the clonality analysis, *TRB* gene rearrangement can complement the *TRG* analysis in certain cases by improving the clinical sensitivity to an overall 94% for detecting T-cell clonal proliferations [11].
- TCR delta (*TRD*), generally together with *TRG*, should only be used as a target in well-defined clinical settings, such as suspected TCRγδ T-cell proliferations or immature (lymphoblastic) T-cell proliferations [1]. The limited use of *TRD* as a target relates to the removal of *TRD* upon rearrangement of the TCRα locus in TCRαβ cells [5, 9].
- Next-generation sequencing (NGS) for analyzing TCR gene rearrangement is a modern technology that can complement PCR. Clonal samples in NGS generate one or two predominant clusters with the same reads that are counted by computer software and expressed as percent of total reads. Hence, NGS allows identification of the junction sequence and Vγ and Jγ segments of the *TRG* clonal rearrangement, in contrast to PCR which only identifies the clone by its size. This allows more accurate clonal detection in follow-up samples, including minimal residual disease monitoring [12, 13].

2. **What are the characteristic genetic alterations seen in T-cell prolymphocytic leukemia (T-PLL)?**
   - T-PLL is an uncommon and aggressive neoplasm of post-thymic T-cell origin with a predilection for elderly males. Small- to medium-sized monoclonal T cells commonly involve the blood, bone marrow, and spleen. A high circulating lymphocyte count (>100 × 10^9/L) can be seen [14]. Nodal and extranodal presentation is also frequent, including skin, pleural, or peritoneal effusions in around 25% of patients [14]. The predominant phenotype of the neoplastic T cells is CD4+CD8-, followed by CD4+CD8+, and CD4-CD8+ [15].

- Consensus guidelines for the diagnosis of T-PLL, which incorporate cytogenetic and molecular data, have been developed by the T-PLL International Study Group [14]. A diagnosis of T-PLL requires all three major criteria, or two major criteria plus at least one minor criterion to be met (Table 18.1).
- About 90% of T-PLL cases harbor abnormalities of the 14q32.1 locus that contains the *TCL1A* (T-cell leukemia/lymphoma 1A or *TCL1*) gene [14], ~80% of which show inv(14)(q11.2;q32.1) and ~10% show t(14;14)(q11.2;q32.1). These alterations lead to the juxtaposition of *TCL1A* and *TCL1B* at 14q32.1 to the TCRα (*TRA*) locus at 14q11.2, which activates the oncogenic properties of *TCL1A* [16]. The 14 kDa protein encoded by *TCL1A* has an adapter-like engagement function in kinase complexes that can lead to enhanced pro-survival signaling [16]. *TCL1A* is the namesake of a 3-paralogue family, which includes the *TCL1B* and *MTCP1* genes [17]. *MTCP1* on chromosome Xp28 is homologous to *TCL1A/B*. A small proportion of T-PLL cases carries the t(X;14)(q28;q11.2) translocation which juxtaposes the *TRA* locus to *MTCP1*.
- Patients with abnormalities of the *ATM* gene at chromosome 11q22.3 (as in ataxia-telangiectasia syndrome) have a higher preponderance for developing T-PLL. Damaging *ATM* aberrations may be one of the initiating leukemogenic events. Dysfunctional *ATM* may be inefficient in alleviating elevated redox burdens and telomere attrition and in evoking a p53-dependent apoptotic response [16].
- A complex karyotype is characteristically seen with numerical and structural abnormalities [15]. Fluorescent in situ hybridization (FISH) can be used to detect recurrent *TCL1A* gene rearrangements, loss of *ATM*, and gains of *MYC* and *AGO2* on chromosome 8q in T-PLL [16].
- Sequencing studies have demonstrated recurrent gain-of-function mutations involving genes of the JAK/STAT signaling pathway, such as *JAK3*, *JAK1*, and *STAT5B* [15].

Table 18.1 T-PLL International Study Group criteria for the diagnosis of T-cell prolymphocytic leukemia

Major criteria (3)
>5 × 10^9/L cells of T-PLL phenotype in peripheral blood or bone marrow
T-cell clonality (by PCR or NGS for *TRB*/*TRG* or by flow cytometry)
Abnormalities of 14q32 or Xq28 or expression of *TCL1A/B* or *MTCP1*
Minor criteria (4)
Abnormalities involving chromosome 11 (11q22.3; *ATM*)
Abnormalities in chromosome 8: idic(8)(p11), t(8;8), or trisomy 8q
Abnormalities in chromosome 5, 12, 13, 22, or complex karyotype
Involvement of T-PLL-specific site (e.g., splenomegaly, effusions)

Note: Diagnosis requires three major criteria or two major criteria plus >one minor criterion [14]
Abbreviations: *T-PLL* T-cell prolymphocytic leukemia, *idic* isodicentric

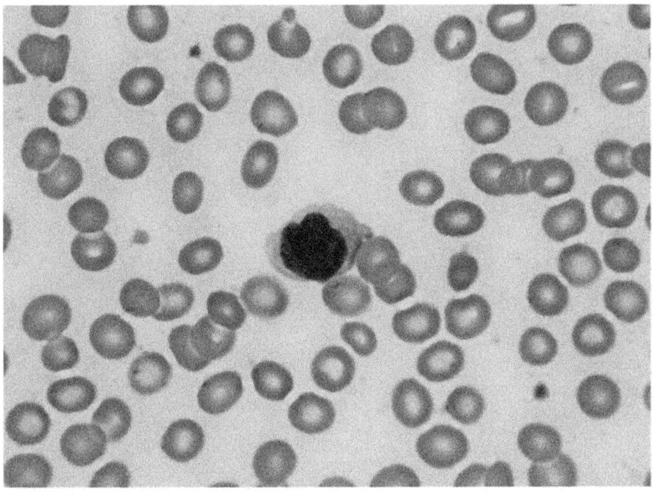

Fig. 18.1 Flower-shaped ATLL cell on peripheral blood smear (×100, oil)

3. **What makes adult T-cell leukemia/lymphoma pathogenically unique among mature T-cell neoplasms?**
   - The casual relationship of HTLV-1 with adult T-cell leukemia/lymphoma (ATLL) makes this lymphoma entity unique. HTLV-1 is necessary for the diagnosis of ATLL, a mature T-cell neoplasm originating predominantly in HTLV-1 endemic areas of the world, such as southwestern Japan, the Caribbean islands, and parts of Central Africa [18].
   - HTLV-1 infection alone is insufficient for malignant transformation of infected T cells. This explains why the lifetime cumulative incidence of developing ATLL is only about 2.5% among HTLV-1 carriers in Japan [19]. Oligoclonal expansion of HTLV-1 infected premalignant cells is often demonstrable in healthy HTLV-1 carriers [18]. However, monoclonal integration of the viral genome into the infected T cells is seen only in the neoplastic setting. In the leukemic phase, HTLV-1-infected neoplastic lymphocytes often appear as multilobed flower-shaped in the blood (Fig. 18.1).
   - Positive HTLV-1 serology in the serum or plasma can be followed by confirmatory testing of the blood sample by real-time DNA PCR which is more reliable than Western blot. PCR testing can also be used to separate HTLV-1 and HTLV-2 infections. The proviral load by quantitative PCR, which indicates the percent of HTLV-1-infected peripheral blood mononuclear cells, can be used to predict the risk of developing ATLL in infected patients [20].

- The HTLV-1 genome encodes three structural proteins (Gag, Pol, Env) as well as complex regulatory proteins (e.g., Tax (p40)) based on parallel sequencing technology [21]. Tax is believed to play a role in leukemogenesis by inducing viral replication and enhancing phosphorylation of *CREB* (cAMP response element-binding transcription factor) [22]. Another HTLV-1 gene implicated in leukemogenesis is *HBZ* (HTLV-1 basic leucine zipper factor) which is the only gene found to be consistently expressed in all ATLL cases [23].
- CCR4 mutations by PCR are detected in ~25% of ATLL, leading to gain of function and increased P13K signaling [24]. Dysregulation of microRNA mediated by HTLV-1 *Tax* and *HBZ* genes may play a role in the pathogenesis of ATLL [25].
- Clonal changes with *TRB* or *TRG* gene rearrangements are associated with transformation from indolent to aggressive disease [26]. Mutations of the *TP53* and *IRF4* genes are seen predominantly in clinically aggressive disease [27].

4. **Given the following scenario, what are the genetic abnormalities commonly associated with this disorder? A young adult male presenting with B symptoms and abdominal pain is found to have hepatosplenomegaly and pancytopenia. The splenic red pulp shows infiltration by atypical medium-sized lymphoid cells with the following flow cytometric phenotype: CD2+, surface and cytoplasmic CD3+, CD4-, CD5-, CD7+, CD8-, CD34-, CD56+, TdT-, TCRαβ-, and TCRγδ+.**
   - The clinicopathologic features described above are typical of hepatosplenic T-cell lymphoma (HSTL), a type of aggressive mature T-cell lymphoma (Fig. 18.2).
   - As in the case scenario above, the vast majority of HSTL originate from TCRγδ cytotoxic T cells that home to the spleen, liver, and bone marrow. A minority of HSTL are of TCRαβ origin which can be demonstrated by flow cytometry or immunohistochemistry using formalin-fixed paraffin-embedded tissue [28]. The αβ subset appears to show a worse prognosis than its γδ counterpart [29].
   - TCR gene rearrangement analysis can be pursued to confirm T-cell clonality. Cases of γδ origin have clonally rearranged *TRG* as well as biallelic rearrangement of the *TRD* gene [28]. Certain γδ cases have shown unproductive rearrangements of *TRB*. The uncommon αβ variant harbors *TRB* clonal gene rearrangement.
   - Isochromosome 7q is the primary karyotypic abnormality seen in ~70% of HSTL, although it is not specific for this entity [30, 31]. The i(7)(q10) abnormality can also be detected in nasal-type extranodal NK/T--cell lymphoma and ALK-negative ALCL. A variety of FISH patterns equivalent to two to five copies of i(7)(q10) can be seen in HSTL, especially in advanced disease [28]. Ring chromosomes resulting in 7q amplification are known to occur. The common gained region has been mapped to 7q22.11q31.1 where increased expression of the *ABCB1* gene encoding a multidrug resistance glycoprotein has been described [32].
   - A distinct gene expression profile is shared by both the gamma delta and alpha beta subtypes, suggesting that they belong to the same disease entity. Genes in the JAK/STAT pathway are often mutated (~40% of HSTL), as are the *STETD2*, *INO80*, and

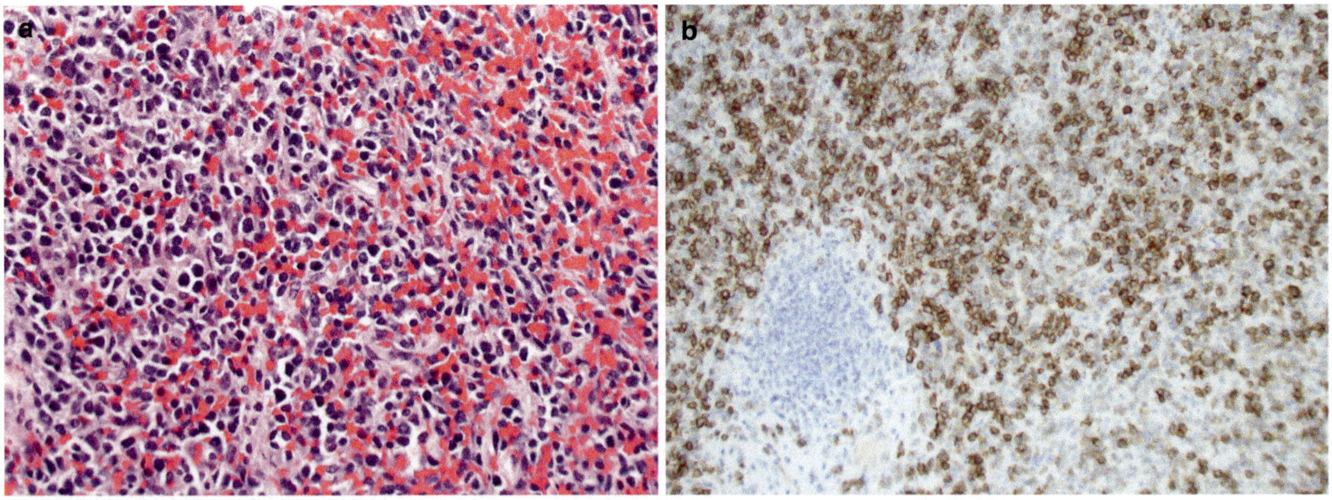

Fig. 18.2 (**a**) Hepatosplenic T-cell leukemia comprises medium-sized cells that infiltrate the cords and sinuses of the spleen (H&E stain, ×40). (**b**) CD56-positive lymphoma cells in the splenic red pulp associated with hypoplastic white pulp near the *lower left* corner (×20)

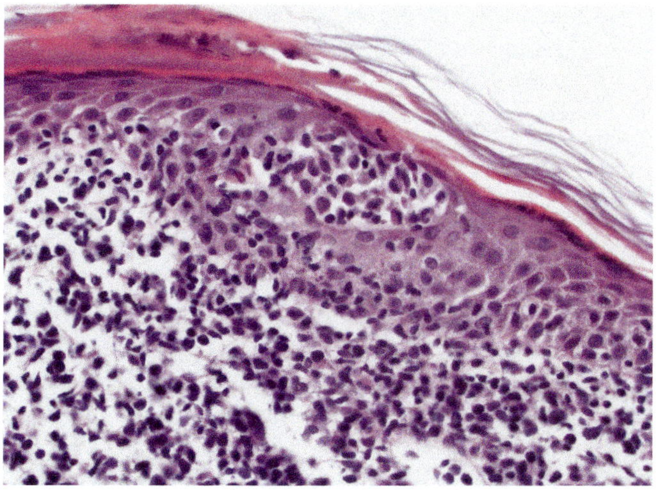

Fig. 18.3 Mycosis fungoides with a Pautrier microabscess in the epidermis of the skin (H&E stain, ×40)

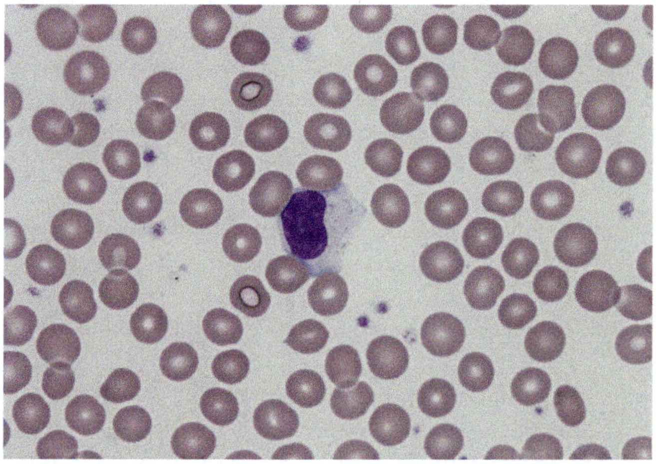

Fig. 18.4 A large granular lymphocyte molds its cytoplasm to the surrounding red blood cells on peripheral blood smear (Wright-Giemsa stain, ×100 oil)

ARIADA1B chromatin-modifying genes (~50% of HSTL) [31, 33].

5. **What is the role of molecular testing in the diagnosis and prognosis of mycosis fungoides?**
   - Mycosis fungoides (MF) is an indolent skin-based T-cell lymphoma, accounting for nearly half of all primary cutaneous lymphomas [34]. Macroscopically, this lymphoma shows stepwise evolution from patches to plagues (palpable lesions) to tumors (skin nodules) [34]. The infiltrates of MF show epidermotropism and are composed of small- to medium-sized T cells (Fig. 18.3). A top differential diagnosis is reactive lymphoid conditions, such as drug reaction and inflammatory dermatoses.
   - TCR gene rearrangement can be used as an adjunctive tool for confirming T-cell clonality in MF. Clonally rearranged *TRG* and *TRB* genes are seen in 50–53% of MF during the patch stage, 73–100% during the plague stage, and 90–100% during the tumor stage [35, 36]. However, false-positive results can be caused by the presence of TCR gene rearrangement reported in as much as 25% to 65% of benign inflammatory dermatoses [37]. If the same T-cell clone can be demonstrated in more than one biopsy specimen, it favors MF over reactive conditions.
   - MicroRNAs (miRNAs) are small noncoding RNAs that regulate gene expression. Using RT-PCR, microRNA (miRNA) profiling may potentially be of diagnostic value as it has been shown to differentiate MF from benign skin conditions [38]. Deregulated miRNAs with increased expression have been reported in MF lesions compared to normal control tissues [39]. Differential miRNA expression has also been demonstrated between early and advanced MF lesions, suggesting that miRNAs may be involved in disease progression [40].
   - Caution is warranted in interpreting monoclonal TCR gene rearrangement in the blood, which is commonly encountered in the early stage of the disease. This finding is not necessarily indicative of blood involvement by MF unless there is morphologic and/or immunophenotypic evidence of disease. Using routine PCR technique, dominant T-cell clones detected in the peripheral blood of MF patients have been found to be rarely malignant, but more often related to aging [41].
   - Complex karyotypes are demonstrable in many patients, especially in advanced disease. Activation of *STAT3* and inactivation of *CDKN2A* and *PTEN* may have prognostic significance as these alterations appear to be associated with aggressive disease [36, 42].
6. **How can T-cell large granular lymphocytic leukemia (T-LGLL) be distinguished from chronic lymphoproliferative disorder of NK cells (CLPD-NK) and reactive large granular lymphocytosis?**
   - Circulating T-LGLL cells and CLPD-NK cells are indistinguishable on peripheral blood smear examination. Under the microscope, both entities are composed of large granular lymphocytes which typically appear as mature, medium-sized lymphocytes with moderate to abundant cytoplasm containing azurophilic granules [43] (Fig. 18.4).
   - Being of T-cell origin, T-LGLL exhibits surface CD3 expression (as demonstrable by flow cytometry) and harbors TCR gene rearrangement by PCR. The *TRG* gene is expected to be rearranged in all cases of T-LGLL, while *TRB* is rearranged in cases express-

ing TCRαβ but not necessarily in those expressing TCRγδ [43].

- Being of natural killer origin, CLPD-NK lacks surface CD3 expression and shows a germline configuration of the TCR genes. Reactive large granular lymphocytes of T-cell or NK-cell origin also lack TCR gene rearrangement.
- *STAT3* has emerged as a key pathogenic driver in T-LGLL and CLPD-NK [43]. Activating mutations in *STAT3* can promote clonal dominance and are associated with a larger clone size [44]. Somatic *STAT3* mutations are observed in about 30%–40% of both T-LGLL [45] and CLPD-NK [46], but not in non-neoplastic large granular lymphocytes. These *STAT3* activating mutations affect mostly exons 21 and 20, which encode the Src homology (SH2) domain, and can lead to transcriptional dysregulation of genes downstream in the JAK/STAT pathway. Identical somatic *STAT3* mutations can be seen in T-LGLL and CLPD-NK, indicating a common pathogenesis for these two entities [46].
- The first evidence of *STAT5B* mutations in human disease was discovered in LGL leukemia, but this mutation is infrequent (2%) [47]. In particular, the N642H mutation was associated with an unusual $CD3^{+}CD8+CD56^{+}$ phenotype and an aggressive clinical course [48].
- Distinguishing CLPD-NK from reactive NK-cell proliferation may pose a dilemma in some cases due to its lack of clonal TCR rearrangement. Besides assessing for *STAT3* mutations by NGS, human androgen receptor X-assay (HUMARA) can be used to demonstrate clonality in female patients with CLPD-NK; polyclonal results are expected in female patients with reactive natural killer cells [49]. The HUMARA gene is located on the X chromosome, and one of the alleles in female normally undergoes inactivation by methylation [50]. Due to the fact that the two alleles often have different CAG repeats, polyclonal female DNA is expected to show two distinct bands after PCR amplification and gel separation. A skewed ratio of X chromosome inactivation restricted to NK cells reflects a clonal population. Since the DNA restriction enzyme *HpaII* preferentially cuts unmethylated DNA, it provides a means to differentiate the methylated from unmethylated allele in the amplicon [50].

7. **What are the characteristic genetic alterations of extranodal NK-/T-cell lymphoma, nasal type (ENKTL-nasal)?**
   - Extranodal NK-/T-cell lymphoma, nasal type (ENKTL-nasal), exhibits angiodestruction and prominent necrosis morphologically, signifying the aggressive nature of the disease [51]. It typically presents in an extranodal site, particularly the nasal cavity and other locations along the upper aerodigestive tract where patients may suffer from a midline destruction lesion.
   - ENKTL-nasal originates predominantly from activated natural killer (NK) cells and less frequently from cytotoxic T cells (25% to 35%) [52]. The lineage derivation of this neoplasm does not appear to impact survival [53]. The subset of cytotoxic T-cell-derived cases expresses either TCRαβ or less commonly, TCRγδ [51]. NK cells are distinguished from cytotoxic T cells by germline configuration of *TRG* and *TRB*, as well as the lack of surface CD3 antigen (as demonstrated by flow cytometry or on frozen tissue). Both NK and T cells express cCD3-epsilon on fixed and frozen tissue and by flow cytometry.
   - EBV is consistently positive within the lesion and likely plays a pathogenic role [51]. EBV is present in a clonal episomal form with type II latency (EBNA1+, EBNA2-, LMP1+) [54]. A 30-bp deletion in the *LMP1* gene is often observed [55]. Peripheral EBV DNA viral load correlates with the lymphoma burden and can be used to monitor disease activity. High EBV DNA is considered a poor prognostic factor.
   - The most common cytogenetic abnormalities are del(6)(q21q25) and i(6)(p10), although these are not specific for ENKTL-nasal. This abnormality results in loss of tumor suppressor genes, including *HACE1*, *PRMD1*, *FOXO3*, and *PTPRK* (receptor-type tyrosine-protein phosphatase κ) [56, 57]. Recurrent mutations and deletions involving multiple genes have been found, such as activating mutations of the JAK/STAT cascade (especially the *STAT3* and *STAT5B* genes), loss-of-function mutations of the RNA helicase *DDX3X* gene (14–20% of cases), loss-of-function mutations of the epigenetic modifier *BCOR* gene (17% of cases), loss-of-function mutations of tumor suppressors *TP53* and *MGA*, and others [58, 59].
   - The gene expression profiles of the NK- and T-cell subtypes of ENKTL-nasal cluster together and are similar to that of non-hepatosplenic gamma delta T-cell lymphomas. Activation of the pro-proliferative JAK/STAT, NF-κB, NOTCH, and Aurora kinase pathways are observed [56, 57]. Gene mutation profiling of this aggressive lymphoma holds promise for identifying potential therapeutic targets or immunotherapy strategies aimed at counteracting these abnormally activated pathways.
8. **What are the molecular genetic links among the following three NK-cell neoplasms – aggressive NK-cell leukemia (ANKL), extranodal NK-/T-cell lymphoma-**

nasal type (ENKTL-nasal), and chronic NK-cell lymphoproliferative disorder (CLPD-NK)?

- All three entities are clonal disorders derived from NK cells. Present in a clonal episomal form, EBV is common to both aggressive NK-cell leukemia (ANKL) (85–100% of cases) and with extranodal NK/T-cell lymphoma (ENKTL-nasal) (close to 100%) [60]. In contrast, EBV is absent in chronic NK-cell lymphoproliferative disorder (CLPD-NK) [51] which is a rare indolent disorder categorized as a provisional entity in the 2016 WHO classification system.
- Somatic alterations in the genes along the JAK/STAT cascade, such as *STAT3*, have been described in all three of these NK-cell entities by next-generation sequencing [61, 62] (Table 18.2). Gain-of-function *STAT3* mutations may represent a common pathogenic link among various NK-cell neoplasms, a link that is shared by T-cell large granular lymphocytic leukemia as well [46].
- It is unclear whether ANKL represents the leukemic counterpart of ENKTL-nasal. Besides showing significant clinicopathologic overlaps, ANKL and ENKTL-nasal harbor a similar set of recurrently mutated genes, including *DDX3X*, *STAT3*, *BCOR*, *KMT2D*, and *FAS*, raising the possibility of similar pathogenetic mechanisms being involved in both diseases [61, 63]. Against this hypothesis, however, are the significant differences in copy number alterations detected by array comparative genomic hybridization between these entities. For instance, losses in 7p and 17p and gains in 1q are much more frequent in ANKL, whereas deletions in 6q are more frequent in ENKTL-nasal but rare in ANKL [63].
- Rare cases of ANKL have been postulated to arise from EBV-negative CLPD-NK, which may partly account for the occasional absence of EBV in ANKL [60]. Both of these conditions are localized to the peripheral blood and bone marrow as their primary sites, but can involve other organs, especially the liver and spleen.

Table 18.2 Clinicopathologic profiles: aggressive NK-cell leukemia (ANKL); extranodal NK/T-cell lymphoma, nasal type (ENKTL-nasal); and chronic NK-cell lymphoproliferative disorder (CPLD-NK)

Feature	ANKL	ENKTL-nasal	CPLD-NK
Sites of distribution	Mostly leukemic; can involve any organ	Extranodal tissues, commonly nasal	Mostly leukemic
Clinical course	Aggressive	Aggressive	Indolent
Clonal EBV	+	+	–
STAT3 (JAK/STAT)	+	+	+
DDX3X	+	+	n.s.
BCOR	+	+	n.s.
KMT2D mutations	+	+	n.s.

Abbreviations: + common or recurrent, – absent, *n.s.* not well studied

9. **What role does the ALK gene play in lymphomagenesis?**
   - *ALK* encodes an oncoprotein known as ALK receptor tyrosine kinase, a member of the insulin receptor superfamily. Its function includes downstream activation of various signaling pathways, including Ras/Raf/MEK/ERK, JAK/STAT, PLC-Y, and PI3K/Akt, which can in turn promote cell proliferation and survival [64].
   - Chromosomal translocations involving *ALK* on chromosome 2p23.2-p23.1 are involved in the lymphomagenesis of a significant proportion of anaplastic large cell lymphomas (ALK+ ALCL) and a small subset of large B-cell lymphomas (ALK+ LBCL). In particular, the dominant t(2;5)(p23;q35);*NPM1-ALK* alteration found in ALCL is rare (~10%) in ALK+ LBCL which is predominated by t(2;17)(p23;q23) [65].
   - *ALK* gene translocation in ALCL appears to confer a favorable prognosis. ALK+ ALCL patients show a relatively high 5-year overall survival of about 70–86% [66].
   - While translocation is the predominant mechanism seen in ALK+ lymphomas, recurrent point mutations within the kinase domain and gene amplifications are more common in certain solid tumors, such as familial neuroblastoma and anaplastic thyroid carcinoma [67].
   - A dual-color break-apart FISH probe set is useful for detecting *ALK* rearrangements without identifying the partner gene which is generally of no clinical significance. A dual-color, dual-fusion FISH strategy can detect specific *ALK* translocations, but it may not be practical due to the large number of potential fusion gene partners [68].
   - Real-time reverse transcription PCR (real-time RT-PCR) for detecting fusion transcripts via cDNA can be used to test for any minimal residual disease in ALK+ ALCL. Patients diagnosed with ALK+ ALCL are treated with crizotinib, a dual ALK/MET inhibitor [69]. Despite the remarkable initial response, resistance to crizotinib can eventually develop. The mechanisms underlying ALK inhibitor resistance are complex and heterogeneous and may involve *ALK* gene amplification, *ALK* kinase domain mutation, and upregulation of various bypass signaling pathways, such as IGF-1R (insulin-like growth factor 1 receptor) [69].

10. **What are the key molecular features that can be used to distinguish primary cutaneous anaplastic large cell lymphoma (PC-ALCL) from systemic anaplastic large cell lymphoma (s-ALCL) with cutaneous involvement?**
    - Both PC-ALCL and s-ALCL (ALK positive or negative) are characteristically composed of cohesive sheets of anaplastic large T cells or null-cells that stain positively for CD30 and cytotoxic markers (granzyme B, TIA1, and perforin) [70] (Fig. 18.5a-c). These morphologic and phenotype overlaps can pose diagnostic challenges.
    - In the 2016 WHO classification of lymphoid neoplasms, PC-ALCL, ALK+ s-ALCL, and ALK-negative s-ALCL represent distinct entities with significantly different prognostic implications. The 10-year disease-free survival rate is 90% for PC-ALCL patients versus only 28% for patients with ALK-negative s-ALCL [66]. Hence, distinguishing PC-ALCL from s-ALCL with cutaneous involvement is of high clinical importance.
    - Located on chromosome 2p, the *ALK* gene is rearranged in about 30–60% of s-ALCL but not in the vast majority of PC-ALCL [70, 71] (Table 18.3). In ALK+ ALCL, t(2;5)(p23;q35) that results in an *NPM1-ALK* fusion protein is the most common alteration (~80% of cases), followed by t(1;2)(q25;p23) with *TPM3-ALK* fusion (~15% of cases) [72]. Less common variant translocations involve *ALK* with other partner genes, such as inv(2)(p23q35) with *ATIC-ALK* fusion, t(2;22)(p23;q11.2) with *MYH9-ALK* fusion, t(2;3)(p23;q12.2) with *TFG-ALK* fusion, and others [68].
    - *DUSP22-IRF4* gene rearrangement on locus 6p25.3 is present in about 25% of PC-ALCL but not in ALK+ ALCL [73, 74]. This *DUSP22-IRF4* rearrangement can also be seen in lymphomatoid papulosis [70] and ALK-negative ALCL, but not typically in

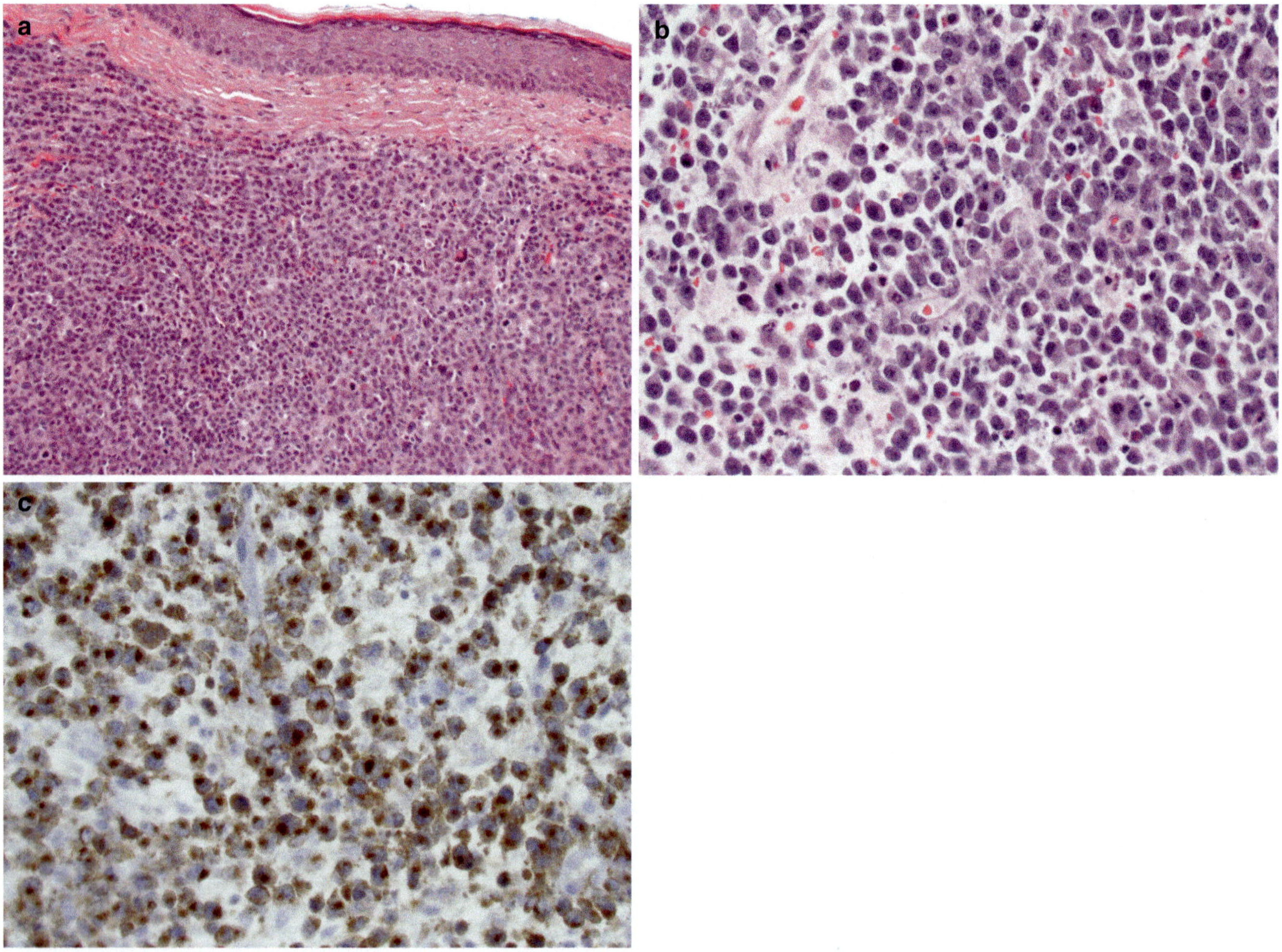

Fig. 18.5 (**a**) Skin: Primary cutaneous anaplastic large cell lymphoma involving dermis of skin. ALK immunostain (not shown) was negative (H&E stain, ×20). (**b**) Lymph node: Systemic ALCL showing characteristic cohesive sheets of large cells (H&E stain, ×40). (**c**) Lymph node: ALK immunostain showing cytoplasmic and membrane positivity in lymph node, consistent with ALK+ ALCL (×40)

Table 18.3 Molecular genetic profiles: primary cutaneous anaplastic large cell lymphoma (PC-ALCL) versus systemic anaplastic large cell lymphoma (s-ALCL)

Feature	PC-ALCL	s-ALCL,ALK-	s-ALCL, ALK+
Clonal *TRG/TRB*	+	+	+
ALK rearrangement	–	–	+
DUSP22-IRF4	~25%	~30%	–
TP63 rearrangement	–	~8%	–
NPM-TYK2	Occasional	–	–

Abbreviations: + mostly present, – absent or not yet known to be present

other T-cell lymphoid neoplasms, including mycosis fungoides/Sézary syndrome, peripheral T-cell lymphoma, and extranodal NK/T-cell lymphoma [75].

- *NPM-TYK2* gene fusion is a recurrent rearrangement seen in occasional cases of PC-ALCL and its related lesion, lymphomatoid papulosis, but is not known to be present in s-ALCL [76]. The corresponding t(5;19) can be detected by FISH. *NPM-TK2* fusion results in downstream activation of STAT signaling.

11. **How does molecular genetic testing play a role in the diagnosis and prognosis of ALK-negative anaplastic large cell lymphoma (ALK-negative ALCL)?**
    - It is important to differentiate ALK-negative ALCL from other T-cell lymphoma entities that may exhibit overlapping features. ALK-negative ALCL is considered as a distinct entity under the 2016 WHO classification system. Its main differential diagnoses include primary cutaneous anaplastic large cell lymphoma (PC-ALCL) and peripheral T-cell lymphoma, not otherwise specified (PTCL-NOS). ALK-negative ALCL tends to affect older patients than its ALK+ counterpart and shows a better 5-year survival rate than PTCL-NOS [77].
    - The majority of ALK-negative ALCL cases show T-cell receptor gene rearrangement even if they exhibit a null-cell phenotype in which T-cell antigens (e.g., CD2, CD3, CD5, CD7) are not expressed.
    - Recurrent gene mutations, including *JAK1, STAT3, PRDM1, TP53, TET2, FAS, and STIM2*, have been reported. In particular, *JAK1* and/or *STAT3* mutations can constitutively activate the JAK/STAT pathway [68].
    - Genetic rearrangements significantly influence the 5-year survival of ALK-negative ALCL: ~90% in cases with *DUSP* rearrangements versus only ~20% in those with *TP63* rearrangements [77, 78]. Patients with no *DUSP22* or *TP63* rearrangements show an intermediate 5-year survival (~40%) [78].
    - *DUSP22* gene rearrangement (in or near the *DUSP22-IRF4* locus on 6p25.3) occurs in about 30% of cases of ALK-negative ALCL and is associated with a favorable prognosis [72]. *DUSP22* encodes a dual-specificity phosphatase that inhibits T-cell receptor signaling and functions as a tumor suppressor by inactivating the mitogen-activated protein kinase (MAPL), ERK2 [74]. The most common translocation partner is the *FRA7H* fragile site on 7q32.3, resulting in t(6;7) as detectable by FISH. *DUSP22-FRA7H* fusion leads to downregulation of *DUSP22* and upregulation of *FRA7H* gene expression [74].
    - Detectable by FISH, *TP63* gene rearrangement on locus 3q28 is reported in about 8% of cases of ALK-negative ALCL and is associated with an unfavorable prognosis [77]. The p63 protein is a transcription factor whose most common fusion gene partner is *TBL1XR1* on 3q26 [79].
    - Gene expression profiling shows both similarities and differences between ALK-negative and ALK+ ALCL cases [78, 80]. The distinction of ALK-negative ALCL from PTCL-NOS is more clear-cut. The characteristic upregulated expression of *BATF*, *TMOD1*, and *TNFRSF8* in ALK-negative ALCL is not seen in PTCL-NOS [81, 82] and can serve as a tool for differentiating challenging cases between ALK-negative ALCL and PTCL-NOS.
12. **What are the characteristic molecular genetic findings associated with breast implant-associated anaplastic large cell lymphoma (i-ALCL)?**
    - As a rare provisional entity in the 2016 WHO classification, breast implant-associated ALCL (i-ALCL) overlaps significantly with ALK-negative systemic ALCL morphologically and phenotypically. However, it is associated with a significantly better overall survival than ALK-negative systemic ALCL, with most i-ALCL patients presenting with stage 1 disease [83]. Hence, it is important to distinguish between i-ALCL and systemic ALCL.
    - Similar to systemic ALCLs, i-ALCL is derived from activated cytotoxic T cells and characteristically shows clonal TCR gene rearrangement. As in systemic ALCL, recurrent mutations of the JAK/STAT pathway genes, particularly *JAK1* and *STAT3*, have been reported [83].
    - Recurrent deletion of chromosomal region 1p21-22 involving loss of the *RPL5* (ribosomal protein L5) gene has been detected [84]. This alteration is not known to be recurrent in systemic ALCL. There is no known association of i-ALCL with *DUSP22* or *TP63* gene rearrangements that are known to significantly influence the prognosis in ALK-negative systemic ALCL [84, 85].
13. **What genetic markers are important in the pathologic evaluation of peripheral T-cell lymphomas, not other specified (PTCLs-NOS)?**

- PTCLs-NOS, an aggressive category of T-cell lymphoma, characteristically harbor complex karyotypes with a variety of recurrent chromosomal aberrations, such as gains in 7q, 8q, and 17q and losses in 4q, 5q, 6q, 9p, and many others [86]. The majority of PTCLs-NOS contain clonal rearrangements of the *TRG* and *TRB* genes.
- Within the category of PTCLs-NOS, the gene expression signatures and microRNA profiles are heterogeneous, reflecting the heterogeneity of these lymphomas. The gene expression profiles of PTCLs-NOS are distinct from those of other T-cell lymphoma entities, including ALCL and AITL [81].
- Gene expression profiling has identified two molecular profiles – *GATA3* and *TBX21* (*T-BET*) – that show distinct genetic aberrations and prognostic implications [87, 88]. *GATA3* and *TBX21* are both transcription factors that regulate gene expression in mostly T helper cells. The PTCL-GATA3 subgroup (~33% of PTCLs-NOS) shows relatively greater genomic complexity that is characterized by frequent loss or mutation of tumor suppressor genes targeting the *CDKN2A/B-TP53* axis and *PTEN*-PI3K pathways [89, 90]. The PTCL-TBX21 subgroup (~49% of PTCLs-NOS) has fewer copy number abnormalities and is enriched in mutations of genes regulating DNA methylation [89].
- The PTCL-GATA3 subgroup shows a worse prognosis than PTCL-TBX21 [89, 91]. A minor subset of PTCL-TBX21 shows a cytotoxic profile and is associated with a worse outcome than the majority of T helper PTCL-TBX21 [87]. Besides a GATA3 or cytotoxic profile, markers of unfavorable prognosis in PTCL-NOS include EBV positivity, NF-kappaB pathway dysregulation, a high proliferation signature by gene expression, and loss of 9p21 which decreases the expression of the cyclin-dependent kinase inhibitors 2A and 2B [86, 92].

14. **What are the molecular genetic characteristics of angioimmunoblastic T-cell lymphoma (AITL) in comparison and contrast to PTCL-NOS?**
    - Despite having substantial morphologic overlaps, PTCL-NOS and AITL exhibit genetic profiles that are distinct from each other. The previously recognized subset of nodal PTCLs with T follicular helper (TFH) features has recently been removed from the category of PTCL-NOS and reclassified under the same diagnostic category as AITL [93].
    - TFH cells represent a subset of effector CD4+ T helper cells that are generated in the germinal centers and display a characteristic CD10+, CXCR5+, BCL6+, ICOS+, and PD1+ phenotype [94]. To qualify a nodal peripheral T-cell lymphoma as having a TFH phenotype typically requires the presence of at least two (ideally three) of the above TFH-associated markers in addition to CD4 expression [93].
    - AITL is derived from TFH cells and, hence, displays a characteristic CD4+, CD10+, CXCR5+, BCL6+, ICOS+, and PD1+ phenotype [94]. It typically shows an expanded follicular dendritic meshwork as demonstrable by CD21 or CD23 staining. Unifying AITL with other nodal lymphomas of TFH cell origin under a single category would render the distinction between PTCL-NOS and AITL more clear-cut [95]. EBV is present in scattered EBER+ B- cells and is observed consistently in AITL (80% to 90% of cases) and only sporadically in PTCL-NOS [93, 96] (Table 18.4).
    - *RHOA* G17V (p.Gly17Val) mutation is found in ~70% of AITL versus ~20% of PTCL-NOS [97]. *RHOA* encodes a small GTPase that regulates the actin cytoskeleton and is involved in cell motility, adhesion, and polarization [98]. This hotspot G17V mutation is a dominant-negative variant that causes loss of function of the GTPase enzyme. In an animal model, *RHOA* G17V in combination with knockout *TET2* mutations as a second hit has been shown to cause AITL [99].
    - Frequently mutated genes in AITL include *TET2* (50–80% of cases), *DNMT3A* (25% of cases), and *IDH2* (25% of cases) [100, 101]. Interestingly, this complement of genes resembles myeloid clonal disorders more than other lymphomas, including PTCL which shows a lower frequency of mutations in these genes [101].
    - The characteristic *IDH2* (isocitrate dehydrogenase 2) mutations found in 25% of AITL involve the arginine-172 codon (R172) [100]. R172 hotspot mutations appear to be largely confined to AITL and lead to a gain of function with increased levels of the

Table 18.4 Pathogenetic profiles: primary peripheral T-cell lymphoma, not otherwise specified (PTCL-NOS), versus angioimmunoblastic T-cell lymphoma (AITL)

Feature	PTCL-NOS	AITL
Clonal *TRG/TRB*	+	+
T follicular helper gene expression profile	–	+
EBV	Rare	~80–90%
RHOA G17V mutation	~20%	~70%
TET2 mutations	Less common	~50–80%
DNMT3A mutations	Less common	~25%
IDH2 mutations	Uncommon	~25%

Abbreviations: + mostly present, – absent

oncometabolite, 2-hydroxyglutarate (2HG) [100, 102].
- Nodal T-cell lymphomas with a TFH phenotype that do not qualify as AITL share a similar tendency as AITL to harbor mutations in the *TET2, DNMT3A*, and *RHOA* genes [93].

15. **What are the characteristic molecular genetic aberrations of the two main subtypes of intestinal T-cell lymphoma – enteropathy-associated T-cell lymphoma (EATL) and monomorphic epitheliotropic intestinal T-cell lymphoma (MEITL)?**
    - While both are associated with poor prognosis, EATL and MEITL (previously, EATL type II) appear to be biologically distinct lymphoma subtypes with divergent clinical, phenotypic, and genetic features, suggesting different pathogenetic pathways being involved [103]. EATL is related to celiac disease (gluten-sensitive enteropathy) and an HLA DQ2 or DQ8 phenotype, while MEITL is characteristically not associated with celiac disease or malabsorption [104]. Morphologically, the lymphoma cells tend to be more pleomorphic and larger in EATL than in MEITL [93].
    - EATL is more likely to express TCRαβ than γ∂, in contrast to MEITL which is more likely to express TCRγ∂ than αβ [105]. Clonal *TRG* or *TRB* rearrangements are demonstrable in the lymphoma cells as well as intraepithelial lymphocytes away from the tumor in both EATL and MEITL.
    - Based on array comparative genomic hybridization, genetic alterations shared by both entities include chromosomal gains of 9q34 which harbors known proto-oncogenes, e.g., *NOTCH1*, *ABL1*, and *VAV2* [103, 106]. Also shared by both entities is deletions in 16q12.1 with a 2.5 megabase loss [103] (Table 18.5).
    - At the molecular level, the JAK/STAT pathway is implicated in the pathogenesis of EATL and MEITL [107]. For instance, *JAK3* and *GNAI2* are mutated in some cases of MEITL [105]. Interestingly, activation of the JAK/STAT cascade has also been described in the CD4+ subset of indolent T-cell lymphoma of the GI tract, a provisional lymphoma entity derived from αβ T cells in mostly the small intestine [108].
    - Genetic alterations that are known to be recurrent in EATL but less common in MEITL include gains of 1q and 5q, loss of 9p (loss of *p16*), and loss of 17p12-13.2 (loss of *TP53*) [103, 107].
    - Genetic alterations that are far more common in MEITL than in EATL include extra signals of *MYC* at 8q24.2 (seen with a FISH break-apart probe), *SETD2* mutation in >90% of MEITL, and activating *STAT5B* mutations in both αβ and γ∂ cases [104, 105, 107].

Table 18.5 Pathogenetic features: enteropathy-associated T-cell lymphoma (EATL) versus monomorphic epitheliotropic intestinal T-cell lymphoma (MEITL)

Feature	EATL	MEITL
Association with celiac disease	Present	Absent
Association with HLA DQ2 or DQ8 phenotype	Present	Absent (same as general population)
Clonal TCR rearrangement	Present (αβ expression > γ∂)	Present (γ∂ expression > αβ)
Gains of 9q34	Common	Common
Losses of 16q12.1	Common	Common
Gains of 1q and 5q	Common	Uncommon
Gains of 8q24/*MYC*	Uncommon	Common
JAK/STAT pathway alterations	Common	Common
STAT5B mutations	Uncommon	Common
SETD2 mutations	Uncommon	Common (>90%)

Abbreviations: *TCR* T-cell receptor

16. **How can subcutaneous panniculitis-like T-cell lymphoma (SPTCL) be distinguished from primary cutaneous gamma delta T-cell lymphoma (PCGD-TCL) at the molecular level?**
    - SPTCL and PCGD-TCL are both T-cell neoplasms that can infiltrate the subcutaneous tissue with a panniculitis-like morphologic pattern. PCGD-TCL is a provisional entity in the 2016 WHO classification system and is grouped together with two other rare primary skin lymphomas under the term, primary cutaneous peripheral T-cell lymphomas, rare subtypes [93]. SPTCL is an indolent disorder with a significantly longer 5-year overall survival (~80%) than PCGD-TCL (~10%) [109, 110].
    - The main difference between SPTCL and PCGD-TCL is that the former originates from alpha beta T cells, while the latter expresses a gamma delta phenotype. This differential expression profile can be demonstrated by flow cytometry or immunohistochemistry [111]. Of note, the previously called subcutaneous panniculitis-like T-cell lymphoma with gamma delta phenotype has been reclassified from originally being a subtype of SPTCL to currently being included in PCGD-TCL [112].
    - By PCR, the majority of SPTCLs (phenotypically αβ) show monoclonal rearrangements of the *TRG*, *TRB*, and *TRG* genes. PCGD-TCLs (phenotypically γ∂) show monoclonal rearrangement of the *TRG* and *TRD* genes, while *TRB* may be rearranged or deleted at the genetic level.
    - About 50% of SPTCLs have *NAV3* (neuron navigator 3) mutations that can be detected by FISH or loss of heterozygosity [111]. These *NAV3* mutations are not specific for SPTCL as they can also be found in

mycosis fungoides and Sézary syndrome [114]. A subset of PCGD-TCL cases harbors mutations in *STAT5B* and, less commonly, in *STAT3* [113, 115]. These mutations activate the JAK/STAT pathway that is implicated widely among cytotoxic T-cell lymphomas.

Gains of chromosomes 5q and 13q seen on array comparative genomic hybridization may be characteristic of SPTCL as they are not usually found in other cutaneous T-cell lymphoma entities [113].

Case Presentations

Case 1

Learning Objective

Understand the prognostic significance of FISH molecular markers in an entity of mature T-cell lymphoma.

Case History

A 51-year-old male complained of worsening dyspnea and was found to have right endobronchial masses and right axillary lymphadenopathy.

Histologic Features

The nodal architecture was diffusely effaced by sheets of atypical medium-sized to large lymphocytes with occasional horseshoe-shaped nuclei (see Fig. 18.6a). Admixed were abundant tingible-body macrophages and occasional small mature lymphocytes. The atypical lymphocytes stained intensely positive for CD3, CD4, CD43, and CD30 (see Fig. 18.6b). The neoplastic cells were focally positive for EMA. Not expressed were CD4, CD5, CD7, ALK-1, cytotoxic markers, EBER, B-cell markers, and histiocytic markers.

Laboratory Findings

Flow cytometric analysis showed no aberrant T-cell or monotypic B-cell phenotype. There was clonal rearrangement of the *TRG* gene.

Molecular Genetic Studies

FISH analysis performed on the formalin-fixed paraffin-embedded tissue showed rearrangement of *DUSP22* and no alteration of the *TP63* gene (see Fig. 18.6c, d).

Final Diagnosis

ALK-negative anaplastic large cell lymphoma

Follow-Up

The patient responded well to systemic chemotherapy and was in disease-free remission at 3 years of follow-up.

Discussion

ALK-negative anaplastic large cell lymphoma (ALCL) overlaps morphologically with its ALK+ counterpart. Hallmark cells, characterized by eccentric, horseshoe-shaped or kidney-shaped nuclei, may be present. The tumor cells characteristically express CD30 and CD43. The expression of T-cell antigens, cytotoxic markers, and EMA is variable. Both the T-cell and null-cell types of ALCL show clonal TCR gene rearrangement in the vast majority of cases. Flow cytometry may yield false-negative results due to underrepresentation of large cells in the sample upon processing.

FISH analysis for *DUSP22* and *TP63* gene rearrangements has become standard practice for the prognostic evaluation of ALK-negative ALCL. The detection of rearrangement of the *DUSP22-IR4* locus and the absence of *TBL1XR1/TP63* gene fusion are associated with a favorable prognosis with a 5-year overall survival of ~90%, in stark contrast to only ~20% in *TP63*-rearranged cases [78]. *DUSP22* rearrangement leads to reduced gene expression and occurs in ~30% of ALK-negative ALCL [72]. This alteration has also been reported in lymphomatoid papulosis and primary cutaneous ALCL, but not in ALK+ ALCL [74, 75].

Case 2

Case History

A 65-year-old female presented with pruritis and weight loss and was found to have generalized lymphadenopathy and hepatosplenomegaly.

Histologic Features

The lymph node showed focally regressed lymphoid follicles and paracortical expansion by an atypical lymphoid infiltrate composed of small- to medium-sized cells, some of which have multiple nuclei (see Fig. 18.7a). There is increased density of high endothelial venules.

Immunohistochemistry highlighted an abnormal CD3+ T-cell population with partial expression of BCL6, PD1, ICOS, CXCL3, and CD10 (see Fig. 18.7c). The dendritic cells associated with the high endothelial venules are highlighted by CD21 (see Fig. 18.7b) and CD23. EBER stains focal large immunoblastic-like cells.

Laboratory Findings

Blood work showed hemolytic anemia with cold agglutinins.

Molecular Genetic Study

PCR and capillary electrophoresis performed on the formalin-fixed paraffin-embedded tissue showed clonal rearrangement of the *TRG*, *IGH*, and *IGK* genes, consistent with the presence of clonal T cells and B cells.

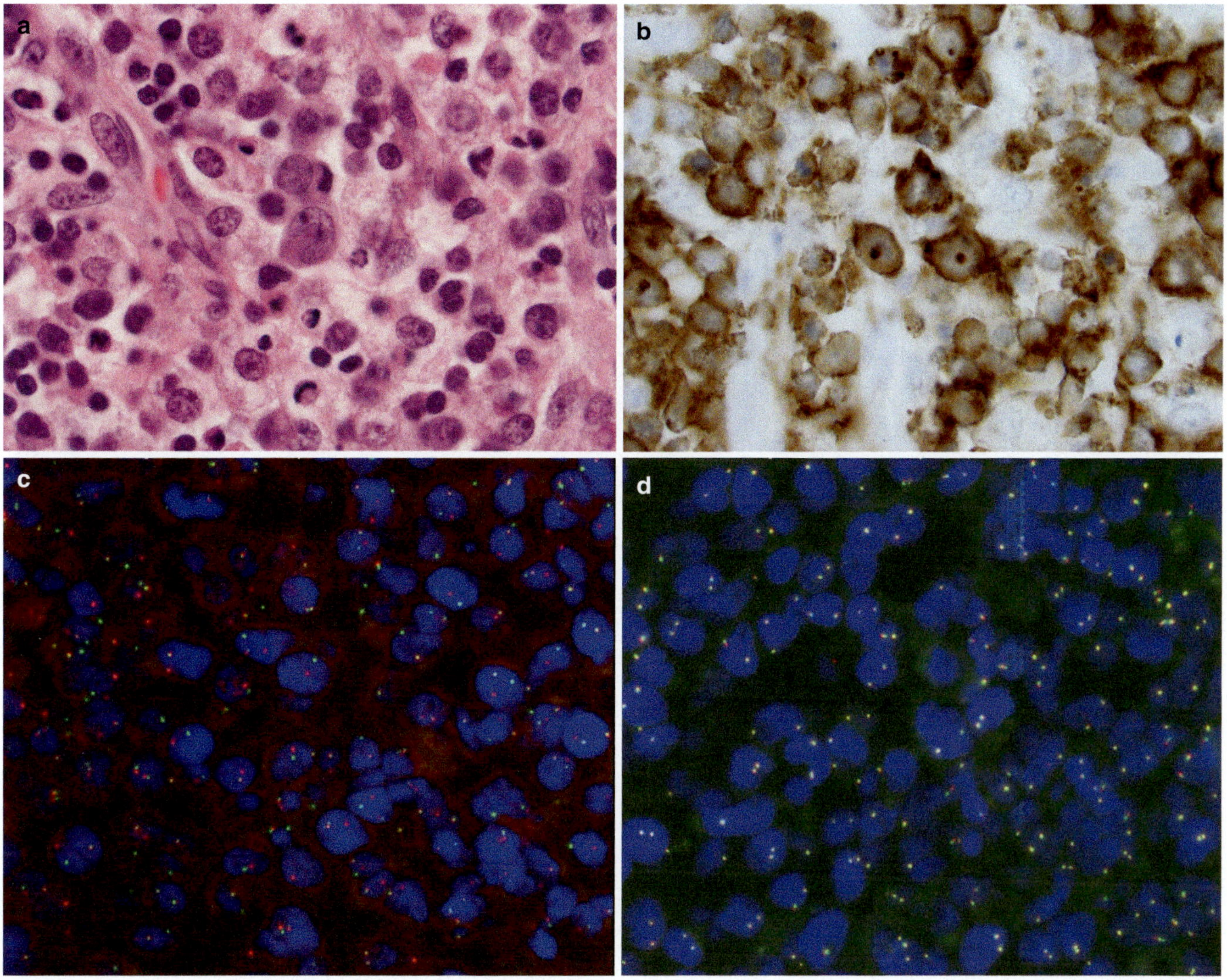

Fig. 18.6 (**a**) ALCL comprising medium-sized to large lymphoma cells with occasional hallmark cells characterized by horseshoe-shaped nuclear contours (H&E stain, ×100 oil). (**b**) Strongly positive CD30 immunostain with a membrane and Golgi pattern in ALCL (×100 oil). (**c**) FISH positive for *DUSP22-IR4* rearrangement with a 1R1G1F signal pattern using a dual-color, break-apart probe set. (**d**) FISH showing a normal 2R2G signal pattern using a dual-color, dual fusion *TBL1XR1/TP63* probe set

Final Diagnosis

Angioimmunoblastic T-cell lymphoma

Follow-Up

The patient was treated with systemic chemotherapy regimen consisting of cyclophosphamide, hydroxydaunorubicin, vincristine, and prednisone (CHOP). She initially showed a good response to treatment with resolution of the lymphadenopathy. However, the patient succumbed to neutropenic sepsis 8 months after diagnosis.

Discussion

Angioimmunoblastic T-cell lymphoma (AITL) is uncommon type of mature T-cell lymphoma that arises from follicular T helper (TFH) cells which represent a crucial checkpoint for B-cell activation and differentiation in the germinal center. AITL is characterized by paracortical proliferation of atypical T cells associated with increased high endothelial venules and follicular dendritic cells [116]. Phenotypically, these CD3+ CD4+ T cells may coexpress CD10, CXCL13, PD1, ICOS, and/or BCL6, which are markers associated with a TFH phenotype [94].

Concurrent *TRG/TRB* and *IGH/IGK* gene rearrangements can be seen in 25–30% of AITL cases, which can potentially cause confusion in its lineage. The immunoglobulin gene rearrangements may be related to EBV infection which is present in ~80–90% of cases and can be detected by EBER in the tissue [93, 115]. Interestingly, gene expression profiling has identified mutations in *TET2, DNMT3A*, and *IDH2*-R172, which share some commonalities with myeloid neoplasms [100, 101].

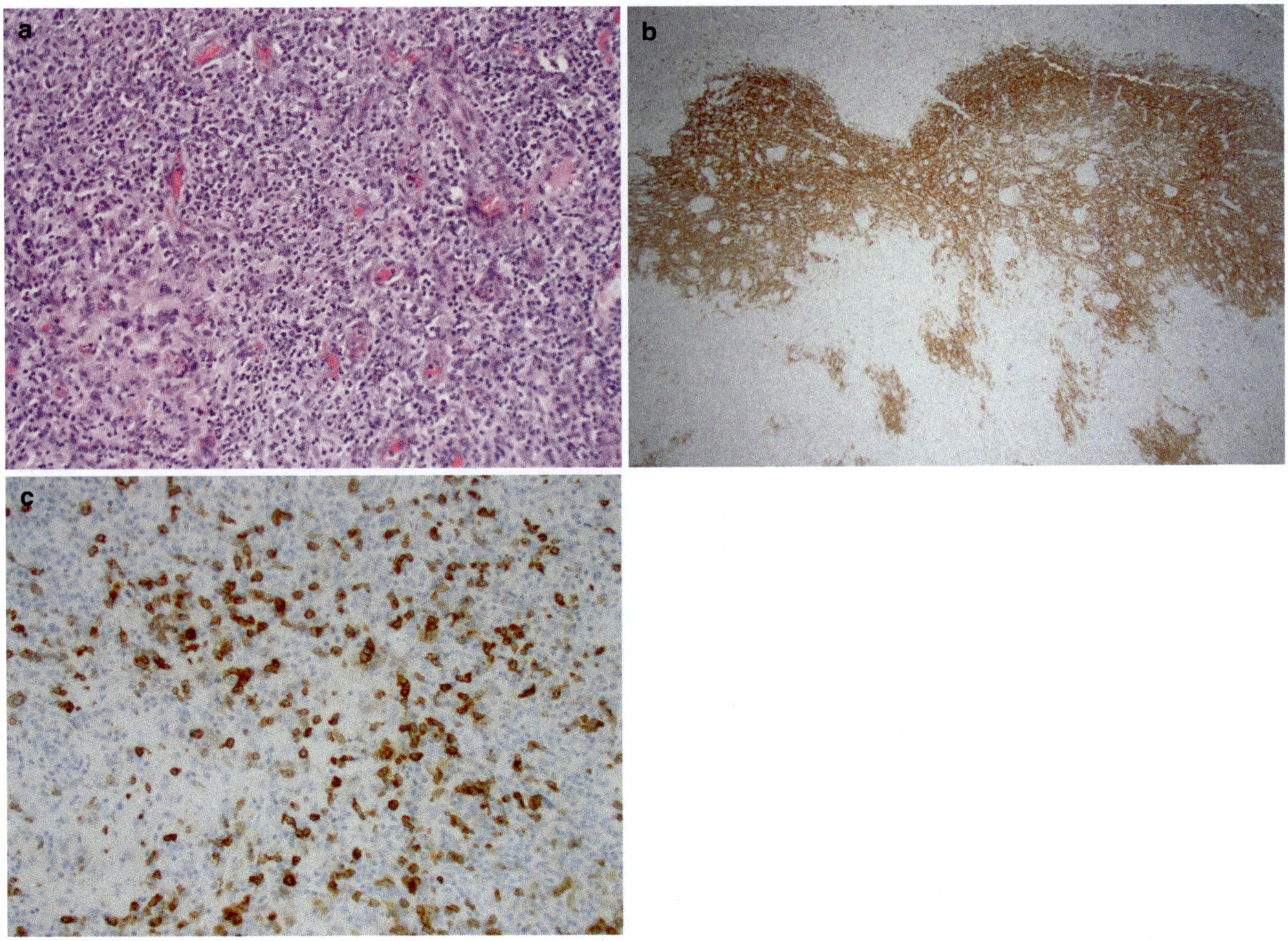

Fig. 18.7 (**a**) Lymph node showing paracortical expansion with prominent vascular proliferation adjacent to a regressed lymphoid follicle near the *lower left* corner (H&E stain, ×20). (**b**) CD23 highlights a markedly expanded follicular dendritic meshwork with extrafollicular extension, entrapping the high endothelial venules (×4). (**c**) A subset of the neoplastic T cells expresses CD10, a TFH marker (×20)

Case 3

Learning Objective

Understand the known etiologic link between a human retrovirus and a mature T-cell lymphoma, which helps to confirm the diagnosis.

Case History

A 49-year-old female from Haiti presented with 1-year history of skin rash and progressive pruritis. Mild axillary lymphadenopathy was found bilaterally.

Histologic Features

The nodal architecture is diffusely effaced by a lymphoid infiltrate composed of variably sized lymphocytes with irregular nuclear contours (see Fig. 18.8a). The proliferative fraction was low and estimated at 10%. Immunohistochemistry revealed an abnormal T-cell phenotype with no coexpression of CD10, BCL6, PD1, CD56, CD57, or CD30. EBER was negative.

Laboratory Findings

CBC was normal except for mild lymphocytosis consisting of some atypical flower-shaped mature lymphocytes (see Fig. 18.8b). Lactate dehydrogenase (LDH) was slightly elevated. Serum calcium was borderline high normal. Serology by enzyme immunoassay was positive for HTLV-1/2 antibody. Flow cytometry of the blood sample showed a proliferation of abnormal CD4+ CD8- T cells with loss of CD7 (see Fig. 18.8c) and coexpression of CD25 and TCRαβ.

Molecular Genetic Studies

The TCRγ and TCRβ genes were clonally rearranged based on PCR and capillary electrophoresis on a lymph node paraffin-embedded tissue block. On the blood sample, real-time PCR for HTLV-1 (targeting the *Pol* gene) was positive, and HTLV-2 was negative, confirming the serological result.

Final Diagnosis

Adult T-cell leukemia/lymphoma, chronic phase

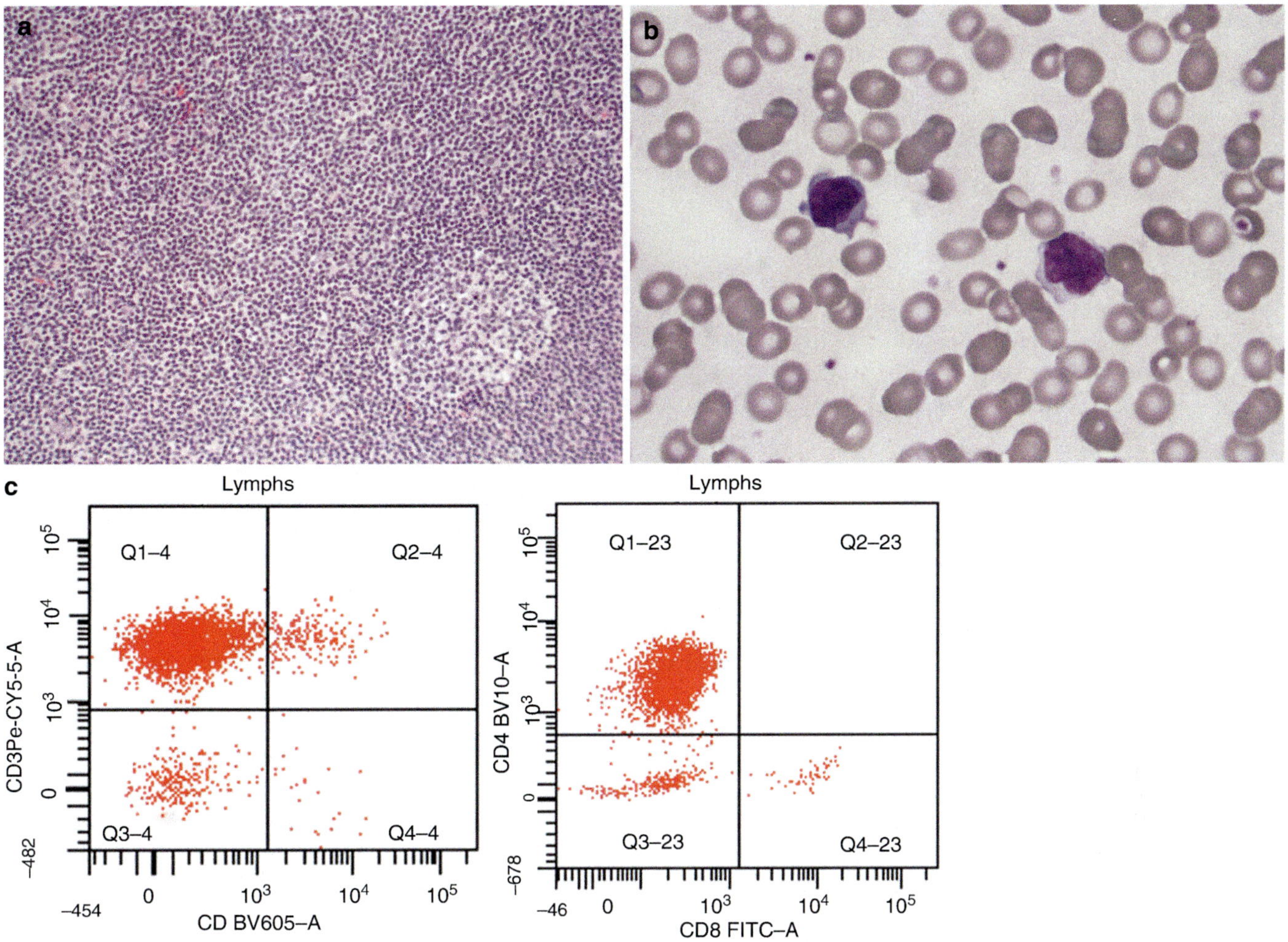

Fig. 18.8 (**a**) ATLL lymphoma cells diffusely expanding the paracortex of the lymph node. A residual lymphoid follicle is seen near the lower right corner (H&E stain, ×20). (**b**) Enlarged lymphocytes with irregular nuclear contours on peripheral blood smear (Wright-Giemsa stain, ×100 oil). (**c**) Abnormal CD4+ CD8- T-cell population (*right panel*) with loss of CD7 (*left panel*) on flow cytometry

Follow-Up

The patient was treated with methotrexate. At 12 months of follow-up, she showed persistent disease by flow cytometry on her peripheral blood. Her disease was clinically nonprogressive. She continued to be monitored closely with CBC and serum chemistry studies, including calcium and LDH.

Discussion

Human T-cell lymphotrophic virus type 1 (HTLV-1) is endemic in Central and South America, the southwestern part of Japan, and parts of Central and West Africa [18]. HTLV-1 is causally related to adult T-cell leukemia/lymphoma (ATLL). The four clinical subtypes of ATLL are: acute, lymphomatous, chronic, and smoldering. The prognosis correlates with the clinical subtype with median survival ranging from ~6 months in the acute subtype to about ~2 years in the chronic subtype and possibly longer in the smoldering subtype [117].

The positive HTLV-1/2 serology using serum or plasma sample can be confirmed by real-time PCR which can also differentiate HTLV-1 from HTLV-2. The genome of HTLV-2 is similar to that of HTLV-1, but is not known to cause human disease. The HTLV-1 genome is monoclonally integrated into the neoplastic T cells and can be demonstrated either by real-time PCR (targeting the *Pol* gene) or conventional PCR (targeting *Tax* and *Pol* genes). The HTLV-1 *Tax* (p40) and *HBZ* genes are believed to play important roles in viral infectivity and leukemogenesis and may potentially be developed into therapeutic targets [118].

Case 4

Case History

A 61-year-old male presented with a fatigue for the past month. He was found to have generalized lymphadenopathy and a rising absolute lymphocyte count that was approaching 60 x 10^9/L.

Histologic Features

The peripheral blood smear showed atypical lymphocytosis with mostly small- to medium-sized mature lymphocytes that were often nucleolated (see Fig. 18.9a). Bone marrow biopsy exhibited an interstitial CD3+ CD4+ lymphoid infiltrate (Fig. 18.9b).

Laboratory Findings

An abnormal lymphocyte population dominated the peripheral blood sample on flow cytometry (>80% of leukocytes). The T cells showed a CD4+ CD8- TCRαβ+ phenotype with a T4:T8 ratio of 80:1 (see Fig. 18.9c). There was loss of CD26 expression on these T cells, which was abnormal. No CD25, CD56, or CD57 coexpression was detectable.

Molecular Genetic Studies

FISH performed on a bone marrow aspirate sample showed an abnormal 1R1G1F signal pattern with a dual-color break-apart probe set, indicative of *TCL1* gene rearrangement at locus 14q32.1 (see Fig. 18.9d). In addition, a gain-of-function mutation of the *JAK3* gene was detected using a 75-gene NGS panel performed on the bone marrow.

Final Diagnosis

T-cell prolymphocytic leukemia

Follow-Up

The patient was treated intravenously with alemtuzumab, an anti-CD52 monoclonal antibody, and showed good response with a reduction in his peripheral lymphocyte count at 4 months of follow-up.

Discussion

T-PLL, a rare type of mature T-cell leukemia, is composed typically of small- to medium-sized non-granular lymphocytes that are commonly found in the blood, bone marrow, spleen, liver, and lymph nodes. It can involve the skin and serous effusions in a minority of cases. International consensus guidelines for the diagnosis of T-PLL have been developed [14] that incorporate clinical and genetic features [see Table 18.1].

This patient satisfied all three major criteria for the diagnosis of T-PLL. He had a circulating T-PLL cell count of >5 × 10^9/L. Clonality was established by flow cytometry based on an abnormal CD4+ CD8- T-cell phenotype with loss of CD26 expression. FISH on the marrow sample demonstrated rearrangement of the *TCL1* gene at 14q32.1 locus, while NGS showed a mutation of the *JAK3* gene.

If only two of the major criteria are represent, at least one of the four clinical/genetic minor criteria should be satisfied in order to establish a diagnosis of T-PLL – abnormalities involving chromosome 11 (11q22.3; *ATM*); abnormalities in chromosome 8 which can include idic(8)(p11), t(8;8), or trisomy 8q; abnormalities in chromosome 5, 12, 13, 22, or complex karyotype; and involvement of a T-PLL-specific site (e.g., splenomegaly, effusions). This patient did not have karyotyping performed in the bone marrow. He had mild borderline splenomegaly and no effusions.

Pathogenetically, the *TCL1* gene is thought to have oncogenic potential [14]. A gain-of-function mutation of the *JAK3* gene activates the JAK/STAT signaling cascade which is a recurrent mechanism of action seen in T-PLL [15].

Case 5

Case History

An 86-year-old male who had been in remission for 11 years from diffuse large B-cell lymphoma presented with B symptoms. PET CT showed extensive hypermetabolic lymphadenopathy, splenomegaly, and marrow activity.

Histologic Features

The lymph node architecture was effaced by a diffuse proliferation of atypical polymorphous lymphocytes (see Fig. 18.10 A1–A8). Immunohistochemistry revealed an aberrant T-cell phenotype (CD3+, double CD4/CD8 negative, CD5 –/+) and a proliferative fraction of ~50%. No coexpression of CD25, EBER, or follicular helper T-cell (TFH) markers with the exception of patchy staining for PD1 is present. Bone marrow biopsy showed interstitial lymphoid aggregates with a similar phenotype as the lymph node, consistent with infiltration by the same T-cell neoplasm with an estimated 20% marrow involvement (see Fig. 18.10 B1–B6). The erythroid series shows nuclear/cytoplasmic dyssynchrony on aspirate smear examination and 4% myeloblasts.

Laboratory Findings

CBC showed neutrophilia, mild lymphopenia, anemia, and thrombocytopenia. Flow cytometric analysis of the marrow sample showed no abnormal B-cell or T-cell population and very low lymphocyte frequency overall. Chromosomal analysis showed del(20)(q11.2q13.1) in 12 of 20 cells.

Molecular Genetic Studies

Clonal *TRG* gene rearrangement was demonstrable in the lymph node. A 75-gene NGS panel performed on the lymph node showed the presence of four mutations involving the

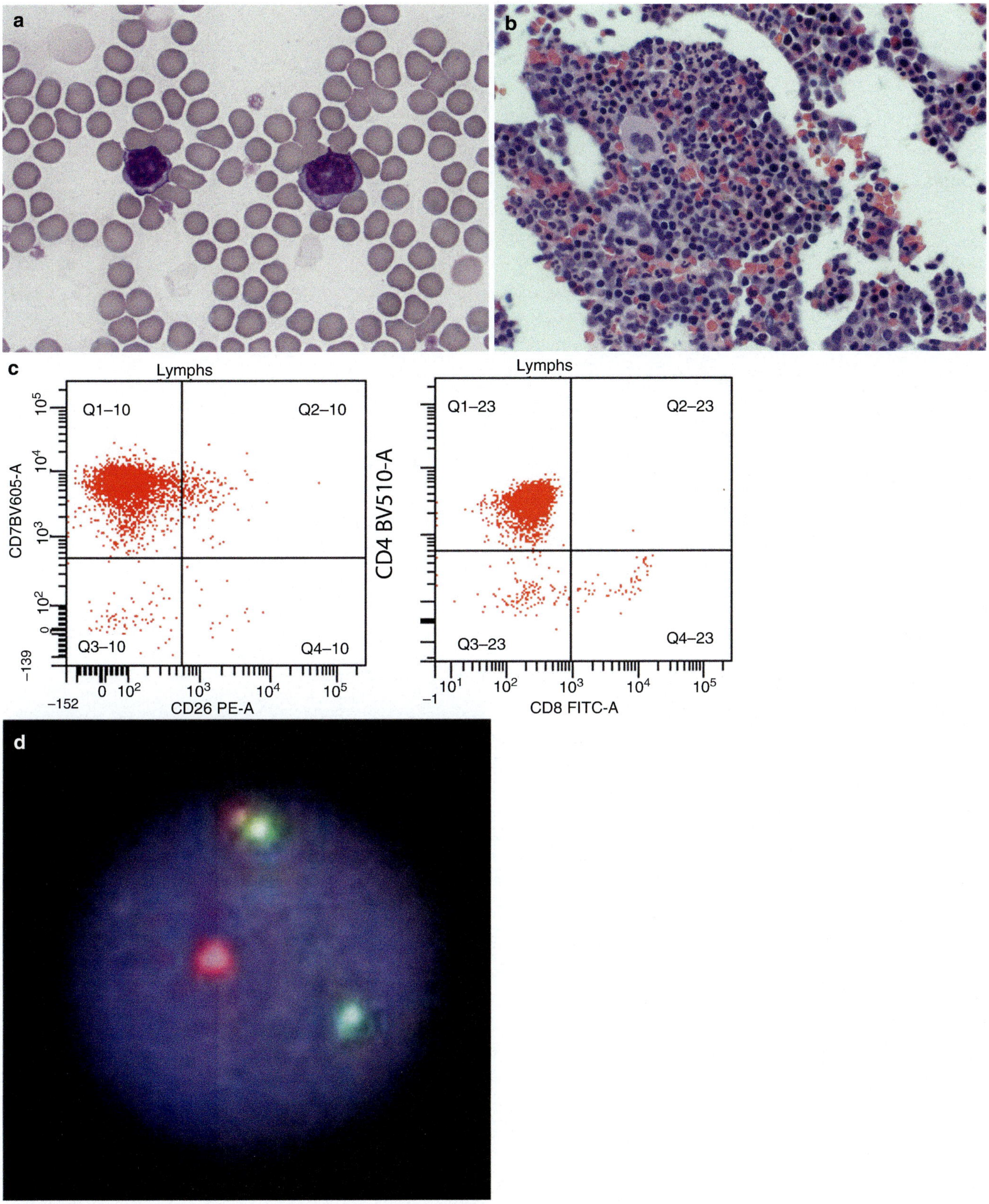

Fig. 18.9 (**a**) T-prolymphocytic leukemia with nucleolated small- to medium-sized lymphocytes on peripheral blood smear (Wright-Giemsa stain, ×100 oil). (**b**) Bone marrow biopsy shows an interstitial lymphoid cell infiltrate. (**c**) Clonal T cells showing a CD4+ CD8- phenotype and loss of CD26 by flow cytometry. (**d**) Abnormal 1R1G1F FISH signal with a dual-color break-apart probe set, indicative of *TCL1* gene rearrangement

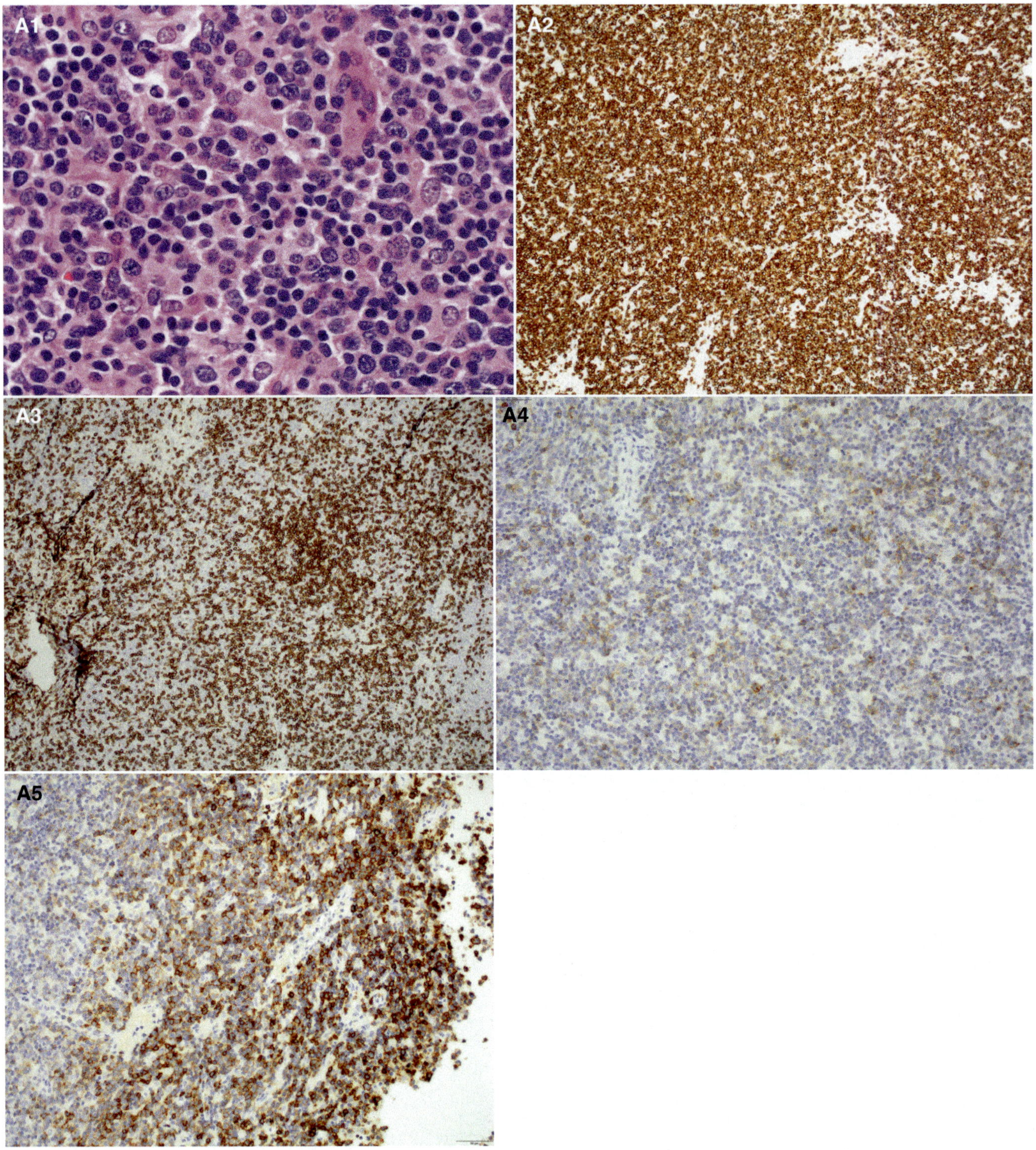

Fig. 18.10 The lymph node (A1–A8) shows diffuse proliferation of variably sized atypical lymphocytes (A1). Immunohistochemistry shows strong CD3 expression (A2) and partial loss of CD5 (A3). A subset of the cells immunoreacts with PD-1 (A4, A5) and no other TFH-associated markers. Flow cytometry shows a dominant T-cell population with cytoplasmic CD3 expression (yellow population in A6). These T cells show partial dim surface CD3 expression but lack other T-cell-associated antigens, including CD4 and CD8 (aqua population in A7). *TRG* gene rearrangement based on a consensus multiplex PCR protocol using standard BIOMED-2 primer sets shows two clonal peaks (214 bp and 241 bp) in the lymph node sample (A8). The staging bone marrow aspirate smear (B1), clot (B2), and biopsy (B3) shows mostly maturing hematopoietic cells. Scattered small interstitial lymphoid aggregates constitute about 20% of the cells in the biopsy and are composed of T cells showing CD3 expression (B4), partial loss of CD5 (B5), and presence of PD-1 (B6)

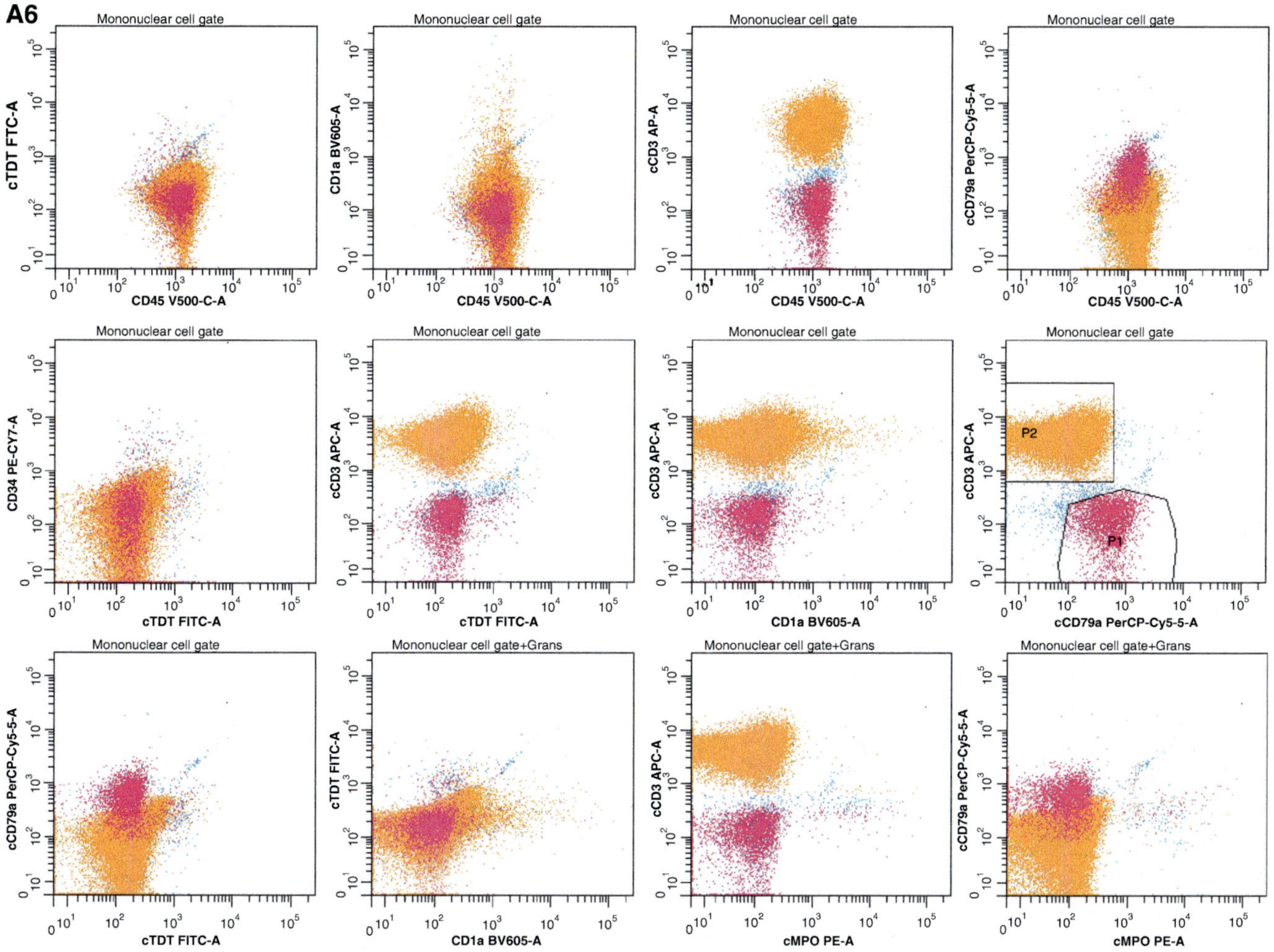

Fig. 18.10 (continued)

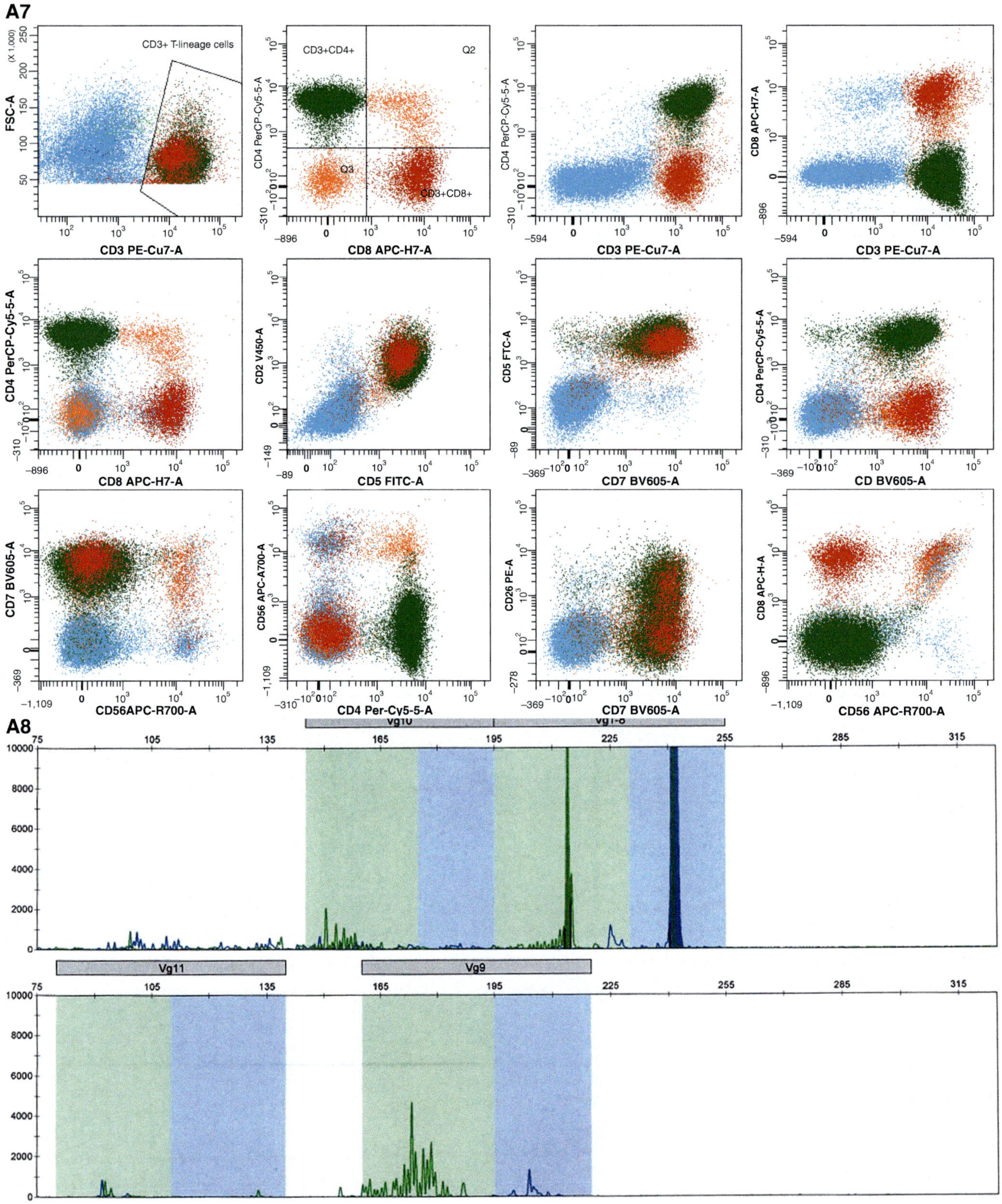

Fig. 18.10 (continued)

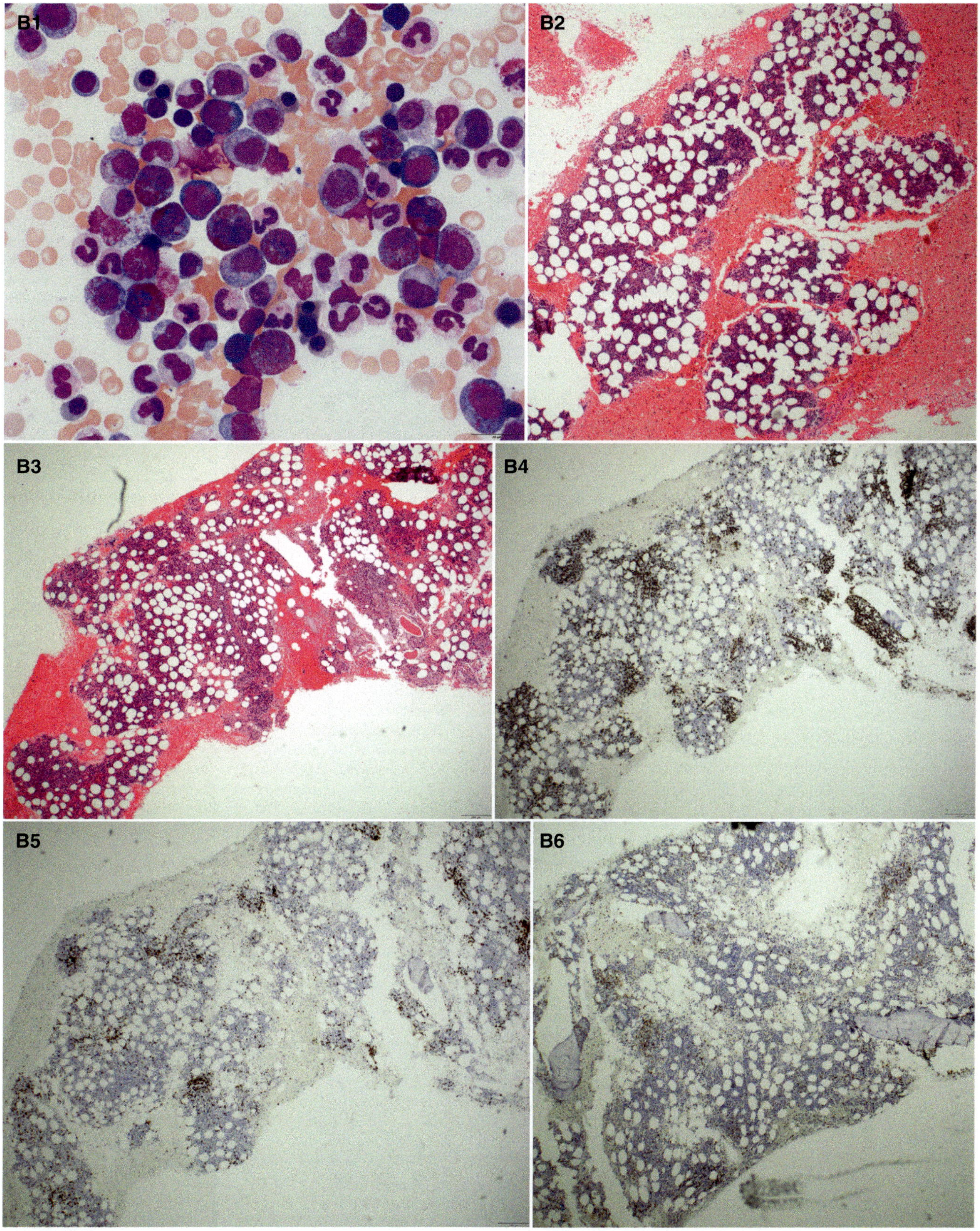

Fig. 18.10 (continued)

Table 18.6 Mutational profiles: lymph node versus bone marrow sample (Case #5)

Mutations	VAF in lymph node (%)	VAF in bone marrow (%)
DNMT3A c.2645G > A (p.R882H)	36	48
TET2 c.3880 T > C (p. Y1294)	31	50
TET2 c.3046delT (p. C1016fs)	20	33
TP53 c.524G > A (p. R175H)	18	2

Note: The VAFs of the first two mutations approached 50%, which was significantly higher than the percentage involvement of lymphoma cells in the bone marrow biopsy, suggesting that these mutations might reside in the myeloid cells
Abbreviation: *VAF* variant allele frequency

DNMT3A, *TET2*, and *TP53* genes (Table 18.6). The same four mutations were detected in the bone marrow sample, two of which had variant allele frequencies that approached 50%.

Final Diagnosis

Peripheral T-cell lymphoma, NOS involving lymph node and bone marrow

Myeloid neoplasm with myelodysplastic features, which may represent therapy-related myeloid neoplasm, in light of the patient's history of chemotherapy

Discussion

The distinction between peripheral T-cell lymphoma, not otherwise specified (PTCL-NOS), and nodal T-cell lymphomas with a TFH phenotype, including AITL, can be challenging at times. TFH cells display a characteristic CD4+, CD10+, CXCR5+, BCL6+, ICOS+, and PD1+ phenotype [94]. However, none of these markers are in and of themselves specific for TFH. In the absence of other morphologic characteristics of AITL, PTCL-NOS can be diagnosed if there is expression of only a single TFH-associated marker in this CD4-negative T-cell lymphoma, as seen in the current case.

Mutations involving the *DNMT3A* and *TET2* genes are seen commonly in AITL and myeloid neoplasms, including myelodysplastic syndrome (MDS). These genes can also be observed in PTCL-NOS, albeit less commonly [101, 102]. Given the relatively low tumor burden in the marrow as demonstrated by immunostains on the biopsy (about 20%) and the negative flow cytometry, the high VAFs (~50%) involving two of the mutations suggested that these mutations were present in the myeloid lineage. The low-level *TP53* mutation (2% VAF) detected in the marrow aspirate probably originated from the small number of lymphoma cells that had escaped entrapment by reticulin fibers. The same *TP53* mutation was detectable in the lymph node. Hence, NGS played an instrumental role in the deduction of a myeloid neoplasm concurrent with PTCL-NOS in the bone marrow.

(Case 5 is contributed by Dr. Linsheng Zhang, Emory University School of Medicine).

References

1. Langerak AW, Groenen PJ, Brüggemann M, et al. EuroClonality/BIOMED-2 guidelines for interpretation and reporting of Ig/TCR clonality testing in suspected lymphoproliferations. Leukemia. 2012;26(10):2159–71.
2. Liu X, He H, Li Y, et al. The application of antigen receptor gene rearrangement of BIOMED-2 in the pathologic diagnosis of 348 cases with non-Hodgkin lymphoma in a single institution in Southwest of China. Pathol Res Pract. 2019;215(11):152615.
3. Tan BT, Seo K, Warnke RA, Arber DA. The frequency of immunoglobulin heavy chain gene and T-cell receptor gamma-chain gene rearrangements and Epstein-Barr virus in ALK+ and ALK- anaplastic large cell lymphoma and other peripheral T-cell lymphomas. J Mol Diagn. 2008;10(6):502–12.
4. Patel KP, Pan Q, Wang Y, et al. Comparison of BIOMED-2 versus laboratory-developed polymerase chain reaction assays for detecting T-cell receptor-gamma gene rearrangements. J Mol Diagn. 2010;12(2):226–37.
5. van Dongen JJ, Langerak AW, Brüggemann M, Evans PA, Hummel M, Lavender FL, et al. Design and standardization of PCR primers and protocols for detection of clonal immunoglobulin and T-cell receptor gene recombinations in suspect lymphoproliferations: report of the BIOMED-2 Concerted Action BMH4-CT98-3936. Leukemia. 2003;17(12):2257–317.
6. Poopak B, Saki N, Purfatholah AA, Najmabadi H, Mortazavi Y, Arzanian MT, et al. Pattern of immunoglobulin and T-cell receptor-δ/γ gene rearrangements in Iranian children with B-precursor acute lymphoblastic leukemia. Hematology. 2014;19(5):259–66.
7. Szczepański T, Beishuizen A, Pongers-Willemse MJ, Hählen K, Van Wering ER, Wijkhuijs AJ, et al. Cross-lineage T cell receptor gene rearrangements occur in more than ninety percent of childhood precursor-B acute lymphoblastic leukemias: alternative PCR targets for detection of minimal residual disease. Leukemia. 1999;13(2):196–205.
8. Havran WL, Boismenu R. Activation and function of gamma delta T cells. Curr Opin Immunol. 1994;6:442–6.
9. Tripodo C, Iannitto E, Florena AM, et al. Gamma-delta T-cell lymphomas. Nat Rev Clin Oncol. 2009;6:707–17.
10. Armand M, Derrieux C, Beldjord K, et al. A new and simple TRG multiplex PCR assay for assessment of t-cell clonality: a comparative study from the EuroClonality Consortium. Hemasphere. 2019;3(3):e255. Published 2019 Jun 4.
11. Fan H, Robetorye RS. Detection of clonal T-cell receptor beta and gamma chain gene rearrangement by polymerase chain reaction and capillary gel electrophoresis. Methods Mol Biol. 2013;999:169–88.
12. Schumacher JA, Duncavage EJ, Mosbruger TL, Szankasi PM, Kelley TW. A comparison of deep sequencing of TCRG rearrangements vs traditional capillary electrophoresis for assessment of clonality in T-cell lymphoproliferative disorders. Am J Clin Pathol. 2014;141(3):348–59.
13. Brüggemann M, Kotrová M, Knecht H, et al. Standardized next-generation sequencing of immunoglobulin and T-cell receptor gene recombinations for MRD marker identification in acute lymphoblastic leukaemia; a EuroClonality-NGS validation study. Leukemia. 2019;33(9):2241–53.

14. Staber PB, Herling M, Bellido M, Jacobsen ED, Davids MS, Kadia TM, et al. Consensus criteria for diagnosis, staging, and treatment response assessment of T-cell prolymphocytic leukemia. Blood. 2019;134(14):1132–43.
15. Sud A, Dearden C. T-cell prolymphocytic leukemia. Hematol Oncol Clin North Am. 2017;31(2):273–83.
16. Schrader A, Crispatzu G, Oberbeck S, Mayer P, Pützer S, von Jan J, et al. Actionable perturbations of damage responses by TCL1/ATM and epigenetic lesions form the basis of T-PLL. Nat Commun. 2018;9(1):697.
17. Teitell MA. The TCL1 family of oncoproteins: co-activators of transformation. Nat Rev Cancer. 2005;5:640–8.
18. Malpica L, Pimentel A, Reis IM, Gotuzzo E, Lekakis L, Komanduri K, Harrington T, Barber GN, Ramos JC. Epidemiology, clinical features, and outcome of HTLV-1-related ATLL in an area of prevalence in the United States. Blood Adv. 2018;2(6):607–20.
19. Satake M, Yamada Y, Atogami S, Yamaguchi K. The incidence of adult T-cell leukemia/lymphoma among human T-lymphotropic virus type 1 carriers in Japan. Leuk Lymphoma. 2015;56(6):1806–12.
20. Kuramitsu M, Okuma K, Yamochi T, Sato T, Sasaki D, Hasegawa H, et al. Standardization of quantitative PCR for human T-cell leukemia virus type 1 in Japan: a collaborative study. J Clin Microbiol. 2015;53(11):3485–91.
21. Martin JL, Maldonado JO, Mueller JD, Zhang W, Mansky LM. Molecular studies of HTLV-1 replication: an update. Viruses. 2016;8(2):31.
22. Lemasson I, Lewis MR, Polakowski N, Hivin P, Cavanagh MH, Thébault S, Barbeau B, Nyborg JK, Mesnard JM. Human T-cell leukemia virus type 1 (HTLV-1) bZIP protein interacts with the cellular transcription factor CREB to inhibit HTLV-1 transcription. J Virol. 2007;81(4):1543–53.
23. Satou Y, Yasunaga J, Yoshida M, Matsuoka M. HTLV-I basic leucine zipper factor gene mRNA supports proliferation of adult T cell leukemia cells. Proc Natl Acad Sci U S A. 2006;103:720–5.
24. Nakagawa M, Schmitz R, Xiao W, Goldman CK, Xu W, Yang Y, et al. Gain-of-function CCR4 mutations in adult T cell leukemia/lymphoma. J Exp Med. 2014;211(13):2497–505.
25. Fochi S, Ciminale V, Trabetti E, Bertazzoni U, D'Agostino DM, Zipeto D, et al. NF-κB and MicroRNA deregulation mediated by HTLV-1 tax and HBZ. Pathogens. 2019;8(4):290.
26. Martin JL, Maldonado JO, Mueller JD, Zhang W, Mansky LM. Molecular studies of HTLV-1 replication: an update. Viruses. 2016;8(2):31.
27. Kataoka K, Iwanaga M, Yasunaga JI, Nagata Y, Kitanaka A, Kameda T, et al. Prognostic relevance of integrated genetic profiling in adult T-cell leukemia/lymphoma. Blood. 2018;131(2):215–25.
28. Gaulard P, Jaffe ES, Krenacs L, Macon WR. Hepatosplenic T-cell lymphoma. In: Swerdlow SH, Campo E, Harris NL, Jaffe ES, Pileri SA, Stein H, Thiele J, editors. WHO classification of tumours of haematopoietic and lymphoid tissues. France: IARC Lyon; 2017. p. 381–2.
29. Yabe M, Medeiros LJ, Tang G, et al. Prognostic factors of hepatosplenic T-cell lymphoma (HSTCL): a clinicopathologic, immunophenotypic, and cytogenetic analysis of 28 patients. Am J Surg Pathol. 2016;40:676–88.
30. Alonsozana EL, Stamberg J, Kumar D, et al. Isochromosome 7q: the primary cytogenetic abnormality in hepatosplenic gamma delta T cell lymphoma. Leukemia. 1997;11:1367–72.
31. Yabe M, Miranda RN, Medeiros LJ. Hepatosplenic T-cell lymphoma: a review of clinicopathologic features, pathogenesis, and prognostic factors. Hum Pathol. 2018;74:5–16.
32. Finalet Ferreiro J, Rouhigharabaei L, Urbankova H, van der Krogt JA, Michaux L, Shetty S, et al. Integrative genomic and transcriptomic analysis identified candidate genes implicated in the pathogenesis of hepatosplenic T-cell lymphoma. PLoS One. 2014;9(7):e102977.
33. McKinney M, Moffitt AB, Gaulard P, et al. The genetic basis of hepatosplenic T cell lymphoma. Cancer Discov. 2017;4:369–79.
34. Jawed SI, Myskowski PL, Horwitz S, Moskowitz A, Querfeld C. Primary cutaneous T-cell lymphoma (mycosis fungoides and Sézary syndrome): part I. Diagnosis: clinical and histopathologic features and new molecular and biologic markers. J Am Acad Dermatol. 2014;70(2):205.e1–16; quiz 221–2.
35. Bergman R, Faclieru D, Sahar D, Sander CA, Kerner H, Ben-Aryeh Y, et al. Immunophenotyping and T-cell receptor gamma gene rearrangement analysis as an adjunct to the histopathologic diagnosis of mycosis fungoides. J Am Acad Dermatol. 1998;39:554–9.
36. Hsiao PF, Hsiao CH, Lin YC, Tseng M, Tsai TF, Jee SH. Histopathologic-molecular correlation in early mycosis fungoides using T-cell receptor gamma gene rearrangement by polymerase chain reaction with laser capture microdissection. J Formos Med Assoc. 2007;106:265–72.
37. Walia R, Yeung CCS. An update on molecular biology of cutaneous T cell lymphoma. Front Oncol. 2020;9:1558.
38. Ralfkiaer U, Lindahl LM, Litman T, Gjerdrum LM, Ahler CB, Gniadecki R, et al. MicroRNA expression in early mycosis fungoides is distinctly different from atopic dermatitis and advanced cutaneous T-cell lymphoma. Anticancer Res. 2014;34(12):7207–17.
39. Garaicoa FH, Roisman A, Arias M, Trila C, Fridmanis M, Abeldaño A, et al. Genomic imbalances and microRNA transcriptional profiles in patients with mycosis fungoides. Tumour Biol. 2016;37(10):13637–47.
40. Manso R, Martínez-Magunacelaya N, Eraña-Tomás I, Monsalvez V, Rodríguez-Peralto JL, Ortiz-Romero PL, et al. Mycosis fungoides progression could be regulated by microRNAs. PLoS One. 2018;13(6):e0198477.
41. Delfau-Larue MH, Laroche L, Wechsler J, Lepage E, Lahet C, Asso-Bonnet M, Bagot M, Farcet JP. Diagnostic value of dominant T-cell clones in peripheral blood in 363 patients presenting consecutively with a clinical suspicion of cutaneous lymphoma. Blood. 2000;96(9):2987–92.
42. Katona TM, O'Malley DP, Cheng L, Hiatt KM, Wang M, Anagnostou JJ Jr, et al. Loss of heterozygosity analysis identifies genetic abnormalities in mycosis fungoides and specific loci associated with disease progression. Am J Surg Pathol. 2007;31(10):1552–6.
43. Lamy T, Moignet A, Loughran TP Jr. LGL leukemia: from pathogenesis to treatment. Blood. 2017;129(9):1082–94.
44. Loughran TP Jr, Zickl L, Olson TL, Wang V, Zhang D, Rajala HL, et al. Immunosuppressive therapy of LGL leukemia: prospective multicenter phase II study by the Eastern Cooperative Oncology Group (E5998). Leukemia. 2015;29(4):886–94.
45. Koskela HL, Eldfors S, Ellonen P, et al. Somatic STAT3 mutations in large granular lymphocytic leukemia. N Engl J Med. 2012;366(20):1905–13.
46. Jerez A, Clemente MJ, Makishima H, et al. STAT3 mutations unify the pathogenesis of chronic lymphoproliferative disorders of NK cells and T-cell large granular lymphocyte leukemia. Blood. 2012;120(15):3048–57.
47. Rajala HL, Eldfors S, Kuusanmäki H, van Adrichem AJ, Olson T, Lagström S, et al. Discovery of somatic STAT5b mutations in large granular lymphocytic leukemia. Blood. 2013;121(22):4541–50.
48. Rajala HL, Porkka K, Maciejewski JP, Loughran TP Jr, Mustjoki S. Uncovering the pathogenesis of large granular lymphocytic leukemia-novel STAT3 and STAT5b mutations. Ann Med. 2014;46(3):114–22.
49. Bárcena P, Jara-Acevedo M, Tabernero MD, López A, Sánchez ML, García-Montero AC, et al. Phenotypic profile of expanded

NK cells in chronic lymphoproliferative disorders: a surrogate marker for NK-cell clonality. Oncotarget. 2015;6(40):42938–51.
50. Allen RC, Zoghbi HY, Moseley AB, Rosenblatt HM, Belmont JW. Methylation of HpaII and HhaI sites near the polymorphic CAG repeat in the human androgen-receptor gene correlates with X chromosome inactivation. Am J Hum Genet. 1992;51(6):1229–39.
51. Haverkos BM, Pan Z, Gru AA, et al. Extranodal NK/T cell lymphoma, nasal type (ENKTL-NT): an update on epidemiology, clinical presentation, and natural history in North American and European cases. Curr Hematol Malig Rep. 2016;11(6):514–27.
52. Tse E, Kwong YL. The diagnosis and management of NK/T-cell lymphomas. J Hematol Oncol. 2017;10(1):85.
53. Hong M, Lee T, Young Kang S, Kim SJ, Kim W, Ko YH. Nasal-type NK/T-cell lymphomas are more frequently T rather than NK lineage based on T-cell receptor gene, RNA, and protein studies: lineage does not predict clinical behavior. Mod Pathol. 2016;29(5):430–43.
54. Ng SB, Khoury JD. Epstein-Barr virus in lymphoproliferative processes: an update for the diagnostic pathologist. Adv Anat Pathol. 2009;16(1):40–55.
55. de Mel S, Hue SS, Jeyasekharan AD, Chng WJ, Ng SB. Molecular pathogenic pathways in extranodal NK/T cell lymphoma. J Hematol Oncol. 2019;12(1):33.
56. Chen YW, Guo T, Shen L, Wong KY, Tao Q, Choi WW, et al. Receptor-type tyrosine-protein phosphatase kappa directly targets STAT3 activation for tumor suppression in nasal NK/T-cell lymphoma. Blood. 2015;125(10):1589–600.
57. Tse E, Kwong YL. NK/T-cell lymphomas. Best Pract Res Clin Haematol. 2019;32(3):253–61.
58. Zhang Y, Li C, Xue W, Zhang M, Li Z. Frequent mutations in natural killer/T cell lymphoma. Cell Physiol Biochem. 2018;49(1):1–16.
59. Jiang L, Gu Z, Yan Z, et al. Exome sequencing identifies somatic mutations of DDX3X in natural killer/T-cell lymphoma. Nat Genet. 2015;47:1061–6.
60. Cohen JI, Iwatsuki K, Ko YH, Kimura H, Manoli I, Ohshima K, et al. Epstein-Barr virus NK and T cell lymphoproliferative disease: report of a 2018 international meeting. Leuk Lymphoma. 2020;61(4):808–19.
61. Dufva O, Kankainen M, Kelkka T, et al. Aggressive natural killer-cell leukemia mutational landscape and drug profiling highlight JAK-STAT signaling as therapeutic target. Nat Commun. 2018;9(1):1567.
62. Huang L, Liu D, Wang N, Ling S, Tang Y, Wu J, et al. Integrated genomic analysis identifies deregulated JAK/STAT-MYC-biosynthesis axis in aggressive NK-cell leukemia. Cell Res. 2018;28(2):172–86.
63. Nakashima Y, Tagawa H, Suzuki R, Karnan S, Karube K, Ohshima K, et al. Genome-wide array-based comparative genomic hybridization of natural killer cell lymphoma/leukemia: different genomic alteration patterns of aggressive NK-cell leukemia and extranodal Nk/T-cell lymphoma, nasal type. Genes Chromosomes Cancer. 2005;44(3):247–55.
64. Ducray SP, Natarajan K, Garland GD, Turner SD, Egger G. The transcriptional roles of ALK fusion proteins in tumorigenesis. Cancers (Basel). 2019;11(8):1074.
65. Pan Z, Hu S, Li M, Zhou Y, Kim YS, Reddy V, et al. ALK-positive large B-cell lymphoma: a clinicopathologic study of 26 cases with review of additional 108 cases in the literature. Am J Surg Pathol. 2017;41(1):25–38.
66. Ferreri AJ, Govi S, Pileri SA, Savage KJ. Anaplastic large cell lymphoma, ALK-negative. Crit Rev Oncol Hematol. 2013;85(2):206–15.
67. Hallberg B, Palmer RH. Mechanistic insight into ALK receptor tyrosine kinase in human cancer biology. Nat Rev Cancer. 2013;13(10):685–700.
68. Tsuyama N, Sakamoto K, Sakata S, Dobashi A, Takeuchi K. Anaplastic large cell lymphoma: pathology, genetics, and clinical aspects. J Clin Exp Hematop. 2017;57(3):120–42.
69. Li Y, Wang K, Song N, Hou K, Che X, Zhou Y, et al. Activation of IGF-1R pathway and NPM-ALK G1269A mutation confer resistance to crizotinib treatment in NPM-ALK positive lymphoma. Investig New Drugs. 2020;38(3):599–609.
70. Prieto-Torres L, Rodriguez-Pinilla SM, Onaindia A, Ara M, Requena L, Piris MÁ. CD30-positive primary cutaneous lymphoproliferative disorders: molecular alterations and targeted therapies. Haematologica. 2019;104(2):226–35.
71. Cao S, Nambudiri VE. Anaplastic lymphoma kinase in cutaneous malignancies. Cancers (Basel). 2017;9(9):123.
72. Montes-Mojarro IA, Steinhilber J, Bonzheim I, Quintanilla-Martinez L, Fend F. The pathological spectrum of systemic Anaplastic Large Cell Lymphoma (ALCL). Cancers (Basel). 2018;10(4):107.
73. Onaindia A, Montes-Moreno S, Rodríguez-Pinilla SM, Batlle A, González de Villambrosía S, Rodríguez AM, et al. Primary cutaneous anaplastic large cell lymphomas with 6p25.3 rearrangement exhibit particular histological features. Histopathology. 2015;66(6):846–55.
74. Feldman AL, Dogan A, Smith DI, et al. Discovery of recurrent t(6;7)(p25.3;q32.3) translocations in ALK-negative anaplastic large cell lymphomas by massively parallel genomic sequencing. Blood. 2011;117(3):915–9.
75. Wada DA, Law ME, Hsi ED, et al. Specificity of IRF4 translocations for primary cutaneous anaplastic large cell lymphoma: a multicenter study of 204 skin biopsies. Mod Pathol. 2011;24(4):596–605.
76. Velusamy T, Kiel MJ, Sahasrabuddhe AA, Rolland D, Dixon CA, Bailey NG, et al. A novel recurrent NPM1-TYK2 gene fusion in cutaneous CD30-positive lymphoproliferative disorders. Blood. 2014;124(25):3768–71.
77. Bennani-Baiti N, Ansell S, Feldman AL. Adult systemic anaplastic large-cell lymphoma: recommendations for diagnosis and management. Expert Rev Hematol. 2016;9(2):137–50.
78. Zeng Y, Feldman AL. Genetics of anaplastic large cell lymphoma. Leuk Lymphoma. 2016;57(1):21–7.
79. Wang X, Boddicker RL, Dasari S, et al. Expression of p63 protein in anaplastic large cell lymphoma: implications for genetic subtyping. Hum Pathol. 2017;64:19–27.
80. Piva R, Agnelli L, Pellegrino E, Todoerti K, Grosso V, Tamagno I, et al. Gene expression profiling uncovers molecular classifiers for the recognition of anaplastic large-cell lymphoma within peripheral T-cell neoplasms. J Clin Oncol. 2010;28(9):1583–90.
81. Mereu E, Pellegrino E, Scarfò I, Inghirami G, Piva R. The heterogeneous landscape of ALK negative ALCL. Oncotarget. 2017;8(11):18525–36.
82. Schleussner N, Merkel O, Costanza M, et al. The AP-1-BATF and -BATF3 module is essential for growth, survival and TH17/ILC3 skewing of anaplastic large cell lymphoma. Leukemia. 2018;32(9):1994–2007.
83. Laurent C, Delas A, Gaulard P, et al. Breast implant-associated anaplastic large cell lymphoma: two distinct clinicopathological variants with different outcomes. Ann Oncol. 2016;27(2):306–14.
84. Blombery P, Thompson E, Ryland GL, Joyce R, Byrne DJ, Khoo C, Lade S, Hertzberg M, Hapgood G, Marlton P, Deva A, Lindeman G, Fox S, Westerman D, Prince M. Frequent activating STAT3 mutations and novel recurrent genomic abnormalities detected in breast implant-associated anaplastic large cell lymphoma. Oncotarget. 2018;9(90):36126–36.
85. Oishi N, Brody GS, Ketterling RP, et al. Genetic subtyping of breast implant-associated anaplastic large cell lymphoma. Blood. 2018;132(5):544–7.
86. Fujiwara SI, Yamashita Y, Nakamura N, Choi YL, Ueno T, Watanabe H, et al. High-resolution analysis of chromosome copy

number alterations in angioimmunoblastic T-cell lymphoma and peripheral T-cell lymphoma, unspecified, with single nucleotide polymorphism-typing microarrays. Leukemia. 2008;22:1891–8.
87. Iqbal J, Wright G, Wang C, Rosenwald A, Gascoyne RD, Weisenburger DD, et al. Lymphoma leukemia molecular profiling project and the international peripheral T-cell lymphoma project. Gene expression signatures delineate biological and prognostic subgroups in peripheral T-cell lymphoma. Blood. 2014;123(19):2915–23.
88. Zhang Y, Lee D, Brimer T, Hussaini M, Sokol L. Genomics of peripheral T-cell lymphoma and its implications for personalized medicine. Front Oncol. 2020;10:898.
89. Amador C, Greiner TC, Heavican TB, Smith LM, Galvis KT, Lone W, et al. Reproducing the molecular subclassification of peripheral T-cell lymphoma-NOS by immunohistochemistry. Blood. 2019;134(24):2159–70.
90. Heavican TB, Bouska A, Yu J, Lone W, Amador C, Gong Q, et al. Genetic drivers of oncogenic pathways in molecular subgroups of peripheral T-cell lymphoma. Blood. 2019;133(15):1664–76.
91. Wang T, Feldman AL, Wada DA, Lu Y, Polk A, Briski R, et al. GATA-3 expression identifies a high-risk subset of PTCL, NOS with distinct molecular and clinical features. Blood. 2014;123(19):3007–15.
92. Cuadros M, Dave SS, Jaffe ES, et al. Identification of a proliferation signature related to survival in nodal peripheral T-cell lymphomas. J Clin Oncol. 2007;25:3321–9.
93. Swerdlow SH, Campo E, Pileri SA, Harris NL, Stein H, Siebert R, et al. The 2016 revision of the World Health Organization classification of lymphoid neoplasms. Blood. 2016;127(20):2375–90.
94. Crotty S. T follicular helper cell differentiation, function, and roles in disease. Immunity. 2014;41:529–42.
95. Jiang M, Bennani NN, Feldman AL. Lymphoma classification update: T-cell lymphomas, Hodgkin lymphomas, and histiocytic/dendritic cell neoplasms. Expert Rev Hematol. 2017;10(3):239–49.
96. Dogan A, Attygalle AD, Kyriakou C. Angioimmunoblastic T-cell lymphoma. Br J Haematol. 2003;121(5):681–91.
97. Palomero T, Couronné L, Khiabanian H, Kim MY, Ambesi-Impiombato A, Perez-Garcia A, et al. Recurrent mutations in epigenetic regulators, RHOA and FYN kinase in peripheral T cell lymphomas. Nat Genet. 2014;46(2):166–70.
98. Sakata-Yanagimoto M, Enami T, Yoshida K, Shiraishi Y, Ishii R, Miyake Y, et al. Somatic RHOA mutation in angioimmunoblastic T cell lymphoma. Nat Genet. 2014;46(2):171–5.
99. Cortes JR, Ambesi-Impiombato A, Couronné L, Quinn SA, Kim CS, da Silva Almeida AC, et al. RHOA G17V induces T follicular helper cell specification and promotes lymphomagenesis. Cancer Cell. 2018;33(2):259–73.
100. Wang C, McKeithan TW, Gong Q, et al. IDH2R172 mutations define a unique subgroup of patients with angioimmunoblastic T-cell lymphoma. Blood. 2015;126(15):1741–52.
101. Odejide O, Weigert O, Lane AA, et al. A targeted mutational landscape of angioimmunoblastic T-cell lymphoma. Blood. 2014;123(9):1293–6.
102. Lemonnier F, Cairns RA, Inoue S, Li WY, Dupuy A, Broutin S, et al. The IDH2 R172K mutation associated with angioimmunoblastic T-cell lymphoma produces 2HG in T cells and impacts lymphoid development. Proc Natl Acad Sci U S A. 2016;113(52):15084–9.
103. Deleeuw RJ, Zettl A, Klinker E, Haralambieva E, Trottier M, Chari R, et al. Whole-genome analysis and HLA genotyping of enteropathy-type T-cell lymphoma reveals 2 distinct lymphoma subtypes. Gastroenterology. 2007;132(5):1902–11.
104. van Vliet C, Spagnolo DV. T- and NK-cell lymphoproliferative disorders of the gastrointestinal tract: review and update. Pathology. 2020;52(1):128–41.
105. Jassim SH, Smith LB. New/revised entities in gastrointestinal lymphoproliferative disorders. Surg Pathol Clin. 2019;12(3):733–43.
106. Zettl A, Ott G, Makulik A, Katzenberger T, Starostik P, Eichler T, et al. A. Chromosomal gains at 9q characterize enteropathy-type T-cell lymphoma. Am J Pathol. 2002;161(5):1635–45.
107. Moffitt AB, Ondrejka SL, McKinney M, et al. Enteropathy-associated T cell lymphoma subtypes are characterized by loss of function of SETD2. J Exp Med. 2017;214:1371–86.
108. Jaffe ES. T-cell and NK-cell neoplasms of the gastrointestinal tract – recurrent themes, but clinical and biological distinctions exist. Haematologica. 2020;105(7):1760–2.
109. Toro JR, Liewehr DJ, Pabby N, Sorbara L, Raffeld M, Steinberg SM, Jaffe ES. Gamma-delta T-cell phenotype is associated with significantly decreased survival in cutaneous T-cell lymphoma. Blood. 2003;101(9):3407–12.
110. Magro CM, Wang X. Indolent primary cutaneous γ/δ T-cell lymphoma localized to the subcutaneous panniculus and its association with atypical lymphocytic lobular panniculitis. Am J Clin Pathol. 2012;138(1):50–6.
111. Rutnin S, Porntharukcharoen S, Boonsakan P. Clinicopathologic, immunophenotypic, and molecular analysis of subcutaneous panniculitis-like T-cell lymphoma: a retrospective study in a tertiary care center. J Cutan Pathol. 2019;46(1):44–51.
112. Damasco F, Akilov OE. Rare cutaneous T-cell lymphomas. Hematol Oncol Clin North Am. 2019;33(1):135–48.
113. Hahtola S, Burghart E, Jeskanen L, Karenko L, Abdel-Rahman WM, Polzer B, Kajanti M, Peltomäki P, Pettersson T, Klein CA, Ranki A. Clinicopathological characterization and genomic aberrations in subcutaneous panniculitis-like T-cell lymphoma. J Invest Dermatol. 2008;128(9):2304–9.
114. Karenko L, Hahtola S, Päivinen S, Karhu R, Syrjä S, Kähkönen M, et al. Primary cutaneous T-cell lymphomas show a deletion or translocation affecting NAV3, the human UNC-53 homologue. Cancer Res. 2005;65(18):8101–10.
115. Küçük C, Jiang B, Hu X, Zhang W, Chan JK, Xiao W, et al. Activating mutations of STAT5B and STAT3 in lymphomas derived from γδ-T or NK cells. Nat Commun. 2015;6:6025.
116. Lunning MA, Vose JM. Angioimmunoblastic T-cell lymphoma: the many-faced lymphoma. Blood. 2017;129(9):1095–102.
117. Katsuya H, Ishitsuka K. Treatment advances and prognosis for patients with adult T-cell leukemia-lymphoma. J Clin Exp Hematop. 2017;57(3):87–97.
118. Enose-Akahata Y, Vellucci A, Jacobson S. Role of HTLV-1 tax and HBZ in the pathogenesis of HAM/TSP. Front Microbiol. 2017;8:2563.

Histiocytic and Dendritic Cell Neoplasms

19

Nathan Paulson, Xi Wang, and Zenggang Pan

List of Frequently Asked Questions

1. What is the origin of histiocytes and dendritic cells?
2. What are the important immunohistochemical markers of non-neoplastic macrophages and dendritic cells?
3. What are the major types of histiocytic and dendritic cell neoplasms?
4. What are the important immunohistochemical markers of neoplastic macrophages and dendritic cell neoplasms?
5. Which histiocytic and dendritic cell neoplasms may be transdifferentiated from B-cell or T-cell lymphomas?
6. Which assays are commonly used to study the molecular genetic changes in the histiocytic and dendritic cell neoplasms?
7. What are the typical clinicopathologic features of Langerhans cell histiocytosis (LCH)?
8. What are the major molecular genetic changes in LCH?
9. What are the major clinicopathologic features of histiocytic sarcoma (HS)?
10. What are the important molecular genetic changes in HS?
11. Which lymphomas may undergo transdifferentiation to HS?
12. How is a clonal relationship established between the lymphoma and transdifferentiated HS?
13. What are the major clinical and radiologic features of Erdheim-Chester disease (ECD)?
14. What are the major morphologic and immunophenotypic features of ECD?
15. What are the major molecular genetic changes in ECD?
16. What are the major clinicopathologic features of disseminated juvenile xanthogranuloma (JXG)?
17. Are there any recurrent molecular genetic changes in disseminated JXG?
18. What are the major clinicopathologic features of follicular dendritic cell sarcoma (FDCS)?
19. How is FDCS distinguished from inflammatory myofibroblastic tumor (IMT)?
20. Are there any recurrent molecular genetic changes in FDCS?
21. What are the major clinicopathologic features of interdigitating dendritic cell sarcoma (iDCS)?
22. What are the major clinicopathologic features of indeterminate dendritic cell tumor (IDCT)?
23. Are there any recurrent molecular genetic changes in IDCT?
24. What are the major clinicopathology features of ALK+ histiocytosis?
25. What are the major molecular genetic changes in ALK+ histiocytosis?

N. Paulson · X. Wang
Department of Pathology and Laboratory Medicine, Yale University School of Medicine, New Haven, CT, USA
e-mail: nathan.paulson@yale.edu; xi.d.wang@yale.edu

Z. Pan (✉)
Department of Pathology, Yale University School of Medicine, New Haven, CT, USA
e-mail: zenggang.pan@yale.edu

Frequently Asked Questions

1. **What is the origin of histiocytes and dendritic cells?**
   - Histiocytes and dendritic cells are part of the mononuclear phagocytic system [1]. Recent discoveries have shown that resident tissue macrophages, including non-neoplastic Langerhans cells, are self-renewing and long-lived cells derived from fetal tissues [2]. Circulating monocytes and dendritic cells subsequently respond to periods of inflammation throughout the body. These circulating monocyte and dendritic cell precursors originate from a common myeloid precursor, which begin as hematopoietic stem cells in the bone marrow [3]. Despite the name, follicular dendritic cells within lymphoid follicles derive from a mesenchymal stem cell and are not part of the hematopoietic system (Fig. 19.1).

Y. Ding, L. Zhang (eds.), *Practical Oncologic Molecular Pathology*, Practical Anatomic Pathology,
https://doi.org/10.1007/978-3-030-73227-1_19

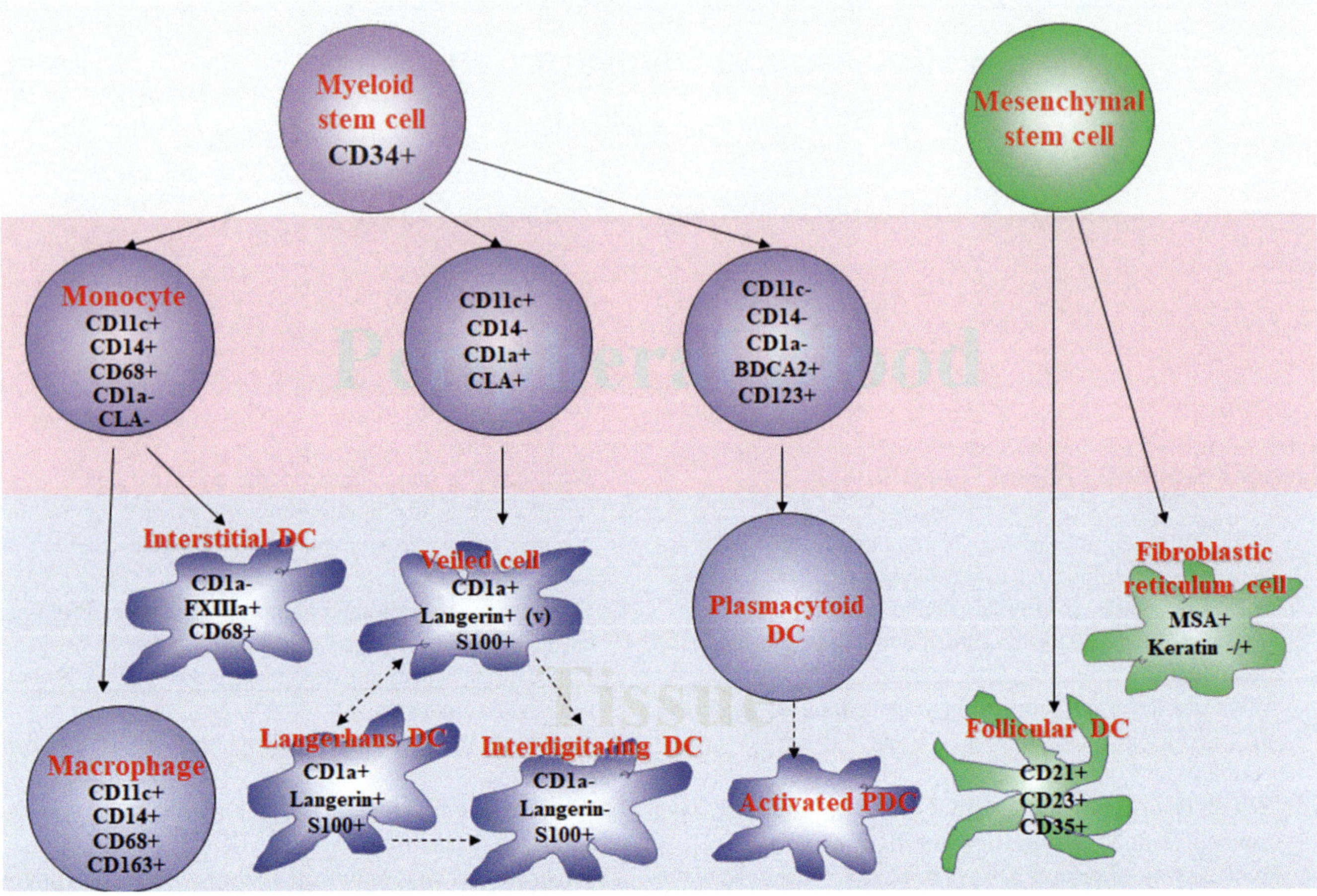

Fig. 19.1 Development of histiocytes and dendritic cells. Macrophages, dendritic cells, and Langerhans cells are derived from marrow myeloid stem cells, whereas follicular dendritic cells are mesenchymal origin

2. **What are the important immunohistochemical markers of non-neoplastic macrophages and dendritic cells?**
   - Immunohistochemical markers play an important role in the distinction of different types of histiocytes and dendritic cells. Macrophages show positive expression of CD68, CD163, CD11c, CD14, and lysozyme, while being negative for S100, CD1a, and langerin. Dendritic cells, on the other hand, do have S100 expression; additional immunohistochemical markers depend on the subtype of dendritic cells. Langerhans cells, for instance, are positive for CD1a and langerin, whereas interdigitating dendritic cells show expression of fascin but not CD1a or langerin. Plasmacytoid dendritic cells are CD123+ but S100-. Indeterminate dendritic cells are S100+ and CD1a + but show no expression of langerin, corresponding to a lack of Birbeck granules by electron microscopy [4, 5]. Follicular dendritic cells, having derived from a separate precursor, show the unique phenotype of CD21, CD23, and CD35 positivity. The important immunohistochemical markers of non-neoplastic macrophages and dendritic cells are summarized in Table 19.1.

3. **What are the major types of histiocytic and dendritic cell neoplasms?**
   - Histiocytic and dendritic cell neoplasms can be separated into categories based on the cells from which they are derived and share a common phenotype [6]. The histiocytic neoplasms derived from macrophages include histiocytic sarcoma, disseminated juvenile xanthogranuloma, Erdheim-Chester disease, and ALK+ histiocytosis [7]. The dendritic cell neoplasms include Langerhans cell histiocytosis, Langerhans cell sarcoma, indeterminate dendritic cell tumor, and interdigitating dendritic cell sarcoma. Follicular dendritic cell sarcoma arises from the follicular dendritic cell [7]. Blastic plasmacytoid dendritic cell neoplasm has a high frequency of skin and bone marrow involvement and leukemic presentation, and it is usually listed under the category of bone marrow neoplasms.

   WHO Classification of Histiocytic and Dendritic Cell Neoplasms

   - Histiocytic sarcoma
   - Langerhans cell histiocytosis
   - Langerhans cell sarcoma

Table 19.1 Immunohistochemical markers of non-neoplastic macrophages and dendritic cells

	CD1a	CD21	CD35	CD45	CD68	Langerin	S100
Follicular DCs	–	+	+	–	–	–	–
Histiocytes	–	–	–	+/–	+	–	–
Langerhans cells	+	–	–	+/–	–/+	+	+
Indeterminate cells	+	–	–	+/–	–/+	–	+
Interdigitating DCs	–	–	–	+/–	–/+	–	+
Plasmacytoid DCs	–	–	–	+/–	+	–	–

- Indeterminate dendritic cell tumor
- Interdigitating dendritic cell sarcoma
- Follicular dendritic cell sarcoma
- Fibroblastic reticular cell tumor
- Disseminated juvenile xanthogranuloma
- Erdheim-Chester disease
- Other histiocytic/dendritic neoplasms

4. **What are the important immunohistochemical markers of neoplastic macrophages and dendritic cell neoplasms?**
   - Neoplastic macrophages and dendritic cell neoplasms are defined by their immunohistochemical expression, which matches the profile of the corresponding type of macrophage or dendritic cell. Immunohistochemical markers can therefore help distinguish between the cells of origin in these neoplastic processes [6, 8]. Most importantly, the histiocytic lesions commonly show an immunohistochemical profile consistent with macrophages, including CD68, CD163, CD4, and lysozyme. Given that there are multiple types of histiocytic neoplasms, there is significant overlap in the immunohistochemical markers seen in these lesions. Dendritic cell neoplasms also show positivity to immunohistochemical markers which correspond to the cell of origin. For instance, neoplastic Langerhans cells stain for S100, CD1a, and langerin, whereas neoplastic follicular dendritic cells stain for CD21, CD23, and CD35. The important immunohistochemical markers of neoplastic macrophages and dendritic cell neoplasms are summarized in Table 19.2.
5. **Which histiocytic and dendritic cell neoplasms may be transdifferentiated from B-cell or T-cell lymphomas?**
   - Transdifferentiation is the process of transformation directly from one cell lineage into another. In the case of histiocytic and dendritic cell neoplasms, there are many examples of transdifferentiation from B- and T-cell neoplasms into Langerhans cell neoplasms, interdigitating dendritic cell sarcoma, histiocytic sarcoma, and even indeterminate cell tumor [9–19]. B-cell neoplasms have shown transdifferentiation ranging from indolent B-cell lymphomas such as small lymphocytic lymphoma [9, 11, 14, 18], splenic marginal zone lymphoma [15], and follicular lymphoma [10, 16, 17] to more aggressive large B-cell lymphomas [12] and even B-lymphoblastic lymphoma/leukemia (Fig. 19.2) [13, 20, 21]. T-cell neoplasms include peripheral T-cell lymphoma, NOS [19], and T-lymphoblastic lymphoma/leukemia [22].
6. **Which assays are commonly used to study the molecular genetic changes in the histiocytic and dendritic cell neoplasms?**
   - The molecular genetic changes found in histiocytic and dendritic cell neoplasms can be detected with a number of assays. Molecular alterations can be seen using broad techniques such as whole exome sequencing, which can also be used for copy number analysis, or with more targeted PCR assays such as pyrosequencing or Sanger sequencing. In the case of *BRAF* V600E mutations, immunohistochemical markers can also be used as a surrogate. For translocations, fluorescence in situ hybridization probes are often used. When transdifferentiation is suspected, T- and B-cell gene rearrangements may be used to determine a clonal relationship between the histiocytic or dendritic cell neoplasm and the original hematopoietic neoplasm.
7. **What are the typical clinicopathologic features of Langerhans cell histiocytosis?**
   - Langerhans cell histiocytosis (LCH) is a neoplastic proliferation of Langerhans cells [7, 23]. It can occur at any age, but is most common in children. Clinically, lesions can be uni- or multifocal and often involve the bone, soft tissue, and skin [24]. In adult smokers, lung lesions are a common presentation. Involvement of the liver, bone marrow, or spleen is rare and associated with a poorer prognosis [25]. Microscopically, LCH is defined by sheets of epithelioid Langerhans cells containing ovoid to folded, often grooved nuclei with fine chromatin, inconspicuous to small nucleoli, and moderate to abundant eosinophilic cytoplasm. Involvement of lymph nodes is defined by a characteristic sinusoidal infiltration, particularly in the early stage of disease. Cytologic atypia and mitoses should be mild. Background eosinophils are variable, but often prominent. Immunohistochemical findings are consistent with non-neoplastic Langerhans cells and show expression of S100, CD1a, and langerin. The latter is a specific marker which corresponds directly to the classic Birbeck granules found by electron microscopy [4, 5].
8. **What are the major molecular genetic changes in LCH?**
   - LCH shows prototypical molecular alterations in the RAS/MAPK pathway, which play a fundamental role

Table 19.2 Immunohistochemical markers of neoplastic macrophages and dendritic cell neoplasms

	CD45	CD68	S100	CD1a	Langerin	CD21, CD23, CD35, D2–40	CD4	CD56, CD123
Follicular dendritic cell sarcoma	–	–	–	–	–	+	–	–
Histiocytic sarcoma	+	+	–	–	–	–	+	–
Langerhans cell histiocytosis	Variable	+	+	+	+	–	+	–
Indeterminate dendritic cell tumor	Variable	Variable	+	+	–	–	Variable	–
Interdigitating dendritic cell sarcoma	Variable	Variable	+	–	–	–	Variable	–
Blastic plasmacytoid dendritic cell neoplasm	–	+	–	–	–	–	+	+

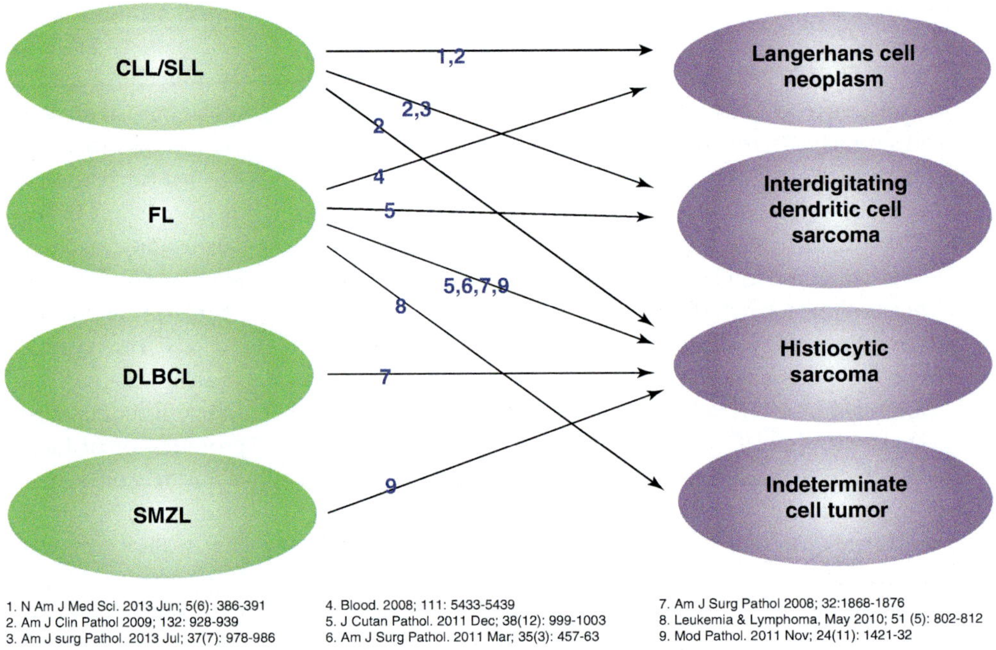

Fig. 19.2 Transdifferentiation of B-cell lymphomas to dendritic or histiocytic neoplasms

in the development of many histiocytic and dendritic cell neoplasms. Mutations in this pathway cause its constitutive activation, leading to cell growth and survival (Fig. 19.3). In particular, *BRAF* V600E and *MAP2K1* are the most commonly mutated genes in LCH, although alterations in *PIK3CA, ERBB3, RAS,* and *ARAF* have also been reported [26–32]. In addition to alterations of the RAS/MAPK pathway, LCH has been described in patients with previous or concomitant B-cell lymphomas [17]. In these cases, LCH may additionally show clonal immunoglobulin gene rearrangement and molecular genetic changes typically seen in the corresponding type of lymphoma.

9. **What are the major clinicopathologic features of histiocytic sarcoma?**
   - Histiocytic sarcoma (HS) is a rare malignant neoplasm of mature macrophages which occurs in nodal or extranodal sites [7, 8, 23, 33, 34]. Lymph node is the most common site of involvement, followed by the GI tract, spleen, skin, and soft tissue. Clinical features are typically non-specific and include B symptoms such as weight loss, fever, and fatigue. HS is most often seen in adults, although pediatric cases have been described, especially in association with lymphoblastic leukemia/lymphoma [33]. Microscopic appearance is variable, but cells typically show morphologic similarity to macrophages with abundant, eosinophilic cytoplasm,

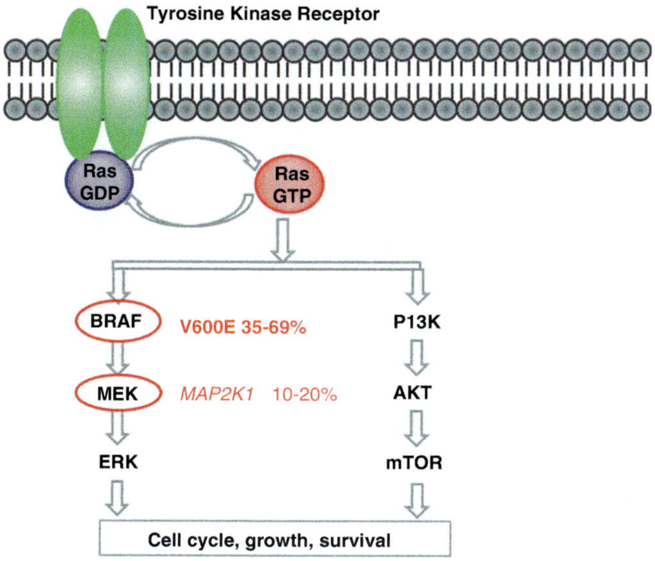

Fig. 19.3 Molecular alterations in Langerhans cell histiocytosis (LCH). LCH commonly shows mutations in the RAS/MAPK pathway, particularly mutations of *BRAF* V600E and *MAP2K1*

often with vacuolization, and large oval, eccentric nuclei with vesicular chromatin and prominent nucleoli. Pleomorphism, cytologic atypia, mitoses, and necrosis are often seen. HS expresses immunohistochemical markers of mature tissue macrophages, including CD68, CD163, lysozyme, and CD4 [6, 7, 23]. In addition, CD11c, CD14, CD45, HLA-DR, and α1-antitrypsin expression is usually seen. Importantly, markers of alternative differentiation should be negative, including B-cell, T-cell, myeloid, melanocytic, epithelial, follicular dendritic cell, Langerhans cell, and other dendritic cell lineages.

10. **What are the important molecular genetic changes in HS?**
    - HS can arise de novo or in association with a previous hematopoietic malignancy via transdifferentiation. In secondary HS cases, the molecular genetic alterations of the original leukemia or lymphoma are seen, usually in conjunction with additional mutations. For instance, HS associated with follicular lymphoma nearly always shows mutations in *CREBBP* or *KMT2D* [19, 35, 36]. In addition, HS arising in patients with mediastinal germ cell tumors is a well-documented phenomenon. In these cases, isochromosome 12p is seen in both HS and germ cell tumor [37]. Recent studies have shown RAS/MAPK pathway alterations in the vast majority of both primary and secondary HS [19, 35]. Commonly described mutations include *KRAS, NRAS, BRAF, MAP2K1, NF1*, and *PTPN11*.
11. **Which lymphomas may undergo transdifferentiation to HS?**
    - Transdifferentiation to HS has been described in chronic lymphocytic leukemia/small lymphocytic lymphoma, follicular lymphoma, diffuse large B-cell lymphoma, B-lymphoblastic leukemia/lymphoma, T-lymphoblastic leukemia/lymphoma, and peripheral T-cell lymphoma, NOS [8, 10, 14, 15, 19–21, 33, 35, 38].
12. **How is a clonal relationship established between the lymphoma and transdifferentiated HS?**
    - A clonal relationship between a lymphoma/leukemia and the transdifferentiated HS can be established through identical clonal immunoglobulin gene rearrangements or T-cell receptor gene rearrangements. In addition, in HS associated with lymphomas with other specific genetic alterations such as *IGH-BCL2* translocation in follicular lymphoma, these can be detected in HS via FISH or PCR assays.
13. **What are the major clinical and radiologic features of Erdheim-Chester disease?**
    - Erdheim-Chester disease (ECD) is a rare non-Langerhans xanthogranulomatous disorder typically seen in adult males [7, 23, 39, 40]. Clinical symptoms vary significantly based on the distribution of organ involvement. Multisystem involvement is seen in the vast majority of patients, with osseous involvement being most common (~96% of cases). Lymph node involvement is extremely rare in ECD. Radiologic findings are characteristic in ECD and include bilateral, symmetric osteosclerotic lesions of the long bones, circumferential thickening of the aorta ("aortic coat"), and perinephric fat stranding ("hairy kidney").
14. **What are the major morphologic and immunophenotypic features of ECD?**
    - Microscopically, ECD shares features with other xanthogranulomatous diseases, including abundant lipid-laden macrophages, Touton giant cells, and fibrosis [7, 39]. Background inflammation is typically lymphoplasmacytic and is variable in intensity. Cytologic atypia is usually minimal, and tumor necrosis and mitoses are rare. By immunohistochemistry, the neoplastic macrophages express CD68, CD163, factor XIIIa, CD14, and fascin [39]. They are negative for S100, CD1a, and langerin.
15. **What are the major molecular genetic changes in ECD?**
    - ECD is characterized by molecular alterations, similar to LCH, in the RAS/MAPK pathway [28, 39, 40]. *BRAF* V600E is the most common mutation and is seen in approximately 65% of cases, followed by mutations involving *PIK3CA* and *MAP2K1* (Fig. 19.4) [28, 40]. For this reason, vemurafenib (an inhibitor of BRAF V600E) has shown promising results. *ARAF, MAP2K2, KRAS*, and *NRAS* mutations have also been described in smaller proportions of cases.
16. **What are the major clinicopathologic features of disseminated juvenile xanthogranuloma?**
    - Juvenile xanthogranulomas (JXG) are lesions with similar xanthogranulomatous appearance to that of

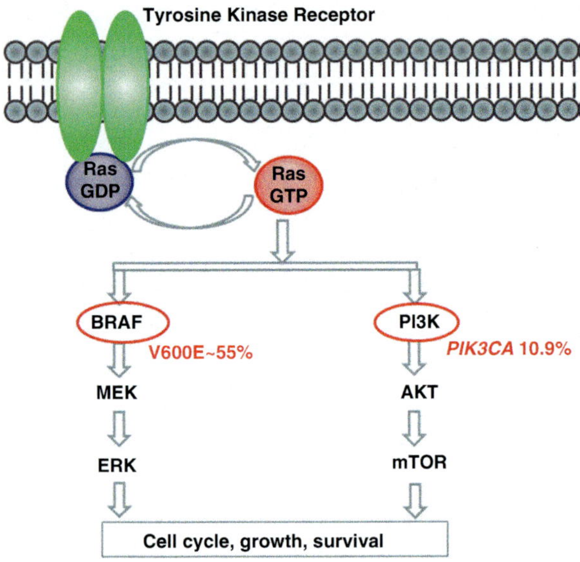

Fig. 19.4 Molecular alterations in Erdheim-Chester disease (ECD). ECD is characterized by molecular alterations in the RAS/MAPK pathway, particularly *BRAF* V600E, followed by mutations of *PIK3CA*

ECD. JXG is typically found as small solitary cutaneous lesions, with presence of non-Langerhans macrophages and Touton giant cells [23, 41, 42]. However, in a small proportion of patients, systemic involvement of JXG can occur. Disseminated JXG occurs almost exclusively in children, with approximately half occurring in patients less than 1 year of age. This form of JXG can involve the skin and soft tissue, liver, spleen, bone, lung, and other organs. Lymph node involvement is extremely rare. Microscopically, the lesions are composed of sheets of macrophages with bland cytology including small round to oval nuclei and abundant, foamy cytoplasm. Touton giant cells are frequent. The immunophenotype is indistinguishable from ECD, with positive staining for CD68, CD163, factor XIIIa, CD14, and fascin and negative staining for S100, CD1a, and langerin [41, 43].

17. **Are there any recurrent molecular genetic changes in disseminated JXG?**
    - Disseminated JXG has shown mutations of RAS/MAPK pathway genes at much lower rates than the other entities discussed herein. In particular, *NRAS, KRAS, MAP2K1*, and *ARAF* mutations have been described [44–46]. Of note, *BRAF* mutations have not been described in disseminated JXG [28].
18. **What are the major clinicopathologic features of follicular dendritic cell sarcoma?**
    - Follicular dendritic cell sarcoma (FDCS) is a rare malignant tumor of mesenchymal origin which occurs primarily in adults [7, 47–49]. Lymph nodes are the most common site of involvement, but extranodal involvement is not uncommon in the skin, soft tissue, GI tract, and spleen. In particular, the inflammatory pseudotumor-like variant of FDCS has a tendency to involve the liver and spleen [50]. Clinical presentation is classically that of a slow-growing mass, although systemic B symptoms can occur, particularly in the inflammatory pseudotumor-like variant. Up to 20% of FDCS occur in association with hyaline-vascular-type Castleman disease, suggesting a possible relation to the follicular dendritic cell hyperplasia [48, 49, 51]. Microscopically, follicular dendritic cell sarcoma is a cellular spindle cell lesion with storiform or whorled appearance. The neoplastic cells have ovoid to elongated nuclei with vesicular chromatin and a small distinct nucleolus. They contain a moderate amount of eosinophilic cytoplasm with indistinct cell borders. Cytologic atypia is typically mild without necrosis or significant mitotic activity. The inflammatory pseudotumor-like variant of FDCS shows a similar neoplastic proliferation with a prominent lymphoplasmacytic inflammatory infiltrate. The immunohistochemical profile of FDCS is identical to its cell of origin, including positivity for CD21, CD23, CD35, clusterin, D2-40, and fascin [6, 52]. EBV positivity is restricted to the inflammatory pseudotumor-like variant, and HHV-8 should always be negative.
19. **How is FDCS distinguished from inflammatory myofibroblastic tumor?**
    - Inflammatory myofibroblastic tumor (IMT) can be a close morphologic mimic of FDCS. Microscopically, it is composed of bland spindle cells with prominent mixed inflammatory infiltrate in a myxoid or collagenous stroma. These findings, especially in IMT with high cellularity, can be difficult to distinguish from FDCS. However, by immunohistochemistry, IMT classically shows expression of smooth muscle actin, desmin, and calponin, but not any of the aforementioned follicular dendritic cell markers such as CD21, CD23, and CD35. In addition, IMT shows ALK positivity in approximately 50% of cases, corresponding to *ALK* rearrangements which can be detected by FISH [53].
20. **Are there any recurrent molecular genetic changes in FDCS?**
    - *BRAF* V600E mutations have been detected in 19% of cases in recent studies [27]. No other recurrent molecular genetic abnormalities have been described.
21. **What are the major clinicopathologic features of interdigitating dendritic cell sarcoma?**
    - Interdigitating dendritic cell sarcoma (iDCS) is a malignant proliferation of interdigitating dendritic cells of the lymph node paracortex [7, 54]. Clinically, iDCS is typically seen in adults and presents as a painless mass, although B symptoms can occur. The most common site of involvement by far is the lymph node,

but extranodal presentations in the skin, soft tissue, GI tract, and nasopharynx have been described. Microscopically, iDCS shows a paracortical proliferation with residual follicles when found in the lymph node, corresponding to the location of its non-neoplastic counterpart. The tumor cells are arranged in a fascicular, storiform, or whorled pattern and contain large spindle to ovoid nuclei with vesicular chromatin and prominent nucleoli (sometimes multiple). In addition, there is abundant eosinophilic cytoplasm with poorly defined cell borders. Prominent background lymphocytes are often present. The immunohistochemical profile is consistent with non-neoplastic interdigitating dendritic cells of the lymph node and shows consistent expression of S100, HLA-DR, and fascin [6]. Staining for macrophage markers such as CD68 and CD163 is variable or absent. The tumor cells are negative for CD1a, langerin, and other specific cell lineage markers. However, cases showing transdifferentiation from a B-cell lymphoma may retain expression of some markers [8, 11, 12, 14].

22. **What are the major clinicopathologic features of indeterminate dendritic cell tumor?**
    - Indeterminate dendritic cell tumor (IDCT) is a particularly rare dendritic cell neoplasm most commonly seen in older individuals [7, 23, 55]. It is classically limited to cutaneous involvement, although lymph node and splenic cases have been rarely reported. Histologically, IDCT is characterized by cells with morphologic similarity to Langerhans cells including oval to reniform nuclei with variably prominent nuclear grooves and prominent eosinophilic cytoplasm. As opposed to LCH, skin involvement typically shows minimal epidermotropism, and the inflammatory infiltrate is lymphoplasmacytic with a minor eosinophil component. By immunohistochemistry, the neoplastic cells are S100 and CD1a positive, but negative for langerin [5, 55]. Expression of other macrophage markers such as lysozyme and CD68 is variable.
23. **Are there any recurrent genetic changes in IDCT?**
    - Indeterminate dendritic cell tumor has recently been described to have a unique *ETV3-NCOA2* translocation which can be detected by FISH [56]. However, not all cases show this translocation [57]. Transdifferentiation from follicular lymphoma has been reported, with retention of clonal immunoglobulin gene rearrangement and *IGH-BCL2* translocation [55]. *BRAF* V600E mutation has also been described in IDCT [58].
24. **What are the major clinicopathology features of ALK+ histiocytosis?**
    - ALK+ histiocytosis is a very rare disease which occurs predominantly in neonates and young children, but cases have recently been described in adult patients as well [59–61]. The most common clinical presentation is hepatosplenomegaly. The skin and liver are the most commonly affected organs. Some cases of ALK+ histiocytosis have a self-limited clinical course, distinct from disseminated JXG. Histologically, the lesions are composed of large histiocytes with abundant, eosinophilic, or vacuolated cytoplasm and folded nuclei with fine chromatin and small nucleoli. The neoplastic cells classically express ALK and macrophage markers including CD68, CD163, and lysozyme. S100 staining is variable and CD1a and langerin are negative.
25. **What are the major molecular genetic changes in ALK+ histiocytosis?**
    - ALK+ histiocytosis is defined by the presence of *ALK* fusions, leading to its distinctive ALK positivity by immunohistochemistry. The most common fusion partner has recently been shown to be *KIF5B* [60]. However, additional partners including *TPM3* and *COLIA2* have also been described.

Case Presentations

Case #1

Learning Objectives

1. To recognize the typical morphology of Langerhans cell histiocytosis (LCH)
2. To generate differential diagnosis based on morphologic features
3. To know the common genetic mutations associated with LCH

Case History

A 9-year-old boy presented with a painful lump on the left parietal region of the skull for 4–6 weeks. A CT scan of the head revealed a 1.0 × 0.9 cm mass with erosion of the underlying left parietal calvarium.

Morphologic and Immunophenotypic Features

- Diffuse infiltration of histiocytic cells in an eosinophil-rich background (Fig. 19.5a)
- Large, epithelioid tumor cells with ovoid or "coffee bean"-shaped nuclei, inconspicuous or small nucleoli, and characteristic nuclear grooves (Fig. 19.5b)
- Tumor cells positive for CD1a (Fig. 19.5c), S100 (Fig. 19.5d), and langerin (not shown)

Molecular Studies

- Positive for *BRAF* V600E mutation in this case by PCR analysis

Diagnosis

Langerhans cell histiocytosis

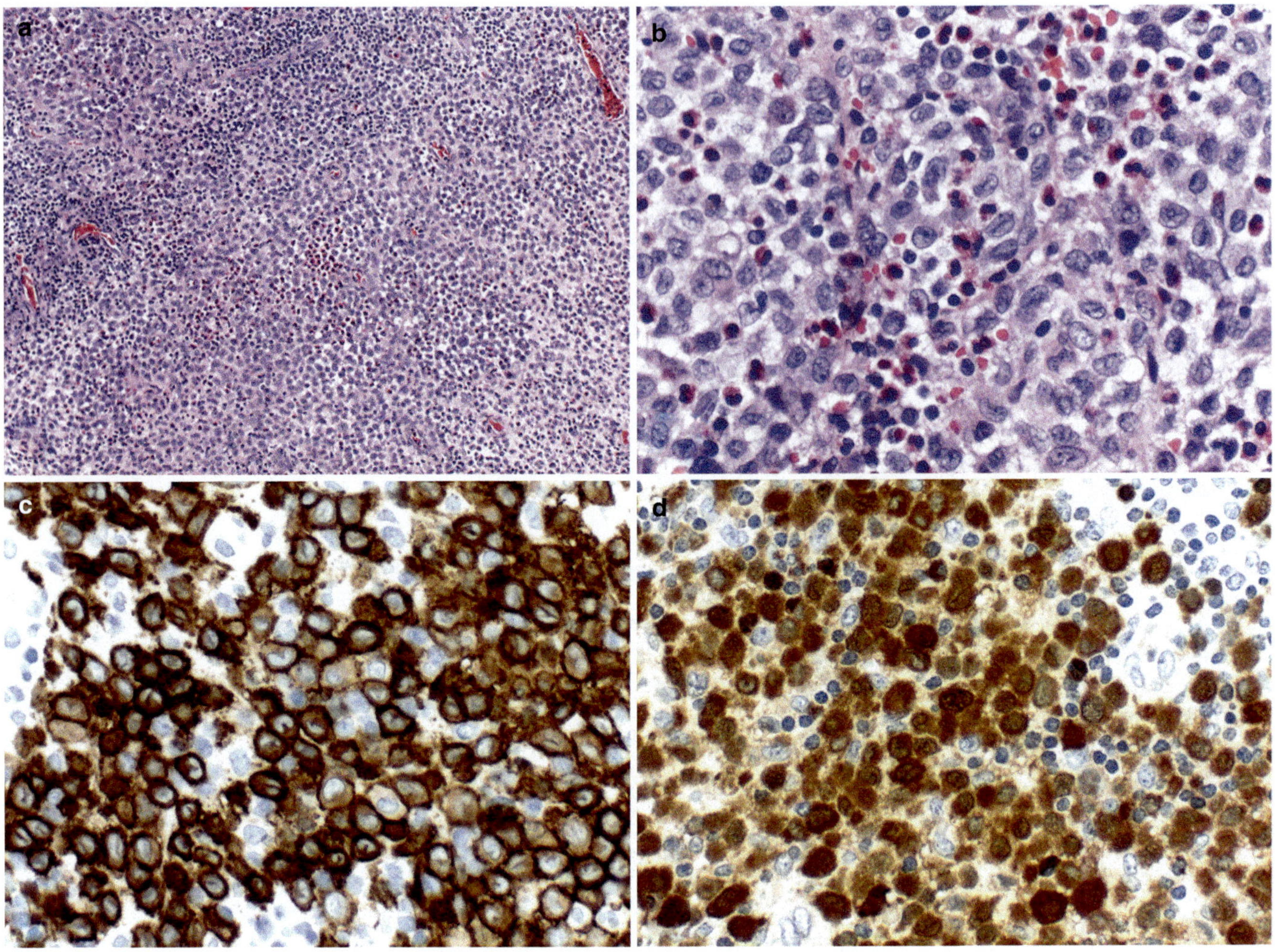

Fig. 19.5 Langerhans cell histiocytosis (LCH). Diffuse infiltration of epithelioid histiocytic cells (**a**) in a background rich in eosinophils, which show ovoid or "coffee bean"-shaped nuclei, inconspicuous nucleoli, and characteristic nuclear grooves (**b**). The tumor cells are positive for CD1a (**c**) and S100 (**d**)

Discussion

1. LCH mostly occurs in pediatric patients as solitary or multifocal lytic lesions in the bone and adjacent soft tissue. Diagnosis of LCH is mainly based on the characteristic morphologic and immunophenotypic features.
2. Differential diagnoses include infections, reactive Langerhans cell proliferation, Langerhans cell sarcoma, and other non-Langerhans cell histiocytic disorders.
3. Diagnosis of LCH prompts additional molecular studies for genetic mutations. Most LCH cases have somatic mutations involving the RAS-RAF-MEK-ERK pathway. The two most common mutations include *BRAF* V600E (50–60% of the cases) and *MAP2K1* (~25%), which are mutually exclusive.
4. In addition, *TP53* and *U2AF1* mutations have been detected in 17% and 19% of LCH cases, respectively, with the *TP53* mutations commonly associated with *BRAF* mutation.

Case #2

Learning Objectives

1. To recognize the typical morphologic and immunophenotypic features of histiocytic sarcoma (HS)
2. To know the differential diagnosis of HS
3. To understand the important genetic changes in HS as well as the clonal relationship between lymphoma and transdifferentiated HS

Case History

A 79-year-old male had a history of low-grade follicular lymphoma 3 years ago. Recently he presented with an enlarged left axillary lymph node, up to 2.8 cm.

Morphologic and Immunophenotypic Features

- The lymph node architecture is effaced by a diffuse proliferation of large tumor cells (Fig. 19.6a).

- The tumor cells are pleomorphic with irregular nuclei, prominent nucleoli, and abundant eosinophilic cytoplasm. Scattered atypical mitotic figures are noted (Fig. 19.6b).
- Focal area of coagulative necrosis is seen. No eosinophils are identified (Fig. 19.6c).
- The atypical cells are positive for CD45, CD68, and CD163 (Fig. 19.6d–f) but are negative for S100, CD1a, and lymphoid markers.

Molecular and Genetic Studies

- FISH studies positive for *BCL2-IGH* rearrangement in the tumor cells
- Molecular studies with PCR assays positive for clonal *IGH* gene rearrangement but negative for clonal *TCR* gene rearrangement

Diagnosis

Histiocytic sarcoma transdifferentiated from follicular lymphoma.

Discussion

1. HS is a malignant neoplasm of mature histiocytes, which may arise *de novo* or in association with lymphoid or myeloid neoplasms.
2. Clonal *IGH* or *TRG* rearrangements can be detected in a subset of *de novo* HS and cases dedifferentiated from lymphomas.
3. *BRAF* V600E mutation is detected in up to 63% of cases.
4. Rare cases associated with mediastinal non-seminomatous germ cell tumors harbor an isochromosome 12p, identical to that seen in germ cell tumors.
5. Differential diagnoses include anaplastic large cell lymphoma, LCH, and metastatic carcinoma with anaplastic features

Case #3

Learning Objectives

1. To know the major clinical and radiologic findings of Erdheim-Chester disease (ECD)
2. To recognize the major morphologic and immunophenotypic features of ECD
3. To understand the major molecular genetic changes of ECD

Case History

A 72-year-old male had a history of coronary arterial disease. Recently he presented with severe aortic stenosis.

Clinical Imaging Studies

CT scans detected moderate to large amount of circumferential pericardial effusion, extensive pericardial fibrosis, extensive bilateral symmetric perinephric fibrosis, 9.2 cm cyst of the left kidney, and periaortic fibrosis (Fig. 19.7). In addition, a bone scan revealed patchy abnormal uptake in bilateral femurs and tibias.

Morphologic and Immunophenotypic Features

- Multiple biopsies were performed from the pericardial tissue. Sections show an atypical histiocytic infiltrate with background inflammatory cells and fibrosis (Fig. 19.8a).
- The histiocytes have round or oval nuclei and abundant foamy cytoplasm. Occasional Touton giant cells are present (Fig. 19.8b).
- The infiltrate is admixed with scattered eosinophils and small lymphocytes (Fig. 19.8c).
- The histiocytes are negative for S100 (Fig. 19.8d) while positive for histiocytic markers CD68 and CD163 (Fig. 19.8e, f).

Molecular and Genetic Studies

- *BRAF* V600E detected in this case by PCR analysis

Diagnosis

Erdheim-Chester disease

Discussion

1. ECD is a rare multisystemic disease characterized by xanthomatous or xanthogranulomatous infiltrates of mature histiocytes. Characteristic bone involvement is noted in ~96% cases of ECD
2. Xanthomatous histiocytic proliferation is also seen in many chronic reactive processes, such as infection and inflammation, which should be considered in the workup for ECD
3. Approximately 55–60% cases of ECD harbor *BRAF* V600E mutation. Cases with wild-type *BRAF* may have mutations in the MAPK signaling pathways, including mutations in *PI3KCA* (10.9% of cases) and *NRAS* (3.7%)

Case #4

Learning Objectives

1. To recognize the typical morphologic features of follicular dendritic cell sarcoma (FDCS)
2. To generate the differential diagnosis based on the morphologic features
3. To know the molecular genetic changes associated with FDCS

Case History

A 48-year-old female presented with a 4.2 cm mediastinal mass.

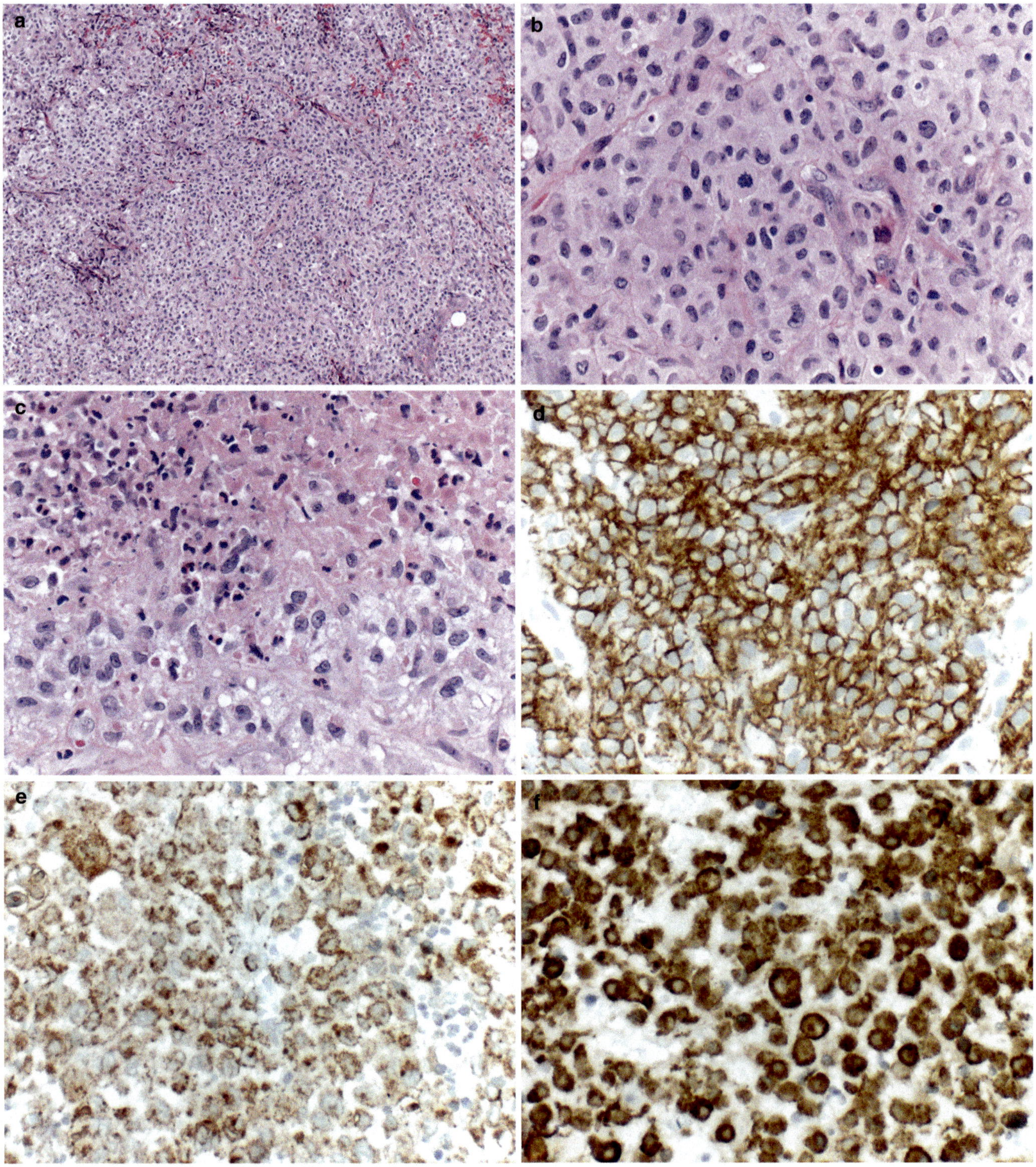

Fig. 19.6 Histiocytic sarcoma (HS). (**a**) HS displays a diffuse infiltrative pattern. (**b**) The tumor cells have abundant pale-pink cytoplasm, and the nuclei reveal variable degrees of pleomorphism. Scattered atypical mitoses are noted. (**c**) Focal necrosis with neutrophils but no eosinophils. The tumor cells are positive for CD45 (**d**), CD68 (**e**), and CD163 (**f**)

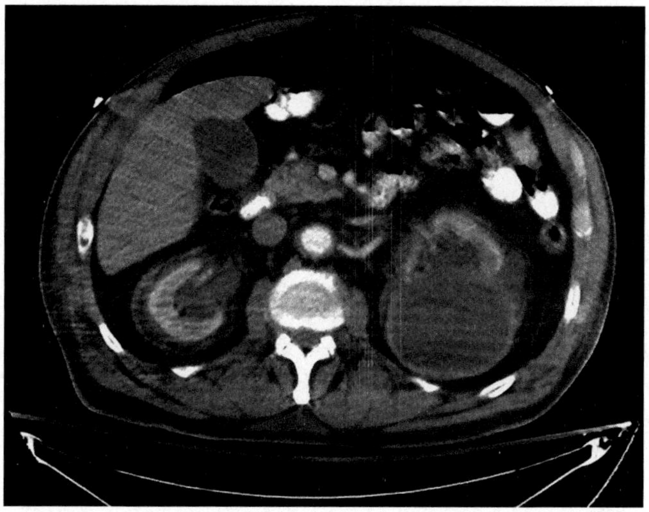

Fig. 19.7 Abdominal CT scan from this 72-year-old male who presented with severe aortic stenosis. Image shows extensive bilateral symmetric perinephric fibrosis, periaortic fibrosis, and a 9.2 cm cyst of the left kidney

Morphologic and Immunophenotypic Features

- The lesion is composed of bland spindle tumor cells in a storiform pattern admixed with frequent small lymphocytes (Fig. 19.9a).
- The tumor cells have oval or elongated nuclei, small but distinct nucleoli, indistinct cell borders, and abundant pale-pink cytoplasm (Fig. 19.9b).
- Positive markers: CD21 (Fig. 19.9c), CD23 (Fig. 19.9d), CD35, and fascin.
- Negative markers: ALK, CD1a, CD3, CD20, CD30, CD45, CD68, CD163, HMB45, cytokeratin, and SMA.

Diagnosis

Follicular dendritic cell sarcoma

Discussion

1. FDC sarcoma mostly presents with a painless, slow-growing mass in the lymph nodes or soft tissue. Approximately 20% cases of FDCS are associated with hyaline-vascular Castleman disease.
2. Indolent T-lymphoblastic proliferation may be noted in association with FDCS (~45% of cases).
3. The major differential diagnosis includes inflammatory myofibroblastic tumor (IMT), spindle cell thymoma, IgG4-related sclerosing disease, melanoma, and rarely large B-cell lymphoma with spindle morphology. The morphologic features and positive stains for FDC markers help with the diagnosis.
4. *BRAF* V600E mutation has been detected in ~19% cases of FDCS. FDCS has no clonal *IGH* or *TRG* gene rearrangements and is usually not transdifferentiated from B-cell or T-cell neoplasms.
5. Approximately 40–50% patients experience local recurrence and ~25% have distant metastases.

Case #5

Learning Objectives

1. To recognize the morphologic and immunophenotypic features of interdigitating dendritic cell sarcoma (iDCS)
2. To generate differential diagnoses of iDCS based on morphology
3. To understand the molecular and genetic changes associated with iDCS

Case History

A 51-year-old male presented with a 3.0 cm submandibular lymph node.

Morphologic and Immunophenotypic Features

- The tumor displays a characteristic paracortical proliferation with scattered residual lymphoid follicles (Fig. 19.10a). The tumor cells have round or ovoid nuclei with vesicular chromatin and a small- to medium-sized nucleolus. The cytoplasm is abundant and pale eosinophilic, with indistinct cell borders (Fig. 19.10b).
- Positive markers: CD45 (weak) and S100 (Fig. 19.10c).
- Negative markers: CD1a, CD3, CD20, CD30, CD68, CD163, HMB45, cytokeratin, melan-A, and SOX10.

Final Diagnosis

Interdigitating dendritic cell sarcoma

Discussion

1. iDCS is very rare and therefore a diagnosis of exclusion. The diagnosis relies on the typical morphologic features of paracortical infiltration, expression of S100, and exclusion of other more common tumors.
2. The differential diagnosis includes FDCS, spindle cell melanoma, spindle cell carcinoma, and high-grade lymphoma. Helpful distinguishing features include clinical history, infiltrative pattern, and immunophenotypes. Rare B-cell or T-cell lymphomas may express S100, and therefore a comprehensive panel of immunostains is recommended.
3. *BRAF* V600E mutation and clonal *IGH* rearrangement have been detected in some cases of iDCS. Transdifferentiation to iDCS has been observed in diffuse large B-cell lymphoma and chronic lymphocytic leukemia/small lymphocytic lymphoma.
4. Both iDCS and spindle cell melanoma express S100 and commonly harbor *BRAF* V600E mutations. Expression of CD68 (KP1) and any evidence of transdifferentiation from clonally related lymphomas suggest iDCS.

Case #6

Learning Objectives

1. To recognize the morphologic and immunophenotypic features of indeterminate dendritic cell tumor (IDCT)

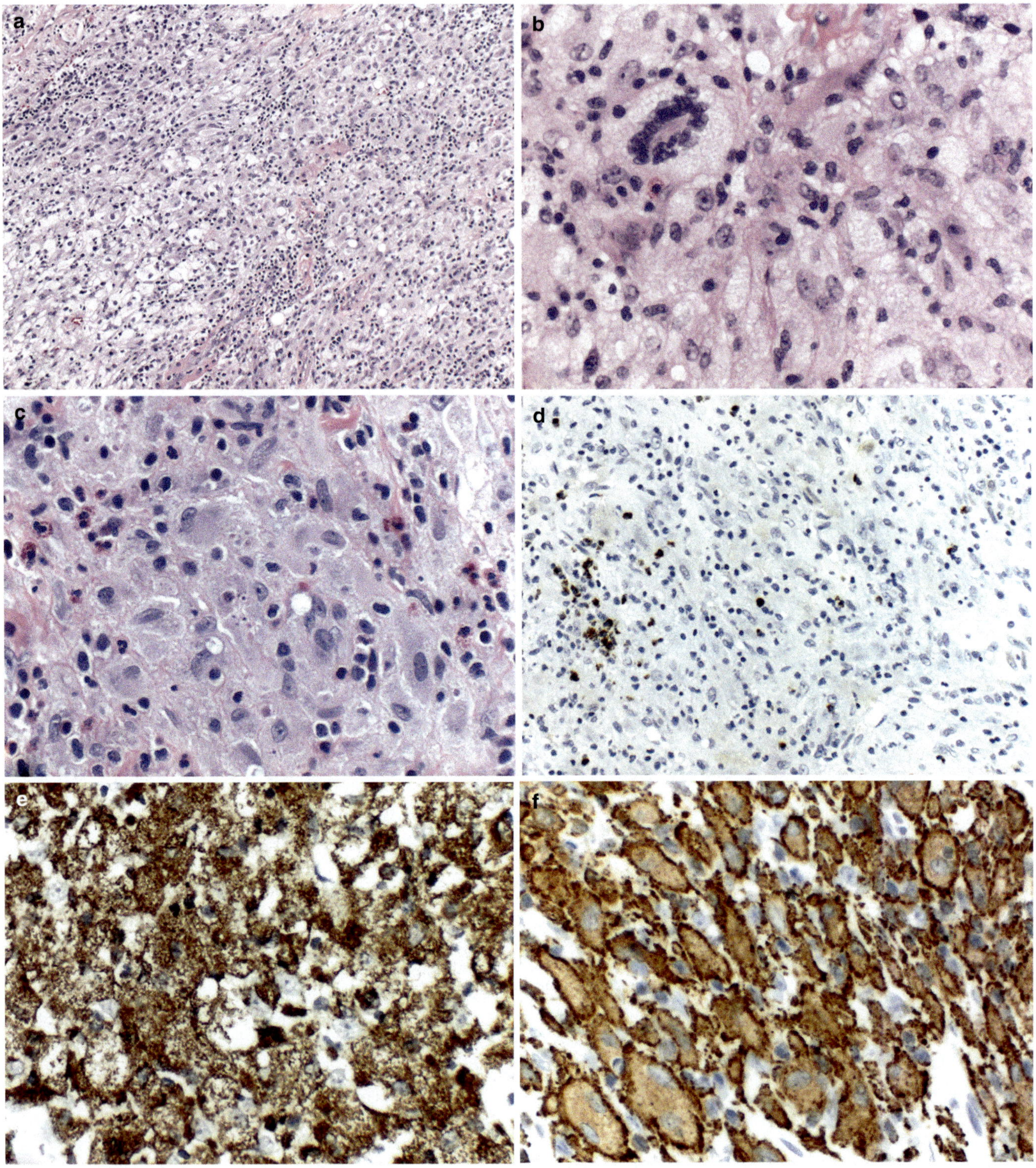

Fig. 19.8 Erdheim-Chester disease (ECD). (**a**), Prominent histiocytic infiltrate with background inflammatory cells and fibrosis. (**b**), Foamy histiocyte and occasional Touton giant cells. (**c**), Background with scattered eosinophils and small lymphocytes. The histiocytes are negative for S100 (**d**) but positive for CD68 (**e**) and CD163 (**f**)

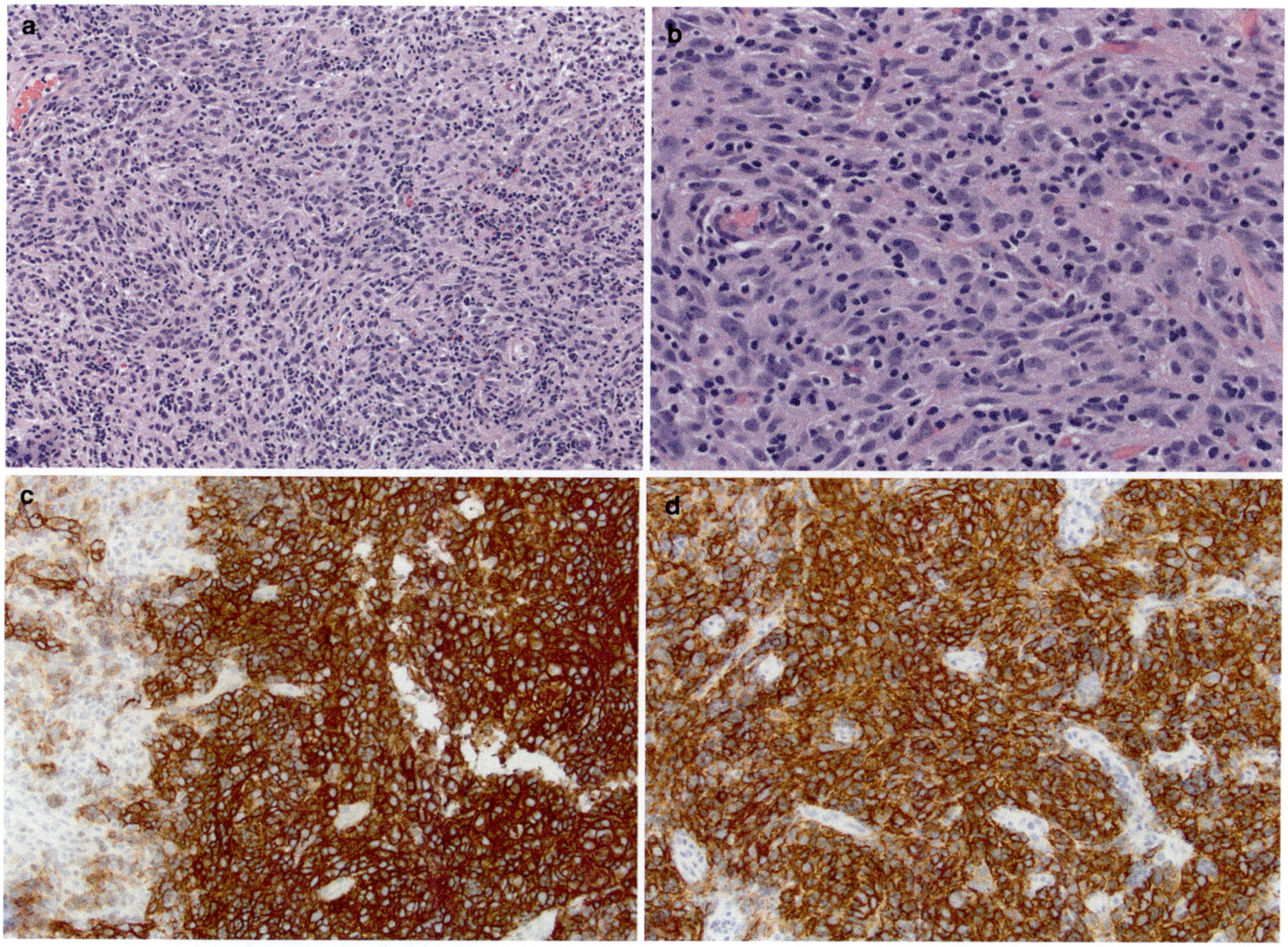

Fig. 19.9 Follicular dendritic cell sarcoma (FDCS). (**a**) Bland spindle tumor cells in a storiform pattern admixed with small lymphocytes. (**b**) The tumor cells have oval or elongated nuclei, small but distinct nucleoli, indistinct cell borders, and pale-pink cytoplasm. CD21 (**c**) and CD23 (**d**) are diffusely positive in FDCS cells

2. To know the differential diagnosis of IDCT
3. To understand the major molecular changes in IDCT

Case History

An 84-year-old female had a large solid splenic mass. A splenectomy was performed. Grossly, the splenic mass measured up to 5.3 cm in greatest dimension.

Morphologic and Immunophenotypic Features

- The mass shows a diffuse infiltration of tumor cells with scattered reactive lymphocytes but no significant eosinophilic infiltrate (Fig. 19.11a). The large tumor cells have bland nuclei and abundant pale eosinophilic cytoplasm (Fig. 19.11b).
- Positive: CD43 (weak), S100, and CD1a.
- Negative: CD3, CD20, CD21, CD23, CD30, CD68, HMB45, cytokeratin, langerin, and SOX10.

Diagnosis

Indeterminate dendritic cell tumor (IDCT)

Discussion

1. Indeterminate dendritic cells are the precursors of Langerhans cells, and the associated IDCT is extraordinarily rare. IDCT usually presents as a solitary skin lesion or less commonly lesions in multiple sites.
2. The key features of IDCT include histiocytic or Langerhans cell-like cytology, positive S100 and CD1a, and negative langerin.
3. The major differential diagnosis is LCH, which usually has abundant reactive eosinophils and positive langerin.
4. *BRAF* V600E mutation has been detected in IDCT. Transdifferentiation from follicular lymphoma has been reported.

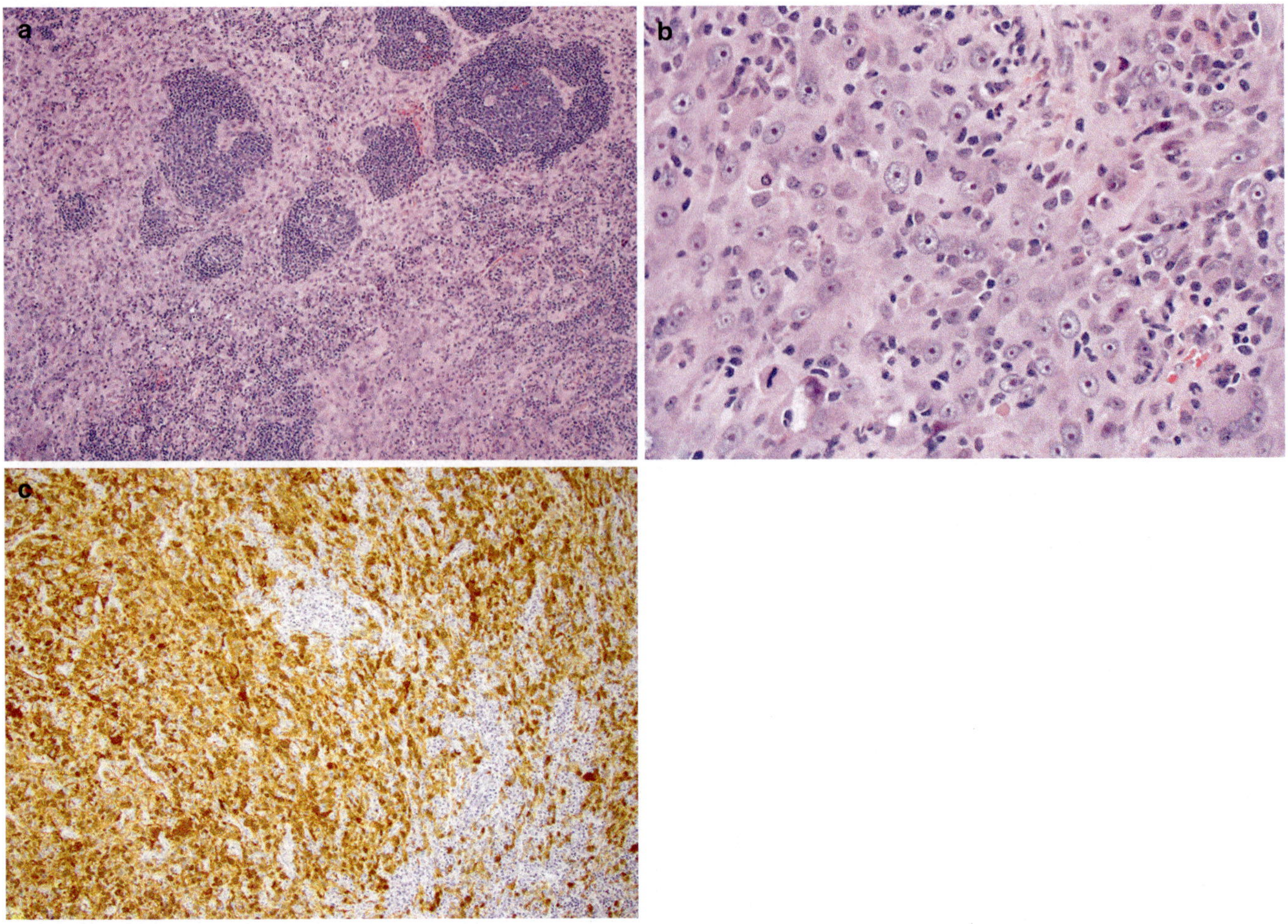

Fig. 19.10 Interdigitating dendritic cell sarcoma. (**a**) Paracortical proliferation with scattered residual lymphoid follicles. (**b**) Tumor cells have round or ovoid nuclei, abundant and eosinophilic cytoplasm, and indistinct cell borders and are strongly positive for S100 (**c**)

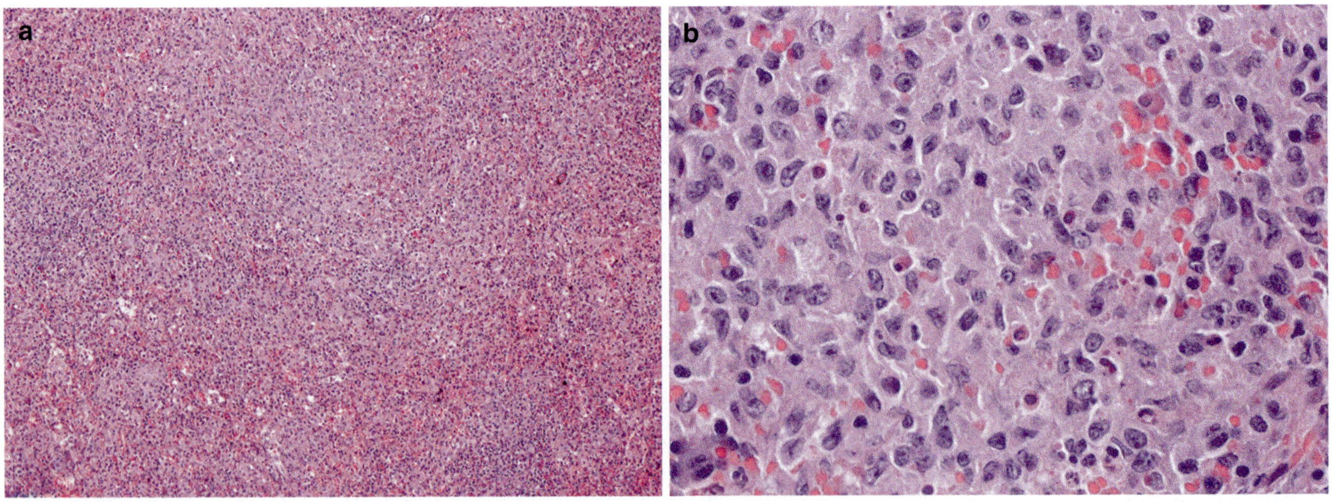

Fig. 19.11 Indeterminate dendritic cell tumor. (**a**) Diffuse infiltration of tumor cells with scattered reactive lymphocytes. (**b**) Large tumor cells with bland nuclei and abundant pale eosinophilic cytoplasm

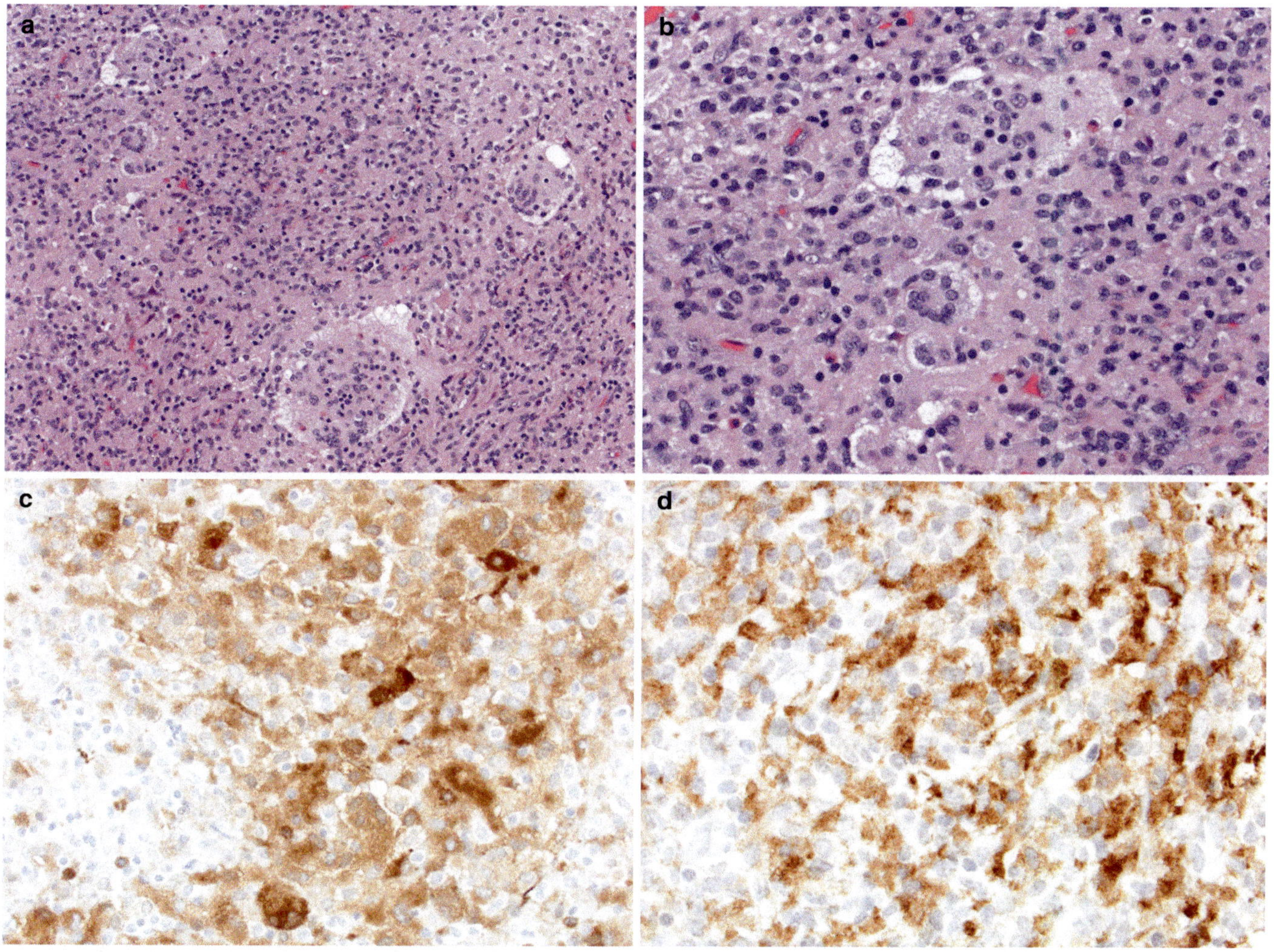

Fig. 19.12 ALK+ histiocytosis. (**a**) Sheets of histiocytes with mixed features of RDD and ECD. (**b**) Large tumor cells with irregular folded nuclei and fine chromatin, scattered Touton giant cells, and emperipolesis of lymphocytes. Tumor cells are positive for ALK (**c**) and S100 (**d**)

Case #7

Learning Objectives

1. To know this novel type of ALK+ histiocytosis and the clinicopathologic features
2. To recognize the morphologic features and molecular genetic findings of ALK+ histiocytosis
3. To understand the integrated approach for the diagnosis of challenging histiocytic disorders

Case History

A 7-year-old female had a cerebellum mass.

Morphologic and Immunophenotypic Features

- The lesion is composed of sheets of histiocytes with mixed features of Rosai-Dorfman disease (RDD) and Erdheim-Chester disease (ECD). There are large epithelioid cells with irregular folded nuclei and fine chromatin, frequent Touton giant cells, and emperipolesis of lymphocytes (Fig. 19.12a, b).
- Immunohistochemical workup shows ALK expression (Fig. 19.12c) and focal S100 positivity (Fig. 19.12d), in addition to positive CD68 and CD163 stains. BRAF VE1 immunostaining is negative on two different platforms.

Molecular and Genetic Studies

- Targeted next-generation sequencing identified in-frame *KIF5B-ALK* gene fusion in this case, which harbors fusions linking exons 1–24 of *KIF5B* to exons 20–29 of *ALK*.
- FISH studies demonstrated the presence of *ALK* rearrangement.

Diagnosis

ALK+ histiocytosis

Discussion

1. ALK+ histiocytosis is one of the newest subtypes of histiocytic disorders which was originally described with predilection for infants.

2. *KIF5B-ALK* fusion has been reported in a few cases of non-Langerhans cell histiocytosis and differs from what has been described in aggressive infantile ALK+ histiocytosis.
3. Our case shows overlapping features of RDD and ECD. Genetic studies identified *ALK* fusion with no additional pathogenic alterations (including mutations of *BRAF*, *MAP2K1*, and *KRAS*) identified. This illustrates an integrated histologic and genetic approach for the diagnosis of challenging histiocytic lesions.

References

1. Guilliams M, Ginhoux F, Jakubzick C, et al. Dendritic cells, monocytes and macrophages: a unified nomenclature based on ontogeny. Nat Rev Immunol. 2014;14(8):571–8.
2. Ginhoux F, Jung S. Monocytes and macrophages: developmental pathways and tissue homeostasis. Nat Rev Immunol. 2014;14(6):392–404.
3. Geissmann F, Manz MG, Jung S, Sieweke MH, Merad M, Ley K. Development of monocytes, macrophages, and dendritic cells. Science. 2010;327(5966):656–61.
4. Chikwava K, Jaffe R. Langerin (CD207) staining in normal pediatric tissues, reactive lymph nodes, and childhood histiocytic disorders. Pediatr Dev Pathol. 2004;7(6):607–14.
5. Lau SK, Chu PG, Weiss LM. Immunohistochemical expression of Langerin in Langerhans cell histiocytosis and non-Langerhans cell histiocytic disorders. Am J Surg Pathol. 2008;32(4):615–9.
6. Pileri SA, Grogan TM, Harris NL, et al. Tumours of histiocytes and accessory dendritic cells: an immunohistochemical approach to classification from the International Lymphoma Study Group based on 61 cases. Histopathology. 2002;41(1):1–29.
7. Swerdlow SH, Campo E, Pileri SA, et al. The 2016 revision of the World Health Organization classification of lymphoid neoplasms. Blood. 2016;127(20):2375–90.
8. Facchetti F, Pileri SA, Lorenzi L, et al. Histiocytic and dendritic cell neoplasms: what have we learnt by studying 67 cases. Virchows Arch. 2017;471(4):467–89.
9. Chen W, Jaffe R, Zhang L, et al. Langerhans cell sarcoma arising from chronic lymphocytic lymphoma/small lymphocytic leukemia: lineage analysis and BRAF V600E mutation study. N Am J Med Sci. 2013;5(6):386–91.
10. Feldman AL, Arber DA, Pittaluga S, et al. Clonally related follicular lymphomas and histiocytic/dendritic cell sarcomas: evidence for transdifferentiation of the follicular lymphoma clone. Blood. 2008;111(12):5433–9.
11. Fraser CR, Wang W, Gomez M, et al. Transformation of chronic lymphocytic leukemia/small lymphocytic lymphoma to interdigitating dendritic cell sarcoma: evidence for transdifferentiation of the lymphoma clone. Am J Clin Pathol. 2009;132(6):928–39.
12. Ochi Y, Hiramoto N, Yoshizato T, et al. Clonally related diffuse large B-cell lymphoma and interdigitating dendritic cell sarcoma sharing MYC translocation. Haematologica. 2018;103(11):e553–6.
13. Ratei R, Hummel M, Anagnostopoulos I, et al. Common clonal origin of an acute B-lymphoblastic leukemia and a Langerhans' cell sarcoma: evidence for hematopoietic plasticity. Haematologica. 2010;95(9):1461–6.
14. Shao H, Xi L, Raffeld M, et al. Clonally related histiocytic/dendritic cell sarcoma and chronic lymphocytic leukemia/small lymphocytic lymphoma: a study of seven cases. Mod Pathol. 2011;24(11):1421–32.
15. Wang E, Hutchinson CB, Huang Q, et al. Histiocytic sarcoma arising in indolent small B-cell lymphoma: report of two cases with molecular/genetic evidence suggestive of a 'transdifferentiation' during the clonal evolution. Leuk Lymphoma. 2010;51(5):802–12.
16. Wang E, Papalas J, Hutchinson CB, et al. Sequential development of histiocytic sarcoma and diffuse large b-cell lymphoma in a patient with a remote history of follicular lymphoma with genotypic evidence of a clonal relationship: a divergent (bilineal) neoplastic transformation of an indolent B-cell lymphoma in a single individual. Am J Surg Pathol. 2011;35(3):457–63.
17. West DS, Dogan A, Quint PS, et al. Clonally related follicular lymphomas and Langerhans cell neoplasms: expanding the spectrum of transdifferentiation. Am J Surg Pathol. 2013;37(7):978–86.
18. Wetzler M, Kurzrock R, Goodacre AM, McLaughlin P, Ku S, Talpaz M. Transformation of chronic lymphocytic leukemia to lymphoma of true histiocytic type. Cancer. 1995;76(4):609–17.
19. Egan C, Lack J, Skarshaug S, et al. The mutational landscape of histiocytic sarcoma associated with lymphoid malignancy. Mod Pathol. 2020;34:336.
20. Feldman AL, Minniti C, Santi M, Downing JR, Raffeld M, Jaffe ES. Histiocytic sarcoma after acute lymphoblastic leukaemia: a common clonal origin. Lancet Oncol. 2004;5(4):248–50.
21. Thakral B, Khoury JD. Histiocytic sarcoma: secondary neoplasm or "transdifferentiation" in the setting of B-acute lymphoblastic leukemia. Blood. 2016;128(20):2475.
22. Castro EC, Blazquez C, Boyd J, et al. Clinicopathologic features of histiocytic lesions following ALL, with a review of the literature. Pediatr Dev Pathol. 2010;13(3):225–37.
23. Emile JF, Abla O, Fraitag S, et al. Revised classification of histiocytoses and neoplasms of the macrophage-dendritic cell lineages. Blood. 2016;127(22):2672–81.
24. Titgemeyer C, Grois N, Minkov M, Flucher-Wolfram B, Gatterer-Menz I, Gadner H. Pattern and course of single-system disease in Langerhans cell histiocytosis data from the DAL-HX 83- and 90-study. Med Pediatr Oncol. 2001;37(2):108–14.
25. Gadner H, Minkov M, Grois N, et al. Therapy prolongation improves outcome in multisystem Langerhans cell histiocytosis. Blood. 2013;121(25):5006–14.
26. Brown NA, Furtado LV, Betz BL, et al. High prevalence of somatic MAP2K1 mutations in BRAF V600E-negative Langerhans cell histiocytosis. Blood. 2014;124(10):1655–8.
27. Go H, Jeon YK, Huh J, et al. Frequent detection of BRAF(V600E) mutations in histiocytic and dendritic cell neoplasms. Histopathology. 2014;65(2):261–72.
28. Haroche J, Charlotte F, Arnaud L, et al. High prevalence of BRAF V600E mutations in Erdheim-Chester disease but not in other non-Langerhans cell histiocytoses. Blood. 2012;120(13):2700–3.
29. Roden AC, Hu X, Kip S, et al. BRAF V600E expression in Langerhans cell histiocytosis: clinical and immunohistochemical study on 25 pulmonary and 54 extrapulmonary cases. Am J Surg Pathol. 2014;38(4):548–51.
30. Jouenne F, Chevret S, Bugnet E, et al. Genetic landscape of adult Langerhans cell histiocytosis with lung involvement. Eur Respir J. 2020;55(2):1901190.
31. McGinnis LM, Nybakken G, Ma L, Arber DA. Frequency of MAP2K1, TP53, and U2AF1 mutations in BRAF-mutated Langerhans cell histiocytosis: further characterizing the genomic landscape of LCH. Am J Surg Pathol. 2018;42(7):885–90.
32. Nelson DS, Quispel W, Badalian-Very G, et al. Somatic activating ARAF mutations in Langerhans cell histiocytosis. Blood. 2014;123(20):3152–5.
33. Takahashi E, Nakamura S. Histiocytic sarcoma : an updated literature review based on the 2008 WHO classification. J Clin Exp Hematop. 2013;53(1):1–8.

34. Hornick JL, Jaffe ES, Fletcher CD. Extranodal histiocytic sarcoma: clinicopathologic analysis of 14 cases of a rare epithelioid malignancy. Am J Surg Pathol. 2004;28(9):1133–44.
35. Egan C, Nicolae A, Lack J, et al. Genomic profiling of primary histiocytic sarcoma reveals two molecular subgroups. Haematologica. 2020;105(4):951–60.
36. Pericart S, Waysse C, Siegfried A, et al. Subsequent development of histiocytic sarcoma and follicular lymphoma: cytogenetics and next-generation sequencing analyses provide evidence for transdifferentiation of early common lymphoid precursor-a case report and review of literature. Virchows Arch. 2020;476(4):609–14.
37. Nichols CR, Roth BJ, Heerema N, Griep J, Tricot G. Hematologic neoplasia associated with primary mediastinal germ-cell tumors. N Engl J Med. 1990;322(20):1425–9.
38. Mori M, Matsushita A, Takiuchi Y, et al. Histiocytic sarcoma and underlying chronic myelomonocytic leukemia: a proposal for the developmental classification of histiocytic sarcoma. Int J Hematol. 2010;92(1):168–73.
39. Goyal G, Heaney ML, Collin M, et al. Erdheim-Chester disease: consensus recommendations for evaluation, diagnosis, and treatment in the molecular era. Blood. 2020;135(22):1929–45.
40. Ozkaya N, Rosenblum MK, Durham BH, et al. The histopathology of Erdheim-Chester disease: a comprehensive review of a molecularly characterized cohort. Mod Pathol. 2018;31(4):581–97.
41. Haroche J, Abla O. Uncommon histiocytic disorders: Rosai-Dorfman, juvenile xanthogranuloma, and Erdheim-Chester disease. Hematology Am Soc Hematol Educ Program. 2015;2015:571–8.
42. Dehner LP. Juvenile xanthogranulomas in the first two decades of life: a clinicopathologic study of 174 cases with cutaneous and extracutaneous manifestations. Am J Surg Pathol. 2003;27(5):579–93.
43. Janssen D, Harms D. Juvenile xanthogranuloma in childhood and adolescence: a clinicopathologic study of 129 patients from the kiel pediatric tumor registry. Am J Surg Pathol. 2005;29(1):21–8.
44. Chakraborty R, Hampton OA, Abhyankar H, et al. Activating MAPK1 (ERK2) mutation in an aggressive case of disseminated juvenile xanthogranuloma. Oncotarget. 2017;8(28):46065–70.
45. Paxton CN, O'Malley DP, Bellizzi AM, et al. Genetic evaluation of juvenile xanthogranuloma: genomic abnormalities are uncommon in solitary lesions, advanced cases may show more complexity. Mod Pathol. 2017;30(9):1234–40.
46. Diamond EL, Durham BH, Haroche J, et al. Diverse and targetable kinase alterations drive histiocytic neoplasms. Cancer Discov. 2016;6(2):154–65.
47. Perez-Ordonez B, Erlandson RA, Rosai J. Follicular dendritic cell tumor: report of 13 additional cases of a distinctive entity. Am J Surg Pathol. 1996;20(8):944–55.
48. Chan JK, Fletcher CD, Nayler SJ, Cooper K. Follicular dendritic cell sarcoma. Clinicopathologic analysis of 17 cases suggesting a malignant potential higher than currently recognized. Cancer. 1997;79(2):294–313.
49. Andriko JW, Kaldjian EP, Tsokos M, Abbondanzo SL, Jaffe ES. Reticulum cell neoplasms of lymph nodes: a clinicopathologic study of 11 cases with recognition of a new subtype derived from fibroblastic reticular cells. Am J Surg Pathol. 1998;22(9):1048–58.
50. Cheuk W, Chan JK, Shek TW, et al. Inflammatory pseudotumor-like follicular dendritic cell tumor: a distinctive low-grade malignant intra-abdominal neoplasm with consistent Epstein-Barr virus association. Am J Surg Pathol. 2001;25(6):721–31.
51. Sun X, Chang KC, Abruzzo LV, Lai R, Younes A, Jones D. Epidermal growth factor receptor expression in follicular dendritic cells: a shared feature of follicular dendritic cell sarcoma and Castleman's disease. Hum Pathol. 2003;34(9):835–40.
52. Grogg KL, Lae ME, Kurtin PJ, Macon WR. Clusterin expression distinguishes follicular dendritic cell tumors from other dendritic cell neoplasms: report of a novel follicular dendritic cell marker and clinicopathologic data on 12 additional follicular dendritic cell tumors and 6 additional interdigitating dendritic cell tumors. Am J Surg Pathol. 2004;28(8):988–98.
53. Coffin CM, Hornick JL, Fletcher CD. Inflammatory myofibroblastic tumor: comparison of clinicopathologic, histologic, and immunohistochemical features including ALK expression in atypical and aggressive cases. Am J Surg Pathol. 2007;31(4):509–20.
54. Pokuri VK, Merzianu M, Gandhi S, Baqai J, Loree TR, Bhat S. Interdigitating dendritic cell sarcoma. J Natl Compr Cancer Netw. 2015;13(2):128–32.
55. Rezk SA, Spagnolo DV, Brynes RK, Weiss LM. Indeterminate cell tumor: a rare dendritic neoplasm. Am J Surg Pathol. 2008;32(12):1868–76.
56. Brown RA, Kwong BY, McCalmont TH, et al. ETV3-NCOA2 in indeterminate cell histiocytosis: clonal translocation supports sui generis. Blood. 2015;126(20):2344–5.
57. Davick JJ, Kim J, Wick MR, Gru AA. Indeterminate dendritic cell tumor: a report of two new cases lacking the ETV3-NCOA2 translocation and a literature review. Am J Dermatopathol. 2018;40(10):736–48.
58. O'Malley DP, Agrawal R, Grimm KE, et al. Evidence of BRAF V600E in indeterminate cell tumor and interdigitating dendritic cell sarcoma. Ann Diagn Pathol. 2015;19(3):113–6.
59. Chan JK, Lamant L, Algar E, et al. ALK+ histiocytosis: a novel type of systemic histiocytic proliferative disorder of early infancy. Blood. 2008;112(7):2965–8.
60. Chang KTE, Tay AZE, Kuick CH, et al. ALK-positive histiocytosis: an expanded clinicopathologic spectrum and frequent presence of KIF5B-ALK fusion. Mod Pathol. 2019;32(5):598–608.
61. Gupta GK, Xi L, Pack SD, et al. ALK-positive histiocytosis with KIF5B-ALK fusion in an adult female. Haematologica. 2019;104(11):e534–6.

20 Bone Marrow Engraftment Analysis

Harold C. Sullivan, Deanna C. Fang, and Jennifer Q. Zhang

List of Frequently Asked Questions

1. What is chimerism? What are the different types of chimerism in relation to hematopoietic progenitor cell transplantation and what is the significance of the different types?
2. What is the clinical utility of chimerism testing?
3. What is the basic principle of chimerism detection, and what parameters are needed for a clinically relevant chimerism test?
4. What cell lineages can be examined by chimerism testing? Which are the more commonly lineages interrogated?
5. What methodologies are used in chimerism testing?
6. What are short tandem repeats (STRs) and how are they used in chimerism testing?
7. How is STR analysis interpreted? How is quantification of donor and recipient DNA performed?
8. What are multiplex STR assays and what are some of their advantages and disadvantages?
9. What are some biological and testing "artifacts" that can be seen in STR analysis?

H. C. Sullivan (✉)
Department of Pathology and Laboratory Medicine, Emory University School of Medicine, Atlanta, GA, USA
e-mail: hcsulli@emory.edu

D. C. Fang
Department of Pathology, UC San Diego School of Medicine, San Diego, CA, USA
e-mail: dfang@health.ucsd.edu

J. Q. Zhang
UCLA Immunogenetics Center, Department of Pathology and Laboratory Medicine, David Geffen School of Medicine at UCLA, Los Angeles, CA, USA
e-mail: JQZhang@mednet.ucla.edu

Frequently Asked Questions

1. **What is chimerism? What are the different types of chimerism in relation to hematopoietic progenitor cell transplantation and what is the significance of the different types?**
   - In genetics, chimerism is defined as the state where an organism is comprised of genetically distinct cell populations that arise from different zygotes.
     - This should be differentiated from mosaicism, which is defined as the state where an organism is comprised of genetically distinct cell populations that arise from the same zygote.
   - In hematopoietic progenitor cell transplantation (HPCT), hematopoietic progenitor cells (HPCs) from a donor are infused into a patient (recipient) with the intention of reconstituting normal hematopoietic function through the donor cells.
   - Donors in HPCT may be autologous (donor and recipient are the same person) or allogeneic (donor and recipient are different persons). Given the definition of chimerism as provided above, the concept of chimerism can only apply in the setting of allogeneic donation.
   - In HPCT, chimerism is further qualified as below [1–3]:
     - Full (or complete) chimerism:
       - 100% of blood and bone marrow cells are of donor origin.
       - Note: other thresholds (>99%, >95%, >90%) have been used for this definition in the literature and may reflect the acknowledged sensitivity of available assays (i.e., a test does not have 100% sensitivity).
     - Mixed (or partial) chimerism:
       - When cells in a particular cellular compartment (e.g., lymphocytes) are comprised of *both* donor and recipient cells.
       - 0% < assessed cells of donor origin <100%.
       - 0% < assessed cells of recipient origin <100%.

Y. Ding, L. Zhang (eds.), *Practical Oncologic Molecular Pathology*, Practical Anatomic Pathology,
https://doi.org/10.1007/978-3-030-73227-1_20

- Mixed chimerism can be further categorized [4–6] and the following qualifiers have been used:
  - Transient/decreasing – recipient cells/DNA detected in the immediate post-transplant period (e.g., first 6 months) before complete chimerism is fully achieved.
  - Stable – the level (%) of mixed chimerism remains stable over time.
  - Progressive – recipient % increases to >10% of cells over time.
  - Increasing – recipient % increases by >5% compared to last sample tested.
- Split chimerism:
  - When cells of donor origin are present in one hematopoietically derived cellular lineage but not in another lineage, e.g.,
    - Myeloid cells = 100% donor origin
    - T cells = 100% recipient origin
- Microchimerism:
  - 0% < blood and bone marrow cells of recipient origin <1%
- Autologous recovery:
  - Where there is recovery of recipient-derived hematopoiesis.
  - Graft failure (graft rejection) is different than autologous recovery in that graft failure is characterized by pancytopenia and autologous recovery is characterized by (recipient) hematopoiesis [7].
  - Note: The exact (%) threshold of recipient cells where this term is applied may vary in the literature, e.g.,
    - 100% [5]
    - >50% [8]

2. **What is the clinical utility of chimerism testing?**
   - One primary goal of HPCT is engraftment, which is characterized by neutrophil (myeloid) engraftment, platelet engraftment, erythroid engraftment, and T-cell (CD3+) engraftment. Chimerism testing is used in assessing T-cell engraftment.
     - The threshold for T-cell engraftment is >5% [complete (full) donor chimerism >95% > mixed (partial) donor chimerism >5%].
     - Donor chimerism <5% defines clinical non-engraftment. Primary graft failure is defined as failure to engraft by day 28 of transplant (or day 42 for umbilical cord transplant). Secondary graft failure is defined as graft loss after having attained engraftment [5, 9, 10].
     - While HPC transplant programs typically assess chimerism at 1-month post-transplant (corresponding to the day 28 temporal landmark), the schedule of follow-up chimerism testing varies between institutions.
     - Note: Graft failure should be distinguished from graft rejection. Graft rejection is a subcategory of graft failure and represents host alloreactivity against the donor. Consequently, graft rejection can only occur in the setting of allogeneic HPCT.
   - Post-transplant monitoring of chimerism has greater clinical utility for allogeneic HPCT patients who undergo nonmyeloablative/reduced intensity conditioning regimens, in contrast to patients who undergo myeloablative/greater intensity regimens where post-transplant hematopoiesis is assumed to be donor-derived.
   - Chimerism testing can be useful in monitoring for risk of relapse in high-risk patients and thereby allowing for preemptive interventions such as donor lymphocyte infusions (DLI) or withdrawal of immunosuppressive therapies (IST). Decreased (or decreasing) % T-cell donor chimerism is associated with increased risk of relapse. Conversely, but not surprisingly, complete % T-cell donor chimerism is not only associated with reduced relapse risk but also with increased risk of graft versus host disease (GVHD) [11].
   - Chimerism testing can also be used in assessing minimal residual disease (MRD), especially if using subset analysis (performing chimerism testing on specific cell lineages). The presence of MRD pre- and/or post-transplant is associated with increased risk of relapse and negative prognosis [12].
   - Donor hematopoietic chimerism (e.g., via HPCT or DLI) is observed to promote tolerance in the solid organ transplant setting. Chimerism testing is involved in these clinical and/or research protocols [3, 13–16].
   - Patients who undergo HPCT from an ABO-incompatible donor are expected to eventually change to the donor's ABO type. Blood bank services may include donor % chimerism results as part of their review before officially changing the ABO typing of an HPCT patient [17].
   - Transfusion-associated graft versus host disease (TA-GVHD) is a rare but highly fatal (>90% mortality) transfusion-associated adverse effect caused by the infusion of viable donor T cells present in a transfused unit [18, 19]. The National Healthcare Safety Network Biovigilance Component Hemovigilance Module Surveillance Protocol v2.5.2 of the Centers for Disease Control and Prevention (CDC) requires the presence of white blood cell (WBC) chimerism for there to be definite imputability of the TA-GHVD diagnosis for biovigilance reporting purposes [20].
     - Note: TA-GVHD should be distinguished from transplant-associated GVHD where the latter is diagnosed clinically or by surgical pathology (biopsy) and does not require chimerism testing, although chimerism testing can help establish diagnosis of transplant-associated GVHD.
   - Because chimerism testing is based on establishing and comparing genetic identities, the testing methods involved can also be used for other identity-related applications, such as:

- Forensic testing to identify suspects, unidentified victims (e.g., in mass disasters), and missing persons [21]
- Parentage and/or kinship testing [22]
- Zygosity testing for twin studies [23]
- Specimen identification (e.g., investigating suspected specimen mix-up)

3. **What is the basic principle of chimerism detection, and what parameters are needed for a clinically relevant chimerism test?**
    - The main objective of chimerism testing is to detect the presence and/or absence of recipient and donor cell populations post-HPC transplantation.
    - In the post-transplantation setting, chimerism testing can determine the proportion of recipient and donor DNA in a given post-transplant sample, whether it be peripheral blood or bone marrow. In order to accomplish this aim, the genomic sequences [e.g., short tandem repeat (STRs), variable number of tandem repeats (VNTRs), single nucleotide polymorphisms (SNPs), microsatellites] that are unique to recipient and donor are amplified and measured to calculate the percent contribution of recipient and donor DNA, respectively.
    - Sensitivity is an important aspect of chimerism testing. Increasing recipient mixed chimerism may herald graft rejection or disease relapse. As such, an assay that has the ability to detect low number of (recipient) cells would be optimal. The overall sensitivity (i.e., limit of detection of a minor cell population) of multiplex STR platforms is reported to be approximately 5% [24], but sensitivity can vary slightly depending on the STR marker examined (1–5%) [25]. Real-time PCR assays generally have far greater sensitivity ranging from 0.01% to 0.5% [26]. Sensitivity of allele detection can be hindered by insufficient DNA input, leading to suboptimal amplification of STR loci. The limit of detection can be enhanced by interrogating cell subsets.
    - Other testing parameters to consider include precision to allow adequate comparison between sequential samples, sequencing resolution that can accommodate large repeat regions of up to 500 bp [27], and turnaround time that permits rapid assessment in situations of clinical urgency. In regard to capillary electrophoresis, considerations include peak sizing of DNA fragment peaks that is based on size standards to ensure reliable quantitation of recipient and donor DNA on capillary electrophoresis [28].
4. **What cell lineages can be examined by chimerism testing? Which are the more commonly lineages interrogated?**
    - Different hematologic cell lineages reconstitute at varying rates post-HPCT [29]; hence, there may be varying percentages of recipient- and donor-derived cells depending on the cell compartment examined.
    - Using chimerism testing, cell subsets (e.g., T cells, myeloid, B cells, NK cells) can be individually analyzed. This first requires sorting cells into subsets by flow cytometry or positive or negative selection using immunomagnetic beads [30, 31].
    - Myeloid cells (e.g., CD33/CD34+ cells, CD13/14+ cells): Monitoring the myeloid compartment post-transplantation can identify residual or recurrent myelogenous leukemia [32]. Studies have shown that increasing mixed chimerism post-transplant places patients at risk for relapse; however, this risk can be mitigated by proper immunotherapeutic interventions [33]. In nonmalignant disorders, increasing recipient chimerism is a risk factor for graft loss [34].
    - T cells (e.g., CD3+ cells) and NK cells (e.g., CD56+ cells): Studies have repeatedly demonstrated that recipient chimerism in the T-cell and NK-cell compartments places patients at risk of graft rejection [35–37]. Additionally, T-cell engraftment kinetics provide prognostic information in regard to development of GVHD with rapid T-cell engraftment placing the patient at risk of acute and chronic GVHD [38, 39].
    - Given that recipient cells may only represent a fraction of a subset of leukocytes, performing STR analysis on whole blood may not be able to detect a small fraction of a minor subset of cells. For example, if NK cells only represent 5% of the cells in peripheral blood and 20% of those cells are of recipient origin, this equates to 1% percent of the total cells in the peripheral blood. Consequently, these recipient-derived cells may be missed on subsequent molecular (e.g., STR) analysis [40]. However, enriching for NK cells first can increase sensitivity. Indeed, subset analysis has been shown to increase the sensitivity of detecting recipient cells in some cases by 2 log [32].
5. **What methodologies are used in chimerism testing?**
    - Chimerism testing can be performed using XY cytogenetics, red cell phenotyping (RCP), fluorescence in situ hybridization (FISH), STR, VNTR, real-time or quantitative PCR (qPCR), and next-generation sequencing. The comparison of these methods is listed in Table 20.1.
    - XY cytogenetics
        - Classic cytogenetic detection of X and Y chromosomes is only useful in the setting of sex-mismatched transplant recipients. It is labor intensive, time-consuming, and limited by the number of cells that can be analyzed. For instance, to detect 1% chimerism, a minimum of 300 or more metaphase cells must be examined which is extremely difficult in the routine cytogenetic clinical laboratory.

Table 20.1 Comparison of chimerism analysis methods

Methods	Advantage	Disadvantage	Sensitivity	Informativity
Erythrocyte phenotyping	Simple, accurate and sensitive	Need to perform before transfusion detects only one cell type	0.004–3%	Low
XY cytogenetics		Sex mismatched transplant	5%	Low
		Labour intensive		
XY-FISH	Fast, high sensitivity	Sex mismatched transplant	0.1–0.5%	High
VNTR		Less sensitive than STR	5%	High
STR	Fast, low input of DNA	Less sensitive than qPCR, NGS	1–5%	Very high
		Problems with stutter peak and preferential amplification		
Real-time PCR	Rapid (3–4 h), high sensitivity	Sensitivity correlates with DNA		
		Require higher input DNA	0.01%	High
		Need pretransplant recipient DNA each time as a control		
NGS	High capacity, high sensitivity, can be used for MRD as the same time	Costly	0.001–0.0001%	Very high
		High complexity work flow		
		Longer turnaround time		

FISH fluorescence in situ hybridization, *STR* short tandem repeat, *VNTR* variable number tandem repeat, *NGS* next-generation sequencing, *MRD* minimal residual disease

- Fluorescence in situ hybridization (FISH)
  - Fluorescence in situ hybridization (FISH) uses DNA fragments incorporated with fluorophore-coupled probes of X and Y chromosomes to examine the presence or absence of complementary sequences in fixed cells or tissues under a fluorescent microscope.
  - FISH is a simple and quantitative method to detect mixed chimerism following sex-mismatched HPCT .
  - Approximately 0.1% of sensitivity can be reached when 500–1000 cells are scored [41].
- Red cell phenotyping (RCP)
  - RCP is a simple, accurate, and very sensitive method for chimerism testing, and the results can be obtained within 24 h. A complete red cell phenotype includes the following blood antigens: A, B, C, c, E, D, K, Fy^a, Fy^b, Jk^a, Jk^b, M, N, S, and s.
  - RCP of patients should be performed before transfusion is given.
    - Note: Patients with autoimmune hemolytic anemia (AIHA) cannot be accurately typed for RBC antigens since patient's red blood cells are coated with IgG.
  - RCP is a lineage-specific detection, and it has been used to determine autologous hematopoiesis mainly in chronic myeloid leukemia (CML) because in CML, at the time of relapse, recipient granulocytes, monocytes, and erythrocytes appear and progressively replace their counterparts of donor origin. Other lineages, such as B and NK cells, remain of donor origin [42]. RCP is a sensitive technique for monitoring CML patients after T-cell-depleted bone marrow transplantation and after donor leukocyte infusion [43].
- STR and VNTR
  - Microsatellite (short tandem repeat) and minisatellite (variable number tandem repeat) genotyping has been the most commonly used assays to assess chimerism status in post HCPT patients. STR will be the focus of the remainder of this chapter.
- qPCR
  - qPCR is based on the detection of single nucleotide polymorphisms (SNP). With only three potential genotypes for most SNP loci (AA, AB, BB), the chance of distinguishing two individuals is much lower than for STR loci, which have 10–20 alleles per locus. Therefore, more SNPs need to be used to find informative markers for donor and recipient pairs compared to STR.
  - The advantage of SNP detection is that SNPs are less susceptible to preferential amplification and stutter peak (see question #9) is not a concern.
  - The amount of input DNA is directly proportional to the sensitivity of qPCR, which, at 100 ng, is more than 2 log higher than that of STR, reaching about 0.01%. The increased sensitivity widens the time period of anticipation of relapse, allowing for early intervention. On the other hand, with a higher sensitivity method, the number of false-positive results increases. The requirement of lager amounts of DNA input compared to STR limits the capability of qPCR in early post-transplant period where leukocyte counts remain low till 2–4 weeks after HPCT [44].
  - qPCR provides sensitive, rapid quantitative results with the possibility of having a report within a few

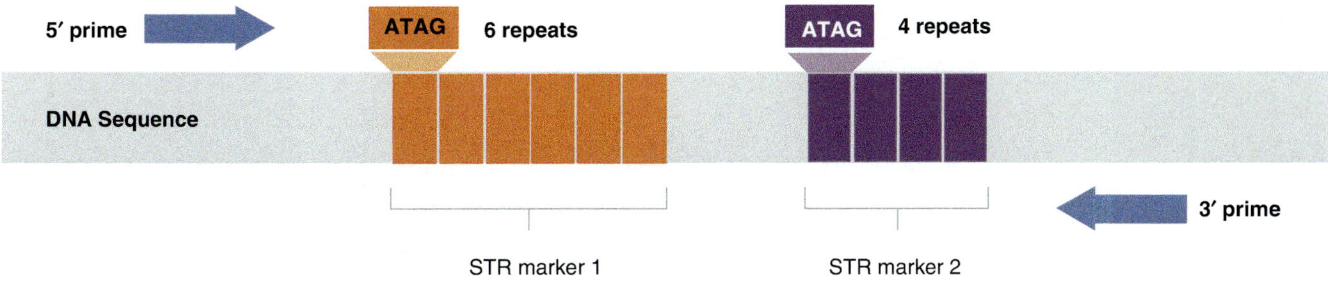

Fig. 20.1 Illustrative examples of STR markers/alleles with six and four repeats of four base pairs

hours from receipt of sample. However, PCR amplification efficiency can dramatically influence the chimerism calculation. To ensure accurate results, pre-transplant patient DNA will be needed as a control, as the result is expressed as higher or lower multiples of the pre-transplant baseline. The use of pre-transplant DNA as a control for each experiment with qPCR raises the concern of pre-transplant DNA sample exhaustion limiting the ability of continual monitoring chimerism post-transplant.

- Next-generation sequencing (NGS)
  - Next-generation sequencing (NGS), also known as "massive parallel sequencing," refers to high-throughput sequencing technologies which enables a large number (millions to billions) of DNA templates to be sequenced in parallel, thereby generating an unprecedented amount of genetic information in a single run. The benefits of NGS include higher sequencing capacity, ability to multiplex samples, and higher diagnostic sensitivity.
  - The advances in NGS made it possible to sequence as many SNPs possible. MRD detection can be performed by amplification of disease-specific markers such as *BCR-ABL1*. MRD detection requires a sensitivity of 0.01% MRD cells (10^{-4}): meaning 1 MRD cell in 10,000 cells out of all bone marrow mononuclear cells can have prognostic value; therefore, STR (sensitivity of 1–5%) is not an ideal test for MRD. As such, qPCR and NGS with higher sensitivity are better suited for MRD testing [45]. NGS offers simultaneous typing of large number of SNP markers as well as multiple disease-specific markers for MRD [46].

6. **What are short tandem repeats and how are they used in chimerism testing?**
   - A locus is defined as polymorphic if the most common allele is present in less than 99% of the population [47]. Polymorphisms (typically) do not have a significant physiologic effect.
   - STRs are a type of polymorphism that is characterized by a short DNA motif (which can be one to several nucleotides long) that is repeated in tandem.
     - Other terminologies for STRs in the literature include "microsatellites" or "simple sequence repeats (SSRs)."
     - STRs are distributed throughout the human genome [48] (Fig. 20.1).
     - Note: VNTRs are highly polymorphic repetitive sequence that are 15–50 nucleotides long [49]. Due to larger amplicon size of VNTR, DNA also has to be better preserved compared to STR. Additionally, due to their larger size, VNTR alleles are more subject to preferential amplification and the sensitivity of VNTR is usually lower compared to STR. Consequently, STR test is used more often than VNTR due to higher sensitivity and availability of commercial reagents on the market.
   - Repeat units can be categorized by the length of the motif, e.g., mono-, di-, tri-, tetra-, penta-, and hepta-nucleotide repeats [50].
     - [AATG] would be an example of a tetra-nucleotide repeat unit [48].
   - The polymorphism of STRs derives primarily from the varying numbers of repeats.
     - For example, one *TPOX* allele might be characterized by six repeats of [AATG], i.e., $[AATG]_6$ = [AATG] [AATG] [AATG] [AATG] [AATG] [AATG], while another *TPOX* allele may characterized by four repeats, i.e., $[AATG]_4$ = [AATG] [AATG] [AATG] [AATG] [51].
   - There are different determinants in the nomenclature of STRs [52, 53].
     - In general, STRs that are located in the intron of a gene are named by the corresponding gene. For example, the STR *TPOX* is located in intron 10 of the human thyroid peroxidase gene, the STR *VWA* is located in intron 40 of the von Willebrand factor (vWF) gene, and the STR *CSF* is located in intron 6 of the CSF-1 receptor gene.

Table 20.2 Different categories of short tandem repeats (STRs)

	Example			
Category	Locus	Repeat structure	Allele designation	Comment/explanation allele designation
Simple	*TPOX*	$[AATG]_4$	4	Repeats of a single motif In this example, there are four repeats of [AATG]
Variant allele	*D2S441*	$[TCTA]_3$ TCA $[TCTA]_8$	11.3	Literature may refer to this as "simple with nonconsensus allele" [55] In this example, there are 11 (3 + 8) repeats of [TCTA] with an interjecting incomplete (imperfect) repeat (TCA) that is three nucleotides long
Compound	*D2S1338*	$[TGCC]_4$ $[TTCC]_6$	10	More than one motif of the same length nucleotide length is present [56] In this example, there are a total of ten (4 + 6) repeats present
Complex	*D21S11*	$[TCTA]_4$ $[TCTG]_6$ $[TCTA]_3$ TA $[TCTA]_3$ TCA $[TCTA]_2$ TCCATA $[TCTA]_6$	24	Motifs of varying lengths are present In this example, there are a total of 24 (4 + 6 + 3 + 3 + 2 + 6) repeats present Note that there are 11 non-repeated nucleotides (TA, TCA, TCCATA) and compare to the example below
Complex	*D21S11*	$[TCTA]_5$ $[TCTG]_6$ [----] -- $[TCTA]_3$ TCA $[TCTA]_2$ TCCATA $[TCTA]_9$	24.2	Motifs of varying lengths are present. In this example, there are a total of 25 (5 + 6 + 3 + 2 + 9) repeats present, but the allele designation is "short of" 25 (i.e., "24.X") because there is also the absence of two non-repeated nucleotides (--, TCA, TCCATA), making it two nucleotides longer than allele 24 in the example above

  - STRs that are not located in genes have a "D#S##" assignment, where "D" refers to DNA, "#" refers to the chromosomal location of the STR, and "S##" refers to a unique segment number. For example, the STR *D2S1338* is located on Chr. 2q35 and the STR *D21S11* is located on Chr. 21q91.1.
  - There are exceptions to the above system. Examples include the STRs *Penta D* and *Penta E* which are both comprised of penta-nucleotide repeats.
  - Of note, some commercial STR kits often include a non-STR markers such as *amelogenin,* which permits gender identification. Amelogenin is a gene that codes for the proteins found in tooth enamel and is present on both the X and Y chromosomes. A commonly used PCR primer set first published by Sullivan et al. [54] targets a 6 bp deletion within intron one of the gene that occurs on the X chromosome, resulting in heterozygosity amplification in males and homozygosity in females.
- There are different categories of STRs [48, 52] (examples are shown in Table 20.2).
  - Simple repeat
  - Simple with nonconsensus alleles
  - Compound repeat
  - Compound with nonconsensus alleles
  - Complex repeats
  - Hypervariable repeats
  - Note: There can be insertions and/or deletions (InDels) in the sequences flanking the repeat sequence resulting in alleles that are "flanking region variants." In these cases, if InDels are within the primer binding sites, the amplicon length will not be a sole reflection of the number of repeats in an STR.
- Allele designation is based on size, which reflects the number of repeats and the presence or absence of other motifs (see Table 20.2 for examples). A person's STR locus genotype indicates the two alleles of an individual.
  - Note: it is possible to encounter alleles of the same size and, therefore, the same allelic designation, but which have different nucleic acid sequences. Table 20.3 demonstrates an example of two alleles of *D1S1656* that have the same size (length), and both have allele designation 10 and, therefore, would not be differentiable by STR. As a result, *D1S1656* is not an informative locus for differentiating recipient from donor in this example. While sequencing could resolve this, it is not necessary for practical purposes to expend the extra cost and effort when there are many other loci one can examine to assess and quantify chimerism.
- Commonly used autosomal loci in for STR testing are shown in Table 20.4 [48].

Table 20.3 Example of two STR alleles of the same size and allelic designation but have different nucleic acid sequences

Example				
Patient	Locus	Allele designation	Repeat structure	STR locus genotype
Recipient	*D1S1656*[a]	10	[TAGA]$_{10}$ [TG]$_{5}$	10, 10 (or 10/10)
		10	[TAGA]$_{10}$ [TG]$_{5}$	
Donor	*D1S1656*[a]	10	[TAGA]$_{9}$ [TAGG] [TG]$_{5}$	10, 18 (or 10/18)
		18	[TAGA]$_{17}$ [TAGG] [TG]$_{5}$	

[a]*D1S1656* would not be a fully informative locus for differentiating recipient from donor in this example

Table 20.4 Commonly used autosomal loci in for STR testing

STR locus	Chromosome position	Repeat region sequences (excluding other variants)	Number of alleles sequenced (as of 2015)
D1S1656	1q42	[TAGA]$_{9–14}$ [TG]$_{5}$ [TAGA]$_{9–17}$ [TAGG] [TG]$_{5}$ [TAGA]$_{1–4}$ [TGA] [TAGA]$_{9–14}$ [TAGG] [TG]$_{5}$	26
TPOX	2p25.3	[AATG]$_{4–14}$	11
D2S441	2p14	[TCTA]$_{8–12}$ [TCTA]$_{2–5}$ [TCAA] [TCTA]$_{4–8}$ [TCTA]$_{11–14}$ [TTTA] [TCTA]$_{2}$ [TCTA]$_{8–10}$ [TCTG] [TCTA] [TCTA]$_{3–4}$ TCA [TCTA]$_{7–11}$	25
D2S1338	2q35	[TGCC]$_{4–9}$ [TTCC]$_{6–19}$ [TGCC]$_{6–8}$ [TTCC]$_{10–17}$ [GTCC] [TTCC]$_{2.}$	51
D3S1358	3p21.31	[TCTA] [TCTG]$_{1–4}$ [TCTA]$_{7–19}$	34
FGA	4q31.3	[TTTC]$_{3}$ [TTTT] [TTCT] [CTTT]$_{5–21}$ [CTCC] [TTCC]$_{2}$ [TTTC]$_{3}$ [TTTT] [TTCT] [CTTT]$_{5–10}$ T [CTTT]$_{3}$ [CTCC] [TTCC]$_{2}$ [TTTC]$_{3}$ [TTTT] [TTCT] [CTTT]$_{1–16}$ [NNNT] [CTTT]$_{1–20}$ [CTCC] [TTCC]$_{2}$ [TTTC]$_{3}$ [TTTT] [TTCT] [CTTT]$_{13}$ TTTCT [CTTT]$_{11–12}$ [CTCC] [TTCC]$_{2}$ [TTTC]$_{3}$ [TTTT] TT [CTTT]$_{11–21}$ [CTCC] [TTCC]$_{2}$ [TTTC]$_{4}$ [TTTT] TT [CTTT]$_{14–18}$ [CTTC]$_{3}$ [CTTT]$_{3}$ [CTCC] [TTCC]$_{4}$ [TTTC]$_{4}$ [TTTT] TT [CTTT]$_{8–11}$ [CTGT]$_{3–5}$ [CTTT]$_{11–15}$ [CTTC]$_{3–4}$ [CTTT]$_{3}$ [CTCC] [TTCC]$_{4.}$	50
D5S818	5q23.2	[AGAT]$_{7–16}$ [AGAT]$_{9–14}$ [ACAT] [AGAT]$_{3}$	6
CSF1PO	5q33.1	[AGAT]$_{5–16}$	14
SE33	6q14	[AAAG]$_{0–2}$ AG [AAAG]$_{0,2–3}$ AG$_{0–1}$ [AAAG]$_{5–22}$ AAAAAG$_{0–1}$ [AG]$_{0, 3, 5, 7, 9}$ AGAAAG$_{0–1}$ [AAAG]$_{0, 5, 8–23}$ AAAAAG$_{0–1}$ [AAAG]$_{0, 3–4. 9, 11, 14, 16–17}$ G [AAGG]$_{0–3}$ [AAAG/ANAG]$_{0–3}$ AG$_{1, 3}$	152
D6S1043	6q15	[AGAT]$_{9–15}$ [AGAT]$_{6,10–17}$ [ACAT] [AGAT]$_{5,11}$	22
D7S820	7q21.11	[GATA]$_{6–14}$	9
D8S1179	8q24.13	[TCTA]$_{7–14}$ [TCTA]$_{1}$ [TCTG]$_{1}$ [TCTA]$_{10–14}$ [TCTA]$_{2}$ [TCTG]$_{1}$ [TCTA]$_{9–15}$ [TCTA]$_{2}$ [TCTG]$_{2}$ [TCTA]$_{11–15}$	26
D10S1248	10q26.3	[GGAA]$_{7–19}$	14
TH01	11p15.5	[AATG]$_{3–12}$ [AATG]$_{3–6}$	15
vWA	12p13.31	[TCTA] [TCTG]$_{3–6}$ [TCTA]$_{7–17}$ TCCA TCTA	38
D12S391	12p13.2	[AGAT]$_{10–18}$ [AGAC]$_{6–11}$ [AGAT]$_{7–18}$ [AGAC]$_{5–10}$ [AGAT]	84
D13S317	13q31.1	[TATC]$_{7–15}$	10
Penta E	15q26.2	[AAAGA]$_{5–32}$ [AAAGA]$_{15–16}$ [AAATA]	30
D16S539	16q24.1	[GATA]$_{5–15}$	11
D18S51	18q21.33	[AGAA]$_{8–40}$ AAAGAGAGAGG [AGAA]$_{13–17, 19}$ AG AGAGAGAGAGG	36

Table 20.4 (continued)

STR locus	Chromosome position	Repeat region sequences (excluding other variants)	Number of alleles sequenced (as of 2015)
D19S433	19q12	[AAGG] [AAAG] [AAGG] [TAGG] [AAGG]$_{2, 6, 8-16}$ [AAGG] AA-- [AAGG] [TAGG] [AAGG]$_{5, 10-17}$	25
D21S11	21q21.1	[TCTA]$_{4-13}$ [TCTG]$_{3-11}$ [TCTA]$_{3}$ TA [TCTA]$_{2-3}$ TCA [TCTA]$_{2}$ TCCATA [TCTA]$_{6-15}$ [TCTA]$_{4-6}$ [TCTG]$_{5-6}$ [TCTA]$_{2-3}$ TA [TCTA]$_{2-3}$ TCA [TCTA]$_{2}$ TCCATA [TCTA]$_{8-16}$ TA [TCTA] [TCTA]$_{5-11}$ [TCTG]$_{6-14}$ [----] -- [TCTA]$_{3}$ TCA [TCTA]$_{2}$ TCCATA [TCTA]$_{9-13}$ [TCTA]$_{5-6}$ [TCTG]$_{5-6}$ [TCTA]$_{3}$ TA [TCTA]$_{3}$ TCA [TCTA]$_{2}$ TCCATA [TCTA]$_{5-10}$ TCA [TCTA]$_{2-6}$ NNN…	91
Penta D	21q22.3	[AAAGA]$_{5-19}$	15
D22S1045	22q12.3	[ATT]$_{5-17}$ ACT [ATT]$_{2.}$	13

Table 20.5 Example of STR locus in which the recipient is heterozygous and the donor is heterozygous

	(a) No shared alleles	(b) One shared allele	(c) Two shared alleles
Scenario	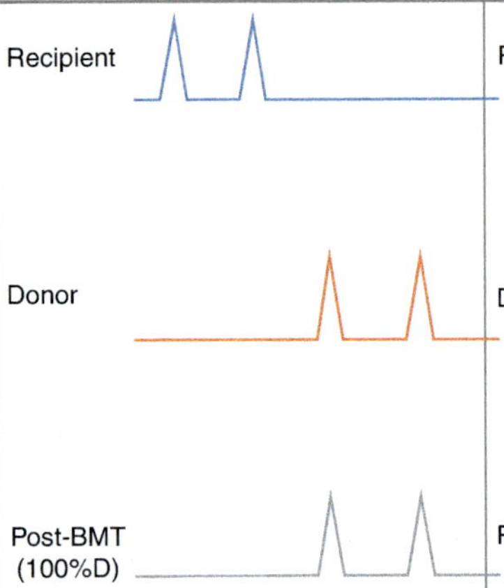	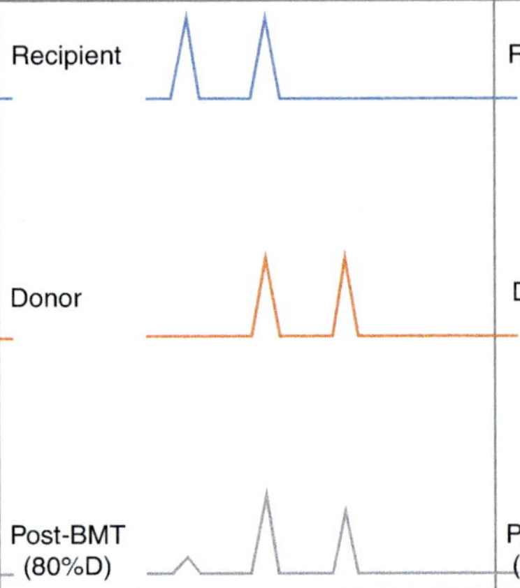	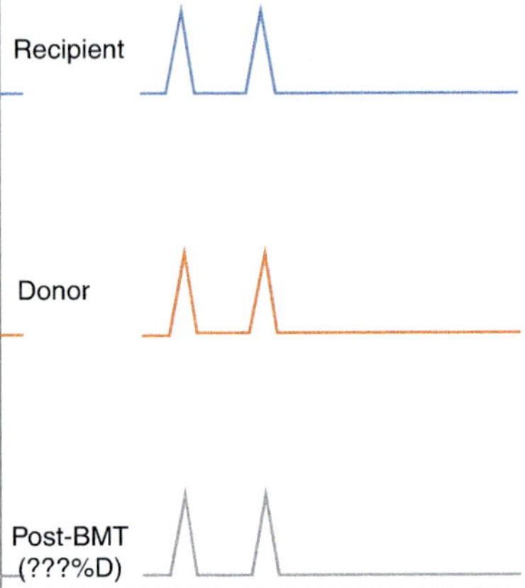
Recipient	R1[a], R2[b]	R1[a], R2[b]	R1[a], R2[b]
Donor	D1[a], D2[b]	D1[a], D2[b]	D1[a], D2[b]
Total number of alleles	Four (4): R1, R2, D1, D2	Three (3): R1, R2 = D1, D2	Two (2): R1 = D1, R2 = D2
Unique alleles	R1, R2, D1, D2	R1, D2	None
Shared alleles	None	R2 = D1	R1 = D1, R2 = D2
Informative?	Fully informative	Fully informative	Uninformative
Calculating post-BMT donor % chimerism	$\frac{(D1+D2)}{(R1+R2+D1+D2)}$	$\frac{D2}{(R1+D2)}$	Not applicable
Should use this locus?	Recommended	Recommended	Not possible

[a]R1 and D1 are the first peaks on the recipient and donor electropherograms, respectively, from left to right
[b]R2 and D2 are the second peaks on the recipient and donor electropherograms, respectively, from left to right

7. **How is STR analysis interpreted? How is quantification of donor and recipient DNA performed?**
   - There are two primary components of STR analysis for chimerism testing. First is the qualitative component of recipient and donor identification. The second is the quantitative component of assessing the percentage (%) of donor chimerism. The latter depends on the ability to distinguish the donor's STR genotype from the recipient's. Therefore, the laboratory needs to be able to perform STR testing on the patient's pretransplant and the donor's samples in order to establish each person's STR identity *before* a patient's post-transplant blood or bone marrow sample can be assessed for donor chimerism.
   - Since allelic designation of STRs is based on size (number of repeats), different alleles can be determined by their migration during electrophoresis which is reflected by the position of the peaks on an electropherogram. When two alleles are the same size (presumably homozygous), they show as a single peak for a designated locus. Heterozygous alleles will show as two peaks.
   - Unique allele peaks are required to distinguish recipient from donor and vice versa.
   - A locus is fully informative when there is at least one unique peak for the recipient and one unique peak for the donor. Fully informative loci are used to calculate the % donor chimerism [57]. For examples, see Tables 20.5a, b, 20.6a, 20.7a, and 20.8a.

Table 20.6 Example of STR locus in which the recipient is heterozygous and donor is homozygous

	(a) No shared alleles	(b) One shared allele
Scenario [20]	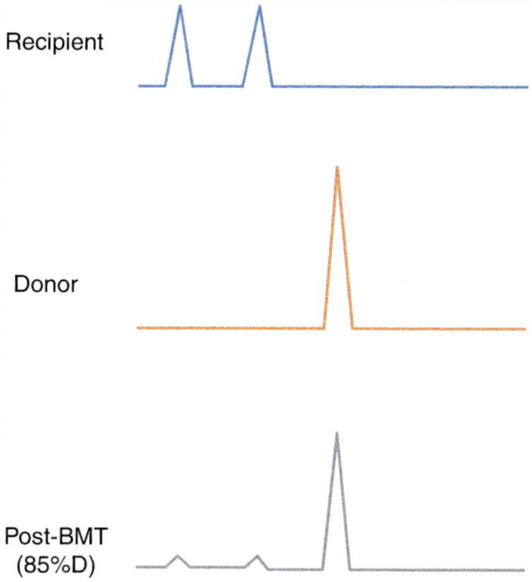	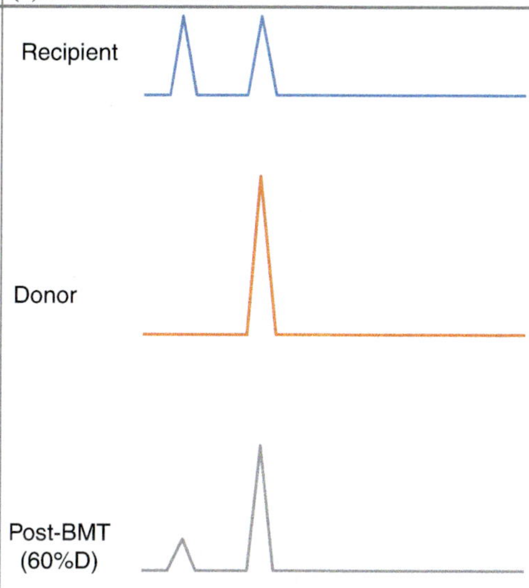
Recipient	R1[a], R2[b]	R1[a], R2[b]
Donor	D1[c]	D1[c]
Total number of alleles	Three (3): R1, R2, D1	Two (2): R1, R2 = D1
Unique alleles	R1, R2, D1	R1
Shared alleles	None	R2 = D1
Informative?	Fully informative	Informative
Calculating post-BMT donor % chimerism	$\frac{D1}{(R1+R2+D1)}$	Not recommended
Should use this locus?	Recommended	Not recommended

[a]R1 is the first peak on the recipient electropherogram from left to right
[b]R2 is the second peak on the recipient electropherogram from left to right
[c]D1 is the homozygous donor allele

  - *Note: Be aware that the term "Informative" in the literature and in clinical labs is generally understood to refer to fully informative loci as opposed to (partially) informative loci (see next bullet point).*
- When only one individual has a unique peak (e.g., recipient) but not the other (e.g., donor) (see Table 20.6b) or vice versa (see Table 20.7b), the locus is technically informative (or partially informative), but not fully informative. It is not recommended that these loci are used in assessing chimerism [57].
- Informative markers can be identified close to 100% of the time with a panel of 12–16 STR markers.
- If there are no unique peaks for the donor and recipient (i.e., recipient and donor share the same peaks), the locus is not informative (see Tables 20.5c) and 20.8b) and cannot be used in assessing chimerism.
- Unique peaks of fully informative loci are quantitated using peak height or area under peak which should correspond to the amount of donor-derived and recipient-derived amplicon. This, in turn, is presumed to correspond to the amount of donor- and recipient-derived DNA, which, in turn, is presumed to correspond to the number of donor-derived and recipient-derived cells [6, 57].
  - A peak that corresponds to a homozygous allele should ideally have approximately twice the height or area of the peaks of heterozygous alleles at the same locus (see Tables 20.6 and 20.7).
  - Also, peaks of heterozygous alleles should ideally have comparable (e.g., 1:1) peak heights or areas under peak to each other.
- In the post-HPCT sample, the % of donor chimerism is calculated by taking the donor's unique peak(s) and dividing its value by the total value of the recipient's and donor's unique peaks.
- The percent donor can be calculated using the following equation [40]:

$$\frac{(D1+D2)}{(D1+D2+R1+R2)}$$

Table 20.7 Example of STR locus in which the recipient is homozygous and donor is heterozygous

	(a) No shared alleles	(b) One shared allele
Scenario	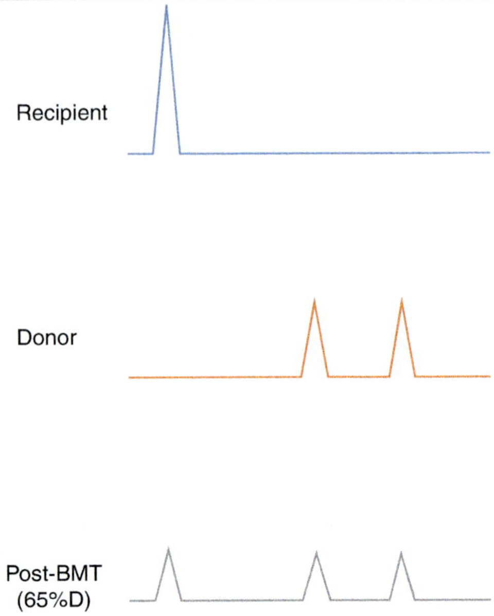	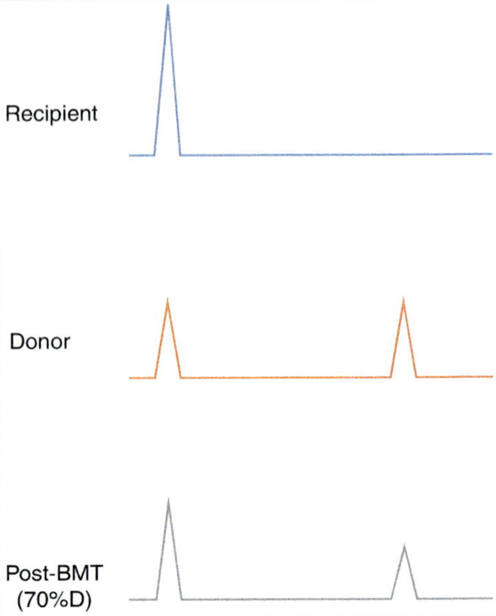
Recipient	R1[a]	R1[a]
Donor	D1[b], D2[c]	D1[b], D2[c]
Total number of alleles	Three (3): R1, D1, D2	Two (2): R1 = D1, D2
Unique alleles	R1, D1, D2	D2
Shared alleles	None	R1 = D1
Informative?	Fully informative	Informative
Calculating post-BMT donor % chimerism	$\frac{(D1+D2)}{(R1+D1+D2)}$	Not recommended
Should use this locus?	Recommended	Not recommended

[a]R1 is the homozygous recipient allele
[b]D1 is the first peak on the donor electropherogram from left to right
[c]D2 is the second peak in the donor electropherogram from left to right

- D1 and D2 are the heights of or the area under the informative donor peaks (if donor is homozygous, D2 = 0).
- R1 and R2 are the heights of or the area under the informative recipient peaks (if recipient is homozygous, R2 = 0).
- Shared peaks between donor and recipient can be omitted from the calculation.

- The exact calculation will depend on whether one is dealing with two, three, or four unique peaks (see Tables 20.5a, b, 20.6a, 20.7a, and 20.8a).
- The % donor chimerism should be calculated for all the fully informative loci. The % values between the different loci should be consistent with each other. The average of these values is reported as the % donor chimerism.
- Recommendations are to use the average of at least three fully informative loci (when possible) and that the coefficient of variance for these loci should be <5% [57].
  - *Note: One could hypothetically use (partially) informative loci to calculate % donor chimerism* [6, 24, 57]. *This assumes ideal amplification circumstances where one assumes that heterozygous alleles are amplified with perfect 1:1 ratio (i.e., no allelic imbalance) and that there is nothing else that interferes with peak height or area under peak (e.g., stutter, split peaks, saturation). Since this is not assured in the "real world" setting, for practical purposes, partially informative loci are generally not recommended for use in calculating % donor chimerism; however, they can be used as long as they have been properly validated.*

Table 20.8 Example of STR locus in which the recipient is homozygous and donor is homozygous

	(a) No shared alleles	(b) One shared allele
Scenario	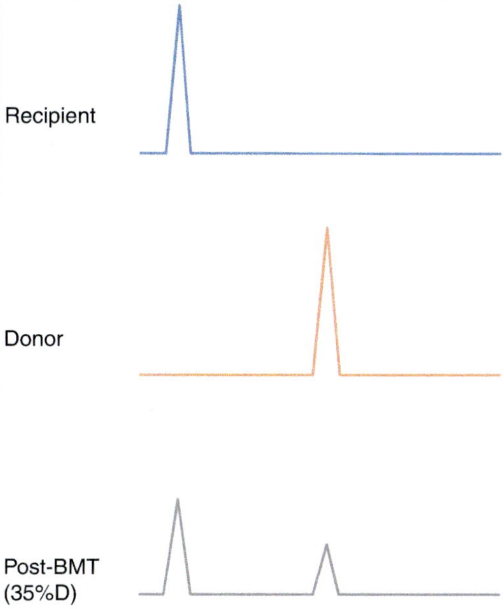	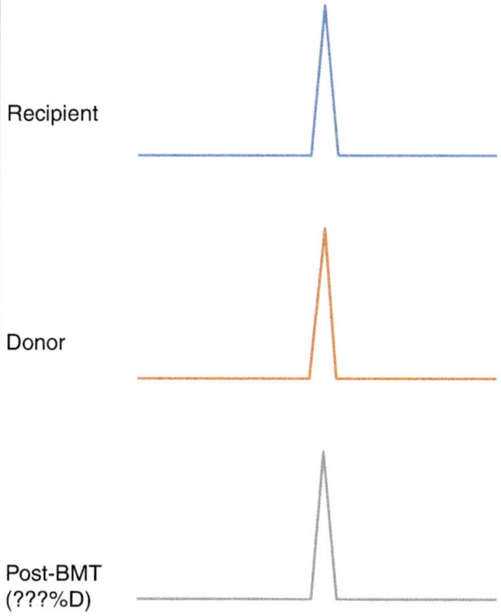
Recipient	R1[a]	R1[a]
Donor	D1[b]	D1[b]
Total number of alleles	Two (2): R1, D1	One (1): R1 = D1
Unique alleles	R1, D1	None
Shared alleles	None	R1 = D1
Informative?	Fully informative	Uninformative
Calculating post-BMT donor % chimerism	$\frac{\text{D1}}{(\text{R1}+\text{D1})}$	Not applicable
Should use this locus?	Recommended	Not possible

[a]R1 is the homozygous recipient allele
[b]D1 is the homozygous donor allele

- Manual calculations can be time-consuming, labor-intensive, and prone to human error. There are analytic software programs that apply algorithms that will select informative loci and automatically result percentage chimerism with minimal data manipulation [58]. Some software program algorithmic equations will compensate for certain artifacts inherent in STR analysis (see question #9).
- One sample only gives the donor and recipient percentages from a single time point. Without reference to transplant timeline or comparison to previous or subsequent samples, a single sample provides limited information. Serial monitoring is important in identifying clinically relevant trends during the engraftment period.
- When umbilical cord blood is used as an HPC cell source for transplantation, due to limited cell dosage, adults will undergo double umbilical/unit cord blood transplantation, where two donor units are infused. While the calculations are not shown here, the principles of establishing informative loci and the calculations in assessing % chimerism are the same, and only now one must account for one recipient and two donors. Chimerism reports should include % values for each donor separately and not as a sum of both donors.

8. **What are multiplex STR assays and what are some of their advantages and disadvantages?**
   - Multiplex STR assays allow multiple loci to be tested simultaneously in a single setup.
   - The advantages include the following [40, 57, 59]:
     - Multiplex assays are particularly useful for chimerism testing because multiple loci are assessed in establishing the genetic identities of the donor and recipient. It is also time-efficient because it precludes the need for add-on testing. For example, if certain loci are determined to be uninformative, other loci have already been tested that can be assessed.

- Because chimerism assessment involves quantitating the % of cells/DNA tested that originate from the donor, having multiple loci tested allows for the averaging of percentages and increased power of analysis. Being able to compare % donor chimerism between loci also provides a form of internal quality reassurance as one would expect the % to be similar across all loci [57].
- It allows for more cost-efficient use of reagents and other consumables.
- It is less laborious and less time-consuming than using monoplex assays.
- It allows amplicons of different loci to all have their sizes assessed against the same DNA size ladder (internal size standard) present in the same single injection [59].

- Disadvantages
  - There can be decreased sensitivity compared to monoplex assays.
  - Spectral overlap can occur if multiple fluorescent markers are involved and must be accounted for. With current assay design and software analysis, this is usually not a significant problem.
  - Testing artifacts (e.g., stutter peak and preferential amplification). See question 9 for detailed description of these artifacts.

9. **What are some biological and testing "artifacts" that can be seen in STR analysis?**
   - The main factor limiting the utility of some informative markers is the presence of stutter peaks. Stutter peaks are generally small peaks at one less repeat from the true allele (Fig. 20.2). Stutter peaks result from strand slippage of polymerase during DNA synthesis (Fig. 20.2) [60]. This results in STR amplicons that are one or more repeats longer or shorter than the actual allele. Stutter peaks can present before (reverse stutter) or after (forward stutter) the STR major peak. Reverse stutter peaks are more common than forward stutter peaks.
   - The size of the stutter peak is usually the allele size ± the nucleotide number of the repeat. For example, the stutter size of trinucleotide repeat will be N ± 3 bp; the stutter size of tetranucleotide repeat will be N ± 4 bp. Stutter peaks can account for 3–15% of the true allelic peak.
   - Stutter peaks can vary depending on any of the following:
     - Repeat size: The amount of stutter product formation is usually reduced when using longer STR repeat markers, e.g., pentanucleotide repeats have less stutter than tetranucleoide repeats, and tetranucleotide repeats have less stutter than trinucleotide repeats.
     - Nucleotide content: STR repeats with higher A and T content are more prone to have stutter likely due to weaker hydrogen bonding between A and T nucleotides (two hydrogen bonds) compared to between C and G nucleotides (three hydrogen bonds).
     - Distance from primary allele: The level of stutter decreases when moving away from the primary allele; therefore, a stutter peak of N ± 6 (2 × 3 bp) or N ± 8 (2 × 4 bp) will be smaller than a stutter peak of N ± 3 (1 × 3 bp) or N ± 4 (1 × 4 bp), respectively.
     - DNA concentration: Stutter can increase when amplifying low levels of DNA template due to stochastic effects.
   - Stutter peaks can complicate STR interpretation particularly when a stutter peak of the recipient falls in the same bin or position as a true donor allele or vice versa. When such colocation of stutter and true informative peaks occurs, discerning the stutter contribution of informative peaks from stutter in a given peak is difficult. For example, post-transplant a minute peak

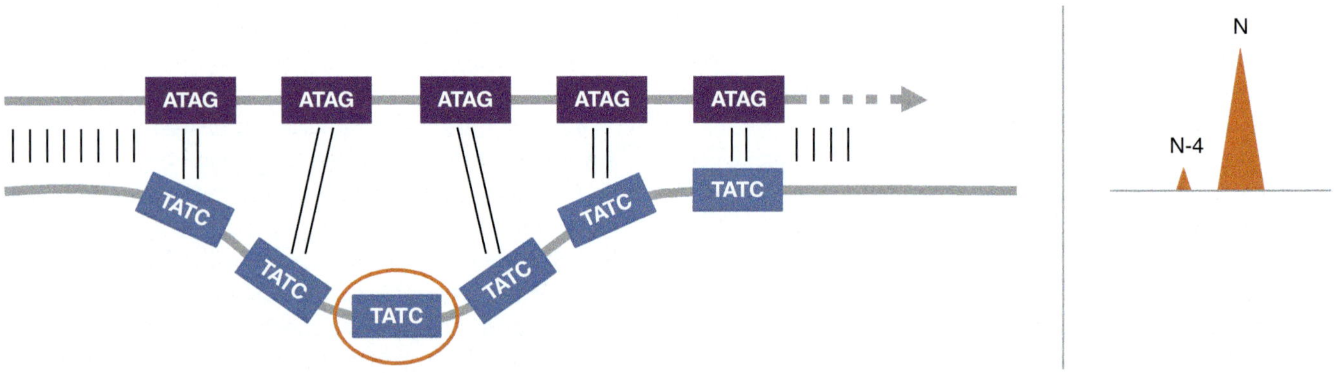

Fig. 20.2 **Left panel**: Illustration demonstrating reverse stutter which is due to slippage of bottom strand (template) that results in deletion of one repeat unit (circle) in the top strand (copy). Note: forward stutter is also possible when there is insertion of unit repeat in the copy strand (not depicted). **Right panel**: Illustration of electropherogram that results from deletion of one repeat unit. N is number of repeats of primary allele; N-4 is the stutter peak with one less repeat than the primary allele

in front of an informative allele could either represent a stutter or could represent a minor component of another informative allele in a mixed chimerism sample if the allele from the minor component and the stutter of the major component colocalize on the electropherogram.

- In order to avoid stutter interference, loci in which stutter peaks and true alleles colocalize should not be included as informative loci in the overall calculation of chimerism percentage [61]. Alternatively, the stutter can be resolved by using adjusted equations that account for the percent stutter contribution at each respective STR marker [62]. See Case 2 for an example.
- Stutter peak correction starts with the calculation of stutter peak percentage. Stutter peak percentage refers to the percentage of stutter peak relative to its primary allele peak and is usually consistent for each locus. The percentage of the stutter peak is determined in the pre-transplant STR test of recipient and donor samples.
- Allelic imbalance results from differential amplification of PCR products of varying lengths [63]. Accordingly, donor and/or recipient alleles can be differentially amplified resulting in one allele at a locus being more efficiently amplified than the other. Preferential amplification tends to be observed with the amplification of shorter products [58]. As such, smaller-sized STR alleles amplify more efficiently than larger-sized alleles and lead to preferential amplification. Consequently, when one allele is preferentially amplified, it may lead to an underestimation of the opposite allele [64].
- Selecting informative loci with alleles with the smallest difference in size (i.e., similar number base pairs) may help avoid the effects of preferential amplification [26]. The peak area ratio (PAR) can be calculated by dividing the weaker intensity allele peak area by the stronger intensity allele peak area (e.g., if $D1 < D2$, then $PAR = D1/D2$). Some laboratory protocols use a predetermined PAR in the selection of informative peaks (e.g., loci are only selected if $PAR > 70\%$). However, some experts recommend selecting recipient loci with shorter recipient allele(s) as to increase the sensitivity of the assay by enhancing the limit of detection of recipient alleles that are preferentially amplified [64].
- Alternatively, the influence of differential amplification on chimerism analysis can be resolved using certain ratio formulas to compensate for the preferential amplification of one of the alleles [58].
- Pull-up peaks are artifactual peaks that occur when there are extremely high signals from fluorescent dyes with overlapping spectral emission that can bleed through to other color channels. These peaks can be resolved by decreasing the PCR amplicon loaded in the capillary by either shortening the injection time or diluting the PCR product [65].
- Non-template nucleotide addition appears as peaks with two spikes. The double peaks result from the preferential 3′ addition of adenosine residues of the amplicon by template-independent means of the Taq polymerase's terminal extendase activity. This artifact can be resolved by concluding PCR amplification with 45 min, 60 °C extension [65].
- Some STR loci can actually contain three alleles, which are known as tri-alleleic bands [66]. There are two types:
  - Type 1 pattern, the more common type, consists of three alleles of uneven heights, generally the sum of two of the peaks equals the height of the third. This type is thought to arise from somatic mutations.
  - Type 2 pattern has peaks of equal heights. Type 2 pattern is thought to arise from chromosomal duplication and/or aneuploidy [67].
- Tri-alleleic bands may confound STR analysis if one or more of the alleles colocalize with the recipient and/or donor alleles.
- Genetic alterations can be seen in malignancies, such as acute myelogenous leukemias, and can result in STR marker length mutations, which can confound chimerism interpretation [68, 69]. Loss of heterozygosity at STR loci can also be seen in malignancies and could result in miscalculation of chimerism post-transplant.

Case Presentations

Case 1

Learning Objective

An assay that reports 100% donor chimerism may miss the presence of recipient-derived cells if the percentage of donor cells present is less than the sensitivity of the assay.

Case History

A 64-year-old female patient is diagnosed with acute myelogenous leukemia (AML) that expressed CD11C, CD13, CD34, CD38, CD117, partial HLA-DR, and CD45. Patient underwent three rounds of induction therapy to achieve complete remission before receiving an HPCT from an unrelated HLA- and ABO-matched donor.

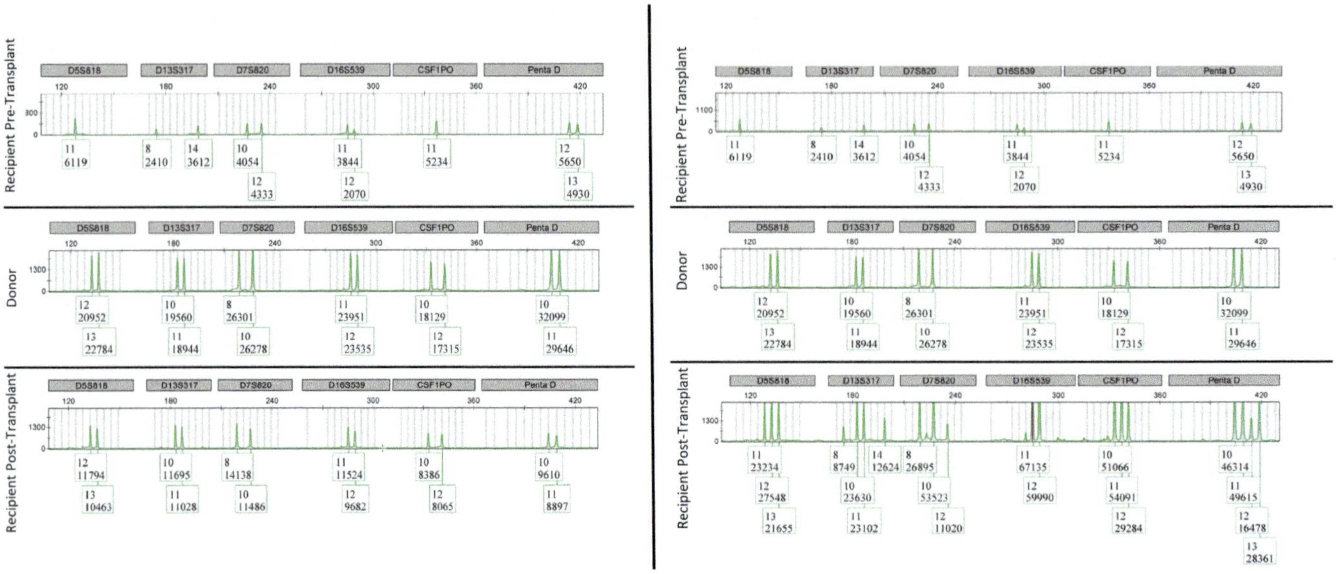

Fig. 20.3 Left panel: STR electropherograms of recipient, pre-transplant [top], donor [middle], and recipient, post-transplant [bottom]. Green boxes show the allele designation on top and peak size on bottom (e.g., recipient, pre-transplant locus D5S818 has an allele designation of 11 and with a peak size of 6119). Informative loci are D5S818, D13S317, D7S820, CSF1PO, and Penta D. D16S539 is not informative. **Right panel**: STR electropherograms of recipient, pre-transplant [top], donor [middle], and recipient, post-transplant – updated [bottom]. This time the updated post-transplant sample is showing three to four allele peaks (corresponding to donor and recipient) at the informative loci

Laboratory Findings

Patient did well post-transplant and STR testing showed 100% donor chimerism in the T-cell (CD3+) and myeloid (CD33+) lineages for the next 3 years (Fig. 20.3). However, because the team became clinically concerned for relapse, a subsequent sample was sent to flow cytometry which showed a 4% population of aberrant myeloblasts expressing partial CD7, CD13, CD34, CD38, dim CD117, and dim CD45. Concurrent STR testing to the flow sample continued to demonstrate 100% donor chimerism.

Final Diagnosis

Relapse of AML

Follow-Up

The patient had a follow-up sample drawn for chimerism testing by STR, this time showing the presence of recipient allele peaks (% donor chimerism <100%), reconfirming the diagnosis of AML relapse (Fig. 20.3).

Discussion

This is a case that demonstrates the potential limitations of sensitivity of multiplex STR testing. This particular STR assay had an established sensitivity of 5% and therefore did not detect the 4% aberrant recipient-derived population. In this particular case, flow cytometry was useful in confirming the clinical suspicion of relapse in this case. Whereas, STR analysis can detect percent recipient, which could be benign or malignant, flow cytometry directly detects aberrant cell population. The United Kingdom National External Quality Assessment Service for Leucocyte Immunophenotyping Chimerism Working Group (UK NEQAS LI) recommends that the limit of detection should be calculated and included on reports that indicate 100% recipient or donor results so that clinicians are not unduly mislead by a "100%" result [57].

Case 2

Learning Objective

To examine STR analysis when stutter peaks are present. Though general recommendations are to avoid loci with stutter peaks, there are calculations that can be performed to account for stutter correction.

Case History

A 40-year-old male received HPCT from his sibling.

Laboratory Testing

STR chimerism testing was performed 30 days post-transplant. The recipient and donor were identical at almost all the STR markers. In fact, only one STR marker was identified as potentially informative (D7S820). The recipient was heterozygous for D7S820 with allele 7 (R1) and 11 (R2), and the donor was heterozygous with allele 8 and 10 (Fig. 20.4).

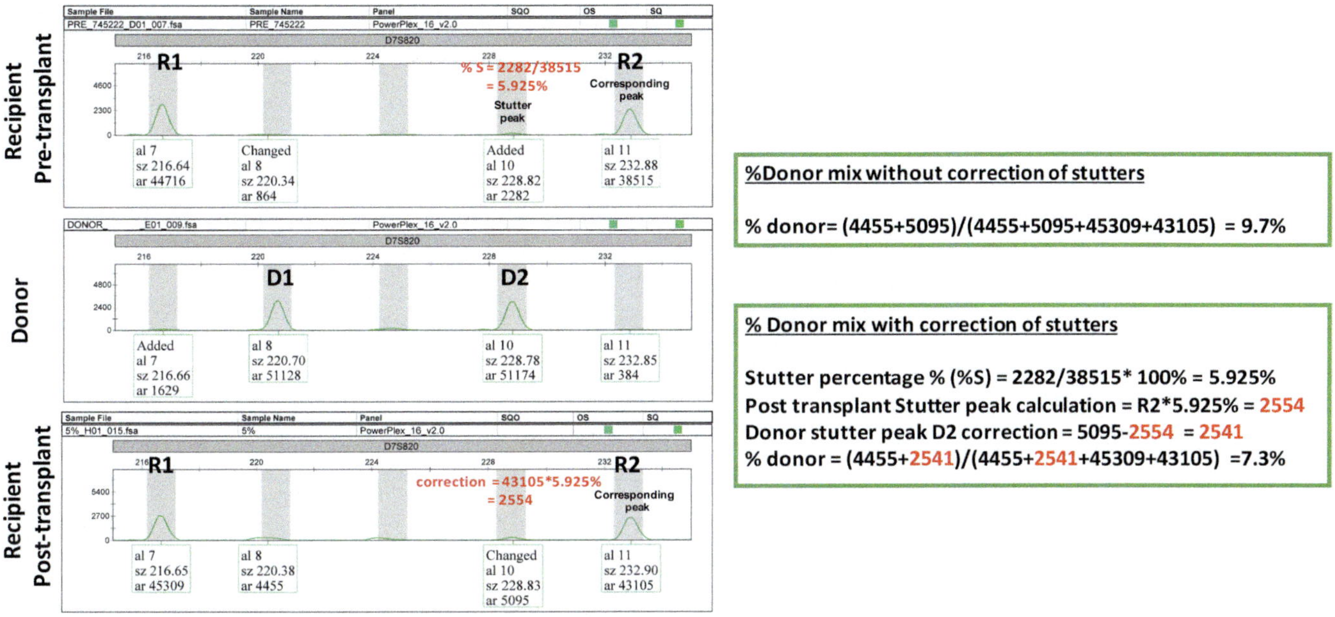

Fig. 20.4 Left panel: STR electropherograms of recipient, pre-transplant [top], donor [middle], and recipient, post-transplant [bottom]. D7S820 allele 10 is indicated as a stutter peak of allele 11 (n − 1) in the recipient pre-transplant specimen. **Right panel**: Calculations demonstrate percent donor chimerism without stutter correction (top box) and with stutter correction (bottom box)

Discussion

D7S820 allele 10 is indicated as a stutter peak of allele 11 (n − 1) in the recipient pre-transplant specimen. Using all peak areas without correction of stutter peak will result in overestimating the percentage of donor DNA. To correct stutter peak, stutter percentage (% Stutter) is calculated by using peak area of allele 10 (stutter peak) divided by the peak area of allele 11 times 100% (in this case 2282/38515 × 100 = 5.925%). The percent of post-transplant stutter is then calculated using the % stutter multiplied by the peak area of allele 11 in the post-transplant sample (5.925% × 43,105 = 2554). The corrected D2 peak area is calculated using D2 peak area (5095) minus the contribution of the stutter peak (2554), and then the corrected D2 (5095 − 2554 = 2541) is used for donor percentage calculation (Fig. 20.4). This case demonstrates the calculation adjustments that must be made in order to use loci in which stutter peak colocalizes with recipient or donor peaks. Though it is generally recommended to avoid using these loci as informative, at times these loci may represent the only available loci that can be used, especially when recipient and donor are identical at most STR markers as seen in this case between siblings.

Case 3

Learning Objective

Explore the uses of chimerism testing beyond HPCT, in particular, how chimerism testing can be used to investigate GVHD post-solid organ transplantation.

Case History

A 53-year-old male with pulmonary fibrosis was transferred from an outside hospital secondary to worsening pulmonary status and increased hypoxia, which was refractory to standard treatment. His workup for an infectious etiology of his pulmonary decline (sputum culture, blood cultures) was negative. Due to worsening respiratory status and hypoxia, he was started on extracorporeal membrane oxygenation and underwent bilateral lung transplant. His postoperative course was notable for cytopenia, transaminitis, diarrhea, and a maculopapular skin rash with desquamation.

Laboratory Findings

- Complete blood count
  - White blood cell count: 2.1 × 10E3/mcL (reference range, 4.2–9.1 × 10E3/mcL)
  - Hemoglobin: 9.2 gm/dL (reference range, 12.9–16.1 gm/dL)
  - Platelet count: 76 × 10E3/mcL (reference range, 150–400 × 10E3/mcL)
- Liver enzymes
  - Alanine aminotransferase: 1420 unit/L (reference range, 7–52 unit/L)
  - Aspartate aminotransferase: 7546 unit/L (reference range, 13–39 unit/L)
  - Alkaline phosphatase: 412 unit/L (reference range, 34–104 unit/L)
- Stool examination
  - No ova or parasites seen on concentrated examination
  - No ova or parasites seen on trichrome stain
  - No cryptosporidium seen

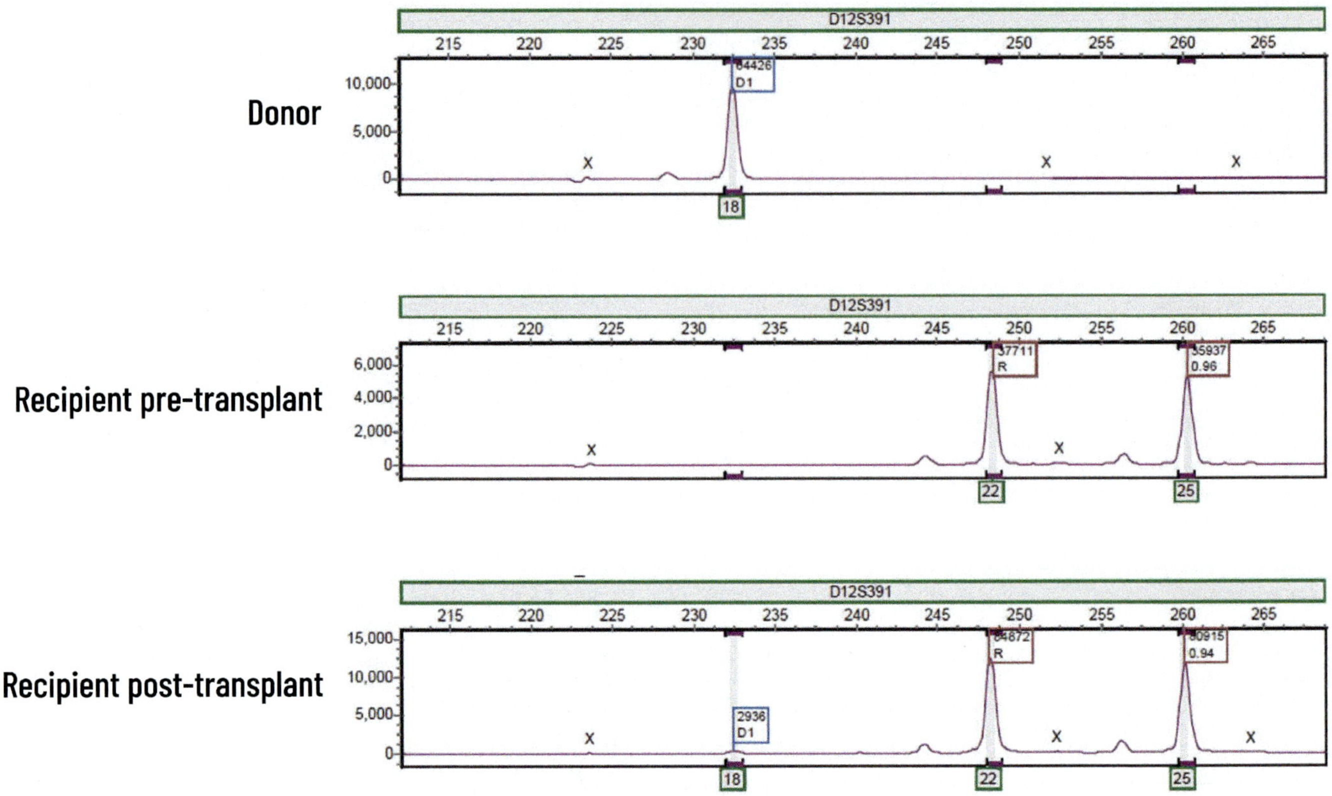

Fig. 20.5 STR electropherograms of recipient (CD3 subset) pre-transplant [middle], donor [top], and recipient post-transplant [bottom]. Post-transplant sample demonstrates a small donor peak (D1), representing approximately 2% of DNA in the sample

  - No cyclospora seen
  - No cystoisospora seen
- Skin biopsy
  - Mild perivascular lymphocytic inflammatory infiltrate, consistent with possible acute graft-versus-host or drug eruption

Genetic Study

- Due to suspicion of GVHD, chimerism testing was performed 3 weeks post-transplant to look for the presence of donor-derived cells in the recipient's peripheral blood.
- The CD33+ fraction showed no chimerism; however the CD3+ fraction showed 2% donor chimerism. A second sample showed similar results (Fig. 20.5).

Final Diagnosis

The clinical team made the presumptive diagnosis of GVHD given the clinical symptoms and the presence of peripheral blood T-cell chimerism, in the absence of another etiology for the pancytopenia and skin rash.

Discussion

While the donor chimerism in the peripheral blood is very suggestive of GVHD, it is a relatively low percentage. It is worth noting that the test sample was from the peripheral blood, and donor chimerism in the transplanted tissue, bone marrow, or GI tract or skin could have been greater as sites of active alloimmunity. GVHD following solid organ transplant has been reported in several patients, predominantly in the small intestine and lung due to the higher lymphoid cell content of these tissues [70, 71]. Mortality in these case reports is very high (85–95% for lungs, up to 77% for small bowel). Fortunately, this patient was able to recover and be discharged from the hospital following this episode of GVHD. Interestingly, the patient developed a donor-specific antibody (DSA) to HLA-C*10, which does not fit well with a GVH immune response, as it instead indicates a host-versus-graft reaction. However, the development of DSA could have been a response to the decrease in immunosuppression in the treatment of presumptive GVHD. In summary, this case highlights an uncommon occurrence of probable GVHD in solid organ transplant, which serves as a reminder that solid organs can contain significant numbers of passenger leukocytes that can mount anti-host responses. Additionally, this case serves to demonstrate the clinical utility of chimerism testing outside its more common uses of monitoring for engraftment and relapse in hematopoietic progenitor cell transplantation.

References

1. Antin JH, Childs R, Filipovich AH, Giralt S, Mackinnon S, Spitzer T, et al. Establishment of complete and mixed donor chimerism after allogeneic lymphohematopoietic transplantation: recommendations from a workshop at the 2001 Tandem Meetings of the

International Bone Marrow Transplant Registry and the American Society of Blood and Marrow Transplantation. Biol Blood Marrow Transplant. 2001;7:473.
2. Khan F, Agarwal A, Agrawal S. Significance of chimerism in hematopoietic stem cell transplantation: new variations on an old theme. Bone Marrow Transplant. 2004;34:1.
3. Scandling JD, Busque S, Lowsky R, Shizuru J, Shori A, Engleman E, et al. Macrochimerism and clinical transplant tolerance. Hum Immunol. 2018;79:266.
4. McCann SR, Crampe M, Molloy K, Lawler M. Hemopoietic chimerism following stem cell transplantation. Transfus Apher Sci. 2005;32:55.
5. Bader P, Niethammer D, Willasch A, Kreyenberg H, Klingebiel T. How and when should we monitor chimerism after allogeneic stem cell transplantation? Bone Marrow Transplant. 2005;35:107.
6. Pindolia K, Janakiraman N, Kasten-Sportes C, Demanet C, Van Waeyenberge C, Pals G, et al. Enhanced assessment of allogeneic bone marrow transplant engraftment using automated fluorescent-based typing. Bone Marrow Transplant. 1999;24:1235.
7. Piccin A, McCann S, Socié G, Oneto R, Bacigalupo A, Locasciulli A, et al. Survival of patients with documented autologous recovery after SCT for severe aplastic anemia: a study by the WPSAA of the EBMT. Bone Marrow Transplant. 2010;45:1008.
8. Quiroga M, Pereira NF, Bitencourt MA, Bonfim C, Monteiro MGM, Pasquini R. Late chimerical status after bone marrow transplantation in severe aplastic anemia according to two different preparatory regimens. Hematol Transfus Cell Ther. 2018;40:112.
9. O'Donnell PV. Chapter 18: Engraftment. In: Wingard JR, Gastineau DA, Leather HL, Snyder EL, Szczepiorkowski ZM, editors. Hematopoietic stem cell transplantation: a handbook for clinicians. 2nd ed. Bethesda: AABB; 2015. p. 255–72.
10. Rezvani AR, Lowsky R, Negrin RS. Chapter 23: Hematopoietic cell transplantation. In: Kaushansky K, Lichtman MA, Prchal JT, Levi MM, Press OW, Burns LJ, Caligiuri MA, editors. Williams hematology. 9th ed. New York: McGraw-Hill Education; 2016. p. 353–82.
11. Tsirigotis P, Byrne M, Schmid C, Baron F, Ciceri F, Esteve J, et al. Relapse of AML after hematopoietic stem cell transplantation: methods of monitoring and preventive strategies. A review from the ALWP of the EBMT. Bone Marrow Transplant. 2016;51:1431.
12. Thomson KJ, Peggs KS. Allogeneic transplantation in the UK: an aggregation of marginal gains? Br J Haematol. 2013;163:149.
13. Leventhal J, Abecassis M, Miller J, Gallon L, Tollerud D, Elliott MJ, et al. Tolerance induction in HLA disparate living donor kidney transplantation by donor stem cell infusion: durable chimerism predicts outcome. Transplantation. 2013;95:169.
14. Leventhal JR, Ildstad ST. Tolerance induction in HLA disparate living donor kidney transplantation by facilitating cell-enriched donor stem cell infusion: the importance of durable chimerism. Hum Immunol. 2018;79:272.
15. Lowsky R, Strober S. Combined kidney and hematopoeitic cell transplantation to induce mixed chimerism and tolerance. Bone Marrow Transplant. 2019;54:793.
16. Sasaki H, Oura T, Spitzer TR, Chen YB, Madsen JC, Allan J, et al. Preclinical and clinical studies for transplant tolerance via the mixed chimerism approach. Hum Immunol. 2018;79:258.
17. Kopko PM. Transfusion support for ABO-incompatible progenitor cell transplantation. Transfus Med Hemother. 2016;43:13.
18. Rühl H, Bein G, Sachs UJ. Transfusion-associated graft-versus-host disease. Transfus Med Rev. 2009;23:62.
19. Kleinman S, Stassinopoulos A. Transfusion-associated graft-versus-host disease reexamined: potential for improved prevention using a universally applied intervention. Transfusion. 2018;58:2545.
20. National Healthcare Safety Network Biovigilance Component Hemovigilance Module Surveillance Protocol v2.5.2 of the Centers for Disease Control (CDC). https://www.cdc.gov/nhsn/pdfs/biovigilance/bv-hv-protocol-current.pdf. Last accessed 26 Oct 2020.
21. Butler JM. Short tandem repeat typing technologies used in human identity testing. BioTechniques. 2007;43:ii.
22. Wenk RE. Testing for parentage and kinship. Curr Opin Hematol. 2004;11:357.
23. Yang MJ, Tzeng CH, Tseng JY, Huang CY. Determination of twin zygosity using a commercially available STR analysis of 15 unlinked loci and the gender-determining marker amelogenin – a preliminary report. Hum Reprod. 2006;21:2175.
24. Thiede C, Florek M, Bornhäuser M, Ritter M, Mohr B, Brendel C, et al. Rapid quantification of mixed chimerism using multiplex amplification of short tandem repeat markers and fluorescence detection. Bone Marrow Transplant. 1999;23:1055.
25. Beck O, Seidl C, Lehrnbecher T, Kreyenberg H, Schwabe D, Klingebiel T, et al. Quantification of chimerism within peripheral blood, bone marrow and purified leukocyte subsets: comparison of singleplex and multiplex PCR amplification of short tandem repeat (STR) loci. Eur J Haematol. 2006;76:237.
26. Gineikiene E, Stoskus M, Griskevicius L. Recent advances in quantitative chimerism analysis. Expert Rev Mol Diagn. 2009;9:817.
27. Fordyce SL, Ávila-Arcos MC, Rockenbauer E, Børsting C, Frank-Hansen R, Petersen FT, et al. High-throughput sequencing of core STR loci for forensic genetic investigations using the Roche Genome Sequencer FLX platform. BioTechniques. 2011;51:127.
28. Butler JM. Forensic DNA typing: biology, technology, and genetics of STR markers. Burlington: Elsevier Academic Press; 2005.
29. Tomblyn MR, Ewell M, Bredeson C, Kahl BS, Goodman SA, Horowitz MM, et al. Autologous versus reduced-intensity allogeneic hematopoietic cell transplantation for patients with chemosensitive follicular non-Hodgkin lymphoma beyond first complete response or first partial response. Biol Blood Marrow Transplant. 2011;17:1051.
30. Willasch A, Eing S, Weber G, Kuçi S, Schneider G, Soerensen J, et al. Enrichment of cell subpopulations applying automated MACS technique: purity, recovery and applicability for PCR-based chimerism analysis. Bone Marrow Transplant. 2010;45:181.
31. Hanson V, Adams B, Lord J, Barker A, Poulton K, Lee H. Assessment of the purity of isolated cell populations for lineage-specific chimerism monitoring post haematopoietic stem cell transplantation. Tissue Antigens. 2013;82:269.
32. Lion T, Daxberger H, Dubovsky J, Filipcik P, Fritsch G, Printz D, et al. Analysis of chimerism within specific leukocyte subsets for detection of residual or recurrent leukemia in pediatric patients after allogeneic stem cell transplantation. Leukemia. 2001;15:307.
33. Bader P, Kreyenberg H, Hoelle W, Dueckers G, Handgretinger R, Lang P, et al. Increasing mixed chimerism is an important prognostic factor for unfavorable outcome in children with acute lymphoblastic leukemia after allogeneic stem-cell transplantation: possible role for pre-emptive immunotherapy? J Clin Oncol. 2004;22:1696.
34. Ozyurek E, Cowan MJ, Koerper MA, Baxter-Lowe LA, Dvorak CC, Horn BN. Increasing mixed chimerism and the risk of graft loss in children undergoing allogeneic hematopoietic stem cell transplantation for non-malignant disorders. Bone Marrow Transplant. 2008;42:83.
35. Breuer S, Preuner S, Fritsch G, Daxberger H, Koenig M, Poetschger U, et al. Early recipient chimerism testing in the T- and NK-cell lineages for risk assessment of graft rejection in pediatric patients undergoing allogeneic stem cell transplantation. Leukemia. 2012;26:509.
36. Matthes-Martin S, Lion T, Haas OA, Frommlet F, Daxberger H, König M, et al. Lineage-specific chimaerism after stem cell transplantation in children following reduced intensity conditioning: potential predictive value of NK cell chimaerism for late graft rejection. Leukemia. 2003;17:1934.
37. Lawler M, McCann SR, Marsh JC, Ljungman P, Hows J, Vandenberghe E, et al. Serial chimerism analyses indicate that mixed haemopoietic chimerism influences the probability of graft

rejection and disease recurrence following allogeneic stem cell transplantation (SCT) for severe aplastic anaemia (SAA): indication for routine assessment of chimerism post SCT for SAA. Br J Haematol. 2009;144:933.
38. Baron F, Baker JE, Storb R, Gooley TA, Sandmaier BM, Maris MB, et al. Kinetics of engraftment in patients with hematologic malignancies given allogeneic hematopoietic cell transplantation after nonmyeloablative conditioning. Blood. 2004;104:2254.
39. Pantin J, Tian X, Shah AA, Kurlander R, Ramos C, Cook L, et al. Rapid donor T-cell engraftment increases the risk of chronic graft-versus-host disease following salvage allogeneic peripheral blood hematopoietic cell transplantation for bone marrow failure syndromes. Am J Hematol. 2013;88:874.
40. Baxter-Lowe LA. Chapter 120: Chimerism. In: Detrick B, Schmitz JL, Hamilton RG, editors. Manual of molecular and clinical laboratory immunology. 8th ed. Washington, DC: ASM Press; 2016. p. 1161–8.
41. Erlecke J, Hartmann I, Hoffmann M, Kroll T, Starke H, Heller A, et al. Automated detection of residual cells after sex-mismatched stem-cell transplantation – evidence for presence of disease-marker negative residual cells. Mol Cytogenet. 2009;2:12.
42. Schaap N, Schattenberg A, Bär B, Mensink E, de Man A, Geurts van Kessel A, et al. Red blood cell phenotyping is a sensitive technique for monitoring chronic myeloid leukaemia patients after T-cell-depleted bone marrow transplantation and after donor leucocyte infusion. Br J Haematol. 2000;108:116.
43. Hendriks EC, de Man AJ, van Berkel YC, Stienstra S, de Witte T. Flow cytometric method for the routine follow-up of red cell populations after bone marrow transplantation. Br J Haematol. 1997;97:141.
44. Bach C, Tomova E, Goldmann K, Weisbach V, Roesler W, Mackensen A, et al. Monitoring of hematopoietic chimerism by real-time quantitative PCR of micro insertions/deletions in samples with low DNA quantities. Transfus Med Hemother. 2015;42:38.
45. Kruse A, Abdel-Azim N, Kim HN, Ruan Y, Phan V, Ogana H, et al. Minimal residual disease detection in acute lymphoblastic leukemia. Int J Mol Sci. 2020;21(3):1054.
46. Lee JM, Kim YJ, Park SS, Han E, Kim M, Kim Y. Simultaneous monitoring of mutation and chimerism using next-generation sequencing in myelodysplastic syndrome. J Clin Med. 2019;8(12):2077.
47. The National Human Genome Research Institute. https://www.genome.gov/10002399/genetic-testing-reportglossary. Last accessed 25 Oct 2020.
48. Gettings KB, Aponte RA, Vallone PM, Butler JM. STR allele sequence variation: current knowledge and future issues. Forensic Sci Int Genet. 2015;18:118.
49. Schichman SA, Suess P, Vertino AM, Gray PS. Comparison of short tandem repeat and variable number tandem repeat genetic markers for quantitative determination of allogeneic bone marrow transplant engraftment. Bone Marrow Transplant. 2002;29:243.
50. Fan H, Chu JY. A brief review of short tandem repeat mutation. Genomics Proteomics Bioinformatics. 2007;5:7.
51. Gettings KB, Borsuk LA, Ballard D, Bodner M, Budowle B, Devesse L, et al. STRSeq: a catalog of sequence diversity at human identification Short Tandem Repeat loci. Forensic Sci Int Genet. 2017;31:111.
52. National Institute of Standards and Techology. Short Tandem Repeat DNA Internet DataBase. https://strbase.nist.gov/intro.htm. Last accessed 27 Oct 2020.
53. Buckingham L. Molecular diagnostics: fundamentals, methods, and clinical applications. 2nd ed. Philadelphia: F. A. Davis; 2012.
54. Sullivan KM, Mannucci A, Kimpton CP, Gill P. A rapid and quantitative DNA sex test: fluorescence-based PCR analysis of X-Y homologous gene amelogenin. BioTechniques. 1993;15:636.
55. Urquhart A, Kimpton CP, Downes TJ, Gill P. Variation in short tandem repeat sequences--a survey of twelve microsatellite loci for use as forensic identification markers. Int J Leg Med. 1994;107:13–20.
56. Tilanus MG. Short tandem repeat markers in diagnostics: what's in a repeat? Leukemia. 2006;20(8):1353–5.
57. Clark JR, Scott SD, Jack AL, Lee H, Mason J, Carter GI, et al. Monitoring of chimerism following allogeneic haematopoietic stem cell transplantation (HSCT): technical recommendations for the use of short tandem repeat (STR) based techniques, on behalf of the United Kingdom National External Quality Assessment Service for Leucocyte Immunophenotyping Chimerism Working Group. Br J Haematol. 2015;168:26.
58. Kristt D, Israeli M, Narinski R, Or H, Yaniv I, Stein J, et al. Hematopoietic chimerism monitoring based on STRs: quantitative platform performance on sequential samples. J Biomol Tech. 2005;16:380.
59. Kimpton CP, Gill P, Walton A, Urquhart A, Millican ES, Adams M. Automated DNA profiling employing multiplex amplification of short tandem repeat loci. PCR Methods Appl. 1993;3:13.
60. Walsh PS, Fildes NJ, Reynolds R. Sequence analysis and characterization of stutter products at the tetranucleotide repeat locus vWA. Nucleic Acids Res. 1996;24:2807.
61. Thiede C, Bornhäuser M, Ehninger G. Evaluation of STR informativity for chimerism testing – comparative analysis of 27 STR systems in 203 matched related donor recipient pairs. Leukemia. 2004;18:248.
62. Chen DP, Tseng CP, Tsai SH, Wu TL, Chang PY, Sun CF. Systematic analysis of stutters to enhance the accuracy of chimerism testing. Ann Clin Lab Sci. 2008;38:264.
63. Walsh PS, Erlich HA, Higuchi R. Preferential PCR amplification of alleles: mechanisms and solutions. PCR Methods Appl. 1992;1:241.
64. Acquaviva C, Duval M, Mirebeau D, Bertin R, Cavé H. Quantitative analysis of chimerism after allogeneic stem cell transplantation by PCR amplification of microsatellite markers and capillary electrophoresis with fluorescence detection: the Paris-Robert Debré experience. Leukemia. 2003;17:241.
65. Schraml E, Lion T. Interference of dye-associated fluorescence signals with quantitative analysis of chimerism by capillary electrophoresis. Leukemia. 2003;17:221.
66. Clayton TM, Guest JL, Urquhart AJ, Gill PD. A genetic basis for anomalous band patterns encountered during DNA STR profiling. J Forensic Sci. 2004;49:1207.
67. Findlay I, Tóth T, Matthews P, Marton T, Quirke P, Papp Z. Rapid trisomy diagnosis (21, 18, and 13) using fluorescent PCR and short tandem repeats: applications for prenatal diagnosis and preimplantation genetic diagnosis. J Assist Reprod Genet. 1998;15:266.
68. Pereira S, Vayntrub T, Hiraki DD, Cherry AM, Arai S, Dvorak CC, et al. Short tandem repeat and human leukocyte antigen mutations or losses confound engraftment and typing analysis in hematopoietic stem cell transplants. Hum Immunol. 2011;72:503.
69. Much M, Buza N, Hui P. Tissue identity testing of cancer by short tandem repeat polymorphism: pitfalls of interpretation in the presence of microsatellite instability. Hum Pathol. 2014;45:549.
70. Bitar C, Olivier K, Lee C, Vincent B, Martin J. Acute graft-vs-host disease following liver transplantation. Cutis. 2019;103:E8.
71. Ganoza A, Mazariegos GV, Khanna A. Current status of graft-versus-host disease after intestinal transplantation. Curr Opin Organ Transplant. 2019;24:199.

Index

Y. Ding, L. Zhang (eds.), *Practical Oncologic Molecular Pathology*, Practical Anatomic Pathology,
https://doi.org/10.1007/978-3-030-73227-1

C

D